Basic Pathology

VINAY KUMAR, M.D.
Vernie A. Stembridge Chair in Pathology
Department of Pathology
The University of Texas
Southwestern Medical School
Dallas, Texas

RAMZI S. COTRAN, M.D.
Frank Burr Mallory Professor of Pathology
Harvard Medical School
Chairman, Department of Pathology
Brigham and Women's Hospital
The Children's Hospital
Boston, Massachusetts

STANLEY L. ROBBINS, M.D.
Consultant in Pathology
Brigham and Women's Hospital
Boston, Massachusetts

With illustrations by
James A. Perkins, M.S., M.F.A.

Basic Pathology

sixth edition

W.B. SAUNDERS COMPANY
A Division of Harcourt Brace & Company

Philadelphia   London   Toronto   Montreal   Sydney   Tokyo

W.B. Saunders Company
A Division of Harcourt Brace & Company

The Curtis Center
Independence Square West
Philadelphia, Pennsylvania 19106

Library of Congress Cataloging-in-Publication Data

Basic pathology / [edited by] Vinay Kumar, Ramzi S. Cotran, Stanley L. Robbins; with illustrations by James A. Perkins.—6th ed.

p. cm.

Rev. ed. of: Basic pathology / Vinay Kumar, Ramzi S. Cotran, Stanley L. Robbins. 5th ed. © 1992.
Includes bibliographical references and index.

ISBN 0-7216-5122-4

1. Pathology.   I. Kumar, Vinay.   II. Cotran, Ramzi S.,
III. Robbins, Stanley L. (Stanley Leonard),   IV. Kumar,
Vinay. Basic pathology.

[DNLM: 1. Pathology.   QZ 4 B3108   1997]
RB111.K895   1997   616.07—dc21

DNLM/DLC   96-46873

Basic Pathology, 6th edition   0-7216-5122-4

Printed in the United States of America.

Last digit is the print number: 9   8   7   6   5   4   3

To
Ambika and Rohit Kumar
and to the
families of Ramzi Cotran and
Stanley Robbins

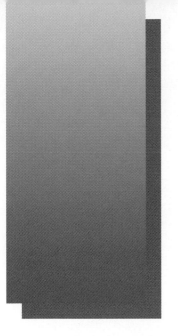

Preface

We launch this sixth edition of *Basic Pathology* with considerable excitement, because in more than one way this is a new book; both the illustrations and the text have been extensively revised, and in some cases the text has been rewritten completely. Changes that are worthy of special mention are as follows:

- The majority of the old black and white photographs, some of which go back to the first edition of this book, have been replaced by over 300 full-color gross and microscopic pictures. In addition, about 200 new pieces of four color art—schematics, flow charts, and diagrammatic representations of diseases—have been added. Most of these appear in chapters devoted to general pathology because of our hope that they will facilitate the understanding of difficult concepts, such as the molecular basis of cancer, interactions of HIV with its receptors, and biochemical basis of apoptotic cell death. In other sections of the book the diagrams have been designed to facilitate the understanding of organ system diseases by providing aesthetically pleasing visual reinforcement. Care has been taken to ensure that the schematic illustrations complement but not replace the text.
- In response to suggestions from many students and instructors, a new chapter that includes selected common disorders of skin has been added. In addition, pediatric disorders previously covered in several different chapters have been consolidated into a new chapter on Genetic and Pediatric Diseases. This reorganization also provided the opportunity to include some general topics in pediatric pathology, such as the principles of teratology, pediatric tumors, and perinatal infections. We hope that these additions will more fully meet the needs of a larger group of readers.
- To achieve a better integration of clinical and anatomic pathology, the discussion of laboratory diagnosis of se-

lected disorders has been expanded. These include syphilis, ischemic heart disease, disorders of the thyroid and adrenal cortex, and genetic disorders. It is hoped that this emphasis will not only provide a more complete discussion of several common disorders but also highlight the importance of laboratory medicine in the practice of medicine. However, no attempt has been made to provide a comprehensive guide to clinical pathology, which is better relegated to specialized texts.

Despite the extensive changes and revisions, our goals remain substantially unaltered. As in previous editions we have strived to provide a balanced, accurate, and up-to-date picture of the central body of pathology. The strong emphasis on clinicopathologic correlations is maintained, and wherever understood the impact of molecular pathology on the practice of medicine is highlighted. Indeed, in the five years since the previous edition, spectacular discoveries relating to the molecular basis of common diseases such as cancer, atherosclerosis, obesity, and diabetes have been made. From the plethora of new findings, we have attempted to restrict our discussion to information that is not only up-to-date but also established, leaving out speculations that may well be exciting for specialists but can be a burden for beginners. We trust that those "breakthroughs" will be incorporated into the teaching by informed instructors.

Finally, we have retained the emphasis on clarity of writing and proper usage of language, in the recognition that lucidity enhances comprehension and facilitates the learning process. Despite the addition of new illustrations and text, we have maintained the text close to its previous size. This required making difficult choices at every step. We trust the readers will agree with our judgments and accept this edition with the same enthusiasm accorded its forebears.

Acknowledgments

We are indebted to many individuals who helped in various ways in the completion of this book. First and foremost, we offer special thanks to our personal editorial assistants: Beverly Shackelford, Paulette Lewis, Marilyn Gibson (at Dallas), Margarita Rosado, Julie Smith, Claudia Davis, and Jackie Davis (at Boston). Beverly not only provided invaluable assistance in editorial matters, as she has done in many previous editions, but also undertook the challenge of preparing the index. In addition, she maintained liaison with the editors at W.B. Saunders, thus ensuring a smooth flow of manuscripts from the authors to the publishers.

Special acknowledgments are owed to Jim Perkins, an outstanding graphic artist, for contributing over 200 new four-color illustrations that have greatly enriched this text. Beni Stewart and her colleagues, Lisa Belser and Jerry Tyson, provided invaluable advice and skillful help in digitizing kodachromes to bring out the best in color and form. We are grateful for their enthusiasm and timely help in meeting numerous deadlines.

Several colleagues have added to the luster of this book by providing their expertise in rewriting or revising some chapters. Their contributions are listed in the Table of Contents, as well as in the chapters themselves. To each of them special thanks. Many others have enchanced the quality of the text by providing helpful critiques in their special areas of expertise. Included among them are Dr. Rakesh K. Kumar (The University of New South Wales, Sydney, Australia) and Dr. Mary F. Lipscomb (University of New Mexico, Albuquerque) for their comments on diseases of the respiratory tract, Dr. Nancy Schneider for assistance with genetic diseases, Dr. Fred Schoen for contributing material for the chapter on blood vessels, and Dr. Andrew Renshaw for his critique of the section on bladder tumors. We are also extremely grateful to many of our colleagues at the University of Texas Southwestern Medical School at Dallas and the Brigham and Women's Hospital at Boston for providing us with photographic gems from their personal collections, and in some instances taking new pictures for specific use in this text. They are individually acknowledged in the credits to their contribution(s). Special thanks are due, however, to Dr. Robert McKenna for providing numerous photographs relating to diseases of red cells and white cells. For any unintended omissions we offer our apologies.

Many at W.B. Saunders deserve recognition for their role in the production of this book. We offer our salute to Hazel Hacker, the finest developmental editor that we have had the privilege to work with. Hazel has the uncanny ability to foresee problems and solve them before they occur; the "well-lubricated" production of this text is owed in no small part to her ability to understand the authors' needs as well as the technicalities of textbook publishing. Her soothing voice and deft interventions provided relief when it was most needed. We were doubly blessed by the teaming together of Hazel Hacker with Lesley Day, our medical editor. Lesley's leadership made it possible for the authors to concentrate on writing the text, without having to worry about the pitfalls that are virtually unavoidable in a task as complex as the publication of a textbook. Others deserving of our thanks are David Harvey (Senior Manuscript Editor), Linda R. Garber (Senior Production Manager), Peg Shaw (Senior Illustration Specialist), Carolyn Naylor (Assistant Director of Production), Pat Morrison (Art/Design Director), Marie Dean (Artist), Karen Giacomucci (Senior Illustrator), and Sharon Iwanczuk (Illustrator). Special mention must be made of Ellen Zanolle (Senior Designer) for giving a fresh look to this edition. Mr. Lewis Reines, President of W.B. Saunders, was supportive as usual and ensured that this text would eventually see the light of day.

Ventures such as this exact a heavy toll from the families of the authors. We thank them for their tolerance of our absences, physically and emotionally. We are blessed and strengthened by their unconditional support and love, and for their sharing with us the belief that our efforts are worthwhile and useful.

And finally, each of us wishes to salute his coauthors for the shared vision, excitement, and dedication to medical education that keep us united despite differences in opinions and individual styles. With each new edition our mutual respect and friendship grows stronger. Vinay Kumar and Ramzi Cotran wish to pay a special tribute to Dr. Stanley Robbins, who started it all and kept it going. Generations of physicians all over the world will continue to owe him a debt, long after he retires.

VK
RC
SLR

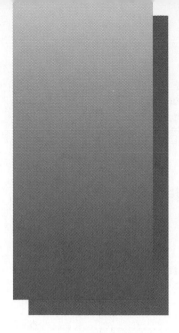

Contents

DISEASES OF ORGAN SYSTEMS

GENERAL PATHOLOGY

1

1

Cell Injury, Death, and Adaptation

RICHARD N. MITCHELL, MD, PhD
RAMZI S. COTRAN, MD

DEFINITIONS

Pathology is a discipline bridging clinical practice and basic science. To render diagnoses and guide therapy, pathologists in clinical practice typically identify changes in the gross or microscopic appearance *(morphology)* of cells and tissues; contemporary molecular, microbiologic, and immunologic techniques are also extensively used. The scientific focus of pathology is on the cause *(etiology)* of disease, the mechanisms of its development *(pathogenesis),* and the pathways by which morphologic changes occur. These fundamental events occur at the molecular and cellular levels, and it is there that we begin our discussion.

Cells are active participants in their environment, constantly adjusting structure and function to accommodate changing demands and extracellular stresses. The cell tends to preserve its intracellular milieu within a relatively narrow range of physiologic parameters—it maintains normal homeostasis. As the cell encounters physiologic stresses or pathologic stimuli, it can undergo adaptation, achieving a new steady state and preserving viability. The principal adaptive responses are atrophy, hypertrophy, hyperplasia, and metaplasia, discussed later in this chapter. If the cell's adaptive capability is exceeded, cell injury develops. Up to a point, cell injury is reversible; however, with severe or persistent stress, the cell suffers irreversible injury and ultimately dies.

There are two principal patterns of cell death:

1. *Necrosis,* most commonly coagulative necrosis, occurs after loss of blood supply or exposure to certain toxins and is characterized by cellular swelling, protein denaturation, and organellar breakdown.
2. *Apoptosis* is a more regulated event, occurring in the normal, or "programmed," death of a specific population under physiologic conditions such as embryogenesis, as well as a variety of pathologic states. The histologic appearance of apoptosis is more subtle than that of necrosis, but there is considerable overlap in the ultimate mechanisms of death in these two conditions (described later).

The relationships among normal, adapted, and reversibly and irreversibly injured cells are demonstrated in Figure 1–1. Myocardium subjected to persistent increased load, as in hypertension or with a stenotic valve, adapts by undergoing *hypertrophy*—an increase in size of the individual cells and ultimately the entire heart—to compensate for the higher pressures it must pump against. Conversely, in periods of prolonged starvation or cachexia (e.g., secondary to malignant tumors), all myocytes (and thus the heart) can undergo *atrophy*—a decrease in size, without appreciable change in cell number. The same myocardium, subjected to ischemia from an occluded coronary artery, may be *reversibly injured* if the occlusion is incomplete or sufficiently brief, or may undergo *irreversible injury* (myocardial infarction) after complete or prolonged occlusion. Whether a specific form of stress induces adaptation or causes reversible or irreversible injury depends not only on the nature and severity of the stress, but also on several other cell-specific variables, including vulnerability, differentiation, blood supply, nutrition, and the previous state of the cell.

The following sections first describe the broad categories of stresses and noxious influences that induce reversible injury, cell death, and adaptation. Second, there are sections describing the mechanisms by which the injury is caused, the morphology of injured cells, and the subcellular and cellular adaptive responses to nonlethal stimuli. Finally, there is a discussion of the processes contributing to cell senescence.

CAUSES OF CELL INJURY

The stresses that can induce cell injury range from the gross physical trauma of a motor vehicle accident to the single gene defect that underlies many metabolic diseases. Most causes can be grouped into the following broad categories.

Hypoxia. Hypoxia, or oxygen deficiency, impinges on aerobic oxidative respiration and is an extremely important and common cause of cell injury and death. Hypoxia should be distinguished from ischemia, which is a loss of blood supply from impeded arterial flow or reduced venous drainage in a tissue. While ischemia is the most common cause of hypoxia, oxygen deficiency may also result from inadequate oxygenation of the blood, for example, as a result of cardiorespiratory failure, or loss of the oxygen-carrying capacity of the blood, as in anemia or carbon monoxide (CO) poisoning (CO produces a stable carbon monoxyhemoglobin that blocks oxygen transport).

Physical Agents. Trauma, extremes of temperatures, radiation, electric shock, and sudden changes in atmospheric pressure all have wide-ranging effects on cells (Chapter 8).

Chemicals and Drugs. Virtually any chemical agent may cause injury; even innocuous substances such as glucose or salt, if sufficiently concentrated, may so derange the osmotic environment that injury or cell death results. Oxygen at sufficiently high partial pressures is also toxic. Agents commonly known as poisons may cause severe damage at the cellular level by altering membrane permeability, osmotic homeostasis, or the integrity of an enzyme or cofactor, potentially culminating in the death of the whole organism. Other agents are those we encounter in our daily environments, including air pollutants, insecticides, carbon monoxide, asbestos, therapeutic drugs, and social "stimuli" such as ethanol.

Microbiologic Agents. These agents range from the submicroscopic viruses to meter-long tapeworms; in between are the rickettsiae, bacteria, fungi, and higher forms of parasites. The diverse ways by which biologic agents cause injury are discussed in Chapter 9.

Immunologic Reactions. Although the immune system serves to defend the body against biologic agents, immune reactions may nevertheless cause cell injury. An anaphylactic reaction to a foreign protein is a prime example, and reactions to self-antigens are responsible for a number of autoimmune diseases (Chapter 5).

Genetic Defects. Genetic defects may result in pathologic changes as conspicuous as the congenital malformations associated with Down syndrome or as subtle as the single amino acid substitution in the hemoglobin S of sickle cell anemia. The major genetic abnormalities are discussed in Chapter 7.

Nutritional Imbalances. Even today, nutritional deficien-

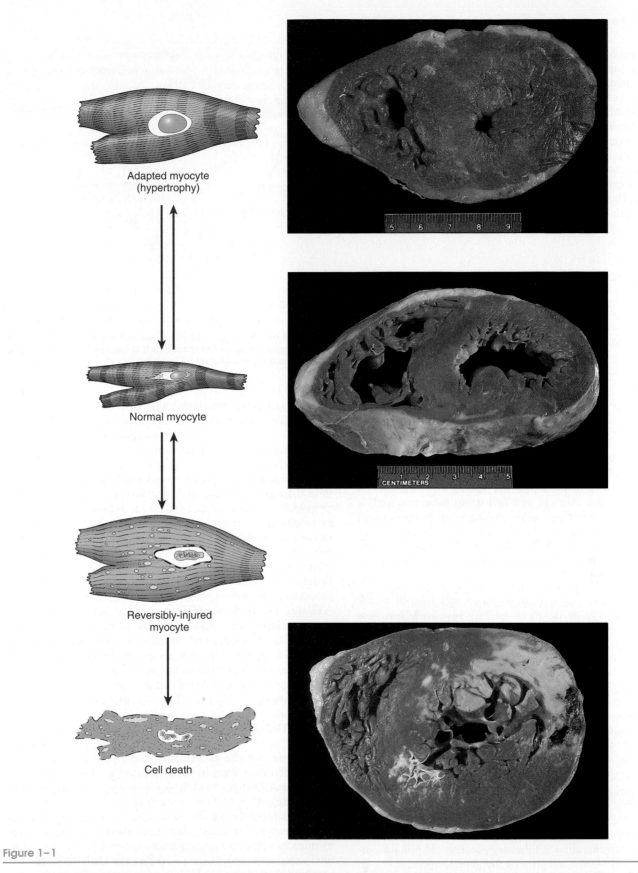

Adapted myocyte
(hypertrophy)

Normal myocyte

Reversibly-injured
myocyte

Cell death

Figure 1-1

The relationship between normal, adapted, reversibly injured, and dead myocardial cells. The cellular adaptation depicted here is hypertrophy, and the type of irreversible cellular injury is ischemic coagulative necrosis. In this example of myocardial hypertrophy, the left ventricular wall is over 2 cm in thickness (normal, 1 to 1.5 cm). In the specimen showing necrosis, the transmural light area in the posterolateral left ventricle represents an acute myocardial infarction. All three have been stained with triphenyltetrazolium chloride, an enzyme substrate, which colors viable myocardium magenta. Failure to stain is due to enzyme leakage following cell death. In reversibly injured myocardium, there are generally only functional effects, without any readily apparent gross or even microscopic changes.

cies are major causes of cell injury. Protein-calorie insufficiency among underprivileged populations is only the most obvious example, and specific vitamin deficiencies are not uncommon even in industrialized nations having relatively high standards of living (Chapter 8). Ironically, excesses in nutrition are also important causes of morbidity and mortality, as in, for example, non–insulin-dependent (adult-onset) diabetes mellitus and the pickwickian syndrome. Moreover, diets rich in animal fats have been strongly implicated in atherosclerosis and increased vulnerability to many disorders.

Aging. The mechanisms of cellular adaptations and injury in aging cells are discussed later in this chapter.

MECHANISMS OF CELL INJURY

With certain injurious agents, the pathogenic mechanisms are well defined; thus, cyanide inactivates cytochrome oxidase in mitochondria, resulting in adenosine triphosphate (ATP) depletion, and certain bacteria can elaborate phospholipases that degrade cell membrane phospholipids. Although there are other examples, the molecular mechanisms connecting most forms of cell injury to ultimate cell death have proved difficult to dissect. First, there are clearly many ways to injure a cell, not all of them invariably fatal. Second, the numerous macromolecules, enzymes, and organelles within the cell are so closely interdependent that it is difficult to distinguish the primary target of injury from any secondary (and not necessarily relevant) ripple effects. Third, the "point of no return," at which *irreversible* damage and cell death have occurred, is still largely undetermined; thus, we have no precise cut-off point to establish cause and effect. Finally, there is probably no common final pathway for cell dying. Given these caveats, there are nevertheless a number of generalizations that can be made:

■ The cellular response to injurious stimuli depends on the type of injury, its duration, and its severity. Thus, low doses of toxins or brief durations of ischemia may lead to reversible cell injury, whereas larger toxin doses or longer ischemic intervals may result in irreversible injury and cell death.

■ The consequences of an injurious stimulus are also dependent on the type of cell being injured, its current status (nutritional, hormonal, and so forth), and its adaptability. For example, striated skeletal muscle in the leg can tolerate complete ischemia for 2 to 3 hours without suffering irreversible injury, whereas cardiac muscle suffers death after only 20 to 30 minutes.

■ The precise biochemical site of injury may be difficult to determine, but four intracellular systems are particularly vulnerable: (1) cell membrane integrity, critical to cellular ionic and osmotic homeostasis; (2) aerobic respiration, important in generating ATP energy stores; (3) protein synthesis; and (4) the integrity of the genetic apparatus.

■ Oxygen and oxygen-derived free radicals and a failure of intracellular calcium homeostatic mechanisms are recurring themes in a wide variety of cell injuries.

Lack of oxygen obviously underlies the pathogenesis of cell

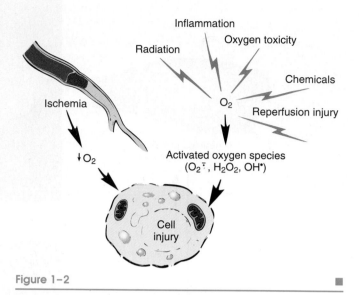

Figure 1–2 ■

The role of oxygen in cell injury. Ischemia causes cell injury by reducing cellular oxygen supplies; other stimuli, such as radiation, induce damage via toxic activated oxygen species.

injury in ischemia, but in addition, partially reduced activated oxygen species are important mediators of cell death (Fig. 1–2). As will be seen, these free radical species cause lipid peroxidation and other deleterious effects on cell structure.

Cytosolic free calcium is normally maintained by ATP-dependent calcium transporters at extremely low concentrations (less than 0.1 μM); this is in the face of sequestered mitochondrial and endoplasmic reticulum calcium stores, and an extracellular calcium typically at 1.3 mM. Ischemia or toxins allow a net influx of extracellular calcium across the plasma membrane, followed by release of calcium from the intracellular stores. Increased cytosolic calcium in turn activates a variety of phospholipases (promoting membrane damage), proteases (catabolizing structural and membrane proteins), ATPases (accelerating ATP depletion), and endonucleases (fragmenting genetic material) (Fig. 1–3). Although cell injury results in increased intracellular calcium, and this in turn mediates a variety of deleterious effects, including cell death, loss of calcium homeostasis is not always a necessary proximate event in irreversible cell injury.

Ischemic and Hypoxic Injury

In this section the mechanisms underlying the sequence of events following acute hypoxic injury (Fig. 1–4) and the ultrastructural changes seen in reversible and irreversible hypoxic injury (Fig. 1–5) are reviewed.

Reversible Injury. The first effect of hypoxia is on the cell's aerobic respiration, that is, oxidative phosphorylation by mitochondria; as a consequence of reduced oxygen tension, the intracellular generation of ATP is markedly reduced. The resulting depletion of ATP has widespread effects on many systems within the cell. As described above, there is an increase in cytosolic free calcium. In addition, the activity of the plasma membrane ATP-driven "sodium pump" is reduced, with subsequent accumulation of intracellular sodium and dif-

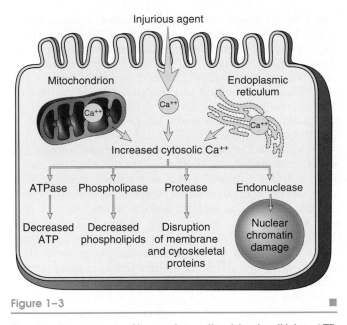

Figure 1–3   ■

Sources and consequences of increased cytosolic calcium in cell injury. ATP, adenosine triphosphate.

fusion of potassium out of the cell. The net gain of sodium solute is accompanied by an isosmotic gain of water, producing *acute cellular swelling.* This is further exacerbated by the increased osmotic load from the accumulation of other metabolites, such as inorganic phosphates, lactic acid, and purine nucleosides.

The decrease in cellular ATP and associated increase in

adenosine monophosphate (AMP) also stimulate the enzyme phosphofructokinase, resulting in an increased rate of anaerobic glycolysis, evolutionarily designed to maintain the cell's energy by generating ATP from glycogen. As a consequence, *glycogen is rapidly depleted;* this can be appreciated histologically by reduced staining for carbohydrates (e.g., the periodic acid–Schiff [PAS] stain). Increased glycolysis also results in accumulation of lactic acid and inorganic phosphates from hydrolysis of phosphate esters, culminating in *reduced intracellular pH.*

The next phenomenon to occur is detachment of ribosomes from the rough endoplasmic reticulum (RER) and dissociation of polysomes into monosomes, with consequent *reduction in protein synthesis.* If hypoxia is not relieved, worsening mitochondrial function and increasing membrane permeability cause further morphologic deterioration. The cytoskeleton disperses, resulting in loss of ultrastructural features such as microvilli, and the formation of cell surface "blebs." Mitochondria, endoplasmic reticulum, and indeed whole cells usually appear swollen owing to loss of osmotic regulation. If oxygen is restored, all the above disturbances are reversible; however, if ischemia persists, irreversible injury follows (Fig. 1–5).

Irreversible Injury. Irreversible injury is associated morphologically with severe vacuolization of the mitochondria and the *accumulation of amorphous, calcium-rich densities in the mitochondrial matrix;* there is also extensive damage to plasma membranes and swelling of lysosomes. Massive calcium influx into the cell occurs, particularly if the ischemic zone is reperfused, and this results in the calcium-mediated insults described above. There is continued loss of proteins, essential coenzymes, and ribonucleic acids from the hyper-

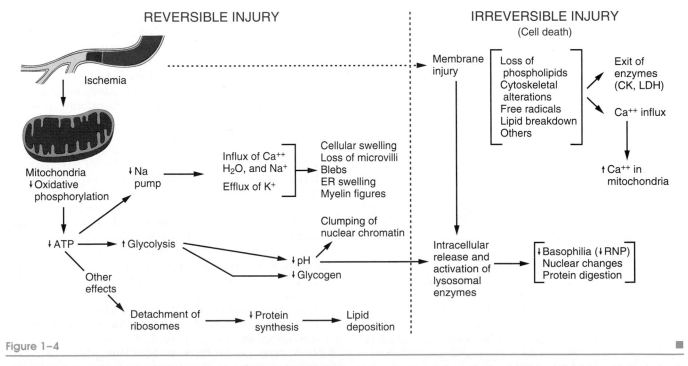

Figure 1–4   ■

Postulated sequence of events in ischemic injury. Note that although diminished oxidative phosphorylation and reduced ATP levels have a central role, ischemia can also directly cause membrane damage. ER, endoplasmic reticulum; CK, creatine kinase; LDH, lactate dehydrogenase; RNP, ribonucleoprotein.

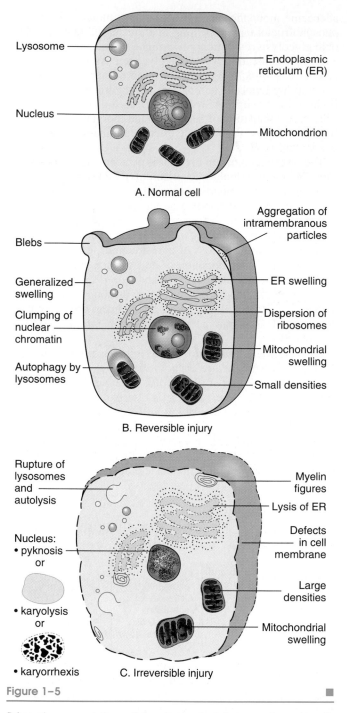

A. Normal cell

- Lysosome
- Nucleus
- Endoplasmic reticulum (ER)
- Mitochondrion

B. Reversible injury

- Blebs
- Generalized swelling
- Clumping of nuclear chromatin
- Autophagy by lysosomes
- Aggregation of intramembranous particles
- ER swelling
- Dispersion of ribosomes
- Mitochondrial swelling
- Small densities

C. Irreversible injury

- Rupture of lysosomes and autolysis
- Nucleus:
  - • pyknosis or
  - • karyolysis or
  - • karyorrhexis
- Myelin figures
- Lysis of ER
- Defects in cell membrane
- Large densities
- Mitochondrial swelling

Figure 1–5 ■

Schematic representations of the ultrastructural features of normal cells (*A*), and those changes seen in reversible (*B*) and irreversible (*C*) cell injury (see text).

permeable membranes, and the cells may also leak metabolites vital for the reconstitution of ATP, thus further depleting intracellular high-energy phosphates (Fig. 1–5). Injury to the lysosomal membranes results in leakage of their enzymes into the cytoplasm; the acid hydrolases are activated in the reduced intracellular pH of the ischemic cell and degrade cytoplasmic and nuclear components.

After cell death, cellular constituents are progressively di-

gested by lysosomal hydrolases; moreover, there is widespread leakage of cellular enzymes into the extracellular space, as well as influx of extracellular macromolecules from the interstitium. The dead cell may ultimately be replaced by large, whorled phospholipid masses described as "myelin figures." These phospholipid precipitates are then either phagocytosed by other cells or further degraded into fatty acids; calcification of such fatty acid residues results in the generation of calcium soaps.

It is also worth noting that leakage of intracellular proteins across the degraded cell membrane into the peripheral circulation provides a means of detecting tissue-specific cellular injury and death in blood serum samples. Cardiac muscle, for example, contains a specific isoform of the enzyme creatine kinase, and of the contractile protein troponins; liver (and specifically bile duct epithelium) contains a temperature-resistant isoform of the enzyme alkaline phosphatase. Irreversible injury and cell death in these tissues is consequently reflected in increased levels of such proteins in the general circulation.

Mechanisms of Irreversible Injury. The sequence of events for hypoxia was described above as a continuum from onset to ultimate digestion of the lethally injured cell by lysosomal enzymes. However, where was the "point of no return" beyond which the cell was irretrievably doomed to destruction? And when did the cell actually die? Two phenomena consistently characterize irreversibility. The first is the inability to reverse mitochondrial dysfunction (lack of oxidative phosphorylation and ATP generation) even after restoration of blood flow and/or oxygen; the second is the development of profound disturbances in membrane function. Although the depletion of ATP in itself might constitute a lethal event, the evidence is conflicting; it has been possible experimentally to dissociate the morphologic changes, as well as ATP depletion, from the inevitability of cell death.

Considerable evidence favors cell membrane damage as a central factor in the pathogenesis of irreversible cell injury. Loss of volume regulation, increased permeability to extracellular molecules, and demonstrable plasma membrane ultrastructural defects occur even in the earliest stages of irreversible injury. There are several potential causes of membrane damage, and all may play a role in certain forms of injury (Fig. 1–6).

1. *Progressive loss of membrane phospholipids.* In ischemic liver, irreversible injury is associated with a marked decrease in membrane phospholipids. One explanation may be increased degradation due to activation of endogenous phospholipases by ischemia-induced increases in cytosolic calcium. Progressive phospholipid loss can also occur secondary to decreased ATP-dependent reacylation or diminished de novo synthesis of phospholipids.

2. *Cytoskeletal abnormalities.* Activation of proteases by increased intracellular calcium may result in damage to the cytoskeleton. In the setting of cell swelling, such injury may cause detachment of the cell membrane from the cytoskeleton, rendering the membrane susceptible to stretching and rupture.

3. *Toxic oxygen radicals.* As detailed later, partially reduced oxygen species are highly toxic and cause injury to cell membranes and other cell constituents. Such oxygen rad-

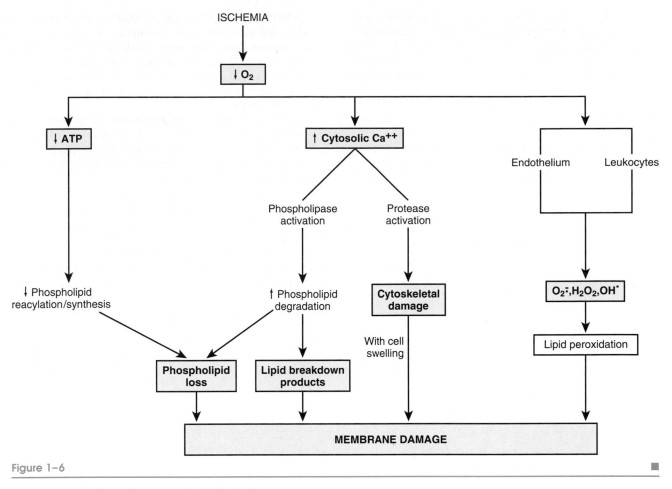

ISCHEMIA

↓ O$_2$

↓ ATP

↑ Cytosolic Ca^{++}

Endothelium   Leukocytes

Phospholipase
activation

Protease
activation

↓ Phospholipid
reacylation/synthesis

↑ Phospholipid
degradation

**Cytoskeletal
damage**

O$_2$$\overline{\cdot}$,H$_2O_2$,OH$^{\cdot}$

With cell
swelling

Lipid peroxidation

**Phospholipid
loss**

**Lipid breakdown
products**

MEMBRANE DAMAGE

Figure 1–6   ■

Mechanisms of membrane damage in ischemia (see text).

icals are increased in ischemic tissues, particularly after restoration of blood flow. The toxic oxygen species are thought to be produced largely (but not exclusively) by infiltrating polymorphonuclear leukocytes introduced during reperfusion. If reperfusion does not occur, lethal ischemic cell injury still eventually ensues, but toxic oxygen species are probably not involved.

4. *Lipid breakdown products.* These catabolic products accumulate in ischemic cells as a result of phospholipid degradation and have a detergent effect on membranes.

Whatever the mechanism(s) of membrane damage, the end result is a massive influx of calcium, with the consequences described above (see Fig. 1–3).

To summarize, hypoxia affects the oxidative phosphorylation and hence the synthesis of vital ATP supplies; membrane damage is critical to the development of lethal cell injury; and calcium is a potential mediator of the morphologic alterations in cell death.

Free Radical Mediation of Cell Injury

As mentioned in the discussion of ischemic reperfusion, free radical–induced injury, particularly that induced by ac-

tivated oxygen species, is an important mechanism of cell damage. Free radical damage contributes to chemical and radiation injury, oxygen and other gaseous toxicity, cellular aging, microbial killing by phagocytic cells (Chapter 2), inflammatory damage, tumor destruction by macrophages, and other injurious processes (see Fig. 1–2).

Free radicals are chemical species with a single unpaired electron in an outer orbital. Such chemical states are extremely unstable and readily react with inorganic or organic chemicals; when generated in cells, they avidly attack and degrade nucleic acids as well as a variety of membrane molecules. In addition, free radicals initiate autocatalytic reactions; molecules that react with free radicals are in turn converted into free radicals, further propagating the chain of damage.

Free radicals may be generated within cells by

1. Absorption of radiant energy (e.g., ultraviolet light, x-rays). For example, ionizing radiation can hydrolyze water into hydroxyl (OH$^{\cdot}$) and hydrogen (H$^{\cdot}$) free radicals.
2. The reduction-oxidation (redox) reactions that occur during normal physiologic processes. During normal respiration, for example, molecular oxygen is sequentially reduced by the addition of four electrons to generate water. In the process, small amounts of toxic intermediate species are generated; these include superoxide radicals (O$_2$$\overline{\cdot}$), hydrogen peroxide (H$_2O_2$), and OH$^{\cdot}$. Further, some intracel-

lular oxidases (such as xanthine oxidase) generate super-oxide radicals as a direct consequence of their activity (Fig. 1–7). Transition metals such as copper and iron also accept or donate free electrons during certain intracellular reactions and thereby catalyze free radical formation, as in the Fenton reaction ($Fe^{++} + H_2O_2 \rightarrow Fe^{+++} + OH^{\cdot} + OH^{-}$). Since most intracellular free iron is in the ferric (Fe^{+++}) state, it must first be reduced to the ferrous (Fe^{++}) form to participate in the Fenton reaction. The reduction is enhanced by superoxide ion, and thus iron and superoxide are both required for maximal oxidative cell injury.

3. The enzymatic metabolism of exogenous chemicals (e.g., carbon tetrachloride; see below).

Three reactions are particularly relevant to cell injury mediated by free radicals:

1. *Lipid peroxidation of membranes.* Double bonds in membrane polyunsaturated lipids are vulnerable to attack by oxygen-derived free radicals. The lipid-radical interactions yield peroxides, which are themselves unstable and reactive, and an autocatalytic chain reaction ensues.

2. *Lesions in deoxyribonucleic acid (DNA).* Free radical reactions with thymine in nuclear and mitochondrial DNA produce single-strand breaks. Such DNA damage has been implicated in both cell killing and malignant transformation of cells.

3. *Cross-linking of proteins.* Free radicals promote sulfhydryl-mediated protein cross-linking, resulting in enhanced rates of degradation or loss of enzymatic activity. Free radical reactions may also directly cause polypeptide fragmentation.

Besides being a consequence of chemical and radiation injury, free radical generation is also a normal part of respiration and other routine cellular activities, including microbial defense. Therefore, it makes sense that cells should have developed mechanisms to degrade free radicals and thereby minimize any injury.

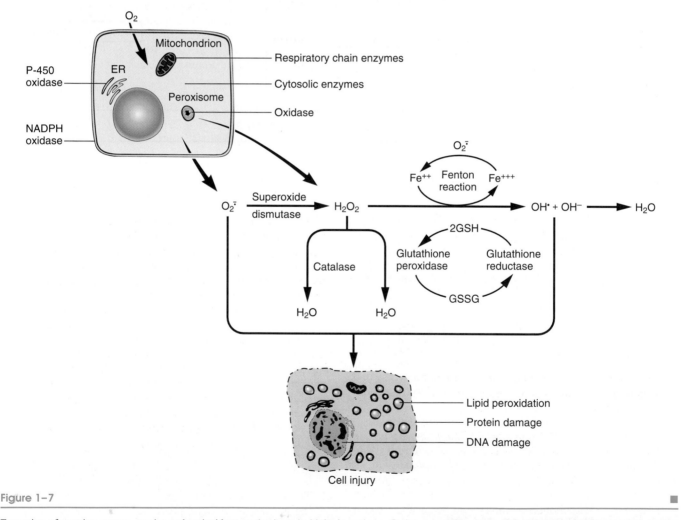

Figure 1–7

Formation of reactive oxygen species and antioxidant mechanisms in biologic systems. O_2 is converted to superoxide ($O_2^{\cdot-}$) by oxidative enzymes in the endoplasmic reticulum (ER), mitochondria, plasma membrane, peroxisomes, and cytosol. $O_2^{\cdot-}$ is converted to H_2O_2 by superoxide dismutase *(SOD)* and then to $OH^{\cdot}$ by the Cu^{++}/Fe^{++} catalyzed Fenton reaction. H_2O_2 is also derived directly from oxidases in peroxisomes. The resultant free radicals can damage lipid (peroxidation), proteins, and DNA. Note that superoxide catalyzes the reduction of Fe^{+++} to Fe^{++}, thus enhancing $OH^{\cdot}$ generation by the Fenton reaction. The major antioxidant enzymes are SOD, catalase, and glutatione peroxidase. GSH, reduced glutathione; GSSG, oxidized glutathione; NADPH, reduced form of nicotinamide-adenine dinucleotide phosphate.

Fortunately, free radicals are inherently unstable and generally decay spontaneously; superoxide, for example, rapidly breaks down in the presence of water into oxygen and hydrogen peroxide. The rate of such decay is significantly increased by the action of superoxide dismutases (SODs) found in many cell types (catalyzing the reaction: $2O_2^- + 2H \rightarrow H_2O_2 + O_2$). Other enzymes (e.g., glutathione [GSH] peroxidase) also protect against injury by catalyzing free radical breakdown ($H_2O_2 + 2GSH \rightarrow 2H_2O + GSSG$ [glutathione homodimer]). Catalase, present in peroxisomes, directs the degradation of hydrogen peroxide ($2H_2O_2 \rightarrow O_2 + 2H_2O$) (Fig. 1–7). In addition, endogenous or exogenous antioxidants (vitamin E and ceruloplasmin) may either block free radical formation or scavenge them once they have formed.

Chemical Injury

Chemicals induce cell injury by one of two general mechanisms:

1. Some chemicals act directly by combining with a critical molecular component or cellular organelle. For example, in mercuric chloride poisoning, mercury binds to the sulfhydryl groups of the cell membrane and other proteins, causing inhibition of ATPase-dependent transport and increased membrane permeability. Many antineoplastic chemotherapeutic agents and antibiotics also induce cell damage by similar direct cytotoxic effects. In such instances, the greatest damage is sustained by the cells that use, absorb, excrete, or concentrate the compounds.
2. Many other toxic chemicals are not intrinsically biologically active but must be first converted to reactive toxic metabolites, which then act on target cells. This modification is usually accomplished by the P-450 mixed function oxidases in the smooth endoplasmic reticulum (SER) of the liver and other organs. Although the metabolites might cause membrane damage and cell injury by direct covalent binding to protein and lipids, the most important mechanism of cell injury involves the formation of reactive free radicals. Carbon tetrachloride (CCl_4, used widely in the dry-cleaning industry) and acetaminophen belong to this category. CCl_4, for example, is converted to the toxic free radical $CCl_3{}^\cdot$, principally in the liver. The free radicals cause autocatalytic membrane phospholipid peroxidation, with rapid breakdown of the endoplasmic reticulum. In less than 30 minutes, there is a decline in hepatic protein synthesis of both enzymes and plasma proteins; within 2 hours, swelling of SER and dissociation of ribosomes from the RER has occurred. There is reduced lipid export from the hepatocytes, owing to their inability to synthesize apoprotein to complex with triglycerides and thereby facilitate lipoprotein secretion; the result is the "fatty liver" of CCl_4 poisoning. Mitochondrial injury follows, with subsequently diminished ATP stores resulting in defective ion transport and progressive cell swelling. The plasma membranes are further damaged by fatty aldehydes resulting from lipid peroxidation in the SER. The end result is a massive calcium influx and cell death.

FORMS AND MORPHOLOGY OF CELL INJURY

All stresses and noxious influences exert their effects first at the molecular level. The time lag required to produce the morphologic changes of cellular adaptation, injury, or death varies with the sensitivity of the methods used to detect these changes. With histochemical or ultrastructural techniques, changes may be seen in minutes to hours after ischemic injury; however, it may take considerably longer (hours to days) before changes can be seen by light microscopy or on gross examination.

In the section below, various forms of cell injury and their morphologic manifestations will be discussed, as follows:

■ Patterns of reversible acute cell injury
■ Patterns of cell death after irreversible injury, called necrosis
■ A pattern of "cell death by suicide," called apoptosis
■ Subcellular alterations that occur largely as a response to more chronic or persistent injurious stimuli
■ Intracellular accumulations of a number of substances—lipids, carbohydrates, proteins—as a result of derangements in cell metabolism or excessive storage

Patterns of Acute Cell Injury

REVERSIBLE INJURY

Two patterns of morphologic changes correlating to reversible injury can be recognized under the light microscope: **cellular swelling** and **fatty change**. Cellular swelling appears whenever cells are incapable of maintaining ionic and fluid homeostasis; the pathogenesis is described above. Fatty change, occurring in hypoxic injury and various forms of toxic or metabolic injury, is manifested by the appearance of lipid vacuoles in the cytoplasm. It is a less universal reaction, principally encountered in cells participating in fat metabolism (e.g., hepatocytes and myocardial cells).

Cellular swelling is the first manifestation of almost all forms of injury to cells. It is a difficult morphologic change to appreciate with the light microscope and may be more apparent at the level of the whole organ. When all cells in an organ are affected, there is pallor, increased turgor, and increased weight. Microscopically, small, clear vacuoles may be seen within the cytoplasm; these represent distended and pinched-off segments of the endoplasmic reticulum. This pattern of nonlethal, reversible injury is sometimes called **hydropic change** or **vacuolar degeneration** (Fig. 1–8).

The ultrastructural changes of reversible cell injury (see Fig. 1–5) include (1) **plasma membrane alterations** such as blebbing, blunting or distortion of microvilli, and loosening of intercellular attachments;

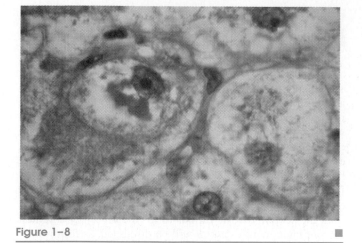

Figure 1–8 ■

Cellular swelling in hepatocytes in alcoholic liver disease. The nuclei and plasma membranes are largely intact, suggesting viability. The swollen hepatocyte on the left also shows eosinophilic intracytoplasmic inclusions just below the nucleus. These are formed by aggregation of intermediate filaments. (Courtesy of Dr. James Crawford, Department of Pathology, Brigham and Women's Hospital, Boston.)

(2) **mitochondrial changes** such as swelling and the appearance of phospholipid-rich amorphous densities; (3) **dilation of the endoplasmic reticulum** with detachment of ribosomes and dissociation of polysomes; and (4) **nuclear alterations**, with disaggregation of granular and fibrillar elements.

NECROSIS

Necrosis refers to a sequence of morphologic changes that follow cell death in living tissue (tissue placed in fixative is dead but not necrotic). As commonly used, necrosis is the gross and histologic correlate of cell death occurring in the setting of irreversible exogenous injury. Its most common manifestation is *coagulative necrosis,* characterized by cell swelling, denaturation of cytoplasmic proteins, and breakdown of cell organelles. Although in a number of pathologic states there is substantial overlap in the mechanisms underlying cell death seen in coagulative necrosis as compared with apoptosis, we will, for simplicity, discuss them separately.

The morphologic appearance of necrosis is the result of two essentially concurrent processes: (1) enzymic digestion of the cell and (2) denaturation of proteins. The hydrolytic enzymes may derive either from the dead cells themselves, in which case the digestion is referred to as *autolysis,* or from the lysosomes of invading inflammatory cells, termed *heterolysis.* These processes require hours to develop, and so there are no detectable changes in cells if, for example, a myocardial infarct causes sudden death. Although subtle ultrastructural changes might be evident 20 to 40 minutes after myocardial cell death, and enzymes leaked from damaged myocardium can be detected in the bloodstream as early as 2 hours after myocardial cell death, the classic histologic features of necrosis are not apparent until 4 to 12 hours after irreversible injury has occurred.

Dead cells show increased eosinophilia (i.e., pink staining from the eosin dye: the "E" in "H & E"). This is attributable in part to increased binding of eosin to denatured intracytoplasmic proteins, and in part to loss of the basophilia (i.e., blue staining from the hematoxylin dye: the "H" in "H & E") which is normally imparted by the RNA in the cytoplasm. The cell may have a more glassy homogeneous appearance than viable cells, due mainly to the loss of glycogen particles. When enzymes have degraded the organelles, the cytoplasm becomes vacuolated and appears moth-eaten. Finally, calcification of the dead cells may occur. Nuclear changes assume one of three patterns (see Fig. 1–5), all due to nonspecific breakdown of DNA. The basophilia of the chromatin may fade (**karyolysis**), presumably secondary to DNAse activity. A second pattern (also seen in apoptotic cell death) is **pyknosis**, characterized by nuclear shrinkage and increased basophilia; the DNA condenses into a solid shrunken mass. In the third pattern, **karyorrhexis**, the pyknotic nucleus fragments. In 1 to 2 days, the nucleus in a dead cell completely disappears.

Once the dead cells have undergone these early changes, the mass of necrotic tissue may exhibit distinctive morphologic patterns depending on whether enzyme catabolism or protein denaturation predominates. Although the terms are somewhat outmoded, they are routinely used and their meanings are understood by pathologists and clinicians. When denaturation is the primary pattern, so-called **coagulative necrosis** develops. In the instance of dominant enzyme digestion, the result is **liquefactive necrosis**; in special circumstances, **caseous necrosis**, or **fat necrosis,** may develop.

Coagulative necrosis implies preservation of the basic structural outline of the coagulated cell or tissue for a span of days. Presumably the injury or the subsequent increasing acidosis denatures not only the structural proteins but also the enzymic proteins, thus blocking cellular proteolysis. Myocardial infarction is a prime example in which acidophilic, coagulated, anucleate cells may persist for weeks. Ultimately, the necrotic myocardial cells are removed by fragmentation and phagocytosis by scavenger white blood cells. The process of coagulative necrosis, with preservation of the general tissue architecture, is characteristic of hypoxic death of cells in all tissues (Fig. 1–9A) except the brain.

Liquefactive necrosis is characteristic of focal bacterial or sometimes fungal infections, since these provide powerful stimuli for the accumulation of white cells (Fig. 1–9B). For unclear reasons, hypoxic death of cells within the central nervous system also results in liquefactive necrosis. Whatever the pathogenesis, liquefaction completely digests the dead cells. Although **gangrenous necrosis** is not a distinctive pattern of cell death, it is still commonly used in

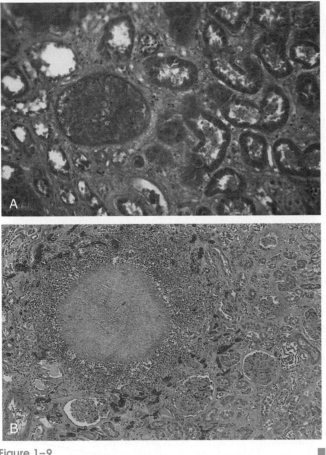

Figure 1-9   ■

A, Kidney infarct exhibiting coagulative necrosis, with loss of nuclei and clumping of the cytoplasm but with preservation of basic outlines of glomerular and tubular architecture. *B*, A focus of liquefactive necrosis in the kidney caused by fungal seeding. The focus is filled with white cells and cellular debris, creating a renal abscess that obliterates the normal architecture.

surgical practice. The term refers to ischemic coagulative necrosis (frequently of a limb); when there is superimposed infection with a liquefactive component, the lesion is called "wet gangrene."

Caseous necrosis is a distinctive form of necrosis encountered most often in foci of tuberculous infection (Chapter 13). The term "caseous" is derived from the cheesy, white gross appearance of the central necrotic area. Microscopically, the necrotic focus is composed of structureless amorphous granular debris enclosed within a distinctive ring of granulomatous inflammation (Chapter 2, see Fig. 2-19). Unlike coagulative necrosis, the tissue architecture is completely obliterated.

Fat necrosis is another well-accepted term that does not really denote a specific pattern of necrosis. Rather, it describes focal areas of fat destruction, typically occurring following pancreatic injury; these result from pathologic release of activated pancreatic enzymes into adjacent parenchyma or

the peritoneal cavity. This occurs in the disastrous abdominal emergency known as acute pancreatitis (Chapter 17); activated pancreatic enzymes escape from acinar cells and ducts, liquefying fat cell membranes and hydrolyzing the triglyceride esters contained within them. The released fatty acids combine with calcium to produce grossly visible chalky white areas (fat saponification), which enable the surgeon or pathologist to identify this disease on simple inspection (Fig. 1-10). Histologically, only shadowy outlines of necrotic fat cells may be seen, with basophilic calcium deposits and a surrounding inflammatory reaction.

Eventually, in the living patient, most necrotic cells and their debris disappear by a combined process of extracellular enzyme digestion and leukocyte phagocytosis. If necrotic cells and cellular debris are not promptly eliminated, they tend to attract calcium salts and other minerals and become calcified. The phenomenon, so-called *dystrophic calcification,* is discussed later in this chapter.

APOPTOSIS

Apoptosis (from root words meaning "a falling away from") is a relatively distinctive and important mode of cell death that should be differentiated from coagulation necrosis (Fig. 1-11, Table 1-1). Apoptosis is responsible for the programmed cell death in several important physiologic (as well as pathologic) processes, including:

1. The programmed destruction of cells during embryogenesis, as occurs in implantation, organogenesis, and developmental involution
2. Hormone-dependent physiologic involution, such as the endometrium during the menstrual cycle, or the lactating breast after weaning; or pathologic atrophy, as in the prostate after castration
3. Cell deletion in proliferating populations, such as intestinal crypt epithelium, or cell death in tumors

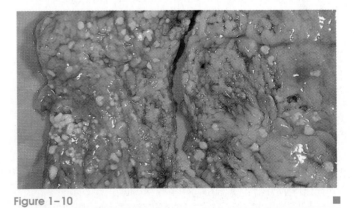

Figure 1-10   ■

Foci of fat necrosis with saponification in the mesentery. The areas of white-yellow chalky deposits represent calcium soap formation at sites of lipid breakdown.

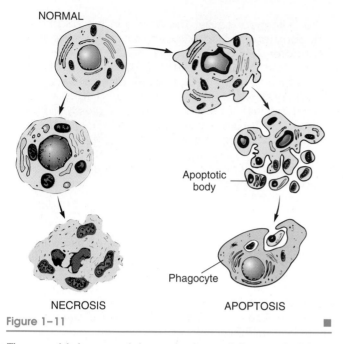

NORMAL

Apoptotic body

Phagocyte

NECROSIS   APOPTOSIS

Figure 1–11 ■

The sequential ultrastructural changes seen in coagulation necrosis *(left)* and apoptosis *(right)*. In apoptosis the initial changes consist of nuclear chromatin condensation and fragmentation, followed by cytoplasmic budding and phagocytosis of the extruded apoptotic bodies. Signs of *coagulation necrosis* include chromatin clumping, organellar swelling, and eventual membrane damage. (Adapted from Walker NI, et al: Patterns of cell death. Methods Achiev Exp Pathol 13:18–32, 1988.)

4. Deletion of autoreactive T cell in the thymus, cell death of cytokine-starved lymphocytes, or cell death induced by cytotoxic T cells

Apoptosis usually involves single cells or clusters of cells that appear on H & E stained sections as round or oval masses with intensely eosinophilic cytoplasm. The nuclear chromatin is condensed, and it aggregates peripherally, under the nuclear membrane, into well-delimited masses of various shapes and sizes. Ultimately, karyorrhexis occurs; at a molecular level, these are reflected in fragmentation of DNA into nucleosome-sized pieces, presumably through the activation of endonucleases (Fig. 1–12). The cells rapidly shrink, form cytoplasmic buds, and fragment into apoptotic bodies composed of membrane-bound vesicles of cytosol and organelles. Because these fragments are quickly extruded and phagocytosed or degraded, substantial apoptosis may occur before the lesion is histologically recognizable. Moreover, apoptosis does not elicit an inflammatory response, further hindering recognition.

Current data suggest that *apoptosis is probably centered on the synthesis and/or activation of a number of cytosolic proteases.* Such induction or activation can be triggered by a va-

riety of stimuli, including withdrawal of growth factors, engagement of specific receptors (e.g., FAS), or initiation of programmed cell death pathways during embryogenesis (Fig. 1–12). The proteases include *calpain I*, a calcium-dependent enzyme (explaining a role for increased cytosolic calcium in the process), and proteases with homology to interleukin-1β converting enzyme (*Ice*). Initial activation of one or more enzymes with broad specificity may then lead to a cascade of activation of other proteases, inexorably culminating in cell suicide. For example, endonuclease activation results in the characteristic DNA fragmentation; cell volume and shape changes may in part be attributable to cleavage of components of the cytoskeleton. The demonstration of apoptosis-specific genes that can stimulate cell death (e.g., the *bax* gene) may explain the requirements for new gene expression in some models of apoptosis. Conversely, the discovery of genes whose products *block* apoptosis (*bcl-2*) suggests why inhibition of protein synthesis, e.g., by sublethal cell injury, might result in apoptotic cell death in other models. Finally, the phagocytosis of apoptotic bodies is facilitated by specific receptors on macrophages or adjacent healthy parenchymal cells. The genes that regulate apoptosis are discussed further in Chapter 6, because they play an important role in neoplastic transformation. A current proposal for the sequence of events leading to apoptosis in different settings is depicted in Figure 1–12.

Subcellular Responses to Injury

Thus far the focus has been largely on the cell as a unit. However, certain conditions are associated with rather distinctive alterations involving only subcellular organelles. Although some of these alterations also occur in acute lethal injury, others represent more chronic forms of cell injury, and

■

Table 1–1.	SIMPLIFIED FEATURES OF COAGULATION NECROSIS VERSUS APOPTOSIS	
	Coagulation Necrosis	**Apoptosis**
Stimuli	Hypoxia, toxins	Physiologic and pathologic
Histology	Cellular swelling Coagulation necrosis Disruption of organelles	Single cells Chromatin condensation Apoptotic bodies
DNA breakdown	Random, diffuse	Internucleosomal
Mechanisms	ATP depletion Membrane injury Free radical damage	Gene activation Endonucleases Proteases
Tissue reaction	Inflammation	No inflammation Phagocytosis of apoptotic bodies

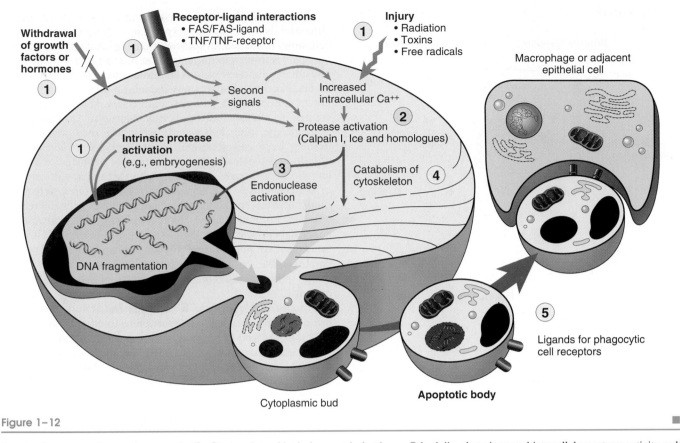

Figure 1-12

Postulated sequence of events in apoptosis (①–⑤). A variety of intrinsic or extrinsic triggers ① lead directly to increased intracellular protease activity and/ or to increased intracellular calcium; these triggers include injurious stimuli such as radiation or free radicals, receptor ligation (e.g., FAS), withdrawal of growth factors, or programmed cell death (e.g., during embryogenesis). ② Increased intracellular calcium also increases intracellular protease activity. The increased protease activity results in a cascade of intracellular degradation, including endonuclease-mediated fragmentation of nuclear chromatin ③ and breakdown of the cytoskeleton ④. The end result is formation of apoptotic bodies containing various intracellular organelles and other cytosolic constituents; these bodies also express new ligands for phagocytic cell binding and uptake ⑤.

still others are adaptive responses. In this section, only some of the more common or interesting of these reactions are discussed.

Cytoskeletal Abnormalities. The cytoskeleton consists of microtubules (20 to 25 nm in diameter), thin actin filaments (6 to 8 nm), thick myosin filaments (15 nm), and various classes of intermediate filaments (10 nm). Several other non-polymerized and nonfilamentous forms of contractile proteins also exist. Cytoskeletal abnormalities may be reflected by (1) defects in cell function, such as cell locomotion and intracellular organelle translocation; or (2) in some instances, intracellular accumulations of fibrillar material.

Intact myofilaments and microtubules are essential for leukocyte migration and phagocytosis; functional deficiencies of the cytoskeleton appear to underlie certain defects in leukocyte movement toward an injurious stimulus (chemotaxis, Chapter 2) or ingestion of pathogens. For example, defective microtubule polymerization in the Chédiak-Higashi syndrome causes delayed or decreased fusion of lysosomes with phagosomes in leukocytes and thus impairs destruction of phagocytosed bacteria. Defects in the organization of microtubules can cause sterility by inhibiting sperm motility, as well as immobilizing cilia of the respiratory epithelium, resulting in

defective clearance of inhaled bacteria and chronic infections (Kartagener's or the immotile cilia syndrome).

Accumulations of intermediate filaments may be seen in certain types of cell injury. For example, the Mallory body, or "alcoholic hyalin," is an eosinophilic intracytoplasmic inclusion in liver cells highly characteristic of alcoholic liver disease (see Fig. 1–8). Such inclusions are now known to be composed predominantly of prekeratin intermediate filaments. The neurofibrillary tangle found in the brain in Alzheimer's disease contains microtubule-associated proteins and neuro-filaments, a reflection of a disrupted neuronal cytoskeleton.

Lysosomal Catabolism. *Primary lysosomes* are 0.2- to 0.8-μm membrane-bound intracellular organelles containing a variety of hydrolytic enzymes; these fuse with membrane-bound vacuoles containing material destined for digestion to form *secondary lysosomes* or *phagolysosomes*. Lysosomes are involved in the breakdown of phagocytosed material in one of two ways: heterophagy and autophagy (Fig. 1–13).

Heterophagy. Materials from the external environment are taken up through a process generically called *endocytosis*; uptake of larger particulate matter is called *phagocytosis*, while uptake of soluble smaller macromolecules is denoted *pinocytosis*. Endocytosed vacuoles and their contents eventually

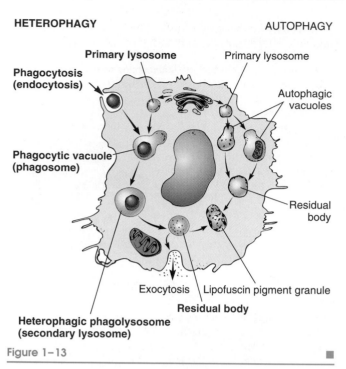

HETEROPHAGY   AUTOPHAGY

Primary lysosome   Primary lysosome

Phagocytosis
(endocytosis)

Autophagic
vacuoles

Phagocytic vacuole
(phagosome)

Residual
body

Exocytosis   Lipofuscin pigment granule

Residual body

Heterophagic phagolysosome
(secondary lysosome)

Figure 1-13   ■

Schematic representation of autophagy *(right)* and heterophagy *(left)*. (Redrawn from Fawcett DW: A Textbook of Histology, 11th ed. Philadelphia, WB Saunders, 1986, p 17.)

fuse with a lysosome, resulting in degradation of the engulfed material. While heterophagy is most conspicuous in the "professional" phagocytes, such as neutrophils and macrophages, it may also occur in other cell types. Examples of heterophagocytosis include the uptake and digestion of bacteria by neutrophils, and the removal of necrotic cells by macrophages.

Autophagy. In this process, intracellular organelles and portions of cytosol are sequestered from the cytoplasm in an *autophagic vacuole* formed from ribosome-free regions of the RER. This then fuses with preexisting primary lysosomes to form an *autophagolysosome.* Autophagy is a common phenomenon involved in the removal of damaged or senescent organelles, and in the cellular remodeling associated with cellular differentiation. It is particularly prominent in cells undergoing atrophy induced by nutrient or hormonal deprivation.

The enzymes in the lysosomes can completely catabolize most proteins and carbohydrates, although some lipids remain undigested. Lysosomes with undigested debris may persist within cells as *residual bodies* or may be extruded. *Lipofuscin pigment* granules (discussed later) represent undigestible material resulting from intracellular lipid peroxidation. Certain indigestible pigments, such as carbon particles inhaled from the atmosphere or inoculated pigment in tattoos, can persist in phagolysosomes of macrophages for decades.

Lysosomes are also repositories where cells sequester materials that cannot be completely metabolized. Hereditary *lysosomal storage disorders*, caused by deficiencies of enzymes that degrade various macromolecules, result in abnormal collections of intermediate metabolites in the lysosomes of cells all over the body; neurons are particularly susceptible to lethal injury from such accumulations (Chapter 7).

Mitochondrial Alterations. As described above, mitochondrial dysfunction clearly plays an important role in acute cell injury and death. In some nonlethal pathologic conditions, however, various alterations in the number, size, shape, and presumably function of mitochondria may also occur. For example, in cellular hypertrophy there is an increase in the number of mitochondria in cells; conversely, mitochondria decrease in number during cellular atrophy (probably via heterophagy, Fig. 1-13). Mitochondria may assume extremely large and abnormal shapes (*megamitochondria*) as seen in hepatocytes in various nutritional deficiencies and alcoholic liver disease. In certain inherited metabolic diseases of skeletal muscle, the *mitochondrial myopathies,* defects in mitochondrial metabolism are associated with increased numbers of unusually large mitochondria containing abnormal cristae. Finally, a type of generally benign tumor called *oncocytoma* (occurring in kidneys, thyroid, parathyroids, or salivary glands) is composed of relatively uniform cells stuffed with abundant, enlarged mitochondria.

Smooth Endoplasmic Reticulum Induction. Protracted use of barbiturates leads to increasing tolerance, so that repeated doses lead to progressively shorter durations of sleep. Patients are therefore said to have "adapted" to the medication. This adaptation is due to induction of an increased volume (hypertrophy) of the hepatocyte SER, which metabolizes the drug (Fig. 1-14). Barbiturates are modified in the liver by oxidative demethylation, which involves the P-450 mixed-function oxidase system found in the SER. The purpose of these enzyme modifications is to increase the solubility of various compounds (e.g., steroids, alcohol, aryl hydrocarbons, insecticides) and thereby facilitate their excretion. Although this is frequently described as "detoxification," many compounds are in fact rendered *more* injurious by P-450 modification. In any event, the barbiturates (and many other substances) stimulate (induce) the synthesis of more enzymes as well as more SER. In this manner, the cell has adapted to be more effective at drug modification. It also follows that cells that have adapted to metabolize one compound frequently are also more effective at metabolizing a number of others. Thus, patients taking phenobarbital for epilepsy who increase their alcohol intake may end up with subtherapeutic levels of the antiseizure medication.

Heat Shock Proteins and Protein Kinesis. One of the most highly conserved biologic responses in the phylogenetic hierarchy is the induction of *stress proteins* in response to potentially injurious stimuli. These were originally called *heat shock proteins (HSPs)* because they were described in fruit fly larvae after slight (4° to 5°C) elevations in temperature; however, the same proteins are elaborated in response to a wide variety of physical and chemical stimuli in all species so far examined.

Many HSPs are constitutively produced in normal cells (e.g., *Hsp 60* and *Hsp 90*) where they presumably play roles in normal intracellular "house-keeping," including protein folding, disaggregation, and intracellular transport (protein kinesis). They are thus also called *chaperonins.* Others, e.g., the *Hsp 70* family of proteins, are primarily seen only after injurious stimuli, where they putatively play a role in refolding denatured polypeptides. The 76-amino acid *ubiquitin* HSP molecule tags irretrievably denatured proteins and thereby tar-

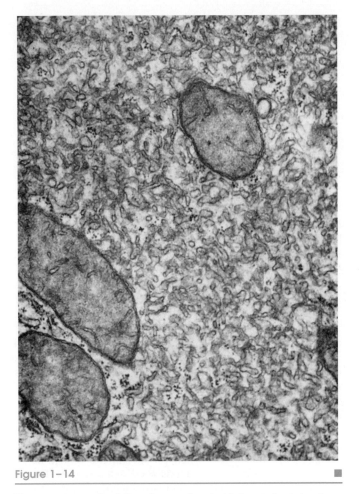

Figure 1–14

Electron micrograph of liver from a phenobarbital-treated rat showing a marked increase in smooth ER. (Reproduced, with permission, from Jones AL, Fawcett DW: Hypertrophy of the agranular endoplasmic reticulum in hamster liver induced by phenobarbital. J Histochem Cytochem 14:215, 1966. Courtesy of Dr. Fawcett.)

gets them for cytosolic catabolism by proteasomes, a particulate cluster of nonlysosomal proteinases.

HSP chaperones have been shown to be induced in myocardial infarcts and neuronal ischemic injury, and their induction appears to limit tissue necrosis in certain models of ischemia and reperfusion. The fact that they are found so ubiquitously, and are up-regulated in the setting of sublethal cellular stresses, strongly suggests that they play a role in cell adaptation to injury. Moreover, there is increasing evidence that misfolded or misdirected proteins may play central roles in a variety of diseases ranging from Creutzfeld-Jakob disease to Alzheimer's disease (Chapter 23).

Intracellular Accumulations

Under some circumstances, normal cells may accumulate abnormal amounts of various substances. These may accumulate either transiently or permanently, and may be harmless or may cause varying degrees of injury. The location of the substance may be in either the cytoplasm (most frequently within lysosomes) or the nucleus. The substance may be synthesized by the affected cells or may be produced elsewhere.

The processes that may result in abnormal intracellular accumulations can be divided into three general types:

1. A normal endogenous substance is produced at a normal or increased rate, but the rate of metabolism is inadequate to remove it. An example of this type of process is fatty change in the liver (see below).
2. A normal or abnormal endogenous substance accumulates because it cannot be metabolized. An important cause is a genetic enzymatic defect in a specific metabolic pathway, so that some metabolite cannot be used. The resulting disorders are referred to as storage diseases (Chapter 7).
3. An abnormal exogenous substance is deposited and accumulates because the cell has neither the enzymatic machinery to degrade the substance nor the ability to transport it to other sites. Accumulations of carbon or silica particles are examples of this type of alteration.

Fatty Change (Steatosis). Fatty change refers to any abnormal accumulation of triglycerides within parenchymal cells. Although itself an indicator of reversible injury, fatty change is sometimes encountered in cells adjacent to those that have undergone necrosis. Fatty change is most often seen in the liver, since this is the major organ involved in fat metabolism, but it may also occur in heart, skeletal muscle, kidney, and other organs. Steatosis may be caused by toxins, protein malnutrition, diabetes mellitus, obesity, and anoxia. However, *alcohol abuse is undoubtedly the most common cause of fatty change in the liver (fatty liver) in industrialized nations.*

Any of a number of steps in liver triglyceride metabolism may be interrupted, thus accounting for the occurrence of fatty liver after diverse hepatic insults. Free fatty acids from adipose tissue or ingested food are normally transported into hepatocytes; there they are esterified to triglycerides, converted into cholesterol or phospholipids, or oxidized to ketone bodies. Some fatty acids are synthesized from acetate within the hepatocytes, as well. Egress of the triglycerides from the hepatocytes requires complexing with apoproteins to form lipoproteins, which may then traverse the circulation (Chapter 7). Excess accumulation of triglycerides may result from defects at any step from fatty acid entry to lipoprotein exit (Fig. 1–15A). Hepatotoxins (e.g., alcohol) alter mitochondrial and SER function; CCl_4 and protein malnutrition decrease synthesis of apoproteins; anoxia inhibits fatty acid oxidation; and starvation increases fatty acid mobilization from peripheral stores.

The significance of fatty change depends on the cause and the severity of accumulation. When mild, it may have no effect on cellular function. More severe fatty change may transiently impair cellular function, but unless some vital intracellular process is irreversibly impaired (e.g., CCl_4 poisoning), fatty change is reversible. In a severe form, fatty change may precede cell death, but it should be emphasized that *cells may die without undergoing fatty change.*

LIVER. In the liver, mild fatty change may not affect the gross appearance. With accumulation, the organ enlarges and becomes progressively

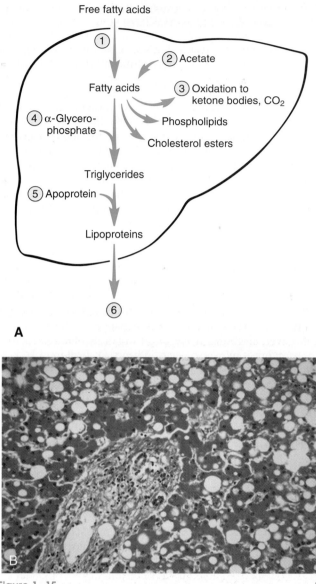

A

Figure 1-15

A, Possible mechanisms leading to accumulation of triglycerides in fatty liver. Defects in any of the six numbered steps of uptake, catabolism, or secretion can result in lipid accumulation. *B*, High-power detail of fatty change of liver. In most cells, the well-preserved nucleus is squeezed into the displaced rim of cytoplasm about the fat vacuole. (*B*, Courtesy of Dr. James Crawford, Department of Pathology, Brigham and Women's Hospital, Boston.)

yellow until, in extreme cases, it may weigh 3 to 6 kg and appear as bright yellow, soft, and greasy.

Fatty change is first seen by light microscopy as small fat vacuoles in the cytoplasm around the nucleus. As the process progresses, the vacuoles coalesce to create cleared spaces that displace the nucleus to the cell periphery (Fig. 1-15*B*). Occasionally, contiguous cells rupture and the enclosed fat globules unite to produce so-called fatty cysts.

HEART. Lipid is found in cardiac muscle in the form of small droplets, occurring in one of two patterns. Prolonged moderate hypoxia (as in profound anemia) results in focal intracellular fat deposits, creating grossly apparent bands of yellowed myocardium alternating with bands of darker, red-brown, uninvolved heart ("tigered effect"). The other pattern of fatty change is produced by more profound hypoxia or by some forms of myocarditis (e.g., diphtheria) and shows more uniformly affected myocytes.

Cholesterol and Cholesterol Esters. Cellular cholesterol metabolism is tightly regulated to ensure normal cell membrane synthesis without significant intracellular accumulation. However, phagocytic cells may become overloaded with lipid (triglycerides, cholesterol, and cholesteryl esters) in several different pathologic processes.

Scavenger macrophages in contact with the lipid debris of necrotic cells or abnormal forms of plasma lipid may become stuffed with lipid because of their phagocytic activities. These macrophages become filled with minute, membrane-bound vacuoles of lipid, imparting a foamy appearance to their cytoplasm (*foam cells*). In *atherosclerosis*, smooth muscle cells and macrophages are filled with lipid vacuoles composed of cholesterol and cholesterol esters; these give atherosclerotic plaques their characteristic yellow color and contribute to the pathogenesis of the lesion (Chapter 10). In hereditary and acquired hyperlipidemic syndromes, macrophages accumulate intracellular cholesterol; when present in the subepithelial connective tissue of skin or in tendons, clusters of these foamy macrophages form masses called *xanthomas*.

Proteins. Morphologically visible protein accumulations are much less common than lipid accumulations; they may occur because excesses are presented to the cells or because the cells synthesize excessive amounts. In the kidney, for example, trace amounts of albumin filtered through the glomerulus are normally reabsorbed by pinocytosis in the proximal convoluted tubules. However, in disorders with heavy protein leakage across the glomerular filter (e.g., glomerulonephritis), there is a commensurately increased pinocytic reabsorption of the protein. Fusion of these pinocytic vesicles with lysosomes results in the histologic appearance of pink, hyaline cytoplasmic droplets. The process is reversible; if the proteinuria abates, the protein droplets are metabolized and disappear. Another example is the marked accumulations of newly synthesized immunoglobulins that may occur in the RER of some plasma cells, resulting in rounded, eosinophilic *Russell bodies*.

Glycogen. Excessive intracellular deposits of glycogen are seen with abnormalities in the metabolism of either glucose or glycogen. In routine histologic preparations, the accumulated glycogen masses appear as vacuoles within the cell. When tissue sections are preserved in nonaqueous fixatives (to prevent solubilization and loss of the water-soluble glycogen) and specifically stained to detect carbohydrate (PAS stain), the glycogen accumulation is highlighted as red-violet globules.

Diabetes mellitus, the prime example of aberrant glucose metabolism, results in glycogen accumulation in renal tubular epithelium, hepatocytes, cardiac myocytes, and beta cells of the islets of Langerhans. Glycogen also accumulates within cells in a group of closely related genetic disorders collectively referred to as *glycogen storage diseases,* or *glycogenoses* (Chapter 7). In these diseases, enzymatic defects in the synthesis or breakdown of glycogen result in massive stockpiling, with secondary injury and cell death.

Pigments. Pigments are colored substances that are either exogenous, coming from outside the body, or endogenous, synthesized within the body itself.

The most common exogenous pigment is carbon or coal dust, which is a ubiquitous air pollutant of urban life. When inhaled, it is phagocytosed by alveolar macrophages and transported through lymphatic channels to the regional tracheobronchial lymph nodes. Aggregates of the pigment grossly blacken the draining lymph nodes and pulmonary parenchyma (anthracosis). Heavy accumulations may induce a fibroblastic reaction or emphysema, resulting in a serious lung disease called coal workers' pneumoconiosis (Chapter 8).

Endogenous pigments include lipofuscin, melanin, and certain derivatives of hemoglobin. *Lipofuscin* or "wear-and-tear pigment" is an insoluble, brownish-yellow granular intracellular material that accumulates in a variety of tissues (particularly the heart, liver, and brain) as a function of age or atrophy. When apparent in tissue grossly, it is called brown atrophy. By electron microscopy, the pigment appears as perinuclear electron-dense granules (Fig. 1–16). Lipofuscin represents complexes of lipid and protein that derive from the free radical–catalyzed peroxidation of polyunsaturated lipids of subcellular membranes. It is not injurious to the cell but is important as a marker of past free radical injury.

Melanin is an endogenous, brown-black pigment formed by melanocytes when the enzyme tyrosinase catalyzes the oxidation of tyrosine to dihydroxyphenylalanine. It is synthesized exclusively by melanocytes, specific cells characteristically found in the epidermis, and acts as an endogenous screen against harmful ultraviolet radiation. Although melanocytes are the only source of melanin, adjacent basal keratinocytes in the skin can accumulate the pigment (e.g., in freckles) or it may be accumulated in dermal macrophages.

Hemosiderin is a hemoglobin-derived granular pigment that is golden-yellow to brown and accumulates in tissues when there is a local or systemic excess of iron. Iron is normally stored in association with the protein apoferritin in the form of ferritin micelles. Hemosiderin pigment represents large aggregates of these ferritin micelles, which are readily seen by light and electron microscopy; the iron can be unambiguously identified by the Prussian blue histochemical reaction. Although usually pathologic, small amounts of hemosiderin are normal in the mononuclear phagocytes of the bone marrow, spleen, and liver, where there is extensive red cell breakdown.

Local excesses of iron, and consequently hemosiderin, result from gross hemorrhages or the myriad minute hemorrhages accompanying severe vascular congestion. The best example is the common bruise. After lysis of the erythrocytes at the site of hemorrhage, the red cell debris is phagocytosed by macrophages; the hemoglobin content is then catabolized by lysosomes with accumulation of the heme iron in hemosiderin. The array of colors through which the bruise passes reflects these transformations. The original red-blue color of hemoglobin is transformed to varying shades of green-blue by the local formation of biliverdin (green bile) and bilirubin (red bile) from the heme moiety; the iron ions of hemoglobin are accumulated as golden-yellow hemosiderin.

Whenever there is systemic overload of iron, hemosiderin is deposited in many organs and tissues, a condition called *hemosiderosis.* It is found at first in the mononuclear phagocytes of the liver, bone marrow, spleen, and lymph nodes and in scattered macrophages throughout other organs. With pro-

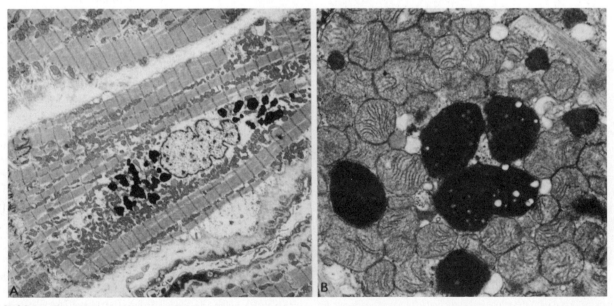

Figure 1–16

Lipofuscin granules in a cardiac myocyte as shown by electron microscopy. *A,* Low magnification. Note the perinuclear, intralysosomal location. *B,* Electron-dense bodies are composed of lipid-protein complexes.

gressive accumulation, parenchymal cells throughout the body (but principally the liver, pancreas, heart, and endocrine organs) become "bronzed" with accumulating pigment. It is seen with (1) increased absorption of dietary iron, (2) impaired utilization of iron, (3) hemolytic anemias, and (4) transfusions (the transfused red cells constitute an exogenous load of iron). These conditions are discussed in Chapter 12. In most instances of systemic hemosiderosis, the pigment does not damage the parenchymal cells or impair organ function. However, more extensive accumulations of iron result in hemochromatosis (Chapter 16), which does result in tissue injury, including liver fibrosis, heart failure, and diabetes mellitus.

Pathologic Calcification

Pathologic calcification is a common process in a wide variety of disease states; it implies the abnormal deposition of calcium salts, together with smaller amounts of iron, magnesium, and other minerals. When the deposition occurs in dead or dying tissues, it is called *dystrophic calcification; it may occur despite normal serum levels of calcium* and in the absence of calcium metabolic derangements. In contrast, the deposition of calcium salts in normal tissues is known as *metastatic calcification and almost always reflects some derangement in calcium metabolism, leading to hypercalcemia.*

Dystrophic Calcification. Dystrophic calcification is encountered in areas of necrosis of any type. It is virtually inevitable in the atheromas of advanced atherosclerosis, which represent areas of intimal injury in the aorta and larger arteries, characterized by accumulated lipids (Chapter 10). Although it may simply represent evidence of previous cell injury, it is also often a cause of organ dysfunction. For example, it commonly develops in aging or damaged heart valves, further hampering their function. Dystrophic calcification of the aor-

tic valves is an important cause of (calcific) aortic stenosis in the elderly (Fig. 1–17).

Regardless of the site, the calcium salts are grossly seen as fine, white granules or clumps, often felt as gritty deposits. Sometimes, a tuberculous lymph node is essentially converted to stone. Histologically, calcification appears as **intracellular** and/or **extracellular** basophilic deposits. In time, **heterotopic bone** may be formed in the focus of calcification.

The pathogenesis of dystrophic calcification involves initiation and propagation, leading ultimately to the formation of crystalline calcium phosphate. Initiation in extracellular sites occurs in membrane-bound vesicles about 200 nm in diameter; in normal cartilage and bone they are known as matrix vesicles, whereas in pathologic calcification they derive from degenerating cells. It is thought that calcium is initially concentrated in these vesicles by its affinity for acidic phospholipids, while phosphates accumulate as a result of the action of membrane-bound phosphatases. Initiation of intracellular calcification occurs in the mitochondria of dead or dying cells that have lost their ability to regulate intracellular calcium. After initiation in either location, propagation of crystal formation occurs. This is dependent on the concentration of Ca^{++} and PO_4 in the extracellular spaces, the presence of mineral inhibitors, and the degree of collagenization. Collagen enhances the rate of crystal growth, and other proteins such as osteopontin (an acidic, calcium-binding phosphoprotein) appear also to be involved.

Metastatic Calcification. Metastatic calcification may occur in normal tissues whenever there is hypercalcemia; clearly, hypercalcemia will also exacerbate dystrophic calcification. The causes of hypercalcemia include primary endocrine dysfunction such as hyperparathyroidism; the effects of tumors, such as in the increased bone catabolism associated with multiple myeloma, metastatic cancer, and leukemia; ingested exogenous substances, resulting in vitamin D intoxication or milk-alkali syndrome; and sarcoidosis. Hypercalcemia may also arise in advanced renal failure, where the resulting phosphate retention leads to secondary hyperparathyroidism.

Metastatic calcification may occur widely throughout the body but principally affects the interstitial tissues of the vasculature, kidneys, lungs, and gastric mucosa. The calcium salts morphologically resemble those described in dystrophic calcification. Although the calcific deposits do not generally cause clinical dysfunction, occasionally extensive involvement of the lungs may produce respiratory deficits (as well as remarkable changes seen in chest radiographs). Massive deposits in the kidney (nephrocalcinosis) may in time also cause renal damage.

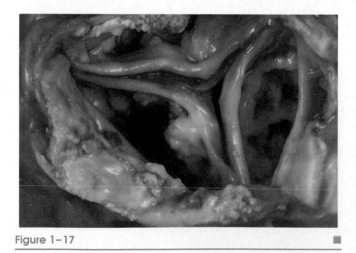

Figure 1–17 ■

A view looking down onto the unopened aortic valve in a heart with calcific aortic stenosis. The semilunar cusps are thickened and fibrotic. Behind each cusp are seen irregular masses of piled-up dystrophic calcification.

CELLULAR ADAPTATIONS OF GROWTH AND DIFFERENTIATION

As described earlier, even under normal conditions, cells must constantly adapt to changes in their environment. These *physiologic adaptations* usually represent responses of cells to normal stimulation by hormones or endogenous chemical mediators (e.g. the enlargement of the breast and induction of lactation by pregnancy). *Pathologic adaptations* often share the same underlying mechanisms, but they allow the cells to modulate their environment and hopefully escape injury. Thus, cellular adaptation is a state that lies between the normal, unstressed cell and the injured, overstressed cell.

Cellular adaptation can proceed by a number of mechanisms. Some adaptive responses involve *up- or down-regulation of specific cellular receptors*; for example, cell surface receptors involved in the uptake of low-density lipoproteins (LDLs) are normally down-regulated when the cells are cholesterol replete (Chapter 7). Other adaptive responses are associated with the *induction of new protein synthesis by the target cell*. These proteins, such as heat shock proteins, may protect cells from certain forms of injury. Still other adaptations involve a switch from producing one type of protein to another, or marked overproduction of a specific protein; such is the case in cells synthesizing various collagens and extracellular matrix proteins in chronic inflammation and fibrosis (Chapter 3). Cellular adaptive responses can thus occur at any of a number of steps, including receptor binding; signal transduction; or protein transcription, translation, or export.

In this section the adaptive changes in cell growth and differentiation that are particularly important in pathologic conditions are considered. These include *atrophy* (decrease in cell size), *hypertrophy* (increase in cell size), *hyperplasia* (increase in cell number), and *metaplasia* (change in cell type).

Atrophy

Shrinkage in the size of the cell by loss of cell substance is known as atrophy. When a sufficient number of cells are involved, the entire tissue or organ diminishes in size, becoming atrophic (Fig. 1–18). It should be emphasized that *although atrophic cells may have diminished function, they are not dead*. In contradistinction, apoptotic death may also be induced by the same signals that cause atrophy, and thus may contribute to loss of cells in "atrophy" of an entire organ.

Causes of atrophy include decreased workload, loss of innervation, diminished blood supply, inadequate nutrition, loss of endocrine stimulation, and aging. Although some of these stimuli are physiologic (e.g., loss of hormone stimulation in menopause) and others pathologic (e.g., denervation), the fundamental cellular changes are identical. They represent a retreat by the cell to a smaller size at which survival is still possible; a new equilibrium is achieved between cell size and diminished blood supply, nutrition, or trophic stimulation.

The biochemical mechanisms of atrophy are varied. In normal cells, there is a finely regulated balance between protein synthesis and degradation, influenced by a number of hormones, including insulin, thyroid-stimulating hormone, and glucocorticoids. Decreased synthesis, increased catabolism, or both may cause atrophy. For example, slight increases of degradation over long periods may result in atrophy, as occurs in some muscular dystrophies.

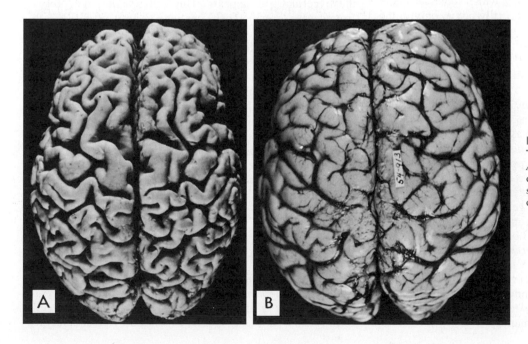

Figure 1–18   ■

A, Atrophy of the brain in an 82-year-old man. The meninges have been stripped. *B*, Normal brain of a 25-year-old man, for comparison.

In many situations, atrophy is accompanied by marked increases in the number of autophagic vacuoles (p 16). Some of the cell debris within the autophagic vacuole may resist digestion and persist as membrane-bound residual bodies (e.g., lipofuscin) described earlier.

Hypertrophy

Hypertrophy constitutes an increase in the size of cells and, with such change, an increase in the size of the organ. Thus, there are no new cells, just larger cells. Moreover, these cells are not enlarged by simple cellular edema but by the increased synthesis of more structural proteins and organelles. Hypertrophy can be *physiologic* or *pathologic* and is caused by increased functional demand or specific hormonal stimulation. The physiologic growth of the uterus during pregnancy involves both smooth muscle hypertrophy and hyperplasia. The cellular hypertrophy is stimulated by estrogen via intracellular estrogen receptors, permitting interaction of the hormone with nuclear DNA, and eventually resulting in increased synthesis of smooth muscle proteins. Adaptive hypertrophy is exemplified by skeletal muscle enlargement in the avid weight lifter, or cardiac enlargement in the chronically hypertensive patient (see Fig. 1–1). The striated muscle cells in both the heart and skeletal muscle undergo hypertrophy because they cannot adapt to increased demands by mitotic division to generate more cells to share the work.

The environmental change that produces hypertrophy of striated muscle appears to be increased workload. Synthesis of more proteins and filaments putatively achieves a balance between the demand and the cell's functional capacity. The greater number of myofilaments permits an increased workload with the same level of metabolic activity per unit volume as the normal cell. However, there may also be a dramatic change in the cell phenotype in response to external stresses. In chronic cardiac volume overload, for example, contractile proteins switch to fetal isoforms (which contract more slowly), and a variety of genes, normally active only in the neonatal heart, are reactivated. The nuclei in nondividing, hypertrophied cells such as cardiac myocytes have a much higher DNA content than normal myocardial cells; this is probably because the cells arrest in the G_2 phase of the cell cycle without undergoing mitosis.

What triggers the changes in gene expression that culminate in hypertrophy? In the heart, there are at least two types of signals: *mechanical triggers*, such as stretch, and *trophic triggers*, such as activation of α-adrenergic receptors. Whatever the exact mechanism(s) of hypertrophy, a limit is reached beyond which enlargement of muscle mass is no longer able to compensate for the increased burden; in the case of the heart, cardiac failure ensues. At this stage a number of "degenerative" changes occur in the myocardial fibers, of which the most important are lysis and loss of myofibrillar contractile elements. The factors that limit continued hypertrophy and cause the regressive changes are incompletely understood. There may be finite limits of the vasculature to adequately supply the enlarged fibers, of the mitochondria to supply ATP, or of the biosynthetic machinery to provide the contractile proteins or other cytoskeletal elements.

Hyperplasia

Hyperplasia constitutes an increase in the number of cells in an organ or tissue. Hypertrophy and hyperplasia are closely related and often develop concurrently in tissues, so that both may contribute to an overall increase in organ size. For example, estrogen-induced growth in the uterus involves increased DNA synthesis, with mitosis, as well as enlargement of smooth muscle and epithelial cells. In certain instances, however, even potentially dividing cells, such as renal epithelial cells, undergo hypertrophy but not hyperplasia.

Hyperplasia can be physiologic or pathologic. *Physiologic hyperplasia* is divided into (1) *hormonal hyperplasia,* exemplified by proliferation of the glandular epithelium of the female breast at puberty and during pregnancy; and (2) *compensatory hyperplasia,* that is, hyperplasia that occurs when a portion of the tissue is removed or diseased. For example, when a portion of the liver is removed, mitotic activity in the remaining cells begins as early as 12 hours later, eventually restoring the liver to its normal weight—at which time cell proliferation ceases. The stimuli for hyperplasia in this setting are polypeptide growth factors, some of which are produced by remnant hepatocytes or nonparenchymal hepatic cells. After restoration of the liver mass, cell proliferation is "turned off" by various growth inhibitors.

Most forms of pathologic hyperplasia are instances of excessive hormonal or growth factor stimulation. For example, after a normal menstrual period there is a burst of proliferative endometrial activity that is essentially physiologic hyperplasia. This proliferation is normally tightly regulated between stimulation by pituitary hormones and ovarian estrogen, and inhibition by progesterone. However, if the balance between estrogen and progesterone is disturbed (e.g., if there are absolute or relative increases in estrogen), hyperplasia results. Endometrial hyperplasia is a common cause of abnormal menstrual bleeding. It is important to note that the hyperplastic process remains controlled; if estrogenic stimulation abates, the hyperplasia disappears. This differentiates the process from cancer, in which cells continue to grow despite the absence of hormonal stimuli. Nevertheless, pathologic hyperplasia constitutes a fertile soil in which cancerous proliferation may eventually arise. Thus, patients with hyperplasia of the endometrium are at increased risk of developing endometrial cancer (Chapter 19).

Hyperplasia is also an important response of connective tissue cells in wound healing, in which proliferating fibroblasts and blood vessels, stimulated by growth factors (Chapter 3), aid in repair. Stimulation by growth factors is also involved in the hyperplasia that is associated with certain virus infections such as by the papillomaviruses that cause the common skin wart.

Metaplasia

Metaplasia is a reversible change in which one adult cell type (epithelial or mesenchymal) is replaced by another adult cell type. This is another cellular adaptation whereby cells sensitive to a particular stress are replaced by other cell types

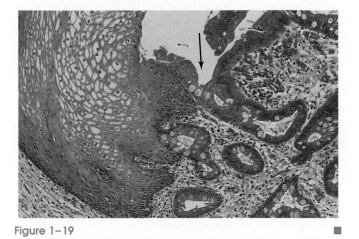

Figure 1–19   ■

Metaplastic transformation *(arrow)* of the normal adult esophageal stratified squamous epithelium to mature columnar epithelium (so-called Barrett's metaplasia).

better able to withstand the adverse environment. It is thought to arise by genetic "reprogramming" of epithelial stem cells, or of undifferentiated mesenchymal cells in connective tissue.

Metaplasia is exemplified by the squamous change that occurs in the respiratory epithelium in habitual cigarette smokers. The normal ciliated columnar epithelial cells of the trachea and bronchi are focally or widely replaced by stratified squamous epithelial cells. A deficiency of vitamin A may also induce squamous metaplasia in the respiratory epithelium. Presumably, the more "rugged" stratified squamous epithelium is able to survive under circumstances that the more fragile specialized epithelium would not tolerate. However, although the adaptive metaplastic epithelium is better able to survive, important protective mechanisms are lost, such as mucus secretion and ciliary clearance of particulate matter. Epithelial metaplasia is therefore a two-edged sword; moreover, the influences that induce metaplastic transformation, if persistent, may induce cancer transformation in the metaplastic epithelium. Thus, the most common form of cancer of the respiratory epithelium is composed of malignant squamous cells. Metaplasia need not always occur in the direction of columnar to squamous epithelium; in chronic gastric reflux, the normal stratified squamous epithelium of the lower esophagus may undergo metaplastic transformation to gastric or intestine-type columnar epithelium (Fig. 1–19).

Metaplasia may also occur in mesenchymal cells but less clearly as an adaptive response. Fibroblasts may be transformed to osteoblasts or chondroblasts to produce bone or cartilage where it is normally not encountered. For example, bone is occasionally formed in soft tissues, particularly (but not always) in foci of injury.

CELLULAR AGING

Cellular aging is discussed here because it probably represents the progressive accumulation over the years of al-

terations in structure and function that may lead to cell death, or at least diminished capacity of the cell to respond to injury.

A number of cell functions decline progressively with age. Mitochondrial oxidative phosphorylation is reduced, as is synthesis of structural, enzymatic, and receptor proteins. Senescent cells have a diminished capacity for nutrient uptake and for repair of chromosomal damage. The morphologic alterations in senescent cells include irregular and abnormal lobed nuclei, pleomorphic vacuolated mitochondria, decreased endoplasmic reticulum, and distorted Golgi apparatus. Concomitantly, there is a steady accumulation of lipofuscin pigment, indicating past membrane injury and lipid peroxidation.

Although a number of theories have been proposed, it is clear that cellular senescence is multifactorial. It involves the cumulative effects of *extrinsic* influences and an *intrinsic* molecular program of cellular aging.

The *wear-and-tear theories* imply that adverse exogenous influences eventually exceed the cells' regenerative potential, thus causing senescence. A favored theory invokes the progressive effects of *free radical damage* throughout life. This damage can occur by repeated environmental exposure to such influences as ionizing radiation, to a progressive reduction of antioxidant defense mechanisms (e.g., vitamin E, glutathione peroxidase), or to both. The accumulation of lipofuscin is consistent with free radical damage, but there is no evidence that the pigment itself is toxic to cells. However, free radicals *can* induce mitochondrial and nuclear DNA damage; free radical injury is estimated to cause some 10,000 base modifications per cell per day. A second wear-and-tear mechanism involves post-translational modifications of intracellular and extracellular proteins. One such modification is free radical oxidation; another is nonenzymatic glycosylation, leading to the formation of advanced glycosylation end products (AGEs) capable of cross-linking adjacent proteins. Such AGEs may well play a role in the pathogenesis of diabetes mellitus (Chapter 17), and age-related glycosylation of lens proteins underlies senile cataracts.

The group of *intrinsic cellular aging* theories hold that progressive cellular damage occurs as a consequence of innate properties of cells conferred by predetermined genetic programming. The theories are lent credence by the old observation that normal human fibroblasts in culture have a finite life span; they stop dividing and become senescent after about 50 doublings (so-called "Hayflick phenomenon"). In contrast, fibroblasts from patients with *progeria*, who age prematurely, have markedly fewer doublings. It is not clear, however, how this concept should apply to postmitotic cells, such as neurons. For mitotically active cells, two hypotheses have been proposed:

■ The somatic mutation hypothesis proposes that errors of DNA replication are not accurately repaired, and the accumulated mistakes ultimately impinge on the viability and survivability of cells.

■ The programmed aging hypothesis assumes a predetermined sequence of events leading ultimately to senescence. Repression and derepression of specific genetic programs are presumably involved. In addition, recent evidence suggests that sequential programmed shortening of *telomeres* (terminal chromosomal structures critical for stabilizing chromosomes) may lead to progressive loss of essential genes, and thus to cell senescence.

Much more might be said about the mechanisms responsible for the alterations that occur in cell senescence. It suffices here to note that, according to the current best evidence, some mechanisms are probably only extensions of those involved in the maturation and differentiation of cells, while others are attributable to environmental influences.

BIBLIOGRAPHY

Chipman JK: Mechanisms of cell toxicity. Curr Opin Cell Biol 1:231, 1989. (A summary of the biochemical mechanisms of cell injury.)

Cristofalo DV, Pignolo RJ: Replicative senescence of human cells in culture. Physiol Rev 73:617, 1993. (A review of current theories of cellular senescence.)

Farber JL: Mechanisms of cell injury by activated oxygen species. Environ Health Perspect 102 (Suppl 10):17, 1994. (An overview of the mechanisms of free radical–induced cell injury.)

Knight JA: Diseases related to oxygen-derived free radicals. Ann Clin Lab Sci 25:111, 1995. (A review of role of oxygen-derived free radicals in cell injury and disease.)

Majno G, Joris I: Apoptosis, oncosis, and necrosis; an overview of cell death. Am J Pathol 146:3, 1995. (A discussion of the historical and pathologic distinctions in the basic modes of cell death.)

Majno G, Joris I: Cells, Tissues and Disease. Principles of General Pathology. Cambridge, MA, Blackwell Science, 1996. (Chapters 2 to 5 clearly cover issues of intracellular pathology and cell death.)

Martin SJ, Green DR: Protease activation during apoptosis: death by a thousand cuts? Cell 82:349, 1995. (A summary of the data regarding intracellular protease activation during apoptosis.)

Mergner WJ, et al (eds): Cell Death. Mechanisms of Acute and Lethal Cell Injury, Vol 1. New York, Field & Wood Medical Publishers, 1990. (A compendium of articles dealing with biochemical mechanisms of cell injury.)

Richter C, et al: Oxidants in mitochondria: from physiology to diseases. Biochim Biophys Acta 1271:67, 1995. (A review of the effects on mitochondrial function of reactive oxygen species; part of a volume with a number of articles covering similar issues.)

Riley PA: Free radicals in biology: oxidative stress and the effects of ionizing radiation. Int J Radiat Biol 65:27, 1994. (A review of causes and mechanisms of free radical injury.)

Schoen FJ, et al: Calcification: pathology, mechanisms and strategies of prevention. J Biomed Mater Res 22:A1, 1988. (A summary of the mechanisms of calcification.)

Science issue devoted to theories of aging. Science 273:54, 1996. (Up-to-date reviews on longevity genes, oxidative injury, and replicative senescence.)

Taubes G: Misfolding the way to disease. Science 271:1493, 1996. (A commentary report on current developments in protein kinesis, as part of an issue devoted to articles on protein folding and intracellular translocation.)

Tomei LD, Cope FO (eds): Apoptosis: The Molecular Basis of Cell Death. New York, Cold Spring Harbor Laboratory Press, 1991. (A compendium of articles relating to various aspects of apoptosis.)

Trump BF, Berezesky IK: Calcium-mediated cell injury and cell death. FASEB J 9:219, 1995. (A review of the current theories regarding cell injury associated with disregulation of intracellular calcium.)

Weinberg JM: The cell biology of ischemic injury. Kidney Int 39:476, 1991. (A discussion of the role of alterations in purine nucleotide metabolism, calcium, phospholipids, and oxidants in ischemic injury in the kidney.)

Welch WJ: Mammalian stress response: cell physiology, structure/function of stress proteins, and implications for medicine and disease. Physiol Rev 72:1063, 1992. (A review of heat shock proteins and cellular response to stress.)

Wolf G, Nielson EG: Molecular mechanisms of renal hypertrophy and hyperplasia. Kidney Int 39:401, 1991. (A review of growth factors and signal mechanisms associated with hypertrophy and hyperplasia.)

2

Acute and Chronic Inflammation

RICHARD N. MITCHELL, MD, PhD
RAMZI S. COTRAN, MD

While various exogenous and endogenous stimuli can cause direct cell injury (Chapter 1), the same stimuli also incite a complex reaction in vascularized connective tissues called *inflammation*. Inflammation is essentially a protective response intended to eliminate both the initial cause of cell injury (e.g., microbes or toxins) and the necrotic cells and tissues arising as a consequence of such injury. As such, inflammation is also intimately interwoven with repair processes (Chapter 3). The inflammatory response dilutes, destroys, or isolates the causative agent, and sets into motion the sequence of events that heal and reconstitute the damaged tissue. During repair, the injured tissue is replaced by regeneration of native parenchymal cells, by filling of the defect with fibroblastic scar tissue (scarring), or most commonly by some combination of these two processes.

Although inflammation helps clear infections and, along with repair, makes wound healing possible, both have considerable potential to cause harm. For example, inflammatory reactions underlie life-threatening anaphylactic responses to insect bites or drugs, as well as chronic diseases such as rheumatoid arthritis and atherosclerosis. Similarly, scarring, such as sometimes follows bacteria-induced inflammation in the pericardial sac, can encase the heart in dense fibrous tissue, permanently impairing cardiac function.

Inflammation is grouped into two basic forms. *Acute* inflammation is of relatively short duration, lasting from a few minutes up to a few days, and is characterized by fluid and plasma protein exudation, and by a predominantly neutrophilic leukocyte accumulation. *Chronic* inflammation is of longer duration (days to years) and is manifested histologically by influx of lymphocytes and macrophages and by tissue destruction and repair; the latter is associated with vascular proliferation and fibrosis.

An initial inflammatory stimulus triggers the release of chemical mediators from plasma or cells, which then regulate the subsequent vascular and cellular responses. Such chemical mediators, acting together or in sequence, amplify the initial inflammatory response and influence its evolution. The inflammatory response is terminated when the injurious stimulus is removed and the inflammatory mediators have been dissipated, catabolized, or inhibited.

ACUTE INFLAMMATION

Acute inflammation is the immediate and early response to injury. A critical function of the response is to deliver leukocytes to the site of injury, where they can help clear invading bacteria (or other infectious agents), as well as degrade necrotic tissues resulting from the damage. Unfortunately, leukocytes themselves may also prolong inflammation and induce tissue damage by releasing enzymes, chemical mediators, and toxic oxygen radicals.

Acute inflammation has three major components: (1) alterations in vascular caliber that lead to a local increase in blood flow (vasodilation), (2) structural changes in the microvasculature that permit plasma proteins to leave the circulation, and (3) emigration of the leukocytes from the microcirculation and accumulation in the focus of injury (Fig. 2–1). These

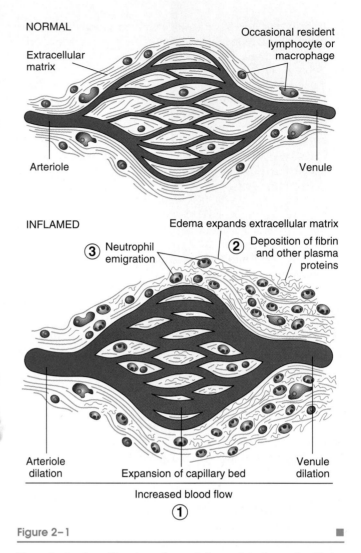

Figure 2–1 ■

The major local manifestations of acute inflammation: ① vascular dilation (causing erythema and warmth), ② extravasation of plasma fluid and proteins (edema), and ③ leukocyte emigration and accumulation in the site of injury.

components account for three of the five classic local signs of acute inflammation: heat (calor), redness (rubor), and swelling (tumor). The two additional cardinal features of acute inflammation, pain (dolor) and loss of function (functio laesa), occur as further consequences of mediator elaboration and of leukocyte emigration in the inflammatory response (see below).

Vascular Changes

CHANGES IN VASCULAR FLOW AND CALIBER

These changes begin relatively quickly after injury but may develop at variable rates, depending on the nature and severity of the original injury.

■ After an inconstant and transient (seconds) vasoconstriction of arterioles, vasodilation occurs. Arterioles are involved first, resulting in the opening of new microvascular beds in the area. The local increased blood flow is the cause of the redness (erythema) and warmth characteristically seen in acute inflammation (Fig. 2–1).

■ Subsequently, the microvasculature becomes more permeable, resulting in the exudation of protein-rich fluid into the extravascular tissues. This causes the red blood cells to become effectively more concentrated, thereby increasing blood viscosity and slowing the circulation. These changes are manifested microscopically by numerous dilated small vessels packed with erythrocytes, a process called *stasis*.

■ As stasis develops, leukocytes (principally neutrophils) begin to settle out of the flowing blood and accumulate along the vascular endothelial surface, a process called *margination*. After adhering to endothelial cells (see below), the leukocytes squeeze between them and migrate through the vascular wall into the interstitial tissue, a process called *emigration*.

INCREASED VASCULAR PERMEABILITY (VASCULAR LEAKAGE)

In the earliest phase of inflammation, the vasodilation and increased blood flow increase intravascular hydrostatic pressure, resulting in increased filtration of fluid from the capillaries. This fluid, called a *transudate*, is essentially an ultrafiltrate of blood plasma and contains little protein. Transudation is soon eclipsed, however, by the increasing vascular permeability, which permits the flow of protein-rich fluid and even cells (called an *exudate*) into the interstitium. The movement of protein-rich fluid from the plasma reduces the intravascular osmotic pressure, at the same time increasing the osmotic pressure of the interstitial fluid. The net result is outflow of water and ions into the extravascular tissues, which accumulation is called *edema* (Fig. 2–2).

How does the normally nonpenetrable endothelial layer become leaky during acute inflammation? At least five mechanisms are known (Fig. 2–3):

1. *Endothelial cell contraction* leads to widened intercellular gaps. Endothelial cell contraction is elicited by histamine, bradykinin, leukotrienes, and many other classes of chemical mediators, and is a reversible process. Cellular contraction occurs rapidly after binding of the mediator to specific receptors and is usually short-lived (15 to 30 minutes); consequently, this is called the *immediate transient response*. Only those endothelial cells lining venules 20 to 60 μm in diameter undergo contraction; endothelium in capillaries and arterioles is unaffected.

2. In experimental in vitro systems, *junctional retraction* is another reversible mechanism resulting in increased vascular permeability. A variety of cytokine mediators (including tumor necrosis factor [TNF] and interleukin 1 [IL-1]) induce a structural reorganization of the cytoskeleton, so that endothelial cells junctions are disrupted. In contrast to the immediate transient response, junctional retraction can occur only some 4 to 6 hours after the initial stimulus, and persists for 24 hours or more.

3. *Direct endothelial injury* results in vascular leakage by causing endothelial cell necrosis and detachment. This effect is usually seen after severe injuries (e.g., burns or in-

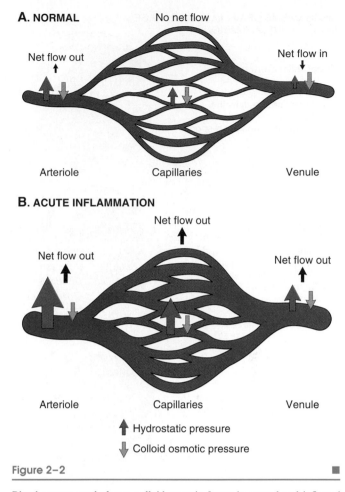

A. NORMAL

No net flow

Net flow out

Net flow in

Arteriole   Capillaries   Venule

B. ACUTE INFLAMMATION

Net flow out

Net flow out

Net flow out

Arteriole   Capillaries   Venule

↑ Hydrostatic pressure

↓ Colloid osmotic pressure

Figure 2–2   ■

Blood pressure and plasma colloid osmotic forces in normal and inflamed microcirculation. *A*, Normal hydrostatic pressure *(red arrows)* is about 32 mm Hg at the arterial end of a capillary bed and 12 mm Hg at the venous end; the mean colloid osmotic pressure of tissues is approximately 25 mm Hg *(green arrows)*, which is equal to the mean capillary pressure. Although fluid tends to leave the precapillary arteriole, it is returned in equal amounts via the postcapillary venule, so that the net flow *(black arrows)* in or out is zero. *B*, Acute inflammation. Arteriole pressure is increased to 50 mm Hg, the mean capillary pressure is increased because of arteriolar dilation, and the venous pressure increases to approximately 30 mm Hg. At the same time, osmotic pressure is reduced (averaging 20 mm Hg) because of protein leakage across the venule. The net result is an excess of extravasated fluid.

fections), and the endothelial cell detachment is often associated with platelet adhesion and thrombosis. In most cases, leakage begins immediately after the injury and persists for several hours (or days) until the damaged vessels are thrombosed or repaired. Thus, the reaction is known as the *immediate sustained response*. Venules, capillaries, and arterioles can all be affected.

Direct injury to endothelial cells may also induce a *delayed prolonged leakage* that begins after a delay of 2 to 12 hours, lasts for several hours or even days, and involves venules and capillaries. Examples include mild to moderate thermal injury, x- or ultraviolet irradiation (i.e., the late-appearing sunburn), and certain bacterial toxins. Although the mechanism is unclear, delayed cell damage attributable to apoptosis and the action of cytokines have both been suggested.

MECHANISMS OF VASCULAR LEAKAGE IN ACUTE INFLAMMATION

Endothelial contraction

- Venules
- Histamine, bradykinins, leukotrienes
- Immediate transient response

Junctional retraction

- Venules
- Cytokines (e.g., interleukin-1 and tumor necrosis factor)
- Onset within 4–6 hours after stimulus

Direct injury

- Arterioles, capillaries, and venules
- Immediate sustained and delayed prolonged leakage

Leukocyte-dependent injury

- Mostly venules
- Pulmonary capillaries
- Late response

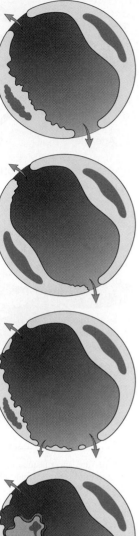

Figure 2–3 ■

Diagrammatic representation of four mechanisms of increased vascular permeability in inflammation. Not shown is the pathway involving increased vesiculovacuolar transcytosis.

4. *Leukocyte-dependent endothelial injury* may occur as a consequence of leukocyte accumulation during the inflammatory response. As discussed below (p 30), such leukocytes may be activated in the process, releasing toxic oxygen species and proteolytic enzymes, which then cause endothelial injury or detachment. This form of injury is largely restricted to those vascular sites (venules and pulmonary capillaries) where leukocytes can adhere to the endothelium.

5. *Increased transcytosis* (not shown in Fig. 2–3), via an intracellular vesiculovacuolar pathway, augments venular permeability, especially following exposure to certain mediators (e.g., vascular endothelial growth factor, VEGF; see later).

Although these mechanisms are separable, they may all participate in response to any particular stimulus. For example, in various stages of a thermal burn, leakage results from chemically mediated endothelial contraction as well as from direct and leukocyte-dependent injury. In addition, different chemical mediators may be produced in consecutive phases of the inflammatory response, resulting in delayed and/or sustained vascular changes.

Leukocyte Cellular Events

The sequence of events in the extravasation of leukocytes from the vascular lumen to the extravascular space is divided into (1) margination and rolling, (2) adhesion and transmigration between endothelial cells, and (3) migration in interstitial tissues toward a chemotactic stimulus (Fig. 2–4).

MARGINATION AND ROLLING

In normal blood flow, red and white blood cells generally travel along the central axis, leaving a cell-poor layer of plasma in contact with endothelium. As vascular permeability increases in early inflammation (as described above), fluid exits the vascular lumen and blood flow slows. As a result, the leukocytes settle out of the central column, marginating to the vessel periphery. Subsequently, the leukocytes tumble on the endothelial surface, transiently sticking along the way, a process called *rolling*. Rolling—as well as leukocyte adhesion and transmigration (described below)—is mediated

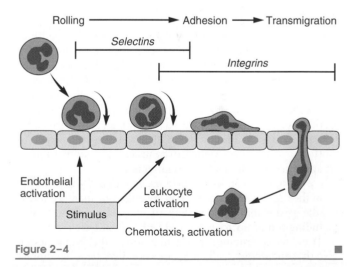

Figure 2–4 ■

Sequence of events in leukocyte emigration in inflammation. The leukocytes (1) roll, (2) arrest and adhere to endothelium, (3) transmigrate through an intercellular junction and pierce the basement membrane, and (4) migrate toward chemoattractants released from the source of injury. The roles of selectins, activating agents, and integrins are also indicated. (Modified and drawn from Travis JT: Biotech gets a grip on cell adhesion. Science 26:906, 1993.)

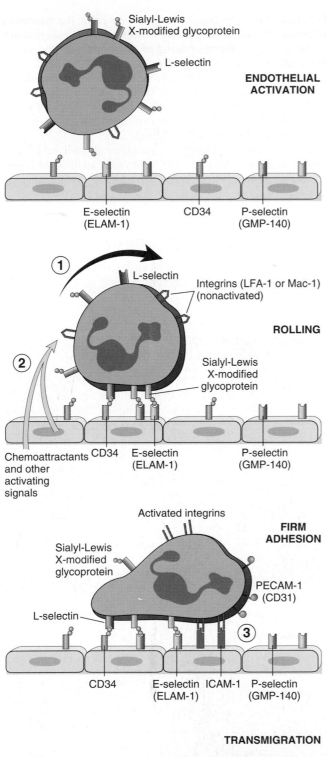

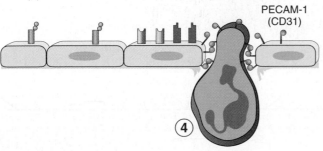

largely by the binding of complementary adhesion molecules on the leukocytes and endothelial surfaces, analogous to a lock and key (Fig. 2–5).

The relatively loose and transient adhesions involved in rolling are accounted for by the *selectin* family of molecules. These receptors are expressed on leukocytes and endothelium. Selectins are characterized by an extracellular domain that binds selected sugars (hence the "lectin" part of the name). These include E-selectin (also called ELAM-1), confined to endothelium; P-selectin (GMP140), present on endothelium and platelets; and L-selectin, studding the surface of most leukocytes. P- and E-selectins bind to sialylated oligosaccharide epitopes of certain leukocyte surface glycoproteins, while L-selectin binds to carbohydrate residues on mucin-like glycoproteins (e.g., GlyCAM-1 and CD34) on the endothelial cell surface. The endothelial selectins are typically at low levels or are not present at all on normal cells, and are up-regulated after stimulation by specific mediators (see Fig. 2–5). This allows a degree of specificity of binding restricted to sites where there is ongoing injury. For example, P-selectin is found at baseline primarily in intracellular Weibel-Palade bodies of endothelial cells; however, within minutes of exposure to mediators such as histamine, thrombin, or platelet-activating factor (PAF), P-selectin is distributed to the cell surface where it can facilitate leukocyte binding. Similarly, E-selectin, which is not present on normal endothelium, is induced after stimulation by inflammatory mediators such as IL-1 and TNF.

ADHESION AND TRANSMIGRATION

Eventually, the leukocytes firmly adhere to the endothelial surface (*adhesion*) before crawling between the cells and through the basement membrane into the extravascular space (*diapedesis*). The adhesion is largely mediated by endothelial adhesion molecules of the immunoglobulin superfamily, binding to various integrins found on the leukocyte cell surfaces (Fig. 2–5). The endothelial adhesion molecules include ICAM-1 (intercellular adhesion molecule 1) and VCAM-1 (vascular cell adhesion molecule 1), both of which have increased surface expression after stimulation of endothelium by various cytokines. Integrins are transmembrane heterodimeric glycoproteins that also function as cell receptors for

Figure 2–5   ■

Molecules mediating endothelial-neutrophil interaction. ① Initial adhesion via the selectins and glycosylated proteins. E- and P-selectins on endothelial cells are upregulated at the inflammatory sites by action of specific mediators. E- and P-selectins bind sialyl-Lewis X oligosaccharide epitopes on certain core glycoproteins on leukocytes, while L-selectins on leukocytes bind sugar moieties on core proteins such as CD34 glycoproteins on endothelial cells. Note that colored balls represent sugar moieties and that the various receptors are consistently color-coded (e.g., L-selectin is orange, CD34 is pink, P-selectin is blue, E-selectin is yellow, and sialyl-Lewis X-linked glycoproteins are green). ② Activation of leukocytes by selectin binding and/or mediators increases integrin avidity. ③ Firm adhesion via integrin-endothelial cell receptor interactions. LFA-1 and Mac-1 integrins are on *all* leukocytes and bind to ICAM-1 on endothelial cells. ④ Homotypic (like-like) interaction of PECAM-1 (CD31) on leukocytes and endothelial cells mediates transmigration between cells.

extracellular matrix (ECM); the principal integrin receptors for ICAM-1 are LFA-1 (CD11a/CD18) and Mac-1 (CD11b/CD18), while VCAM-1 binds to the integrin VLA-4. These are normally expressed on leukocyte plasma membranes, but they do not adhere to their appropriate ligands until the leukocytes are activated by chemotactic agents or other stimuli (often produced by the endothelium or other cells at the site of injury). Only then do the integrins undergo the conformational change necessary to confer high binding affinity for the endothelial adhesion molecules.

After stable binding to the endothelial surface (primarily LFA-1/Mac-1 binding to ICAM-1), the leukocytes transmigrate between cells along the intercellular junction. As mentioned previously, this leukocyte diapedesis (like increased vascular permeability) occurs predominantly in the venules of the systemic vasculature, and in the capillaries of the lungs. PECAM-1 (platelet endothelial cell adhesion molecule 1, also called CD31), a cell-cell adhesion molecule, is a likely candidate for mediating this process. After traversing the endothelial junctions, leukocytes are able to cross the basement membrane by focally degrading it with secreted collagenases.

The identity of the emigrating leukocytes varies depending on the nature of the inciting stimulus, and also changes as the inflammatory site ages. Thus, in most forms of acute inflammation, neutrophils predominate for the first 6 to 24 hours and are followed by monocytes in the subsequent 24 to 48 hours (Fig. 2–6). The pattern is best explained by the sequential expression of different adhesion molecules and chemotactic factors. In addition, neutrophils are rather short-lived, undergoing apoptosis within 24 to 48 hours after exiting the blood stream, while monocytes survive substantially longer and may persist for long periods as tissue macrophages.

CHEMOTAXIS AND ACTIVATION

After extravasation, leukocytes emigrate toward the site of injury along a chemical gradient, in a process called *chemo-*

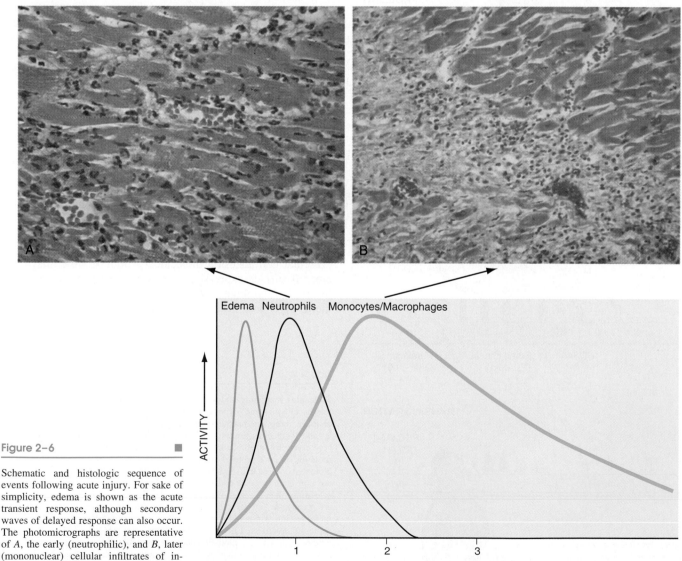

Figure 2–6 ■

Schematic and histologic sequence of events following acute injury. For sake of simplicity, edema is shown as the acute transient response, although secondary waves of delayed response can also occur. The photomicrographs are representative of *A,* the early (neutrophilic), and *B,* later (mononuclear) cellular infiltrates of infarcted myocardium.

taxis (see Fig. 2–4). Both exogenous and endogenous substances can act as chemotactic agents for leukocytes, including: (1) soluble bacterial products, particularly peptides with *N*-formyl-methionine termini; (2) components of the complement system, particularly C5a (p 36); (3) products of the lipoxygenase pathway of arachidonic acid (AA) metabolism, particularly leukotriene B$_4$ (LTB$_4$) (p 37); and (4) cytokines especially those of the *chemokine* family (e.g., IL-8, see later).

Chemotactic agents bind to specific receptors on the leukocyte cell surface and induce an intracellular cascade of phospholipid metabolites, eventually culminating in increased intracellular calcium (both from intracellular stores and from extracellular influx) (Fig. 2–7 and see also Chapter 3). The increased cytosolic calcium triggers the assembly of cytoskeletal contractile elements necessary for movement. The leukocytes move by extending *pseudopods* that anchor themselves to the extracellular matrix and then pull the remainder of the cell after. The direction of such movement is specified, in all likelihood by a higher density of receptor-chemotactic ligand interactions on one side of the cell. Locomotion involves assembling actin monomers into cross-linked polymers at the pseudopod's leading edge, while disassembling such actin filaments elsewhere within the cell.

Besides stimulating locomotion, chemotactic factors also induce other leukocyte responses, generically referred to as *leukocyte activation* (Fig. 2–7):

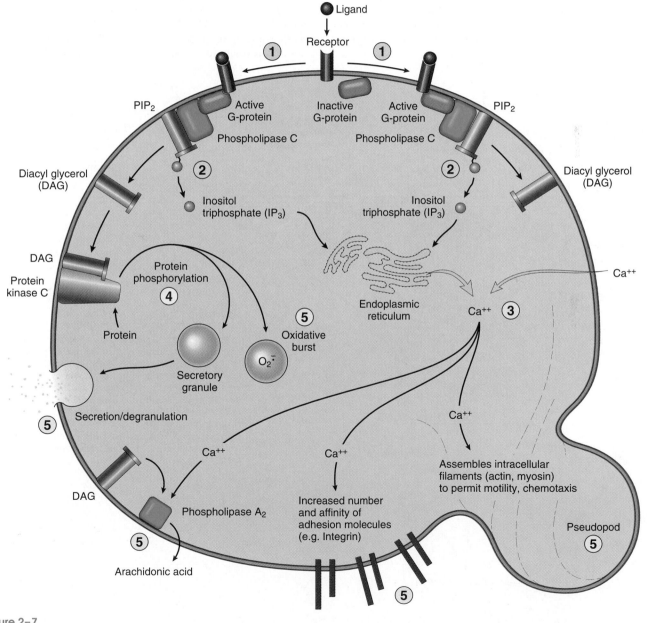

Figure 2–7

Biochemical events in leukocyte activation. The key events are ① receptor-ligand binding, ② phospholipase-C activation, ③ increased intracellular calcium, and ④ activation of protein kinase C. The biologic activities ⑤ resulting from leukocyte activation include chemotaxis, modulation of adhesion molecules, elaboration of arachidonic acid metabolites, secretion/degranulation, and the oxidative burst. PIP$_2$, phosphatidylinositol bisphosphate.

■ Production of AA metabolites from phospholipids (p 37)
■ Degranulation and secretion of lysosomal enzymes, and generation of the oxidative burst (see below)
■ Modulation of leukocyte adhesion molecules, including increased (or decreased) numbers and increased (or decreased) affinities

PHAGOCYTOSIS AND DEGRANULATION

Phagocytosis and the release of lysosomal enzymes are two of the major benefits accruing from the accumulation of leukocytes at the site of inflammation. Phagocytosis consists of three distinct but interrelated steps (Fig. 2–8A): (1) recognition and attachment of the particle to the ingesting leukocyte; (2) engulfment, with subsequent formation of a phagocytic vacuole; and (3) killing or degradation of the ingested material.

Recognition and attachment of most microorganisms is facilitated by coating them with serum proteins generically called *opsonins*, which in turn bind to specific receptors on the leukocytes. The most important opsonins are the immunoglobulin G (IgG) molecule (and specifically the Fc portion of the molecule) and the C3b fragment of complement (and its stable C3bi form). In many cases the binding of IgG is responsible for triggering the activation of the complement cascade that results in deposition of the C3b fragments on the targeted particle; however, a number of stimuli (e.g., microbial surfaces) can directly induce complement activation by an IgG-independent *alternative pathway* (p 36). In either event, the corresponding receptors on leukocytes are the Fc receptor (FcR) and the complement receptors 1, 2, and 3 (CR1, 2, and 3).

Binding of the opsonized particles triggers engulfment. Pseudopods are extended around the object to be engulfed, eventually forming a phagocytic vacuole. The membrane of the vacuole then fuses with the membrane of a lysosomal

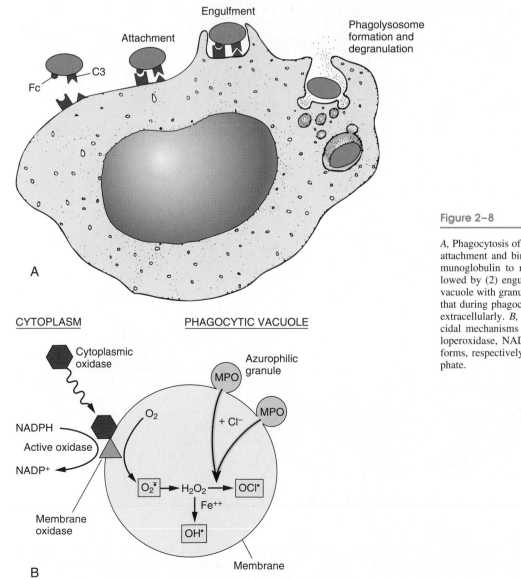

Figure 2–8 ■

A, Phagocytosis of a particle (e.g., a bacterium) involves (1) attachment and binding of C3b and the Fc portion of immunoglobulin to receptors on the leukocyte surface, followed by (2) engulfment and (3) fusion of the phagocytic vacuole with granules (lysosomes), and degranulation. Note that during phagocytosis, granule contents may be released extracellularly. *B,* Summary of oxygen-dependent bactericidal mechanisms within the phagolysosome. MPO, myeloperoxidase, NADP$^+$ and NADPH, oxidized and reduced forms, respectively, of nicotine adenine dinucleotide phosphate.

granule, resulting in discharge of the granule's contents into the phagolysosome and degranulation of the leukocyte (Fig. 2–8A).

The ultimate step in phagocytosis of microbes is killing and degradation. Bacterial and other microbial killing is accomplished largely by reactive oxygen species (Fig. 2–8B). Phagocytosis stimulates an oxidative burst characterized by a sudden increase in oxygen consumption, glycogen catabolism (glycogenolysis), increased glucose oxidation, and production of reactive oxygen metabolites. The generation of the oxygen metabolites is due to rapid activation of a leukocyte NADPH oxidase, which oxidizes NADPH (reduced nicotinamide adenine dinucleotide phosphate), and in the process reduces oxygen to superoxide ion ($O_2^{\cdot-}$).

$$2O_2 + NADPH \xrightarrow[\text{NADPH oxidase}]{} 2O_2^{\cdot-} + NADP^+ + H^+$$

Superoxide is then converted, mostly by spontaneous dismutation ($O_2^{\cdot-} + 2H^+ \rightarrow H_2O_2$) into hydrogen peroxide. The quantities of hydrogen peroxide produced are insufficient to effectively kill most bacteria. However, the lysosomes of neutrophils (called *azurophilic granules*) contain the enzyme myeloperoxidase (MPO), and in the presence of a halide such as Cl^-, MPO converts H_2O_2 to $HOCl^{\cdot}$ (hypochlorous radical). $HOCl^{\cdot}$ is a powerful oxidant and antimicrobial agent (NaOCl is the active ingredient in chlorine bleach) that kills bacteria by halogenation, or by protein and lipid peroxidation. Fortunately, since NADPH oxidase is active only after translocation of a cytosolic subunit to the membrane of the phagolysosome, the reactive end products are generated only within that compartment (Fig. 2–8B). After the oxygen burst, H_2O_2 is eventually broken down to water and O_2 by the actions of catalase. The dead microorganisms are then degraded by the action of the lysosomal acid hydrolases.

It is important to note that even in the absence of an oxidative burst (see below), other constituents of the leukocyte granules are capable of killing bacteria and other infectious agents. These include *bactericidal permeability increasing protein (BPI)*, *lysozyme, lactoferrin,* and the so-called *defensins,* a group of peptides that apparently kill microbes by forming holes in their membranes.

LEUKOCYTE-INDUCED TISSUE INJURY

Phagocytosis results in the release of lysosomal enzymes not only within the phagolysosome but also potentially into the extracellular space where cell injury and matrix degradation result (Fig. 2–8A). This may occur by premature degranulation of lysosomes before complete closure of the phagocytic vacuole, or during attempts by the leukocyte to phagocytose large, flat surfaces (*frustrated phagocytosis*), or potentially membranolytic substances (such as urate crystals in gout). In addition, activated leukocytes release reactive oxygen species (see above) and products of AA metabolism (see below), which are potent mediators capable of causing direct endothelial injury and tissue damage. Indeed, leukocyte-dependent tissue injury from persistent and/or runaway leukocyte activation underlies many human diseases, including rheumatoid arthritis and certain forms of chronic lung disease (Chapters 3 and 13).

DEFECTS IN LEUKOCYTE FUNCTION

Since leukocytes play a central role in host defense, it is not surprising that defects in leukocyte function, both genetic and acquired, lead to increased vulnerability to infections, often recurrent and life threatening. Although individually rare, these disorders underscore the importance of the complex series of events that must occur in vivo to protect the human body after invasion by microorganisms.

1. *Defects in adhesion.* In leukocyte adhesion deficiency I (LAD-I), defective synthesis of the CD18 subunit of the leukocyte integrins LFA-1 and Mac-1 leads to impaired endothelial adhesion. LAD-2 is caused by a general defect in fucose metabolism resulting in the absence of sialyl–Lewis X, the oligosaccharide epitope that binds E- and P-selectins.
2. *Defects in chemotaxis or phagocytosis.* One such disorder, Chédiak-Higashi syndrome, is suspected to result from disordered assembly of microtubules, impairing locomotion as well as lysosomal degranulation into phagosomes.
3. *Defects in microbicidal activity.* An example is chronic granulomatous disease (CGD), a genetic deficiency in one of the several components of the NADPH oxidase responsible for generating superoxide (see above). In these patients, engulfment of bacteria does not result in activation of oxygen-dependent killing mechanisms, despite the fact that the MPO activity of the cells is normal. Interestingly, this is true even in infections by bacteria that produce hydrogen peroxide, in part because many of them (e.g., *Staphylococcus aureus*) also possess their own catalase, which degrades the H_2O_2 and thus prevents its utilization by the neutrophils.

SUMMARY OF THE ACUTE INFLAMMATORY RESPONSE

To review (see Fig. 2–1), the vascular changes in acute inflammation are characterized by increased blood flow secondary to arteriolar and capillary bed dilation (erythema and warmth). Increased vascular permeability, either through widened interendothelial cell junctions of the venules or by direct endothelial cell injury, results in an exudate of protein-rich extravascular fluid (tissue edema). The leukocytes, predominantly neutrophils, first adhere to the endothelium via adhesion molecules, then leave the microvasculature and migrate to the site of injury under the influence of chemotactic agents. Phagocytosis of the offending agent follows, which may lead to the death of infectious microorganisms. During chemotaxis and phagocytosis, activated leukocytes may release toxic metabolites and proteases extracellularly, potentially causing endothelial and tissue damage (pain and loss of function).

Chemical Mediators of Inflammation

We can now turn to a discussion of the chemical mediators that account for the vascular and cellular events in acute inflammation. While the plethora of mediators described to date may have survival value for the organism, it is neither desirable to review, nor possible to remember, every mediator in detail. Instead, we will review general principles and highlight only some of the more important molecules.

■ Mediators derive from plasma or by local production from cells (Fig. 2–9). Plasma-derived mediators (complement, kinins, coagulation factors) are present as circulating precursors that must be activated, usually by proteolytic cleavage, to acquire their biologic properties. Cell-derived mediators are normally sequestered in intracellular granules (e.g., histamine in mast cells) that are subsequently secreted, or are synthesized de novo (e.g., prostaglandins) in response to a stimulus.

■ Most mediators perform their biologic activity by initially binding to specific receptors on target cells. However, some have direct enzymatic and/or toxic activities (e.g., lysosomal proteases or reactive oxygen species).

■ Mediators may stimulate target cells to release secondary effector molecules. These secondary mediators may have activities similar to the initial effector molecule, in which case they may amplify a particular response. On the other hand, they may have opposing activities, and thereby function to counter-regulate the initial stimulus.

■ Mediators may act on only one or a very few targets, or may have widespread activity, and may have widely differing outcomes depending on which cell type they affect.

■ Mediator function is generally tightly regulated. Once activated and released from the cell, most mediators quickly decay (e.g., AA metabolites), are inactivated by enzymes (e.g., kininase inactivates bradykinin), or are eliminated (e.g., antioxidants scavenge toxic oxygen metabolites).

■ A major reason for the checks and balances is that most mediators have the potential to cause harmful effects.

VASOACTIVE AMINES

Histamine is widely distributed in tissues, particularly in mast cells adjacent to vessels, as well as in circulating basophils and platelets. Preformed histamine is present in mast cell granules that are released in response to a variety of stimuli: (1) physical injury such as trauma or heat; (2) immune reactions involving binding of IgE antibodies to Fc receptors on mast cells; (3) C3a and C5a fragments of complement (see below), the so-called *anaphylatoxins;* (4) leukocyte-derived histamine-releasing proteins; (5) neuropeptides (e.g., substance P); and (6) certain cytokines (e.g., IL-1 and IL-8).

In humans, histamine causes arteriolar dilation and is the principal mediator of the immediate phase of increased vascular permeability, causing venular endothelial contraction and widening of the interendothelial cell junctions. Soon after its release, histamine is inactivated by histaminase.

Serotonin (5-hydroxytryptamine) is also a preformed vasoactive mediator, with effects similar to histamine. It is found primarily within platelet-dense body granules (along with histamine, adenosine diphosphate, and calcium), and release is stimulated by platelet aggregation (see Chapter 4).

PLASMA PROTEASES

Many of the effects of inflammation are mediated by three interrelated plasma-derived factors—the clotting system, complement, and the kinins—all linked by the initial activation of Hageman factor (Fig. 2–10).

The clotting system (see also Chapter 4) is a cascade of plasma proteases, which can be triggered by the proteolytic action of activated Hageman factor (Fig. 2–10). Hageman factor (also known as *factor XII* of the *intrinsic coagulation cascade*) is a protein synthesized by the liver that circulates

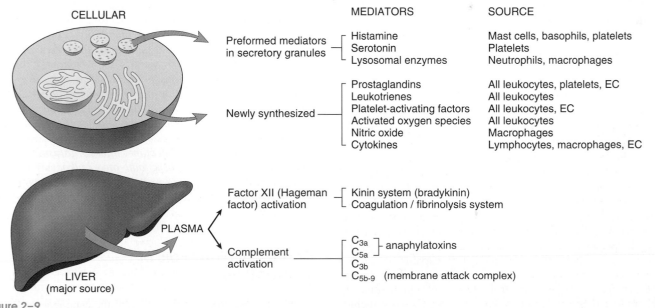

CELLULAR		MEDIATORS	SOURCE
	Preformed mediators in secretory granules	Histamine	Mast cells, basophils, platelets
		Serotonin	Platelets
		Lysosomal enzymes	Neutrophils, macrophages
	Newly synthesized	Prostaglandins	All leukocytes, platelets, EC
		Leukotrienes	All leukocytes
		Platelet-activating factors	All leukocytes, EC
		Activated oxygen species	All leukocytes
		Nitric oxide	Macrophages
		Cytokines	Lymphocytes, macrophages, EC

LIVER (major source)

PLASMA

Factor XII (Hageman factor) activation ⎱ Kinin system (bradykinin) / Coagulation / fibrinolysis system

Complement activation ⎱ C3a / C5a ⎰ anaphylatoxins / C3b / C5b-9 (membrane attack complex)

Figure 2–9

Chemical mediators of inflammation. EC, endothelial cells.

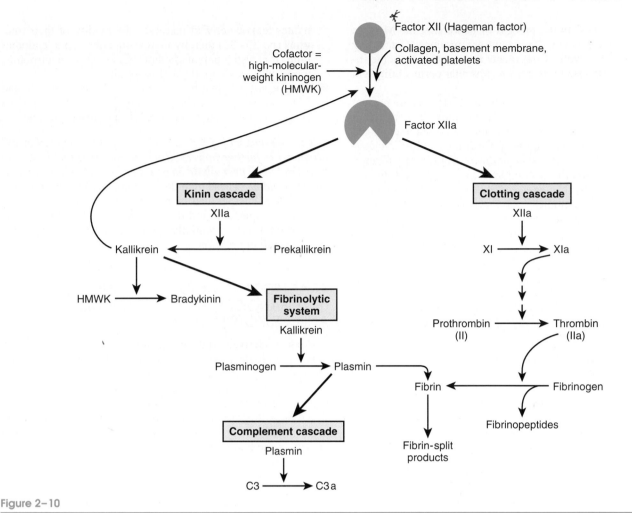

Figure 2–10

Plasma mediator systems triggered by activation of factor XII (Hageman factor): their interrelationships and major effects.

in an inactive form until it encounters collagen, basement membrane, or activated platelets (as at a site of endothelial injury). Factor XII then undergoes a conformational change (becoming factor XIIa), exposing an active serine center that can subsequently cleave a number of protein substrates (see below). In the clotting system, the resultant proteolytic cascade results in activation of thrombin (factor IIa) from precursor prothrombin (factor II), which in turn cleaves circulating soluble fibrinogen to generate an insoluble fibrin clot. Thrombin also enhances leukocyte adhesion to endothelium, and fibrinopeptides resulting from fibrinogen cleavage increase vascular permeability and are chemotactic for leukocytes.

At the same time that factor XIIa is inducing clotting, it can also activate the *fibrinolytic system.* This mechanism exists to carefully counter-regulate clotting by causing further cleavage of the fibrin molecule and thereby solubilizing the fibrin clot. Without fibrinolysis and other regulatory mechanisms, initiation of the coagulation cascade, even by trivial injury, would culminate in continuous and irrevocable clotting of the entire vasculature. In addition, the process of fibrinolysis also contributes to the vascular phenomena of inflammation (see Fig. 2–1). Plasminogen activator (released from endothelium, leu-

kocytes, and other tissues) cleaves plasminogen, a plasma protein bound up in the evolving fibrin clot. This generates plasmin, a multifunctional protease that degrades fibrin to fibrin split products and is therefore important in lysing fibrin clots. However, in the context of inflammation, fibrin split products also increase vascular permeability, while plasmin cleaves the complement C3 component to C3a, resulting in vasodilation and increased vascular permeability (see below).

Kinin system activation leads ultimately to the formation of bradykinin from its circulating precursor, high molecular weight kininogen (HMWK). The intermediate steps in the formation of bradykinin are illustrated in Figure 2–10. Like histamine, bradykinin causes increased vascular permeability, arteriolar dilation, and extravascular smooth muscle contraction (e.g., in bronchial smooth muscle). It also causes pain when injected into the skin. The actions of bradykinin are short-lived because it is rapidly inactivated by degradative kininases present in plasma and tissues.

The complement system consists of a cascade of plasma proteins that play an important role in both immunity and inflammation. They function in immunity primarily by ultimately generating a porelike membrane attack complex (MAC) that effectively punches holes in the membranes of invading microbes. In the process of generating the MAC, a number of complement fragments are produced, including C3b opsonins, as well as fragments that contribute to the inflammatory response by increasing vascular permeability and leukocyte chemotaxis.

Complement components (numbered C1 to C9) are present in plasma as inactive forms. Briefly, the most critical step in the elaboration of the biologic functions of complement is the activation of the third component, C3 (Fig. 2–11). C3 cleavage can occur (1) via the *classic pathway,* triggered by fixation of C1 to antigen-antibody complexes; or (2) through the *alternative pathway*, triggered by bacterial polysaccharides (e.g., endotoxin), complex polysaccharides, or aggregated IgA. Parenthetically, the alternative pathway involves a distinct set of serum components, including properdin and factors B and D. Whichever pathway is involved, C3 convertase cleaves C3 to C3a and C3b. C3b then binds to the C3 convertase complex to form C5 convertase; this complex cleaves C5 to generate C5a and initiate the final stages of assembly of the C5 to C9 MAC. The various other complement-derived factors generated along the way affect a variety of phenomena in acute inflammation:

■ *Vascular effects.* C3a and C5a (also called *anaphylatoxins*) increase vascular permeability and cause vasodilation by inducing mast cells to release their histamine. C5a also activates the lipoxygenase pathway of AA metabolism in neutrophils and monocytes (see below), causing further release of inflammatory mediators.
■ *Leukocyte activation, adhesion, and chemotaxis.* C5a activates leukocytes and increases the avidity of their integrins (pp 30–31) thereby increasing adhesion to endothelium. It is also a potent chemotactic agent for neutrophils, monocytes, eosinophils, and basophils.
■ *Phagocytosis.* When fixed to a microbial surface, C3b and C3bi act as opsonins, augmenting phagocytosis by cells bearing C3b receptors (neutrophils and macrophages).

The significance of C3 and C5 (and their activation by-products) is further increased by the fact that they can also be activated by proteolytic enzymes present within the inflammatory exudate. These include lysosomal hydrolases released from neutrophils, as well as plasmin. Thus, the chemotactic effect of complement and the complement-activating effects of neutrophils can potentially set up a self-perpetuating cycle of neutrophil emigration.

ARACHIDONIC ACID METABOLITES (EICOSANOIDS): PROSTAGLANDINS AND LEUKOTRIENES

Products derived from the metabolism of AA affect a variety of biologic processes including inflammation and hemostasis. They can be thought of as short-range hormones that act locally at the site of generation and then rapidly spontaneously decay, or are enzymatically destroyed.

AA is a 20-carbon polyunsaturated fatty acid (4 double bonds) derived primarily from dietary linoleic acid and present in the body only in esterified form as a component of

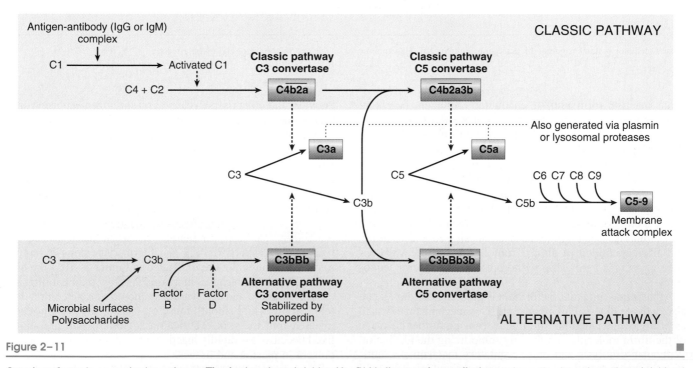

Figure 2–11

Overview of complement activation pathways. The classic pathway is initiated by C1 binding to antigen-antibody complexes; the alternative pathway is initiated by C3b binding to various activating surfaces, such as microbial cell walls. The C3b involved in alternative pathway initiation may be generated in several ways, including spontaneously, by the classic pathway, or by the alternative pathway itself (see text). Both pathways converge and lead to the formation of inflammatory complement mediators (C3a and C5a) and the membrane attack complex. Bars over the letter designations of complement components indicate enzymatically active forms; dashed lines indicate proteolytic activities of various components. (Modified from Abbas AK, et al: Cellular and Molecular Immunology, 2nd ed. Philadelphia, WB Saunders, 1994.)

cell membrane phospholipids. It is released from these phospholipids via cellular phospholipases that have been activated by mechanical, chemical, or physical stimuli, or by inflammatory mediators such as C5a. AA metabolism proceeds along one of two major pathways (Fig. 2–12), named for the enzymes that initiate the reactions.

Cyclooxygenase Pathway. These include PGE_2, PGD_2, $PGF_{2\alpha}$, PGI_2 (prostacyclin), and thromboxane (TXA_2), each of which is derived by the action of a specific enzyme. Some of these enzymes have a restricted tissue distribution. For example, platelets contain the enzyme thromboxane synthetase, and hence TXA_2, a potent platelet-aggregating agent and vasoconstrictor, is the major prostaglandin product in these cells. Endothelium, on the other hand, lacks thromboxane synthetase but possesses prostacyclin synthetase, which leads to the formation of PGI_2, a vasodilator and a potent inhibitor of platelet aggregation. The opposing roles of TXA_2 and PGI_2 in hemostasis are further discussed in Chapter 4. PGD_2 is the major metabolite of the cyclooxygenase pathway in mast cells; along with PGE_2 and $PGF_{2\alpha}$ (which are more widely distributed), it causes vasodilation and potentiates edema formation. Aspirin and nonsteroidal anti-inflammatory agents (NSAIDs) such as ibuprofen inhibit the proximal cyclooxygenase activity and thus inhibit all prostaglandin synthesis. Lipoxygenase, however, is not affected by these anti-inflammatory agents.

Recent studies have revealed that there are two forms of cyclooxygenases (COX), called COX-1 and COX-2. Of interest, COX-1 but not COX-2 is expressed in the gastric mucosa. At this site the mucosal prostaglandins generated by the actions of COX-1 are protective because they prevent acid-induced damage. While inhibition of cyclooxygenases by aspirin and NSAID reduces inflammation by blocking prostaglandin synthesis, these drugs also predispose to gastric ulceration. To preserve the anti-inflammatory effects and prevent the harmful effects on the gastric mucosa, several highly selective COX-2 inhibitors are being developed. These are expected to exert anti-inflammatory effects without predisposing the gastric mucosa to ulceration.

Lipoxygenase Pathway. 5-Lipoxygenase is the predominant AA-metabolizing enzyme in neutrophils, and the products of its actions are the best characterized. The 5-hydroperoxy derivative of AA, 5-HPETE, is quite unstable and is either reduced to 5-HETE (which is chemotactic for neutrophils) or converted into a family of compounds collectively called *leukotrienes*. The first leukotriene generated from 5-HPETE is called leukotriene A_4 (LTA_4), which in turn gives rise to LTB_4 by enzymatic hydrolysis or to LTC_4 by addition of glutathione. *LTB_4 is a potent chemotactic agent and causes aggregation of neutrophils. LTC_4, and its subsequent metabolites LTD_4 and LTE_4, cause vasoconstriction, bronchospasm, and increased vascular permeability.*

In summary, the eicosanoids can participate in every aspect of acute inflammation (Fig. 2–12), including pain and fever. The fact that eicosanoids hold a central role in inflammatory processes is borne out by the clinical anti-inflammatory utility

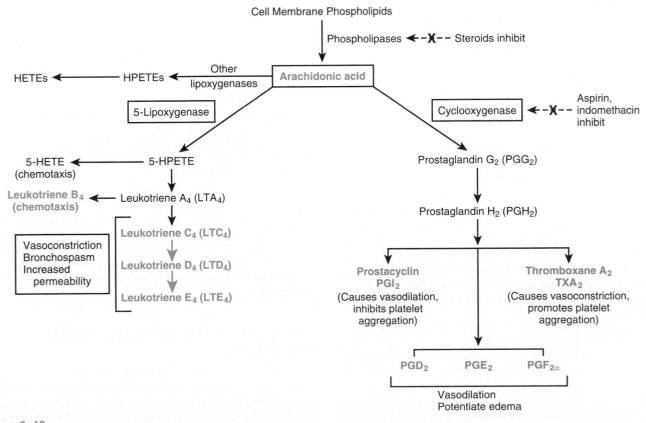

Figure 2–12

Generation of arachidonic acid metabolites and their roles in inflammation.

of agents that suppress cyclooxygenase activity (e.g., aspirin and NSAIDs). Glucocorticoids, which are powerful anti-inflammatory agents, may act in part by inhibiting the activity of phospholipase A$_2$ (recall that phospholipases are required for the generation of AA from the membrane phospholipids).

PLATELET-ACTIVATING FACTOR

Originally named for its ability to aggregate platelets and cause degranulation, PAF is another phospholipid-derived mediator with a broad spectrum of inflammatory effects. Formally, PAF is acetyl glycerol ether phosphocholine; it is derived from the membrane phospholipids of neutrophils, monocytes, basophils, endothelium, and platelets (and other cells) by the action of phospholipase A$_2$. Besides platelet stimulation, PAF causes vasoconstriction and bronchoconstriction and is 100 to 10,000 times more potent than histamine in inducing vasodilation and increased vascular pemeability. PAF also causes enhanced leukocyte adhesion (via integrin conformational changes), chemotaxis, leukocyte degranulation, and the oxidative burst. PAF acts directly on target cells via specific receptors, and it also stimulates the synthesis of other mediators, particularly eicosanoids.

CYTOKINES

Cytokines are polypeptide products of many cell types (but principally activated lymphocytes and macrophages) that modulate the function of other cell types. Cytokines can act on the same cell that produces them (*autocrine* effect), on other cells in the immediate vicinity (*paracrine* effect), or systemically (*endocrine* effect). Although historically associated with cellular immune responses, various cytokines, in particular *interleukin-1 (IL-1), tumor necrosis factor-α and -β (TNF-α and -β), interferon-γ (IFN-γ), and the chemokines,* have additional effects that are important in the inflammatory response. These cytokines can exert local effects on endothelium, leukocytes, and fibroblasts, as well as induce systemic acute-phase reactions (Fig. 2–13).

Both IL-1 and TNF-α are produced by activated macrophages; TNF-β and IFN-γ are secreted by T cells, and IL-1 by additional other cell types. Secretion is stimulated by endotoxin, immune complexes, toxins, physical injury, or a variety of inflammatory mediators. In endothelium, IL-1 and TNF both induce a spectrum of changes, denoted *endothelial activation.* These include increased expression of adhesion molecules, secretion of additional cytokines and growth factors, production of eicosanoids and nitric oxide (NO) (see below), and increased endothelial thrombogenicity. TNF also causes aggregation and activation of neutrophils, and the release of proteolytic enzymes from mesenchymal cells, thus contributing to tissue damage.

IL-1 and TNF also induce the systemic acute-phase responses typically associated with infection or injury. These include fever, lethargy, hepatic synthesis of various proteins, metabolic wasting (cachexia), neutrophil release into the circulation, and release of adrenocorticotropic hormone (inducing corticosteroid synthesis and release). TNF also induces NO synthesis (see below), which may play a major role in mediating the hypotensive effects of septic shock, including diminished myocardial contractility and vascular smooth mus-

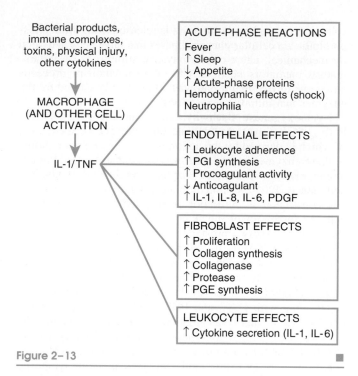

Figure 2–13

Major effects of interleukin 1 (IL-1) and tumor necrosis factor (TNF) in inflammation.

cle relaxation. IFN-γ is a potent activator of macrophages and neutrophils, up-regulating the enzymes responsible for their oxidative burst, and enabling them to kill phagocytosed microbes; it is also one of the most important stimuli for the synthesis of NO synthase (see below).

The *chemokines* are a family of proteins that share similar patterns of paired cysteine repeats and two internal disulfide-bridged loops. They are called chemokines because they are chemoattractant molecules for inflammatory cells and because they also exert selected cytokine effects. Interleukin-8 (IL-8), one of the first described chemokines, is a powerful chemotactic agent and activator primarily of neutrophils; it is produced by activated macrophages, endothelium, or fibroblasts, mainly in response to IL-1 and TNF. Other chemokines include platelet factor 4 (chemotactic for neutrophils, monocytes, and eosinophils), monocyte chemoattractant protein-1 (MCP-1) (chemotactic for monocytes), RANTES (chemotactic for memory CD4+ T cells and monocytes), and eotaxin (chemotactic for eosinophils). Current evidence suggests that unique combinations of chemokines may act to recruit the particular cell populations present in a given inflammatory site.

NITRIC OXIDE AND OXYGEN-DERIVED FREE RADICALS

NO is a short-acting, soluble free radical gas produced by a variety of cells and capable of mediating a bewildering number of effector functions. In the central nervous system, it regulates neurotransmitter release, as well as blood flow. Macrophages use it as a cytotoxic metabolite for microbes and tumor cells. When produced by endothelium (where it was originally named *endothelium-derived relaxation factor* or *EDRF*), it activates guanylyl cyclase in vascular smooth muscle, resulting in increased cyclic guanosine monophosphate (cGMP) and ultimately smooth muscle relaxation (vasodilation). Although we are primarily interested here in the effects of NO relevant to the inflammatory response (Fig. 2–14), its ubiquitous generation and diverse effects make it an important mediator in a vast number of physiologic and pathologic states.

Since the half-life of NO is measured in seconds, it can affect only those cells in near proximity to the source where it is generated. Moreover, the short half-life of NO dictates that its effects are regulated primarily by the rate of synthesis. NO is synthesized de novo from L-arginine, molecular oxygen, and NADPH by the enzyme nitric oxide synthase (NOS). There are three isoforms of NOS, with different tissue distributions, dependence on Ca^{++}, and constitutive versus inducible modes of expression. Type I (ncNOS) is a *neuronal con*stitutive NOS, whose enzyme activity is dependent on elevated intracellular Ca^{++}. Type II (iNOS) is an *in*ducible enzyme present in many cell types, including hepatocytes, cardiac myocytes, and respiratory epithelium; its activity is independent of intracellular Ca^{++} concentrations. Of significance in inflammation, iNOS is also present in endothelium, smooth muscle cells, and macrophages; it is induced by a number of inflammatory cytokines and mediators, most notably by IL-1, TNF-α, and IFN-γ, and by lipopolysaccharide (LPS) present in the cells walls of gram-negative bacteria. Type III (ecNOS) is a *c*onstitutively synthesized NOS found primarily (but not exclusively) within *e*ndothelium, with activity that is also dependent on intracellular Ca^{++}. Calcium-elevating agonists of ecNOS activity include bradykinin, or thrombin (see above), as well as increased shear stress on the endothelial surface.

NO plays multiple roles in inflammation (Fig. 2–14), including (1) vascular smooth muscle relaxation (vasodilation), (2) antagonism of all stages of platelet activation (adhesion, aggregation, and degranulation), and (3) acting as a microbicidal agent (with or without superoxide radicals) in activated macrophages.

Oxygen-derived free radicals are synthesized via the NADPH oxidase pathway (see above) and are released from neutrophils and macrophages after stimulation by chemotactic agents, immune complexes, or phagocytic activity. Superoxide (O_2^{-}) is subsequently converted to H_2O_2, $OH\cdot$, and toxic NO derivatives. These short-lived mediators have been implicated in a variety of tissue injuries, including (1) endothelial damage, with thrombosis and increased permeability; (2) protease activation and antiprotease inactivation, with a net increase in breakdown of the extracellular matrix; and (3) direct injury to other cell types (e.g., tumor cells, erythrocytes, parenchymal cells). Fortunately, a variety of antioxidant protective mechanisms (e.g, catalase, superoxide dismutase, and glutathione) are present in tissues and serum to minimize the toxicity of the oxygen metabolites (see Chapter 1).

LYSOSOMAL CONSTITUENTS

The lysosomal granules of neutrophils and monocytes contain a number of molecules that can potentially act as mediators of acute inflammation. These may be released after cell death, by leakage during the formation of the phagocytic vacuole, or by frustrated phagocytosis against large surfaces, as described previously (p 33).

While *acid proteases* have acidic pH optima and are generally active only within phagolysosomes, *neutral proteases,* including enzymes such as elastase, collagenase, and cathepsin, are active in the extracellular matrix and cause destructive,

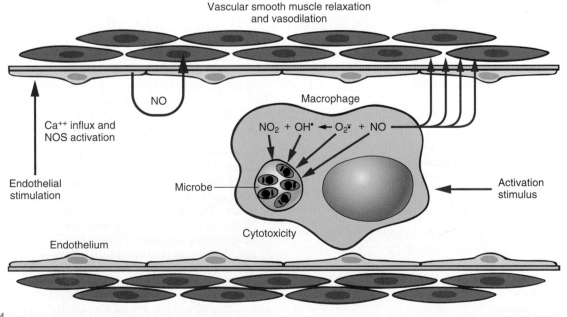

Figure 2–14

Sources and effects of nitric oxide (NO) in inflammation. Note NO synthesis by endothelial cells (mostly via ecNOS, *left*) and by macrophages (mostly via iNOS, *right*). NO causes vasodilation, and NO free radicals are cytotoxic to microbial and mammalian cells. (Courtesy of Dr. Jeffrey Joseph.)

deforming tissue injury by degrading elastin, collagen, basement membrane, and other matrix proteins. Neutral proteases can also cleave C3 and C5 directly to generate the C3a and C5a anaphylatoxins, and can promote the generation of bradykinin-like peptides from kininogen.

Thus, if the initial leukocyte infiltration is left unrestrained, substantial vascular permeability and tissue damage may result. These effects are checked, however, by a series of *antiproteases* present in the serum and extracellular matrix. These include α_2-macroglobulin (in the serum), as well as the archetypal antiprotease α_1-antitrypsin, which is the major inhibitor of neutrophil elastase. Deficiencies of these inhibitors may result in sustained activation of leukocyte proteases, and severe tissue destruction in the lung, giving rise to emphysema (Chapter 13).

SUMMARY OF THE CHEMICAL MEDIATORS OF ACUTE INFLAMMATION

Table 2–1 represents an attempt to abstract the most relevant mediators *in vivo* of acute inflammation. Vasodilation is predominantly regulated by the prostaglandins (PGI_2 and TXA_2) and NO, while increased vascular permeability is probably mediated via histamine, the anaphylotoxins (C3a and C5a), the kinins, PAF, and leukotrienes C, D, and E. Chemotaxis is strongly driven by C5a, LTB_4, and the chemokines. Cytokines and prostaglandins also play a major role in leukocyte and endothelial activation, as well as the systemic manifestations of acute inflammation. Finally, tissue damage is in large part attributable to the effects of NO, oxygen-derived free radicals, and leukocyte lysosomal enzymes.

■

Table 2–1.	MOST LIKELY MEDIATORS IN INFLAMMATION

Vasodilation
 Prostaglandins
 Nitric oxide

Increased vascular permeability
 Vasoactive amines
 C3a and C5a (through liberating amines)
 Bradykinin
 Leukotrienes C_4, D_4, E_4
 Platelet-activating factor

Chemotaxis, leukocyte activation
 C5a
 Leukotriene B_4
 Bacterial products
 Chemokines (e.g., IL-8)

Fever
 IL-1, IL-6, TNF-α
 Prostaglandins

Pain
 Prostaglandins
 Bradykinin

Tissue damage
 Neutrophil and macrophage lysosomal enzymes
 Oxygen metabolites
 Nitric oxide

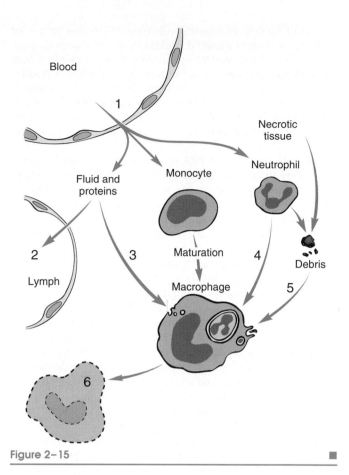

Figure 2–15 ■

Events in the complete resolution of inflammation: (1) return to normal vascular permeability; (2) removal of edema fluid and proteins by drainage into lymphatics or (3) by macrophage pinocytosis; (4) phagocytosis of apoptotic neutrophils and (5) necrotic debris by macrophages; and (6) removal of macrophages. Note the central role of macrophages in resolution. (Modified from Haslett C, Henson PM: In Clark R, Henson PM (eds): The Molecular and Cellular Biology of Wound Repair. New York, Plenum Press, 1988.)

Outcomes of Acute Inflammation

Although the consequences of acute inflammation are modified by the nature and intensity of the injury, the site and tissue affected, and the ability of the host to mount a response, acute inflammation generally has one of four outcomes:

1. *Complete resolution.* When the injury is limited or short-lived, when there has been little tissue destruction, and when the tissue is capable of *regeneration*, the most usual outcome is restoration to histologic and functional normalcy. This resolution involves neutralization or removal of the chemical mediators, with subsequent normalization of vascular permeability and halting of leukocyte emigration. Eventually, the combined efforts of lymphatic drainage and macrophages lead to the clearance of the edema fluid, inflammatory cells, and necrotic debris from the battlefield (Fig. 2–15).

2. *Scarring* or *fibrosis* (Chapter 3) results when inflammation occurs in tissues that do not regenerate, or after substantial tissue destruction. In addition, extensive fibrinous exudates that cannot be completely absorbed are organized by in-

growth of connective tissue elements, resulting in the formation of a mass of fibrous tissue.

3. *Abscess formation* may occur in the setting of certain bacterial or fungal infections (these organisms are then said to be *pyogenic*, or "pus forming").

4. *Progression to chronic inflammation* may follow acute inflammation (see below).

CHRONIC INFLAMMATION

In contrast to acute inflammation, which is distinguished by vascular changes, edema, and a largely neutrophilic infiltrate, *chronic inflammation is characterized by* (1) *infiltration with mononuclear ("chronic inflammatory") cells,* including macrophages, lymphocytes, and plasma cells; (2) *tissue destruction,* largely induced by the inflammatory cells; and (3) *repair involving new vessel proliferation (angiogenesis) and fibrosis* (Fig. 2–16). Chronic inflammation can be considered to be inflammation of prolonged duration (weeks to months to years) in which active inflammation, tissue injury, and healing proceed simultaneously.

Chronic inflammation may follow acute inflammation. This transition occurs when the acute response cannot be resolved, either because of the persistence of the injurious agent or because of interference in the normal process of healing. For example, a peptic ulcer of the duodenum initially shows acute inflammation followed by the beginning stages of resolution. However, recurrent bouts of duodenal epithelial injury interrupt this process and result in a lesion characterized by both acute and chronic inflammation (Chapter 16). Alternatively, some forms of injury (e.g., viral infections) engender a response that involves chronic inflammation essentially from the beginning. Although the injurious agents mediating chronic inflammation may be less noxious than those that cause acute inflammation, the overall failure to resolve the process may lead to substantially more long-term injury. Fibrosis—the proliferation of fibroblasts and accumulation of excess extracellular matrix—is also a common feature of many chronic inflammatory diseases and is an important cause of organ dysfunction (Chapter 3).

Chronic inflammation arises in the following settings:

■ *Persistent infections*, most characteristically by a selected set of microorganisms including mycobacteria (tubercle bacilli), *Treponema pallidum* (causative organism of syphilis), and certain fungi. These organisms are of low direct pathogenicity, but typically evoke an immune response called *delayed hypersensitivity* (Chapter 5) that may culminate in a granulomatous reaction (see below).

■ *Prolonged exposure to potentially toxic agents.* Examples include nondegradable exogenous material such as inhaled particulate silica, which can induce a chronic inflammatory response in the lungs (silicosis, Chapter 13); and endogenous agents such as chronically elevated plasma lipid components, which may contribute to atherosclerosis (Chapter 10).

■ *Autoimmune diseases*, in which an individual develops an immune response to self-antigens and tissues (Chapter 5). Because the antigens putatively causing the response are in most instances constantly renewed, a self-perpetuating immune reaction results (e.g., rheumatoid arthritis).

Chronic Inflammatory Cells

Macrophages are but one component of the *mononuclear phagocyte system*, consisting of closely related cells of bone marrow origin, including the circulating blood monocytes, and tissue macrophages. Macrophages are diffusely scattered in connective tissues, or clustered in organs such as the liver (Kupffer cells), spleen and lymph nodes (sinus histiocytes), central nervous system (microglia), and lungs (alveolar macrophages).

The half-life of circulating monocytes is about 1 day; under the influence of adhesion molecules and chemotactic factors, they begin to emigrate at a site of injury within the first 24 to 48 hours after onset of acute inflammation, as described previously. When monocytes reach the extravascular tissue, they undergo transformation into larger, phagocytic cells called macrophages. Macrophages may also become activated, a process resulting in increased cell size, increased content of lysosomal enzymes, more active metabolism, and greater ability to kill ingested organisms, and some tumor cells. Activation signals include cytokines secreted by sensitized T lymphocytes (in particular IFN-γ), bacterial endotoxins, various mediators produced during acute inflammation, and extracellular matrix proteins such as fibronectin. After activation, macrophages secrete a wide variety of biologically active products listed below. They are important in mediating the tissue destruction, angiogenesis, and fibrosis characteristic of chronic inflammation (Fig. 2–17):

■ *Acid and neutral proteases.* Recall that the latter were also implicated as mediators of tissue damage in acute inflammation. Other enzymes, such as plasminogen activator, greatly amplify the generation of proinflammatory substances.

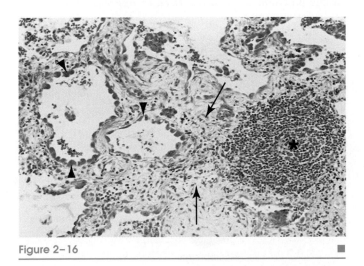

Figure 2–16 ■

Chronic inflammation in the lung, showing the three characteristic histologic features: (1) collection of chronic inflammatory cells (*), (2) destruction of parenchyma (normal alveoli are replaced by spaces lined by cuboidal epithelium, *arrowheads*), and (3) replacement by connective tissue (fibrosis, *arrows*).

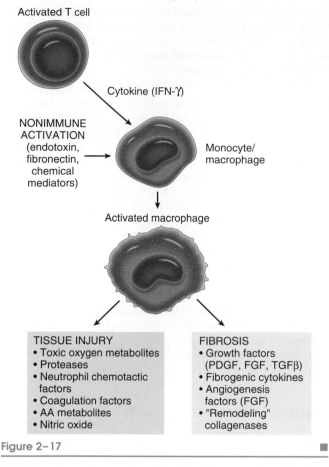

Activated T cell

Cytokine (IFN-γ)

NONIMMUNE
ACTIVATION
(endotoxin,
fibronectin,
chemical
mediators)

Monocyte/
macrophage

Activated macrophage

TISSUE INJURY	FIBROSIS
• Toxic oxygen metabolites	• Growth factors
• Proteases	(PDGF, FGF, TGFβ)
• Neutrophil chemotactic	• Fibrogenic cytokines
factors	• Angiogenesis
• Coagulation factors	factors (FGF)
• AA metabolites	• "Remodeling"
• Nitric oxide	collagenases

Figure 2–17 ■

Activation of macrophages via cytokines from immune-activated T cells or by nonimmunologic stimuli such as endotoxin. The products made by activated macrophages that also mediate tissue injury and fibrosis are indicated. AA, arachidonic acid; PDGF, platelet-derived growth factor; FGF, fibroblast growth factor; TGFβ, transforming growth factor β (see Chapter 3).

■ *Complement components and coagulation factors.* Although hepatocytes are the major source of these proteins in plasma, activated macrophages may make locally significant amounts of these proteins in the extracellular matrix. These include complement proteins C1 to C5; properdin; and coagulation factors V, VIII, and tissue factor.
■ *Reactive oxygen species and NO*
■ *Eicosanoids*
■ *Cytokines,* such as IL-1 and TNF, as well as a variety of *growth factors* that influence the proliferation of, for example, smooth muscle cells and fibroblasts, and production of extracellular matrix.

At sites of acute inflammation where the the irritant is cleared and the process is resolved, macrophages eventually die or wander off into lymphatics. In chronic inflammatory sites, however, macrophage accumulation persists. Steady release of lymphocyte-derived factors (see later) is an important mechanism by which macrophages are recruited to or immobilized in inflammatory sites. IL-4 or IFN-γ can also induce macrophages to fuse into large, multinucleated cells called *giant cells* (p 43). Under appropriate conditions, macrophages also have the capacity to proliferate.

Other types of *cells present in chronic inflammation are lymphocytes, plasma cells, and eosinophils.* Both T and B lymphocytes migrate into inflammatory sites via adhesion molecules and chemokines similar to those used to recruit monocytes. They are mobilized in any immune reaction, as well as in non–immune-mediated inflammation. T lymphocytes have a reciprocal relationship to macrophages in chronic inflammation (Fig. 2–18); they are activated by interaction with antigen presenting cells (primarily macrophages and dendritic cells) expressing partially degraded antigen fragments on their cell surface in association with histocompatibility antigens (Chapter 5). The activated lymphocytes in turn produce a variety of cytokines, including IFN-γ, a major stimulator for monocytes and macrophages. Activated macrophages in turn release cytokines, including IL-1 and TNF; these can further activate lymphocytes, as well as other cell types (as we have seen). The end result is an inflammatory focus where macrophages and T cells can persistently stimulate one another until the triggering antigen is removed, or some modulatory event occurs.

Plasma cells are the terminally differentiated end product of B-cell activation; they can produce antibodies directed against antigens in the inflammatory site or sometimes against altered tissue components. *Eosinophils are characteristically found in inflammatory sites around parasitic infections, or as part of immune reactions mediated by immunoglobulin E* (IgE), typically associated with allergies. Their emigration is driven by adhesion molecules similar to those used by neutrophils, and by specific chemokines (e.g., *eotaxin*), derived from leukocytes or epithelial cells. Eosinophil-specific granules contain major basic protein (MBP), a highly charged cationic protein that is toxic to parasites but also causes epithelial cell lysis.

Granulomatous Inflammation

Granulomatous inflammation is a distinctive pattern of chronic inflammation *characterized by aggregations of acti-*

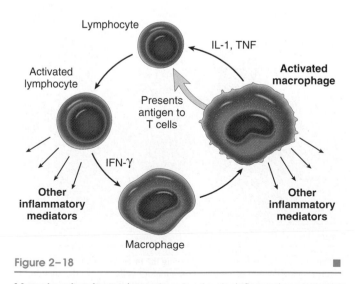

Lymphocyte

IL-1, TNF

Activated
lymphocyte

**Activated
macrophage**

Presents
antigen to
T cells

IFN-γ

**Other
inflammatory
mediators**

**Other
inflammatory
mediators**

Macrophage

Figure 2–18 ■

Macrophage-lymphocyte interactions in chronic inflammation. Activated lymphocytes and macrophages influence each other, and both cell types release inflammatory mediators that affect other cells.

Table 2–2. EXAMPLES OF GRANULOMATOUS INFLAMMATION

Bacterial
   Tuberculosis *(Mycobacterium tuberculosis)*
   Leprosy *(M. leprae)*
   Syphilitic gumma *(Treponema pallidum)*
   Cat-scratch disease (gram-negative bacillus)

Parasitic
   Schistosomiasis *(Schistosoma mansoni, S. haemotobium, S. japon-
      icum)*

Fungal
   Histoplasma capsulatum
   Blastomycosis
   Cryptococcus neoformans
   Coccidioides immitis

Inorganic metals or dusts
   Silicosis
   Berylliosis

Foreign body
   Suture, breast prosthesis, vascular graft

Unknown
   Sarcoidosis

*vated macrophages that have acquired an enlarged, squa-
mous cell–like (called epithelioid) appearance.* Granulomas
are encountered in relatively few pathologic states, tuberculosis being the archetypal granulomatous disease; therefore,
recognition of the granulomatous pattern is important because
of the limited number of conditions (some life threatening)
that cause it (Table 2–2).

In the usual H & E preparations (Fig. 2–19), the
enlarged macrophages have pale pink granular
cytoplasm with indistinct cell boundaries. The nodules of epithelioid macrophages are surrounded
by a collar of lymphocytes that are presumably
secreting the cytokines responsible for macro-

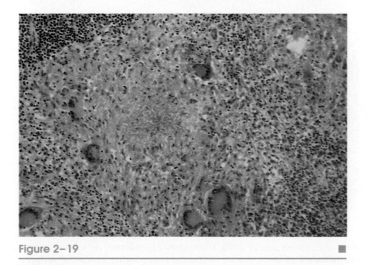

Figure 2–19

A typical tuberculous granuloma showing an area of central necrosis, epithelioid macrophages, multiple giant cells, and lymphocytes.

phage activation. Older granulomas also develop
a surrounding rim of fibroblasts and connective tissue, conceivably to help contain the injurious
agent that caused formation of the granuloma in
the first place. Frequently, but not invariably, multinucleated giant cells 40 to 50 μm in diameter are
also found in granulomas. They consist of a large
mass of cytoplasm and multiple nuclei, and derive
from the fusion of 20 or more macrophages.

Granulomas may occur in response to relatively inert foreign bodies (e.g., suture, splinter, breast implant), forming so-
called *foreign body granulomas*. Granulomas also form in the
setting of T cell–mediated immune responses to organisms
(e.g., the tubercle bacillus) or indigestible particles, where T
cell–derived cytokines are responsible for transforming macrophages into activated epithelioid cells and giant cells. They
are discussed further in Chapter 5.

■ **ROLE OF LYMPHATICS AND
LYMPH NODES IN
INFLAMMATION**

The system of lymphatics and lymph nodes serves to drain
and sample fluid accumulated in the extravascular matrix. In
concert with the mononuclear phagocyte system, it represents
a secondary line of defense utilized whenever a local inflammatory response fails to contain and neutralize injurious
agents. Lymphatics are also used to deliver antigens and lymphocytes from peripheral sites to more central lymph nodes
where T cells, B cells, and the appropriate antigen-presenting
cells can all gather to mount an immune response.

Lymphatics are almost as abundant as capillaries. They are
difficult to visualize in typical tissue sections, however, because they are delicate, thin-walled channels that readily collapse. They are lined with continuous endothelium having
loose, overlapping cell junctions, scant basement membrane,
and no muscular support, except in the larger ducts. Lymphatic valves ensure that lymph flows only in a distal to proximal direction, and delicate fibrils tether the lymphatic walls
to the extracellular matrix, helping to maintain patency.

Lymph flow is increased in inflammation and is important
in the resolution of the inflammatory response, helping to
drain the edema fluid, extravasated leukocytes, and cellular
debris from the extravascular space (see Fig. 2–15). Unfortunately, lymphatic drainage can also provide channels for
dissemination of the injurious agent. As a result, secondary
inflammatory involvement of lymphatic channels *(lymphangitis)* or the regional filtering lymph nodes *(reactive lymphadenitis)* may develop. In an infection of the hand, for example, red lymphangitic streaking may extend up the arm,
accompanied by tender, enlarged axillary lymph nodes. Reactive lymphadenitis is histologically characterized by hyperplasia of the lymphoid follicles and of the macrophages lining
the sinuses *(sinus histiocytosis)*, often with associated phagocytosis of cell debris (Chapter 12).

Fortunately, these secondary lines of defense are often able to contain the infection. However, they are occasionally overwhelmed, and infectious organisms can then drain through progressively larger lymphatics until they gain access to the bloodstream, resulting in *bacteremia*. The mononuclear phagocytes of the liver, spleen, and bone marrow are the next fall-back position, but even these may be breached in sufficiently massive infections. At that point, various tissues in the body may become seeded with microbes; heart valves, kidneys, joints, and meninges are favored sites.

MORPHOLOGIC PATTERNS IN ACUTE AND CHRONIC INFLAMMATION

The severity of the inflammatory response, its specific cause, and the particular tissue involved can all modify the basic morphologic patterns of acute and chronic inflammation. Such patterns, which frequently have clinical significance, are as follows:

SEROUS INFLAMMATION. This is characterized by the outpouring of a watery, relatively protein-poor fluid (*effusion*) that, depending on the site of injury, derives either from the serum or from the secretions of mesothelial cells lining the peritoneal, pleural, and pericardial cavities. The skin blister resulting from a burn or viral infection is a good example of a serous effusion accumulated either within or immediately beneath the epidermis of the skin (Fig. 2–20A).

FIBRINOUS INFLAMMATION. This occurs as a consequence of more severe injuries, with the resultant greater vascular permeability allowing larger molecules (specifically, *fibrinogen*) to pass the endothelial barrier. Histologically, the accumulated extravascular fibrin appears as an eosinophilic meshwork of threads, or sometimes as an amorphous coagulum (Fig. 2–20B). Fibrinous exudates may be degraded by fibrinolysis and the accumulated debris may be removed by macrophages, resulting in restoration of the normal tissue struc-

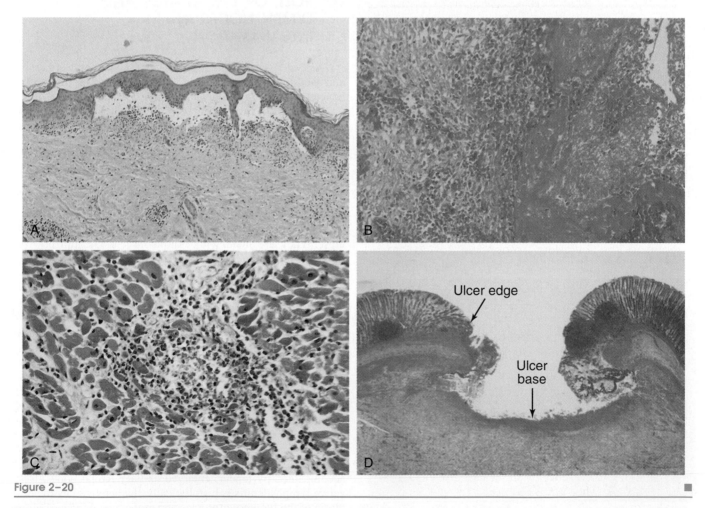

Figure 2–20 ■

Histologic patterns of acute inflammation. *A,* Serous inflammation. Low-power view of a cross-section of a skin blister showing epidermis separated from the dermis by a focal collection of serous effusion. *B,* Fibrinous inflammation. A pink meshwork of fibrin exudate (on the right) overlies the pericardial surface. *C,* Suppurative inflammation. A bacterial abscess in myocardium. *D,* Ulceration. A low-power cross-section of duodenal ulcer crater with an acute inflammatory exudate in the base.

ture *(resolution)*. However, failure to completely remove the fibrin results in the ingrowth of fibroblasts and blood vessels, leading ultimately to scarring *(organization)*. For example, organization of a fibrinous pericardial exudate to form scar tissue can lead to the development of fibrous strands that bridge the pericardial space and restrict myocardial function.

SUPPURATIVE (PURULENT) INFLAMMATION. This is manifested by the presence of large amounts of purulent exudate (pus) consisting of neutrophils, necrotic cells, and edema fluid. Certain organisms (e.g., staphylococci) are more likely to induce this localized suppuration and are therefore referred to as pyogenic. Abscesses are focal collections of pus that may be caused by deep seeding of pyogenic organisms into a tissue, or by secondary infections of necrotic foci. Abscesses typically have a central, largely necrotic region rimmed by a layer of preserved neutrophils (Fig. 2–20C), with a surrounding zone of dilated vessels and fibroblastic proliferation indicative of early repair. In time, the abscess may become completely walled off and eventually replaced by connective tissue.

ULCERATION. This refers to a site of inflammation where an epithelial surface (skin, gastric epithelium, colonic mucosa, bladder epithelium) has become necrotic and eroded, often with associated subepithelial acute and chronic inflammation. This can occur as a consequence of toxic or traumatic injury to the epithelial surface (e.g., peptic ulcers, Chapter 15) or may be due to vascular compromise (as in foot ulcers associated with the vasculopathy of diabetes, Chapter 17). The peptic ulcer of the stomach or duodenum (Fig. 2–20D) illustrates the typical findings. There is usually an early intense neutrophilic infiltrate with associated vascular dilation. In chronic lesions where there has been repeated insult, the area surrounding the ulcer develops fibroblastic proliferation, scarring, and the accumulation of chronic inflammatory cells.

SYSTEMIC EFFECTS OF INFLAMMATION

Fever is only one of the more obvious of the systemic effects of inflammation, collectively identified as *acute-phase reactions*. These include increased slow-wave sleep, anorexia, accelerated degradation of skeletal muscle proteins, hypotension, hepatic synthesis of a variety of acute-phase proteins (e.g., complement and coagulation proteins), and alterations in the circulating white blood cell pool.

The cytokines IL-1, IL-6, and TNF are the most important mediators of the acute-phase reactions. These cytokines are produced by leukocytes (and other cell types) in response to infection, or to immune and toxic injury, and are released systemically, frequently in a sort of cytokine cascade. TNF can induce the production of IL-1, which in turn induces the production of IL-6 (Chapter 3). IL-6 stimulates the hepatic synthesis of several plasma proteins, most notably fibrinogen; elevated fibrinogen levels cause erythrocytes to agglutinate more readily, which may explain why inflammation is associated with a higher *erythrocyte sedimentation rate* by objective testing. Although IL-1 and TNF induce other consequences (see Fig. 2–13), their effects are similar to one another. For example, they both act on the thermoregulatory center of the hypothalamus, most likely via local prostaglandin E production, to induce fever (hence the efficacy of aspirin and NSAIDs in reducing fever).

Leukocytosis (increased white blood cell count) is a common feature of inflammatory reactions, especially those induced by bacterial infection. The leukocyte count usually increases to 15,000 or 20,000 cells/μl (normal = 4000 to 10,000 cells/μl), but exceptionally may climb as high as 40,000 to 100,000 cells/μl, a so-called *leukemoid reaction*. Leukocytosis initially results from the release of cells from the bone marrow (caused by IL-1 and TNF) and is associated with an increased number of relatively immature neutrophils in the blood ("left-shift"). Prolonged infection, however, also induces proliferation of precursors in the bone marrow, caused by IL-1 and TNF-driven increases in the production of colony-stimulating factors.

Most bacterial infections induce a relatively selective increase in polymorphonuclear cells (*neutrophilia*), while parasitic infections (as well as allergic responses) characteristically induce eosinophilia. Certain viruses, such as infectious mononucleosis (Chapter 12), mumps, and rubella, engender selective increases in lymphocytes (*lymphocytosis*). However, most viral infections, as well as rickettsial, protozoal, and certain types of bacterial infections (typhoid fever), are associated with a decreased number of circulating white cells (*leukopenia*). Leukopenia is also encountered in infections that overwhelm patients debilitated by, for example, disseminated cancer.

Although this concludes our discussion of the cellular and molecular events in acute and chronic inflammation, we still need to consider the changes induced by the body's attempts to heal the damage, the process of *repair*. As described next in Chapter 3, the repair begins almost as soon as the inflammatory changes have started and involves several processes, including cell proliferation, differentiation, and extracellular matrix deposition.

BIBLIOGRAPHY

Baggiolini M, et al: Interleukin-8 and the chemokine family. Int J Immunopharmacol 17:103, 1995. (A good summary of the chemokines.)

Butcher EC, Picker LJ: Lymphocyte homing and homeostasis. Science 272:60, 1996. (A review of adhesion molecules.)

Cotran RS, Briscoe DM: Endothelial cells in inflammation. In Kelley, W, et al (eds): Textbook of Rheumatology, 5th ed. Philadelphia, WB Saunders, 1996. (An overview of inflammatory cells and adhesion molecules.)

Dray A: Inflammatory mediators of pain. Br J Anaesthesiol 75:125, 1995. (Current concepts of pain in inflammation.)

Dvorak, AM, et al: The vesiculo-vacuolar organelle (VVO): A distinct endothelial cell structure that provides a transcellular pathway for macromolecular extravasation. J Leuko Biol 59:100, 1996. (A description of the transcytosis pathway for increased vascular permeability.)

Goetzl EJ, et al: Specificity of expression and effects of eicosanoid mediators in normal physiology and human diseases. FASEB J 9:1051, 1995. (A review of the various eicosanoids and their most significant effects.)

Imhof BA, Dunon D: Leukocyte migration and adhesion. Adv Immunol 58: 345, 1995. (A comprehensive review of adhesion molecules and mechanisms of leukocyte migration.)

Kagan BL, et al: Defensins: a family of antimicrobial and cytotoxic peptides. Toxicology 87:131, 1994. (A summary of the nonoxidative mechanisms of microbial killing.)

Kaufmann SH: Immunity to intracellular bacteria. Annu Rev Immunol 11: 129, 1993. (A thorough, comprehensive review of the basic immunology related to intracellular bacterial pathogens, and the role of granulomatous inflammation in normal defense.)

Liles WC, VanVoorhis WC: Review: nomenclature and biologic significance of cytokines involved in inflammation and host immune response. J Infect Dis 172:1573, 1995. (A well-organized, largely tabular compilation of information on 42 different cytokines, including cell distribution and effects.)

Moilanen E, Vapaatalo H: Nitric oxide in inflammation and immune response. Ann Med 27:359, 1995. (An overview of the roles of nitric oxide in inflammation.)

Morgan BP: Physiology and pathophysiology of complement: progress and trends. Crit Rev Clin Lab Sci 32:265, 1995. (An excellent review of the various aspects of complement.)

Premack BA, Schall TJ: Chemokine receptors: Gateways to inflammation and infection. Nat Med 2:1174, 1996. (A lucid review of chemokines and their receptors; also includes the current nomenclature of this expanding universe of molecules.)

Schmidt HHHW, Walter U: NO at work. Cell 78:919, 1994. (A brief overview of the effects of nitric oxide, in an issue covering several aspects of the molecule.)

Stewart RJ, Marsden PA: Biologic control of the tumor necrosis factor and interleukin-1 signaling cascade. Am J Kidney Dis 25:954, 1995. (A review of the mechanisms of action and effects of IL-1 and TNF.)

Stossel TP: On the crawling of animal cells. Science 260:1045, 1993. (A brief summary of the mechanisms and significance of cell locomotion.)

Streiter RM, Kunkel SL: Acute lung injury: the role of cytokines in the elicitation of neutrophils. J Invest Med 42:640, 1994. (A good review of the interplay between soluble mediators and leukocytes in acute inflammation.)

Tedder TF, et al: The selectins: vascular adhesion molecules. FASEB J 9: 866, 1995. (A review of the structure, distribution, and function of selectins.)

Tracey KJ, Cerami A: Tumor necrosis factor, cytokines and disease. Annu Rev Cell Biol 9:317, 1993. (An overview of the effects and mechanisms of action.)

Tsokos GC: Lymphocytes, cytokines, inflammation, and immune trafficking. Curr Opin Rheumatol 7:376, 1995. (Cytokine and adhesion molecule interplay in inflammation and pathologic states.)

3

Repair: Cell Regeneration, Fibrosis, and Wound Healing

RICHARD N. MITCHELL, MD, PhD
RAMZI S. COTRAN, MD

Even as cells and tissues are being injured, events that contain the damage and prepare the surviving cells to replicate are set into motion. In general, the number of cells in a given tissue is a cumulative function of the rates at which new cells enter and exit the population. Entry of new cells into a tissue population is largely determined by their proliferation rates, while cells can leave the population either by cell death or differentiation into another cell type. As shown in Figure 3–1, increased cell number in a particular population may therefore result from either increased proliferation or decreased cell death or differentiation.

Repair begins very early in the process of inflammation and involves two dichotomous processes: (1) *regeneration of injured tissue by parenchymal cells of the same type,* and (2) *replacement by connective tissue (fibroplasia),* resulting in a permanent scar. Commonly, tissue repair involves some combination of the two. Interestingly, both regeneration and scarring are directed by similar mechanisms including cell growth and differentiation, as well as cell-matrix interactions.

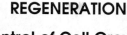

REGENERATION

Control of Cell Growth and Differentiation at Sites of Injury

Cellular proliferation is largely regulated by biochemical factors produced in the local microenvironment that can either stimulate or inhibit cell growth. Thus, an excess of stimulators

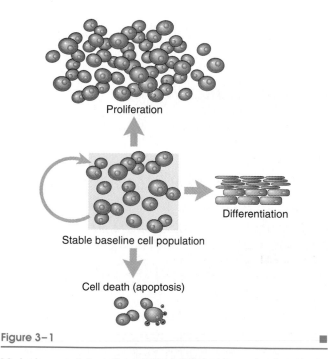

Figure 3–1 ■

Mechanisms regulating cell populations. Cell numbers can be altered by increased or decreased rates of cell death (apoptosis) or by changes in the rates of proliferation or differentiation. (Modified from McCarthy NJ, et al: Apoptosis in the development of the immune system: growth factors, clonal selection and *bcl-2.* Cancer Metastasis Rev 11:157, 1992.)

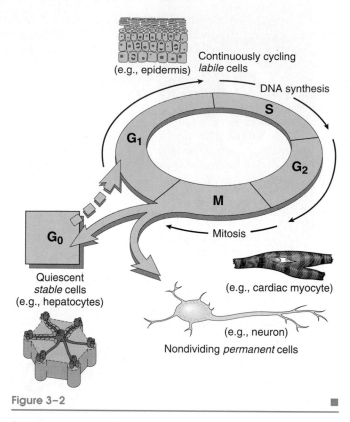

Figure 3–2 ■

Cell populations and cell cycle phases. Constantly dividing labile cells continuously cycle from one mitosis to the next. Nondividing permanent cells have exited the cycle and are destined to die without further division. Quiescent stable cells in G_0 are neither cycling nor dying and can be induced to re-enter the cycle by an appropriate stimulus.

or a deficiency of inhibitors results in net cell growth. Although growth can be accomplished by shortening the length of the cell cycle or decreasing the rate of cell loss, *the most important regulatory control is the induction of resting cells (in G_0) to enter the cell cycle* (see below).

CELL CYCLE AND THE PROLIFERATIVE POTENTIAL OF DIFFERENT CELL TYPES

The cell growth cycle (Fig. 3–2) consists of G_1 (presynthetic), S (DNA synthesis), G_2 (premitotic), and M (mitotic) phases. Quiescent cells are in a physiologic state called G_0. The cells of the body are divided into three groups on the basis of their regenerative capacity and their relationship to the cell cycle. With the exception of tissues composed primarily of nondividing permanent cells, most mature tissues contain variable proportions of continuously dividing cells, quiescent cells that occasionally go back to the cell cycle, and nondividing cells.

■ *Continuously dividing (labile) cells* proceed through the cell cycle from one mitosis to the next and proliferate throughout life, replacing cells that are continuously dying. Labile cells include many epithelia such as the stratified squamous surfaces of the skin, oral cavity, vagina, and cervix; the cuboidal epithelia of the ducts draining exocrine organs (e.g., salivary glands, pancreas, biliary tract); the columnar epithelium of the gastrointestinal tract, uterus, and fallopian tubes; and the transitional epithelium of the urinary tract. The hematopoietic cells of the bone marrow are also continuously replenishing the circulating peripheral blood cell elements.

■ *Quiescent (stable) cells* usually demonstrate a low level of replication. At baseline, they are considered to be in G_0, but after cell loss they can be driven into G_1 by an appropriate stimulus leading to rapid increases in division and tissue reconstitution. The growth capacity of stable cells is best exemplified by the ability of the liver to regenerate after hepatectomy or following toxic, viral, or chemical injury. Included in the category of stable cells are the parenchymal cells of liver, kidney, and pancreas, as well as vascular endothelial cells and mesenchymal cells such as fibroblasts and smooth muscle.

■ *Nondividing (permanent) cells* exited the cell cycle at some point in intrauterine development and cannot undergo further mitotic division in postnatal life. These include nerve cells and cardiac myocytes, where irreversible injury results in only scarring. Skeletal muscle is also generally placed in this category, although this tissue does have a limited regenerative capacity, largely owing to the proliferation and differentiation of immature stem cells associated with endomysial sheaths.

MOLECULAR EVENTS IN CELL GROWTH

Although many chemical mediators affect cell growth, the most important are *polypeptide growth factors* circulating in the serum or produced locally by cells in a paracrine fashion. Most growth factors have *pleiotropic effects*; that is, in addition to stimulating cellular proliferation, they mediate a wide variety of other activities, including cell migration, differentiation, and tissue remodeling, and are therefore involved in various stages of wound healing. The growth factors induce cell proliferation by affecting the expression of genes involved in normal growth control pathways, the so-called *protooncogenes*. The expression of these genes is tightly regulated during normal regeneration and repair. Alterations in the structure or expression of protooncogenes can convert them into *oncogenes*, which contribute to uncontrolled cell growth characteristic of cancers; thus, normal and abnormal cellular proliferation may follow similar pathways (Chapter 6). Here we shall review the normal proteins and molecular events (Fig. 3–3) that result in cell division because these are critical to an understanding of regeneration and repair.

■ *Ligand-receptor binding.* Cell growth is typically initiated by the binding of a growth factor to its specific receptors either at the cell surface or within the cell. Although most receptors are expressed on the plasma membrane, steroid receptors are intracellular (in either the cytoplasm or the

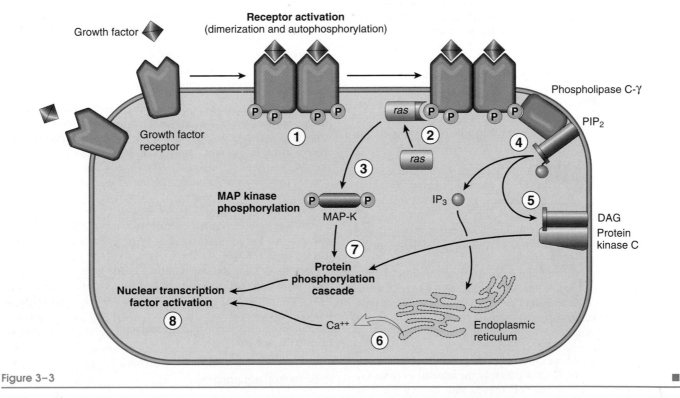

Figure 3–3   ■

Cellular events initiated by interaction of growth factors and their receptors. Most growth factor receptors have intrinsic tyrosine kinase activity, which is activated by receptor dimerization and autophosphorylation (with conformational change) after ligand binding ①. Phosphorylated receptor tyrosine kinases can activate *ras* ②, which eventually results in phosphorylation of the MAP kinases (MAP-K) ③. Activated receptors can also activate phospholipase C-γ, which catabolizes PIP_2 to DAG and IP_3 ④; DAG recruits and activates protein kinase C, which phosphorylates additional proteins. IP_3 releases intracellular calcium from the endoplasmic reticulum ⑥. Together the increased intracellular calcium and the kinase-mediated phosphorylation cascade ⑦ eventually result in activation of nuclear transcription factors and cellular proliferation ⑧. PIP_2, IP_3, DAG: see text (p 50).

nucleus) and interact with lipophilic steroid ligands that cross the cell membrane.

■ *Receptor activation.* Most growth factor receptors are cell surface protein monomers with intrinsic cytoplasmic domain tyrosine kinase activity (Fig. 3–3). Ligand binding typically causes receptor dimerization, which in turn leads to autophosphorylation of specific tyrosines on the dimer partners. The resultant activated phosphoproteins may then set up a cascade of signals either by binding to secondary effector molecules (see below) or by phosphorylating other proteins. Some transmembrane growth factor receptors lack kinase activity and instead mediate signaling by recruiting intracellular protein kinases after ligand binding.

■ *Signal transduction and second messengers.* Activated receptors bind either to additional protein kinases or to adapter proteins capable of coupling receptors to further signaling molecules. The bound proteins may then be phosphorylated or otherwise undergo conformational changes to acquire new activities. Secondary signaling proteins include

1. *GTP-binding proteins,* including G proteins and the *ras* family of proteins. These proteins couple activated membrane receptors to intracellular effectors. *Ras* activation, for example, leads to a phosphorylation cascade that eventually affects numerous cytoplasmic enzymes called *mitogen-activated protein (MAP) kinases* (Fig. 3–3).

2. *Phospholipase C-γ (PLC-γ).* This protein catalyzes the degradation of phosphatidyl 4,5-bisphosphate (PIP_2) into inositol 1,4,5-trisphosphate (IP_3) and diacylglycerol (DAG). IP_3 then mobilizes intracellular calcium stores, and DAG induces the membrane translocation and activation of protein kinase C (PKC), a member of a family of serine/threonine kinases. The net result is elevated intracellular calcium and further phosphorylation of intracellular proteins (Fig. 3–3). The protein phosphorylation initiated by such receptor-ligand interactions is counter-regulated by intracellular *phosphatases.* They can terminate signal transduction by removing phosphates from a variety of proteins.

■ *Transcription factors.* The cascade of MAP kinases and other second messengers (e.g., calcium) eventually transmit growth signals to the nucleus, inducing expression of a large number of growth regulatory genes. Some of these genes, such as *myc, fos,* and *jun,* code for transcription factors and are involved in the regulation of DNA synthesis, and cell division.

■ *Cell cycle and cyclins.* The entry and progression of cells through the cell cycle are controlled by changes in the intracellular concentrations and activity of a group of proteins called *cyclins.* Cyclins regulate cell division by forming activated complexes with a group of constitutively expressed protein kinases called *cyclin-dependent kinases (cdk)* that regulate specific steps in the cell cycle. Cdc-2, for example, is a cdk that controls the transition from G_2 to M (Fig. 3–4); as the cell moves into G_2, cyclin B is synthesized and it binds to cdc-2. This complex is activated by phosphorylation and the active kinase then phosphorylates a variety of proteins involved in mitosis, including those involved in DNA replication, depolymerization of nuclear lamina, and mitotic spindle formation. After cell

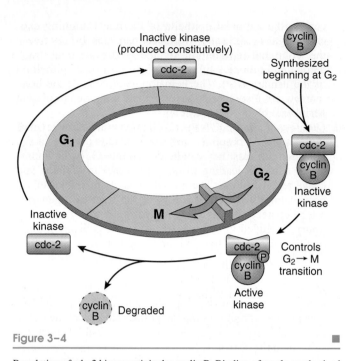

Figure 3–4 ■

Regulation of cdc-2 kinase activity by cyclin B. Binding of newly synthesized cyclin B to inactive cdc-2 kinase at the beginning of G_2 results in a complex that can be activated by phosphorylation. This active kinase complex then phosphorylates a number of proteins important in regulating the $G_2 \rightarrow$ M transition. Following mitosis, the cyclin B dissociates from the complex and is degraded, leaving behind the inactive cdc-2 kinase, which can re-enter the cycle at the next G_2 stage. (Adapted from Dr. Anindya Dutta.)

division, the relevant cyclins are degraded; until there is a new growth stimulus and synthesis of new cyclins, the cells cannot undergo further mitosis.

To summarize, polypeptide growth factors bind to and activate their receptors, many of which possess intrinsic kinase activity. They subsequently phosphorylate a number of substrates involved in signal transduction and the generation of second messengers, including PLC-γ and ras. The resultant kinase cascade leads to the activation of nuclear transcription factors, initiates DNA synthesis, and ultimately culminates in cell division. The process of cell proliferation is directed by a family of proteins called cyclins that, when complexed with cdk, control the phosphorylation of proteins involved in mitosis.

As mentioned at the outset, many of the genes that regulate normal cell growth, including those that encode growth factors, their receptors, signal-transduction proteins, transcription factors, and cyclins and cdk can be converted into oncogenes by mutations that derail the normal regulation of their functions (Chapter 6).

GROWTH INHIBITION

In addition to specific signals that stimulate and positively regulate growth, cells and tissues are also subject to a number of negative, growth inhibitory signals. Contact inhibition of growth in confluent cultures is one such example. Growth suppression in vivo is also evident, for example, in the model of partial hepatectomy in which, quite remarkably, hepatocytes stop proliferating when the liver has attained its normal preoperative size and configuration. The discovery that loss of tumor suppressor genes occurs in certain cancers suggests that such genes encode components of cellular inhibitory pathways (Chapter 6). Polypeptide factors that function as growth inhibitors include transforming growth factor-β (TGF-β) and tumor necrosis factor (TNF). Insoluble extracellular matrix molecules may also suppress cellular responses to stimulatory mediators in the local tissue microenvironment (see below).

GROWTH FACTORS

Polypeptide growth factors may act on a variety of cell types or may have a rather limited target population. Besides promoting growth, these mediators may also influence cell locomotion, contractility, and differentiation, all of which bear on repair and wound healing. The various growth factors may work by endocrine, paracrine, or autocrine pathways, although wound healing and repair in connective tissues are most commonly achieved by one cell in a tissue secreting a factor that regulates the activities of adjacent cells (*paracrine stimulation*). Cells that carry receptors for their own endogenously produced factors also exhibit *autocrine stimulation*, important in compensatory epithelial hyperplasia at sites of injury (e.g., hepatic regeneration). Although there is an impressive and ever-widening array of growth factors, we shall review here only those that have a broad target action or are involved in important pathologic processes. Table 3–1 summarizes some of the growth factors involved in mediating the angiogenesis, fibroblast migration, proliferation, and collagen deposition in healing wounds.

■ *Epidermal growth factor (EGF)* is mitogenic for a variety of epithelial cells and fibroblasts. It stimulates cell division by binding to a tyrosine kinase receptor on the cell membrane (c-*erb* B1), followed by phosphorylation and other activation events, as described earlier. Transforming growth factor-α (TGF-α) shares homology with EGF, binds to the EGF receptor, and exerts similar biologic activities as EGF.

■ *Platelet-derived growth factor (PDGF)* is a highly cationic A- and B-chain heterodimer. While it is released from platelet α granules following activation, it is also produced by activated macrophages, endothelial and smooth muscle cells, and a variety of tumors. PDGF induces fibroblast, smooth muscle cell, and monocyte migration and proliferation, but has other proinflammatory properties as well. It binds to two types of specific receptors (α and β) that have intrinsic protein kinase activity.

■ *Fibroblast growth factors (FGFs)* are a family of polypeptides that bind tightly to heparin and other anionic molecules (and thus have a strong affinity for basement membranes); they exhibit a number of activities in addition to growth stimulation. Basic FGF (b-FGF), in particular, has the ability to induce all the steps necessary for new blood vessel formation (angiogenesis, see below); it is elaborated by activated macrophages and other cells.

■ *TGF-β* has pleiotropic and often conflicting effects. It is produced in an inactive form by a variety of cell types, including platelets, endothelium, T cells, and activated macrophages, and must be proteolytically cleaved (e.g., by plasmin) to become functional. Although TGF-β is a growth inhibitor for most epithelial cell types in culture, it has variable effects on the proliferation of mesenchymal cells. In low concentrations it induces the synthesis and secretion of PDGF, and is therefore indirectly mitogenic. However, at high concentrations it is growth inhibitory because it blocks the expression of PDGF receptors. TGF-β also stimulates fibroblast chemotaxis and the production of collagen and fibronectin by cells, while at the same time inhibiting degradation of the extracellular matrix by metalloproteinases. All these effects tend to favor fibrogenesis, and *TGF-β is increasingly implicated in the fibrosis elicited in chronic inflammatory states.*

■ *Vascular endothelial growth factor (VEGF)* is actually a series of dimeric glycoprotein isoforms with partial homology to PDGF. VEGF activity was originally isolated from tumors where it has a central role in the growth of new blood vessels *(angiogenesis);* it also promotes angiogenesis in normal embryonic development, in healing wounds, and in chronic inflammatory states, and is re-

■

Table 3–1.   MAJOR GROWTH FACTORS IN WOUND HEALING

	EGF or (TGF-α)	PDGF	b-FGF	TGF-β	VEGF	IL-1 or TNF
Angiogenesis	+	0	++	+	++	+
Chemotaxis						
Monocytes	0	+	+	+	0	+
Fibroblasts	0	+	+	+	0	0
Endothelial Cells	+	0	+	−	+	0
Proliferation						
Fibroblasts	+	+	+	±	0	+
Endothelial Cells	+	0	++	−	++	0 or −
Collagen Synthesis	+	+	+	++	0	+
Collagenase Secretion	+	+	+	+	0	+

++, major role; +, stimulates; −, inhibits; ±, variable (dose-dependent) effect; 0, no effect; EGF, epidermal growth factor; TGF-β, transforming growth factor-β; PDGF, platelet-derived growth factor; b-FGF, basic fibroblast growth factor; VEGF, vascular endothelial growth factor.

sponsible for a marked increase in vascular permeability. It is this latter activity, that leads to increased deposition of plasma proteins (e.g., fibrinogen) in the extracellular matrix and provides a provisional stroma for fibroblast and endothelial cell ingrowth. The receptors for VEGF are expressed only on endothelial cells, so that effects on other cell types are all indirect.

■ *Cytokines* are also in many cases growth factors. IL-1 and TNF, for example, induce fibroblast proliferation. They are also chemotactic for fibroblasts, and stimulate the synthesis of collagen and collagenase by these cells. The net results of their actions tend to be fibrogenic.

Extracellular Matrix and Cell-Matrix Interactions

The extracellular matrix (ECM) comprises a significant proportion of any tissue. Besides providing turgor to soft tissues and rigidity to bone, ECM supplies a substratum for cell adhesion and critically regulates the growth, movement, and differentiation of the cells living within it. Moreover, although labile and stable cells are capable of complete regeneration, reconstitution of normal structure requires an intact ECM. ECM consists of *fibrous structural proteins* and an *interstitial matrix* composed of adhesive glycoproteins embedded in a proteoglycan and glycosaminoglycan gel. The fibrous structural proteins are the collagens and elastin. The seemingly random array of interstitial matrix in connective tissues becomes highly organized around epithelial cells, endothelial cells, and smooth muscle cells, forming the specialized *basement membrane (BM)*. BM directs cell polarity and is required for the orderly renewal of an epithelial tissue. In the absence of an intact BM, cells proliferate in a haphazard fashion, producing disorganized masses bearing no morphologic or functional resemblance to the original tissue.

There are three components in most ECMs.

Collagen. The collagens are proteins composed of three protein α chains braided into a ropelike triple helix; the individual chains are able to tightly intertwine because each α polypeptide has glycines present at every third position. More than 30 distinct α chains form approximately 18 different collagen types, some of which may be unique to specific cells and tissues. Some collagen types (e.g., types I, III, and V) form fibrils by virtue of lateral cross-linking of the triple helices; other collagens (e.g., type IV) are nonfibrillar and are components of BMs. The fibrillar collagens form a major proportion of the connective tissue in healing wounds and particularly in scars, and are discussed further in that context below.

Adhesive Glycoproteins. These are structurally diverse proteins whose major role is to link ECM components to one another and to cells. They include fibronectin, laminin, and thrombospondin; fibronectin, described here, is prototypical for these molecules.

Fibronectin is a large (400-kD) disulfide-linked heterodimer (Fig. 3–5) synthesized by a variety of cells, including fibroblasts, monocytes, and endothelium, and associated with cell surfaces, BMs, and pericellular matrix. It has specific domains that bind to a wide spectrum of ECM components (e.g., collagen, fibrin, heparin, and proteoglycans) and can

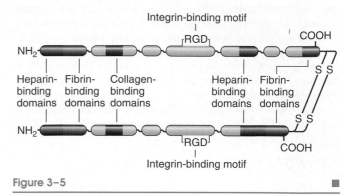

Figure 3–5 ■

The fibronectin molecule. Note the various domains that bind to extracellular matrix (ECM) components, as well as the cell surface integrin-binding domain containing the Arg-Gly-Asp (RGD) motif.

also attach to cell integrins via a tripeptide arginine-glycine–aspartic acid (RGD) motif.

Integrins are a family of transmembrane α/β heterodimeric glycoproteins whose intracellular domains associate with cytoskeletal elements (e.g., vinculin and actin at focal adhesion complexes). Recall that in Chapter 2 we earlier encountered some of the integrins as leukocyte surface molecules that mediate firm adhesion and transmigration across endothelium at sites of inflammation. Integrins on epithelial or mesenchymal cells also bind to ECM; these interactions signal cell attachment and can affect cell locomotion, proliferation, or differentiation (Fig. 3–6). Integrin-ECM interactions can utilize the same intracellular signaling pathways used by growth factor receptors; for example, integrin-mediated adhesion to fibronectin triggers PIP_2 synthesis and enhances its subsequent hydrolysis in response to various growth factors.

Thus, adhesive matrix proteins such as fibronectin can directly mediate the attachment, spreading, and migration of cells. By activating intracellular signaling pathways, fibronectin also enhances the sensitivity of certain cells (e.g., endothelium) to the proliferative effects of growth factors. In the early stages of healing skin wounds, large quantities of fibronectin, mostly plasma derived, accumulate in the ECM and act as an initial scaffolding for the ingrowth of endothelium and fibroblasts. After 2 or 3 days, the fibronectin is actively synthesized by proliferating endothelial cells (see below).

Proteoglycans. These molecules consist of glycosaminoglycans (e.g., dermatan sulfate and heparan sulfate) linked to a protein backbone much like bristles on a test-tube brush; they help regulate ECM structure and permeability. Proteoglycans can also be integral cell membrane proteins and in that capacity modulate cell growth and differentiation. For example, the proteoglycan *syndecan* binds ECM collagen, fibronectin, thrombospondin, and b-FGF and associates with the intracellular actin cytoskeleton to maintain normal epithelial sheet morphology. Glycosaminoglycans without a protein core (e.g., hyaluronic acid) are also important constituents of the ECM.

To summarize, cell growth and differentiation involve at least two types of signals acting in concert. One derives from soluble molecules such as polypeptide growth factors and

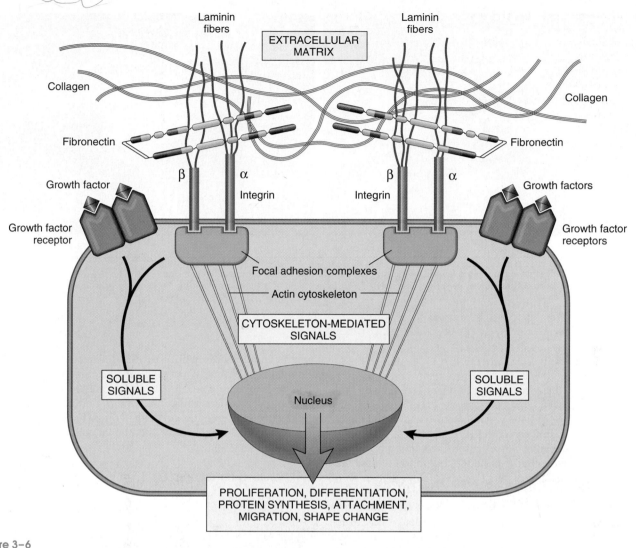

Figure 3-6   ■

Schematic showing mechanisms by which ECM (e.g., fibronectin and laminin) and growth factors can influence cell growth, motility, differentiation, and protein synthesis. Integrins bind ECM and interact with the cytoskeleton at focal adhesion complexes (protein aggregates that include vinculin, α-actinin, and talin). This can initiate the production of intracellular second messengers, or can directly mediate nuclear signals. Cell surface receptors for growth factors also initiate second signals. Together, these are integrated by the cell to yield various responses, including changes in cell growth, locomotion, and differentiation.

growth inhibitors. The other involves insoluble elements of the ECM such as laminin, fibronectin, and collagens.

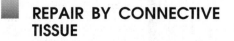

REPAIR BY CONNECTIVE TISSUE

Severe or persistent tissue injury and inflammation with damage both to parenchymal cells and to the stromal framework leads to a situation where repair cannot be accomplished by parenchymal regeneration alone. Under these conditions, the nonregenerated parenchymal cells begin being replaced within 24 hours by proliferating fibroblasts and vascular en-

dothelial cells. By 3 to 5 days, granulation tissue, indicative of healing, is well established. The term *granulation tissue* derives from the pink, soft, granular gross appearance, such as that seen beneath the scab of a skin wound. Its histologic appearance is characterized by proliferation of fibroblasts and new thin-walled, delicate capillaries, in a loose ECM (Fig. 3–7A). Granulation tissue then progressively accumulates connective tissue matrix and eventually results in fibrosis (scarring; Fig. 3–7B). There are three components to this process; the first leads to the formation of the granulation tissue scaffolding on which the final scar will develop and mature:

1. Formation of new blood vessels (angiogenesis)
2. Fibrosis
3. Maturation and organization of the scar (remodeling).

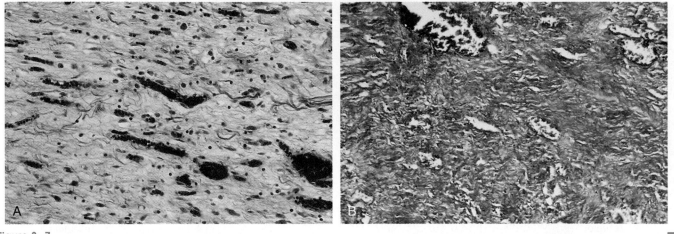

Figure 3–7 ■

A, Granulation tissue showing numerous blood vessels, edema, and a loose ECM containing occasional inflammatory cells. This is a trichrome stain that stains collagen blue; minimal mature collagen can be seen at this point. *B*, Trichrome stain of mature scar, showing dense collagen, with only scattered vascular channels.

Angiogenesis

New vessels in the evolving site of repair originate by budding from preexisting vessels, a process called *angiogenesis* or *neovascularization*. Four general steps occur in the development of a new capillary vessel (Fig. 3–8): (1) proteolytic degradation of the parent vessel basement membrane, allowing formation of a capillary sprout; (2) migration of endothelial cells toward the angiogenic stimulus; (3) proliferation of the endothelial cells behind the leading front of migrating cells; and (4) maturation of endothelial cells with organization into capillary tubes. These new vessels are leaky due to incompletely formed interendothelial junctions and increased transcytosis (Chapter 2). Indeed, this leakiness explains why granulation tissue is often edematous and accounts in part for edema that may persist in healing wounds long after the acute inflammatory response has resolved.

Several factors induce angiogenesis, notably b-FGF and VEGF. Both can bind to proteoglycans in the basement membrane and can presumably be released when such structures are damaged. Directly or indirectly they also induce endothelial cells to secrete proteinases to degrade the basement membrane, promote endothelial cell migration and proliferation, and direct (in conjunction with laminin) vascular tube formation from the expanding endothelial cell population.

Fibrosis (Fibroplasia)

Fibrosis or *fibroplasia* occurs on the granulation tissue framework of new vessels and loose ECM that develop early at the repair site. The process of fibrosis occurs in two steps: (1) emigration and proliferation of fibroblasts in the site of injury, and (2) deposition of ECM by these cells. The recruitment and stimulation of fibroblasts is driven by the various growth factors described previously. The sources of these growth factors include activated endothelium, but perhaps more importantly, they also include a variety of inflammatory

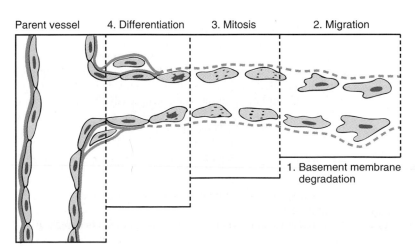

Parent vessel 4. Differentiation 3. Mitosis 2. Migration

1. Basement membrane degradation

Figure 3–8 ■

Four steps in angiogenesis. The parent mature vessel is on the left. 1, Basement membrane and ECM matrix degradation. 2, Endothelial migration. 3, Endothelial proliferation (mitosis). 4, Organization and maturation. (Adapted from Ausprunk DH: In Houck JC (ed): Chemical Messengers of the Inflammatory Process. Amsterdam, Elsevier/North Holland, 1979.)

cells. Macrophages, for example, are important cellular constituents of granulation tissue, responsible for clearing extracellular debris, fibrin, and other foreign matter at the site of injury; they also elaborate PDGF, b-FGF, and TGF-β and therefore promote fibroblast migration and proliferation. If the appropriate chemotactic stimuli are present, lymphocytes may also be present, and mast cells are increased in number; each of these can contribute directly or indirectly to fibroblast proliferation and activation.

As healing progresses, the number of proliferating fibroblasts and new vessels decreases; however, the fibroblasts progressively assume a more synthetic phenotype, and hence there is increased deposition of ECM. Collagen synthesis, in particular, is critical to the development of strength in a healing wound site. As described below, collagen synthesis by fibroblasts begins early in wound healing (days 3 to 5) and continues for several weeks, depending on the size of the wound. Many of the same growth factors that regulate fibroblast proliferation also participate in stimulating ECM synthesis. Collagen synthesis, for example, is induced by a number of the molecules, including growth factors (PDGF, b-FGF, and TGF-β) and cytokines (IL-1 and TNF) secreted by leukocytes and fibroblasts. *Net collagen accumulation, however, depends not only on increased synthesis but also on diminished collagen degradation* (discussed below). Ultimately, the granulation tissue scaffolding evolves into a scar composed of largely inactive, spindle-shaped fibroblasts, dense collagen, fragments of elastic tissue, and other ECM components (see Fig. 3–7B).

Scar Remodeling

Collagens (and other ECM components) are degraded by a family of *metalloproteinases* that are dependent on zinc ions for their activity; these should be distinguished from neutrophil elastase, cathepsin G, plasmin, and other *serine proteinases* that can also degrade ECM but are not metalloenzymes. Metalloproteinases include *interstitial collagenases,* which cleave the fibrillar collagen types I, II, and III; *gelatinases* (or *type IV collagenases*), which degrade amorphous collagen and fibronectin; and *stromelysins,* which catabolize a variety of ECM constituents, including proteoglycans, laminin, fibronectin, and amorphous collagen.

These enzymes are produced by a variety of cell types (fibroblasts, macrophages, neutrophils, synovial cells, and some epithelial cells), and their synthesis and secretion are regulated by growth factors, cytokines, and phagocytic stimuli (Fig. 3–9). Given their potential to wreak havoc in tissues, the activity of the metalloproteinases is tightly controlled. Thus, they are typically elaborated as inactive (zymogen) precursors that must be first activated; this is accomplished by certain chemicals (e.g., HOCl) or proteases (e.g., plasmin) likely to be present only at sites of injury. In addition, activated collagenases can be rapidly inhibited by specific *tissue inhibitors of metalloproteinase (TIMPs),* produced by most mesenchymal cells (Fig. 3–9). In sites of inflammation and wound healing, collagen degradation aids in the debridement of injured sites and also in the remodeling of connective tissues necessary to repair the defect. Indeed, collagenases and

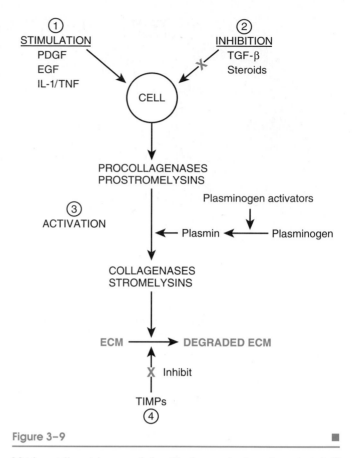

Figure 3–9

Matrix metalloproteinase regulation. The four mechanisms shown include ① regulation of synthesis by a variety of growth factors or cytokines, ② inhibition of synthesis by corticosteroids or TGF-β, ③ regulation of the activation of the secreted but inactive precursors, and ④, blockade of the enzymes by specific tissue inhibitors of metalloproteinases (TIMPs). (Modified from Matrisian LM: Metalloproteinases and their inhibitors in matrix remodelling. Trends Genet 6:122, 1990.)

their inhibitors are spatially and temporally regulated in healing wounds.

■ WOUND HEALING

Wound healing is a complex but systematic process (Fig. 3–10). Soluble growth factors regulate the orderly migration, proliferation, and differentiation of cells, as well as the synthesis and degradation of ECM proteins. The ECM in turn directly affects cellular events and modulates cell responsiveness to the growth factors. Physical factors, including the forces generated by changes in cell shape, also contribute to the total process. Wound healing involves processes that have been well-described previously, namely: (1) induction of an acute inflammatory response by the initial injury, (2) parenchymal cell regeneration, (3) migration and proliferation of both parenchymal and connective tissue cells, (4) synthesis of ECM proteins, (5) remodeling of parenchymal elements to

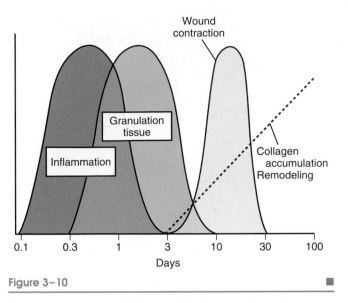

Figure 3-10 ■

The orderly phases of wound healing. (Modified from Clark RA: In Goldsmith LA (ed): Physiology, Biochemistry, and Molecular Biology of the Skin, 2nd ed, Vol I. New York, Oxford University Press, 1991, p 577.)

restore tissue function, and (6) remodeling of connective tissue to achieve wound strength. Here, we will briefly describe the healing of skin wounds, a process involving both epithelial regeneration and the formation of connective tissue scar.

Healing by First Intention

One of the simplest examples of wound repair is the healing of a clean, uninfected surgical incision approximated by surgical sutures (Fig. 3–11). This is referred to as *primary union* or *healing by first intention.* The incision causes only focal disruption of epithelial basement membrane continuity and death of a relatively few epithelial and connective tissue cells. As a result, epithelial regeneration predominates over fibrosis. The narrow incisional space rapidly fills with fibrin-clotted blood; dehydration at the surface produces a scab to cover and protect the healing repair site.

Day 1. Neutrophils are seen at the incision margin, migrating toward the fibrin clot. Basal cells at the cut edge of the epidermis begin to exhibit increased mitotic activity. Within 24 to 48 hours, epithelial cells from both edges have begun to migrate and proliferate along the dermis, depositing basement membrane components as they progress. The cells meet in the midline beneath the surface scab, yielding a thin but continuous epithelial layer.

Days 2–3. Neutrophils have been largely replaced by macrophages, and granulation tissue progressively invades the incision space. Collagen fibers are now evident at the incision margins, but these are vertically oriented and do not bridge the incision. Epithelial cell proliferation continues, yielding a thickened epidermal covering layer.

Days 4–5. Neovascularization reaches its peak as granulation tissue fills the incisional space. Collagen fibrils become more abundant and begin to bridge the incision. The epidermis

recovers its normal thickness as differentiation of surface cells yields a mature epidermal architecture with surface keratinization.

Second Week. There is continued collagen accumulation and fibroblast proliferation. The leukocyte infiltrate, edema, and increased vascularity are substantially diminished. The long process of "blanching" begins, accomplished by increasing collagen deposition within the incisional scar and the regression of vascular channels.

First Month. The scar comprises a cellular connective tissue largely devoid of inflammatory cells and covered by an essentially normal epidermis. However, the dermal appendages destroyed in the line of the incision are permanently lost. The tensile strength of the wound increases with time, as described below.

Healing by Second Intention

When cell or tissue loss is more extensive, as in infarction, inflammatory ulceration, abscess formation, or even just large wounds, the reparative process is more complex. In these situations, regeneration of parenchymal cells alone cannot restore the original architecture. As a result, there is extensive ingrowth of granulation tissue from the wound margin, followed in time by accumulation of ECM and scarring. This form of healing is referred to as *secondary union* or *healing by second intention* (Fig. 3–11).

Secondary healing differs from primary healing in several respects:

1. Large tissue defects intrinsically have a greater volume of necrotic debris, exudate, and fibrin that must be removed. Consequently, the inflammatory reaction is more intense with greater potential for secondary inflammation-mediated injury (Chapter 2).
2. Much larger amounts of granulation tissue are formed. Larger defects accrue a greater volume of granulation tissue to fill in the gaps in the stromal architecture and provide the underlying framework for the regrowth of tissue epithelium. A greater volume of granulation tissue generally results in a greater mass of scar tissue.
3. Secondary healing exhibits the phenomenon of wound contraction. Within 6 weeks, for example, large skin defects may be reduced to 5% to 10% of their original size, largely by contraction. This process has been ascribed to the presence of myofibroblasts, modified fibroblasts exhibiting many of the ultrastructural and functional features of contractile smooth muscle cells.

Wound Strength

Carefully sutured wounds have approximately 70% of the strength of unwounded skin, largely because of the placement of the sutures. When sutures are removed, usually at 1 week, wound strength is approximately 10% of unwounded skin, but this increases rapidly over the next 4 weeks. The recovery of tensile strength results from collagen synthesis exceeding degradation during the first 2 months, and from structural modifications of collagen (e.g., cross-linking and increased fiber

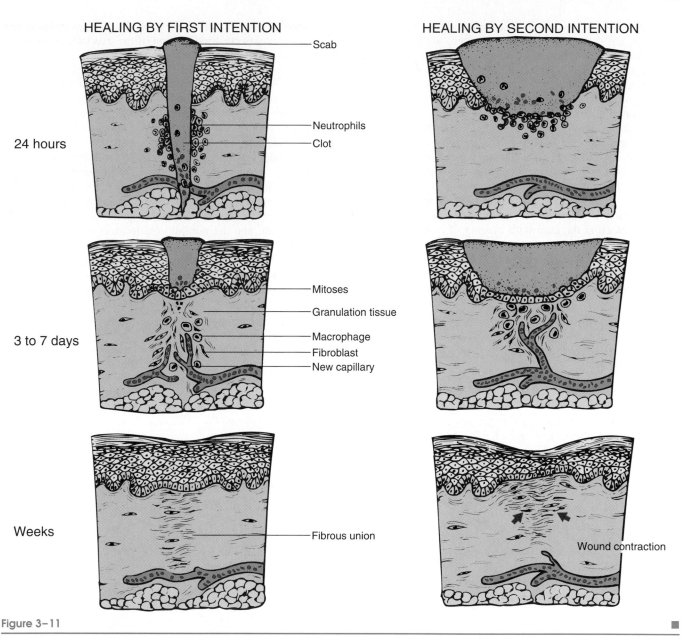

HEALING BY FIRST INTENTION

HEALING BY SECOND INTENTION

24 hours

Scab

Neutrophils

Clot

3 to 7 days

Mitoses

Granulation tissue

Macrophage

Fibroblast

New capillary

Weeks

Fibrous union

Wound contraction

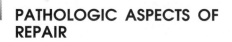

Figure 3–11

Steps in wound healing by first intention *(left)* and second intention *(right)*. In the latter, the resultant scar is much smaller than the original wound, owing to wound contraction.

size) when synthesis declines at later times. Wound strength reaches approximately 70% to 80% of normal by 3 months but usually does not substantially improve beyond that point.

PATHOLOGIC ASPECTS OF REPAIR

In wound healing, normal cell growth and fibrosis may be altered by a variety of influences, frequently reducing the quality and adequacy of the reparative process. These factors may be extrinsic (e.g., infection) or intrinsic to the injured tissue:

■ *Infection* is the single most important cause of delay in healing, by prolonging the inflammation phase of the process and potentially increasing the local tissue injury. *Nutrition* has profound effects on wound healing; protein deficiency, for example, and particularly vitamin C deficiency, inhibit collagen synthesis and retard healing. *Glucocorticoids* have well-documented anti-inflammatory effects and their administration may result in poor wound strength owing to diminished fibrosis. In some instances, however, the anti-inflammatory effects of glucocorticoids are desirable. For example, in corneal infections glucocorticoids are sometimes prescribed (along with antibiotics) to reduce the likelihood of opacity that may result from laying down of collagen. *Mechanical factors* such as increased local pressure or torsion may cause wounds to pull apart, or *dehisce*. *Poor perfusion*, due either to arteriosclerosis or to obstructed venous drainage, also impairs healing. Finally, *foreign bodies* such as fragments of steel, glass, or even bone impede healing.

■ *The type of tissue injured* is also an important factor. Complete repair occurs only in tissues composed of stable and labile cells; injury to tissues composed of permanent cells must inevitably result in scarring with, at most, attempts at functional compensation by the remaining viable elements. Such is the case with healing of a myocardial infarction.

■ *The location of the injury,* or the character of the tissue in which the injury occurs, is also important. For example, inflammations arising in tissue spaces (pleural, peritoneal, synovial cavities) develop extensive exudates. Subsequent repair may occur by digestion of the exudate, initiated by the proteolytic enzymes of leukocytes and resorption of the liquefied exudate. This is called *resolution*, and in the absence of cellular necrosis, the normal tissue architecture is generally restored. However, in the setting of significant necrosis, granulation tissue grows into the exudate, ultimately resulting in fibrous tissue, a process referred to as *organization*.

■ Aberrations of cell growth and ECM production may occur even in what begins as normal wound healing. For example, the accumulation of exuberant amounts of collagen can give rise to prominant, raised scars known as *keloids*. There appears to be a heritable predisposition to keloid formation, and the condition is more common in blacks. Healing wounds may also generate excessive granulation tissue that protrudes above the level of the surrounding skin and in fact hinders re-epithelialization. Called *exuberant granulation*, or *proud flesh*, restoration of epithelial

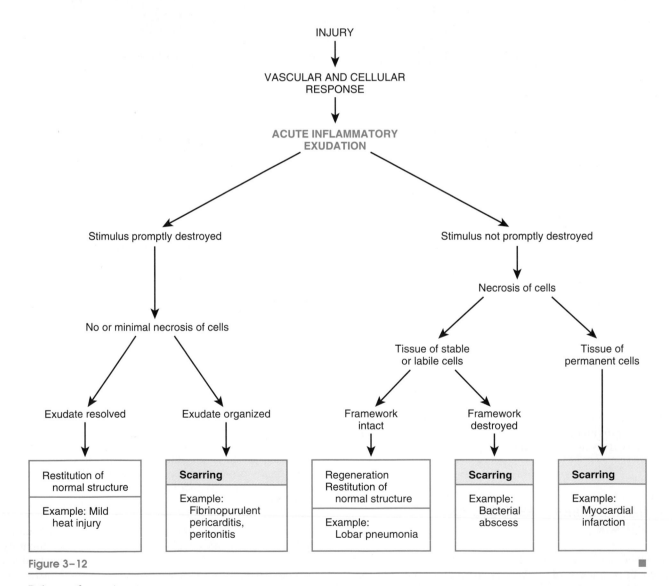

Figure 3–12

Pathways of reparative responses.

continuity requires cautery or surgical resection of the granulation tissue.

■ The mechanisms underlying the disabling fibrosis associated with chronic inflammatory diseases such as rheumatoid arthritis, pulmonary fibrosis, and cirrhosis are essentially identical to those that are involved in normal wound healing. However, in these diseases persistent stimulation of fibrogenesis results from chronic immune/autoimmune reactions that sustain the synthesis and secretion of growth factors, fibrogenic cytokines, or proteases. For example, collagen degradation by collagenases, normally important in wound remodeling, is responsible for much of the joint destruction seen in rheumatoid arthritis (Chapter 5).

OVERVIEW OF THE INFLAMMATORY-REPARATIVE RESPONSE

Figure 3–12 is an overview of the possible repair pathways, which can vary depending on the type and extent of injury, the nature of the injured tissue, and persistence of inflammatory stimuli. Clearly, not all injuries result in permanent damage: many are resolved with almost perfect repair. More often, however, an injury and subsequent inflammatory response leave residual scarring. Although functionally imperfect, the scarring patches the tissue defect and allows the residual parenchyma to continue functioning. Occasionally, however, the scarring may be so large or so situated that it causes permanent dysfunction. In a healed myocardial infarct, for example, the fibrous tissue not only represents a loss of functioning muscle, but may also serve as a nidus for arrhythmias or a focus for thrombus formation.

BIBLIOGRAPHY

Baramova E, Foidart JM: Matrix metalloproteinase family. Cell Biol Int 19: 239, 1995. (Chemistry and biology of collagen degradation pathways.)

Berridge MJ: Calcium signaling and cell proliferation. Bioessays 17:491, 1995. (Intracellular signaling pathways regulating cell cycle events.)

Birchmeier C, et al: Factors controlling growth, motility, and morphogenesis of normal and malignant epithelial. Int Rev Cytol 160:221, 1995. (A detailed overview of growth factors and their down-stream effects.)

Boulikas T: Phosphorylation of transcription factors and control of the cell cycle. Crit Rev Eukaryot Gene Expr 5:1, 1995. (A detailed overview of cell cycle regulation, emphasizing cyclins and cyclin-dependent kinases.)

Clark RAF, Henson PM (eds): The Molecular and Cellular Biology of Wound Repair. New York, Plenum, 1996. (A comprehensive volume on wound repair.)

Dvorak HF, et al: Vascular permeability factor/vascular endothelial growth factor, microvascular hyperpermeability, and angiogenesis. Am J Pathol 146:1029, 1995. (A good summary of the chemistry and biology of VPF/VEGF.)

Fantl WJ, et al: Signaling by receptor tyrosine kinases. Annu Rev Biochem 62:453, 1993. (Intracellular signaling pathways.)

Faull RJ, Ginsberg MH: Inside-out signaling through integrins. Am J Soc Nephrol 1996 (in press). (A review of the roles and functional activities of integrins.)

Folkman J: Tumor angiogenesis. In Mendelsohn J, et al (eds): The Molecular Basis of Cancer. Philadelphia, WB Saunders, 1995, pp 206–232. (An excellent review of angiogenic factors in normal and neoplastic states.)

Jans DA: Nuclear signaling pathways for polypeptide ligands and their membrane receptors. FASEB J 8:841, 1994. (Signal transduction from the plasma membrane to the cytosol and into the nucleus.)

Mignatti P: Extracellular matrix remodeling by metalloproteinases and plasminogen activators. Kidney Int (Suppl) 49:S12, 1995. (How ECM accumulation is regulated by degradation.)

Morgan DO: Principles of CDK regulation. Nature 374:131, 1995. (An elegant description of the interconnected regulatory mechanisms controlling cellular proliferation.)

Nigg EA: Cyclin-dependent protein kinases: key regulators of the eukaryotic cell cycle. Bioessays 17:471, 1995. (A readable and concise review of cyclin-cdk cell cycle control.)

Postlethwaite AE: Role of T cells and cytokines in effecting fibrosis. Int Rev Immunol 12:247, 1995. (How inflammation can affect fibroblast growth and differentiation.)

Prockop DJ, Kivirikko KI: Collagens: molecular biology, diseases and potentials for therapy. Annu Rev Biochem 64:403, 1995. (A detailed description of the chemistry and biology of ECM.)

Sanchez Y, Elledge SJ: Stopped for repairs. Bioessays 17:545, 1995. (A brief overview of the p53 regulation of cell cycle in the setting of DNA damage.)

Slavin J: Fibroblast growth factors: at the heart of angiogenesis. Cell Biol Int 19:431, 1995. (A good review of the biology and chemistry of the FGFs.)

Vernon RB, Sage EH: Between molecules and morphology. Extracellular matrix and creation of vascular form. Am J Pathol 147:873, 1995. (A description of how ECM and growth factors may direct the morphology of growing endothelium.)

Weber KT, et al: Connective tissue and repair in the heart. Potential regulatory mechanisms. Ann NY Acad Sci 752:286, 1995. (ECM deposition and remodeling in nonregenerating tissues.)

4

Hemodynamic Disorders, Thrombosis, and Shock

RICHARD N. MITCHELL, MD, PhD
VINAY KUMAR, MD

The health and well-being of cells and tissue depend not only on an intact circulation for delivery of oxygen, but also on normal fluid homeostasis. Edema, vascular congestion, hemorrhage, or shock, as well as thrombosis, embolism, and infarction, may all be precipitated by abnormalities in either blood supply or fluid balance. Pulmonary edema, for example, is sometimes the terminal event in heart disease. Hemorrhage and shock may be the sequelae of injuries as diverse as trauma or infection. Thrombosis, embolism, and infarction underlie three of the most important caues of morbidity and mortality in Western society: myocardial infarction, pulmonary embolism, and cerebrovascular accident (stroke). Thus, the hemodynamic disorders described in this chapter are important in a wide spectrum of human disease.

EDEMA

Approximately 60% of lean body weight is water, two thirds of which is intracellular with the remainder being in the extracellular compartments, mostly as interstitial fluid (only about 5% of total body water is in blood plasma). The term *edema* signifies increased fluid in the interstitial tissue spaces. In addition, depending on the site, collections of fluid in the different body cavities are variously designated *hydrothorax, hydropericardium,* or *hydroperitoneum* (the last is more commonly called *ascites*). *Anasarca* is a severe and generalized edema with profound subcutaneous tissue swelling.

In general, the opposing effects of vascular hydrostatic pressure and plasma colloid osmotic pressure are the major factors that govern movement of fluid between vascular and interstitial spaces. Normally the outflow of fluid from the arteriolar end of the microcirculation is nearly balanced by inflow at the venular end; a small amount of interstitial fluid is drained by the lymphatics. Either increased capillary pressure or diminished colloid osmotic pressure can result in increased interstitial fluid (Fig. 4–1, and see Fig. 2–2). In addition, as discussed in Chapter 2, edema can also result from local effects of inflammatory mediators on vascular permeability (see Fig. 2–3). As extravascular fluid accumulates in either case, the increased tissue hydrostatic and plasma colloid osmotic pressures eventually achieve a new equilibrium, and water reenters the venules. Edema fluid is also removed via the lymphatics, ultimately returning to the bloodstream via the thoracic duct (Fig. 4–1); clearly, lymphatic obstruction (e.g., that due to scarring or tumor) can also impair fluid drainage and cause edema. The edema fluid occurring in hydrodynamic derangements is typically a protein-poor *transudate,* with a specific gravity below 1.012. Conversely, because of the increased vascular permeability, inflammatory edema is a protein-rich *exudate* with a specific gravity usually over 1.020.

Table 4–1 lists the pathophysiologic categories of edema; the noninflammatory causes are described in further detail below.

Increased Hydrostatic Pressure. Local increases may result from impaired venous outflow, for example, secondary to *deep venous thrombosis* in the lower extremities with edema restricted to the affected leg. *Generalized increases* in venous pressure, with resultant systemic edema, occur most com-

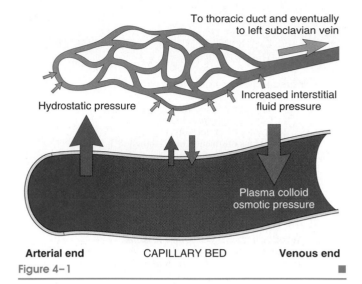

Figure 4–1 ■

Factors affecting fluid transit across capillary walls (see also Fig. 2–2). Capillary hydrostatic and osmotic forces are normally balanced so that there is no *net* loss or gain of fluid across the capillary bed. However, *increased* hydrostatic pressure or *diminished* plasma osmotic pressure leads to a net accumulation of extravascular fluid (edema). As the interstitial fluid pressure increases, tissue lymphatics remove much of the excess volume, eventually returning it to the circulation via the thoracic duct. If the ability of the lymphatics to drain tissue is exceeded, persistent tissue edema results.

monly in *congestive heart failure* (Chapter 11) affecting right ventricular cardiac function. Although increased venous hydrostatic pressure is important, the pathogenesis of cardiac edema is more complex (Fig. 4–2). Congestive heart failure is associated with reduced cardiac output and therefore reduced renal perfusion. Renal hypoperfusion in turn triggers the renin-angiotensin-aldosterone axis, inducing sodium and water retention by the kidneys (*secondary aldosteronism*). This is intended to increase intravascular volume and thereby improve cardiac output with restoration of normal renal perfusion. However, if the failing heart cannot increase cardiac output, the extra fluid load only results in increased venous pressure, and eventually edema. Unless cardiac output is restored or renal water retention reduced (e.g., by salt restriction, diuretics, and/or aldosterone antagonists), a vicious cycle of renal fluid retention and worsening edema ensues. Although discussed here in the context of edema in congestive heart failure, it should be understood that salt restriction, diuretics, and aldosterone antagonists are of value in the management of generalized edema resulting from a variety of other causes.

Reduced Plasma Osmotic Pressure. This can result from excessive loss or reduced synthesis of albumin, the serum protein most responsible for maintaining colloid osmotic pressure. An important cause of albumin loss is the *nephrotic syndrome* (Chapter 14), characterized by a leaky glomerular basement membrane and generalized edema. Reduced albumin synthesis occurs in the setting of diffuse liver diseases (e.g., cirrhosis, Chapter 16), or as a consequence of protein malnutrition (Chapter 8). In each case, reduced plasma osmotic pressure leads to a net movement of fluid into the interstitial tissues and a resultant plasma volume contraction. Predictably, with reduced intravascular volume, renal hypo-

■

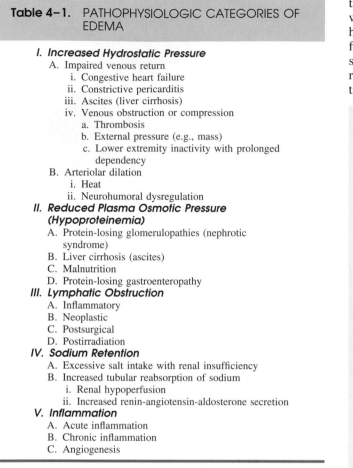

Table 4–1. PATHOPHYSIOLOGIC CATEGORIES OF EDEMA

I. Increased Hydrostatic Pressure
 A. Impaired venous return
  i. Congestive heart failure
  ii. Constrictive pericarditis
  iii. Ascites (liver cirrhosis)
  iv. Venous obstruction or compression
   a. Thrombosis
   b. External pressure (e.g., mass)
   c. Lower extremity inactivity with prolonged dependency
 B. Arteriolar dilation
  i. Heat
  ii. Neurohumoral dysregulation
II. Reduced Plasma Osmotic Pressure (Hypoproteinemia)
 A. Protein-losing glomerulopathies (nephrotic syndrome)
 B. Liver cirrhosis (ascites)
 C. Malnutrition
 D. Protein-losing gastroenteropathy
III. Lymphatic Obstruction
 A. Inflammatory
 B. Neoplastic
 C. Postsurgical
 D. Postirradiation
IV. Sodium Retention
 A. Excessive salt intake with renal insufficiency
 B. Increased tubular reabsorption of sodium
  i. Renal hypoperfusion
  ii. Increased renin-angiotensin-aldosterone secretion
V. Inflammation
 A. Acute inflammation
 B. Chronic inflammation
 C. Angiogenesis

Modified from Leaf, A, and Cotran RS: Renal Pathophysiology, 3rd ed. New York, Oxford University Press, 1985, p 146.

perfusion with secondary aldosteronism follows. Unfortunately, the retained salt and water cannot correct the plasma volume deficit, because the primary defect of low serum proteins persists. As with congestive heart failure, edema precipitated by one mechanism is exacerbated by secondary salt and fluid retention.

Lymphatic Obstruction. Impaired lymphatic drainage and consequent *lymphedema* is usually localized; it can result from inflammatory or neoplastic obstruction. For example, the parasitic infection *filariasis* often causes massive lymphatic and lymph node fibrosis in the inguinal region. The resultant edema of the external genitalia and lower limbs is so extreme that it is called *elephantiasis*. Cancer of the breast may be treated by removal and/or irradiation of the breast and the associated axillary lymph nodes. Resection of the lymphatic channels as well as scarring related to the surgery and radiation can result in severe edema of the arm. In carcinoma of the breast, infiltration and obstruction of superficial lymphatics can cause edema of the overlying skin, giving rise to the so-called "peau d'orange" (orange peel) appearance. Such a finely pitted appearance results from an accentuation of depressions in the skin at the site of hair follicles.

Sodium and Water Retention. These are clearly contrib-

utory factors in several forms of edema; however, salt retention may also be a primary cause of edema. Increased salt, with the obligate accompanying water, causes both increased hydrostatic pressure (due to expansion of the intravascular fluid volume) and diminished vascular colloid osmotic pressure. Salt retention may occur with any acute reduction of renal function, including poststreptococcal glomerulonephritis, and acute renal failure (Chapter 14).

MORPHOLOGY. Edema is most easily recognized grossly; microscopically, edema fluid generally is manifest only as clearing and separation of the extracellular matrix elements. Although any organ or tissue in the body may be involved, edema is most commonly encountered in subcutaneous tissues, lungs, and brain. Severe, generalized edema is also called **anasarca.**

Subcutaneous edema may have different distributions depending on the cause. It can be diffuse or may be more prominent in the regions with the highest hydrostatic pressures. In the latter case, the edema distribution is influenced by gravity and is termed dependent. **Edema of the dependent parts of the body** (e.g., the legs when standing, the sacrum when recumbent) **is a prominent feature of cardiac failure, particularly of the right ventricle.** Edema due to **renal dysfunction** or **nephrotic syndrome** is generally more severe than cardiac edema **and affects all parts of the body equally.** However, it may be initially manifest in tissues with a loose connective tissue matrix, such as the eyelids, causing periorbital edema. Finger pressure over significantly edematous subcutaneous tissue displaces the interstitial fluid and leaves a finger-shaped depression, so-called **pitting edema.**

Pulmonary edema is a common clinical problem (Chapter 11) most frequently seen in the setting of left ventricular failure (where it often has a dependent distribution in the lungs), but also occurring in renal failure, adult respiratory distress syndrome (ARDS, Chapter 13), pulmonary infections, and hypersensitivity reactions. The lungs are typically two to three times their normal weight, and sectioning reveals frothy, sometimes blood-tinged fluid representing a mixture of air, edema fluid, and extravasated red cells.

Edema of the brain may be localized to sites of focal injury (e.g., abscesses or neoplasm) or may be generalized, as in encephalitis, hypertensive crises, or obstruction to the brain's venous outflow. Trauma may result in local or generalized edema, depending on the nature and extent of the injury. With generalized edema, the brain is grossly swollen with narrowed sulci and distended gyri showing signs of flattening against the unyielding skull (see also Chapter 23).

Clinical Correlation. The effects of edema may range

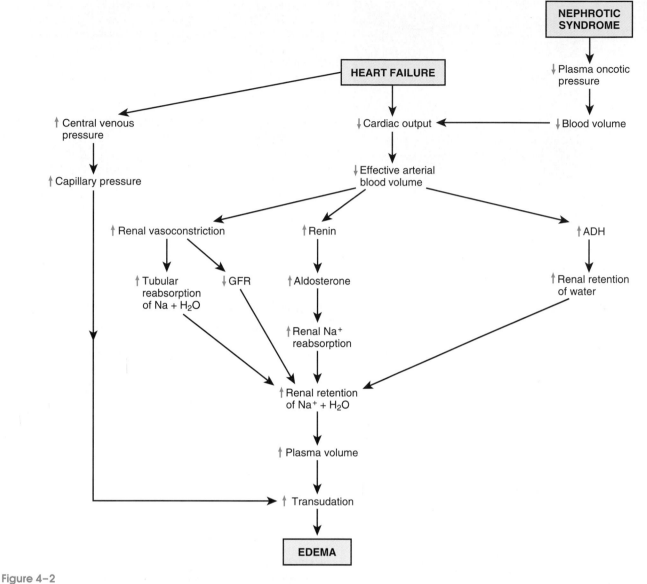

Figure 4–2   ■

Sequence of events leading to systemic edema in heart failure, or with reduced plasma osmotic pressure, as in the nephrotic syndrome. ADH, antidiuretic hormone; GFR, glomerular filtration rate.

from merely annoying to fatal. Subcutaneous tissue edema in cardiac or renal failure is important primarily because it points to underlying disease; however, when significant, it can impair wound healing or the clearance of infection. On the other hand, pulmonary edema can cause death by interfering with normal ventilatory function. Not only does fluid collect in the alveolar septa around capillaries and impede oxygen diffusion, but edema fluid in the alveolar spaces also creates a favorable environment for bacterial infection. Brain edema is serious and can be rapidly fatal; if severe, brain substance can herniate (be pushed out) through, for example, the foramen magnum, or the brainstem vascular supply can be compressed. Either condition can injure the medullary centers and cause death (Chapter 23).

 HYPEREMIA AND CONGESTION

Both terms indicate a local increased volume of blood in a particular tissue. Hyperemia is an *active process* resulting from augmented tissue inflow due to arteriolar dilation, for example, skeletal muscle during exercise or at sites of inflammation. The affected tissue is redder owing to the engorgement with oxygenated blood. Congestion is a *passive process* resulting from impaired outflow from a tissue. It may occur systemically, as in cardiac failure, or may be local, resulting from an isolated venous obstruction. The tissue has a blue-red

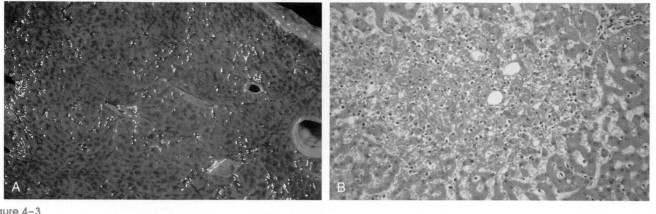

Figure 4–3

Liver with chronic passive congestion and hemorrhagic necrosis. *A*, Central areas are red and slightly depressed compared with the surrounding tan viable parenchyma, forming the so-called "nutmeg liver" pattern. *B*, Centrilobular necrosis with degenerating hepatocytes and hemorrhage. (Courtesy of Dr. James Crawford, Department of Pathology, Brigham and Women's Hospital, Boston.)

color (cyanosis), especially as worsening congestion leads to accumulation of deoxygenated hemoglobin in the affected tissues.

Congestion of capillary beds is closely related to the development of edema, so that congestion and edema commonly occur together. In long-standing congestion, called *chronic passive congestion*, the stasis of poorly oxygenated blood causes chronic hypoxia, which can result in parenchymal cell degeneration or death, sometimes with microscopic scarring. Capillary rupture at these sites of chronic congestion may also cause small foci of hemorrhage; breakdown and phagocytosis of the red cell debris can eventually result in small clusters of hemosiderin-laden macrophages.

MORPHOLOGY. Cut surfaces of hyperemic or congested tissues are hemorrhagic and wet. Microscopically, **acute pulmonary congestion** is characterized by alveolar capillaries engorged with blood; there may also be associated alveolar septal edema and/or focal minute intra-alveolar hemorrhage. In **chronic pulmonary congestion** the septa have become thickened and fibrotic, and the alveolar spaces may contain numerous hemosiderin-laden macrophages ("heart failure cells"). In **acute hepatic congestion** the central vein and sinusoids are distended with blood, and there may even be central hepatocyte degeneration; the periportal hepatocytes, better oxygenated because of their proximity to hepatic arterioles, experience less severe hypoxia and may only develop fatty change. In **chronic passive congestion of the liver** the central regions of the hepatic lobules are grossly red-brown and slightly depressed (owing to a loss of cells), and are accentuated against the surrounding zones of uncongested tan, sometimes fatty, liver ("nutmeg liver," Fig. 4–3*A*). Microscopically, there is evidence of centrilobular necrosis with hepatocyte drop-out and

hemorrhage, including hemosiderin-laden macrophages (Fig. 4–3*B*). In severe and long-standing hepatic congestion (most commonly associated with heart failure), there may even be grossly evident hepatic fibrosis ("cardiac cirrhosis"). It is important to note that because the central portion of the hepatic lobule is the last to receive blood, centrilobular necrosis can also occur whenever there is reduced hepatic blood flow (including shock from any cause); there need not be previous hepatic congestion.

HEMORRHAGE

Hemorrhage generally indicates extravasation of blood due to rupture of blood vessels. As described above, capillary bleeding can occur under conditions of chronic congestion, and an increased tendency to hemorrhage from usually insignificant injury is seen in a wide variety of clinical disorders collectively called *hemorrhagic diatheses* (Chapter 12). However, rupture of a large artery or vein is almost always due to vascular injury, including trauma, atherosclerosis, or inflammatory or neoplastic erosion of the vessel wall.

Hemorrhage may be external or may be enclosed within a tissue; the accumulation is referred to as a *hematoma*. Hematomas may be relatively insignificant (as in a bruise) or may accumulate sufficient blood to cause death (e.g., a massive retroperitoneal hematoma resulting from rupture of a dissecting aortic aneurysm, Chapter 10). Minute hemorrhages into skin, mucous membranes, or serosal surfaces are denoted as *petechiae*, while slightly larger hemorrhages are called *purpura*. Larger (over 1 to 2 cm) subcutaneous hematomas (bruises) are called *ecchymoses*. The erythrocytes in these local hemorrhages are degraded and phagocytosed by macrophages; the hemoglobin (red-blue color) is then enzymatically converted into bilirubin (blue-green color) and eventually into hemosiderin (golden-brown), accounting for the characteristic color changes in a hematoma. Large accumulations of blood in one or another of the body cavities are called *hemothorax, hemopericardium, hemoperitoneum,* or *hemarthrosis.* Patients with extensive hemorrhages occasionally develop jaundice from the massive breakdown of red cells and systemic release of bilirubin.

The clinical significance of hemorrhage depends on the volume and rate of blood loss. Rapid removal of up to 20% of the blood volume or slow losses of even larger amounts may have little impact in healthy adults; greater losses, however, may result in *hemorrhagic (hypovolemic) shock* (discussed later). The site of hemorrhage is also important; bleeding that would be trivial in the subcutaneous tissues may cause death if located in the brain stem. Finally, loss of iron, and subsequent iron deficiency anemia, occurs in the setting of chronic or recurrent external blood loss (e.g., a peptic ulcer or menstrual bleeding). In contrast, when red cells are retained, as in hemorrhage into body cavities or tissues, the iron can be reutilized for hemoglobin synthesis.

HEMOSTASIS AND THROMBOSIS

Normal hemostasis results from a set of well-regulated processes that maintain blood in a fluid, clot-free state in normal vessels, while inducing the rapid formation of a localized hemostatic plug at the site of vascular injury. The pathologic flip side to hemostasis is thrombosis, which represents the formation of a blood clot (thrombus) within the noninterrupted vascular system, and can be understood as inappropriate activation of normal hemostatic processes. Both hemostasis and thrombosis are dependent on three general components: *the vascular wall, platelets, and the coagulation cascade.* We begin our discussion with the process of normal hemostasis and follow it with a description of the three components that regulate hemostasis.

Normal Hemostasis

The general sequence of events in hemostasis is shown in Figure 4–4.

1. After initial injury, there is a brief period of *arteriolar vasoconstriction,* largely attributable to reflex neurogenic mechanisms, and augmented by the local secretion of factors such as endothelin (a potent endothelium-derived vasoconstrictor). The effect is transient, however, and bleeding would resume were it not for activation of the platelet and coagulation systems.

A. VASOCONSTRICTION

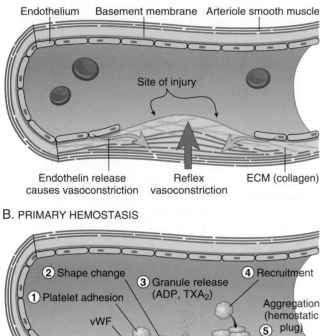

B. PRIMARY HEMOSTASIS

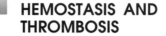

C. SECONDARY HEMOSTASIS

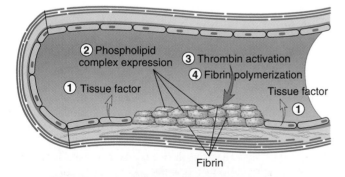

D. ANTITHROMBOTIC COUNTER-REGULATION

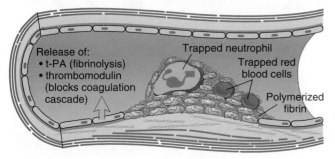

Figure 4–4 ■

Diagrammatic representation of the normal hemostatic process. *A,* After vascular injury, local neurohumoral factors induce a transient vasoconstriction. *B,* Platelets adhere to exposed extracellular matrix via von Willebrand factor (vWF), and are activated, undergoing a shape change and granule release; released adenosine diphosphate (ADP) and thromboxane A₂ (TXA₂) lead to further platelet aggregation, to form the primary hemostatic plug. *C,* Local activation of the coagulation cascade (involving tissue factor and platelet phospholipids) results in fibrin polymerization, "cementing" the platelets into a definitive secondary hemostatic plug. *D,* Counter-regulatory mechanisms, such as release of t-PA (fibrinolytic) and thrombomodulin (interfering with the coagulation cascade), limit the hemostatic process to the site of injury.

2. *Endothelial injury* also exposes highly thrombogenic sub-endothelial extracellular matrix (ECM), which allows platelets to adhere and become activated, that is, undergo a shape change and release secretory granules. Within minutes, the secreted products have recruited additional platelets *(aggregation)* to form a hemostatic plug; this is the process of *primary hemostasis.*

3. Tissue factor is also released at the site of injury; it acts in conjunction with the secreted platelet factors to activate the coagulation cascade, culminating in *fibrin deposition.* Thrombin activated in the coagulation sequence also induces further platelet recruitment and granule release. This sequence, *secondary hemostasis,* takes longer than the formation of the initial platelet plug.

4. Polymerized fibrin and platelet aggregates form a solid, permanent plug to prevent any further hemorrhage. At this stage, counter-regulatory mechanisms (e.g., tissue plasminogen activator [t-PA]) are set into motion to limit the hemostatic plug to the site of injury.

The following sections review the components of normal hemostasis.

ENDOTHELIUM

Endothelial cells modulate several, and frequently opposing, aspects of normal hemostasis. On the one hand, they normally possess antiplatelet, anticoagulant, and fibrinolytic properties; on the other hand, they are capable (after injury or activation) of exerting procoagulant functions (Fig. 4–5). Recall that endothelium may be activated by infectious agents, hemodynamic factors, plasma mediators, and (most significantly) cytokines (Chapter 2). The balance between endothelial anti- and prothrombotic activities determines whether thrombus formation, propagation, or dissolution occurs.

Antithrombotic Properties

■ *Antiplatelet effects.* An intact endothelium prevents platelets from meeting the highly thrombogenic subendothelial ECM. Nonactivated platelets do not adhere to the endothelium, a property intrinsic to the plasma membrane of endothelium. Moreover, if platelets are activated (e.g., after focal endothelial injury), they are inhibited from adhering to the surrounding uninjured endothelium by endothelial prostacyclin (PGI_2) and nitric oxide. Both mediators are potent vasodilators and inhibitors of platelet aggregation; their synthesis by endothelial cells is stimulated by a number of factors (e.g., thrombin) produced during coagulation.

■ *Anticoagulant properties.* These are mediated by membrane-associated, heparin-like molecules and thrombomodulin, a specific thrombin receptor (Fig. 4–5). The heparin-like molecules act indirectly; they are cofactors allowing antithrombin III to inactivate thrombin, factor Xa, and several other coagulation factors (see below). Thrombomodulin also acts indirectly; it binds to thrombin, converting it from a procoagulant to an anticoagulant capable of activating the anticoagulant protein C. Activated protein C inhibits clotting by proteolytic cleavage of factors Va and VIIIa; it requires protein S, synthesized by endothelial cells, as a cofactor.

■ *Fibrinolytic properties.* Endothelial cells synthesize tissue type plasminogen activator (t-PA), promoting fibrinolytic activity to clear fibrin deposits from endothelial surfaces (see Fig. 4–4D).

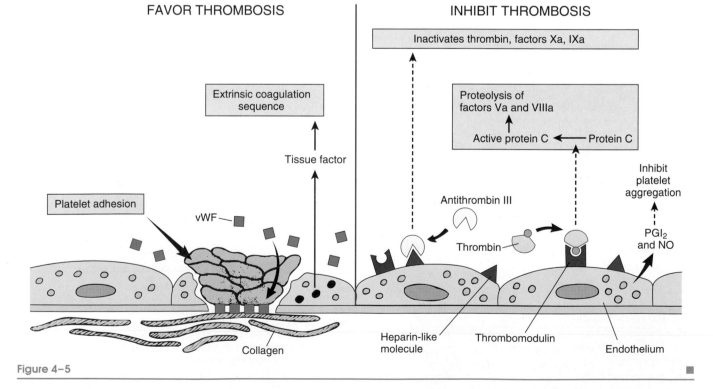

Figure 4–5

A schematic illustration of some of the pro- and anticoagulant activities of endothelial cells. Not shown are the pro- and antifibrinolytic properties. vWF, von Willebrand factor; PGI_2, prostacyclin; NO, nitric oxide.

Prothrombotic Properties

While endothelial cells have activities that can limit blood clotting, they are also prothrombotic, affecting platelets, coagulation proteins, and the fibrinolytic system. Recall that endothelial injury leads to adhesion of platelets to subendothelial collagen; this is facilitated by *von Willebrand factor (vWF)*, an essential cofactor for platelet binding to collagen and other surfaces. It should be noted that vWF is a product of normal endothelium, found in the plasma; it is not synthesized after endothelial injury. Endothelial cells are also induced by cytokines (e.g., tumor necrosis factor [TNF] or interleukin 1 [IL-1]) or bacterial endotoxin to secrete tissue factor, which, as we shall see, activates the extrinsic clotting pathway. By binding to activated factors IX and X, endothelial cells further augment the catalytic activities of these coagulation factors. Finally, endothelial cells also secrete inhibitors of plasminogen activator (PAIs), which depress fibrinolysis.

In summary, intact endothelial cells serve primarily to inhibit platelet adherence and blood clotting. However, injury or activation of endothelial cells results in a procoagulant phenotype that contributes to localized clot formation.

PLATELETS

Platelets play a central role in normal hemostasis. When circulating, they are membrane-bound smooth discs expressing a number of glycoprotein receptors of the integrin family. Platelets contain two specific types of granules. *Alpha granules* express the adhesion molecule P-selectin on their membranes and contain fibrinogen, fibronectin, factors V and VIII, platelet factor 4 (a heparin-binding chemokine), platelet-derived growth factor (PDGF), and transforming growth factor β (TGF-β). The other granules are *dense bodies* or *delta granules*, which contain adenine nucleotides (ADP and ATP), ionized calcium, histamine, serotonin, and epinephrine.

After vascular injury, platelets encounter ECM constituents that are normally sequestered beneath an intact endothelium; these include collagen (most important), proteoglycans, fibronectin, and other adhesive glycoproteins. On contact with ECM, platelets undergo three general reactions: (1) adhesion and shape change, (2) secretion (release reaction), and (3) aggregation (see Fig. 4–4B).

■ *Platelet adhesion* to ECM is mediated largely via interactions with vWF, which acts as a bridge between platelet surface receptors (e.g., glycoprotein Ib) and exposed collagen. Genetic deficiency of vWF (von Willebrand disease, Chapter 12) or of its receptors results in defective platelet adhesion and bleeding disorders.

■ *Secretion (release reaction)* of the contents of both types of granules occurs soon after adhesion. The process is initiated by binding of agonists to platelet surface receptors followed by an intracellular phosphorylation cascade. The release of the dense body contents is especially important because calcium is required in the coagulation cascade, and ADP is a potent mediator of *platelet aggregation* (platelets adhering to other platelets, see below), as well as augmenting ADP release from other platelets. In addition, platelet activation leads to the surface expression of a *phospholipid complex* that provides a critical nucleation

and binding site for calcium and coagulation factors in the *intrinsic clotting pathway* (see below).

■ *Platelet aggregation* follows adhesion and secretion. Besides ADP, the vasoconstrictor thromboxane A$_2$ (TXA$_2$, Chapter 2), secreted by platelets, is also an important stimulus for platelet aggregation. ADP and TXA$_2$ set up an autocatalytic reaction leading to build-up of an enlarging platelet aggregate, the *primary hemostatic plug*. This primary aggregation is reversible, but with activation of the coagulation cascade, *thrombin* is generated. Thrombin binds to a platelet surface receptor, and with ADP and TXA$_2$ causes further aggregation. This is followed by *platelet contraction*, creating an irreversibly fused mass of platelets ("viscous metamorphosis") constituting the definitive *secondary hemostatic plug*. At the same time, thrombin converts fibrinogen to *fibrin* within and about the platelet plug, essentially cementing the platelets in place (see below).

It is worth emphasizing that the prostaglandin PGI$_2$ (synthesized by endothelium) is a vasodilator and inhibits platelet aggregation, whereas TXA$_2$ is a platelet-derived prostaglandin that activates platelet aggregation and is a potent vasoconstrictor. The interplay of PGI$_2$ and TXA$_2$ constitutes an exquisitely balanced mechanism for modulating human platelet function: in the normal state it prevents intravascular platelet aggregation, but after endothelial injury it favors the formation of hemostatic plugs. The clinical use of aspirin (a cyclooxygenase inhibitor) in patients at risk for coronary thrombosis is related to its ability to inhibit the synthesis of TXA$_2$.

Both erythrocytes and leukocytes are also found in hemostatic plugs; leukocytes adhere to platelets and endothelium via adhesion molecules (Chapter 2) and contribute to the inflammatory response that accompanies thrombosis. Thrombin also contributes by directly stimulating neutrophil and monocyte adhesion, and by generating chemotactic *fibrin split products* from the cleavage of fibrinogen.

In summary (see Fig. 4–4), (1) platelets adhere to the ECM at sites of endothelial injury and become activated; (2) upon activation, they secrete granule products (e.g., ADP) and synthesize TXA$_2$; (3) platelets also expose phospholipid complexes important in the intrinsic caoagulation pathway; (4) injured cells release tissue factor to activate the extrinsic coagulation cascade; (5) released ADP stimulates formation of a primary hemostatic plug, which is eventually converted (via ADP, thrombin and TXA$_2$) into a larger definitive secondary plug; and (6) fibrin deposition stabilizes and anchors the aggregated platelets.

COAGULATION CASCADE

This constitutes the third component of the hemostatic process and is a major contributor to thrombosis. The details are schematically presented in Figure 4–6; only general principles and newer concepts are discussed below.

■ The coagulation cascade is essentially a series of conversions of inactive proenzymes to activated enzymes, culminating in the formation of *thrombin*. Thrombin then converts the soluble plasma protein *fibrinogen* into the insoluble fibrous protein *fibrin*.

■ Each reaction in the pathway results from the assembly of

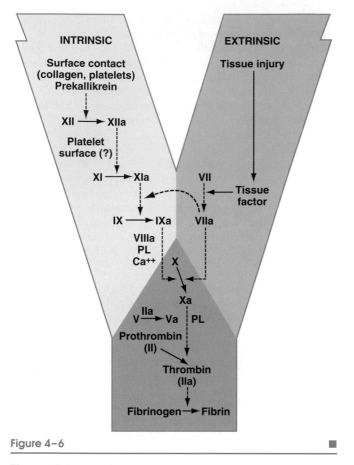

Figure 4–6 ■

The coagulation cascade. Note the common links between the intrinsic and extrinsic pathways. The lower case "a" represents activated factor; PL is the phospholipid surface.

1. *Antithrombins* (e.g., antithrombin III) are characterized by their ability to inhibit the activity of thrombin and other serine proteases—factors IXa, Xa, XIa, and XIIa. Antithrombin III is activated by binding to heparin-like molecules on endothelial cells; hence, the usefulness of administering heparin in clinical situations to minimize thrombosis.

2. *Proteins C and S* are two vitamin K–dependent proteins characterized by their ability to inactivate the cofactors Va and VIIIa. The activation of protein C by thrombomodulin was described above.

3. The *plasminogen-plasmin* system breaks down fibrin and interferes with fibrin polymerization. The fibrin split products, once released, also serve as potent anticoagulants. Plasminogen is proteolytically cleaved to its active form, plasmin, either by a factor XII–dependent pathway or by plasminogen activators (PAs). There are two groups of these: (1) *urokinase-like* PA is present in plasma and various tissues and activates plasminogen in the fluid phase, and (2) *tissue-type PA (t-PA)*, synthesized principally by endothelial cells and active when attached to fibrin. The affinity for fibrin makes t-PA a much more useful therapeutic reagent since it targets the t-PA to sites of recent clotting.

■ Endothelial cells further modulate the coagulation/anticoagulation balance by releasing plasminogen activator inhibitors (PAIs); these block fibrinolysis and confer an overall procoagulation effect. The PAIs are increased by certain cytokines and probably play a role in the intravascular thrombosis accompanying severe inflammations.

a complex composed of an *enzyme* (activated coagulation factor), a *substrate* (proenzyme form of coagulation factor), and a *cofactor* (reaction accelerator). These components are assembled on a *phospholipid complex* and held together by *calcium ions.* Thus, clotting tends to remain localized to sites where such an assembly can occur, for example, on the surface of activated platelets. One such reaction, conversion of factor X to factor Xa, is illustrated in Figure 4–7.

■ Traditionally, the blood coagulation scheme has been divided into *extrinsic* and *intrinsic* pathways, converging where factor X is activated (see Fig. 4–6). The intrinsic pathway is initiated in vitro by activation of Hageman factor (factor XII), while the extrinsic pathway is activated by *tissue factor*, a cellular lipoprotein present at sites of tissue injury. However, such a division is only an artifact of in vitro testing; there are, in fact, several interconnections between the two pathways. For example, tissue factor is also involved in the "intrinsic pathway" activation of factor IX (see Fig. 4–6).

■ Once activated, the coagulation cascade must be restricted to the local site of vascular injury to prevent clotting of the entire vascular tree. Besides the localization of factor activation to sites of exposed phospholipids, clotting is controlled by three groups of natural anticoagulants:

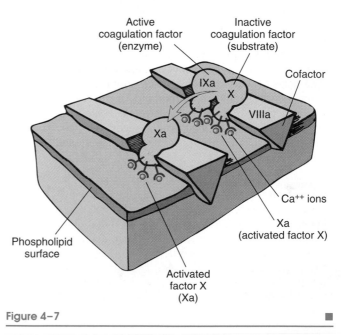

Figure 4–7 ■

Schematic illustration of the conversion of factor X to factor Xa. The reaction complex, consisting of an enzyme (factor IXa), a substrate (factor X), and a reaction accelerator (factor VIIIa), is assembled on the phospholipid surface of platelets. Calcium ions hold the assembled components together and are essential for reaction. Activated factor Xa then becomes the enzyme part of a second adjacent complex in the coagulation cascade. (Modified from Mann KG: Clin Lab Med 4:217, 1984.)

Thrombosis

Having discussed the process of normal hemostasis, we can now turn our attention to the dysregulation that underlies thrombus formation.

PATHOGENESIS

Three primary influences predispose to thrombus formation, the so-called *Virchow's triad*: (1) endothelial injury, (2) stasis *or* turbulence of blood flow, and (3) blood hypercoagulability (Fig. 4–8).

■ *Endothelial injury* is the dominant influence, and by itself can lead to thrombosis. It is particularly important in thrombus formation in the heart and arterial circulation, for example within the cardiac chambers when there has been endocardial injury (e.g., myocardial infarction or valvulitis), over ulcerated plaques in severely atherosclerotic arteries, or at sites of traumatic or inflammatory vascular injury. Injury may occur from hemodynamic stresses of hypertension, turbulent flow over scarred valves, or bacterial endotoxins. Even subtle influences such as homocystinuria, hypercholesterolemia, radiation, or products absorbed from cigarette smoke may be sources of endothelial injury. Regardless of the cause of endothelial damage, the end results include exposure of subendothelial collagen (and other platelet activators), adherence of platelets, release of tissue factor, and local depletion of prostacyclin and PA (see Figs. 4–4 and 4–5).

■ *Alterations in normal blood flow. Turbulence* contributes to arterial and cardiac thrombosis by causing endothelial injury or dysfunction, as well as by forming countercurrents and local pockets of stasis; *stasis* is a major factor in the development of venous thrombi. Normal blood flow is *laminar;* that is, the cellular elements flow centrally in the vessel lumen, separated from the endothelium by a slower-moving clear zone of plasma. Stasis and turbulence there-

Table 4–2.	CONDITIONS ASSOCIATED WITH AN INCREASED RISK OF THROMBOSIS

Primary (Genetic)
  Mutations in factor V
  Antithrombin III deficiency
  Protein C or S deficiency
  Fibrinolysis defects
Secondary (Acquired)
  High risk for thrombosis
    Prolonged bed rest or immobilization
    Myocardial infarction
    Tissue damage (surgery, fracture, burns)
    Cancer
    Prosthetic cardiac valves
    Disseminated intravascular coagulation
    Lupus anticoagulant
  Low risk for thrombosis
    Atrial fibrillation
    Cardiomyopathy
    Nephrotic syndrome
    Hyperestrogenic states
    Oral contraceptive use
    Sickle cell anemia
    Smoking

fore (1) disrupt laminar flow and bring platelets into contact with the endothelium; (2) prevent dilution of activated clotting factors by fresh-flowing blood; (3) retard the inflow of clotting factor inhibitors and permit the build-up of thrombi; and (4) promote endothelial cell activation, predisposing to local thrombosis, leukocyte adhesion, and a variety of other endothelial cell effects.

Turbulence and stasis contribute to thrombosis in a number of clinical settings. Ulcerated atherosclerotic plaques not only expose subendothelial ECM, but also generate local turbulence. Abnormal aortic and arterial dilations called *aneurysms* cause local stasis and are favored sites of thrombosis (Chapter 10). Myocardial infarctions not only have associated endothelial injury, but also have regions of noncontractile myocardium, adding an element of stasis in the formation of mural thrombi. Mitral valve stenosis (e.g., after rheumatic heart disease) results in left atrial dilation, which in the setting of atrial fibrillation exhibits profound stasis and is a prime location for development of thrombi. Hyperviscosity syndromes (such as polycythemia, Chapter 12) increase resistance to flow and cause small vessel stasis; the deformed red cells in sickle cell anemia (Chapter 12) cause vascular occlusions, with the resultant stasis predisposing to thrombosis.

■ *Hypercoagulability* is an uncommon and poorly understood cause of thrombosis; it is loosely defined as any alteration of the coagulation pathways that predisposes to thrombosis, and can be divided into *primary* (genetic) and *secondary* (acquired) disorders (Table 4–2). Of the inherited causes of hypercoagulability, mutations in the factor V gene are the most common; approximately 2% to 15% of the Caucasian population carries a factor V mutation (referred to as the Leiden mutation, after the Dutch city in which it was first discovered). Among patients with recurrent deep vein thrombosis, the frequency is much higher, approaching 60% in some studies. *Mutant factor V is re-*

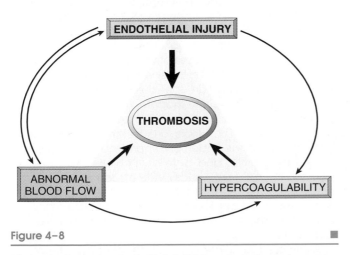

Figure 4–8   ■

Virchow's triad in thrombosis. Endothelial integrity is the single most important factor. Moreover, injury to endothelial cells can alter local blood flow and/or coagulability; abnormal blood flow (stasis or turbulence), in turn, can cause endothelial injury. The factors may act independently or may combine to cause thrombus formation.

sistant to the anticoagulant effect of activated protein C, and hence there is functional deficiency of protein C. Patients with primary hypercoagulable states associated with an inherited lack of anticoagulants (e.g., antithrombin III, protein C, or protein S) typically present with venous thrombosis and recurrent thromboembolism in adolescence or early adult life. Although these hereditary disorders are uncommon, the basis of the thrombotic tendencies is understood.

The pathogenesis of the thrombotic diathesis in a number of common clinical settings is more complicated and multifactorial. In some of the acquired conditions (e.g., cardiac failure or trauma), factors such as stasis or vascular injury may be most important. In other cases (oral contraceptive use and the hyperestrogenic state of pregnancy), hypercoagulability may be partly caused by increased hepatic synthesis of many coagulation factors and reduced synthesis of antithrombin III (Chapter 9). In disseminated cancers, release of procoagulant tumor products predisposes to thrombosis. The hypercoagulability seen with advancing age may be due to increasing platelet aggregation and reduced PGI_2 release by endothelium. Smoking and obesity promote hypercoagulability by unknown mechanisms. Among the acquired causes of thrombotic diathesis, the so-called *lupus anticoagulant* deserves special mention. These patients have high titers of autoantibodies directed against anionic phospholipids and a high frequency of arterial and venous thrombosis. Some of them have manifestations of a well-defined autoimmune disease such as systemic lupus erythematosus (Chapter 5), but in others, thrombosis is the major or only clinical manifestation. The mechanism by which antiphospholipid antibodies promote thrombosis in vivo are unknown. Possibilities include induction of platelet aggregation, inhibition of prostacyclin production by endothelial cells, or interference in the generation of protein C. In vitro, these antibodies inhibit clotting by interfering with the assembly of phospholipid complex, and hence their designation as lupus anticoagulant.

MORPHOLOGY OF THROMBI. Thrombi may develop anywhere in the cardiovascular system: within the cardiac chambers; on valve cusps; or in arteries, veins, or capillaries. They are of variable size and shape, depending on the site of origin and the circumstances leading to their development. Arterial or cardiac thrombi usually begin at a site of endothelial injury (e.g., atherosclerotic plaque) or turbulence (vessel bifurcation); venous thrombi characteristically occur in sites of stasis. An area of attachment to the underlying vessel or heart wall, frequently firmest at the point of origin, is characteristic of all thrombi. Arterial thrombi tend to grow in a retrograde direction from the point of attachment; venous thrombi extend in the direction of blood flow, that is, toward the heart. The propagating tail may not be well attached and, particularly in veins, is prone to fragment, creating an **embolus.**

When formed in the heart or aorta, thrombi may have grossly (and microscopically) apparent laminations called **lines of Zahn;** these are produced by alternating pale layers of platelets admixed with some fibrin, and darker layers containing more red cells. Lines of Zahn are significant only in that they imply thrombosis at a site of blood flow; in veins or in smaller arteries, the laminations are typically not as apparent, and, in fact, thrombi formed in the sluggish venous flow usually resemble statically coagulated blood (much like blood clotted in a test tube). Nevertheless, careful evaluation generally reveals irregular, somewhat ill-defined laminations.

When arterial thrombi arise in heart chambers or in the aortic lumen, they are usually applied to the wall of the underlying structure and are termed **mural thrombi.** Abnormal myocardial contraction (arrythmias, dilated cardiomyopathy, or myocardial infarction) leads to the formation of cardiac mural thrombi (Fig. 4–9A), while ulcerated atherosclerotic plaques and aneurysmal dilation are the precursors of aortic thrombus formation (Fig. 4–9B).

Arterial thrombi are usually **occlusive;** the most common sites, in descending order, are coronary, cerebral, and femoral arteries. The thrombus is usually superimposed on an atherosclerotic plaque, although other forms of vascular injury (vasculitis, trauma) may be involved. The thrombi typically are firmly adherent to the injured arterial wall and are gray-white and friable, composed of a tangled mesh of platelets, fibrin, erythrocytes, and degenerating leukocytes.

Venous thrombosis, or **phlebothrombosis,** is almost invariably occlusive; the thrombus often creates a long cast of the vein lumen. Because these thrombi form in the slowly moving venous blood, they tend to contain more enmeshed erythrocytes and are therefore known as **red,** or **stasis, thrombi. Phlebothrombosis most commonly (90% of cases) affects the veins of the lower extremities.** Less commonly, venous thrombi may develop in the upper extremities, periprostatic plexus, or ovarian and periuterine veins; under special circumstances they may be found in the dural sinuses, portal vein, or hepatic vein (Chapter 16). At autopsy, postmortem clots may be confused for venous thrombi. Postmortem clots are gelatinous with a dark red dependent portion where red cells have settled by gravity, and a yellow "chicken fat" supernatant; they are usually not attached to the underlying wall. In contrast, red thrombi are more firm, almost always have a point of attachment, and on transection reveal vague strands of pale gray fibrin.

Under special circumstances, thrombi may form on heart valves. Bacterial or fungal blood-borne infections may lead to valve damage and the development of large thrombotic masses or vegetations

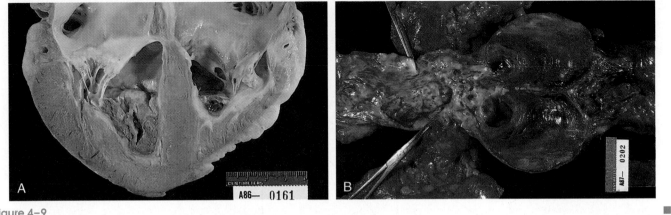

Figure 4–9

Mural thrombi. *A*, Thrombus in the left and right ventricular apices, overlying a white fibrous scar. *B*, Laminated thrombus in a dilated abdominal aortic aneurysm. Numerous friable mural thrombi are also superimposed on advanced atherosclerotic lesions of the more proximal aorta *(left side of picture)*.

(**infective endocarditis,** Chapter 11). Sterile vegetations can also develop on noninfected valves in patients with hypercoagulable states, so-called **nonbacterial thrombotic endocarditis** (Chapter 11). Less commonly, noninfective, **verrucous (Libman-Sacks) endocarditis** may occur in patients who have systemic lupus erythematosus (Chapter 5).

FATE OF THE THROMBUS

If a patient survives the immediate effects of a thrombotic vascular obstruction, thrombi undergo some combination of the following four events in the ensuing days or weeks (Fig. 4–10):

■ *Propagation.* The thrombus may accumulate more platelets and fibrin (propagate), eventually obstructing some critical vessel.
■ *Embolization.* Thrombi may dislodge and be transported to other sites in the vasculature.
■ *Dissolution.* Thrombi may be removed by fibrinolytic activity.
■ *Organization and recanalization.* Thrombi may induce inflammation and fibrosis (*organization*) and may eventually become *recanalized*, that is, may re-establish vascular flow.

Propagation and embolization are discussed further below. As for dissolution, activation of the fibrinolytic pathways can lead to rapid shrinkage and even total lysis of *recent* thrombi. With older thrombi, extensive fibrin polymerization renders the thrombus substantially more resistant to proteolysis, and lysis is ineffectual. This is important, because therapeutic infusions of fibrinolytic agents such as t-PA (e.g., for pulmonary thromboemboli or coronary thrombosis) are likely to be effective only for a short period after the formation of thrombi.

Older thrombi tend to become *organized*. This refers to the ingrowth of endothelial cells, smooth muscle cells, and fibroblasts into the fibrin-rich thrombus. In time, capillary channels are formed that may anastomose to create conduits from one end of the thrombus to the other, re-establishing to some ex-

tent the continuity of the original lumen. This *recanalization* (Fig. 4–11) essentially converts the thrombus into a vascularized subendothelial mass of connective tissue that is eventually incorporated into the vessel wall. With time and contraction of the mesenchymal cells, only a fibrous lump may remain to mark the original thrombus site. Occasionally, instead of organizing, the center of a thrombus undergoes enzymatic digestion, presumably because of the release of lysosomal enzymes from trapped leukocytes and platelets. This is particularly likely in large thrombi within aneurysmal dilations or the cardiac chambers. If bacterial seeding occurs, such degraded thrombus is an ideal culture medium, resulting for example in a so-called *mycotic aneurysm* (Chapter 10).

Clinical Correlation. Thrombi are significant because (1) they cause obstruction of arteries and veins and (2) they are possible sources of emboli. The importance of each is dependent on where the thrombus occurs. Thus, while venous thrombi may cause congestion and edema in vascular beds distal to an obstruction, a far graver consequence is that thrombi, most frequently those occurring in deep leg veins, are responsible for a major cause of death, namely, pulmonary embolization (p 73). Conversely, although arterial thrombi can embolize, their role in vascular obstruction at critical sites, such as coronary or cerebral vessels, is much more important.

Venous Thrombosis (Phlebothrombosis). The great preponderance of venous thrombi occur in either the superficial or the deep veins of the leg. Superficial venous thrombi usually occur in the saphenous system, particularly when there are varicosities. Such thrombi may cause local congestion, and swelling, pain, and tenderness along the course of the involved vein, but rarely embolize. However, the local edema and impaired venous drainage do predispose the overlying skin to infections from slight trauma and to the development of varicose ulcers. Deep thrombi in the *larger leg veins at or above the knee joint* (e.g., popliteal, femoral, and iliac veins) are more serious because they may embolize. They may also cause edema of the foot and ankle and produce pain and tenderness. However, in approximately half of the patients such thrombi are entirely asymptomatic and are recognized only after they have embolized. The venous obstruction is rapidly compensated for by opening collateral bypass channels of drainage.

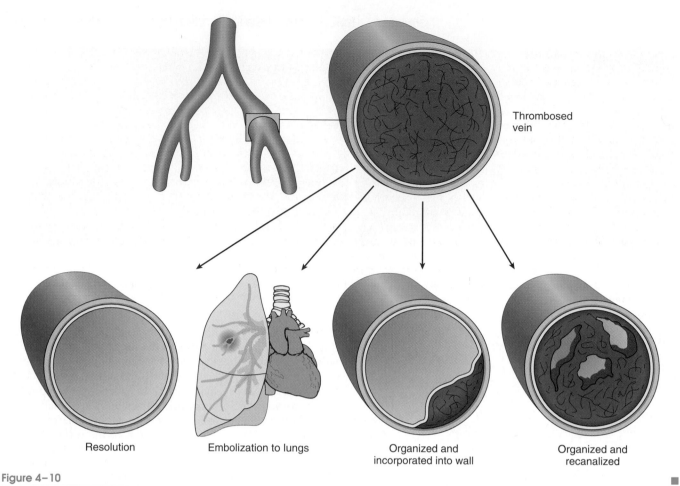

Thrombosed vein

Resolution

Embolization to lungs

Organized and incorporated into wall

Organized and recanalized

Figure 4–10 ▪

Potential outcomes of venous thrombosis.

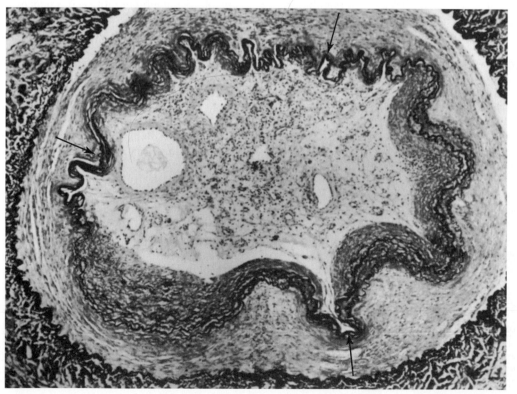

Figure 4–11 ▪

Low-power view of a thrombosed artery. The original lumen is delineated by the internal elastic lamina *(arrows)* and is totally filled with organized thrombus, now punctuated by a number of recanalized channels.

Deep venous thrombosis may occur in a variety of clinical settings, as described above. Cardiac failure is an obvious reason for stasis in the venous circulation. Trauma, surgery, and burns usually result in reduced physical activity, injury to vessels, release of procoagulant substances from tissues, and/or reduced t-PA activity. Many factors act in concert to predispose to thrombosis in the puerperal and postpartum states. Besides the potential for amniotic fluid infusion into the circulation at the time of delivery (p 74), late pregnancy and the postpartum period are associated with hypercoagulability. Tumor-associated procoagulant release is largely responsible for the increased risk of evanescent thromboses seen in disseminated cancers, giving rise to the pattern known as *migratory thrombophlebitis* (Trousseau's syndrome). Regardless of the specific clinical setting, advanced age, bed rest, and immobilization increase the risk of deep venous thrombosis; reduced physical activity diminishes the milking action of muscles in the lower leg and so slows venous return.

Cardiac and Arterial Thrombosis. *Myocardial infarction* is frequently associated with dyskinetic contraction of the myocardium as well as damage to the adjacent endocardium, providing a site for the origin of a mural thrombus (see Fig. 4–9A). *Rheumatic heart disease* may result in mitral valve stenosis, followed by left atrial dilation; concurrent atrial fibrillation augments atrial blood stasis and formation of mural thrombi. *Atherosclerosis* is a prime initiator of thromboses, related to loss of endothelial integrity and abnormal vascular flow (see Fig. 4–9B). In addition to the obstructive consequences, cardiac and aortic mural thrombi can also embolize peripherally. Virtually any tissue may be affected, but the brain, kidneys, and spleen are prime targets because of their large flow volume.

Disseminated Intravascular Coagulation

A variety of disorders ranging from obstetric complications to advanced malignancy may be complicated by disseminated intravascular coagulation (DIC), the sudden or insidious onset of widespread fibrin thrombi in the microcirculation. While these thrombi are not usually visible on gross inspection, they are readily apparent microscopically and can cause diffuse circulatory insufficiency, particularly in the brain, lungs, heart, and kidneys. With the development of the multiple thrombi, there is a rapid concurrent consumption of platelets and coagulation proteins (hence the synonym *consumption coagulopathy*); at the same time, fibrinolytic mechanisms are activated, and as a result an initially thrombotic disorder can evolve into a serious bleeding disorder. *It should be emphasized that DIC is not a primary disease, but rather a potential complication of any condition associated with widespread activation of thrombin.* It is discussed in greater detail along with other bleeding diatheses in Chapter 12.

■ EMBOLISM

An embolus is a detached intravascular solid, liquid, or gaseous mass that is carried by the blood to a site distant from its point of origin. Virtually 99% of all emboli represent some part of a dislodged thrombus, hence the commonly used term *thromboembolism.* Rare forms of emboli include droplets of fat, bubbles of air or nitrogen, atherosclerotic debris (*cholesterol emboli*), tumor fragments, bits of bone marrow, or foreign bodies such as bullets. However, unless otherwise specified, an embolism should be considered to be thrombotic in origin. Inevitably, emboli lodge in vessels too small to permit further passage, resulting in partial or complete vascular occlusion. The potential consequence of such thromboembolic events is the ischemic necrosis of distal tissue, known as *infarction.* Thromboembolic infarctions of the lungs and brain are important causes of morbidity and mortality in industrialized nations. Depending on the site of origin, emboli may lodge anywhere in the vascular tree; the clinical outcomes are best understood from the standpoint of whether emboli lodge in the pulmonary or systemic circulations.

Pulmonary Thromboembolism

Pulmonary embolism is the cause of death in 10% to 15% of hospitalized patients and results in about 50,000 deaths per year in the United States. In more than 95% of instances, thromboemboli originate from deep leg veins above the level of the knee, as described previously. They are carried through progressively larger channels and usually pass through the right heart into the pulmonary vasculature. Depending on the size of the embolus, it may occlude the main pulmonary artery, impact across the bifurcation (*saddle embolus*), or pass out into the smaller, branching arterioles (Fig. 4–12). Frequently, there are multiple emboli, perhaps sequentially, or a shower of smaller emboli from a single large mass; in general,

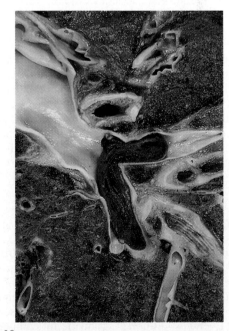

Figure 4–12   ■

Large embolus derived from a lower extremity deep venous thrombosis, and now impacted in a pulmonary artery branch.

the patient who has had one pulmonary embolus is at high risk of having more. Rarely, an embolus may pass through an interatrial or interventricular defect to gain access to the systemic circulation (*paradoxical embolism*). The clinical consequences of pulmonary embolism are discussed in Chapter 13; some general comments are offered here:

■ Most pulmonary emboli (60% to 80%) are clinically silent because they are small. With time they undergo organization and become incorporated into the vascular wall; in some cases organization of the thromboembolus leaves behind a delicate, bridging fibrous *web.*

■ Sudden death, right heart failure (*cor pulmonale*), or cardiovascular collapse occur when 60% or more of the pulmonary circulation is obstructed with emboli.

■ Embolic obstruction of medium-sized arteries may result in pulmonary hemorrhage but usually does not cause pulmonary infarction because of blood flow into the area from an intact bronchial circulation. However, a similar embolus in the setting of left-sided cardiac failure (and resultant sluggish bronchial artery blood flow) may result in a large infarct.

■ Embolic obstruction of small end-arteriolar pulmonary branches usually does result in associated infarction.

■ Multiple emboli over time may cause pulmonary hypertension with right heart failure.

Systemic Thromboembolism

Systemic thromboembolism refers to emboli traveling within the arterial circulation. Most (80%) arise from intracardiac mural thrombi, with the rest originating from thrombi associated with ulcerated atherosclerotic plaques or aortic aneurysms, or from fragmentation of a valvular vegetation (Chapter 11). In contrast to venous emboli, which tend to lodge primarily in one vascular bed (the lung), arterial emboli can travel to a wide variety of sites; the site of arrest depends on the point of origin of the thromboembolus and the volume of blood flow through the down-stream tissues. The major sites for arteriolar embolization are the lower extremities (75%) and the brain (10%), with the intestines, kidneys, and spleen involved to a lesser extent. The consequences of systemic emboli depend on the extent of collateral vascular supply in the affected tissue, the tissue's vulnerability to ischemia, and the caliber of the vessel occluded; in general, however, arterial emboli cause infarction of tissues that are perfused by the vessel.

Fat Embolism

Microscopic fat globules may be found in the circulation after fractures of long bones (which have fatty marrows) or, rarely, in the setting of soft tissue trauma and burns. Presumably the fat is released by marrow or adipose tissue injury and enters the circulation by rupture of the marrow vascular sinusoids or of venules. Although traumatic fat embolism occurs in some 90% of individuals with severe skeletal injuries, only 1% of such patients show any clinical findings. *Fat embolism syndrome is characterized by pulmonary insufficiency,* *neurologic symptoms, anemia, and thrombocytopenia and is fatal in about 10% of cases.* Typically the symptoms appear 1 to 3 days after injury, with sudden onset of tachypnea, dyspnea, and tachycardia. Neurologic symptoms include irritability and restlessness, with progression to delirium or coma.

The pathogenesis of this syndrome probably involves both mechanical obstruction and chemical injury. While microemboli of neutral fat cause occlusion of pulmonary or cerebral microvasculature, free fatty acids released from fat globules also cause local toxic injury to endothelium. A characteristic petechial skin rash is related to rapid onset of thrombocytopenia, presumably caused by platelets adhering to the myriad fat globules and being removed from the circulation.

Air Embolism

Gas bubbles within the circulation can obstruct vascular flow (and cause distal ischemic injury) almost as readily as thrombotic masses. Air may enter the circulation during obstetric procedures or as a consequence of chest wall injury. Generally in excess of 100 ml of air is required to produce a clinical effect; the bubbles act like physical obstructions and may coalesce to form frothy masses sufficiently large to occlude major vessels.

A particular form of gas embolism called *decompression sickness* occurs when individuals are exposed to sudden changes in atmospheric pressure. Scuba and deep sea divers, underwater construction workers, and individuals in unpressurized aircraft in rapid ascent are all at risk. When air is breathed at high pressure (e.g., during a deep sea dive), increased amounts of gas (particularly nitrogen) become dissolved in the blood and tissues. If the diver then ascends (depressurizes) too rapidly, the nitrogen expands in the tissues, and bubbles out of solution in the blood to form gas emboli.

The rapid formation of gas bubbles within skeletal muscles and supporting tissues in and about joints is responsible for the painful condition called *the bends.* Gas emboli may also induce focal ischemia in a number of tissues, including brain and heart. In the lungs, edema, hemorrhages, and focal atelectasis or emphysema may appear, leading to respiratory distress, the so-called *chokes.* Treatment of gas embolism consists of placing the individual in a compression chamber where the barometric pressure may be raised, thus forcing the gas bubbles back into solution. It is then hoped that subsequent slow decompression will permit gradual resorption and exhalation of the gases so that obstructive bubbles do not reform.

A more chronic form of decompression sickness is called *caisson disease,* in which persistence of gas emboli in the bones leads to multiple foci of ischemic necrosis; the more common sites are the heads of the femora, tibiae, and humeri.

Amniotic Fluid Embolism

Amniotic fluid embolism is a grave but fortunately uncommon complication of labor and the immediate postpartum period (1 in 50,000 deliveries). It has a mortality rate in excess of 80%, and as other obstetric complications (e.g., eclampsia, pulmonary embolism) have been better controlled, amniotic fluid embolism has become an important cause of maternal mortality. The onset is characterized by sudden severe dyspnea, cyanosis, and hypotensive shock, followed by seizures and coma. If the patient survives the initial crisis, pulmonary edema typically develops, along with (in half the patients) disseminated intravascular coagulation, due to release of thrombogenic substances from amniotic fluid.

The underlying cause is the infusion of amniotic fluid (and all of its contents) into the maternal circulation via a tear in the placental membranes and rupture of uterine veins. The classic findings are therefore the presence in the pulmonary microcirculation of squamous cells shed from fetal skin, lanugo hair, fat from vernix caseosa, and mucin derived from the fetal respiratory or gastrointestinal tracts. There is also marked pulmonary edema and changes of diffuse alveolar damage (Chapter 13), as well as systemic fibrin thrombi, indicative of disseminated intravascular coagulation.

INFARCTION

An infarct is an area of ischemic necrosis caused by occlusion of either the arterial supply or the venous drainage in a particular tissue. Tissue infarction is a common and extremely important cause of clinical illness. More than half of all deaths in the United States are caused by cardiovascular disease, and most of these are attributable to myocardial or cerebral infarction. Pulmonary infarction is a common complication in a number of clinical settings, bowel infarction is frequently fatal, and ischemic necrosis of the extremities (gangrene) is a serious problem in the diabetic population.

Nearly 99% of all infarcts result from thrombotic or embolic events, and almost all result from arterial occlusion. Occasionally, infarction may also be caused by other mechanisms, such as local vasospasm, swelling of an atheroma secondary to hemorrhage within a plaque, or extrinsic compression of a vessel, for example, by tumor. Other uncommon causes include twisting of the vessels (e.g., in testicular torsion or bowel volvulus), compression of the blood supply by edema or by entrapment in a hernial sac, and traumatic rupture of the blood supply. Although venous thrombosis may cause infarction, it more often merely induces venous obstruction and congestion. Usually, bypass channels then rapidly open, providing some outflow from the area, which in turn improves the arterial inflow. Infarcts caused by venous thrombosis are more likely in organs with a single venous outflow channel, such as the testis and ovary.

TYPES OF INFARCTS. Infarcts can be classified on the basis of their color (really reflecting the amount of hemorrhage), and the presence or absence of microbial infection. Therefore, infarcts may be either **red (hemorrhagic)** or **white (anemic),** and may be either **septic** or **bland.**

■ **Red infarcts** occur (1) with venous occlusions (such as in ovarian torsion); (2) in loose tissues (such as lung) that allow blood to collect in the infarcted zone; (3) in tissues with dual circulations such as lung and small intestine, permitting flow of blood from the unobstructed vascular channel into the necrotic area (obviously such perfusion is not sufficient to rescue the ischemic tissues); (4) in tissues that were previously congested because of sluggish venous outflow; and (5) when flow is re-established to a site of previous arterial occlusion and necrosis (e.g., fragmentation of an occlusive embolus or angioplasty of a thrombotic lesion) (Fig. 4–13A).

■ **White or pale infarcts** occur with arterial occlusions, or in solid organs (such as heart, spleen, and kidney), where the solidity of the tissue limits the amount of hemorrhage that can seep into the area of ischemic necrosis from adjoining capillary beds (Fig. 4–13B).

All infarcts tend to be wedge shaped, with the occluded vessel at the apex and the periphery of the organ forming the base (Fig. 4–13A and B); when the base is a serosal surface, there is often an overlying fibrinous exudate. The lateral margins may be irregular, reflecting the pattern of vascular supply

---

Figure 4–13 ■

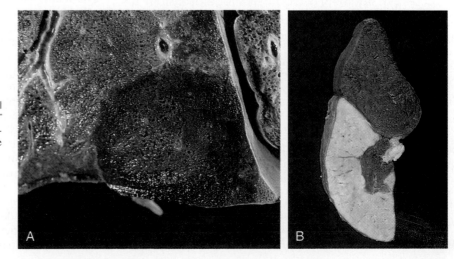

Examples of infarcts. *A,* Hemorrhagic, roughly wedge-shaped pulmonary infarct. *B,* Sharply demarcated pale infarct in the spleen.

from adjacent vessels. At the outset, all infarcts are poorly defined and slightly hemorrhagic. The margins of both types of infarcts tend to become better defined with time by a narrow rim of hyperemia attributable to inflammation at the edge of the lesion.

In solid organs, the relatively few extravasated red cells are lysed, with the released hemoglobin remaining in the form of hemosiderin. Thus, infarcts resulting from arterial occlusions typically become progressively more pale and sharply defined with time (Fig. 4–13B). In spongy organs, by comparison, the hemorrhage is too extensive to permit the lesion ever to become pale (Fig. 4–13A). Over the course of a few days, however, it does become more firm and brown, reflecting the development of hemosiderin pigment.

The dominant histologic characteristic of infarction is **ischemic coagulative necrosis** (Chapter 1). It is important to recall that if the vascular occlusion has occurred shortly (minutes to hours) before the death of the patient, no demonstrable histologic changes may be evident; if the patient survives even 12 to 18 hours, the only change present may be a hemorrhagic suffusion.

An inflammatory response begins to develop along the margins of infarcts within a few hours and is usually well defined within 1 or 2 days. Inflammation at these sites is incited by the necrotic tissue, and ultimately, in all forms of infarcts, there is gradual degradation of the dead tissue with phagocytosis of the tissue debris by incoming inflammatory cells. Eventually, the inflammatory response is followed by a reparative response beginning in the preserved margins. In stable or labile tissues, some parenchymal regeneration may occur at the periphery where the underlying stromal architecture has been spared. However, most infarcts are ultimately replaced by scar tissue (Fig. 4–14).

The brain is an exception to these generalizations; like other causes of necrosis, ischemic tissue injury in the central nervous system results in **liquefactive necrosis** (Chapter 1).

Septic infarctions may arise when embolization occurs by a fragment of a bacterial vegetation from a heart valve, or when microbes seed an area of necrotic tissue. In these cases, the infarct is converted into an **abscess,** with a correspondingly greater inflammatory response. The eventual sequence of organization, however, follows the pattern already described above.

Factors That Influence Development of an Infarct. The consequences of a vascular occlusion can range from no or minimal effect, all the way up to death of a tissue or even the individual. *The major determinants include (1) the nature of the vascular supply, (2) the rate of development of the occlusion, (3) the vulnerability of a given tissue to hypoxia, and (4) the blood oxygen content.*

■ *Nature of the vascular supply.* The availability of an al-

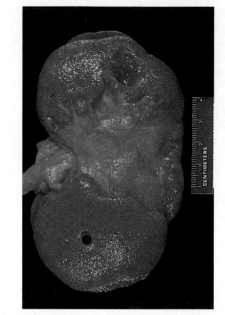

Figure 4–14 ■

An old kidney infarct, now represented by a large depressed fibrotic cortical scar.

ternative blood supply is the most important factor in determining whether occlusion of a vessel will cause damage. For example, since lungs have a dual pulmonary and bronchial artery blood supply, obstruction of small pulmonary arterioles does not cause infarction in an otherwise healthy individual with an intact bronchial circulation. Similarly, the liver, with its dual hepatic artery and portal vein circulation, is relatively resistant to infarction, as are the hand and forearm owing to the double arterial supply through the radial and ulnar arteries. In contrast, renal and splenic circulations are end-arterial, and obstruction of such vessels generally causes infarction.

■ *Rate of development of occlusion.* Slowly developing occlusions are less likely to cause infarction because they provide time for the development of alternative pathways of flow. For example, small inter-arteriolar anastomoses, normally with minimal functional flow, interconnect the three major coronary arteries in the heart. If one of the coronaries is only slowly occluded (e.g., by an encroaching atherosclerotic plaque), flow within this collateral circulation may increase sufficiently to prevent infarction, even though the major coronary artery is eventually occluded.

■ *Vulnerability to hypoxia.* The susceptibility of a tissue to hypoxia influences the likelihood of infarction. Neurons undergo irreversible damage when deprived of their blood supply for only 3 to 4 minutes. Myocardial cells, although hardier than neurons, are also quite sensitive and die after only 20 to 30 minutes of ischemia. In contrast, fibroblasts within myocardium remain viable after many hours of ischemia.

■ *Oxygen content of blood.* The partial pressure of oxygen in blood also determines the outcome of vascular occlusion. Partial flow obstruction of a small vessel in an anemic or cyanotic patient might lead to tissue infarction, whereas it would be without effect under conditions of normal oxygen tension. In this way, congestive heart failure, with compromised flow and ventilation, could cause infarction in the setting of an otherwise inconsequential blockage.

■ SHOCK

Shock, or "cardiovascular collapse," is the final common pathway for a number of potentially lethal clinical events, including severe hemorrhage, extensive trauma or burns, large myocardial infarction, massive pulmonary embolism, and microbial sepsis. Regardless of the underlying pathology, *shock constitutes systemic hypoperfusion due to reduction either in cardiac output or in the effective circulating blood volume.* The end results are *hypotension,* followed by *impaired tissue perfusion* and *cellular hypoxia.* Although the hypoxic and metabolic effects of hypoperfusion initially cause only reversible cellular injury, persistence of the shock eventually causes irreversible tissue injury and can culminate in the death of the patient.

Shock may be grouped into three general categories: cardiogenic, hypovolemic, and septic (Table 4–3). The mechanisms underlying cardiogenic and hypovolemic shock are fairly straightforward; essentially they involve *low cardiac output.* Septic shock, by comparison, is substantially more complicated and is discussed in further detail below.

■ *Cardiogenic shock* results from myocardial pump failure. This may be caused by intrinsic myocardial damage (infarction), ventricular arrhythmias, extrinsic compression (cardiac tamponade, Chapter 11), or outflow obstruction (pulmonary embolism).

■ *Hypovolemic shock* results from loss of blood or plasma volume. This may be caused by hemorrhage, fluid loss from severe burns, or trauma.

■ *Septic shock* is caused by systemic microbial infection. Most commonly this occurs in the setting of gram-negative infections (*endotoxic shock*), but it can also occur with gram-positive and fungal infections.

Less commonly, shock may occur in the setting of an anesthetic accident or a spinal cord injury (*neurogenic shock*), due to loss of vascular tone and peripheral pooling of blood. *Anaphylactic shock,* initiated by a generalized IgE-mediated hypersensitivity response, is associated with systemic vasodilation and increased vascular permeability (Chapter 5). In these instances, widespread vasodilation causes a sudden increase in the capacity of the vascular bed, which cannot be filled adequately by the normal circulating blood volume. Thus, tissue hypoperfusion and cellular anoxia result.

Pathogenesis of Septic Shock

Septic shock is currently the most common cause of death in intensive care units, accounting for some 100,000 deaths annually in the United States. It often results from dissemination of an initially localized infection (e.g., abscess, peritonitis, pneumonia) into the vasculature. Most cases of septic shock are caused by endotoxin-producing gram-negative bacilli (Chapter 9), hence the term *endotoxic shock.* Endotoxins are bacterial wall lipopolysaccharides (LPS) released when the cell walls are degraded (e.g., in an inflammatory response); LPS consists of a toxic fatty acid (*lipid A*) core and a complex polysaccharide coat (including O antigens) unique to each bacterial species. Analogous molecules in the walls of gram-positive bacteria and fungi, as well as certain bacterial proteins (called *superantigens*), can also elicit a syndrome similar to septic shock.

All the cellular and associated hemodynamic effects of septic shock can be reproduced by injection of LPS alone. At low dosage, LPS predominantly serves to activate monocytes and macrophages, with effects presumably intended to enhance its ability to eliminate invading bacteria. LPS can also directly activate complement, which likewise contributes to local bacterial eradication. The mononuclear phagocytes respond to LPS by producing TNF, which in turn induces IL-1 synthesis. TNF and IL-1 both act on endothelial cells to produce further cytokines (e.g., IL-6 and IL-8), as well as induce adhesion molecules (Chapter 2). Thus, the initial release of LPS results in a circumscribed cytokine cascade (Fig. 4–15) doubtless intended to enhance the *local* acute inflammatory response and improve clearance of the infection.

With moderately severe infections, and therefore with higher levels of LPS (and a consequent augmentation of the cytokine cascade), cytokine-induced secondary effectors (e.g., nitric oxide and platelet-activating factor, Chapter 2) become significant. In addition, systemic effects of TNF and IL-1 may begin to be seen, including fever and increased synthesis of acute-phase reactants (Chapter 2, and Fig. 4–16). LPS at higher doses also causes direct endothelial cell injury, which in turn triggers the coagulation cascade.

Finally, at still higher levels of LPS, the syndrome of septic

Table 4–3. THE THREE MAJOR TYPES OF SHOCK

Type of Shock	Clinical Examples	Principal Mechanisms
Cardiogenic	Myocardial infarction Ventricular rupture Arrhythmia Cardiac tamponade Pulmonary embolism	Failure of myocardial pump due to intrinsic myocardial damage or extrinsic pressure or obstruction to outflow
Hypovolemic	Hemorrhage Fluid loss, e.g., vomiting, diarrhea, burns, or trauma	Inadequate blood or plasma volume
Septic	Overwhelming microbial infections; endotoxic shock, gram-positive septicemia, or fungal sepsis	Peripheral vasodilation and pooling of blood; endothelial activation/injury; leukocyte-induced damage; disseminated intravascular coagulation

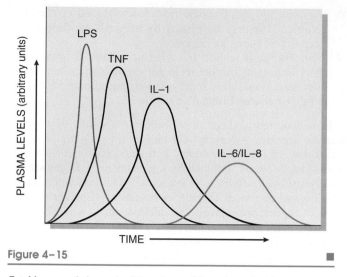

Figure 4–15

Cytokine cascade in sepsis. After release of lipopolysaccharide (LPS), there are successive waves of tumor necrosis factor (TNF), interleukin 1 (IL-1), and IL-6 secretion. (Modified from Abbas AK, et al: Cellular and Molecular Immunology, 2nd ed. Philadelphia, WB Saunders, 1994.)

shock supervenes (Fig. 4–16); the same cytokine and secondary mediators now at high levels result in

■ Systemic vasodilation (hypotension)
■ Diminished myocardial contractility
■ Widespread endothelial injury and activation, causing systemic leukocyte adhesion and diffuse alveolar capillary damage in the lung (Chapter 13)
■ Activation of the coagulation system, culminating in DIC

The hypoperfusion resulting from the combined effects of widespread vasodilation, myocardial pump failure, and DIC causes *multiorgan system failure* that affects the liver, kidneys, and central nervous system, among others. Unless the underlying infection (and LPS overload) is rapidly brought under control, the patient usually dies. In some experimental models, antibodies to IL-1 or TNF (or their receptors), or pharmacologic inhibitors of the secondary mediators (e.g., nitric oxide synthesis), have demonstrated some efficacy in protecting against septic shock; unfortunately, these reagents have not yet proved of significant clinical benefit in patients.

Stages of Shock

Shock is a progressive disorder that, if uncorrected, leads to death. Unless the insult is massive and rapidly lethal (e.g., a massive hemorrhage from a ruptured aortic aneurysm), shock tends to evolve through three general (albeit somewhat arbitrary) stages. These stages have been documented most clearly in hypovolemic shock but are common to other forms also:

■ An initial *nonprogressive stage* during which reflex compensatory mechanisms are activated and perfusion of vital organs is maintained
■ A *progressive stage* characterized by tissue hypoperfusion and onset of worsening circulatory and metabolic imbalances

■ An *irreversible stage* that sets in after the body has incurred cellular and tissue injury so severe that even if the hemodynamic defects are corrected, survival is not possible.

In the early nonprogressive phase of shock, a variety of *neurohumoral mechanisms* help maintain cardiac output and blood pressure. These include baroreceptor reflexes, release of catecholamines, activation of the renin-angiotensin axis, antidiuretic hormone release, and generalized sympathetic stimulation. The net effect is *tachycardia, peripheral vasoconstriction,* and *renal conservation of fluid.* Cutaneous vasoconstriction, for example, is responsible for the characteristic coolness and pallor of skin in shock. Coronary and cerebral vessels are less sensitive to the sympathetic response and thus maintain relatively normal caliber, blood flow, and oxygen delivery to their respective vital organs. It should be noted, however, that in *septic shock with early vasodilation the skin may feel warm and flushed rather than cold and clammy.*

If the underlying causes are not corrected, shock passes imperceptibly to the progressive phase, during which there is widespread tissue hypoxia. In the setting of persistent oxygen deficit, intracellular aerobic respiration is replaced by anaerobic glycolysis with excessive production of lactic acid. The resultant metabolic *lactic acidosis lowers the tissue pH and blunts the vasomotor response;* arterioles dilate and blood begins to pool in the microcirculation. Peripheral pooling not only worsens the cardiac output but also puts endothelial cells at risk of developing anoxic injury with subsequent DIC. With widespread tissue hypoxia, vital organs are affected and begin to fail; *clinically, the patient may become confused and the urinary output declines.*

Unless there is intervention, the process eventually enters an irreversible stage. Widespread cell injury is reflected in lysosomal enzyme leakage, further aggravating the shock state. A poorly characterized myocardial depressant factor exacerbates the already compromised myocardial contractile function. Also, if ischemic bowel allows intestinal flora to enter the circulation, endotoxic shock may be superimposed. At this point the patient has complete renal shutdown due to acute tubular necrosis (Chapter 14), and despite heroic measures the downward clinical spiral almost inevitably culminates in death.

MORPHOLOGY. The cellular and tissue changes induced by shock are essentially those of hypoxic injury (Chapter 1); since shock is characterized by **failure of multiple organ systems,** the cellular changes may appear in any tissue. Nevertheless, they are particularly evident in the brain, heart, lungs, kidneys, adrenals, and gastrointestinal tract.

The **brain** may develop so-called ischemic encephalopathy, discussed in Chapter 23. The **heart** may undergo focal and widespread coagulation necrosis, or may exhibit subendocardial hemorrhage and/or contraction band necrosis (Chapter 11). While these changes are not diagnostic of shock (they may also be seen in the setting of cardiac reperfusion after irreversible injury, or after catecholamine administration), they are usually much more

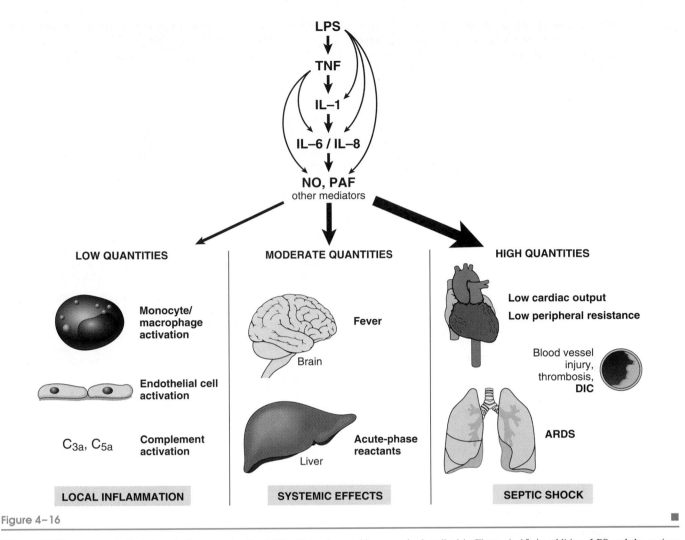

LPS

TNF

IL–1

IL–6 / IL–8

NO, PAF
other mediators

LOW QUANTITIES

Monocyte/
macrophage
activation

Endothelial cell
activation

C₃ₐ, C₅ₐ   Complement
activation

LOCAL INFLAMMATION

MODERATE QUANTITIES

Fever

Brain

Acute-phase
reactants

Liver

SYSTEMIC EFFECTS

HIGH QUANTITIES

Low cardiac output

Low peripheral resistance

Blood vessel
injury,
thrombosis,
DIC

ARDS

SEPTIC SHOCK

Figure 4–16   ■

Effects of LPS and secondarily-induced effector molecules. LPS initiates the cytokine cascade described in Figure 4–15; in addition, LPS and the various factors can also directly stimulate down-stream cytokine production, as indicated. Secondary effectors that become important include nitric oxide (NO) and platelet-activating factor (PAF). At low levels, only local inflammatory effects are seen. With moderate levels, more systemic events occur in addition to the local vascular effects. At high concentrations, the syndrome of septic shock is seen. DIC, disseminated intravascular coagulation; ARDS, adult respiratory distress syndrome. (Modified from Abbas AK, et al: Cellular and Molecular Immunology, 2nd ed. Philadelphia, WB Saunders, 1994.)

extensive in the setting of shock. The **kidneys** typically exhibit extensive tubular ischemic injury (acute tubular necrosis, Chapter 14), so that oliguria, anuria, and electrolyte disturbances constitute major clinical problems. The **lungs** are seldom affected in pure hypovolemic shock because they are somewhat resistant to hypoxic injury. However, when shock is caused by bacterial sepsis or trauma, changes of diffuse alveolar damage (Chapter 13) may appear, the so-called **shock lung.** The **adrenal** changes in shock are those seen in all forms of stress; essentially there is cortical cell lipid depletion. This does not reflect adrenal exhaustion but rather conversion of the relatively inactive vacuolated cells to metabolically active cells that utilize stored lipids for the synthesis of steroids. The **gastrointestinal tract** may suffer patchy mucosal hemorrhages and necroses, referred to as hemorrhagic enteropathy. The **liver** may develop fatty change and, with se-

vere perfusion deficits, central hemorrhagic necrosis (Chapter 16).

With the exception of neuronal and myocyte loss, virtually all of these tissue changes may revert to normal if the patient survives. Unfortunately, most patients with irreversible changes due to severe shock succumb before the tissues get an opportunity to recover.

Clinical Course. The clinical manifestations depend on the precipitating insult. In hypovolemic and cardiogenic shock the patient presents with hypotension; a weak, rapid pulse; tachypnea; and cool, clammy, cyanotic skin. In septic shock, however, the skin may be warm and flushed owing to peripheral vasodilation. The initial threat to life stems from the underlying catastrophe that precipitated the shock state: the myocardial infarct, severe hemorrhage, or uncontrolled bacterial infection. Rapidly, however, the cardiac, cerebral, and pulmonary changes secondary to the shock state materially worsen the problem. Eventually, electrolyte disturbances and metabolic acidosis also exacerbate the situation. If the patients survive the initial complications, they enter a second phase dominated by renal insufficiency and marked by a progressive fall in urine output, as well as severe fluid and electrolyte imbalances.

The prognosis varies with the origin of shock and its duration. Thus, 80% of young, otherwise healthy patients with hypovolemic shock survive with appropriate management, whereas cardiogenic shock associated with extensive myocardial infarction or gram-negative shock carries mortality rates of 70% to 80%, even with the best care currently available.

BIBLIOGRAPHY

Bell WR: Thrombolytic therapy. Agents, indications, and laboratory monitoring. Med Clin North Am 78:745, 1994. (A primer on the utility and use of thrombolytic agents.)

Bick RL: Disseminated intravascular coagulation. Objective laboratory diagnostic criteria and guidelines for management. Clin Lab Med 14:729, 1994. (An exhaustive and comprehensive review of DIC, including etiology and pathophysiology; the same volume has other reviews concerning hemostasis and thrombosis.)

Brady AJ: Nitric oxide, myocardial failure, and septic shock. Int J Cardiol 50:269, 1995. (A brief review describing the role of nitric oxide in mediating the profound hypotension in septic shock.)

Burrell R: Human responses to bacterial endotoxin. Circ Shock 43:137, 1994. (A critical review of the literature examining the systemic and specific tissue effects of lipopolysaccharide administration.)

Chesebro JH, et al: Evolving concepts in the pathogenesis and treatment of arterial thrombosis. Mt Sinai J Med 62:275, 1995. (An excellent and up-to-date overview of the clinical and pathophysiologic issues in thrombosis.)

Dahlback B, et al: Resistance to activated protein C, the FV:Q506 allele, and venous thrombosis. Annals Hematol 72:166, 1996. (A brief review of the mutations in factor V that lead to hypercoagulability and venous thrombosis.)

Dudney TM, Elliott CG: Pulmonary embolism from amniotic fluid, fat, and air. Prog Cardiovasc Dis 36:447, 1994. (A comprehensive review of nonthrombotic pulmonary emboli, including the mechanisms of injury.)

Fiore LD, Deykin D: Mechanisms of hemostasis and arterial thrombosis. Cardiol Clin 12:399, 1994. (A highly readable summary of the mechanisms underlying physiologic and pathologic blood clotting.)

Goldhaber SZ: Venous thrombosis: prevention, treatment, and relationship to paradoxical embolus. Cardiol Clin 12:505, 1994. (An excellent and thorough review of the pathophysiologic and clinical issues regarding deep venous thrombosis.)

Macik BG, Ortel TL: Clinical and laboratory evaluation of the hypercoagulable states. Clin Chest Med 16:375, 1995. (A good summary of the mechanisms and clinical findings in the various hypercoagulable states.)

Packham MA: Role of platelets in thrombosis and hemostasis. Can J Physiol Pharmacol 72:278, 1994. (Principles of normal and pathologic regulation of platelet hemostasis.)

Pearson JD: Endothelial cell function and thrombosis. Baillieres Clin Haematol 7:441, 1994. (A concise review of the roles played by endothelium in hemostasis and thrombosis.)

Resnick N, Gimbrone MA Jr: Hemodynamic forces are complex regulators of endothelial gene expression. FASEB J 9:874, 1995. (A review examining the role of hemodynamic forces in modifying and regulating endothelial cell function.)

Sriskandan S, Cohen J: The pathogenesis of septic shock. J Infect 30:201, 1995. (A nice review describing the pathologic mechanisms underlying septic shock; additional articles in the same volume cover management and other therapeutic issues.)

5

Disorders of the Immune System

The immune system is like the proverbial two-edged sword. On the one hand, humans are dependent on the immune system for survival; on the other hand, they are vulnerable to disorders in its function ranging from immunodeficiency states to hypersensitivity disorders. Put more succinctly, the disorders range from those caused by "too little" to those caused by "too much or inappropriate" immunoreactivity. To encompass this spectrum, the various disorders of immune function are considered under the following headings:

■ Immune mechanisms of tissue injury
■ Autoimmune diseases
■ Immunodeficiency diseases

We will also consider amyloidosis, a disease characterized by deposition of an abnormal protein (amyloid) in the tissues. Although not an immunologic disease in the traditional sense, it is clear that amyloidosis is associated with derangements of the immune apparatus.

Because abnormalities of lymphocyte function are fundamental to immunologic disease, some salient aspects of lymphocyte biology are reviewed first and are followed by a brief description of the histocompatibility genes, because their products are relevant to both normal and abnormal immune responses.

CELLS OF THE IMMUNE SYSTEM

T Lymphocytes

T lymphocytes are the mediators of cellular immunity and are essential for induction of humoral immunity to most naturally encountered antigens. They circulate in blood, where they make up 60% to 70% of peripheral lymphocytes. T lymphocytes are also found in the *paracortical areas of lymph nodes and periarteriolar sheaths of the spleen.* Each T cell is genetically programmed to recognize a specific cell-bound antigen by means of an antigen-specific T-cell receptor (TCR). In approximately 95% of T cells, the TCR consists of a disulfide-linked heterodimer made up of an $\alpha\beta$ polypeptide chain (Fig. 5–1), each having a variable (antigen-binding) and a constant region. In a minority of peripheral blood T cells, another type of TCR, composed of $\gamma\delta$ polypeptide chains, is found. The TCR $\gamma\delta$ cells tend to aggregate at epithelial interfaces such as the mucosa of the respiratory, gastrointestinal, and genitourinary tracts. Both the $\alpha\beta$ and $\gamma\delta$ TCRs are noncovalently linked to a cluster of five polypeptide chains, referred to as the CD3 molecular complex. The CD3 proteins are nonvariable. They do not bind antigen but are involved in transduction of signals into the T cell after it has bound the antigen. TCR diversity is generated by somatic rearrangement of the genes that encode the α, β, γ, and δ TCR chains. As might be expected, every somatic cell has TCR genes from the germ line. During ontogeny, somatic rearrangements of

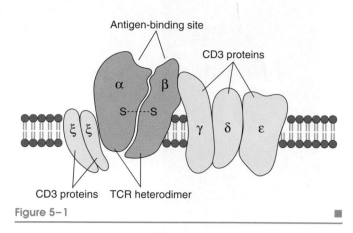

Antigen-binding site

CD3 proteins

CD3 proteins   TCR heterodimer

Figure 5–1 ■

The T-cell receptor (TCR) complex: a schematic illustration of TCRα and TCRβ polypeptide chains linked to the CD3 molecular complex.

these genes occur only in T cells; hence, the *demonstration of TCR gene rearrangements by Southern blot analysis is a molecular marker of T-lineage cells.* Such analyses are utilized in classification of lymphoid malignancies (Chapter 12). Furthermore, because each T cell has a unique DNA rearrangement (and hence a unique TCR), *it is possible to distinguish polyclonal (non-neoplastic) T-cell proliferations from monoclonal (neoplastic) T-cell proliferations.*

In addition to CD3 proteins, T cells express a variety of other nonpolymorphic function-associated molecules, including CD4 and CD8. These two molecules serve as coreceptors and are expressed on two mutually exclusive subsets of T cells. CD4 is expressed on approximately 60% of mature CD3+ T cells, whereas CD8 is expressed on about 30% of T cells. Thus, in normal healthy persons, the CD4-CD8 ratio is about 2:1. During antigen presentation, CD4 molecules on T cells bind to the nonpolymorphic portions of class II major histocompatibility complex (MHC) molecules (discussed later) expressed on antigen-presenting cells. In contrast, CD8 molecules bind to class I MHC molecules during antigen presentation. Because of these properties, CD4+ helper/inducer T cells can recognize antigen only in the context of class II MHC antigens, whereas the CD8+ cytotoxic/suppressor T cells recognize cell-bound antigens only in association with class I MHC antigens.

The CD4+ and CD8+ T cells perform distinct but somewhat overlapping functions. CD4+ T cells are often called "helper" T cells because the soluble molecules (cytokines) secreted by them influence virtually all other cells of the immune system, including B cells, natural killer (NK) cells, and macrophages. The central role of CD4+ helper cells is tragically illustrated when this subset is selectively destroyed by the human immunodeficiency virus (HIV). Recent studies have revealed two functionally distinct subsets of CD4+ T cells that are of clinical relevance. The so-called T_H1 CD4+ cells secrete primarily interleukin-2 (IL-2) and interferon-γ (IFN-γ) and thereby help in the induction of cell-mediated immunity. By contrast, the T_H2 subset of CD4+ cells secretes other cytokines such as IL-4 and IL-5, which help in the induction of humoral immunity. As discussed later, these cytokines are pivotal in the pathogenesis of type I hypersensitivity reactions, including bronchial asthma. The CD8+ T cells, like CD4+ cells, can secrete cytokines, but they are best known for their ability to kill virus-infected or tumor cells by direct cytotoxicity.

B Lymphocytes

B lymphocytes constitute 10% to 20% of the circulating peripheral lymphocyte population. They are also present in bone marrow; in peripheral lymphoid tissues such as lymph nodes, spleen, and tonsils; and in extralymphatic organs such as the gastrointestinal tract. In lymph nodes they are found in the superficial cortex. In the spleen they are found in the white pulp. *At both sites they are aggregated in the form of lymphoid follicles, which upon activation develop pale-staining germinal centers.*

Upon antigenic stimulation, B cells form plasma cells that secrete immunoglobulins, which in turn are the mediators of humoral immunity. Of the five immunoglobulin isotypes, IgG, IgM, and IgA constitute 95% of serum immunoglobulins; IgE occurs in traces; and IgD occurs predominantly in a cell-bound form on the B-cell membrane. Monomeric IgM, present on the surface of all B cells, constitutes the antigen receptor on B cells. As with T cells, each B-cell receptor has a unique antigen specificity, derived in part from somatic rearrangements of immunoglobulin genes. *Thus, the presence of rearranged immunoglobulin genes in a lymphoid cell is used as a molecular marker of B-lineage cells.* In addition to surface IgM, several nonpolymorphic molecules are also expressed on B cells. These include CD19 and CD20, which are restricted to B cells and hence are of practical value in the classification of lymphoid malignancies. CD21, a B cell–associated molecule, serves as a complement receptor, and also binds to Epstein-Barr virus (EBV). Hence, human B cells are readily infected by EBV.

Macrophages

Macrophages are a part of the mononuclear phagocyte system, and as such their role in inflammation was discussed in Chapter 2. Here we need only to emphasize that macrophages play several roles in the immune response.

■ First, they are required to process and present antigen to immunocompetent T cells. The presence of class II MHC antigens (p 85) on macrophages is considered critical for their antigen-presenting function. Because T cells (unlike B cells) cannot be triggered by free antigen, presentation of antigens by macrophages or other antigen-presenting cells (e.g., Langerhans' cells, discussed below) is obligatory for induction of cell-mediated immunity.

■ They produce a whole array of cytokines, which not only influence the function of T and B cells, but also affect other cell types, including endothelial cells and fibroblasts.

■ Macrophages lyse tumor cells by secreting toxic metabolites and proteolytic enzymes, and as such may play a role in immunosurveillance.

■ Macrophages are important effector cells in certain forms of cell-mediated immunity, such as the delayed hypersensitivity reaction.

Dendritic and Langerhans' Cells

Dendritic and Langerhans' cells make up a population of cells that have dendritic cytoplasmic processes and large amounts of class II molecules on their cell surfaces. Dendritic cells are found in lymphoid tissues, and Langerhans' cells occur in the epidermis. Both of these cell types are extremely efficient in antigen presentation. Unlike macrophages, they are poorly phagocytic, and hence they do not exhibit antimicrobial or scavenger cell activities. Another type of dendritic cell, distinct from the cells described above, is found primarily in the germinal centers of lymphoid follicles in the lymph nodes and spleen. The Fc receptors on these cells trap antigens complexed to their antibodies by binding to the Fc portion of antibodies. This provides a mechanism whereby, after an initial antibody response, antigens can persist in the lymphoid tissue and facilitate the maintenance of immunologic memory. Tragically, in patients with acquired immunodeficiency syndrome (AIDS), the HIV uses the same trick to persist within lymph nodes.

Natural Killer (NK) Cells

These cells make up approximately 10% to 15% of the peripheral blood lymphocytes and do not bear T-cell receptors or cell surface immunoglobulins. Morphologically, NK cells are somewhat larger than small lymphocytes, and they contain abundant azurophilic granules. Hence, they are also called large granular lymphocytes. NK cells are endowed with an innate ability to lyse a variety of tumor cells, virally infected cells, and some normal cells, *without previous sensitization.* These cells are believed to be a part of the "natural" (as opposed to adaptive) immune system that may be the first line of defense against neoplastic or virus-infected cells. Although they share some surface markers with T cells (e.g., CD2), NK cells do not rearrange T-cell receptor genes and are CD3 negative. Two cell surface molecules, CD16 and CD56, are widely utilized to identify NK cells. Of these, CD16 is of functional significance. It represents the Fc receptor for IgG and hence endows NK cells with another function—the ability to lyse IgG-coated target cells. This phenomenon, known as antibody-dependent cell-mediated cytotoxicity (ADCC), is described in greater detail later in this chapter. NK cells express two types of receptors on their cell membrane. One type activates NK-cell killing by recognizing ill-defined molecules on target cells; the other type inhibits the lytic pathway by recognition of self class I MHC molecules. These class I–recognizing receptors on NK cells are biochemically distinct from T-cell receptors. It is believed that NK cells are inhibited from killing normal cells because all nucleated normal cells express self class I MHC molecules. If virus infection or neoplastic transformation perturbs or reduces normal expression of class I molecules, inhibitory signals delivered to NK cells are interrupted, and lysis occurs (Fig. 5–2). NK cells also secrete cytokines and are believed to be an important source of IFN-γ.

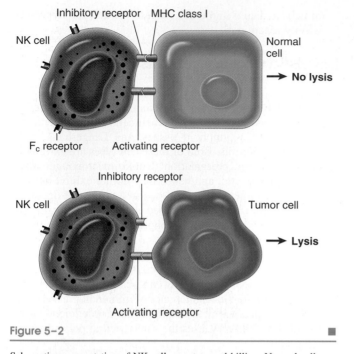

Inhibitory receptor · MHC class I

NK cell · Normal cell · **No lysis**

F_c receptor · Activating receptor

Inhibitory receptor

NK cell · Tumor cell · **Lysis**

Activating receptor

Figure 5–2 ■

Schematic representation of NK cell receptors and killing. Normal cells are not killed because inhibitory signals from normal MHC class I molecules override activating signals. In tumor cells, or virus-infected cells, reduced expression or alteration of MHC molecules interrupts the inhibitory signals, allowing activation of NK cells and lysis of target cells.

CYTOKINES: MESSENGER MOLECULES OF THE IMMUNE SYSTEM

It is well known that the induction and regulation of the immune responses involve multiple interactions among lymphocytes, monocytes, inflammatory cells (e.g., neutrophils), and endothelial cells. Many such interactions are mediated by short-acting soluble mediators. Depending on the source, mediators are called *lymphokines* (lymphocyte derived, such as the T cell–derived factor IL-2) or *monokines* (monocyte derived, such as TNF-α). Because of an increasing awareness that many such factors have a wide spectrum of effects and that a given factor may be produced by several cell types, it is now customary to group these polypeptide mediators under the single rubric of "cytokines."

We will not attempt to list the currently well-characterized and molecularly cloned cytokines, because new cytokines are being discovered rapidly by toiling armies of scientists. Instead, we will classify the currently known cytokines into five categories on the basis of their general properties:

■ Cytokines that mediate natural immunity. Included in this group are IL-1, TNF-α, IL-6, and type 1 interferons. Certain of these cytokines (e.g., interferons) protect against viral infections, while others (e.g., IL-1, TNF-α, IL-6) initiate nonspecific inflammatory responses.
■ Cytokines that regulate lymphocyte growth, activation, and differentiation. Within this category are IL-2, IL-4,

IL-5, IL-12, IL-15, and transforming growth factor-β (TGF-β). Some, such as IL-2 and IL-4, usually favor lymphocyte growth and differentiation; others, such as IL-10 and TGF-β, down-regulate immune responses.
■ Cytokines that activate inflammatory cells. In this category are interferon-γ (IFN-γ), TNF-α, lymphotoxin (TNF-β), and migration inhibitory factor. Most of these cytokines, derived from T cells, serve to activate the functions of nonspecific effector cells.
■ Cytokines that affect leukocyte movements (chemotaxis and chemokinesis) are also called chemokines (Chapter 2). Some important members of this family are IL-8, eotaxin, and macrophage inflammatory protein-1α).
■ Cytokines that stimulate hematopoiesis by acting on hematopoietic progenitor cells. Several members of this family are called colony-stimulating factors (CSFs) because they were initially detected by their ability to promote the growth of hematopoietic cell colonies from the bone marrow. Examples include granulocyte-macrophage (GM) CSF, granulocyte (G) CSF, and stem cell factor. Two other cytokines in this group, IL-3 and IL-7, affect the growth of lymphocyte progenitor cells.

It should be noted that this subdivision of cytokines into functional groups, although convenient, is somewhat arbitrary because many cytokines such as IL-1 and TNF-α are pleotropic in their effects.

HISTOCOMPATIBILITY GENES (ANTIGENS)

Although initially despised by immunologists and surgeons because they evoke rejection of transplanted organs, histocompatibility molecules are physiologically important regulators of the immune response. *The principal function of the cell surface histocompatibility molecules is to bind peptide fragments of foreign proteins for presentation to appropriate antigen-specific T cells.* Recall that T cells (unlike B cells) can recognize only membrane-bound antigens. The histocompatibility molecules and the corresponding genes are complex in structure and organization and are still incompletely understood. Here we summarize only the salient features of human histocompatibility antigens, primarily to facilitate understanding of their role in rejection of organ transplants and in disease susceptibility. Several genes code for histocompatibility antigens, but those that code for the most important transplantation antigens are clustered on a small segment of chromosome 6. This cluster constitutes the human major histocompatibility complex (MHC) and is also known as the HLA complex (Fig. 5–3). It is equivalent to the murine H-2 complex. The initials HLA stand for human leukocyte antigens, as MHC-encoded antigens were initially detected on the white cells. The HLA system is highly polymorphic; that is, there are several alternative forms (alleles) of a gene at each locus. This, as we shall see, constitutes a formidable barrier in organ transplantation.

On the basis of their chemical structure, tissue distribution,

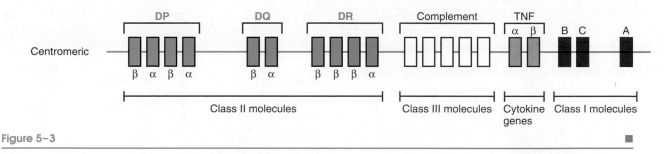

Figure 5-3   ■

Schematic representation of the HLA complex and its subregions. The relative distances between various genes and regions are not drawn to scale.

and function, the MHC gene products are classified into three categories:

■ Class I antigens are coded by three closely linked loci designated HLA-A, HLA-B, and HLA-C (Fig. 5-3). Each of these molecules is a heterodimer, consisting of a polymorphic glycoprotein of 45,000 daltons (heavy chain or α chain) linked noncovalently to a smaller nonpolymorphic peptide called β_2-microglobulin. The latter is encoded by a gene on chromosome 15. *The extracellular portion of the α chain contains a cleft where foreign peptides bind to MHC molecules for presentation to T cells.* Class I antigens are present on virtually all nucleated cells and platelets.

■ Class II antigens are coded for in a region known as HLA-D. There are at least three subregions, DP, DQ, and DR, within the originally defined HLA-D region. Class II antigens differ from class I antigens in several respects. Chemically, they exist as heterodimers of noncovalently associated α and β subunits. Both of these chains are polymorphic. Like class I molecules, the extracellular portion of the class II heterodimer contains a cleft for the binding of antigenic peptides. Unlike class I antigens, their tissue distribution is quite restricted; they are found mainly on antigen-presenting cells (monocytes and macrophages, dendritic cells), B cells, and some activated T cells. However, several other cell types, such as vascular endothelial cells, fibroblasts, and renal tubular epithelial cells, can be induced to express class II antigens by IFN-γ, a lymphokine produced by activated T cells.

■ Class III proteins are those components of the complement system (C2, C3, and Bf) that are coded within the MHC. Genes for the cytokines TNF-α and TNF-β are also encoded within the MHC. Although genetically linked to class I and II antigens, class III molecules and the cytokine genes do not act as histocompatibility (transplantation) antigens and will not be discussed further.

Because HLA antigens form an allelic series, an individual inherits only one determinant from each parent and can have no more than two different antigens for every locus. Thus, cells of a heterozygous individual express six different class I HLA antigens, three of maternal origin and three of paternal origin. Owing to the polymorphism at the major HLA loci, innumerable combinations of antigens can exist, and therefore each individual in a non-inbred population is likely to have a more or less unique antigenic profile, like a fingerprint on the cell surface.

SIGNIFICANCE OF HLA COMPLEX

Organ Transplantation. HLA antigens were discovered in the course of transplantation studies, and they continue to present formidable barriers to the success of clinical organ transplantation. HLA antigens of the graft evoke both humoral and cell-mediated responses, which lead eventually to graft destruction, as discussed later in this chapter. Because the severity of the rejection reaction is related to the degree of HLA disparity between donor and recipient, HLA typing is of clinical significance in the selection of donor-recipient combinations.

Induction of Immune Responses. As mentioned in the introduction to this section, the major physiologic function of the HLA molecules is to present antigens to T cells. Thus, histocompatibility molecules play an important role in the induction of both cellular and humoral immunity.

Class I MHC molecules bind to intracellularly synthesized peptides (e.g., viral antigens) and present them to CD8+ cytotoxic T lymphocytes. In this interaction, the T-cell receptor recognizes the MHC-peptide complex, and the CD8 coreceptor binds to the nonpolymorphic portion of the class I molecule (Fig. 5-4). It is important to note that *CD8+ cytotoxic T cells can recognize viral (or other) peptides only if presented as a complex with class I self-antigens. This phenomenon is referred to as HLA restriction.* Because one of the important functions of CD8+ cytotoxic T cells is to eliminate virus-infected cells, and viral antigens can be recognized only when complexed to class I MHC molecules, it makes "good sense" to have widespread expression of class I HLA antigens.

In contrast to class I MHC molecules, class II molecules are important for the presentation of antigens to CD4+ helper T cells. The nature of antigens presented in association with class II molecules also differs. In general, class II molecules present exogenous antigens that are first internalized and processed by antigen-presenting cells, and then the class II-peptide complex is transported to the cell surface. Because CD4+ T cells can recognize foreign antigens only in the context of class II self-molecules, they are referred to as being "class II restricted."

Regulation of Immune Responses. The role of class II antigens in the induction of helper T cells has an important bearing on the genetic regulation of the immune response.

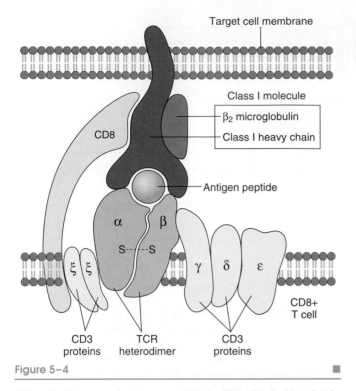

Target cell membrane

Class I molecule
- β₂ microglobulin
- Class I heavy chain

CD8

Antigen peptide

α β

S----S

ξ ξ

γ δ ε

CD8+ T cell

CD3 proteins TCR heterodimer CD3 proteins

Figure 5–4 ■

Schematic illustration of antigen recognition by CD8+ T cells. Note that the TCR (TCR heterodimer) recognizes a complex formed by the peptide fragment of the antigen and class I MHC molecule. The CD8 molecule binds to the nonpolymorphic portion of the class I molecule and thus acts as an accessory structure during antigen recognition.

How class II antigens influence the magnitude of the immune response is not fully understood. One possibility is that different antigenic peptides bind to different alleles of class II molecules. It follows, then, that an individual will recognize and mount an immune response against a given antigen only if he or she inherits those class II molecules that can bind the antigenic peptide and present it to T-helper cells. The consequence of inheriting such a class II gene would depend on the nature of the antigen and the type of immune response generated. For example, if the antigen were ragweed pollen and the response were production of IgE antibody, the individual would be genetically prone to type I hypersensitivity disease. On the other hand, good responsiveness to a viral antigen may be beneficial for the host.

HLA and Disease Association. A variety of diseases has been found to be associated with certain HLA types (Table 5–1). The best known is the association between ankylosing spondylitis and HLA-B27; individuals who possess this antigen have a 90-fold greater chance (relative risk) of developing the disease than do those who are negative for HLA-B27. The diseases that show association with HLA can be broadly grouped into the following categories: (1) *inflammatory diseases,* including ankylosing spondylitis and several postinfectious arthropathies, all associated with HLA-B27; (2) *inherited errors of metabolism,* such as hemochromatosis (HLA-A3) and 21-hydroxylase deficiency (HLA-BW47); and (3) *autoimmune diseases,* including autoimmune endocrinopathies, associated with alleles at the DR locus. The mechanisms underlying all these associations are not understood at

Table 5–1. ASSOCIATION OF HLA WITH DISEASE

Disease	HLA Allele	Relative Risk
Ankylosing spondylitis	B27	87.4
Postgonococcal arthritis	B27	14.0
Acute anterior uveitis	B27	14.6
Rheumatoid arthritis	DR4	5.8
Chronic active hepatitis	DR3	13.9
Primary Sjögren's syndrome	DR3	9.7
Insulin-dependent diabetes	DR3	5.0
	DR4	6.8
	DR3/DR4	14.3
Hemochromatosis	A3	8.2
21-Hydroxylase deficiency	BW47	15.0

present. In view of the physiologic role of the HLA complex in regulation of the immune response, it is somewhat easier to speculate on the possible mechanisms that may underlie the associations with immunologically mediated diseases. As discussed above, HLA class II genes can regulate immune responsiveness. Accordingly, an association between certain autoimmune diseases and HLA-DR antigens may result from an inappropriate immune response to autoantigens.

IMMUNE MECHANISMS OF TISSUE INJURY

Immune responses (humoral or cell mediated) to antigens of either endogenous or exogenous sources can cause tissue-damaging reactions. Classically, these are called *hypersensitivity reactions* and the resultant tissue lesions *hypersensitivity disease.* The term hypersensitivity, however, is somewhat misleading because it implies abnormal or excessive sensitivity to an antigen. Hypersensitivity disease may result from perfectly usual or normal immune responses to an antigen (e.g., the rejection of tissue grafts from antigenically dissimilar donors). A better designation for hypersensitivity disease might be "diseases resulting from immune-mediated tissue-damaging reactions," but, alas, this is too cumbersome a designation.

Hypersensitivity diseases (Table 5–2) are best classified on the basis of the immunologic mechanism mediating the disease. This approach is of great value, because it clarifies the manner in which the immune response ultimately causes tissue injury and disease.

■ In type I disease, the immune response releases vasoactive amines and other mediators that are derived from the mast cells or basophils affecting vascular permeability and smooth muscle in various organs. Eosinophils also play a role.

■ In the type II disorder, humoral antibodies participate directly in injuring cells by predisposing them to phagocytosis or to lysis.

■ Type III disorders are best remembered as "immune complex diseases"; here humoral antibodies bind antigens and

Table 5–2.   MECHANISMS OF IMMUNOLOGICALLY MEDIATED DISORDERS

Type	Prototype Disorder	Immune Mechanism
I Anaphylactic Type	Anaphylaxis, some forms of bronchial asthma	Formation of IgE (cytotropic) antibody → release of vasoactive amines and other mediators from basophils and mast cells followed by recruitment of other inflammatory cells
II Cytotoxic Type	Autoimmune hemolytic anemia, erythroblastosis fetalis, Goodpasture's disease, pemphigus vulgaris	Formation of IgG, IgM → binds to antigen on target cell surface → phagocytosis of target cell or lysis of target cell by C8, C9 fraction of activated complement or ADCC
III Immune Complex Disease	Arthus reaction, serum sickness, SLE, certain forms of acute glomerulonephritis	Antigen-antibody complexes → activated complement → attracted neutrophils → release of lysosomal enzymes and other toxic moieties
IV Cell-Mediated (Delayed) Hypersensitivity	Tuberculosis, contact dermatitis, transplant rejection	Sensitized T lymphocytes → release of lymphokines and T cell–mediated cytotoxicity

activate complement. The fractions of complement then attract neutrophils. Ultimately, it is the activated complement and the release of neutrophilic enzymes and other toxic moieties (e.g., oxygen metabolites) that produce the tissue damage.

■ Type IV disorders are examples of tissue injury in which cell-mediated immune responses with sensitized lymphocytes are the ultimate cause of the cellular and tissue injury. Each of these immune mechanisms is discussed in the succeeding sections.

TYPE I HYPERSENSITIVITY (ANAPHYLACTIC TYPE)

Type I hypersensitivity is a rapidly occurring reaction that follows the combination of an antigen with antibody previously bound to the surface of mast cells and basophils. Many type I reactions have two well-defined phases. The initial response, characterized by vasodilatation, vascular leakage, and smooth muscle spasm, usually becomes evident within 5 to 30 minutes after exposure to an allergen and tends to subside in 60 minutes. A second, *late-phase* reaction sets in 2 to 8 hours later without additional exposure to antigen and lasts for several days. This late-phase reaction follows in only about 50% of individuals; it is characterized by increasingly intense infiltration of tissues with eosinophils, neutrophils, basophils, and monocytes, as well as tissue destruction in the form of mucosal epithelial cell damage.

Because *mast cells* and *basophils* are central to the development of type I hypersensitivity, we will first review some of their salient characteristics and then discuss the immune mechanisms that underlie this form of hypersensitivity. Mast cells are widely distributed in the tissues; they are found predominantly near blood vessels and nerves and in subepithelial sites. Their cytoplasm contains membrane-bound granules that possess a variety of biologically active mediators. As detailed below, mast cells and basophils are activated by cross-linking of high-affinity IgE Fc receptors; mast cells may also be triggered by several other stimuli, such as complement

components C5a and C3a (anaphylatoxins), both of which act by binding to their receptors on mast cell membrane. Other mast cell secretagogues include macrophage-derived cytokines (e.g., IL-8), some drugs such as codeine and morphine, mellitin (present in bee venom), and physical stimuli (e.g., heat, cold, sunlight). Basophils are similar to mast cells in many respects, but unlike mast cells they are not normally present in tissues. Instead, they circulate in the blood in extremely small numbers. Like other granulocytes, they can be recruited to inflammatory sites.

In humans, type I reactions are mediated by IgE antibodies (also called reaginic antibodies); in other species, IgG antibodies can mediate anaphylactic reactions. The basic sequence of events in the pathogenesis of this form of hypersensitivity begins with the initial exposure to certain antigens (often called allergens). *The allergen stimulates the induction of CD4+ T cells of the T_H2 type. These CD4+ cells play a pivotal role in the pathogenesis of type I hypersensitivity* because the cytokines secreted by them cause IgE production by B cells, act as growth factors for mast cells, and recruit and activate eosinophils. IgE antibodies bind to the high-affinity receptors specific for the Fc portion of IgE molecule, expressed on mast cells and basophils. Once IgE is bound to the surface of mast cells, the individual is primed to develop type I hypersensitivity. Re-exposure to the same antigen results in fixing of the antigen to cell-bound IgE, initiating a series of reactions that lead to the release of several powerful mediators that are responsible for the tissue changes and clinical features of type I hypersensitivity (Fig. 5–5). The mediator release requires that adjacent IgE molecules on the surface of mast cells and basophils be cross-linked by binding to a multivalent antigen. The cross-linking of cell-bound IgE induces a membrane signal that initiates several parallel and independent processes (Fig. 5–6): one leads to mast cell degranulation with discharge of preformed, or *primary, mediators;* the other involves de novo synthesis and release of *secondary mediators* such as arachidonic acid metabolites and cytokines.

Primary Mediators. Primary mediators, or preformed mediators, are contained within mast cell granules. Upon de-

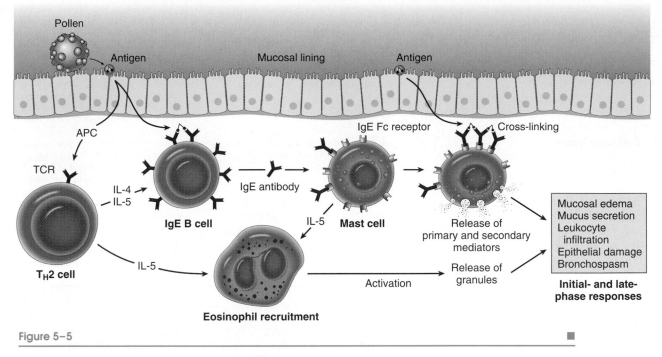

Figure 5-5 ■

Sequence of events leading to type I hypersensitivity. TCR, T-cell receptor; APC, antigen-presenting cell; T_H2, T-helper 2; CD4+ cells.

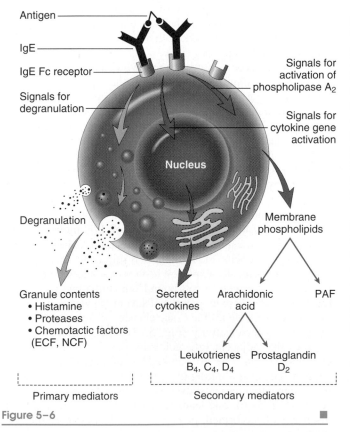

Figure 5-6 ■

Activation of mast cells in type I hypersensitivity and release of their mediators. ECF, eosinophil chemotactic factor; NCF, neutrophil chemotactic factor; PAF, platelet activating factor.

granulation of mast cells, they are rapidly released and thus act early in the course of type I hypersensitivity reactions. *Histamine* is the most important preformed mediator. It is known to cause increased vascular permeability, vasodilatation, bronchospasm, and increased secretion of mucus. Other rapidly released mediators are factors that are *chemotactic for neutrophils and eosinophils.* Accumulation of eosinophils is often prominent in these allergic reactions. Other mediators make up the granule matrix; they include heparin and neutral proteases (e.g., tryptase). The neutral proteases can cleave complement components to generate additional chemotactic and inflammatory factors. C3a, for example, can cause further mast cell degranulation.

Secondary Mediators. These include two classes of compounds: (1) lipid mediators and (2) cytokines. The lipid mediators are generated by sequential reactions in the mast cell membranes that lead to activation of phospholipase A_2, an enzyme that acts on membrane phospholipids to yield *arachidonic acid.* This, you may recall, is the parent compound from which leukotrienes and prostaglandins are derived by the 5-lipoxygenase and cyclooxygenase pathways, respectively (Chapter 2).

■ Leukotrienes are extremely important in the pathogenesis of type I hypersensitivity. Leukotrienes C_4 and D_4 are the most potent vasoactive and spasmogenic agents known. On a molar basis, they are several thousand times more active than histamine in increasing vascular permeability and causing bronchial smooth muscle contraction. Leukotriene B_4 is highly chemotactic for neutrophils, eosinophils, and monocytes.

■ Prostaglandin D_2 is the most abundant mediator derived by the cyclooxygenase pathway in mast cells. It causes intense bronchospasm as well as increased mucus secretion.

■ Platelet-activating factor (PAF, Chapter 2), another secondary mediator, causes platelet aggregation, release of histamine, and bronchospasm. It is also chemotactic for neutrophils and eosinophils, causing their accumulations and subsequent degranulation. Although its production is also initiated by the activation of phospholipase A_2, it is not a product of arachidonic acid metabolism.

■ Mast cells can produce a variety of cytokines, including TNF-α, IL-1, IL-4, IL-5, and IL-6. IL-4 and IL-5 are also released by the T_H2 cells that initiate IgE synthesis. IL-4 is a mast cell growth factor, and along with IL-5 it is required for IgE synthesis by B cells. Mast cell and T_H2 cell–derived cytokines also contribute to the accumulation and activation of eosinophils and other inflammatory cells late in the course of immediate hypersensitivity.

In summary, a variety of chemotactic, vasoactive, and spasmogenic compounds (Table 5–3) mediate type I hypersensitivity reactions. Some of these compounds are released rapidly from sensitized mast cells and are believed to be responsible for the intense immediate reactions associated with conditions such as systemic anaphylaxis. Others, such as cytokines, are probably responsible for the late-phase reactions. Eosinophils are important effectors of tissue injury in the late-phase response because they produce major basic protein and eosinophil cationic protein, which are toxic to epithelial cells. Major basic protein also induces activation of mast cells, neutrophils, and platelets. Recent studies indicate that accumulation of eosinophils is not only dependent on the release of mast cell–derived mediators, but also caused by the release of a chemokine called *eotaxin*. This specific chemoattractant for eosinophils is released by epithelial cells and endothelial cells under the influence of cytokines such as TNF-α that are abundant at sites of type I hypersensitivity reactions. Because inflammation is a major component of the late-phase reaction,

its control usually requires broad-spectrum anti-inflammatory drugs such as glucocorticosteroids.

Clinical Manifestations. A type I reaction may occur as a systemic disorder or as a local reaction. Often this is determined by the route of antigen exposure. Systemic (parenteral) administration of protein antigens (such as antisera) and drugs (such as penicillin) results in *systemic anaphylaxis*. Within minutes after re-exposure, itching, hives, and skin erythema appear, followed shortly thereafter by striking respiratory difficulty, resulting presumably from constriction of respiratory bronchioles. Thus, the principal organ affected is the lung, more specifically the smooth musculature of the pulmonary blood vessels and the respiratory passages. Pulmonary obstruction is accentuated by hypersecretion of mucus. Laryngeal edema may cause obstruction of the upper airway. In addition, the musculature of the entire gastrointestinal tract may be affected, with resultant vomiting, abdominal cramps, and diarrhea. The patient may go into shock and even die within minutes.

Local reactions generally occur on the skin or mucosal surfaces when these are the sites of antigenic exposure. In the skin, they may take the form of *urticaria* (hives). The common forms of skin and food allergies, hay fever, and certain forms of asthma are examples of localized anaphylactic reactions. Susceptibility to localized type I reactions appears to be genetically controlled, and the term "atopy" is used to imply familial predisposition to such localized reactions. Patients who suffer from nasobronchial allergy (including hay fever and some forms of asthma) often have a family history of similar conditions. The genetic basis of atopy is not clearly understood; it seems, however, that these individuals have higher-than-normal levels of circulating IgE, which may be linked to a gene mapped on chromosome 5q.

Before we close the discussion of type I hypersensitivity, it should be noted that these reactions did not evolve only to cause much human discomfort and diseases. Type I hypersensitivity, particularly the late-phase inflammatory reactions, plays an important protective role in several parasitic infections. IgE antibodies are regularly produced in response to

■

Table 5–3.   SUMMARY OF THE ACTION OF MAST CELL MEDIATORS IN TYPE I HYPERSENSITIVITY*

Action	Mediator	Source
Cellular Infiltration	Leukotriene B_4	Membrane phospholipids
	Eosinophil chemotactic factor of anaphylaxis	Mast cell granules
	Neutrophil chemotactic factor of anaphylaxis	Mast cell granules
	*Cytokines	Mast cells
Vasoactive (Vasodilatation, Increased Vascular Permeability)	Histamine	Mast cell granules
	*Platelet-activating factor (PAF)	Membrane lipids
	Leukotrienes C_4, D_4, E_4	Membrane lipids
	Neutral proteases that activate complement	Mast cell granule matrix
	Prostaglandin D_2	Membrane lipids
Smooth Muscle Spasm	Leukotrienes C_4, D_4, E_4	Membrane lipids
	Histamine	Mast cell granules
	Prostaglandins	Membrane lipids
	PAF	Membrane lipids

* Important for late-phase reactions.

many helminthic infections. Figure 5–7 provides a schematic illustration of the process by which IgE antibodies serve to inflict damage on the schistosome larvae by recruiting inflammatory cells and causing antibody-dependent cell-mediated cytotoxicity (described later).

TYPE II HYPERSENSITIVITY (ANTIBODY DEPENDENT)

In type II hypersensitivity, antibodies are formed against target antigens that are either normal or altered cell membrane components. *Unlike type III hypersensitivity reactions, discussed later, the antigens in this type of reaction are intrinsic to the cell or tissue that is damaged.* Three different antibody-

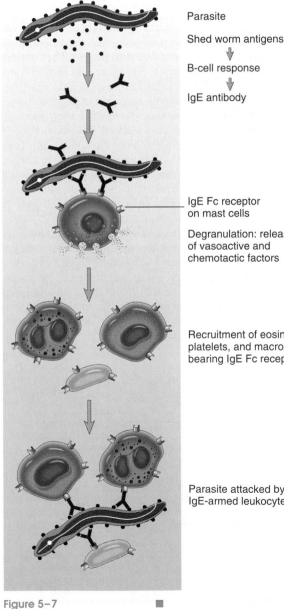

Figure 5–7 ■

IgE-mediated destruction of parasites.

- Parasite
- Shed worm antigens
- B-cell response
- IgE antibody
- IgE Fc receptor on mast cells
- Degranulation: release of vasoactive and chemotactic factors
- Recruitment of eosinophils, platelets, and macrophages bearing IgE Fc receptors
- Parasite attacked by IgE-armed leukocytes

dependent mechanisms are involved in this type of hypersensitivity (Fig. 5–8).

Complement-Mediated Reactions. In complement-mediated cytotoxicity, antibody reacts with a cell surface antigen, leading to fixation of complement and to cell lysis. In addition, cells coated with antibodies become susceptible to phagocytosis (opsonization), a process also favored by fixation of complement. Blood cells are the ones most commonly damaged by this mechanism. Clinically, antibody-mediated reactions against blood cells occur in the following situations:

- Transfusion reactions, in which red cells from an incompatible donor are destroyed after being coated with antibodies normally present in the recipient. Such antibodies are directed against blood group antigens.
- Rhesus incompatibility, in which an Rh-negative mother is sensitized by red cells from an Rh-positive baby. The maternal Rh antibodies can cross the placenta and cause destruction of the Rh-positive fetal red cells. The resulting syndrome is called erythroblastosis fetalis (Chapter 7).
- Some persons develop antibodies against their own blood elements, resulting in autoimmune hemolytic anemia, agranulocytosis, or thrombocytopenia. The possible reasons for such autoantibody formation are discussed in a later section. In addition to blood cells, antibodies may form against other tissue components, for example, basement membrane collagen, causing Goodpasture's syndrome, and desmosomes, resulting in pemphigus vulgaris.

Antibody-Dependent Cell-Mediated Cytotoxicity (ADCC). This is the second possible mechanism involved in type II reactions. Many cell types that bear receptors for the Fc portion of IgG cause the lysis of target cells coated with IgG antibody. This interaction involves the Fc receptors of the killer cells, which engage the Fc portion of the antibody coating the target cell (Fig. 5–8). *Lysis of the target cell requires contact but does not involve phagocytosis or fixation of complement.* ADCC can be mediated by a variety of cell types bearing Fc-IgG receptors. These include neutrophils, eosinophils, macrophages, and NK cells. In most cases IgG antibodies are involved in ADCC, but in certain instances (e.g., eosinophil-mediated ADCC against parasites, see Fig. 5–7) IgE antibodies are utilized.

Antibody-Mediated Cellular Dysfunction. In some cases, antibodies directed against cell surface receptors impair or dysregulate function without causing cell injury or inflammation. For example, in myasthenia gravis antibodies reactive with acetylcholine receptors in the motor end plates of skeletal muscles impair neuromuscular transmission and therefore cause muscle weakness. The converse, antibody-mediated stimulation of cell function, is noted in Graves' disease. In this disorder, antibodies against the thyroid-stimulating hormone receptor on thyroid epithelial cells stimulate the cells, resulting in hyperthyroidism.

TYPE III HYPERSENSITIVITY (IMMUNE COMPLEX MEDIATED)

Type III hypersensitivity is mediated by antigen-antibody (immune) complexes, which initiate an acute inflammatory reaction in the tissues. *Activation of complement and accu-*

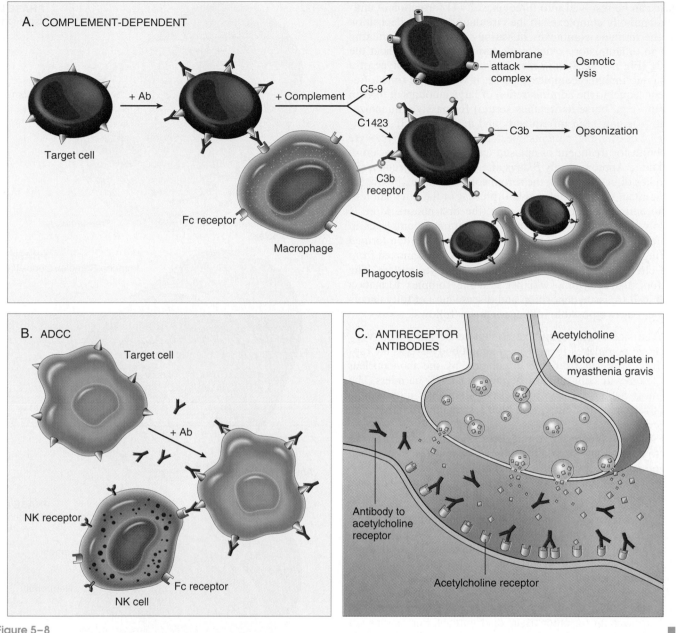

Figure 5–8   ■

Schematic illustration of three different mechanisms of antibody-mediated injury in type II hypersensitivity. *A*, Complement-dependent reactions that lead to lysis of cells or render them susceptible to phagocytosis. *B*, Antibody-dependent cell-mediated cytotoxicity (ADCC). IgG-coated target cells are killed by cells that bear Fc receptors for IgG (e.g., NK cells, macrophages). *C*, Antireceptor antibodies disturb the normal function of receptors. In this example, acetylcholine receptor antibodies impair neuromuscular transmission in myasthenia gravis.

mulation of polymorphonuclear leukocytes are important components of immune complex–mediated tissue injury. The formation of immune complexes can be initiated by exogenous antigens such as bacteria and viruses or by endogenous antigens such as DNA. Pathogenic immune complexes either are formed in the circulation and then deposited in the tissues, or are formed at extravascular sites where antigen may have been planted (in situ immune complexes). Some forms of glomerular diseases in which immune complexes are formed in situ on the glomerular basement membrane are discussed in Chapter 14.

There are two patterns of immune complex–mediated injury. In one, the complexes are deposited in various tissues of the body, thus causing a systemic pattern of injury. In the other, the injury is localized to the site of formation, within a tissue or organ, of the complexes. Although the mechanism of tissue injury is the same, the sequence of events and the conditions leading to the formation of the immune complexes are different. We will therefore consider these two patterns separately.

Systemic Immune Complex Disease (Serum Sickness Type). The pathogenesis of systemic immune complex disease can be resolved into three phases: (1) formation of antigen-antibody complexes in the circulation and (2) deposition of the immune complexes in various tissues, thus initiating (3) an inflammatory reaction in various sites throughout the body (Fig. 5–9). *Acute serum sickness* is the prototype of a systemic immune complex disease; it was at one time a frequent sequel to the administration of large amounts of foreign serum (e.g., horse antitetanus serum) for passive immunization. It is now seen infrequently and in different clinical settings. For example, patients injected with horse antithymocyte globulin for treatment of aplastic anemia can develop serum sickness. Approximately 5 days after the serum injection, antibodies directed against the serum components are produced; these react with the antigen still present in the circulation to form antigen-antibody complexes (the first phase). More is involved than the mere formation of immune complexes in the circulation; indeed, immune complexes are often formed during many immune responses, and they are removed from the circulation by the mononuclear phagocyte system. The factors that determine whether immune complex formation will lead to tissue deposition and disease are not fully understood, but two possible influences are as follows:

■ The size of the complexes seems to be important. Very large complexes formed in great antibody excess are rapidly removed from the circulation by the mononuclear phagocytic cells and are therefore relatively harmless. The most pathogenic complexes are of small or intermediate size, circulate longer, and bind less avidly to phagocytic cells.

■ Since the mononuclear phagocyte system normally serves to filter out the circulating immune complexes, its overload or intrinsic dysfunction increases the probability of persistence of immune complexes in the circulation and tissue deposition.

Tissue injury does not occur unless the circulating immune complexes are extravasated into various tissues (second phase) by an increase in vascular permeability. This is thought to be mediated by local secretions of cytokines and other mediators released from inflammatory cells, which bind the complexes via their Fc and C3b receptors. Although this mechanism explains the vascular localization of the complexes, it fails to account for other tissue distributions. For reasons not entirely clear, *the favored sites of immune complex deposition are kidneys, joints, skin, heart, serosal surface, and small vessels.* Localization in the kidney could be explained in part by the filtration function of the glomerulus, with trapping of the circulating complexes in the glomeruli. Other factors that influence renal disposition are discussed later, in the context of glomerular diseases (Chapter 14). There is at present no satisfactory explanation for the peculiar localization of immune complexes in the other sites of predilection.

Once complexes are deposited in the tissues, they initiate an acute inflammatory reaction (third phase). It is during this phase (approximately 10 days after antigen administration) that clinical features such as fever, urticaria, arthralgias, lymph node enlargement, and proteinuria appear. Central to the pathogenesis of tissue injury is the fixation of complement by the complexes, activation of the complement cascade, and release of biologically active fragments (Chapter 2), notably the anaphylatoxins (C3a and C5a), which increase vascular

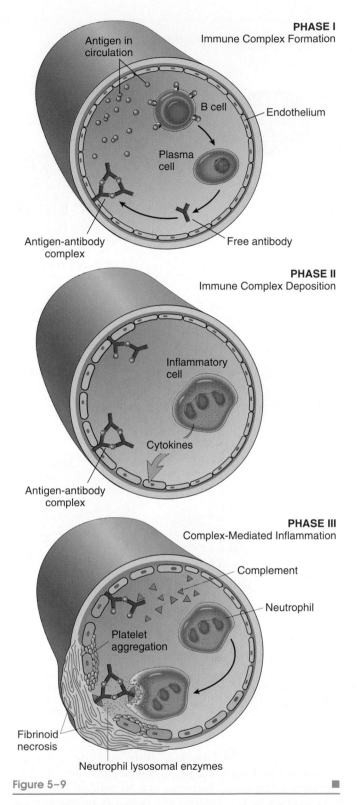

PHASE I
Immune Complex Formation

Antigen in circulation

B cell

Endothelium

Plasma cell

Antigen-antibody complex

Free antibody

PHASE II
Immune Complex Deposition

Inflammatory cell

Cytokines

Antigen-antibody complex

PHASE III
Complex-Mediated Inflammation

Complement

Neutrophil

Platelet aggregation

Fibrinoid necrosis

Neutrophil lysosomal enzymes

Figure 5–9 ■

Schematic illustration of the three sequential phases in the induction of systemic type III (immune complex) hypersensitivity.

permeability and yield chemotactic factors for polymorphonuclear leukocytes. Phagocytosis of immune complexes by the accumulated neutrophils results in the release of lysosomal enzymes, such as neutral proteases, which can digest base-

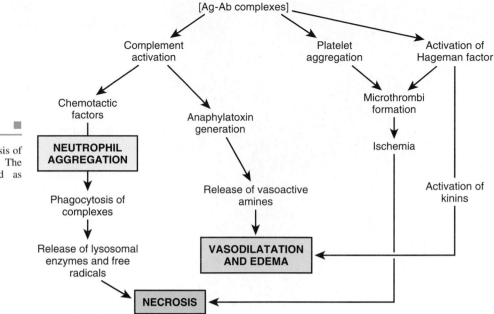

Figure 5–10 ■

Schematic representation of the pathogenesis of immune complex–mediated tissue injury. The morphologic consequences are depicted as boxed areas.

ment membranes, collagen, elastin, and cartilage. Tissue damage may also be mediated by free oxygen radicals produced by activated neutrophils. The released lysosomal enzymes serve to perpetuate the inflammatory process. Immune complexes lead to other effects also: aggregation of platelets and activation of Hageman factor, both of which augment the inflammatory process (Fig. 5–10). Microthrombi formed by platelet aggregation and initiation of clotting also contribute to the tissue injury by producing local ischemia.

It should be clear from the discussion above that only those antibodies that activate complement by the classic pathway (IgG, IgM) or alternative pathway (IgA) can mediate type III hypersensitivity. The important role of complement in the pathogenesis of the tissue injury is supported by the fact that, during the active phase of the disease, consumption of complement induces low serum levels.

The morphologic consequences of immune complex injury are dominated by acute necrotizing vasculitis, microthrombi, and superimposed ischemic necrosis accompanied by acute inflammation of the affected organs. The necrotic vessel wall takes on a smudgy eosinophilic appearance called "fibrinoid necrosis" (Fig. 5–11). Immune complexes can be visualized in the tissues, usually in the vascular wall, by both electron microscopy (Fig. 5–12) and immunofluorescence (Fig. 5–13). In due course the lesions tend to resolve, especially when they were brought about by a single large exposure to antigen (e.g., acute serum sickness and acute poststreptococcal glomerulonephritis, Chapter 14). However, chronic immune complex disease develops when there is persistent antigenemia or repeated exposure to the antigen. This occurs in some human diseases, such as systemic lupus erythematosus (SLE). Often, however, despite the fact that the morpho-

logic changes and other findings suggest immune complex disease, the inciting antigens are unknown. Included in this category are rheumatoid arthritis, polyarteritis nodosa, membranous glomerulonephritis, and several vasculitides.

Local Immune Complex Disease (Arthus Reaction). The Arthus reaction may be defined as a localized area of tissue necrosis resulting from acute immune complex vasculitis. The reaction can be produced experimentally by injecting an antigen into the skin of a previously immunized animal. Antibodies against the antigen are therefore already present in the circulation. Because of the large excess of antibodies, immune complexes are formed; these are precipitated at the site of

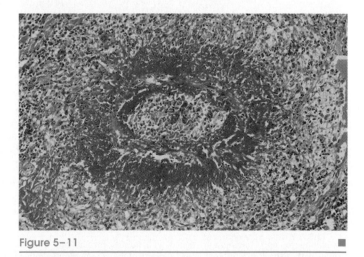

Figure 5–11 ■

Immune complex vasculitis. The necrotic vessel wall is replaced by smudgy, pink "fibrinoid" material. (Courtesy of Dr. Trace Worrell, Department of Pathology, University of Texas Southwestern Medical School, Dallas.)

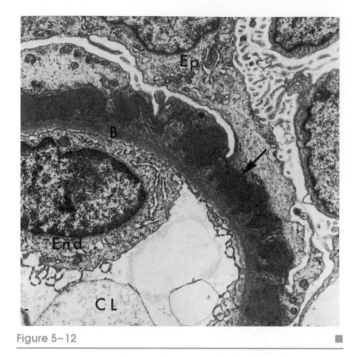

Figure 5-12 ■

Membranous glomerulonephritis. Electron micrograph showing electron-dense deposits *(arrow)* along the epithelial side of the basement membrane (B). CL, capillary lumen; End, endothelium; Ep, epithelium.

injection, especially within vessel walls, where the injected antigen is immediately bound to the circulating antibodies. Once the complexes are formed, the subsequent events are very similar to those described in the systemic pattern. Histologically, there is severe necrotizing vasculitis and intense accumulation of neutrophils. Intrapulmonary Arthus-type reactions seem to be responsible for a number of diseases in humans, including *farmer's lung,* a hypersensitivity reaction to molds that grow on hay (Chapter 13).

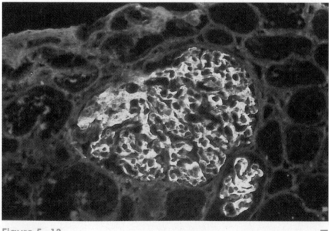

Figure 5-13 ■

Immunofluorescence micrograph stained with fluorescent anti-IgG from a patient with diffuse proliferative lupus nephritis. One complete glomerulus and part of another one are seen. Note the mesangial and capillary wall deposits of IgG. (Courtesy of Dr. Helmut Renké, Department of Pathology, Brigham and Women's Hospital, Boston.)

TYPE IV HYPERSENSITIVITY (CELL MEDIATED)

Type IV hypersensitivity is mediated by T cells rather than by antibodies. *Two types of reactions mediated by different T cell subsets are involved in type IV hypersensitivity:* (1) delayed-type hypersensitivity, initiated by CD4+ T cells; and (2) cellular cytotoxicity, mediated by CD8+ T cells. In both cases the reaction is initiated by the exposure of sensitized T cells to specific antigenic peptides bound to self-MHC molecules, but the subsequent events are different. In delayed hypersensitivity T_H1-type CD4+ T cells secrete cytokines, leading to recruitment of other cells, especially macrophages, which are the major effector cells. In cell-mediated cytotoxicity, on the other hand, cytotoxic CD8+ T cells themselves assume the effector function.

Delayed-Type Hypersensitivity. The classic example of a delayed hypersensitivity reaction is a positive Mantoux reaction (tuberculin test) elicited in an individual already sensitized to the tubercle bacillus by a previous infection (Chapter 13). After intracutaneous injection of tuberculin, a local area of erythema and induration begins to appear at 8 to 12 hours, reaches a peak (approximately 1 to 2 cm in diameter) in 2 to 7 days, and thereafter slowly subsides. Histologically, cutaneous delayed hypersensitivity in humans is characterized by emigration of lymphocytes and monocytes from dermal venules, producing perivascular "cuffing" (Fig. 5-14). An associated increased microvascular permeability results from the local secretion of cytokines with escape of plasma proteins, giving rise to dermal edema and deposition of fibrin. With

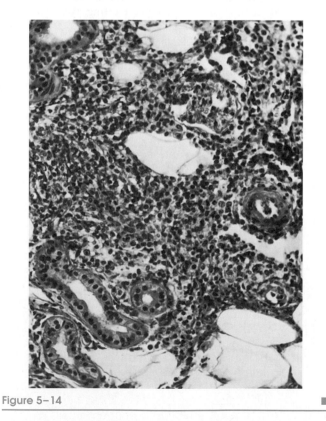

Figure 5-14 ■

A tuberculin reaction in the dermis. There is infiltration of lymphocytes and macrophages about the small vessels and skin adnexa.

certain persistent or nondegradable antigens, the initial perivascular mononuclear cell infiltrate is replaced by macrophages over a period of 2 to 3 weeks. The accumulated macrophages often undergo a morphologic transformation into epithelium-like cells and are then referred to as epithelioid cells. *A microscopic aggregation of epithelioid cells, usually surrounded by a collar of lymphocytes, is referred to as a granuloma.* The epithelioid cells often fuse to give rise to multinucleated giant cells. If the nuclei are dispersed to the periphery of the cells, the giant cells are referred to as Langerhans' type. This pattern of inflammation that is characteristic of type IV hypersensitivity is called granulomatous inflammation. Recognition of a granuloma is of great importance because of the limited number of possible conditions that can cause it. In the usual hematoxylin and eosin preparations, the epithelioid cells have a pale pink granular cytoplasm with indistinct cell boundaries, often appearing to merge into one another. The nucleus is less dense (vesicular) than that of a lymphocyte, is oval or elongated, and may show folding of the nuclear membrane. Older granulomas develop an enclosing rim of fibroblasts and connective tissue. Although some observers rely heavily on the finding of giant cells, the *identification of a granulomatous reaction actually rests on the recognition of epithelioid cells.*

The sequence of events in delayed hypersensitivity, as exemplified by the tuberculin reaction, begins with the first exposure of the individual to tubercle bacilli. CD4+ lymphocytes recognize peptide antigens of tubercle bacilli in association with class II antigens on the surface of monocytes or cutaneous dendritic (Langerhans') cells that have processed mycobacterial antigens. This process leads to the formation of sensitized CD4+ cells of the T_H1 type that remain in the circulation for long periods, sometimes years. Upon intracutaneous injection of tuberculin into such an individual, the memory T_H1 cells interact with the antigen on the surface of antigen-presenting cells and are activated (i.e., they undergo blast transformation and proliferation). These changes are accompanied by the secretion of a number of cytokines, which are responsible for the expression of delayed-type hypersensitivity (Fig. 5–15). Cytokines most relevant to this reaction and their actions are as follows:

■ IL-12, a cytokine produced by macrophages, acts early during the induction of delayed hypersensitivity. It is critical for the differentiation of T_H1 cells, which are the source of other cytokines, listed below. IL-12 is also a potent stimulator of IFN-γ secretion by T cells and NK cells.

■ IFN-γ is the most important mediator of delayed-type hypersensitivity. It is an extremely potent activator of macrophages. Activated macrophages are altered in several ways: their ability to phagocytose and kill microorganisms is markedly augmented; they express more class II molecules on the surface, thus facilitating further antigen presentation; their capacity to kill tumor cells is enhanced; and they secrete several polypeptide growth factors, such as platelet-derived growth factor (PDGF) and TGF-β, which stimulate fibroblast proliferation and augment collagen synthesis. Thus activated, macrophages serve to eliminate the offending antigen, and if the activation is sustained, fibrosis results.

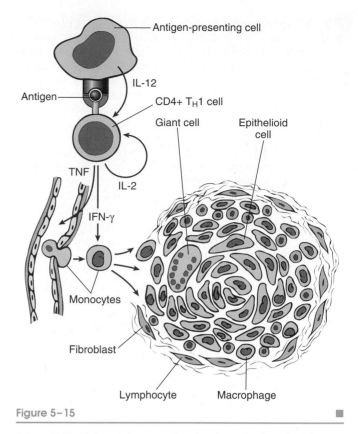

Figure 5–15 ■

Schematic illustration of the events that give rise to the formation of granuloma in type IV hypersensitivity reactions. Note the role played by T cell–derived cytokines.

■ IL-2 causes autocrine and paracrine proliferation of T cells, which accumulate at sites of delayed hypersensitivity; included in this infiltrate are some antigen-specific CD4+ T_H1 cells and many more bystander T cells activated by IL-2.

■ TNF-α and lymphotoxin are two cytokines that exert important effects on endothelial cells: (1) increased secretion of nitric oxide and prostacyclin, which in turn favors increased blood flow by causing local vasodilatation; (2) increased expression of E-selectin (Chapter 2), an adhesion molecule that promotes attachment of the passing lymphocytes and monocytes; and (3) induction and secretion of low-molecular-weight chemotactic factors such as IL-8. Together, all of these changes in the endothelium facilitate the extravasation of lymphocytes and monocytes at the site of the delayed hypersensitivity reaction.

This type of hypersensitivity is a major mechanism of defense against a variety of intracellular pathogens, including mycobacteria, fungi, and certain parasites, and may also be involved in transplant rejection and tumor immunity. The central role of CD4+ T cells in delayed hypersensitivity is manifested in patients with AIDS. Because of the loss of CD4+ cells, the host response against intracellular pathogens such as *Mycobacterium tuberculosis* is markedly impaired. The bacteria are engulfed by macrophages but are not killed, and instead of granuloma formation, there is accumulation of unactivated macrophages.

T Cell–Mediated Cytotoxicity. In this variant of type IV hypersensitivity, sensitized CD8+ T cells kill antigen-bearing target cells. Such effector cells are called cytotoxic T lymphocytes (CTLs). CTLs, directed against cell surface histocompatibility antigens, play an important role in graft rejection, to be discussed next in this chapter. They also play a role in resistance to virus infections. As discussed earlier, class I MHC molecules bind to and present viral peptides to CD8+ T lymphocytes. It is this peptide-MHC complex that is recognized by cytotoxic T lymphocytes. The lysis of infected cells before viral replication is completed leads in due course to elimination of the infection. In addition to their ability to lyse target cells, cytotoxic CD8+ cells can also secrete cytokines such as IFN-γ, which inhibits virus replication. It is believed that many tumor-associated peptides (Chapter 6) are also presented on the cell surface, and hence CTLs are also involved in tumor immunity. The mechanisms by which CD8+ cells kill their targets are beginning to be understood. Two pathways are involved. In one, the CD8+ T cells deliver the lethal hit by secreting perforin molecules that drill holes in the target cell, thus causing osmotic lysis. In the other, Fas ligands expressed on the membrane of CTLs bind to Fas molecules on the target cells, and this interaction induces apoptosis of the target cell (Chapter 1).

TRANSPLANT REJECTION

Rejection of organ transplants is a complex immunologic phenomenon that involves cell-mediated and antibody-mediated responses, both of which are targeted on the HLA antigens in the graft.

T Cell–Mediated Rejection. The classic acute rejection, which occurs within 10 to 14 days in nonimmunosuppressed recipients, is largely the result of cell-mediated immunity. As already mentioned, this involves delayed hypersensitivity and T cell–mediated cytotoxicity. The generation of CTL in response to HLA-incompatible organ grafts starts when the recipient's lymphocytes encounter foreign HLA antigens on the surface of cells in the graft. It is believed that the donor lymphoid cells ("passenger lymphocytes"), especially dendritic cells contained within the grafts, are the most important immunogens, because they are rich in both class I and class II antigens, and they also express costimulatory molecules such as B7. The generation of a T cell–mediated response against an allograft involves recognition of allogeneic class I and class II HLA molecules expressed on dendritic cells contained within the graft. Donor class I and class II molecules with their associated peptides are recognized by the T-cell receptors of host CD8+ and CD4+ cells, respectively. In addition, nonpolymorphic costimulatory molecules (e.g., the B7 protein) expressed on the antigen-presenting dendritic cells must also be recognized by their receptors (e.g., CD28 and CTLA-4) expressed on host T cells. Failure to receive the costimulatory signals leads to apoptosis of effector T cells or tolerance, rather than to an immune response, an observation that can be exploited for preventing graft rejection in animal models. The sequence of events that leads to the generation of mature CD8+ cytotoxic T lymphocytes is complex and not fully understood. A widely accepted model is presented in Figure 5–16. Once mature CTLs are generated, they lyse the grafted tissue. In addition to the specific cytotoxic T cells, lympho-

kine-secreting CD4+ T cells are also generated, as occurs in the delayed hypersensitivity reaction. This leads to increased vascular permeability and local accumulation of mononuclear cells (lymphocytes and macrophages), as previously described. The delayed hypersensitivity, with its attendant microvascular injury, produces tissue ischemia, which, along with the destruction mediated by accumulated macrophages, is an important mechanism of graft destruction.

Antibody-Mediated Rejection. Although T cells are of paramount importance in the rejection of organ transplants, antibodies also mediate rejection under two conditions:

■ *Hyperacute rejection* occurs when preformed antidonor antibodies are present in the circulation of the recipient. Such antibodies may be present in a recipient who has already rejected an organ transplant. Multiparous women who develop anti-HLA antibodies against paternal antigens shed from the fetus may also have preformed antibodies to grafts taken from their husbands or children. Previous blood transfusions from HLA-nonidentical donors can also lead to presensitization, because platelets and white cells are particularly rich in HLA antigens. In such circumstances, rejection occurs immediately after transplantation, because the circulating antibodies react with and deposit rapidly on the vascular endothelium of the grafted organ. Complement fixation occurs and an Arthus-type reaction follows.
■ Even in nonsensitized individuals, anti-HLA humoral antibodies develop concurrently with T cell–mediated rejection. The major target of antibody-mediated damage in this setting is also the vascular endothelium. Superimposed on the immunologically mediated vascular damage are platelet aggregation and coagulation, adding ischemic insult to the injury.

MORPHOLOGY OF REJECTION REACTIONS. On the basis of morphology and the mechanisms involved, rejection reactions have been classified as hyperacute, acute, and chronic.

The morphologic changes in these patterns are described as they relate to renal transplants. Similar changes would be encountered in any other vascularized visceral organ transplant.

Hyperacute Rejection. Hyperacute rejection may occur within minutes or a few hours in presensitized persons. **Basically, it is characterized by widespread acute arteritis and arteriolitis, thrombosis of vessels, and ischemic necrosis,** all of which result from reaction with preformed humoral antibodies. As a consequence of the vascular damage, the graft never becomes vascularized and it undergoes ischemic necrosis. Virtually all arterioles and arteries exhibit characteristic acute fibrinoid necrosis of their walls, with narrowing or complete occlusion of the lumina by precipitated fibrin and cellular debris. It should be noted that with the current practice of cross-matching (testing recipients for the presence of antibodies di-

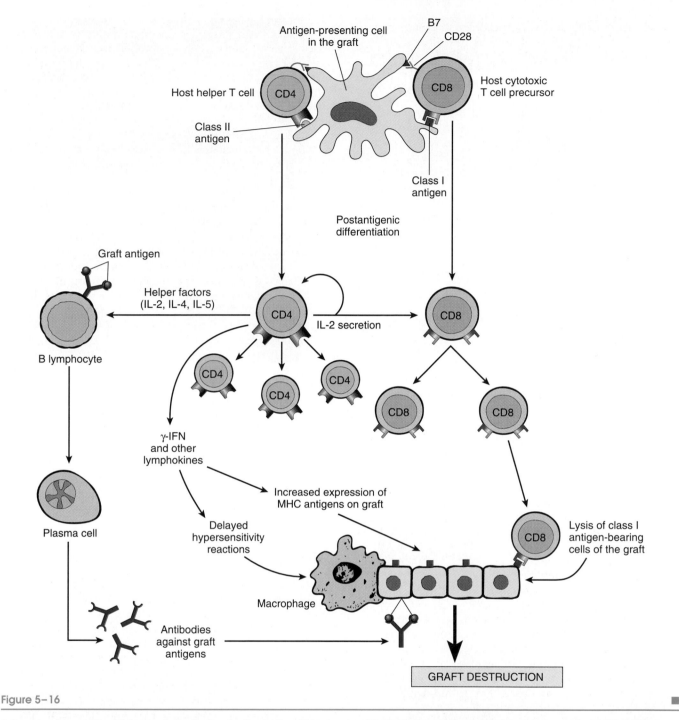

Figure 5–16 ■

Schematic representation of the events that lead to the destruction of histoincompatible grafts. Donor class I and class II antigens along with costimulatory (B7) molecules are recognized by CD8+ cytotoxic T cells and CD4+ helper T cells, respectively, of the host. The interaction of the CD4+ cells with peptides presented by class II antigens leads to proliferation of CD4+ cells and the release of interleukin 2 (IL-2) from the cells. IL-2 further augments the proliferation of CD4+ cells and also provides helper signals for the differentiation of class I-specific CD8+ cytotoxic cells. In addition to IL-2, a variety of other soluble mediators (lymphokines) that promote B-cell differentiation and participate in the induction of a local delayed hypersensitivity reaction are produced by CD4+ helper cells. Eventually, several mechanisms converge to destroy the graft: (1) lysis of cells that bear class I antigens by CD8+ cytotoxic T cells, (2) antigraft antibodies produced by sensitized B cells, and (3) nonspecific damage inflicted by macrophages and other cells that accumulate as a result of the delayed hypersensitivity reaction. MHC, major histocompatibility complex.

rected against donors' lymphocytes), hyperacute rejection is no longer a significant clinical problem. **_Acute Rejection._** Acute rejection may occur within days of transplantation in the untreated recipient or may appear suddenly months or even years later, after immunosuppression has been employed and terminated. As suggested earlier, acute graft rejection is a combined process in which both cellular and humoral tissue injuries play parts. In any one patient, one or the other mechanism may predominate. Histologically, humoral rejection is associated with vasculitis, whereas cellular rejection is marked by an interstitial mononuclear cell infiltrate.

Acute cellular rejection is most commonly seen within the initial months after transplantation and is often accompanied by the abrupt onset of clinical signs of failure of renal function. Histologically, there may be extensive interstitial mononuclear cell infiltration by CD4+ and CD8+ T cells, and edema may occur (Fig. 5–17). Plasma cells are also seen in long-standing cases. Glomerular and peritubular capillaries contain large numbers of mononuclear cells, which may also invade the tubules and cause focal tubular necrosis. In the absence of accompanying arteritis, these cellular rejections respond promptly to immunosuppressive therapy.

Acute rejection vasculitis (humoral rejection) may also be present in acute graft rejection. The histologic lesions consist of vascular (endothelial) damage due to deposition of immunoglobulins and complement. Thrombosis of damaged vessels ensues, with areas of infarction. More common than this acute type of vasculitis is so-called subacute vasculitis, characterized by marked thickening of the intima by a cushion of proliferating fibroblasts, myocytes, and foamy macrophages,

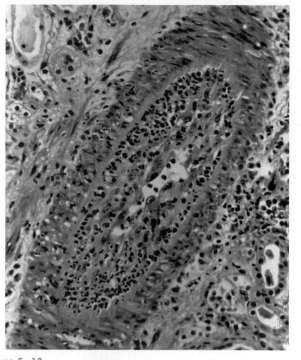

Figure 5–18

Acute humoral rejection of a renal allograft manifested by subacute vasculitis. The vascular intima is markedly thickened and inflamed. (Courtesy of Dr. Helmut Renké, Department of Pathology, Brigham and Women's Hospital, Boston.)

often leading to luminal narrowing or obliteration (Fig. 5–18). Almost all of the patients so affected also show evidence of acute cellular rejection.

Chronic Rejection. Because most instances of acute graft rejection can usually be controlled by immunosuppressive therapy, chronic changes are commonly seen in the renal allograft. Patients with chronic rejection present clinically with a progressive rise in serum creatinine levels (an index of renal dysfunction) over a period of 4 to 6 months. The vascular changes consist of dense intimal fibrosis, resulting possibly from recurrent antibody-mediated injury. These vascular lesions result in renal ischemia manifested by loss or hyalinization of glomeruli, interstitial fibrosis, and tubular atrophy and shrinkage of the renal parenchyma. The kidneys also have interstitial mononuclear cell infiltrates containing large numbers of plasma cells and numerous eosinophils.

Methods of Increasing Graft Survival. Because HLA antigens are the major targets in transplant rejection, better matching of the donor and the recipient improves graft survival. The benefits of HLA matching are most dramatic in intrafamilial (living, related donor) kidney transplants. However, the effects of HLA matching on graft survival in renal transplants from cadavers are less dramatic, possibly because of differences at other (non-HLA) minor histocompatibility antigens. Matching is more predictive of graft survival in rel-

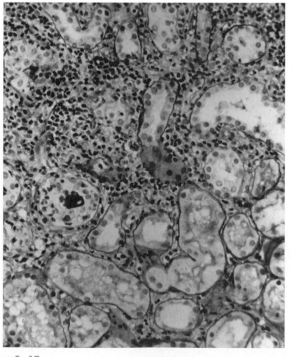

Figure 5–17

Acute cellular rejection of renal allograft manifested by a diffuse mononuclear cell infiltrate and interstitial edema. (Courtesy of Dr. Helmut Renké, Department of Pathology, Brigham and Women's Hospital, Boston.)

atively homogeneous populations such as Europeans than in extensively outbred populations such as that of the United States.

Immunosuppression of the recipient is a practical necessity in all organ transplantation except in the case of identical twins. Drugs that inhibit T cell–mediated immunity, such as cyclosporine, are a powerful and effective means of blunting the rejection reactions. However, the use of cyclosporine is limited by its significant renal toxicity. Another avenue for immunosuppression is the administration of polyclonal anti–T cell antibodies or monoclonal anti-CD3 antibodies that react with all T cells. Immunosuppression definitely improves graft survival, but it renders the individual vulnerable to opportunistic fungal, viral, and bacterial infections, and *EBV-induced lymphoid tumors*. Often, an immunosuppressed patient dies of disseminated and refractory infections rather than of organ failure. To circumvent the untoward effects of immunosuppression, much effort is devoted to producing donor-specific tolerance of host T cells. One such avenue involves preventing the activation of costimulatory pathways by the administration of antibodies against the CD28/CTLA-4 coreceptors. With such intervention, at least in experimental animals, T-cell tolerance, rather than activation, occurs.

Transplantation of Other Solid Organs. Although the kidney is the most frequently transplanted solid organ, transplantation of liver, heart, lungs, and pancreas is rapidly increasing. Liver transplantation is indicated for extrahepatic biliary atresia, certain forms of cirrhosis, and inborn errors of metabolism such as α_1-antitrypsin deficiency. Cardiac transplantation is performed most commonly in patients with cardiomyopathies. Unlike the case with kidney transplantation, in liver and heart transplantation no effort is made to match the HLA antigens of the donor and host. This peculiarity is related to the fact that compatibility of size is very important (e.g., a child cannot receive a heart transplant from an adult), and the window of time during which the harvested liver or heart retains viability is too short to allow tissue typing by currently used methods.

Transplantation of Allogeneic Hematopoietic Cells. Transplantation of bone marrow is a form of therapy increasingly employed for hematopoietic malignancies, aplastic anemias, certain immune deficiency states, and certain nonhematopoietic malignancies. The recipient is given large doses of irradiation either to destroy the malignant cells (e.g., as in leukemia) or to create a graft bed (as in aplastic anemia), and the destroyed bone marrow is replaced by marrow transplantation. *Two major problems complicate this form of transplantation: graft-versus-host disease (GVH) and transplant rejection.* GVH disease occurs when immunologically competent cells or their precursors are transplanted into recipients who are immunologically compromised because of the primary disease or from previous treatment with drugs or irradiation. When such recipients receive normal bone marrow cells from allogeneic donors, the immunocompetent T cells derived from the donor marrow recognize the recipient's tissue as "foreign" and react against it. This results in the generation of cytotoxic lymphocytes and lymphokine-secreting T cells, which are detrimental to the recipient's tissues. The resultant acute GVH syndrome causes *epithelial cell necrosis in three principal target organs: liver, skin, and gut.* Destruction of small bile ducts gives rise to jaundice, and mucosal

ulceration of the gut results in bloody diarrhea. Cutaneous involvement is manifested by a generalized rash. In addition, the host bone marrow is also severely suppressed, rendering the patient prey to infections. *Chronic GVH disease* may follow the acute syndrome or may occur insidiously. These patients may develop skin lesions resembling those of systemic sclerosis (SS) and manifestations mimicking autoimmune disorders. GVH disease is a potentially lethal complication that can be minimized but not eliminated by HLA matching. As a possible solution to this problem, T cells are depleted from the donor marrow. This protocol has proved to be a mixed blessing: the risk of GVH disease is reduced, but the incidence of graft failures and the recurrence of leukemia increase. It seems that the multifunctional T cells not only mediate GVH but also are required for the engraftment of the transplanted bone marrow stem cells and elimination of leukemia cells.

Rejection of allogeneic bone marrow transplants is mediated by both the radiation-resistant T cells and NK cells of the host. T cell–mediated rejection occurs by the same general mechanisms that were described earlier—host T cells recognize and react against alloantigens on the grafted hematopoietic cells. NK cells, by contrast, are triggered to destroy the grafted cells because the allogeneic cells fail to engage the inhibitory receptors on NK cells that are specific for self class I molecules (see Fig. 5–2). *Thus, the absence of normal self class I MHC molecules, rather than the presence of non-self MHC antigens, seems to underlie NK cell–mediated rejection of bone marrow transplants.*

■ AUTOIMMUNE DISEASES

An immune reaction against "self-antigens"—autoimmunity—is now a well-established cause of disease. In recent years a growing list of diseases have been attributed to autoimmunity, although in many instances the target antigens and the precise sequence of events leading to organ injury have not been identified. Presumed autoimmune diseases (Table 5–4) range from *single organ* (or *single cell*) *type disorders,* which involve specific immune reactions directed against one particular organ or cell type, to *multisystem diseases,* characterized by lesions in many organs and associated usually with a multiplicity of autoantibodies or cell-mediated reactions, or both. In most of the latter diseases the pathologic changes are found principally within the connective tissue and blood vessels of the various organs involved. Thus, these were once called "collagen vascular diseases" or "connective tissue diseases." As will be seen, the autoimmune reactions in these systemic diseases are not specifically directed against the constituents of connective tissue or blood vessels, but these older designations remain useful because they connote widespread lesions affecting many organs and systems.

The immunologic evidence that the diseases listed in Table 5–4 are indeed the result of autoimmune reactions is more compelling for some than for others. With SLE, the presence of a multiplicity of autoantibodies logically explains many of the observed changes. Moreover, the autoantibodies can be identified within the lesions by immunofluorescence and electron microscopic techniques. In many other disorders, such as polyarteritis nodosa, an immune-mediated basis of tissue in-

Table 5-4. AUTOIMMUNE DISEASES

Single Organ or Cell Type	Systemic
Probable	*Probable*
Hashimoto's thyroiditis	Systemic lupus ery-
Autoimmune hemolytic anemia	thematosus
Autoimmune atrophic gastritis of	Rheumatoid arthritis
pernicious anemia	Sjögren's syndrome
Autoimmune encephalomyelitis	Reiter's syndrome
Autoimmune orchitis	*Possible*
Goodpasture's syndrome*	
Autoimmune thrombocytopenia	Inflammatory myopathy
Insulin-dependent diabetes mellitus	Systemic sclerosis
Myasthenia gravis	(scleroderma)
Graves' disease	Polyarteritis nodosa
Possible	
Primary biliary cirrhosis	
Chronic active hepatitis	
Ulcerative colitis	
Membranous glomerulonephritis	

* Target is basement membrane of glomeruli and alveolar walls.

jury is suspected, but the nature of the antigen is not established. Indeed, in some cases of polyarteritis nodosa an exogenous antigen derived, for example, from hepatitis B virus may initiate the immune attack.

Only the systemic autoimmune diseases are considered in this chapter. The single-target involvements are more appropriately discussed in the chapters that deal with specific organs. Before describing individual disorders, we will consider the general nature of self-tolerance and theories about its loss.

Self-Tolerance

Immune tolerance is defined as a state in which the individual is incapable of developing an immune response against a specific antigen. *Self-tolerance refers to a lack of immune responsiveness to the individual's own tissue antigens.* Obviously, self-tolerance is necessary if our tissues are to live harmoniously with an army of lymphocytes.

Three major mechanisms are believed to prevent antiself reactivity in healthy individuals: clonal deletion, clonal anergy, and peripheral suppression (mediated, for example, by suppressor T cells). Some of these pathways of self-tolerance are illustrated in Figure 5–19 and briefly described below.

Clonal Deletion. Clonal deletion is the loss or deletion of self-reactive clones of T lymphocytes, B lymphocytes, or both during their maturation. Indeed, there is abundant evidence that *T lymphocytes bearing receptors for self-antigens are deleted within the thymus during the process of T-cell maturation.* Many autologous protein antigens are expressed in the thymus in association with MHC self-molecules. The developing T cells that express high-affinity receptors for such self-antigens are "negatively selected," or deleted, by apoptosis triggered by the activation of fas-ligand on T-cell precursors (see Fig. 1–12). Hence the peripheral T-cell pool lacks potentially self-reactive cells. Whereas clonal deletion may also

affect self-reactive B cells, this mechanism plays a less important role in B-cell tolerance.

Clonal Anergy. Many, but not all, self-reactive T cells undergo apoptosis in the thymus. Those that escape this major checkpoint are rendered inactive outside the thymus by a process known as clonal anergy. This refers to prolonged or irreversible functional inactivation of lymphocytes, induced by encounter with antigens under certain conditions. It is well established that activation of antigen-specific T cells requires two signals: recognition of peptide antigen in association with MHC molecules on the surface of antigen-presenting cells (APCs) and a set of second signals delivered by recognition of costimulatory molecules (e.g., B7-1 and B7-2) expressed by APCs. If the antigen is presented by cells that do not express costimulators, a negative signal is delivered and the cell becomes anergic. Such a cell then fails to be activated even if the relevant antigen is presented by competent APCs (e.g., macrophages, dendritic cells) that express costimulatory molecules. Autoreactive T cells may undergo anergy when they encounter self-antigens on somatic tissues that, unlike APC, do not express costimulatory molecules. Clonal anergy affects

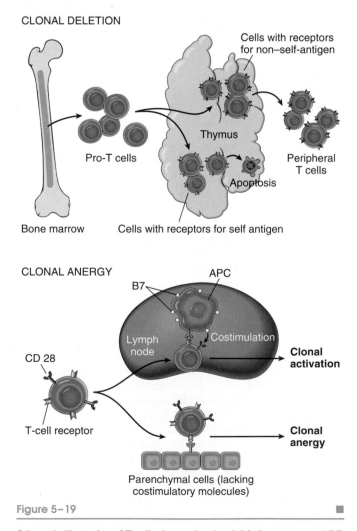

CLONAL DELETION

Cells with receptors for non–self-antigen

Thymus

Pro-T cells

Peripheral T cells

Apoptosis

Bone marrow   Cells with receptors for self antigen

CLONAL ANERGY

B7   APC

Lymph node   Costimulation

CD 28   Clonal activation

T-cell receptor

Clonal anergy

Parenchymal cells (lacking costimulatory molecules)

Figure 5–19   ■

Schematic illustration of T-cell tolerance by clonal deletion or anergy. APC, antigen-presenting cells.

B cells as well and is probably the major mechanism for B-cell tolerance to self-antigens.

Peripheral Suppression by T Cells. Although clonal deletion and anergy are the primary mechanisms of self-tolerance, it is believed that additional fail-safe mechanisms must also exist. Many factors, both cellular and humoral, that can actively suppress lymphocytes have been described. However, most interest has focused on suppressor T cells. These cells, like cytotoxic T cells, are CD8+ but are believed to comprise a distinct subset. In experimental models it is possible to demonstrate inactivation of both helper T cells and B cells by suppressor T cells. These effects may be mediated by the secretion of inhibitory cytokines such as IL-10. At present, however, the molecular basis of suppressor cell action remains mysterious.

In summary, prevention of autoimmunity is so vital to survival that several mechanisms have evolved to protect us from our "protectors." Because helper T cells are critical control elements for both cellular and humoral immunity, *tolerance of self-reactive T cells is a major mechanism for prevention of autoimmune diseases.* Most self-antigens are T cell dependent; therefore, autoantibody formation may be prevented by tolerance of either hapten-specific B cells or the relevant helper T cells, or both. Lymphocytes (both T and B cells) that "leak" through the barriers of clonal deletion or anergy are restrained by suppressor mechanisms.

Mechanisms of Autoimmune Disease

Breakdown of one or more of the mechanisms of self-tolerance can unleash an immunologic attack on tissues that leads to the development of autoimmune diseases. Although immunocompetent cells are undoubtedly involved in mediating the tissue injury, we do not know the precise influences that initiate their reactions against self, but genetic factors and infectious agents are thought to be important. First, the mechanisms involved in the breakdown of self-tolerance will be discussed, followed by the genetic and microbial factors.

LOSS OF SELF-TOLERANCE

Bypass of Helper T-Cell Tolerance. Many self-antigens have multiple determinants, some recognized by B cells (called haptens), others by T cells (called carriers). Antibody response occurs only when potentially self-reactive B cells receive help from T cells. Tolerance to such antigens is often associated with clonal deletion or clonal anergy of helper T cells in the presence of fully competent specific B cells. Therefore, this form of tolerance may be overcome if the need for tolerant helper T cells is bypassed or substituted. This can be accomplished by at least two mechanisms:

1. *Modification of the molecule.* If the T-cell epitope of a self-antigen is modified, it may be recognized as foreign by clones of helper T cells that were not deleted (Fig. 5–20). These could then cooperate with the B cells, leading to the formation of autoantibodies. Such modification of the T-cell determinants of an autoantigen may result from complexing with drugs or microorganisms. For example, autoimmune hemolytic anemia, which occurs after the administration of certain drugs, may result from drug-induced alterations in the red cell surface that create antigens that can be recognized by T-helper cells (Chapter 12).

2. *Expression of costimulatory molecules.* As mentioned earlier, autoreactive T cells become anergic if they are exposed to self-antigens on parenchymal cells that do not express costimulatory molecules. Infections and the resultant inflammation can activate macrophages to express costimulatory molecules, and also present self-antigen, thereby triggering the activation of autoreactive T cells.

Molecular Mimicry. Some infectious agents share epitopes with self-antigens. An immune response against such

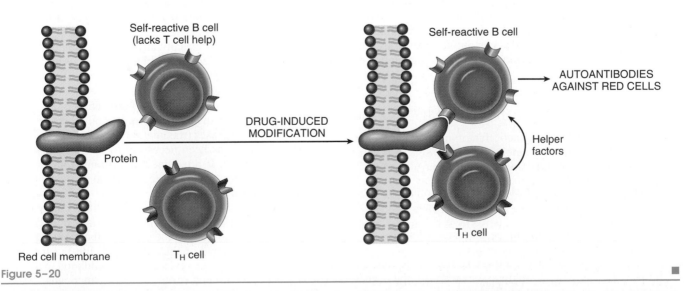

Figure 5–20

Schematic representation of how drug-induced modification of a red cell membrane protein may be recognized by T-helper cells and lead to formation of anti-red antibodies.

microbes may produce a tissue-damaging reaction against the cross-reacting self-antigen. Such a scenario is considered likely in the pathogenesis of rheumatic heart disease, which follows infection with certain streptococci. Antibodies against streptococcal antigens apparently recognize and damage cardiac valves and myocardium (see Fig. 11–11 in Chapter 11). Type I diabetes, characterized by immunologically mediated destruction of pancreatic islet beta cells, is sometimes associated with infection with Coxsackie virus. Apparently T cells directed against certain viral antigens cross-react with glutamic decarboxylase, a protein expressed by beta cells of the islets (Chapter 17).

Polyclonal Lymphocyte Activation. It was mentioned earlier that in some instances self-tolerance may be maintained by anergy of autoreactive lymphocytes that were not deleted during development. Autoimmunity may occur if such self-reactive but anergic clones are stimulated and reactivated by antigen-independent mechanisms. In the case of B cells, several microbial products, especially endotoxins, can act as powerful polyclonal stimulants. Mice injected with endotoxins produce antibodies of many specificities, including autoantibodies. In humans, infection of B cells with EBV could also achieve the same effects because all human B cells are activated by EBV. T cells, on the other hand, may be stimulated by bacterial superantigens that can bind to MHC class II molecules and activate a large number of T cells independent of specific antigens.

Imbalance of Suppressor-Helper T-Cell Function. It may be expected from our discussion of suppressor T cells that any loss of their function will contribute to autoimmunity and, conversely, that excessive T-cell help may drive B cells to extremely high levels of autoantibody production. Experimental evidence supporting both of these possibilities is derived from the study of murine models of SLE.

Emergence of Sequestered Antigens. Certain antigens are anatomically segregated from the developing immune system, and hence clonal deletion or anergy fails to occur. If they are released into the circulation after trauma or infection, they induce an immune response, just as any non–self-antigen would. An example in this category is sympathetic ophthalmitis, an immunologically mediated inflammation of the eyes following trauma to one of the eyes. Presumably, an immune response against the sequestered ocular antigens develops, followed by immunologically mediated damage to the target antigen in both of the eyes.

GENETIC FACTORS IN AUTOIMMUNITY

There is little doubt that genetic factors play a significant role in the predisposition to autoimmune diseases. This conclusion is derived from three lines of evidence:

■ Familial clustering of several human autoimmune diseases such as SLE, autoimmune hemolytic anemia, and autoimmune thyroiditis.
■ Linkage of several autoimmune diseases with HLA, especially class II antigens.
■ Induction of autoimmune diseases in transgenic rats. In humans, HLA-B27 is strongly associated with the occurrence of certain autoimmune diseases such as ankylosing spondylitis. When cloned human HLA-B27 gene is introduced into the germ line of rats, the transgenic rats develop ankylosing spondylitis. This model provides direct evidence for genetic regulation of autoimmunity.

The precise role of MHC genes in autoimmunity is not entirely clear. As discussed earlier, it is likely that the MHC class II alleles influence the presentation of autoantigenic peptides to T cells. It should be noted, however, that genes outside the MHC also influence predisposition to autoimmunity, by mechanisms that are unclear.

MICROBIAL AGENTS IN AUTOIMMUNITY

A variety of microbes, including bacteria, mycoplasmas, and viruses, have been implicated in the triggering of autoimmunity at one time or another.

Microbes may trigger autoimmune reactions in several ways. First, microbial antigens and autoantigens may become associated to form immunogenic units and bypass T-cell tolerance, as described earlier. Second, some viruses (such as EBV) and bacterial products are nonspecific polyclonal B-cell mitogens and thus may induce formation of autoantibodies. Third, infection may result in loss of suppressor T-cell function by mechanisms that at present are not entirely clear. Viruses and other microbes, particularly certain bacteria such as streptococci and *Klebsiella* organisms, may share cross-reacting epitopes with self-antigens, as discussed earlier. Despite much suggestive data, at present there is no clear evidence to implicate any microbe in the causation of human autoimmune disease.

Against this general background we turn to the individual systemic autoimmune diseases. Although each disease is discussed separately, it will be apparent that there is considerable overlap in clinical, serologic, and morphologic features.

Systemic Lupus Erythematosus

SLE is an autoimmune, multisystem disease of protean manifestations and variable behavior. *Clinically,* it is an unpredictable, remitting, relapsing disease of acute or insidious onset that may involve virtually any organ in the body; however, it principally affects the skin, kidneys, serosal membranes, joints, and heart. *Immunologically,* the disease involves a bewildering array of autoantibodies, especially antinuclear antibodies. The clinical presentation of SLE is so variable and bears so many similarities to other autoimmune connective tissue diseases (rheumatoid arthritis, polymyositis, and others) that it has been necessary to develop diagnostic criteria (Table 5–5). If a patient demonstrates four or more of the criteria during any interval of observation, the diagnosis of SLE is established.

SLE is a fairly common disease; its incidence may be as high as one case per 2500 persons in certain populations. There is a strong female preponderance—about 10:1. It usually arises in the second or third decade of life but may become manifest at any age, even in early childhood. The disease is more common and severe in black Americans.

Etiology and Pathogenesis. The fundamental defect in SLE seems to be a failure to maintain self-tolerance. As a

Table 5-5. THE 1982 REVISED CRITERIA FOR THE CLASSIFICATION OF SLE*

1. Butterfly rash
2. Discoid lupus
3. Photosensitivity
4. Oral ulcers
5. Arthritis
6. Serositis
   a. Pleuritis: rub heard by a physician or pleural effusion, *or*
   b. Pericarditis: documented by ECG or rub, or evidence of pericardial effusion
7. Renal disorder
   a. Persistent proteinuria >0.5 gm/dl/day
   b. Cellular casts: may be red cell, hemoglobin, granular, tubular, or mixed
8. Neurologic disorder
   a. Seizures: in the absence of offending drugs or known metabolic derangements
   b. Psychosis: in the absence of offending drugs
9. Hematopoietic disorder
   a. Hemolytic anemia: with reticulocytosis *or*
   b. Leukopenia: 4000 cells/μl on two or more occasions *or*
   c. Lymphopenia: 1500 cells/μl on two or more occasions *or*
   d. Thrombocytopenia: 100,000/μl in the absence of offending drugs
10. Immunologic disorder
    a. Positive LE cell preparation *or*
    b. Anti-DNA: presence of antibody to untreated DNA in abnormal titer *or*
    c. Anti-Sm: presence of antibody to Sm nuclear antigen *or*
    d. False-positive STS known to be positive for at least 6 months and confirmed by TPI or FTA tests
11. Antinuclear antibody. An abnormal titer of antinuclear antibody by immunofluorescence or an equivalent assay at any point in time and in the absence of drugs known to be associated with "drug-induced lupus" syndrome

STS, serologic test for syphilis; TPI, treponemal inhibition; FTA, fluorescent treponemal antibody.

* The proposed classification is based on 11 criteria. For the purpose of identifying patients in clinical studies, a person shall be said to have SLE if any four or more of the 11 criteria are present serially or simultaneously, during any interval of observation.

Modified from Tan EM, et al: The 1982 revised criteria for the classification of systemic lupus erythematosus. Arthritis Rheum 25:1271, 1982. Reprinted from Arthritis and Rheumatism Journal, copyright 1982. Used by permission of the American Rheumatism Association.

consequence, a wide array of autoantibodies that damage tissues is produced. The cellular and molecular basis of antoimmunity in SLE is still not clear. The spectrum of autoantibodies will be described first, followed by a brief review of the theories that attempt to explain their origins.

Antinuclear Antibodies (ANAs). ANAs are directed against several nuclear antigens and can be grouped into four categories: (1) antibodies to DNA, (2) antibodies to histones, (3) antibodies to nonhistone proteins bound to RNA, and (4) antibodies to nucleolar antigens. Several techniques are employed to detect ANAs. Clinically, the most commonly utilized method is indirect immunofluorescence, which detects a variety of nuclear antigens, including DNA, RNA, and proteins *(generic ANA)*. The pattern of nuclear fluorescence suggests the type of antibody present in the patient's serum. Four basic patterns are recognized:

■ Homogeneous or diffuse staining usually reflects antibodies to chromatin, histones, and double-stranded DNA.

■ Rim or peripheral staining patterns are most commonly indicative of antibodies to double-stranded DNA.
■ Speckled pattern refers to the presence of uniform or variable-sized speckles. It reflects the presence of antibodies to non-DNA nuclear constituents such as antibodies to histones and ribonucleoproteins. These components are easily extracted with salt solutions, and hence are sometimes called extractable nuclear antigens (ENAs). Examples include Sm antigen and SS-A and SS-B antigens (Table 5-6).
■ Nucleolar pattern refers to the presence of a few discrete spots of fluorescence within the nucleus that represent antibodies to nucleolar RNA. This pattern is reported most often in patients with systemic sclerosis.

It must be emphasized, however, that the patterns are not absolutely specific for the type of antibody. The immunofluorescence test for ANA is quite *sensitive* for the detection of SLE, but it is not *specific*. Table 5-6 shows that the ANAs detected by this technique are present not only in SLE but also in several other related autoimmune diseases. Furthermore, approximately 10% of normal persons have low titers of these antibodies, the incidence increasing with age. Some clinically useful ANAs are listed in Table 5-6. It will be noted that antibodies to double-stranded DNA and the so-called Smith (Sm) antigen are virtually diagnostic of SLE.

Antibodies against blood cells, including red cells, platelets, and lymphocytes, are found in many patients. Antiphospholipid antibodies are present in 30% to 40% of lupus patients and react with a wide variety of anionic phospholipids. Some bind to cardiolipin antigen, used in serologic tests for syphilis, and therefore lupus patients may have a false-positive test (e.g., VDRL test) result for syphilis. Because phospholipids are required for blood clotting, patients with antiphospholipid antibodies may display prolongation of in vitro clotting tests, such as partial thromboplastin time, that are not corrected by mixing with normal plasma (Chapter 12). Therefore, these antibodies are sometimes referred to as "lupus anticoagulant." Despite having a circulating anticoagulant that delays clotting in vitro, these patients have complications associated with a *pro*coagulant state. They tend to have venous and arterial thromboses, thrombocytopenia, and recurrent spontaneous miscarriages. The pathogenesis of thrombosis in patients with antiphospholipid antibodies is unknown. Proposed mechanisms include direct endothelial cell injury, antibody-mediated platelet activation, and inhibition of endogenous anticoagulants such as protein C.

Genetic Factors. The evidence supporting a genetic predisposition to SLE takes many forms.

■ There is a high rate of concordance (30%) in monozygotic twins.
■ Family members have an increased risk of developing SLE, and clinically unaffected first-degree relatives may reveal autoantibodies.
■ In North American Caucasian populations there is a positive association between SLE and class II HLA genes, particularly at the HLA-DQ locus.
■ Some lupus patients (about 6%) have inherited deficiencies of complement components. Lack of complement presumably impairs removal of immune complexes from the cir-

Table 5–6. PREVALENCE OF ANTINUCLEAR ANTIBODIES IN VARIOUS AUTOIMMUNE DISEASES

		Disease				
Nature of Antigen	*Antibody System*	*SLE (%)*	*Systemic Sclerosis Diffuse (%)*	*Limited Scleroderma (%)*	*Sjögren's Syndrome (%)*	*Polymyositis (%)*
Many nuclear antigens (DNA, RNA, proteins)	Generic ANA (indirect IF)	>95	70–90	70–90	50–90	40–60
Native DNA	Anti–double-stranded DNA	40–70	<5	<5	<5	<5
Ribonucleoprotein (Smith antigen)	Anti-Sm	15–30	<5	<5	<5	<5
Ribonucleoprotein	SS-A(Ro)	25–60	<5	<5	85–95	10
Ribonucleoprotein	SS-B(La)	10–35	<5	<5	70–90	<5
DNA topoisomerase I	Scl-70	<5	70–75	10–15	<5	<5
Centromeric proteins	Anticentromere	<5	<10	60–80	<5	<5
Histidyl-tRNA synthetase (Cytoplasmic)	Jo-1	<5	<5	<5	<5	20–40

Boxed entries indicate high correlation.
Data modified from von Mühlen CA, Tan EM: Autoantibodies in diagnosis of systemic rheumatic diseases. Semin Arthritis Rheum 24:323, 1995.

culation and favors tissue deposition, giving rise to tissue injury.

Nongenetic Factors. The role of nongenetic factors in initiating autoimmunity is best exemplified by the occurrence of an SLE-like syndrome in patients receiving certain *drugs,* such as procainamide and hydralazine. Most patients treated with procainamide for more than 6 months develop ANAs, and clinical features of SLE appear in 15% to 20%. *Sex hormones* seem to exert an important influence on the occurrence of SLE. Androgens appear to protect, whereas estrogens seem to favor the development of SLE: witness the overwhelming female preponderance of the disease. Exposure to ultraviolet light is another environmental factor that exacerbates the disease in many individuals. Ultraviolet light may trigger formation of *DNA–anti-DNA immune complexes* by damaging DNA, or may possibly modulate immune responses.

Immunologic Factors. With the host of autoantibodies that have been described, it will come as no surprise that *B-cell hyperactivity is a feature of SLE.* There is overwhelming evidence that B cells are "turned on" in these patients, but the basis of this B-cell hyperactivity is not entirely clear. In theory, excessive B-cell activation could result from an intrinsic defect in B cells, excessive stimulation by helper T cells, or a defect in suppressor T cells that fails to dampen the B-cell response. Recent studies lay the blame squarely on the shoulders of CD4+ helper T cells that drive self-reactive B cells to make autoantibodies. The mechanisms by which T cells lose self-tolerance are shrouded in mystery. It is clear, however, that the basis of immunologic dysregulation is multifac-

torial, conditioned by the genetic background of the host as well as some environmental triggers (Fig. 5–21).

Mechanisms of Tissue Injury. Regardless of the exact sequence by which autoantibodies are formed, they are clearly the mediators of tissue injury. Most of the visceral lesions are mediated by immune complexes (type III hypersensitivity). DNA–anti-DNA complexes can be detected in the glomeruli. It is believed that free DNA binds first to the basement membrane, followed by the formation of DNA–anti-DNA complexes in situ. Low levels of serum complement and granular deposits of complement and immunoglobulins in the glomeruli further support the immune complex nature of the disease. On the other hand, autoantibodies against red cells, white cells, and platelets mediate their effects via type II hypersensitivity. There is no evidence that ANAs, which are involved in immune complex formation, can permeate intact cells. However, if cell nuclei are exposed, the ANAs can bind to them. In tissues, nuclei of damaged cells react with ANAs, lose their chromatin pattern, and become homogeneous, to produce so-called *LE bodies* or *hematoxylin bodies.* Related to this phenomenon is the *LE cell, which is seen only in vitro.* Basically, the LE cell is any phagocytic leukocyte (neutrophil or macrophage) that has engulfed the denatured nucleus of an injured cell. When blood is withdrawn and agitated, a sufficient number of leukocytes can be damaged to thus expose their nuclei to ANAs. The LE cell test is positive in up to 70% of patients with SLE. However, with newer techniques for detection of ANA, this test is now largely of historical interest.

To summarize, SLE appears to be a multifactorial disease involving complex interactions among genetic, hormonal, and

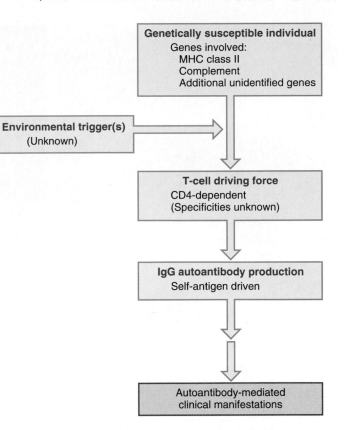

Figure 5–21   ■

Model for the pathogenesis of systemic lupus erythematosus. (From Drake CG, Kotzin BL: Genetic and immunologic mechanisms in the pathogenesis of systemic lupus erythematosus. Curr Opin Immunol 4: 733, 1992.)

environmental factors, all of which presumably act in concert to produce pronounced B-cell activation, resulting in the production of several autoantibodies. Each factor may be necessary but not enough for the expression of disease, and the relative importance of various factors may vary in different individuals.

MORPHOLOGY. The morphologic changes in SLE result largely from the formation of immune complexes in a variety of tissues. SLE is therefore a systemic disease with protean manifestations. Although many organs may be involved, some are affected more than others (Table 5–7). We will first discuss changes in small blood vessels that may be present in any tissue and then the specific anatomic lesions in the organs most frequently involved.

An **acute necrotizing vasculitis** affecting small arteries and arterioles may be present in any tissue, although skin and muscles are most commonly affected. The arteritis is characterized by necrosis and fibrinoid deposits within the vessel walls, which contain immunoglobulins, DNA, the third component of complement (C3), and fibrinogen. At a later stage, the involved vessels undergo fibrous thickening with luminal narrowing. Frequently, a perivascular lymphocytic infiltrate is present.

Skin lesions are prominent clinical findings in these patients. Classically, the lesion is an erythematous or maculopapular eruption over the malar eminences and bridge of the nose, creating a butterfly pattern. A similar rash may be present elsewhere on the extremities and trunk. It is usually **exacerbated by exposure to sunlight** or **ultraviolet light** in tanning parlors. Microscopically, the areas of involvement show liquefactive de-

■

Table 5–7.   DISTRIBUTION OF LESIONS IN SLE

Site of Lesion	Approximate Percentage of Cases
Joints*	95
Kidneys*	60
Heart*	50
Serous membranes*	40
Skin	80
Lymph node enlargement	60
Gastrointestinal tract	30
Central nervous system	30
Liver	25
Spleen	20
Eyes	20
Lungs	15
Peripheral nervous system	10

* Lesions cause major clinical findings.

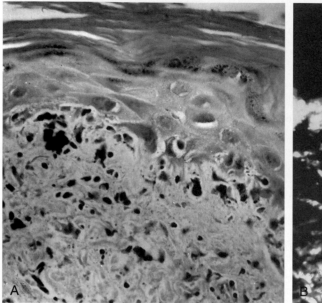

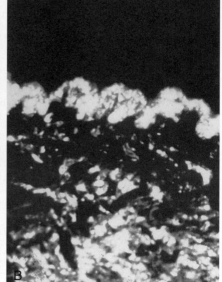

Figure 5-22 ■

Systemic lupus erythematosus involving the skin. *A*, Hematoxylin and eosin-stained section shows liquefactive degeneration of the basal layer of epidermis and edema at the dermoepidermal junction. *B*, Immunofluorescence micrograph stained for IgG reveals deposits of immunoglobulin along the dermoepidermal junction. (Courtesy of Dr. Candace Kasper, Department of Pathology, University of Texas Southwestern Medical School, Dallas.)

generation of the basal layer of the epidermis, edema at the dermoepidermal junction, and mononuclear infiltrates around blood vessels and appendages (Fig. 5–22).

Deposits of immunoglobulin and complement can be seen along the dermoepidermal junction, in both involved and uninvolved skin. In 20% to 30% of patients, so-called **discoid lupus** develops. This takes the form of coin-shaped or disc-like erythematous raised patches with adherent keratotic scaling, which may progress to atrophic scarring. These lesions may be present anywhere on the body. Discoid lesions may be present without the characteristic systemic involvement of SLE, but approximately 5% to 10% of such cases eventually progress to SLE.

Serosal membranes, particularly the pericardium and pleura, may exhibit a variety of changes ranging from serous effusions or fibrinous exudation in acute cases to fibrous opacification in chronic cases.

Cardiovascular system involvement is manifested primarily in the form of pericarditis. Symptomatic or asymptomatic pericardial involvement is present in most patients. Myocarditis, manifested as nonspecific mononuclear cell infiltration, may also be present but is less common. Valvular endocarditis, sometimes called Libman-Sacks endocarditis, may occur, but with widespread use of steroids its incidence has declined. This **nonbacterial verrucous endocarditis** takes the form of single or multiple, irregular, 1- to 3-mm warty deposits on any valve in the heart, distinctively on **either surface of the leaflets** (i.e., on the surface exposed to the forward flow of the blood or on the underside of the leaflet) (Fig. 5–23). By contrast, an increasing number of patients show clinical and anatomic manifestations of coro-

nary artery disease. The basis of accelerated atherosclerosis is not fully understood, but it seems to be multifactorial. Glucocorticoid treatment causes alterations in lipid metabolism and renal disease causes hypertension—both of these are risk factors for atherosclerosis (Chapter 10).

Kidney involvement is one of the most important anatomic features of SLE, and renal failure is an important cause of death. Although the kidney appears normal by light microscopy in 25% to 30% of cases, almost all cases of SLE show some renal abnormality if examined by immunofluorescence and electron microscopy. According to the World Health Organization morphologic classification, five patterns are recognized: (1) normal by light, electron, and immunofluorescent microscopy (class I), which is quite rare; (2) mesangial lupus glomerulonephritis (class II); (3) focal glomerulonephritis (class III); (4) diffuse proliferative glomerulonephritis (class IV); and (5) membranous glomerulonephritis (class V). The pathogenesis of all forms of glomerulonephritis involves deposition of DNA–anti-DNA complexes within the glomeruli. These evoke an inflammatory response that may cause proliferation of the endothelial, mesangial, and epithelial cells and, in severe cases, necrosis of the glomeruli.

Mesangial lupus nephritis is seen in 20% of cases and is associated with mild clinical symptoms. Immune complexes deposit in the mesangium, with a slight increase in the mesangial matrix and cellularity.

Focal proliferative glomerulonephritis implies involvement of portions of less than 50% of glomeruli. It is seen in approximately 25% of cases. Typically, one or several glomerular lobules within an otherwise normal glomerulus exhibit swelling and proliferation of endothelial and mesangial cells, foci of acute

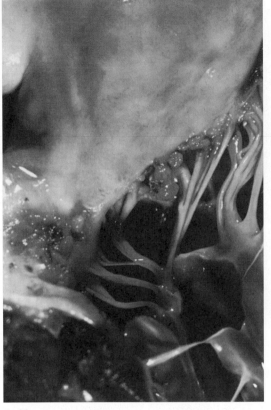

Figure 5–23   ■

Libman-Sacks endocarditis of the mitral valve in lupus erythematosus. The small vegetations attached to the margin of the valve leaflet are easily seen.

capillary necrosis infiltrated with neutrophils, and sometimes fibrinoid deposits and intracapillary thrombi. Focal lesions are usually associated with mild clinical manifestations such as microscopic hematuria and proteinuria. Transitions to more serious forms of renal involvement may occur in some patients.

Diffuse proliferative glomerulonephritis is the most common form of renal lesion, affecting 45% to 50% of patients. Most of the glomeruli show proliferation of endothelial and mesangial cells affecting the entire glomerulus. Thus, there is diffuse hypercellularity of the glomeruli (Fig. 5–24). Sometimes macrophages and proliferated epithelial cells fill Bowman's space to create crescent-shaped masses of cells, not surprisingly referred to as "crescents." Electron microscopy reveals subendothelial immune complexes (between endothelium and basement membrane) (Fig. 5–25). Immune complexes can also be visualized by staining with fluorescent antibodies directed against immunoglobulins or complement. As described earlier, a granular fluorescent staining pattern is seen (see Fig. 5–13). When extensive, immune complexes create a peculiar thickening of the capillary wall, which appears to resemble rigid wire loops on routine light microscopy (Fig. 5–26). In

due course, glomerular injury gives rise to scarring (glomerulosclerosis). These patients are overtly symptomatic. Most have hematuria with moderate to severe proteinuria, hypertension, and renal insufficiency.

Membranous glomerulonephritis is the designation given to glomerular disease in which the principal histologic change consists of widespread thickening of the capillary wall. It occurs in 15% of cases. Membranous glomerulonephritis associated with SLE is very similar, if not identical, to that encountered in idiopathic membranous glomerulopathy, and is described more fully in Chapter 14. Thickening of glomerular capillary walls is the consequence of both the increased deposition of basement membrane–like material and the accumulation of immune complexes between the basement membrane and the visceral epithelium (subepithelial). This form of glomerular lesion is almost always associated with severe proteinuria or the overt nephrotic syndrome (Chapter 14).

Interstitial and tubular lesions are also seen in SLE. In approximately 50% of patients, granular deposits composed of immunoglobulin and complement are present around the tubules. Immune complex—mediated tubule injury leads to diffuse interstitial fibrosis.

Joint involvement, although very common clinically, **is usually not associated with striking anatomic changes nor with joint deformity.** When present, it consists of swelling and a nonspecific mononuclear cell infiltration in the synovial membranes. Erosion of the membranes and destruction of articular cartilage, such as occurs with RA, is exceedingly rare.

Central nervous system involvement is common, resulting from microvascular injury that gives rise to multifocal cerebral microinfarcts. Neuronal damage may also be caused by antineuronal antibodies.

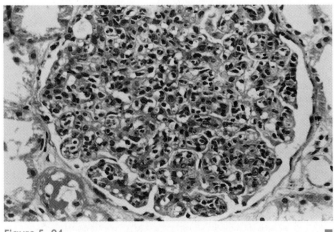

Figure 5–24   ■

Lupus nephritis, diffuse proliferative type. Note the marked increase in cellularity throughout the glomerulus. Hematoxylin and eosin stain. (Courtesy of Dr. Helmut Renké, Department of Pathology, Brigham and Women's Hospital, Boston.)

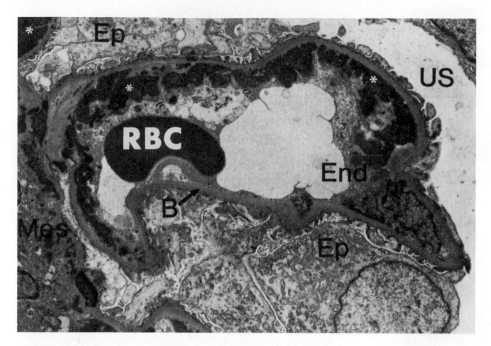

Figure 5–25 ■

Electron micrograph of a renal glomerular capillary loop from a patient with systemic lupus erythematosus nephritis. Subendothelial dense deposits correspond to "wire loops" seen by light microscopy. End, endothelium; Mes, mesangium; Ep, epithelial cell with foot processes; RBC, red blood cell in capillary lumen; B, basement membrane; US, urinary space; *, electron-dense deposits in subendothelial location. (Courtesy of Dr. Edwin Eigenbrodt, Department of Pathology, University of Texas Southwestern Medical School, Dallas.)

The **spleen** may be of normal size or moderately enlarged. Capsular fibrous thickening is common, as is follicular hyperplasia. One of the most constant alterations in spleens of both normal and abnormal size consists of a marked perivascular fibrosis, producing so-called **onion-skin lesions** around the central penicilliary arteries.

Many **other organs and tissues** may be involved. The changes consist essentially of acute vasculitis of the small vessels, foci of mononuclear infiltrations, and fibrinoid deposits. In addition, lungs may reveal interstitial fibrosis, along with pleural inflammation; the liver shows nonspecific inflammation of the portal tracts.

Clinical Manifestations. The diagnosis of SLE may be obvious in a young woman with a classic butterfly rash over the face, fever, pain but no deformity in one or more peripheral joints (feet, ankles, knees, hips, fingers, wrists, elbows, shoulders), pleuritic chest pain, and photosensitivity. However, in many patients the presentation of SLE is subtle and puzzling, taking forms such as a febrile illness of unknown origin, abnormal urinary findings, or neuropsychiatric manifestations, including psychosis. A variety of clinical findings may point toward renal involvement, including hematuria, red cell casts, proteinuria, and, in some cases, the classic nephrotic syndrome (Chapter 14). Renal failure may occur, especially in patients with diffuse proliferative or membranous glomerulonephritis, or both. The hematologic derangements mentioned (see Table 5–5) may in some cases be the presenting manifestation as well as the dominant clinical problem. ANAs can be found in virtually 100% of patients, but they can also be found in patients with other autoimmune disorders. As mentioned earlier, anti–double-stranded DNA antibodies are considered highly diagnostic of SLE. Serum complement levels are low, either because of an inherited deficiency or, more commonly, as a result of deposition in immune complexes. The titer of anti–double-stranded DNA antibodies and the level of serum complement are correlated with the severity of renal disease.

The course of SLE is extremely variable. Some unfortunate individuals follow a progressively downhill course to death within months. More often the disease is characterized by flare-ups and remissions. Acute attacks are usually controlled by adrenocortical steroids or immunosuppressive drugs. Overall, the 10-year survival rate is approximately 70%. Renal fail-

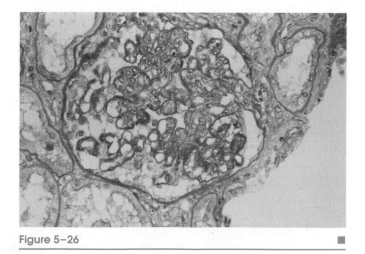

Figure 5–26 ■

Lupus nephritis. A glomerulus with several "wire loop" lesions representing extensive subendothelial deposits of immune complexes. PAS stain. (Courtesy of Dr. Helmut Renké, Department of Pathology, Brigham and Women's Hospital, Boston.)

ure, intercurrent infections, and diffuse central nervous system involvement are the major causes of death.

Rheumatoid Arthritis

Rheumatoid arthritis (RA) is a systemic, chronic inflammatory disease that affects principally the joints and sometimes many other organs and tissues throughout the body as well. More specifically, *the disease is characterized by a nonsuppurative proliferative synovitis, which in time leads to the destruction of articular cartilage and progressive disabling arthritis.* When extra-articular involvement develops—for example, of the skin, heart, blood vessels, muscles, and lungs—RA assumes more than a passing resemblance to SLE and scleroderma and, along with these entities, is sometimes referred to as a connective tissue disease.

RA is a very common condition, with a prevalence of approximately 1%. It usually has its onset in the fourth or fifth decade but may begin at any age. It is three to five times more common in women than in men. Because the pathogenesis of this condition is facilitated by a knowledge of the morphologic changes, these are reviewed first.

MORPHOLOGY. RA is a systemic disease that can cause significant damage to many organs. Its most destructive effects are seen in the joints. It produces **symmetric arthritis, which affects principally the small joints** of the hands and feet, ankles, knees, wrists, elbows, and shoulders. Typically, the proximal interphalangeal and metacarpophalangeal joints are affected, but distal interphalangeal joints are spared. Axial involvement, when it occurs, is limited to the upper cervical spine; similarly, hip joint involvement is extremely uncommon. Histologically, the affected joints show chronic synovitis. There is proliferation and hypertrophy of synovial lining cells, resulting sometimes in the formation of finger-like (villous) projections. The subsynovial connective tissue is heavily infiltrated by lymphocytes, macrophages, and plasma cells; often there is formation of lymphoid nodules. Neovascularization is prominent, with plump endothelial cells that express high levels of adhesion molecules (Fig. 5–27). The highly vascularized, inflammatory, reduplicated synovium that covers the articular cartilaginous surfaces is known as a **pannus** (mantle). With full-blown inflammatory joint involvement, periarticular soft tissue edema usually develops, which is classically manifested first by fusiform swelling of the proximal interphalangeal joints. With progression of the disease, the articular cartilage subjacent to the pannus is eroded and in time virtually destroyed. The subarticular bone may also be attacked and eroded. Eventually the pannus fills the joint space, and subsequent **fibrosis and calcification** may cause **permanent ankylosis**.

Early in the disease the synovial fluid is increased in volume, becomes turbid because of an inflammatory infiltrate, and loses some of its mucin content (thus forming a poor mucin clot when mixed with dilute acetic acid). Although the synovial membrane is infiltrated by chronic inflammatory cells, **the synovial fluid contains acute inflammatory cells.** The contained neutrophils exhibit granular inclusions of phagocytized immune complexes.

Rheumatoid subcutaneous nodules eventually appear in about one quarter of patients; the nodules usually occur along the extensor surface of the forearm or other areas subjected to mechanical pressure. They are firm, nontender, oval or rounded masses up to 2 cm in diameter. Less commonly, these nodules appear in the Achilles tendons, on the back of the skull, overlying the ischial tuberosities, or along the tibia. They are characterized by a central focus of fibrinoid necrosis surrounded by a palisade of macrophages, which in turn is rimmed by granulation tissue. Rheumatoid nodules may also involve the viscera, including lung, spleen, pericardium, aorta, and the heart valves.

Since RA is a systemic disease, a number of other structures may be affected. Acute necrotizing vasculitis may involve small or large arteries. Serosal involvement may manifest itself as fibrinous pleuritis or pericarditis, or both. Lung parenchyma may be damaged by progressive interstitial fibrosis. Ocular changes such as uveitis and keratoconjunctivitis (similar to those seen in Sjögren's syndrome) may be prominent in some cases.

Etiology and Pathogenesis. There is little doubt that there is a genetic predisposition to RA and that the joint inflammation is immunologically mediated; however, the initiating agent(s) and the precise interplay between genetic and environmental factors remain to be clarified.

In all likelihood the disease is initiated, in a genetically predisposed individual, by activation of helper T cells responding to some arthritogenic agent, possibly a microbe. Activated CD4+ cells produce a number of cytokines that have two principal effects: (1) activation of macrophages and other cells in the joint space, which release tissue-destructive enzymes and other factors that perpetuate inflammation; and (2) activation of the B-cell system, resulting in the production of antibodies, some of which are directed against self-constituents. The resultant autoimmune reactions damage the joints and are believed to play an important role in disease progression. In the context of this general scheme, we can now discuss the roles of genetic factors, T cells, cytokines, B cells, and infectious agents (Fig. 5–28).

The importance of genetic factors in the pathogenesis of RA is supported by the increased frequency of this disease among first-degree relatives and a high concordance rate in monozygotic twins. The role of genetic factors is further strengthened by the association of RA with HLA-DR4 or HLA-DR1 or both of these class II MHC genes. It is of interest

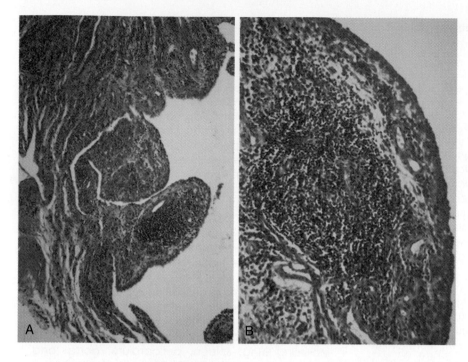

Figure 5–27 ■

Rheumatoid arthritis. *A,* Low magnification reveals marked synovial hypertrophy with formation of villi. *B,* At higher magnification, subsynovial tissue containing a dense lymphoid aggregate is seen. (Courtesy of Dr. Jim Richardson, Department of Pathology, University of Texas Southwestern Medical School, Dallas.)

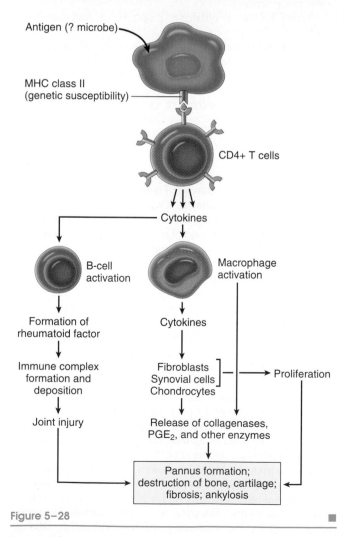

Figure 5–28 ■

Immunopathogenesis of rheumatoid arthritis.

that the susceptibility-associated DR alleles share a common stretch of four amino acids, located in the antigen-binding cleft of the DR molecule. Thus, it seems that the association between certain DR molecules and RA may be explained by the capacity of individuals carrying these DR determinants to bind an arthritogenic antigen, which in turn activates helper T cells and initiates disease.

As mentioned earlier, rheumatoid synovium is heavily infiltrated with lymphocytes. Most of these are activated CD4+ helper T cells. Activated CD4+ cells are a well-known source of cytokines, which activate other immune cells (e.g., B cells, other T cells) as well as macrophages. The latter in turn themselves secrete a variety of proinflammatory and tissue-degrading factors. The rheumatoid synovium is embarrassingly rich in both lymphocyte- and monocyte-derived cytokines. The activity of these cytokines can account for many features of rheumatoid synovitis. Not only are the cytokines proinflammatory, but some, such as IL-1 and TGF-β, cause proliferation of synovial cells and fibroblasts. They also stimulate synovial cells and chondrocytes to secrete proteolytic and matrix-degrading enzymes.

Although T cells play a primary role in the pathogenesis of RA, B cells are also involved. Approximately 80% of patients have rheumatoid factors (RFs), which are autoantibodies directed against the Fc portion of IgG, present in serum and synovial fluid. The significance of *circulating* RFs in the pathogenesis of RA is uncertain, but their presence in the joints is believed to contribute to the inflammatory reaction. Synovial fluid IgG rheumatoid factors self-associate (IgG–anti-IgG) to form immune complexes that fix complement, attract polymorphonuclear leukocytes, and lead to tissue injury by a type III hypersensitivity reaction. Why antibodies against autologous IgG are formed remains unclear. Finally, we come to the elusive infectious agent(s) whose antigens activate T cells. Many candidates have been considered, but none have been chosen. Included in the category of suspects are EBV, mycoplasmas, parvoviruses, and mycobacteria.

There is circumstantial evidence implicating each of these, but in no case has a causal relationship been established. So we must leave it that, although *joint damage in RA is of immune origin and appears to occur in genetically predisposed individuals, the precise trigger that initiates these reactions is still unknown.*

Clinical Course. Although RA is basically a symmetric polyarticular arthritis, the joint involvement may be associated with constitutional symptoms such as weakness, malaise, and low-grade fever. Many of these systemic manifestations result from the same mediators that cause joint inflammation (e.g., IL-1 and TNF-α). The arthritis first appears insidiously, with aching and stiffness of the joints, particularly in the morning. As the disease advances the joints become enlarged, motion is limited, and in time complete ankylosis may appear. The fingers may become virtually immobilized in a clawlike position with ulnar deviation. At this stage of the disease, anemia of chronic disease is common (Chapter 12). The vasculitis may give rise to Raynaud's phenomenon (p 114) and chronic leg ulcers. It is obvious that with such multisystem involvement RA must be differentiated from SLE, scleroderma, polymyositis, dermatomyositis, and Lyme disease, as well as other forms of arthritis. Helpful in differential diagnosis are (1) characteristic radiographic findings; (2) sterile, turbid synovial fluid with decreased viscosity, poor mucin clot formation, and inclusion-bearing neutrophils; and (3) RF (60% to 80% of patients). It must be appreciated, however, that RF may also be present with SLE, sarcoidosis, leprosy, syphilis, tuberculosis, bacterial endocarditis, and other diseases associated with persistent antigenemia.

The clinical course of RA is highly variable. In a minority of patients the disease may become stabilized or may even regress; most of the remainder pursue a chronic, remitting, relapsing course. After 15 to 20 years, the majority of patients become permanently and severely crippled. Life expectancy is reduced by 4 to 10 years. RA is an important cause of reactive amyloidosis, which develops in 5% to 10% of these patients, particularly those with long-standing severe disease.

JUVENILE RHEUMATOID ARTHRITIS

Juvenile RA refers to chronic idiopathic arthritis that occurs in children. It is not a single disease but a heterogeneous group of disorders, most of which differ significantly from the adult form of RA. Some variants involve few large joints such as knees, elbow, and ankles and are hence called *pauciarticular* types. RF is absent. Some are associated with HLA-B27, and their clinical features overlap with the spondyloarthropathies described below. Extra-articular inflammatory manifestations such as uveitis may be present. One variant, previously called Still's disease, has an acute febrile onset and systemic manifestations, including leukocytosis (15,000 to 25,000 cells per microliter), hepatosplenomegaly, lymphadenopathy, and skin rash.

Spondyloarthropathies

For years, several entities in this group of disorders were considered variants of RA; however, careful clinical, morpho-logic, and genetic studies have revealed fundamental differences that distinguish these disorders from RA, and hence they are segregated from it. The spondyloarthropathies are characterized by the following features:

■ Pathologic changes that begin in the ligamentous attachments to bone rather than in the synovium
■ Frequent involvement of the sacroiliac joints along with peripheral inflammatory arthropathy
■ Absence of RF (hence the name seronegative spondyloarthropathies)
■ Association with HLA-B27

This group of disorders includes several clinical subsets, of which ankylosing spondylitis is the prototype (Table 5–8). Others in this category are Reiter's syndrome, psoriatic arthropathy, spondylitis associated with inflammatory bowel diseases, and reactive arthropathies (which follow infections by *Yersinia, Shigella, Salmonella, Helicobacter,* and *Campylobacter* organisms). There is a considerable overlap in these conditions, and they are distinguished from each other according to the particular peripheral joint involved and associated extraskeletal manifestations (e.g., urethritis, conjunctivitis, and uveitis are characteristic of Reiter's syndrome). It will be noted that sacroiliitis is common to all. Although these seronegative spondyloarthropathies are believed to be caused by immune mechanisms, their pathogenesis remains obscure. As mentioned earlier, clinical features of most of the spondyloarthropathies have been reproduced in HLA-B27 transgenic rats, clearly implicating the B27 gene in the pathogenesis of these conditions.

Sjögren's Syndrome

Sjögren's syndrome is a clinicopathologic entity characterized by dry eyes (keratoconjunctivitis sicca) and dry mouth (xerostomia) resulting from immune-mediated destruction of the lacrimal and salivary glands. It occurs as an isolated disorder (primary form), also known as the *sicca syndrome,* or more often in association with another autoimmune disease (secondary form). Among the associated disorders, RA is the most common, but some patients have SLE, polymyositis, systemic sclerosis, vasculitis, or thyroiditis.

Etiology and Pathogenesis. Several lines of evidence suggest that Sjögren's syndrome is an autoimmune disease in which the ductal epithelial cells of the exocrine glands are the primary target. Nevertheless, there is evidence of a systemic B-cell hyperactivity manifested by hypergammaglobulinemia and the presence of antinuclear antibodies and RF (even in the absence of associated RA). As with SLE, it is suspected that the primary defect is in T-helper cells. Activated CD4+ cells dominate the lymphocytic infiltrate in the salivary and lacrimal glands. Most patients with primary Sjögren's syndrome possess autoantibodies to two nuclear antigens, designated SS-A and SS-B. Those with anti–SS-A antibodies are more likely to have systemic (extraglandular) manifestations.

Genetic factors also play a role in the pathogenesis of Sjögren's syndrome. Patients with the primary form of the disease have an increased frequency of HLA-DR3, whereas those

Table 5-8. SOME FEATURES OF SPONDYLOARTHROPATHIES

Feature	Ankylosing Spondylitis	Reiter's Syndrome	Psoriatic Arthropathy	Spondylitis With Inflammatory Bowel Disease	Reactive Arthropathy
HLA-B27	95%	80%	20%–50%	50%	80%
Sacroiliitis	Always	Often	Often	Often	Often
Peripheral joints	Lower > upper (Often)	Lower usually	Upper > lower	Lower > upper	Lower > upper
Uveitis	++	++	+	+	+
Conjunctivitis	−	+	−	−	−
Urethritis	−	+	−	−	+/−
Skin involvement	−	+	++	−	−
Mucosal involvement	−	+	−	+	+

Modified from Wyngaarden, J, et al.: Cecil Textbook of Medicine, 19th ed. Philadelphia, WB Saunders, 1992, p 1517.

with associated RA are more likely to have HLA-DR4. These genetic studies suggest that despite several clinical similarities, patients with primary and secondary forms of Sjögren's syndrome constitute distinct subsets.

MORPHOLOGY. Lacrimal and salivary glands are the primary targets, but other secretory glands, including those in the nose, pharynx, larynx, trachea, bronchi, and vagina, may also be involved. When they are so involved, all reveal an intense lymphocytic and plasma cell infiltration and destruction of the native architecture, similar to the changes encountered in Hashimoto's thyroiditis (Chapter 20). Sometimes the lymphoid infiltrates create germinal follicles.

The lack of tears in the eyes, resulting from the destruction of lacrimal glands, leads to drying of the corneal epithelium, which becomes inflamed, eroded, and ulcerated **(keratoconjunctivitis)**. The oral mucosa may atrophy, with inflammatory fissuring and ulceration **(xerostomia)**. Dryness and crusting of the nose may lead to ulcerations and even perforation of the nasal septum. When the respiratory passages are involved, secondary laryngitis, bronchitis, and pneumonitis may appear. Approximately 25% of the patients (especially those with anti–SS-A antibodies) develop extraglandular disease affecting the central nervous system, skin, kidneys, and muscles. Renal lesions take the form of mild interstitial nephritis associated with tubular transport defects. Unlike the situation in SLE, glomerulonephritis is rare. Skin involvement is manifested by widespread vasculitis.

Clinical Course. Sjögren's syndrome predominantly affects women over 40 years of age. Patients present with dry mouth, lack of tears, and the resultant complications described earlier. Salivary glands are often enlarged owing to lympho-

cytic infiltrates, especially in the primary form. In about 60% of patients, Sjögren's syndrome is associated with other "connective tissue diseases." Of particular interest is the development of B-cell lymphomas in approximately 1% of patients. In addition, about 10% of patients have had lesions designated as "pseudolymphomas." These consist of marked inflammatory hyperplastic changes within the salivary glands, bordering on the appearance of lymphoid cancer. It would therefore appear that in this disorder of probable immune origin, lymphoid hyperactivity may in time give rise to abnormal pseudolymphomatous proliferations and in some cases to true malignant lymphoid tumors.

Systemic Sclerosis

Although the designation *scleroderma* is time honored, this disorder is better called systemic sclerosis (SS) because it is characterized by inflammatory and fibrotic changes throughout the interstitium of many organs in the body. Although skin involvement is the usual presenting symptom and eventually appears in approximately 95% of cases, it is the visceral involvement—of the gastrointestinal tract, lungs, kidneys, heart, and striated muscles—that produces the major disabilities and threatens life. The disease may begin at any age, from infancy to the advanced years, but it most often commences in the third to fifth decades. Women are affected about three times more often than men.

SS can be classified into two groups on the basis of its clinical course:

■ Diffuse scleroderma, characterized by widespread skin involvement at onset, with rapid progression and early visceral involvement.
■ Limited scleroderma, with relatively limited skin involvement, often confined to the fingers and face. Involvement of the viscera occurs late, and hence the disease in these patients generally has a relatively benign course. This is also called the CREST syndrome (described later).

Etiology and Pathogenesis. SS is a disease of unknown cause. Fibrosis, the hallmark of SS, seems to be related to activation of the immune system, vascular injury, and activation of fibroblasts. How these three are related is not clear, but a possible scenario is presented in Figure 5–29.

Activation of the immune system involves both T and B cells. It is proposed that CD4+ cells responding to an as yet unidentified antigen accumulate in the skin and release cytokines that activate mast cells and macrophages, which in turn release fibrogenic cytokines such as IL-1, PDGF, and fibroblast growth factors. The possibility that activated T cells play a role in the pathogenesis of SS is supported by the observation that several features of this disease (including the cutaneous sclerosis) are seen in chronic GVH disease, a disorder that results from sustained activation of T cells in recipients of allogeneic bone marrow transplants. The activation of B cells, although not linked to fibrosis, is manifested by the presence of hypergammaglobulinemia and antinuclear antibodies. Two antinuclear antibodies more or less unique to SS have been described. *One of these, directed against DNA topoisomerase I (Scl-70), is highly specific; it is present in 70% to 75% of patients with diffuse scleroderma and in less than 1% of patients with other connective tissue diseases.* This gives rise to a nucleolar pattern fluorescence characteristic of SS. The other, *an anticentromere antibody*, is found in 60% to 80% of patients with limited scleroderma (i.e., the CREST syndrome).

Microvascular disease is consistently present early in the course of SS. Intimal fibrosis is evident in 100% of digital arteries of patients with SS. It is proposed that repeated cycles of endothelial injury followed by platelet aggregation lead to release of platelet factors (e.g., PDGF, TGF-β) that trigger periadventitial fibrosis and eventual ischemic injury caused by widespread narrowing of the microvasculature. The factor that incites endothelial injury remains mysterious. It is possible that endothelial injury is not the primary event, but that instead endothelial cells activated by T cell–derived cytokines release PDGF and factors chemotactic for fibroblasts. Thus, a primary immunologic abnormality may result in vascular damage and fibrosis.

MORPHOLOGY. Virtually any organ may be affected in SS, but the most prominent changes are found in the skin, musculoskeletal system, gastrointestinal tract, lungs, kidneys, and heart.

The changes in the **skin** almost always begin in the fingers and distal regions of the upper extremities and extend proximally to involve the upper arm, shoulders, neck, and face. In advanced cases the entire back and abdomen as well as the lower extremities may be affected. The earliest changes consist only of some dermal edema and perivascular infiltrates of CD4+ T cells. As the disease advances, there is considerable increase in dermal collagen, with epidermal atrophy and loss of skin adnexa (Fig. 5–30). The walls of dermal capillaries and arterioles are markedly thickened and hyalinized. The fingers may take on a tapered, clawlike appearance and the dermal fibrosis may limit motion in the joints. The sclerotic atrophy of the tips of the fingers often causes resorption of the terminal phalanges of the fingers. Focal and sometimes diffuse subcutaneous calcifi-

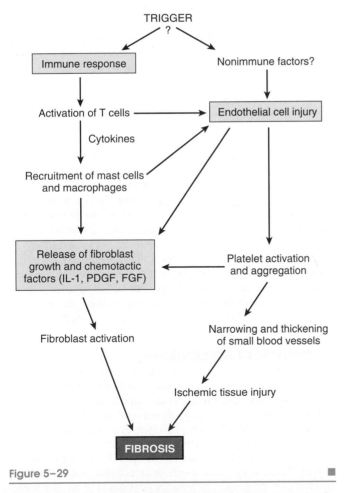

TRIGGER
?

Immune response

Nonimmune factors?

Activation of T cells ⟶ Endothelial cell injury

Cytokines

Recruitment of mast cells and macrophages

Release of fibroblast growth and chemotactic factors (IL-1, PDGF, FGF)

Platelet activation and aggregation

Fibroblast activation

Narrowing and thickening of small blood vessels

Ischemic tissue injury

FIBROSIS

Figure 5–29　■

Schematic illustration of the possible mechanisms leading to systemic sclerosis. PDGF, platelet-derived growth factor; FGF, fibroblast growth factor.

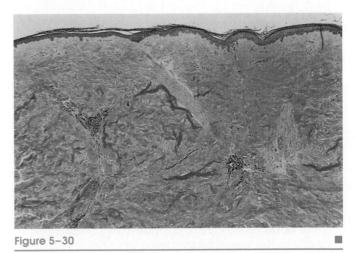

Figure 5–30　■

Systemic sclerosis. Note the extensive deposition of dense collagen in the dermis with virtual absence of appendages and thinning of epidermis. (Courtesy of Dr. Trace Worrell, Department of Pathology, University of Texas Southwestern Medical School, Dallas.)

cations may develop, especially in patients with limited scleroderma (CREST syndrome). Recurrent traumatic ulcerations associated with chronic ischemia due to vascular occlusion may progress to autoamputation of the fingers. The face may take on the appearance of a drawn mask.

The **gastrointestinal tract** is affected in approximately 80% of patients. The most common manifestation consists of progressive atrophy and fibrosis of the esophageal wall, involving principally the submucosa and muscularis of the lower two thirds. This may be accompanied by atrophy and ulceration of the overlying mucosa. Almost invariably the small vessels in these areas show progressive thickening of their walls, accompanied by a perivascular infiltrate of lymphocytes. Similar atrophy and fibrosis may occur in the stomach, small bowel, and colon.

In the **musculoskeletal system,** both joints and muscles are affected. Early in the disease a nonspecific inflammatory synovitis may appear, resembling the early stages of RA. With progression, the synovium undergoes collagenous sclerosis, followed in some cases by some bony resorption of the subjacent bone. At the same time, sclerosis in the periarticular connective tissues limits joint motion. Destruction of joints, such as occurs with RA, is rare. Focal inflammatory infiltrates followed by fibrosis may appear in the skeletal muscles, and many of these patients develop muscle atrophy.

The **lungs** often develop diffuse interstitial fibrosis of the alveolar septa, accompanied by progressive thickening of the walls of the smaller pulmonary vessels. The fibrosis may lead to the production of microcysts. Thus, patients with SS may develop lesions indistinguishable from those of idiopathic pulmonary fibrosis (honeycomb lung, Chapter 13).

The **kidneys** are frequently damaged by a variety of lesions (66% of cases). The principal changes are found in small arteries, which show concentric intimal proliferation, deposition of acid mucopolysaccharides, reduplication of the internal elastic lamina, and hyalinization. Although these vascular changes resemble those found in malignant hypertension, it should be noted that in SS they are restricted to vessels 150 to 500 μm in diameter, and moreover they are not always associated with hypertension. Indeed, hypertension is seen in only 30% of cases; in 20% it takes the form of malignant hypertension. In patients with hypertension the lesions in the kidney are more severe and often include fibrinoid necrosis of arterioles, focal necrosis of glomeruli, and microinfarcts. About half of the patients die of renal failure.

The **heart** may have focal interstitial fibrosis, principally in the perivascular areas, and occasionally there are perivascular infiltrates of lymphocytes and macrophages. Small intramyocardial arteries and arterioles may show vascular thickening. Be-

cause of the changes in the lungs, right-sided cardiac hypertrophy and failure (cor pulmonale, Chapter 11) is often present.

Other sites may be affected, particularly nerve trunks; this is possibly related to microvascular lesions with ischemic and fibrotic alterations in the perineurium.

Clinical Course. It must be apparent from the described anatomic changes that SS has many of the features of RA, SLE, and (as will be described) dermatomyositis. It is, however, distinctive because of the striking cutaneous changes. Almost all patients develop *Raynaud's phenomenon,* a vascular disorder characterized by reversible vasospasm of the arteries. Typically the hands turn white on exposure to cold, reflecting vasospasm, followed by a blue color as capillaries and venules dilate and blood stagnates. Finally, the color changes to red as reactive vasodilatation occurs. The progressive collagenization of the skin leads to atrophy of the hands, with increasing stiffness and eventually complete immobilization of the joints. *Difficulty in swallowing results from esophageal fibrosis and resultant hypomotility.* Eventually, destruction of the esophageal wall leads to atony and dilatation. Malabsorption may appear if the submucosal and muscular atrophy and fibrosis involve the small intestine. Dyspnea and chronic cough reflect the pulmonary changes. With advanced pulmonary involvement, secondary pulmonary hypertension may develop, leading in turn to right-sided cardiac dysfunction. Renal functional impairment secondary to both the advance of SS and the concomitant malignant hypertension is frequently marked.

Limited scleroderma, or the so-called CREST syndrome, is characterized by **c**alcinosis, **R**aynaud's phenomenon, **e**sophageal dysmotility, **s**clerodactyly, and **t**elangiectasia. Raynaud's phenomenon is frequently the presenting feature and is associated with limited skin involvement confined to the fingers and face. These two features may be present for decades before the appearance of distinctive visceral lesions.

The course of diffuse SS is difficult to predict. In most patients the disease pursues a steady, slow, downhill course over the span of many years. In the absence of renal involvement, the life span may be normal. The overall 10-year survival rate ranges from 35% to 70%. The chances of survival are significantly better for patients with localized scleroderma than for those with the usual diffuse progressive disease.

Inflammatory Myopathies

Inflammatory myopathies make up a heterogeneous group of extremely uncommon disorders characterized by immunologically mediated muscle injury and inflammation. Depending on the clinical, morphologic, and immunologic features, three relatively distinct disorders—*polymyositis, dermatomyositis*, and *inclusion body myositis*—have been described. These may occur alone or in conjunction with other autoimmune diseases, such as SS. Women with dermatomyositis have a slightly increased risk of developing visceral cancers (lung, ovary, stomach). Because these disorders are rare, only a few salient features will be summarized.

■ Clinically, they are characterized by muscle weakness, usually bilaterally symmetric, that initially affects large muscles of the trunk, neck, and limbs. Thus, tasks such as getting up from a chair or climbing steps become increasingly difficult. In dermatomyositis an associated skin rash affects the upper eyelids and causes periorbital edema.
■ Histologically, there is infiltration by lymphocytes, and both degenerating and regenerating muscle fibers are seen. The pattern of muscle injury and the location of the inflammatory infiltrates are somewhat distinctive for each subtype.
■ Immunologically, evidence supports antibody-mediated tissue injury in dermatomyositis, whereas polymyositis and inclusion body myositis appear to be mediated by cytotoxic T cells. Antinuclear antibodies are present in most patients. Of these, only Jo-1 antibodies, directed against t-RNA synthetase, are specific for this group of disorders.

The diagnosis of these myopathies is based on clinical features, laboratory evidence of muscle injury (e.g., increased levels of creatine kinase), electromyography, and biopsy.

Mixed Connective Tissue Disease

Mixed connective tissue disease is a term used to describe patients who present with features of SLE, inflammatory myopathy, and SS. They are distinguished from these disorders serologically by high titers of antibodies to a ribonucleoprotein antigen called U1RNP, and clinically by the paucity of renal disease and an excellent therapeutic response to corticosteroids. Many rheumatologists do not recognize this disease as a separate entity and believe that in most such patients it evolves into SS.

IMMUNODEFICIENCY DISEASES

Immunodeficiency diseases may develop because of inherited defects in the development of the immune system, or they may be secondary to the effects of diseases that affect the normal immune system. Clinically, they present with increased susceptibility to infections and, sometimes, cancer. The type of infections in a given patient depend largely on the component of the immune system that is deficient. Patients with *defects in immunoglobulin, complement, or phagocytic cells typically suffer from recurrent infections with pyogenic bacteria*; on the other hand, those with *defects in cell-mediated immunity are prone to infections caused by viruses, fungi, and intracellular bacteria*. Our discussion will begin with a brief account of the primary immunodeficiencies, to be followed by a detailed description of the acquired immunodeficiency syndrome (AIDS), the most devastating example of secondary immunodeficiency.

Primary Immunodeficiency States

Primary immunodeficiency states are experiments of nature that have greatly helped our understanding of the ontogeny and regulation of the immune system (Fig. 5–31). They usually come to attention early in life because of the vulnerability of the child to recurrent infections. Although these immune disorders are relatively uncommon, they are often devastating because many affected patients develop fatal infections. A few of the more common syndromes will be characterized.

X-LINKED AGAMMAGLOBULINEMIA: BRUTON'S DISEASE

Bruton's disease is one of the more common forms of primary immunodeficiency. It is *characterized by the failure of pre-B cells to differentiate into B cells*. During normal B-cell differentiation, the immunoglobulin heavy chain genes are rearranged first, followed by rearrangement of the light chains. In Bruton's agammaglobulinemia, B-cell maturation stops after the rearrangement of heavy-chain genes. Because light chains are not produced, the complete immunoglobulin molecule containing heavy and light chains cannot be assembled and transported to the cell membrane. Free heavy chains can be found in the cytoplasm. This block in differentiation is due to mutations in a tyrosine kinase, appropriately called Bruton's tyrosine kinase (*btk*).

As an X-linked disease, this disorder is seen almost entirely in males, but sporadic cases have been described in females. *It usually does not become apparent until about 6 months of age, when maternal immunoglobulins are depleted.* In most cases, recurrent bacterial infections such as acute and chronic pharyngitis, sinusitis, otitis media, bronchitis, and pneumonia call attention to the underlying immune defect. Almost always the causative organisms are *Haemophilus influenzae, Streptococcus pneumoniae,* or *Staphylococcus aureus*. Because antibodies are important for neutralizing infectious viruses, these patients are also susceptible to certain viral infections, especially those caused by enteroviruses. For similar reasons, *Giardia lamblia*, an intestinal protozoon that is normally resisted by secreted IgA, causes persistent infections in these cases. In general, however, most viral, fungal, and protozoal infections are handled normally owing to intact T cell–mediated immunity. The classic form of this disease has the following characteristics:

■ B cells are absent or remarkably decreased in the circulation, and the serum levels of all classes of immunoglobulins are depressed. Pre-B cells are found in normal numbers in bone marrow.
■ Germinal centers of lymph nodes, Peyer's patches, the appendix, and tonsils are underdeveloped or rudimentary.
■ There is remarkable absence of plasma cells throughout the body.
■ T cell– and cell-mediated reactions are entirely normal.

Autoimmune diseases occur with increased frequency in patients with Bruton's disease. Nearly half of these children develop a condition similar to rheumatoid arthritis that clears remarkably with restitutive immunoglobulin therapy. Similarly, SLE, dermatomyositis, and other autoimmune disorders

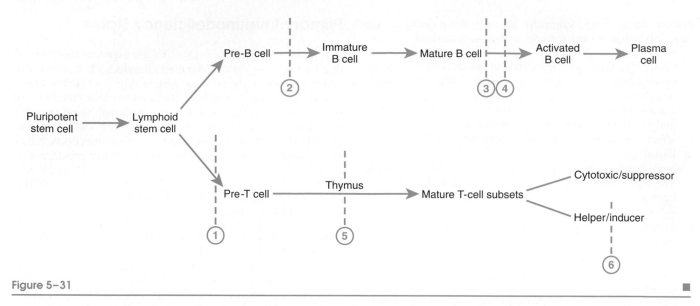

Figure 5–31

Simplified scheme of lymphocyte development. Numbers indicate cells or steps affected in various immunodeficiency states. 1, Severe combined immunodeficiency. In most cases there is a defect in the development of T cells with secondary loss of B-cell function. The lymphoid stem cell is rarely affected. 2, Bruton's agammaglobulinemia. 3, Isolated IgA deficiency, which affects only IgA-secreting B cells. 4, Common variable immunodeficiency affects secretion of several Ig classes. 5, DiGeorge's syndrome. 6, Acquired immunodeficiency syndrome (AIDS).

are more common in these patients. The basis of these peculiar associations is not known.

ISOLATED DEFICIENCY OF IMMUNOGLOBULIN A

The most common of all the primary immunodeficiency diseases, IgA deficiency affects about one in 700 individuals of Caucasian descent. It should be recalled that IgA is the major immunoglobulin in external secretions and is thus involved in mucosal defense. In patients with IgA deficiency a marked IgA decrease occurs both in serum and in secretions. Although most persons with this condition are asymptomatic, weakened mucosal defenses predispose some individuals to *recurrent sinopulmonary infections and diarrhea.* There is also a significant association with autoimmune diseases, the basis of which is not entirely clear. Some individuals with IgA deficiency are also deficient in IgG2 and IgG4 subclasses of immunoglobulin G. This subgroup of patients is particularly prone to develop infections. The pathogenesis of IgA deficiency seems to involve a block in the terminal differentiation of IgA-secreting B cells to plasma cells. Although the molecular basis of this defect is not understood, there seems to be a linkage to an unidentified gene within the class III (complement) region of MHC.

COMMON VARIABLE IMMUNODEFICIENCY

This relatively common but poorly defined derangement probably represents a heterogeneous group of disorders. It may be congenital or acquired, sporadic or familial (with an inconstant mode of inheritance). The feature *common to all patients is hypogammaglobulinemia,* generally affecting all antibody classes, but sometimes only IgG. Hence, the clinical manifestations are similar to those of Bruton's agammaglobulinemia. However, in contrast to Bruton's disease, both sexes are affected equally, and the onset of symptoms is much later, in the second or third decade of life. The cellular basis of immunoglobulin deficiency is not fully understood and is likely to differ among patients. In general, most patients have normal numbers of B cells, which fail to mature into antibody-secreting cells. It is suspected that defective T-cell help or excessive T-cell suppression may account for poor B-cell functions. As with isolated IgA deficiency, a linkage with class III (complement) genes of the HLA has been noted, suggesting that these two disorders may be related. Paradoxically, these patients are prone to develop a variety of autoimmune disorders (hemolytic anemia, pernicious anemia), as well as lymphoid tumors. Perhaps all of these are manifestations of a dysregulated immune system.

THYMIC HYPOPLASIA (DiGEORGE'S SYNDROME)

DiGeorge's syndrome results from a lack of thymic influence on the immune system. The thymus is usually rudimentary, and T cells are deficient or absent in the circulation. They are similarly depleted in the thymus-dependent areas of the lymph nodes and spleen. Thus, *infants with this defect are extremely vulnerable to viral, fungal, and protozoal infections.* Susceptibility to intracellular bacteria is also increased, because phagocytic cells that eliminate them require T cell–derived signals for activation. The B-cell system and serum immunoglobulins are generally unaffected.

This disorder results from a congenital malformation affecting the third and fourth pharyngeal pouches. These structures give rise to the thymus, parathyroid glands, and portions of the lips, ears, and aortic arch. Hence, in addition to thymic hypoplasia the parathyroid glands are also either hypoplastic or totally absent, often leading to *tetany from hypocalcemia.* Most of these infants have additional developmental defects affecting the face, ears, heart, and great vessels. Transplantation of thymus tissue has been successful in some of these infants. In others (with partial defects), immunity may improve spontaneously with age.

SEVERE COMBINED IMMUNODEFICIENCY (SCID)

SCID represents a constellation of genetically distinct syndromes all having in common variable defects in both humoral and cell-mediated immune responses. Affected infants are susceptible to recurrent, severe infections by a wide array of pathogens, including bacteria, viruses, fungi, and protozoa. Opportunistic infections with *Candida*, *P. carinii*, cytomegalovirus, and *Pseudomonas* cause serious, often lethal, disease. Despite common clinical features, the underlying defects in individual patients are quite different. The so-called classic form, resulting from a combined deficiency of T and B cells, is rare. More commonly, SCID results from a severe defect in the T-cell compartment, with secondary impairment of humoral immunity.

The most common form, accounting for 50% to 60% of cases, is X-linked, and hence SCID is more common in boys than in girls. The X-linked form results from a mutation in the common γ chain, which forms a subunit of several cytokine receptors, including receptors for IL-2, IL-4, IL-7, IL-11, and IL-15. Thus, patients have a functional deficiency of all these cytokines. Many of these are required for normal T-cell development, and hence these patients lack T cells.

The remaining cases of SCID are inherited as autosomal recessive disorders. Most of these result from a lack of adenosine deaminase (ADA), an enzyme involved in purine metabolism. It is believed that a deficiency of ADA leads to accumulation of adenosine and deoxyadenosine triphosphate, which are toxic to lymphocytes, especially T cells. A smaller number of autosomal recessive cases of SCID result from failure of expression of class II MHC molecules. This in turn severely impairs the function of CD4+ helper T cells because they can recognize antigens only if presented by class II molecules. Consequently, both cell-mediated immunity and T-dependent antibody responses are impaired.

In the two most common forms of SCID (cytokine receptor mutation and ADA deficiency), the thymus is hypoplastic and fetal in type. Lymph nodes are difficult to find and are markedly reduced in size; they lack both germinal centers, which normally contain B cells, and the paracortical T cells. The lymphoid tissues of the tonsils, gut, and appendix are also markedly hypoplastic. Most affected persons have marked lymphopenia, with a deficiency of both T and B cells. Others have normal numbers of B cells, which are nonfunctional owing to lack of T-cell help. Still others have normal numbers of circulating lymphocytes that bear the cell surface markers of very immature intrathymic T cells. Patients with SCID are treated by bone marrow transplantation. Gene therapy, wherein the normal ADA gene is introduced into the patient's own bone marrow, is also being attempted.

GENETIC DEFICIENCIES OF THE COMPLEMENT SYSTEM

The various components of the complement system play a critical role in inflammatory and immunologic responses. As might be expected, hereditary deficiency of complement components, especially C3, which is critical for both the classic and alternative pathways, results in an increased susceptibility to infection with pyogenic bacteria. Inherited deficiencies of C1q, C2, and C4 increase the risk of immune complex–mediated disease (e.g., SLE), possibly by impairing the clearance of immune complexes from circulation. The absence of C1 esterase inhibitor allows uncontrolled C1 esterase activation with the generation of vasoactive C2 kinin. These patients develop *hereditary angioedema,* characterized by recurrent episodes of localized edema affecting skin and mucous membranes. The deficiences of the later-acting components of the classic pathway (C5 to C8) result in recurrent neisserial (gonococcal, meningococcal) infections.

Secondary Immunodeficiencies

Secondary immunodeficiencies are sometimes encountered in patients with malnutrition, infection, cancer, renal disease, Hodgkin's disease, or sarcoidosis. They also occur commonly in patients receiving immunosuppressive drugs for prevention of graft rejection or treatment of autoimmune diseases. Many of these secondary states can be accounted for by loss of immunoglobulins (as in proteinuric renal diseases), inadequate synthesis of immunoglobulins (as in malnutrition), or loss of lymphocytes (as may occur with drugs and systemic infections), but other mechanisms may also be operative. *As a group, the secondary immunodeficiencies are more common than the disorders of genetic origin.* Here we discuss only AIDS, which has assumed epidemic proportions in the last 10 years and has terrorized the entire world.

ACQUIRED IMMUNODEFICIENCY SYNDROME (AIDS)

AIDS can best be characterized as an epidemic of a *retroviral disease characterized by profound immunosuppression associated with opportunistic infections, secondary neoplasms, and neurologic manifestations.* As of late 1996, a little over 500,000 patients with AIDS had been reported in the United States. On the basis of serologic data, it is estimated that approximately 1.5 million individuals have been infected with HIV, the agent that causes AIDS. Worldwide, an estimated 13 million people are infected, with Africa bearing the largest burden of some 7.5 million cases. Some measure of the impact of the AIDS epidemic is provided by the mortality data. In the United States, AIDS is the leading cause of death in men between 25 and 44 years of age, and the fourth ranking cause of death in women in the same age group. No less impressive is the explosion of new knowledge relating to this modern plague. So rapid is the pace of research on the molecular biology of HIV and its effects that any textbook covering this topic is doomed to be out of date by the time it is published. It is with this sobering realization that an attempt will be made to summarize the currently available data on the epidemiology, etiology, pathogenesis, and clinical features of HIV infection.

Epidemiology. Although AIDS was first described in the United States, which has 40% of the reported cases, AIDS has now been reported from over 173 countries around the world. Although the largest number of people infected with HIV are in Africa, the most rapid increase of HIV infection in the 1990s has been in Southeast Asian countries, including Thailand, India, and Indonesia.

Epidemiologic studies in the United States have identified five groups of adults at risk for developing AIDS. The case distribution in these groups is as follows:

1. Homosexual or bisexual males constitute by far the largest group, accounting for 60% of reported cases. This includes 6% who were also intravenous drug abusers. However, transmission of AIDS in this category is on the decline; currently, less than 50% of new cases can be attributed to male homosexual contacts.
2. Intravenous drug abusers with no history of homosexuality compose the next largest group, representing about 24% of all patients. They represent the majority of all cases among heterosexuals.
3. Hemophiliacs, especially those who received large amounts of factor VIII concentrates before 1985, make up 1% of all cases.
4. Recipients of blood and blood components who are not hemophiliacs but who received transfusions of HIV-infected whole blood or components (e.g., platelets, plasma) account for 2% of patients.
5. Heterosexual contacts of members of other high-risk groups (chiefly intravenous drug abusers) constitute 7% of the patient population.

In the remaining cases, no obvious risk factors can be detected.

The epidemiology of HIV infection and AIDS is quite different in children under 13 years of age. Close to 2% of all AIDS cases occur in this population, the vast majority resulting from transmission of virus from mother to infant. Approximately 10% of children with AIDS are hemophiliacs and others who received blood or blood products before 1985.

On the basis of epidemiologic studies and laboratory investigations, it is now established that transmission of HIV may occur through three routes: *sexual contact, parenteral inoculation,* and *passage of the virus from infected mothers to their newborns.*

Venereal transmission is clearly the predominant mode of infection worldwide. Currently, most U.S. patients are homosexual or bisexual males, and hence most sexual transmission has occurred among homosexual men. The virus is carried in the lymphocytes present in the semen and enters the recipient's body through abrasions in rectal mucosa. Heterosexual transmission, although initially of less quantitative importance in the United States, is the most common mode by which HIV is spread outside this country. Currently, even in the United States, *the rate of increase of heterosexual transmission has outpaced transmission by other means.* Such spread is occurring most rapidly in female sex partners of male intravenous drug abusers. As such, the number of women with AIDS is increasing rapidly. In addition to male-to-female transmission, HIV can also be transmitted from females to

males, albeit much less efficiently. HIV is present in the vaginal and cervical secretions of infected women. All forms of sexual transmission are aided and abetted by the concomitant presence of other sexually transmitted diseases that cause genital ulcerations. Examples of such "co-factors" include infections with *Treponema pallidum, Haemophilus ducreyi,* and herpes simplex virus.

Parenteral transmission of HIV has occurred in three groups of individuals: intravenous drug abusers, hemophiliacs who received factor VIII concentrates, and random recipients of blood transfusion. Of these three, intravenous drug abusers constitute by far the largest group. Transmission occurs by sharing of needles, syringes, and other paraphernalia contaminated with HIV-containing blood. This group occupies a pivotal position in the AIDS epidemic because it represents the principal link in the transmission of HIV to other adult populations through heterosexual activity.

Transmission of HIV by transfusion of blood or blood products such as lyophilized factor VIII concentrates has been virtually eliminated in recent years. This happy outcome resulted from three public health measures: screening of donated blood and plasma for antibody to HIV, heat treatment of clotting factor concentrates, and screening of donors on the basis of history. There is, however, an extremely small risk of acquiring HIV through transfusion of contaminated but seronegative blood, because a newly infected individual may not develop antibodies for the first few weeks.

As alluded to earlier, mother-to-infant transmission is the major cause of pediatric AIDS. Infected mothers transmit HIV by three routes—transplacental, in utero; intrapartum, during delivery; and via breast milk, in the perinatal period. Of these, the transplacental and intrapartum routes account for most cases. Together, vertical transmission by these routes occurs in 12% to 30% of infants at risk.

Because of the uniformly fatal outcome of AIDS, there has been much concern in the lay public and among health care workers regarding the spread of HIV infection outside the high-risk groups. Extensive studies indicate that *HIV infection cannot be transmitted by casual personal contact in the home, workplace, or school.* No convincing evidence for spread by insect bites has been obtained. Regarding transmission of HIV infection to health care workers, there seems to be an extremely small but definite risk. Seroconversion has been documented after accidental needlestick injury or exposure of nonintact skin to infected blood in laboratory accidents. After such accidents the risk of seroconversion is believed to be about 0.3%. By comparison, the rate of seroconversion after accidental exposure to hepatitis B–infected blood is about 30%. Transmission of HIV from an infected health care worker to a patient is extremely uncommon, with risk estimates varying from 0.0024% to 0.000024%.

Etiology. There is little doubt that AIDS is caused by HIV, a human retrovirus belonging to the lentivirus family. Included in this group are feline immunodeficiency virus, simian immunodeficiency virus, visna virus of sheep, and the equine infectious anemia virus. These nontransforming retroviruses have several features in common:

■ A long incubation period, followed by a slowly progressive fatal outcome
■ Tropism for hematopoietic and nervous systems

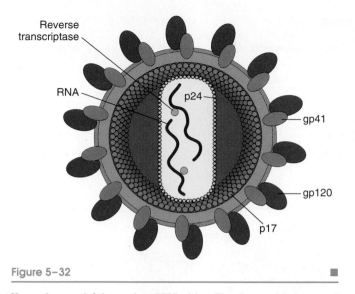

Figure 5–32 ■

Human immunodeficiency virus (HIV) virion. The virus particle is covered by a membrane that is derived from the host cell. Studding the membrane are viral glycoproteins, gp41 and gp120. Inside there is a core made up of proteins designated p17 and p24. The viral RNA and the enzyme reverse transcriptase are carried in the core.

■ An ability to cause immunosuppression
■ Cytopathic effects in vitro

Two genetically different but closely related forms of HIV, HIV-1 and HIV-2, have been isolated from patients with AIDS. HIV-1 is the most common type associated with AIDS in the United States, Europe, and Central Africa, whereas HIV-2 causes a similar disease principally in West Africa. The ensuing discussion relates primarily to HIV-1 and diseases caused by it; however, it is generally applicable to HIV-2 as well.

Like most C-type retroviruses, the HIV-1 virion is spherical and contains an electron-dense core surrounded by a lipid envelope derived from the host cell membrane. The virus core contains several core proteins, two strands of genomic RNA, and the enzyme reverse transcriptase (Fig. 5–32). Studding the viral envelope are two viral glycoproteins, gp120 and

gp41, that are critical for HIV infection of cells. The HIV-1 proviral genome contains the *gag, pol,* and *env* genes, which code for the core proteins, reverse transcriptase, and envelope proteins, respectively (Fig. 5–33). In addition to these three standard retroviral genes, HIV and other lentiviruses contain several other genes that exert regulatory functions. By using genetically manipulated viruses it has been found that some of these genes, such as *tat* (transactivator), *rev* (regulator of expression of virus), and *nef* (erroneously called negative factor), enhance or promote virus replication; others, such as *vif* (viral infectivity factor), promote the infectivity of cell-free virus. Recently, some patients were found who had been transfused many years earlier with blood contaminated with an HIV strain lacking the *nef* gene. Surprisingly, they did not develop AIDS, suggesting that viral regulatory proteins such as *nef* may be suitable targets for potential anti-HIV drugs, or that HIV mutants lacking critical regulatory proteins may be used for vaccination.

Pathogenesis. There are two major targets of HIV: the immune system and the central nervous system. The effects of HIV infection on each of these will be discussed separately.

Immunopathogenesis of HIV Disease. Profound immunosuppression, primarily affecting cell-mediated immunity, is the hallmark of AIDS. This results chiefly from a severe loss of CD4+ T cells as well as an impairment in the function of surviving helper T cells. Because depletion of CD4+ T cells is critical to the pathogenesis of AIDS, we focus our attention first on the events that lead to the infection and destruction of T cells, after which HIV infection of monocytes and its consequences are discussed.

There is abundant evidence that *the CD4 molecule is in fact a high-affinity receptor* for HIV. This explains the selective tropism of the virus for CD4+ T cells and its ability to infect other CD4+ cells, particularly macrophages (Fig. 5–34). The initial step in infection is the binding of gp120 envelope glycoprotein to CD4 molecules that serve as the primary receptors for HIV. However, binding to CD4 is not sufficient for infection. HIV must also bind to other cell surface molecules (coreceptors) for entry into the cell. Recent studies indicate that membrane proteins called CXCR4 and CCR5 that are receptors for chemokines (Chapter 2) serve this role. Thus, HIV must bind to its primary receptor CD4, and its coreceptors before fusion with the cell membrane and internalization.

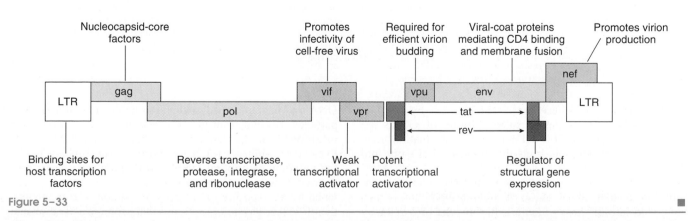

Figure 5–33 ■

HIV proviral genome. Several genes and their recognized functions are illustrated. The genes outlined in red are unique to HIV; others are shared by all retroviruses.

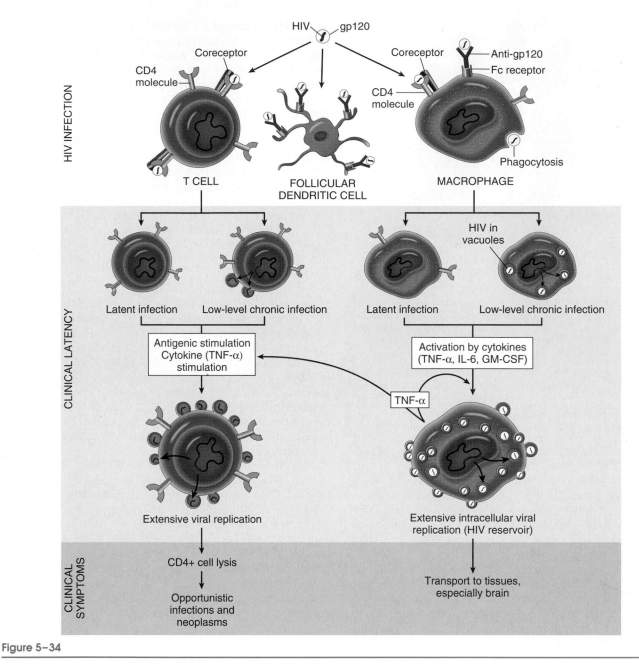

Figure 5–34

Immunopathogenesis of HIV infection. CD4+ T cells and macrophages are the major targets of HIV. Infection of these two cell types leads to somewhat distinctive events that eventually lead to a marked loss of CD4+ T cells and dissemination of HIV into various tissues, especially the central nervous system. Note that dendritic cells carry antibody-coated virus, and along with macrophages act as reservoirs of HIV. Viral replication continues unabated in both T cells and macrophages during the clinical latent phase. Although the coreceptors on CD4+ T cells and macrophages are made to look alike, their chemical nature may be different on these two cell types. There is also evidence for two types of coreceptors on CD4+ T cells.

The importance of coreceptors is highlighted by the fact that individuals who inherit mutant forms of CCR5 are resistant to infection by HIV-1. This information may be useful for developing drugs that prevent viral entry into cells.

Once internalized, the viral genome undergoes reverse transcription, leading to formation of proviral DNA that is then integrated into the host genome. After this the provirus may remain locked into the chromosome for months or years, and hence the infection may become latent. Alternatively, proviral DNA may be transcribed, with the formation of complete viral particles that bud from the cell membrane. Such productive infection,when associated with extensive viral budding, leads to cell death (Fig. 5–34). It is important to note that in T cells the initiation of proviral DNA transcription (and hence productive infection) occurs only when the infected cell is activated by an exposure to antigens or cytokines. It is obvious therefore that physiologic stimuli that promote activation and growth of normal T cells lead to the death of HIV-infected T cells.

It might be surmised from the preceding discussion that productive infection of T cells is the mechanism by which HIV causes lysis of CD4+ T cells. It is interesting to note, however, that in the peripheral blood of patients with AIDS the overwhelming majority of CD4+ cells do not show evidence of active virus production. This paradox is not completely resolved, but recent studies indicate that early in the course of infection the virus is localized primarily in the lymphoid organs (lymph nodes, tonsils, and spleen) and infects T cells that reside at these locales. Many CD4+ cells in the lymph nodes are latently infected, but productive infection is continually activated, leading to an erosion of CD4+ T cells. *For several years after infection, the rate of CD4+ cell loss appears to be deceptively slow, because of compensatory expansion of uninfected cells.* Hence, despite considerable destruction of CD4+ cells, their numbers in the peripheral blood may remain steady during the period of clinical latency (discussed below), and the viral burden in the blood appears low. In addition to cell death resulting from productive infection, several indirect mechanisms exist that could contribute to the loss of helper T cells are:

■ Loss of immature precursors of CD4+ T cells, either by direct infection of thymic progenitor cells or by infection of accessory cells that secrete cytokines essential for CD4+ T-cell differentiation.
■ Fusion of infected and uninfected cells, with formation of syncytia (giant cells) (Fig. 5–35). In tissue culture the gp120 expressed on productively infected cells binds to CD4 molecules on uninfected T cells, followed by cell fusion. Fused cells develop "ballooning" and usually die within a few hours.

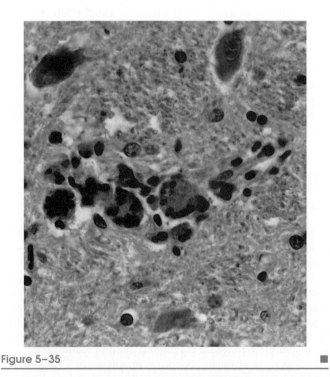

Figure 5–35   ■

HIV infection. Formation of giant cells in the brain. (Courtesy of Dr. Dennis Burns, Department of Pathology, University of Texas Southwestern Medical School, Dallas.)

■ Apoptosis of uninfected CD4+ cells by binding of gp120 to the CD4+ molecule, followed by activation through the T-cell receptor. Apoptosis may also result from aberrant immune activation.

Loss of CD4+ cells by direct and indirect mechanisms leads to an inversion of the CD4-CD8 ratio in the peripheral blood. It may be recalled that the normal CD4-CD8 ratio is close to 2, whereas in patients with AIDS a ratio close to 0.5 is not uncommon. Such an inversion, although a consistent finding in AIDS, should not be considered diagnostic, because it may also occur with certain other viral infections.

Although marked reduction in CD4+ T cells, a hallmark of AIDS, can account for most of the immunodeficiency late in the course of HIV infection, there is compelling evidence for *qualitative defects in T cells that can be detected even in asymptomatic HIV-infected persons.* Such defects include a reduction in antigen-induced T-cell proliferation, impaired production of cytokines, defects in intracellular signaling, and many more. In particular, it seems that there is an imbalance between the functions of CD4+ $T_H 1$ cells and $T_H 2$ cells. Thus, production of IL-2 and IFN-γ is impaired, but IL-4 and IL-10 are unaffected. Such an imbalance favors humoral immune responses over cell-mediated responses, thus accounting for the presence of anti-HIV antibodies in virtually every infected individual. There is also a selective loss of the memory subset of CD4+ helper T cells early in the course of the disease. This observation explains the inability of peripheral blood T cells to be activated when challenged with common recall antigens.

In addition to infection and loss of CD4+ T cells, *infection of monocytes and macrophages is also extremely important in the pathogenesis of HIV infection.* Like T cells, *most of the macrophages that are infected by HIV are found in the tissues and not in peripheral blood.* A relatively high frequency (10% to 50%) of productively infected macrophages are detected in certain tissues such as brain, lymph nodes, and lungs. Several important differences between HIV infection of T cells and macrophages need to be emphasized:

■ Because many macrophages express low levels of CD4, HIV may infect these cells by the gp120-CD4 pathway; in addition, HIV may enter macrophages by phagocytosis or by Fc receptor–mediated endocytosis of antibody-coated HIV particles (see Fig. 5–34).
■ Infected macrophages bud relatively small amounts of virus from the cell surface, but these cells contain large numbers of virus particles located exclusively in intracellular vacuoles. Despite the fact that macrophages allow viral replication, they are quite resistant to the cytopathic effects of HIV, unlike CD4+ T cells.

HIV infection of macrophages has two important implications. First, monocytes and macrophages represent a veritable virus factory and reservoir, whose output remains largely protected from host defenses. Second, macrophages provide a safe vehicle for HIV to be transported to various parts of the body, particularly the nervous system. Although macrophages are resistant to the lytic effects of HIV, their function is often impaired in HIV-infected individuals. These defects include impaired chemotaxis, decreased secretion of IL-1, and (most important) poor capacity to present antigens to T cells.

Recent studies have documented that, in addition to macrophages, *follicular dendritic cells (FDCs) in the germinal centers of lymph nodes are also important reservoirs of infectious HIV virions.* The dendritic processes of these cells express receptors for the Fc portion of IgG, and hence they trap HIV virions coated with IgG anti-HIV antibodies. Thus, the antibodies formed early in response to HIV infections can not only neutralize cell-free virus, but they also facilitate viral localization to the FDC. Surprisingly, the antibody-coated virus localized to the FDC retains the ability to infect CD4+ cells as they traverse the intricate meshwork formed by the dendritic processes of the FDC. *Together, these studies provide clear evidence that the macrophages, FDCs, and CD4+ T cells contained in the lymphoid tissues are the major sites of HIV infection and peristence.*

Low-level chronic or latent infection of T cells and macrophages is an important feature of HIV infection. It is widely believed that integrated provirus, without virus expression (latent infection), could remain in the cells from months to years. Completion of the viral life cycle in latently infected cells occurs only after cell activation, which in the case of CD4+ T cells results in cell lysis. When a latently infected CD4+ cell encounters an antigen (environmental or HIV derived), it undergoes a series of activation steps that include up-regulation of cytokine secretion and expression cytokine receptors. These physiologic responses also activate transcription of HIV proviral DNA, resulting in the production of virions and cell lysis. Furthermore, TNF-α, a cytokine produced by activated macrophages, also leads to transcriptional activation of HIV-mRNA in T-helper cells. In effect, HIV thrives when the host macrophages and T cells are physiologically activated, an act that can be best described as "subversion from within." Such activation in vivo may result from antigenic stimulation, especially by other infecting microorganisms such as cytomegalovirus, EBV, hepatitis B virus, or herpes simplex virus. The life style of most HIV-infected patients in the United States places them at increased risk of recurrent exposure to other sexually transmitted diseases, and in Africa the socioeconomic conditions probably impose a higher burden of chronic microbial infections. It is easy to visualize how a vicious cycle of cell destruction may be set up in patients with AIDS. The multiple infections to which these individuals are prone because of diminished helper T-cell function lead to increased TNF-α production, which in turn stimulates more HIV production, followed by infection and loss of additional CD4+ T cells.

Although much attention has been focused on T cells and macrophages because they can be infected by HIV, virtually no arm of the immune system remains unaffected in AIDS patients. Polyclonal B-cell activation results in hypergammaglobulinemia, perhaps because of multiple interacting factors such as infection with cytomegalovirus and EBV, both of which are polyclonal B-cell activators. gp120 itself can cause B-cell proliferation, and HIV-infected macrophages produce increased amounts of IL-6, which favors activation of B cells. *Despite the presence of spontaneously activated B cells, patients with AIDS are unable to mount an antibody response to a new antigen.* This could in part be due to lack of T-cell help, but antibody responses against T-independent antigens are also suppressed, and hence there may be other defects in B cells as well. Impaired humoral immunity renders these patients prey to disseminated infections caused by encapsulated bacteria such as *S. pneumoniae* and *H. influenzae,* both of which require antibodies for effective opsonization.

As we close this discussion of immunopathogenesis, it must be recalled that CD4+ T cells play a pivotal role in regulating the immune response: they produce a plethora of cytokines such as IL-2, IL-4, IL-5, and IFN-γ; macrophage chemotactic factors; and hematopoietic growth factors such as GM-CSF. Therefore, loss of this "master cell" has ripple effects on virtually every other cell of the immune system, including NK cells, as illustrated in Figure 5–36 and summarized in Table 5–9.

Pathogenesis of Central Nervous System Involvement. The pathogenesis of neurologic manifestations deserves special mention because, in addition to the lymphoid system, the nervous system is a major target of HIV infection. Only macrophages and cells belonging to the monocyte and macrophage lineage (microglia) in the brain are infected with HIV. The virus is carried into the brain by infected monocytes contained in the peripheral blood. Neural damage is believed to result from cytotoxic factors released by infected macrophages. HIV-infected macrophages produce cytokines such as TNF-α and other factors that injure neurons, in large part by increasing intracellular calcium. Among the toxic substances produced in this manner are nitric oxide and platelet-activating factor.

Natural History of HIV Infection. The course of HIV infection can best be understood in terms of an interplay between HIV and the immune system. Three phases reflecting the dynamics of virus-host interaction can be recognized: an early, acute phase; a middle, chronic phase; and a final, crisis phase (Fig. 5–37). The four clinical subgroups of HIV infection, proposed by the Centers for Disease Control (CDC), can be reasonably assigned to the three phases of infection, as noted in Table 5–10.

The *early, acute phase* represents the initial response of an immunocompetent adult to HIV infection. Clinically, this phase is associated with self-limited acute illness (CDC group I: Acute infection) that develops in 50% to 70% of adults infected with HIV. Nonspecific symptoms such as sore throat, myalgias, fever, rash, and sometimes aseptic meningitis develop 3 to 6 weeks after infection and resolve spontaneously 2 to 3 weeks later. This phase is characterized initially by high levels of virus in the plasma. Usually there is an abrupt, sometimes severe, reduction in CD4+ T cells. Soon, however, a virus-specific immune response develops, evidenced by seroconversion (usually within 3 to 17 weeks of presumed exposure), and, more importantly, by the development of virus-specific CD8+ cytotoxic T cells. HIV-specific cytotoxic T cells are detected in blood at about the time viral titers begin to fall and are most likely responsible for the containment of HIV infection. As viremia abates, CD4+ T cells return to nearly normal numbers, signaling the end of the early acute phase. It should be noted, however, that reduction in plasma virus does not signal the end of viral replication. During the initial viremic phase, there is widespread seeding of lymphoid organs with HIV, where it remains within macrophages and CD4+ cells, and on the dendritic processes of FDC, in the form of immune complexes.

The *middle, chronic phase* represents a stage of immune containment of the virus. The immune system is largely intact,

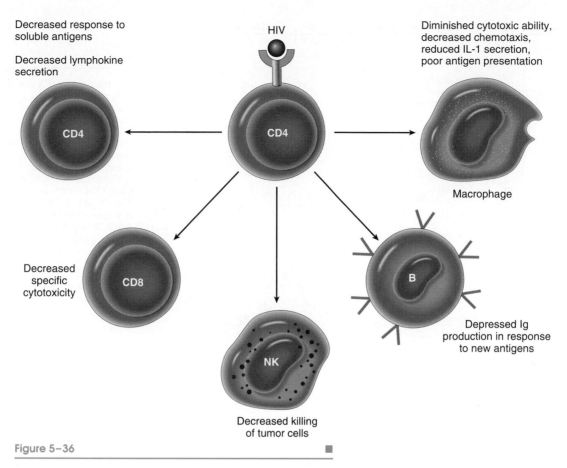

Decreased response to soluble antigens

Decreased lymphokine secretion

HIV

Diminished cytotoxic ability, decreased chemotaxis, reduced IL-1 secretion, poor antigen presentation

CD4

CD4

Macrophage

Decreased specific cytotoxicity

CD8

B

NK

Depressed Ig production in response to new antigens

Decreased killing of tumor cells

Figure 5–36 ■

The multiple effects of loss of CD4+ T cells as a result of HIV infection.

■

Table 5–9. MAJOR ABNORMALITIES OF IMMUNE FUNCTION IN AIDS

Lymphopenia

Predominantly due to selective loss of CD4+ helper-inducer T-cell subset; inversion of CD4-CD8 ratio

Decreased T-Cell Function in Vivo

Susceptibility to opportunistic infections
Susceptibility to neoplasms
Decreased delayed type hypersensitivity

Altered T-Cell Function in Vitro

Decreased proliferative response to mitogens, alloantigens, and soluble antigens
Decreased specific cytotoxicity
Decreased helper function for pokeweed mitogen–induced B-cell immunoglobulin production
Decreased IL-2 and IFN-γ production

Polyclonal B-Cell Activation

Hypergammaglobulinemia and circulating immune complexes
Inability to mount de novo antibody response to a new antigen
Refractoriness to normal signals for B-cell activation in vitro

Altered Monocyte or Macrophage Functions

Decreased chemotaxis
Decreased HLA class II antigen expression
Diminished capacity to present antigen to T-cells

and *continued HIV replication may last for several years.* During this phase, there is a continuing battle between HIV and the host immune system. The CD8+ cytotoxic T-cell response remains activated, and (contrary to earlier reports) viral replication in the lymphoid tissues continues unabated. The extensive viral turnover is associated with continued loss of large numbers of CD4+ cells. However, because of the immense regenerative capacity of the immune system, a large proportion of the CD4+ cells that were lost is replenished. Thus, the decline of CD4+ cells in the peripheral blood is modest. After an extended and variable period, host defense begins to wane, the number of CD4+ cells begins to decline, and the proportion of the surviving CD4+ cells infected with HIV increases, as does the viral burden per CD4+ cell. Not unexpectedly, HIV spillover into the plasma increases. During the middle, chronic phase, patients are either asymptomatic (CDC group II) or develop persistent generalized lymphadenopathy (CDC group III). Constitutional symptoms are usually absent or mild. Persistent lymphadenopathy with significant constitutional symptoms (fever, rash, fatigue) reflects the onset of immune system decompensation, escalation of viral replication, and the onset of the "crisis" phase.

The *final, crisis phase* is characterized by a serious breakdown of host defense, a marked increase in viremia, and clinical disease. Typically, patients present with fever of more than 1 month's duration, fatigue, loss of weight, and diarrhea.

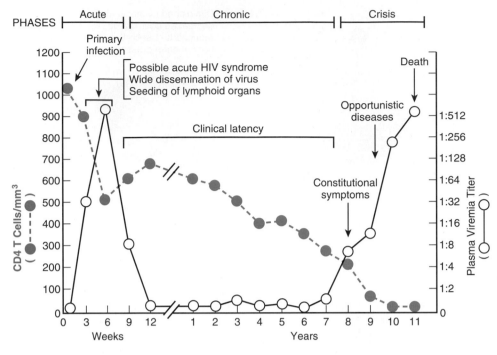

Figure 5–37 ■

Typical course of HIV infection. During the early period after primary infection, there is widespread dissemination of virus and a sharp decrease in the number of CD4+ T cells in peripheral blood. An immune response to HIV ensues, with a decrease in detectable viremia followed by a prolonged period of clinical latency during which viral replication and CD4 cell loss continues. Because CD4+ cells are replenished, the decline in their numbers is slow. Ultimately, after years it reaches a critical level below which there is a substantial risk of opportunistic diseases. (Redrawn from Pantaleo G, Graziosi C, Fauci AS: The immunopathogenesis of human immunodeficiency virus infection. N Engl J Med 328:327, 1993. Reprinted by permission of The New England Journal of Medicine. Copyright 1993, Massachusetts Medical Society.)

The CD4+ cell count is reduced, and patients develop opportunistic infections, secondary neoplasms, and neurologic manifestations. At this point the patient is said to have developed full-blown AIDS. According to current CDC guidelines, any HIV-infected individual whose CD4+ cell count drops below $200/\mu$l is said to have AIDS, even if the usual AIDS-defining conditions are not manifest. In the absence of treatment, most if not all patients with HIV infection will progress to AIDS after a chronic phase lasting 7 to 10 years. This period, often referred to as the *clinical latent phase,* is shorter in those who receive a large parenteral inoculum of HIV, as occurs with blood transfusions, or may be especially long in those who receive prophylactic antiretroviral therapy.

From a practical standpoint, CD4+ T-cell counts in the blood are reasonably accurate prognosticators of disease progression. Therefore, the CDC recommends stratification of

HIV infection into three categories on the basis of CD4+ cell counts: CD4+ counts greater than or equal to 500 cells/μl; 200 to 499 cells/μl; and fewer than 200 cells/μl. Patients in the first group are usually asymptomatic; counts below 500/μl are associated with the early symptoms, and decline of CD4+ levels below 200/μl is associated with severe immunosuppression and recurrent opportunistic infections.

It should be evident from our discussion that in each of the three phases of HIV infection viral replication continues to occur at a fairly brisk rate. Even in the middle, chronic phase, before the severe decline in the CD4+ cell count, there is extensive turnover of virus. In other words, *HIV infection lacks a phase of true microbiologic latency,* that is, a phase during which *all* the HIV is in the form of proviral DNA and no cell is productively infected. In keeping with this, recent studies indicate that, in addition to CD4+ cell counts, the amount of virus in the blood is also useful in determining the prognosis. Furthermore, because continued viral replication favors the emergence of mutant viruses, some of which are drug resistant, a strong case has been made for starting antiretroviral therapy, with multiple drugs, early in the course of HIV infection before the onset of clinical symptoms.

Clinical Features. The clinical manifestations of HIV infection can be readily surmised from the foregoing discussion. They range from a mild acute illness to severe disease. Because the salient clinical features of the acute early and chronic middle phases of HIV infection were described earlier, we will here summarize the clinical manifestations of the terminal phase, commonly known as AIDS.

In the United States the typical adult patient with AIDS is a young homosexual male or an intravenous drug abuser who presents with fever, weight loss, diarrhea, generalized lymphadenopathy, multiple opportunistic infections, neurologic disease, and (in many cases) secondary neoplasms. The infections and neoplasms listed in Table 5–11 are included in the

Table 5–10. PHASES OF HIV INFECTION AND CORRESPONDING CDC CLASSIFICATION CATEGORIES

Phase	CDC Classification	
Early, acute	Group I:	Acute infection
Middle, chronic	Group II:	Asymptomatic infection
	Group III:	Persistent generalized lymphadenopathy
Final, crisis	Group IV	
	Subgroup A:	Constitutional disease
	Subgroup B:	Neurologic disease
	Subgroup C:	Secondary infection
	Subgroup D:	Secondary neoplasm
	Subgroup E:	Other conditions

Table 5–11.   AIDS-DEFINING OPPORTUNISTIC INFECTIONS AND NEOPLASMS FOUND IN PATIENTS WITH HIV INFECTION

INFECTIONS
Protozoal and Helminthic Infections
Cryptosporidiosis or isosporidiosis (enteritis)
Pneumocystosis (pneumonia or disseminated infection)
Toxoplasmosis (pneumonia or CNS infection)

Fungal Infections
Candidiasis (esophageal, tracheal, or pulmonary)
Cryptococcosis (CNS infection)
Coccidioidomycosis (disseminated)
Histoplasmosis (disseminated)

Bacterial Infections
Mycobacteriosis ("atypical," e.g., *Mycobacterium avium-intracellulare,* disseminated or extrapulmonary; *M. tuberculosis,* pulmonary or extrapulmonary)
Nocardiosis (pneumonia, meningitis, disseminated)
Salmonella infections, disseminated

Viral Infections
Cytomegalovirus (pulmonary, intestinal, retinitis, or CNS infections)
Herpes simplex virus (localized or disseminated)
Varicella-zoster virus (localized or disseminated)
Progressive multifocal leukoencephalopathy

NEOPLASMS
Kaposi's sarcoma
Non-Hodgkin's lymphomas (Burkitt's, immunoblastic)
Primary lymphoma of brain
Invasive cancer of uterine cervix

CNS, central nervous system.

surveillance definition of AIDS. Pneumonia caused by the opportunistic fungus *P. carinii* (representing reactivation of a previous latent infection) is the presenting feature in many cases, although its incidence is declining thanks to effective prophylactic regimens. The risk of developing this infection is extremely high in individuals with fewer than 200 CD4+ cells per microliter. Approximately 12% of patients present with an opportunistic infection other than *P. carinii* pneumonia (Table 5–11). Among the most common are recurrent mucosal candidiasis, disseminated cytomegalovirus infection (particularly enteritis and retinitis), severe ulcerating oral and perianal herpes simplex, and disseminated infection with *M. tuberculosis* and atypical mycobacteria *(Mycobacterium avium-intracellulare)*. The AIDS epidemic has caused a resurgence of active tuberculosis in the United States. While in most cases it represents reactivation, the frequency of new infections is also increasing. Whereas *M. tuberculosis* manifests itself early in the course of AIDS, infections with atypical mycobacteria are seen late in the course of HIV disease, usually occurring in patients with fewer than 100 CD4+ cells/ μl. Toxoplasmosis is the most common secondary infection of the central nervous system. Cryptococcal meningitis is also quite frequent. Persistent diarrhea, so common in patients with AIDS, is often caused by *Cryptosporidium* or *Isospora belli* infections, but bacterial pathogens such as *Salmonella* and *Shigella* may also be involved. Because of depressed humoral immunity, AIDS patients are susceptible to infections with *S. pneumoniae* and *H. influenzae.*

Patients with AIDS have a high incidence of certain tumors, particularly Kaposi's sarcoma, non-Hodgkin's lymphomas, and cervical cancer in women. Kaposi's sarcoma is a vascular tumor otherwise rare in the United States. Although in recent years there has been a definite and unexplained decline in its incidence in the AIDS population, it remains the most common neoplasm in AIDS patients. Several features are peculiar to this tumor in these patients. It is far more common among homosexual or bisexual males than in intravenous drug abusers or patients belonging to other risk groups. The lesions can arise early, before the immune system is compromised, or in advanced stages of HIV infection. Unlike the lesions in sporadic cases of Kaposi's sarcoma, those that occur in AIDS patients are multicentric and tend to be more aggressive. Both the cause and pathogenesis of AIDS-associated Kaposi's sarcoma are still unclear. It arises from primitive mesenchymal cells that form vascular channels. The abnormal growth of these cells seems to result from the action of autocrine and paracrine growth factors, including fibroblast growth factor, IL-6, and oncostatin. The HIV-associated *tat* protein also plays a role, because mice transgenic for this protein develop vascular lesions. Recently, a novel human herpes virus called HHV-8 has also been implicated. Thus, the origin of Kaposi's sarcoma in patients seems to be a multifactorial event in which HIV proteins, cytokines, and HHV-8 act in concert.

Non-Hodgkin's lymphomas constitute the second most common type of AIDS-associated tumors. These tumors are highly aggressive, occur most frequently in severely immunosuppressed patients, and involve many extranodal sites. Brain is the most common extranodal site, and hence primary lymphoma of the brain is considered an AIDS-defining conditon. In keeping with their aggressive clinical course, most such lymphomas have a high-grade histologic picture (Chapter 12). As with other high-grade lymphomas, those that occur in the setting of AIDS are primarily of B-cell origin. At least in some cases (up to 50%), these lymphomas are associated with EBV and progress from polyclonal to monoclonal B-cell lesions. Because of an increased susceptibility to infection with human papillomavirus, women with AIDS are at increased risk for dysplastic changes in the cervical epithelium, with a concomitant increase in the incidence of invasive cervical cancer.

Involvement of the central nervous system is a common and important manifestation of AIDS. *In 70% to 90% of patients there is some form of neurologic involvement at autopsy, and 30% to 50% have clinically manifest neurologic dysfunction.* Significantly, in some patients neurologic manifestations may be the sole or earliest presenting feature of HIV infection. In addition to opportunistic infections and neoplasms, several virally determined neuropathologic changes occur. These include an aseptic meningitis occurring at the time of seroconversion, vacuolar myelopathy, peripheral neuropathies, and (most commonly) a progressive encephalopathy clinically designated the AIDS-dementia complex (Chapter 23).

MORPHOLOGY. The anatomic changes in the tissues (with the exception of lesions in the brain) are neither specific nor diagnostic. In general the pathologic features of AIDS are those characteristic of widespread opportunistic infections, Kaposi's sarcoma, and lymphoid tumors. Most of these lesions have been discussed elsewhere, because they also occur in patients who do not have HIV infection. To appreciate the distinctive nature of lesions in the central nervous system, they are discussed in the context of other disorders affecting the brain (Chapter 23). Here we concentrate on changes in the lymphoid organs.

Biopsy specimens from enlarged lymph nodes in the early stages of HIV infection reveal a marked follicular hyperplasia (Chapter 12). The medulla shows intense plasmacytosis. These changes, affecting primarily the B-cell areas of the node, are the morphologic counterparts of the polyclonal B-cell activation and hypergammaglobulinemia seen in patients with AIDS. In addition to changes in the follicles, the sinuses show increased cellularity due primarily to an increase in histiocytes, but contributed to also by immunoblasts (B cells) and plasma cells. Under the electron microscope and by in situ hybridization, HIV particles can be detected within the germinal centers, concentrated on the villous processes of the follicular dendritic cells. As will be evident from our earlier discussion, viral DNA can also be detected in macrophages and CD4+ cells.

With the onset of full-blown AIDS, the frenzy of B-cell proliferation subsides and gives way to a pattern of severe follicular involution and generalized lymphocyte depletion. The organized network of follicular dendritic cells is disrupted and the follicles may even become hyalinized. These "burnt-out" lymph nodes are atrophic and small and may harbor numerous opportunistic pathogens. Because of profound immunosuppression, the inflammatory response to infections both in the lymph nodes and at extranodal sites may be sparse or atypical. For example, with severe immunosuppression mycobacteria do not evoke granuloma formation because CD4+ cells are deficient. In the empty-looking lymph nodes and in other organs the presence of infectious agents may not be readily apparent without the application of special stains. As might be expected, lymphoid depletion is not confined to the nodes; in the later stages of AIDS, the spleen and thymus also appear to be "wastelands."

Non-Hodgkin's lymphomas, involving the nodes as well as extranodal sites such as liver, gastrointestinal tract, and bone marrow, are primarily high-degree diffuse B-cell neoplasms (Chapter 12).

Since the discovery of AIDS in 1981, the concerted efforts of epidemiologists, immunologists, and molecular biologists have resulted in spectacular advances in our understanding of this disorder. Despite all this progress, however, the prognosis of AIDS patients remains dismal. Of the 500,000 patients reported, over 300,000 were dead by late 1996. With time, true mortality figures are likely to be much higher, perhaps approaching 100%. However, approximately 5% of patients with documented HIV infection do not develop progressive disease. Their CD4+ counts remain above $500/\mu l$. Such long-term nonprogressors are under intense scrutiny, for they may provide clues to the control of HIV infection. Some seem to have been infected by mutant viruses lacking the *nef* regulatory protein, thus exposing the Achilles heel of HIV. Others develop a vigorous immune response, the analysis of which will be useful in vaccine development. At present, however, prevention and public health measures remain the mainstay of control.

AMYLOIDOSIS

Amyloid is an abnormal proteinaceous substance that is deposited between cells in many tissues and organs of the body in a variety of clinical disorders. Since its first recognition, it has been delineated by its morphologic appearance on light microscopy. With usual tissue stains, *amyloid appears as an intercellular pink translucent material*. At one time it was thought to be starchlike, hence the designation "amyloid"; however, it is now known to be composed largely of protein.

Despite the striking morphologic uniformity of amyloid in all cases, *it is quite clear that amyloid is not a single chemical entity*. Two major and several minor biochemical forms exist. These are deposited by several different pathogenetic mechanisms, and therefore amyloidosis should not be considered a single disease; rather, it is a group of diseases that share in common the deposition of similar-appearing proteins. At the heart of the morphologic uniformity is the remarkably uniform physical organization of amyloid protein, which we will consider first. This will be followed by a discussion of the chemical nature of amyloid.

Physical Nature of Amyloid. By electron microscopy, amyloid appears to be made up largely of nonbranching fibrils with a width of approximately 7.5 to 10 nm. X-ray crystallography and infrared spectroscopy demonstrate a characteristic pattern described as a "β-pleated sheet conformation," which is unique among fibrillar mammalian proteins. This conformation (Fig. 5–38), seen regardless of the clinical setting or the chemical composition, is responsible for the distinctive staining and optical properties of amyloid (discussed later). In other words, any fibrillar protein deposited in tissues that yields a β-pleated sheet will be recognized as amyloid. In addition to the fibrils, a nonfibrillar pentagonal substance (P component) is a minor component of all amyloid deposits.

Chemical Nature of Amyloid. Two major chemical classes of amyloid have been identified: *one composed of immunoglobulin light chains called AL (amyloid light chain), the other made up of a nonimmunoglobulin protein designated AA (amyloid associated)*. These proteins are antigenically distinct and, as discussed later, are deposited in different clinical settings. Immunoglobulin amyloid fibril protein (AL) is made up of complete immunoglobulin light chains, the N-terminal fragment of light chains, or both. Most frequently it is the λ light chain that gives rise to AL. The AL amyloid protein is associated with B-cell dyscrasias and is produced by immunoglobulin-secreting cells. The other major form of amyloid

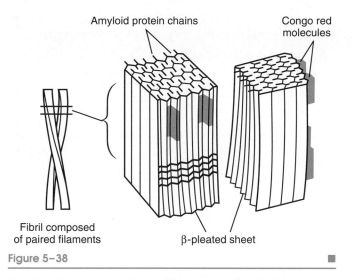

Amyloid protein chains

Congo red molecules

Fibril composed of paired filaments

β-pleated sheet

Figure 5–38   ■

Structure of an amyloid fibril, depicting the β-pleated sheet structure and binding sites for the Congo red dye, which is used for diagnosis of amyloidosis. (After Glenner GD: Amyloid deposit and amyloidosis. The β-fibrilloses. N Engl J Med 302:1283, 1980. Reprinted by permission of The New England Journal of Medicine. Copyright 1980, Massachusetts Medical Society.)

fibril protein, AA, can be described as a unique nonimmunoglobulin protein with a molecular weight of 8500 daltons. AA fibrils are derived from a larger precursor protein in the serum called SAA (serum amyloid-associated protein), which serves as the protein component (apoprotein) of a high-density lipoprotein. SAA behaves as an acute-phase reactant, its serum concentration increasing 1000-fold within 24 hours of an inflammatory stimulus. As will be pointed out, AA protein is the major component of the amyloid deposited secondary to chronic inflammatory diseases.

Several other biochemically distinct proteins have been found in amyloid deposits in a variety of clinical settings:

■ Transthyretin is a normal serum protein that binds and *trans*ports *thy*roxine and *retin*ol, hence the name. A mutant form of transthyretin (and its fragments) is deposited in a group of genetically determined disorders referred to as familial amyloid polyneuropathies. Another variant form of transthyretin is deposited in amyloidosis associated with aging.

■ β_2-microglobulin, a normal serum protein that is a component of the MHC class I molecules, has been identified as the amyloid fibril subunit in the amyloidosis that complicates the course of patients receiving long-term hemodialysis.

■ β_2-amyloid protein ($A\beta_2$), a 4000-dalton peptide, constitutes the core of cerebral plaques found in Alzheimer's disease as well as the amyloid deposited in walls of cerebral blood vessels of patients with Alzheimer's disease. The $A\beta_2$ protein is derived from a much larger transmembrane glycoprotein, called amyloid precursor protein (APP).

■ In addition to the foregoing types, amyloid deposits derived from diverse precursors such as hormones (procalcitonin, proinsulin) and keratin have also been reported.

The nonfibrillar P component described earlier is a normal serum α_1-glycoprotein that bears a striking structural homology to C-reactive protein, a well-known acute-phase reactant. Serum P component has an affinity for purified amyloid fibrils, and its presence in amyloid deposits is responsible for the staining with periodic acid–Schiff (PAS) that led early observers to believe that amyloid was a saccharide.

Classification. Classification of amyloidoses is based on the associated clinical setting, anatomic distribution, and chemical composition of amyloid (Table 5–12).

Immunocyte Dyscrasias With Amyloidosis. Amyloidosis in this category is systemic in distribution and results from deposition of immunoglobulin light chains (AL) or their fragments, produced by aberrant clones of B cells. *In the United States this is the most common form of amyloidosis.* The best example in this category is amyloidosis associated with multiple myeloma, a malignant neoplasm of plasma cells (Chapter 12). This disorder is characterized by proliferation of neoplastic B cells in the bone marrow, often producing multiple osteolytic lesions in the skeleton. The malignant plasma cells are monoclonal and therefore secrete a single species of immunoglobulin (monoclonal gammopathy), producing an M (myeloma) protein spike on serum electrophoresis. In addition to complete immunoglobulin molecules, the plasma cells may also synthesize and secrete only the λ or κ light chains, also known as Bence Jones proteins. These are present in the blood of up to 70% of patients with multiple myeloma, but amyloidosis develops in only 6% to 15% of cases of myeloma. Most patients who develop amyloidosis do have Bence Jones proteins. However, it is clear that free light-chain production, although necessary, is not by itself sufficient to produce amyloidosis. It is believed that the quality of the light chain produced (amyloidogenic potential) and the subsequent handling (degradation?) are important factors that determine whether the Bence Jones proteins are deposited as amyloid.

Most patients with AL amyloidosis (also called primary amyloidosis) do not have multiple myeloma. However, like multiple myeloma, primary amyloidosis is a disorder of immunoglobulin-secreting cells. Monoclonal immunoglobulins, free light chains, or both can be found in serum or urine. Most patients have a modest increase in the number of plasma cells in the bone marrow, but the destructive skeletal lesions seen in multiple myeloma are not present.

Reactive Systemic Amyloidosis. The amyloid deposits in this group are systemic in distribution and are composed of AA protein. This category is commonly referred to as "secondary amyloidosis" because it is believed to be secondary to chronic inflammatory conditions. *The unifying feature of various conditions that predispose to reactive systemic amyloidosis is the protracted breakdown of cells, resulting in most cases from a chronic inflammatory disorder.* Before the advent of antimicrobial chemotherapy, diseases such as tuberculosis, chronic osteomyelitis, and bronchiectasis were the common culprits, and in many parts of the world infectious disease is still the number one cause of amyloidosis. In the United States, however, it more commonly complicates rheumatoid arthritis, other connective tissue disorders, ulcerative colitis, neoplasms (e.g., Hodgkin's disease), and chronic skin infections associated with intravenous drug abuse. As mentioned, AA protein, which is deposited as amyloid, is derived from SAA, a precursor protein in the serum.

Heredofamilial Amyloidosis. This group includes several mendelian disorders characterized by widespread deposits of

Table 5-12. CLASSIFICATION OF AMYLOIDOSIS

Clinicopathologic Category	Associated Diseases	Major Fibril Protein	Chemically Related Precursor Protein
Systemic (Generalized) Amyloidosis			
Immunocyte dyscrasias with amyloidosis (primary amyloidosis)	Multiple myeloma and other monoclonal B-cell proliferations	AL	Immunoglobulin light chains, chiefly λ type
Reactive systemic amyloidosis (secondary amyloidosis)	Chronic inflammatory conditions	AA	SAA
Hemodialysis-associated amyloidosis	Chronic renal failure	β_2-microglobulin	β_2-microglobulin
Hereditary amyloidosis			
(1) Familial Mediterranean fever	—	AA	SAA
(2) Familial amyloidotic neuropathies (several types)	—	Transthyretin*	Transthyretin
Localized Amyloidosis			
Senile cardiac	—	Transthyretin	Transthyretin
Senile cerebral	Alzheimer's disease	$A\beta_2$	APP
Endocrine (e.g., medullary carcinoma of thyroid)	—	Procalcitonin	Calcitonin

* Transthyretin is also known as prealbumin. The transthyretins deposited as amyloid are mutant forms of normal transthyretin except in senile cardiac amyloidosis. AL, amyloid light chain; AA, amyloid-associated (protein); SAA, serum amyloid-associated (protein).

amyloid in the tissues. Best characterized is familial Mediterranean fever, which is inherited as an autosomal recessive trait. Affected persons are of Armenian, Sephardic Jewish, or Arabic origins. The amyloid fibrils are composed of AA protein. This may be related to the recurrent bouts of inflammation of the joints and serosal surfaces that characterize this condition. Several other heredofamilial forms characterized by deposition of amyloid in the nerves have been recognized but are extremely rare. As mentioned earlier, in these neuropathic forms, mutant transthyretins are deposited as amyloid fibrils (Table 5-12).

Localized Amyloidosis. Localized amyloidosis is a heterogeneous group, in terms of both chemical composition of amyloid and clinical presentation. Sites that may be involved in the form of nodular deposits include lungs, larynx, skin, urinary bladder, and tongue. Often, infiltrates of plasma cells are found around the nodules, and in at least some cases the amyloid consists of AL protein. Local deposits of amyloid are also sometimes found within tumors of the endocrine system. Medullary carcinoma of the thyroid is one such example in which the amyloid is chemically related to calcitonin, a hormone secreted by the tumor cells.

Amyloid of Aging. Two well-documented forms of amyloidosis occur in aging persons. Senile cardiac amyloidosis affects elderly patients, most often in the eighth and ninth decades of life. In many cases the amyloid fibrils are formed of transthyretin. Senile cardiac amyloidosis may be asymptomatic or may produce serious cardiac dysfunction. Senile cerebral amyloidosis refers to the deposition of $A\beta_2$ protein in the cerebral blood vessels and plaques of patients with Alzheimer's disease (Chapter 23).

Pathogenesis. Although the precursors of the two major amyloid proteins have been identified, several aspects of their origins are still not clear. In reactive systemic amyloidosis, it appears that long-standing tissue destruction and inflamma-

tion lead to elevated SAA levels (Fig. 5-39). SAA is synthesized by the liver cells under the influence of cytokines such as IL-6 and IL-1; however, increased production of SAA by itself is not sufficient for the deposition of amyloid. Elevation of serum SAA levels is common to inflammatory states but in most instances does not lead to amyloidosis. It is believed that SAA is normally degraded to soluble end products by the action of monocyte-derived enzymes. Conceivably, individuals who develop amyloidosis have an enzyme defect that results in the incomplete breakdown of SAA, thus generating insoluble AA molecules. In the case of immunocyte dyscrasias, the source of the precursor proteins is well defined, and amyloid material can be derived in vitro by proteolysis of immunoglobulin light chains. However, we still do not know why only a fraction of persons who have circulating Bence Jones proteins develop amyloidosis. Again, defective proteolytic degradation has been invoked, but firm evidence is lacking.

MORPHOLOGY. There are no consistent or distinctive patterns of organ or tissue distribution of amyloid deposits in any of the categories cited. Nonetheless, a few generalizations can be made. In amyloidosis secondary to chronic inflammatory disorders, kidneys, liver, spleen, lymph nodes, adrenals, and thyroid, as well as many other tissues, are typically affected. Although immunocyte-associated amyloidosis cannot reliably be distinguished from the secondary form by its organ distribution, it more often involves the heart, gastrointestinal tract, respiratory tract, peripheral nerves, skin, and tongue. However, the same organs affected by reactive systemic amyloidosis (secondary amyloidosis), including kidneys, liver,

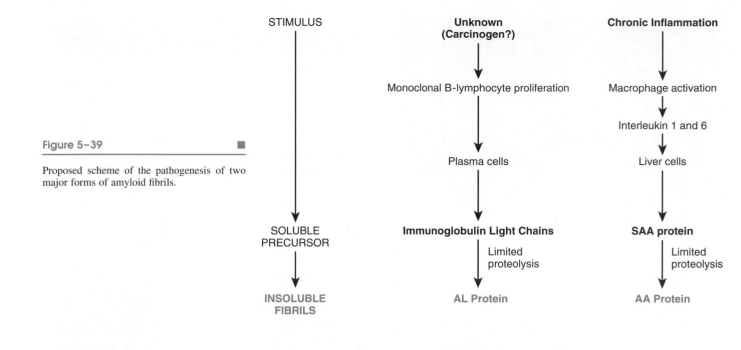

Figure 5–39 ■

Proposed scheme of the pathogenesis of two major forms of amyloid fibrils.

and spleen, may also contain deposits in the immunocyte-associated form of the disease.

The localization of amyloid deposits in the **heredofamilial syndromes** is varied. In familial Mediterranean fever the amyloidosis may be widespread, involving the kidneys, blood vessels, spleen, respiratory tract, and (rarely) liver. The localization of amyloid in the remaining hereditary syndromes can be inferred from the designation of these entities. **Localized organ amyloidosis** has already been characterized.

Whatever the clinical disorder, the amyloidosis may or may not be apparent on macroscopic examination. Often, small amounts are not recognized until the surface of the cut organ is painted with iodine and sulfuric acid. This yields mahogany brown staining of the amyloid deposits. When amyloid accumulates in larger amounts, the organ is frequently enlarged and the tissue appears gray with a waxy, firm consistency. **Histologically, the deposition always begins between cells,** often closely adjacent to basement membranes. As the amyloid accumulates, it encroaches on the cells. In time the depositions surround and destroy the trapped native cells. In the immunocyte-associated form, perivascular and vascular localizations are common.

The histologic diagnosis of amyloid is based almost entirely on its staining characteristics. The most commonly used staining technique utilizes the dye Congo red, which under ordinary light imparts a pink or red color to amyloid deposits. Under polarized light the Congo red–stained amyloid shows green birefringence. This reaction is shared by all forms of amyloid and is due to the crossed β-pleated configuration of amyloid fibrils. AA and AL amyloid can be distinguished in histo-

logic sections. AA protein loses affinity for Congo red after incubation of tissue sections with potassium permanganate, whereas AL proteins and most other chemical forms of amyloid do not. Immunoperoxidase staining with monoclonal antibodies directed toward various chemical forms of amyloid is also useful in diagnosis.

Because the pattern of organ involvement in different clinical forms of amyloidosis is variable, each of the major organ involvements is described separately.

Amyloidosis of the kidney is the most common and most serious involvement in the disease. Grossly, the kidney may appear unchanged, or it may be abnormally large, pale, gray, and firm. In long-standing cases the kidney may be reduced in size. Microscopically, the amyloid deposits are found principally in the glomeruli, but they are also present in the interstitial peritubular tissue as well as in the walls of the blood vessels. The glomerulus first develops focal deposits within the mesangial matrix and diffuse or nodular thickenings of the basement membranes of the capillary loops. With progression, the deposition encroaches on the capillary lumina and eventually leads to total obliteration of the vascular tuft (Fig. 5–40). The interstitial peritubular deposits are frequently associated with the appearance of amorphous pink casts within the tubular lumina, presumably of proteinaceous nature. Amyloid deposits may develop in the walls of blood vessels of all sizes, often causing marked vascular narrowing. It is this vascular narrowing that presumably leads to the contracture of the kidneys, mentioned previously.

Amyloidosis of the spleen often causes moderate or even marked enlargement (200 to 800 gm). For obscure reasons, one of two patterns may de-

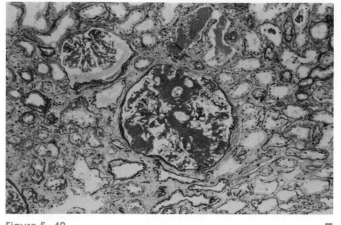

Figure 5–40 ■

Amyloidosis of the kidney. The glomerular architecture is almost totally obliterated by the massive accumulation of amyloid.

velop. The deposits may be virtually limited to the splenic follicles, producing tapioca-like granules on gross examination ("sago spleen"), or the involvement may affect principally the splenic sinuses and eventually extend to the splenic pulp, forming large, sheetlike deposits ("lardaceous spleen"). In both patterns, the spleen appears firm in consistency and often reveals on the cut surface the pale, gray, waxy deposits in the distribution described.

Amyloidosis of the liver may cause massive enlargement, up to such extraordinary weights as 9000 gm. In such advanced cases the liver is extremely pale, grayish, and waxy on both the external surface and the cut section. Histologically, the deposits appear first in the space of Disse and then progressively enlarge to encroach on the adjacent hepatic parenchyma and sinusoids. The trapped liver cells are literally squeezed to death and are eventually replaced by sheets of amyloid.

Amyloidosis of the heart may occur either as an isolated organ involvement or as part of a systemic distribution. When accompanied by systemic involvement, it is usually associated with immunocyte dyscrasias. The isolated form **(senile amyloidosis)** is usually confined to individuals of advanced age. The deposits may not be evident on gross examination, or they may cause minimal to moderate cardiac enlargement. The most characteristic gross findings are gray-pink, dewdrop-like subendocardial elevations, particularly in the atrial chambers. However, on histologic examination, in addition to these focal subendocardial accumulations, deposits are frequently found throughout the myocardium, beginning between myocardial fibers and eventually causing their pressure atrophy.

Amyloidosis of the endocrine organs, particularly of the adrenals, thyroid, and pituitary, is common in advanced systemic distributions. In this case also the amyloid deposition begins in relation to stromal and endothelial cells and progressively encroaches on the parenchymal cells. Surprisingly, large amounts of amyloid may be present in any of these endocrine glands without apparent disturbance of function.

Other organs may be involved. Indeed, no organ or tissue of the body is exempt. Deposits may be encountered in the upper and lower respiratory passages, sometimes in nodular masses. The gastrointestinal tract is a relatively favored site, in which amyloid may be found at all levels, sometimes producing tumorous masses that must be distinguished from neoplasms. Depositions in the tongue may produce macroglossia. On the basis of the frequent involvement of the gastrointestinal tract in systemic cases, gingival, intestinal, and rectal biopsies are employed in the diagnosis of suspected cases. Congo red staining and polarization microscopy should be used in all cases to detect trace amounts, which may be limited to the vascular walls within the tissue examined. The skin, eye, and nervous system are also affected. Deposition of β_2-microglobulin amyloid in patients receiving long-term dialysis occurs most commonly in the carpal ligaments of the wrist, resulting in compression of the median nerve (carpal tunnel syndrome).

Clinical Correlation. Amyloidosis may be an unsuspected finding at autopsy in a patient who has no apparent related clinical manifestations, or it may be responsible for serious clinical dysfunction and even death. All depends on the particular sites or organs affected and the severity of the involvement. Nonspecific complaints such as weakness, fatigue, and weight loss are the most common initial symptoms. Later in the course, amyloidosis tends to manifest itself in one of several ways: by renal disease, hepatomegaly, splenomegaly, or cardiac abnormalities. Renal involvement giving rise to severe proteinuria (nephrotic syndrome) is often the major cause of symptoms in reactive systemic amyloidosis (secondary amyloidosis). Advancement of the renal disease may lead to renal failure, which is an important cause of death in these patients. The hepatosplenomegaly rarely causes significant clinical dysfunction, but it may be the presenting finding. Cardiac amyloidosis may manifest itself as conduction disturbances or an apparent cardiomyopathy. Cardiac arrhythmias are an important cause of death in cardiac amyloidosis. In one large series, 40% of the patients with AL amyloid died of cardiac disease.

The diagnosis of amyloidosis may be suspected from the clinical signs and symptoms and from some of the findings mentioned; however, more specific tests must often be employed for definitive diagnosis. *Biopsy followed by Congo red staining is the most important tool in the diagnosis of amyloidosis.* In general, biopsy is taken from the organ suspected to be involved. For example, renal biopsy is useful in the presence of urinary abnormalities. Rectal and gingival biopsy specimens contain amyloid in up to 75% of cases with generalized amyloidosis. Examination of abdominal fat aspirates stained with Congo red is a simple, low-risk method that is finding widespread use. In suspected cases of immunocyte-associated amyloidosis, serum and urinary protein electrophoresis and immunoelectrophoresis should be performed. Bone marrow in such cases usually shows plasmacytosis, even if skeletal lesions of multiple myeloma are not present.

The outlook for patients with generalized amyloidosis is poor, and the mean survival time after diagnosis ranges from 1 to 3 years. When the disease is associated with immunocytic dyscrasias, cytotoxic drugs have been used to treat the underlying disorder.

BIBLIOGRAPHY

Abbas AK, Murphy KM, Sher A: Functional diversity of helper T lymphocytes. Nature 383:787, 1996. (An excellent review of T_H1 and T_H2 lymphocytes and the implications of this dichotomy.)

Akil M, Amos RS: Rheumatoid arthritis. I: Clinical features and diagnosis. BMJ 310:587, 1995. (A short and easy-to-read article summarizing clinical aspects of rheumatoid arthritis.)

Boumpas DT, et al: Systemic lupus erythematosus: emerging concepts. Part 1: Renal, neuropsychiatric, cardiovascular, pulmonary, and hematologic disease. Ann Intern Med 122:940, 1995. (Review of literature relating to the pathogenesis of organ injury in lupus.)

Chadwick EG, Yogev R: Pediatric AIDS. Pediatr Clin North Am 42:969, 1995. (A review covering various aspects of AIDS in children.)

Dalakas MC: Polymyositis, dermatomyositis, and inclusion-body myositis. N Engl J Med 325:1487, 1991. (An excellent review of the current thinking on the etiology, pathogenesis, and clinical aspects of inflammatory myopathies.)

Feldman M, Brennan FM, Maini RN: Rheumatoid arthritis. Cell 85:307, 1996. (A short review of the immunopathogenesis of rheumatoid arthritis.)

Garcia-Zepeda EA, et al: Human eotaxin is a specific chemoattractant for eosinophil cells and provides a new mechanism to explain tissue eosinophilia. Nature Med 2:449, 1996. (Isolation and characterization of human eotaxin.)

Golbus J, McCune WJ: Lupus nephritis: classification, prognosis, immunopathogenesis, and treatment. Rheum Dis Clin North Am 20:213, 1994. (A scholarly and detailed discussion of the renal disease in lupus.)

Herndier BG, et al: Pathogenesis of AIDS lymphomas. AIDS 8:1025, 1994.

(A scholarly review of the factors that are critical to the causation of B cell lymphomas in AIDS.)

Ho D: Viral counts count in HIV infection. Science 272:1124, 1996. (A short editorial on the relevance of plasma viral load in the prognosis of AIDS.)

Huang Y, et al: The role of mutant CCR5 allele in HIV-1 transmission and disease progression. Nat Med 2:1240, 1996. (Role of chemokine receptors in pathogenesis of AIDS.)

Kotzin BL: Systemic lupus erythematosus. Cell 85:303, 1996. (An in depth discussion of the immunologic derangements in SLE.)

Panayi GS: The immunopathogenesis of rheumatoid arthritis. Br J Rheumatol 32 (Suppl 1):4, 1993. (A review of the role of T lymphocytes in the pathogenesis of rheumatoid arthritis.)

Quinn TC: The epidemiology of the acquired immunodeficiency syndrome in the 1990s. Emerg Med Clin North Am 13:1, 1995. (A review of the changing patterns of the epidemiology of HIV infection.)

Roizman B: New viral footprints in Kaposi's sarcoma. N Engl J Med 332:1227, 1995. (An editorial that summarizes the possible role of a herpes virus in the causation of AIDS-related Kaposi's sarcoma.)

Rosen FS, et al: The primary immunodeficiences. N Engl J Med 333:431, 1995. (An extremely lucid review of the molecular basis of primary immunodeficiency.)

Schrager LK, Fauci AS: Trapped but still dangerous. Nature 377:680, 1995. (A short commentary on the infectious nature of HIV trapped on dendritic cells.)

Steinman L: Escape from "horror autotoxicus": pathogenesis and treatment of autoimmune disease. Cell 80:7, 1995. (A short review of the relevant factors in the pathogenesis of autoimmune disease.)

Suthanthiran M, Strom TB: Renal transplantation. N Engl J Med 331:365, 1994. (A very readable review of the modern view of the immunobiology and clinical aspects of renal transplantation.)

Theofilopoulos AN: The basis of autoimmunity. Part I: Mechanisms of aberrant self-recognition. Immunol Today 16:90, 1995. (A scholarly and detailed discussion of the cellular and genetic basis of autoimmunity.)

von Mühlen CA, Tan EM: Autoantibodies in the diagnosis of systemic rheumatic diseases. Semin Arthritis Rheum 24:323, 1995. (A scholarly discussion of the various autoantibodies in a wide variety of autoimmune diseases.)

Wain-Hobson S: Virological mayhem. Nature 373:102, 1995. (A short commentary on the revelation that there is extensive viral replication during all phases of HIV infection.)

Weiss RA: HIV receptors and the pathogenesis of AIDS. Science 272:1885, 1996. (A brief commentary on the nature and significance of HIV coreceptors.)

Wigley FM: Clinical aspects of systemic and localized scleroderma. Curr Opin Rheumatol 6:628, 1994. (An update on the clinical manifestations of scleroderma.)

6

Neoplasia

Cancer is the second leading cause of death in the United States; only cardiovascular diseases exact a higher toll. Even more agonizing than the mortality rate is the emotional and physical suffering inflicted by these neoplasms. The only hope for controlling this dreadful scourge lies in learning more about its etiology and pathogenesis, and indeed great strides have been made in understanding the etiology and molecular basis of cancer. This chapter deals with the basic biology of neoplasia—namely, the nature of benign and malignant neoplasms as well as the molecular basis of neoplastic transformation. We will also discuss the host response to tumors and the clinical features of neoplasia.

DEFINITIONS

"Neoplasia" literally means "new growth." A neoplasm, as defined by Willis, is "an abnormal mass of tissue the growth of which exceeds and is uncoordinated with that of the normal tissues and persists in the same excessive manner after the cessation of the stimuli which evoked the change." *Fundamental to the origin of all neoplasms is loss of responsiveness to normal growth controls.* Neoplastic cells are said to be transformed because they continue to replicate, apparently oblivious to the regulatory influences that control normal cell growth. In addition, neoplasms seem to behave as parasites and compete with normal cells and tissues for their metabolic needs. Thus, tumors may flourish in patients who are otherwise wasting. Neoplasms also enjoy a certain degree of autonomy and more or less steadily increase in size regardless of their local environment and the nutritional status of the host. Their autonomy, however, is by no means complete. Some neoplasms require endocrine support, and indeed such dependencies can sometimes be exploited to the disadvantage of the neoplasm. Moreover, all are critically dependent on the host for their nutrition and blood supply.

In common medical usage a neoplasm is often referred to as a *tumor*, and the study of tumors is called *oncology* (from *oncos,* tumor, and *logos,* study of). Strictly speaking, a tumor is merely a swelling that could be produced by, among other things, edema or hemorrhage into a tissue. Currently, the term *tumor* is applied almost solely to neoplastic masses that may cause swellings on or within the body; use of the term for non-neoplastic lesions has almost disappeared. In oncology the division of neoplasms into benign and malignant categories is most important. This categorization is based on a judgment of a neoplasm's potential clinical behavior.

A tumor is said to be "benign" when its microscopic and gross characteristics are considered relatively innocent, implying that it will remain localized, cannot spread to other sites, and is therefore generally amenable to local surgical removal and survival of the patient. It should be noted, however, that benign tumors can produce more than localized lumps, and sometimes they are responsible for serious disease, as will be pointed out later.

Malignant tumors are collectively referred to as *cancers*, derived from the Latin word for crab—they adhere to any part that they seize on in an obstinate manner, like a crab. "Malignant," as applied to a neoplasm, implies that the lesion can invade and destroy adjacent structures and spread to distant sites (metastasize) to cause death. Obviously, not all cancers pursue so deadly a course. Some are discovered early and are successfully treated, but the designation *malignant* constitutes a red flag.

NOMENCLATURE

All tumors, benign and malignant, have two basic components: (1) the parenchyma, made up of transformed or neoplastic cells; and (2) the supporting, host-derived, non-neoplastic stroma, made up of connective tissue and blood vessels. Obviously, it is the parenchyma of the neoplasm that determines its biologic behavior, and it is this component from which the tumor derives its name. The stroma, however, carries the blood supply and provides support for the growth of parenchymal cells and is therefore crucial to the growth of the neoplasm.

Benign Tumors. In general, these are designated by attaching the suffix "-oma" to the cell type from which the tumor arises. A benign tumor arising in fibrous tissue is a *fibroma;* a benign cartilaginous tumor is a *chondroma.* The nomenclature of benign epithelial tumors is more complex. They are classified sometimes on the basis of their microscopic pattern and sometimes on the basis of their macroscopic pattern. Others are classified by their cells of origin. Some examples follow:

■ *Adenoma.* This term is applied to benign epithelial neoplasms producing gland patterns and to those derived from glands but not necessarily exhibiting gland patterns. A benign epithelial neoplasm arising from renal tubule cells and growing in glandlike patterns would be termed an adenoma, as would a mass of benign epithelial cells that produces no glandular patterns but has its origin in the adrenal cortex.
■ *Papilloma.* Papillomas are benign epithelial neoplasms, growing on any surface, that produce microscopic or macroscopic finger-like fronds (Fig. 6–1).
■ *Polyp.* A polyp is a mass that projects above a mucosal surface, as in the gut, to form a macroscopically visible structure. Although this term is commonly used for benign tumors, some malignant tumors may also appear as polyps. Sometimes, especially in the colon, the term is also applied to non-neoplastic growths that form polypoid masses.
■ *Cystadenomas.* Cystadenomas are hollow cystic masses; typically they are seen in the ovary.

Malignant Tumors. The nomenclature of malignant tumors essentially follows that of benign tumors, with certain additions and exceptions.

Malignant neoplasms arising in mesenchymal tissue or its derivatives are called *sarcomas.* A cancer of fibrous tissue origin is a *fibrosarcoma,* and a malignant neoplasm composed of chondrocytes is a *chondrosarcoma.* Thus, sarcomas are designated by their histogenesis (i.e., the cell type of which they are composed). Malignant neoplasms of epithelial cell origin are called *carcinomas.* It must be remembered that the epithelia of the body are derived from all three germ layers;

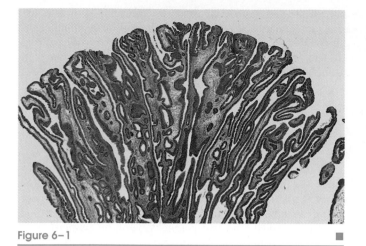

Figure 6-1 ■

Papilloma of the colon with finger-like projections into the lumen. (Courtesy of Dr. Trace Worrell, Department of Pathology, University of Texas Southwestern Medical School, Dallas.)

thus, a malignant neoplasm arising in the renal tubular epithelium (mesoderm) is a carcinoma, as are the cancers arising in the skin (ectoderm) and lining epithelium of the gut (endoderm). It is evident, then, that mesoderm may give rise to carcinomas (epithelial) and sarcomas (mesenchymal). Carcinomas may be further qualified. *Squamous cell carcinoma* would denote a cancer in which the tumor cells resemble stratified squamous epithelium, and *adenocarcinoma* a lesion in which the neoplastic epithelial cells grow in gland patterns. Sometimes the tissue or organ of origin can be identified, as for instance in the designation of renal cell adenocarcinoma or in cholangiocarcinoma, which implies an origin from bile ducts. Sometimes the tumor grows in a very undifferentiated pattern and must be called *poorly differentiated carcinoma.*

The parenchymal cells in a neoplasm, whether benign or malignant, more or less resemble each other, as though all had been derived from a single progenitor. Indeed, it appears that most neoplasms are of monoclonal origin, as will be documented later. However, in some instances, the stem cell may undergo *divergent differentiation,* creating so-called *mixed tumors.* The best example is the mixed tumor of salivary gland origin. These tumors have obvious epithelial components dispersed throughout an apparent fibromyxoid stroma, sometimes harboring islands of cartilage or bone (Fig. 6–2). All of these diverse elements are thought to derive from epithelial or myoepithelial cells, or both, in the salivary glands, and hence the preferred designation of these neoplasms is *pleomorphic adenoma.* Fibroadenoma of the female breast is another common mixed tumor. This benign tumor contains a mixture of proliferated ductal elements (adenoma) embedded in a loose fibrous tissue (fibroma). Although recent studies suggest that only the fibrous component is neoplastic, the term *fibroadenoma* remains in common usage. The multifaced mixed tumors should not be confused with a *teratoma,* which contains recognizable mature or immature cells or tissues representative of more than one germ layer and sometimes all

three. Teratomas take origin from totipotential cells such as are normally present in the ovary and testis and sometimes abnormally present in sequestered midline embryonic rests. Such cells obviously have the capacity to differentiate into any of the cell types to be found in the adult body and so, not surprisingly, may give rise to neoplasms that mimic, in a helter-skelter fashion, bits of bone, epithelium, muscle, fat, nerve, and other tissues. When all the component parts are well differentiated, it is a *benign (mature) teratoma;* when less well differentiated, it is an immature, potentially or overtly, malignant teratoma.

The specific names of the more common forms of neoplasms are presented in Table 6–1. Some glaring inconsistencies may be noted. For example, the terms *lymphoma, mesothelioma, melanoma,* and *seminoma* are used for malignant neoplasms. These inappropriate usages are firmly entrenched in medical terminology; perhaps it is irrational to expect humans to be rational.

There are other instances of confusing terminology. The *hamartoma* is a malformation that presents as a mass of disorganized tissue indigenous to the particular site. Thus, one may see a mass of mature but disorganized hepatic cells, blood vessels, and possibly bile ducts within the liver, or there may be a hamartomatous nodule in the lung containing islands of cartilage, bronchi, and blood vessels. Another misnomer is the term *choristoma.* This congenital anomaly is better described as a *heterotopic rest* of cells. For example, a small nodule of very well developed and normally organized pancreatic substance may be found in the submucosa of the stomach, duodenum, or even small intestine. This heterotopic rest may be replete with islets of Langerhans as well as exocrine glands. The term *choristoma,* connoting a neoplasm, imparts to the heterotopic rest a gravity far beyond its usual trivial significance. Regrettably, neither life nor the terminology of neoplasms is simple, but the terminology has importance because it is the language by which the nature and significance of tumors are categorized.

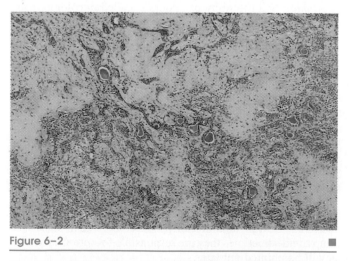

Figure 6-2 ■

Mixed tumor of the parotid gland contains epithelial cells forming ducts and myxoid stroma that resembles cartilage. (Courtesy of Dr. Trace Worrell, Department of Pathology, University of Texas Southwestern Medical School, Dallas.)

Table 6–1. NOMENCLATURE OF TUMORS

Tissue of Origin	Benign	Malignant
Composed of one parenchymal cell type		
Tumors of mesenchymal origin		
Connective tissue and derivatives	Fibroma	Fibrosarcoma
	Lipoma	Liposarcoma
	Chondroma	Chondrosarcoma
	Osteoma	Osteogenic sarcoma
Endothelial and related tissues		
Blood vessels	Hemangioma	Angiosarcoma
Lymph vessels	Lymphangioma	Lymphangiosarcoma
Synovium		Synovial sarcoma
Mesothelium		Mesothelioma
Brain coverings	Meningioma	Invasive meningioma
Blood cells and related cells		
Hematopoietic cells		Leukemias
Lymphoid tissue		Malignant lymphomas
Muscle		
Smooth	Leiomyoma	Leiomyosarcoma
Striated	Rhabdomyoma	Rhabdomyosarcoma
Tumors of epithelial origin		
Stratified squamous	Squamous cell papilloma	Squamous cell or epidermoid carcinoma
Basal cells of skin or adnexa		Basal cell carcinoma
Epithelial lining		
Glands or ducts	Adenoma	Adenocarcinoma
	Papilloma	Papillary carcinomas
	Cystadenoma	Cystadenocarcinoma
Respiratory passages		Bronchogenic carcinoma
		Bronchial "adenoma"
Neuroectoderm	Nevus	Malignant melanoma
Renal epithelium	Renal tubular adenoma	Renal cell carcinoma
Liver cells	Liver cell adenoma	Hepatocellular carcinoma
Urinary tract epithelium (transitional)	Transitional cell papilloma	Transitional cell carcinoma
Placental epithelium	Hydatidiform mole	Choriocarcinoma
Testicular epithelium (germ cells)		Seminoma
		Embryonal carcinoma
More than one neoplastic cell type— mixed tumors, usually derived from one germ layer		
Salivary glands	Pleomorphic adenoma (mixed tumor of salivary origin)	Malignant mixed tumor of salivary gland origin
Breast	Fibroadenoma	Malignant cystosarcoma phyllodes
Renal anlage		Wilms' tumor
More than one neoplastic cell type derived from more than one germ layer—teratogenous		
Totipotential cells in gonads or in embryonic rests	Mature teratoma, dermoid cyst	Immature teratoma, teratocarcinoma

CHARACTERISTICS OF BENIGN AND MALIGNANT NEOPLASMS

Nothing is more important to the patient with a tumor than being told "It is benign." In most instances such a prediction can be made with remarkable accuracy based on long-established clinical and anatomic criteria, but some neoplasms defy easy characterization. Certain features may point to innocence and others to malignancy. Moreover, in a few instances there is not perfect concordance between the appearance of a neoplasm and its biologic behavior. However, these problems are not the rule, and there are generally reliable criteria by which benign and malignant tumors can be differentiated. They can be distinguished on the basis of differentiation and anaplasia, rate of growth, local invasion, and metastasis.

Differentiation and Anaplasia

Differentiation and anaplasia refer only to the parenchymal cells that constitute the transformed elements of neoplasms. The stroma carrying the blood supply is critical to the growth of tumors but does not aid in the separation of benign from malignant ones. The amount of stromal connective tissue does, however, determine the consistency of a neoplasm. Certain cancers induce a dense, abundant fibrous stroma (desmoplasia), making them hard, so-called scirrhous tumors. *The differentiation of parenchymal cells refers to the extent to which they resemble their normal forebears, both morphologically and functionally.*

Benign neoplasms are composed of well-differentiated cells that resemble very closely their normal counterparts. Thus, the lipoma is made up of mature fat cells laden with cytoplasmic lipid vacuoles and the chondroma of mature cartilage cells that synthesize their usual cartilaginous matrix, evidence of both morphologic and functional differentiation. In well-differentiated benign tumors, mitoses are extremely scant in number and are of normal configuration.

Malignant neoplasms are characterized by a wide range of parenchymal cell differentiation, from surprisingly well differentiated to completely undifferentiated (Fig. 6–3). Malignant neoplasms that are composed of undifferentiated cells are said to be "anaplastic." Indeed, lack of differentiation, or anaplasia, is considered a hallmark of malignancy. The term *anaplasia* literally means "to form backward." It implies dedifferentiation, or loss of the structural and functional differentiation of normal cells. However, it is now known that cancers arise from stem cells in tissues, so failure of differentiation, rather than dedifferentiation of specialized cells, accounts for undifferentiated tumors.

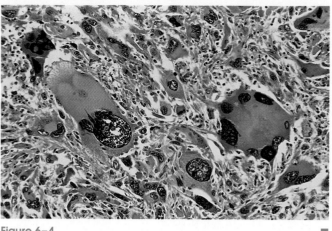

Figure 6–4 ■

Anaplastic tumor of the skeletal muscle (rhabdomyosarcoma). Note the marked cellular and nuclear pleomorphism, hyperchromatic nuclei, and tumor giant cells. (Courtesy of Dr. Trace Worrell, Department of Pathology, University of Texas Southwestern Medical School, Dallas.)

Anaplastic cells display marked *pleomorphism* (i.e., marked variation in size and shape) (Fig. 6–4). Characteristically the *nuclei are extremely hyperchromatic* and large. The nuclear-cytoplasmic ratio may approach 1:1 instead of the normal 1:4 or 1:6. *Giant cells* may be formed that are considerably larger than their neighbors and possess either one enormous nucleus or several nuclei. *Anaplastic nuclei are variable and bizarre in size and shape.* The chromatin is coarse and clumped, and nucleoli may be of astounding size. More important, *mitoses are often numerous and distinctly atypical;* anarchic multiple spindles may be seen that sometimes can be resolved as tripolar or quadripolar forms (Fig. 6–5). Also, anaplastic cells usually fail to develop recognizable patterns of orientation to each other, i.e., they lose normal polarity. They may grow in sheets, with total loss of communal structures, such as gland formations or stratified squamous archi-

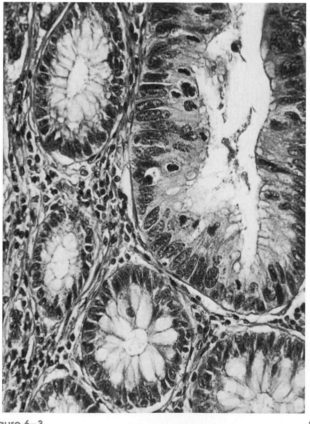

Figure 6–3 ■

Histologic detail of well-differentiated adenocarcinoma of the colon. The normal colonic glands are at left and below, and the cancerous gland is at upper right. Compare the normal cells' basal small nuclei and apical vacuoles with the cancerous cells' pleomorphic nuclei and virtual lack of secretory vacuoles.

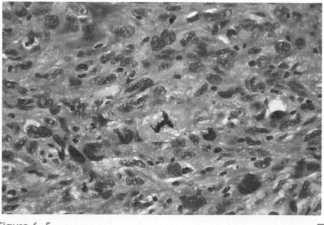

Figure 6–5 ■

High-power detail of anaplastic tumor cells to show cellular and nuclear variation in size and shape. The prominent cell in the center field has an abnormal tripolar spindle.

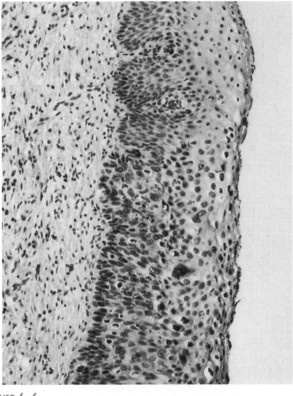

Figure 6–6   ■

Carcinoma in situ of the uterine cervix. In the lower part of the section, the entire thickness of the epithelium is replaced by atypical, dysplastic cells, with loss of orderly differentiation. The basement membrane is intact, and there is no evidence of tumor cells in the subepithelial stroma.

tecture. Thus, anaplasia is the most extreme disturbance in cell growth encountered in the spectrum of cellular proliferations. As mentioned at the outset, malignant tumors differ widely with respect to differentiation. At one extreme are extremely undifferentiated, anaplastic tumors, and at the other extreme are cancers that bear striking resemblance to their tissue of origin. Well-differentiated adenocarcinomas of the prostate, for example, may contain normal-looking glands. Such tumors may sometimes be difficult to distinguish from benign proliferations. Between the two extremes lie tumors loosely referred to as "moderately well differentiated."

Before we leave the subject of differentiation and anaplasia, we should discuss *dysplasia,* a term used to describe disorderly but non-neoplastic proliferation. Dysplasia is encountered principally in the epithelia. It is a *loss in the uniformity of the individual cells, as well as a loss in their architectural orientation.* Dysplastic cells exhibit considerable pleomorphism (variation in size and shape) and often possess deeply stained (hyperchromatic) nuclei, which are abnormally large for the size of the cell. Mitotic figures are more abundant than usual. Frequently the mitoses appear in abnormal locations within the epithelium. Thus, in dysplastic stratified squamous epithelium, mitoses are not confined to the basal layers, where they normally occur, but may appear at all levels and even in surface cells. There is considerable architectural anarchy. For example, the usual progressive maturation of tall cells in the

basal layer to flattened squames on the surface may be lost and replaced by a disordered scrambling of dark basal-appearing cells (Fig. 6–6). When dysplastic changes are marked and involve the entire thickness of the epithelium, the lesion is referred to as *carcinoma in situ,* a preinvasive stage of cancer (Chapter 19). Although dysplastic changes are often found adjacent to foci of cancerous transformation and, in long-term studies of cigarette smokers, epithelial dysplasia almost invariably antedates the appearance of cancer, the term *dysplasia without qualifications does not indicate cancer, nor do dysplasias necessarily progress to cancer.* Mild to moderate changes that do not involve the entire thickness of epithelium may be reversible, and with removal of the putative inciting causes, the epithelium may revert to normal.

Turning to the functional differentiation of neoplastic cells, as might be presumed, the better the differentiation of the cell, the more completely it retains the functional capabilities found in its normal counterparts. Thus, benign neoplasms and even well-differentiated cancers of endocrine glands frequently elaborate the hormones characteristic of their origin. Well-differentiated squamous cell carcinomas elaborate keratin (Fig. 6–7), just as well-differentiated hepatocellular carcinomas elaborate bile. However, in some instances unanticipated functions emerge. Some cancers may elaborate fetal proteins (antigens) not produced by comparable cells in the adult. On the other hand, cancers of nonendocrine origin may assume hormone synthesis to produce so-called ectopic hormones. For example, bronchogenic carcinomas may produce adrenocorticotropic hormone, parathyroid-like hormone, insulin, and glucagon, as well as others. More will be said about these phenomena later in this chapter. Despite exceptions, *the more rapidly growing and the more anaplastic a tumor, the less likely it is to have specialized functional activity.*

In summary, the cells in benign tumors are almost always well differentiated and resemble their normal cells of origin; the cells in cancers are more or less differentiated, but some loss of differentiation is always present.

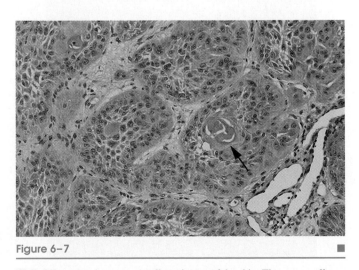

Figure 6–7   ■

Well-differentiated squamous cell carcinoma of the skin. The tumor cells are strikingly similar to normal squamous epithelial cells, with intercellular bridges and nests of keratin pearls *(arrow)*. (Courtesy of Dr. Trace Worrell, Department of Pathology, University of Texas Southwestern Medical School, Dallas.)

Rate of Growth

It is common knowledge that most benign tumors grow slowly and that most cancers grow much faster to eventually spread locally and to distant sites (metastasize) and thereby cause death. There are many exceptions to this generalization, however, and some benign tumors grow more rapidly than some cancers. For example, the rate of growth of leiomyomas (benign smooth muscle tumors) of the uterus is influenced by the circulating levels of estrogens. Thus, they may rapidly increase in size during pregnancy and conversely cease growing or even atrophy and become largely fibrocalcific after menopause. Other influences such as adequacy of blood supply, and possibly pressure constraints, also may affect the growth rate of benign tumors. Adenomas of the pituitary gland locked into the sella turcica have been observed to suddenly shrink in size. Presumably they undergo a wave of necrosis as progressive enlargement compresses their blood supply. Noting these variables, it is nonetheless true that most benign tumors under clinical observation for long periods of time increase in size slowly over the span of months to years, but there is some variation in rate of growth from one neoplasm to another.

The rate of growth of malignant tumors correlates in general with their level of differentiation. Thus, there is wide variation. Some grow slowly for years and then enter a phase of rapid growth, signifying the emergence of an aggressive subclone of transformed cells. Others grow relatively slowly, and indeed, there are exceptional instances when growth comes almost to a standstill. Even more exceptionally, cancers (particularly choriocarcinomas) have spontaneously disappeared as they have become totally necrotic, leaving only secondary metastatic implants. With the exception of these rarities, most cancers progressively enlarge over time, some slowly, others rapidly, but the notion that they "emerge out of the blue" is not true. Many lines of experimental and clinical evidence document that most, perhaps all, cancers take years, and sometimes decades, to evolve into clinically overt lesions. Rapidly growing malignant tumors often contain central areas of ischemic necrosis because the tumor blood supply, derived from the host, fails to keep pace with the oxygen needs of the expanding mass of cells.

Local Invasion

A benign neoplasm remains localized at its site of origin. It does not have the capacity to infiltrate, invade, or metastasize to distant sites, as do cancers. As fibromas and adenomas, for example, slowly expand, *most develop an enclosing fibrous capsule* that separates them from the host tissue. This capsule is probably derived from the stroma of the native tissue as the parenchymal cells atrophy under the pressure of the expanding tumor. The stroma of the tumor itself may also contribute to the capsule (Figs. 6–8 and 6–9). However, it should be emphasized that *not all benign neoplasms are encapsulated.* The leiomyoma of the uterus, for example, is quite discretely demarcated from the surrounding smooth muscle by a zone of compressed and attenuated normal myometrium, but there is no well-developed capsule. Nonetheless, a well-

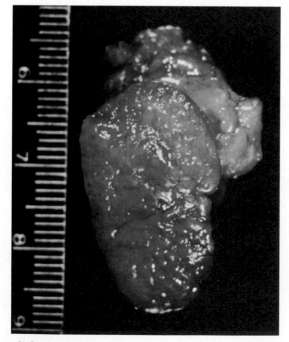

Figure 6–8 ■

Gross view of fibroadenoma of the breast. The discrete tumor bulges above the level of the surrounding breast substance as it extrudes from its tight encapsulation.

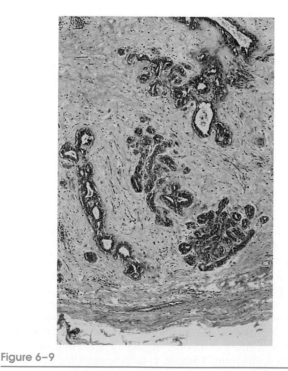

Figure 6–9 ■

Microscopic view of the fibroadenoma of the breast seen in Figure 6–8. The fibrous capsule *(below)* sharply delimits the tumor from the surrounding tissue. (Courtesy of Dr. Trace Worrell, Department of Pathology, University of Texas Southwestern Medical School, Dallas.)

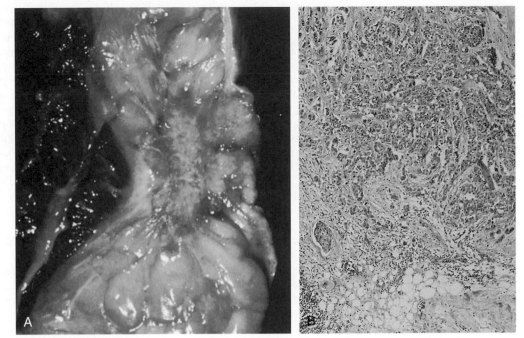

Figure 6–10　■

A, Close-up view of the cut surface of cancer of the female breast. The tumor has infiltrated and eroded through the skin *(right),* and its crablike extensions pull on the adjacent fat and dark pectoral muscles. *B,* Microscopic view of the breast carcinoma seen in *A,* illustrating the invasion of breast stroma and fat by nests and cords of tumor cells (compare with Fig. 6–9). The absence of a well-defined capsule should be noted. (Courtesy of Dr. Trace Worrell, Department of Pathology, University of Texas Southwestern Medical School, Dallas.)

defined cleavage plane exists around these lesions. A few benign tumors are neither encapsulated nor discretely defined. This is particularly true of some vascular benign neoplasms of the dermis. These exceptions are pointed out only to emphasize that although encapsulation is the rule in benign tumors, the lack of a capsule does not imply that a tumor is malignant.

Cancers grow by progressive infiltration, invasion, destruction, and penetration of the surrounding tissue (Fig. 6–10). They do not develop well-defined capsules. There are, however, occasional instances in which a slowly growing malignant tumor deceptively appears to be encased by the stroma of the surrounding native tissue, but usually microscopic examination reveals tiny, crablike feet penetrating the margin and infiltrating adjacent structures. The infiltrative mode of growth makes it necessary to remove a wide margin of surrounding normal tissue when surgical excision of a malignant tumor is attempted. The surgeon must have knowledge of the invasive potential of the various forms of cancer, because there are striking differences among them.

Next to the development of metastases, local invasiveness is the most reliable feature that distinguishes malignant from benign tumors.

Metastasis

The term *metastasis* connotes the development of secondary implants (metastases) discontinuous with the primary tumor, possibly in remote tissues (Fig. 6–11). *The properties of invasiveness and, even more so, metastasis more unequivocally identify a neoplasm as malignant than any of the other neoplastic attributes.* However, not all cancers have equivalent ability to metastasize. At one extreme are basal cell car-

cinomas of the skin and most primary tumors of the central nervous system that are highly invasive in their primary sites of origin, but they rarely metastasize. At the other extreme are osteogenic (bone) sarcomas, which have usually metastasized to the lungs at the time of initial discovery.

Approximately 30% of newly diagnosed patients with solid tumors (excluding skin cancers other than melanomas) present with metastases. An additional 20% have occult metastases at the time of diagnosis.

In general, the more anaplastic and the larger the primary neoplasm, the more likely is metastatic spread. However, exceptions abound. For example, extremely small cancers have been known to metastasize, and conversely, some large, ugly lesions may not have spread. Dissemination strongly prejudices, if it does not preclude, the possibility of cure of the disease, so it is obvious that, short of prevention of cancer,

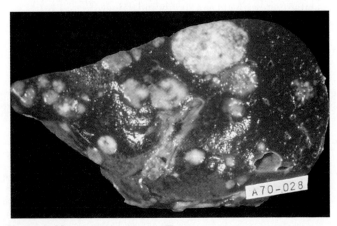

Figure 6–11　■

A liver studded with metastatic cancer.

no achievement would confer greater benefit on patients than methods to prevent metastasis.

Malignant neoplasms disseminate by one of three pathways: (1) seeding within body cavities, (2) lymphatic spread, or (3) hematogenous spread. Although direct transplantation of tumor cells (as, for example, on surgical instruments or on the surgeon's gloves) may theoretically occur, happily, in clinical practice it is exceedingly rare and in any event is an artificial mode of dissemination.

Seeding of cancers occurs when neoplasms invade a natural body cavity. Carcinoma of the colon may penetrate the wall of the gut and reimplant at distant sites in the peritoneal cavity. A similar sequence may occur with lung cancers in the pleural cavities. This mode of dissemination is particularly characteristic of cancers of the ovary, which often cover the peritoneal surfaces widely. Strangely, the implants may literally glaze all peritoneal surfaces and yet not invade the underlying parenchyma of the abdominal organs. Here is an instance of the ability to reimplant elsewhere that appears to be separable from the capacity to invade. Neoplasms of the central nervous system, such as a medulloblastoma or ependymoma, may penetrate the cerebral ventricles and be carried by the cerebrospinal fluid to reimplant on the meningeal surfaces, either within the brain or in the spinal cord.

Lymphatic spread is more typical of carcinomas, whereas the hematogenous route is favored by sarcomas. However, there are numerous interconnections between the lymphatic and vascular systems, and so all forms of cancer may disseminate through either or both systems. The pattern of lymph node involvement depends principally on the site of the primary neoplasm and the natural lymphatic pathways of drainage of the site. Thus, lung carcinomas arising in the respiratory passages metastasize first to the regional bronchial lymph nodes and then to the tracheobronchial and hilar nodes. Carcinoma of the breast usually arises in the upper outer quadrant and first spreads to the axillary nodes. Medial lesions may drain through the chest wall to the nodes along the internal mammary artery. Thereafter, in both instances the supra- and infraclavicular nodes may be seeded. In some cases the cancer cells appear to traverse the lymphatic channels within the immediately proximate nodes to be trapped in subsequent lymph nodes, producing so-called skip metastases. Indeed, the cells may traverse all of the lymph nodes to ultimately reach the vascular compartment via the thoracic duct.

It should be noted that although enlargement of nodes in proximity to a primary neoplasm should arouse strong suspicions of metastatic spread, it does not always imply cancerous involvement. The necrotic products of the neoplasm and tumor antigens often evoke reactive changes in the nodes, such as enlargement and hyperplasia of the follicles (lymphadenitis) and proliferation of macrophages in the subcapsular sinuses (sinus histiocytosis).

Hematogenous spread is the most feared consequence of a cancer. It is the favored pathway for sarcomas, but carcinomas are by no means shy about using it. As might be expected, arteries are less readily penetrated than are veins. With venous invasion, the blood-borne cells follow the venous flow draining the site of the neoplasm. Understandably, *the liver and lungs are the most frequently involved secondary sites in such hematogenous dissemination.* All portal area drainage flows to the liver, and all caval blood flows to the lungs. Cancers arising in close proximity to the vertebral column often embolize through the paravertebral plexus; this pathway is probably involved in the frequent vertebral metastases of carcinomas of the thyroid and prostate.

Certain carcinomas have a propensity for invasion of veins. The renal cell carcinoma often invades the renal vein to grow in a snake-like fashion up the inferior vena cava, sometimes reaching the right side of the heart. Hepatocellular carcinomas often penetrate portal and hepatic radicles to grow within them into the main venous channels. Remarkably, such intravenous growth may not be accompanied by widespread dissemination.

Many observations suggest that mere anatomic localization of the neoplasm and natural pathways of venous drainage do not wholly explain the systemic distributions of metastases. For example, prostatic carcinoma preferentially spreads to bone, bronchogenic carcinomas tend to involve the adrenals and the brain, and neuroblastomas spread to the liver and bones. Conversely, skeletal muscles are rarely the site of secondary deposits. The probable basis of such tissue-specific homing of tumor cells is discussed in a later section.

In conclusion, the various features discussed in the preceding sections, as summarized in Table 6–2 and Figure 6–12, permit the differentiation of benign and malignant neoplasms. Against this background of the structure and behavior of neoplasms, we can turn to some considerations of their nature and origins.

Table 6–2. COMPARISON OF BENIGN AND MALIGNANT TUMORS

Characteristics	Benign	Malignant
Differentiation/anaplasia	Well-differentiated; structure may be typical of tissue of origin	Some lack of differentiation with anaplasia; structure is often atypical
Rate of growth	Usually progressive and slow; may come to a standstill or regress; mitotic figures are rare and normal	Erratic and may be slow to rapid; mitotic figures may be numerous and abnormal
Local invasion	Usually cohesive and expansile, well-demarcated masses that do not invade or infiltrate the surrounding normal tissues	Locally invasive, infiltrating the surrounding normal tissues; sometimes may seem cohesive and expansile
Metastasis	Absent	Frequently present; the larger and less differentiated the primary, the more likely are metastases

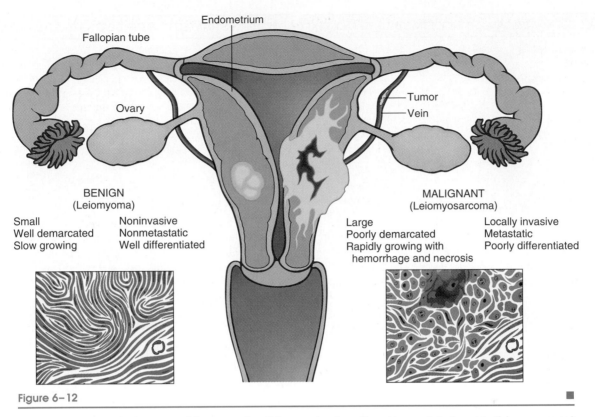

Figure 6-12

Comparison between a benign tumor of the myometrium (leiomyoma) and a malignant tumor of similar origin (leiomyosarcoma.)

EPIDEMIOLOGY

Because cancer is a disorder of cell growth and behavior, its ultimate cause has to be defined at the cellular and molecular levels. However, cancer epidemiology can contribute substantially to knowledge about the origin of cancer. For example, the now well-established concept that cigarette smoking is causally associated with lung cancer arose primarily from epidemiologic studies. A comparison of the incidence of colon cancer and dietary patterns in the Western world and Africa led to the recognition that dietary fat and fiber content are important factors in the causation of this cancer. Thus, major insights into the causes of cancer can be obtained by epidemiologic studies that relate particular environmental, racial (hereditary?), and cultural influences to the occurrence of specific neoplasms. In addition, certain diseases associated with an increased risk of developing cancer (preneoplastic disorders) also provide clues to the pathogenesis of cancer. In the following discussion we first summarize the overall incidence of cancer to gain an insight into the magnitude of the cancer problem and then review some factors relating to the patient and environment that influence the predisposition to cancer.

Cancer Incidence

Some perspective on the likelihood of developing a specific form of cancer can be gained from national incidence and mortality data. Overall, it is estimated that about 1.3 million new cancer cases occurred in 1996, and 554,000 deaths were caused by cancer in the United States. The incidence of the most common forms of cancer and the major killers is presented in Figure 6-13.

The death rates of many forms of malignant neoplasia have changed in the past few decades (Fig. 6-14). Particularly notable is the significant increase in the overall cancer death rate among males that was attributable largely to lung cancer but has finally begun to drop. In contrast, the overall death rate among females has fallen slightly, owing mostly to the decline in death rates from cancers of the uterus, stomach, and large bowel. These welcome trends have more than counterbalanced the striking climb in the rate of lung cancer among females, which not long ago was a relatively uncommon form of neoplasia in this sex. The declining death rate from uterine cancer can reasonably be attributed to the gratifying control of cervical carcinoma, made possible by the widespread use of cytologic smear studies for early detection of carcinoma while it is still curable. The causes of decline in death rates for cancers of the large bowel and stomach are, however, obscure, but there have been speculations about decreasing exposure to dietary carcinogens.

Geographic and Environmental Factors

Data on the death rates for specific forms of cancer among the nations of the world are also interesting; sometimes there

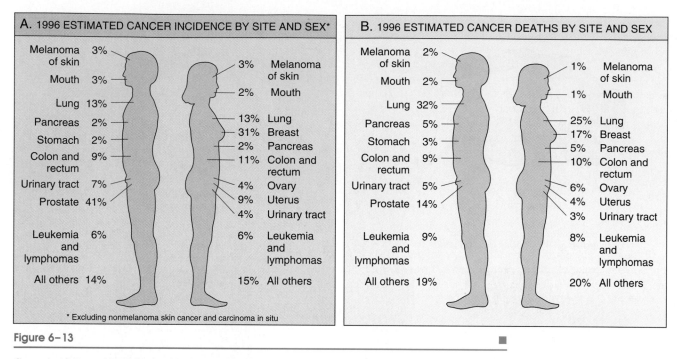

Figure 6–13

Cancer incidence and mortality by site and sex. (Adapted from Parker SL, et al: Cancer statistics. CA 46:5, 1996.)

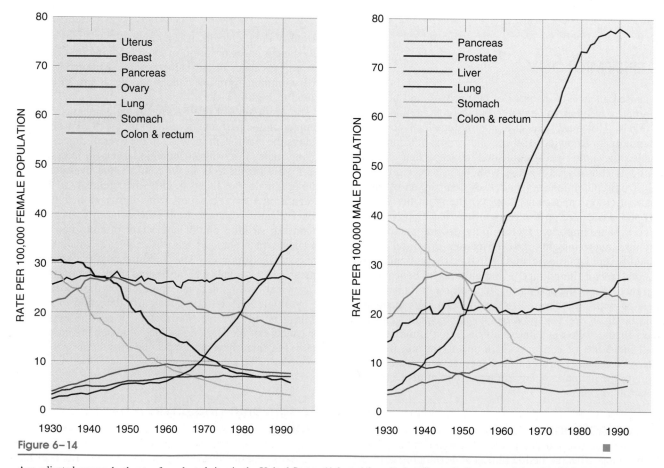

Figure 6–14

Age-adjusted cancer death rates for selected sites in the United States. (Adapted from Parker SL, et al: Cancer statistics. CA 46:5, 1996.)

are striking differences. For example, the age-adjusted death rate in 1986 for cancer of the breast per 100,000 women was 27 in the United States, 36 in England and Wales, and 32 in the Netherlands, but, in contrast, only seven in Japan. Conversely, the death rate for stomach carcinoma in both males and females is about seven times higher in Japan than in the United States. Liver cell carcinoma is relatively infrequent in the United States but is the number one lethal cancer among many African native populations. Nearly all the evidence indicates that these geographic differences are environmental rather than genetic in origin. For example, Nisei (second-generation Japanese living in the United States) have mortality rates for certain forms of cancer that are intermediate between those of natives of Japan and of Americans of native lineage, and the two rates come closer with each passing generation.

There is no paucity of environmental carcinogens. They lurk in the ambient environment, in the workplace, in food, and in personal practices. They can be as universal as sunlight, found particularly in urban settings (as, for example, asbestos), or limited to a certain occupation (Table 6–3). Certain features of diet have also been implicated as possible predisposing influences. Among the possible environmental influences, the most distressing are those incurred in personal practices, notably cigarette smoking and chronic alcohol consumption. The risk of cervical cancer is also linked to age at first intercourse and the number of sex partners (pointing to a possible causal role for venereal transmission of an oncogenic virus). Thus, there is no escape; it seems that everything one does to earn a livelihood, to subsist, or for pleasure, turns out to be fattening, immoral, illegal, or—more disturbing—possibly carcinogenic.

Age

In general, the frequency of cancer increases with age. Most of the mortality occurs between ages 55 and 75 years and then declines, along with the population base, after age 75. The rising incidence with age may be explained by the accumulation of somatic mutations associated with the emergence of malignant neoplasms (discussed later). The decline in immune competence that accompanies aging may also be a factor. However, cancer is no stranger among young people: it causes slightly more than 10% of all deaths among children younger than 15 years (Chapter 7). The major lethal cancers in children are lymphoblastic leukemia, tumors of the central nervous system, lymphomas, soft tissue sarcomas, and bone sarcomas. As discussed later, study of several childhood tumors, particularly retinoblastoma and Wilms' tumor, has provided novel insights into the pathogenesis of malignant transformation.

Heredity

Because cancer is estimated to occur in one of every four or five individuals, nearly all families have at least one afflicted first- or second-degree relative. Understandably, a question often asked is, "Is cancer an inherited disease?" Re-

grettably, there is no simple answer. A predisposition to a few uncommon forms of cancer can be hereditary, transmitted in mendelian fashion (Table 6–4), and the suspicion grows that inherited susceptibility may also play a role in the genesis of several common cancers.

Childhood retinoblastoma is the most striking example of the role of heredity. Approximately 40% of the retinoblastomas are familial. The predisposition to this tumor shows an autosomal dominant pattern of inheritance. Carriers of this gene have a 10,000-fold greater risk of developing retinoblastoma, usually bilateral. They also have a greatly increased risk of developing a second cancer, particularly osteogenic sarcoma. As discussed later, a "cancer suppressor" gene has been implicated in the pathogenesis of retinoblastoma. Adenomatous polyposis coli is another hereditary disorder marked by an extraordinarily high risk of cancer. Individuals who inherit the autosomal dominant mutation have at birth, or soon thereafter, innumerable polypoid adenomas of the colon and in virtually 100% of cases are fated to develop a carcinoma of the colon by age 50 years. In addition to the dominantly inherited cancerous or precancerous disorders, there is a small group of autosomal recessive conditions collectively characterized by some defect in DNA repair. Homozygotes with xeroderma pigmentosum, for example, have a strong predisposition to sunlight-induced melanomas and basal cell and squamous cell carcinomas of the skin in addition to other non-neoplastic cutaneous and ocular abnormalities. All the well-defined conditions already discussed account for only a small fraction of the total burden of malignant neoplasia. What can be said about the influence of heredity on the large preponderance of malignant neoplasms? To begin with, as we point out in subsequent sections, the evidence is strong that carcinogenesis involves mutations in the genome. One or more such mutations may be inherited in germ line. Such individuals are likely to be more predisposed to cancer than others. It is not surprising, therefore, that familial predisposition has also been noted with common neoplasms such as carcinoma of the breast, colon, ovary, prostate, and uterus and with melanomas. Indeed, with each of these types of neoplasia, specific families have been identified in which there appear to be mendelian patterns of inheritance. Rare families have an increased predisposition to diverse forms of cancer, ranging from sarcomas of soft tissues and bone to breast carcinoma. However, *with most forms of malignancy, well-defined genetic influences can be identified in only a few instances.* Most seem to develop spontaneously, following mutations in somatic cells, and are therefore presumed to be largely of environmental origin.

There is increasing evidence, however, that genetic predisposition contributes to at least a proportion of the so-called environmental or spontaneous cancers. The converse is equally true: environmental factors contribute to the development of many hereditary neoplasms. For example, individuals with xeroderma pigmentosum develop primarily cancers of the skin, a tissue exposed to radiant energy.

Heredity and environment can be viewed, then, as the two ends of a spectrum of predisposing influences. At the extremes are neoplasms that develop because of a strong hereditary component and those related to heavy exposure to environmental carcinogens, but in between are the great majority that

Table 6–3. OCCUPATIONAL CANCERS

Agents or Groups of Agents	Human Cancer Site for Which Reasonable Evidence is Available	Typical Use or Occurrence
Arsenic and arsenic compounds	Lung, skin, hemangiosarcoma	By-product of metal smelting. Component of alloys, electrical and semiconductor devices, medications and herbicides, fungicides, and animal dips.
Asbestos	Lung, mesothelioma; gastrointestinal tract (esophagus, stomach, large intestine)	Formerly used for many applications because of fire, heat, and friction resistance; will still be found in existing construction, as well as fire-resistant textiles, friction materials (i.e., brake linings), underlayment and roofing papers, and floor tiles.
Benzene	Leukemia, Hodgkin's disease	Principal component of light oil. Although use as solvent is discouraged, many applications exist in printing and lithography, paint, rubber, dry cleaning, adhesives and coatings, and detergents. Formerly widely used as solvent and fumigant.
Beryllium and beryllium compounds	Lung	Missile fuel and space vehicles. Hardener for lightweight metal alloys, particularly in aerospace applications and nuclear reactors.
Cadmium and cadmium compounds	Prostate	Uses include yellow pigments and phosphors. Found in solders. Used in batteries and as alloy and in metal platings and coatings.
Chromium compounds	Lung	Component of metal alloys, paints, pigments, and preservatives.
Ethylene oxide	Leukemia	Ripening agent for fruits and nuts. Used in rocket propellant and chemical synthesis, in fumigants for foodstuffs and textiles, and in sterilants for hospital equipment.
Nickel compounds	Nose, lung	Nickel plating. Component of ferrous alloys, ceramics, and batteries. By-product of stainless steel arc welding.
Radon and its decay products	Lung	From decay of minerals containing uranium. Can be serious hazard in quarries and underground mines.
Vinyl chloride	Angiosarcoma, liver	Refrigerant. Monomer for vinyl polymers. Adhesive for plastics. Formerly "inert" aerosol propellant in pressurized containers.

Modified from Stellman JM, Stellman SD. Cancer and workplace. CA 46:70, 1996.

result from varying contributions of heredity and environment.

Acquired Preneoplastic Disorders

In addition to the genetic influences described earlier, certain clinical conditions are well-recognized predispositions to the development of malignant neoplasia and are therefore referred to as *preneoplastic disorders*. This designation is unfortunate, because it implies a certain inevitability, but in fact, although such conditions may increase the likelihood, in most instances cancer does not develop. A brief listing of the chief conditions follows:

■ Persistent regenerative cell replication (e.g., squamous cell carcinoma in the margins of a chronic skin fistula or in a long-unhealed skin wound; hepatocellular carcinoma in cirrhosis of the liver).

■ Hyperplastic and dysplastic proliferations (e.g., endometrial carcinoma in atypical endometrial hyperplasia; bronchogenic carcinoma in the dysplastic bronchial mucosa of habitual cigarette smokers).

■ Chronic atrophic gastritis (e.g., gastric carcinoma in pernicious anemia).

■ Chronic ulcerative colitis (e.g., an increased incidence of colorectal carcinoma in long-standing disease).

■ Leukoplakia of the oral cavity, vulva, or penis (e.g., increased risk of squamous cell carcinoma).

■ Villous adenomas of the colon (e.g., high risk of transformation to colorectal carcinoma).

In this context it may be asked, "What is the risk of malignant change in a benign neoplasm?" or, stated differently, "Are benign tumors precancerous?" In general the answer is no, but inevitably there are exceptions, and perhaps it is better to say that each type of benign tumor is associated with a particular level of risk, ranging from high to virtually non-

Table 6–4. HEREDITARY NEOPLASMS AND PRENEOPLASTIC CONDITIONS

Disorder	Inheritance	Features
Hereditary neoplasms		
Retinoblastoma	AD	Often bilateral; susceptible to second tumors, especially osteosarcoma
Familial adenomatous polyposis coli	AD	Multiple adenomatous polyps and adenocarcinomas of the colon
Multiple endocrine neoplasia I	AD	Adenomas of the pituitary, parathyroid, and pancreatic islet cells
Multiple endocrine neoplasia II	AD	Medullary carcinoma of the thyroid, pheochromocytoma, and parathyroid tumors
Neurofibromatosis type I (von Recklinghausen's disease)	AD	Gliomas of the brain and optic nerve, acoustic neuroma, meningioma, pheochromocytoma
Wilms' tumor	AD	Wilms' tumor of kidney; other congenital malformations
Li Fraumeni Syndrome	AD	Multiple: breast, colon, sarcomas
Hereditary preneoplastic conditions		
Defective DNA repair–chromosomal instability		
Xeroderma pigmentosum	AR	Basal and squamous cell carcinoma of skin; malignant melanomas in patients exposed to UV light
Bloom's syndrome	AR	Acute leukemias, various carcinomas
Fanconi's anemia	AR	Acute leukemias, squamous cell carcinomas, and liver cell cancer
Ataxia-telangiectasia	AR	Acute leukemia, lymphoma, breast cancer in females
Immune deficiency syndromes		
X-linked agammaglobulinemia	XR	Lymphomas and leukemia
Wiskott-Aldrich syndrome	XR	Acute leukemias and lymphoma
X-linked lymphoproliferative syndrome	XR	Abnormal response to EBV; EBV-induced B-cell immunoblastic lymphomas

AD, autosomal dominant; AR, autosomal recessive; EBV, Epstein-Barr virus; UV, ultraviolet; XR, X-linked recessive.

existent. For example, adenomas of the colon as they enlarge undergo malignant transformation in up to 50% of cases; in contrast, malignant change is extremely rare in leiomyomas of the uterus.

CARCINOGENESIS: THE MOLECULAR BASIS OF CANCER

It could be justifiably argued that the proliferation of literature on the molecular basis of cancer has outpaced the growth of even the most malignant of tumors! Understandably, therefore, it is easy to get lost in the growing forest of information. It might then be profitable to list some fundamental principles before we delve into the details of the genetic basis of cancer.

■ *Nonlethal genetic damage lies at the heart of carcinogenesis.* Such genetic damage (or mutation) may be acquired by the action of environmental agents such as chemicals, radiation, or viruses, or it may be inherited in the germ line. The genetic hypothesis of cancer implies that a tumor mass results from the clonal expansion of a single progenitor cell that has incurred the genetic damage (i.e., tumors are monoclonal). This expectation has been realized in most tumors that have been analyzed. Clonality of tumors is assessed quite readily in women who are heterozygous for polymorphic X-linked markers such as the enzyme glucose-6-phosphate dehydrogenase (G6PD) or X-linked restriction fragment length polymorphisms (RFLPs). The principle underlying such an analysis is illustrated in Figure 6–15.

■ *Three classes of normal regulatory genes—the growth-promoting protooncogenes, the growth-inhibiting cancer suppressor genes (antioncogenes), and genes that regulate programmed cell death, or apoptosis—are the principal targets of genetic damage.* Mutant alleles of protooncogenes are considered dominant because they transform cells despite the presence of their normal counterpart. In contrast, both normal alleles of the tumor suppressor genes must be damaged for transformation to occur, so this family of genes is sometimes referred to as *recessive oncogenes.* Genes that regulate apoptosis may be dominant, as are protooncogenes, or they may behave as cancer suppressor genes.

■ In addition to the three classes of genes mentioned earlier, a fourth category of genes, those that regulate repair of damaged DNA, are also pertinent in carcinogenesis. *The DNA repair genes affect cell proliferation or survival indirectly by influencing the ability of the organism to repair nonlethal damage in other genes, including protooncogenes, tumor suppressor genes, and genes that regulate apoptosis.* A disability in the DNA repair genes can predispose to widespread mutations in the genome and hence to neoplastic transformation.

■ *Carcinogenesis is a multistep process at both the phenotypic and genetic level.* A malignant neoplasm has several phenotypic attributes, such as excessive growth, local invasiveness, and the ability to form distant metastases. These characteristics are acquired in a stepwise fashion, a phenomenon called *tumor progression.* At the molecular level, progression results from accumulation of genetic lesions that in some instances are favored by defects in DNA repair.

With this overview (Fig. 6–16) we can now address in

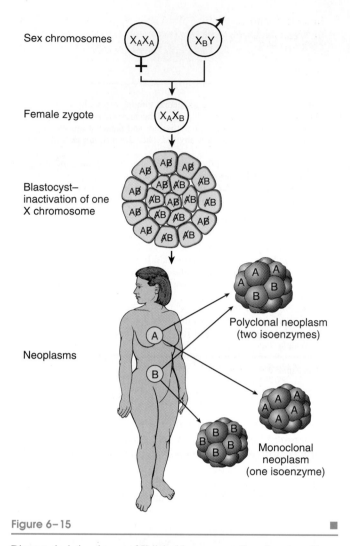

Figure 6–15 ■

Diagram depicting the use of X-linked isoenzyme cell markers as evidence of the monoclonality of neoplasms. Because of random X inactivation, all females are mosaics with two cell populations (with G6PD isoenzyme A or B in this case). When neoplasms that arise in women who are heterozygous for X-linked markers are analyzed, they are made up of cells that contain the active maternal (X_A) or the paternal (X_B) X chromosome but not both.

some detail the molecular pathogenesis of cancer and then discuss the carcinogenic agents that inflict genetic damage.

Oncogenes and Cancer

As often happens in science, the discovery of protooncogenes was not straightforward. These cellular genes were first discovered by the Nobel laureates Michael Bishop and Harold Varmus as "passengers" within the genome of acute transforming retroviruses, which cause rapid induction of tumors in animals and can also transform animal cells in vitro. Molecular dissection of their genomes revealed the presence of unique transforming sequences (viral oncogenes or v-*oncs*) not found in the genomes of nontransforming retroviruses. Most surprisingly, molecular hybridization revealed that the v-*onc* sequences were almost identical to sequences found in the normal cellular DNA. From this evolved the concept that

during evolution retroviral oncogenes were *transduced* (captured) by the virus through a chance recombination with the DNA of a (normal) host cell that had been infected by the virus. Because they were discovered initially as "viral genes," protooncogenes are named after their viral homologs. Each v-*onc* is designated by a three-letter word that relates the oncogene to the virus from which it was isolated. Thus, the v-*onc* contained in *fe*line *s*arcoma virus is referred to as v-*fes*, whereas the oncogene in *si*mian *s*arcoma virus is called v-*sis*. The corresponding protooncogenes are referred to as *fes* and *sis* by dropping the prefix.

Although the study of transforming animal retroviruses provided the first glimpse of protooncogenes, these investigations did not explain the origin of human tumors, which (with rare exceptions) are not caused by infection with retroviruses. Hence the question was raised: do nonviral tumors contain oncogenic DNA sequences? The answer was provided by experiments involving DNA-mediated gene transfer (DNA transfection). When DNA extracted from several different human tumors was transfected into mouse fibroblasts in vitro, the recipient cells underwent malignant transformation. The conclusion from such experiments was inescapable: DNA of spontaneously arising cancers contains oncogenic sequences, or oncogenes. Many of these transforming sequences have turned out to be homologous to the *ras* protooncogenes that are the forebears of v-*oncs* contained in Harvey (H) and Kir-

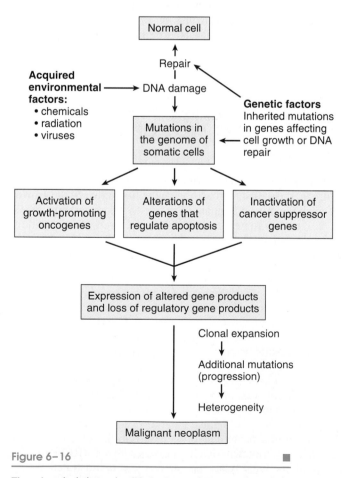

Figure 6–16 ■

Flow chart depicting a simplified scheme of cancer pathogenesis.

sten (K) sarcoma viruses. Others, such as the c-*erb B* onco-gene, represent novel transforming sequences that have never been detected in retroviruses. To summarize, protooncogenes may become oncogenic by retroviral transduction (v-*onc*s) or by influences that alter their behavior in situ, thereby con-verting them into cellular oncogenes (c-*onc*s). Two questions follow: (1) What are the functions of oncogene products? and (2) How do the normally "civilized" protooncogenes turn into "enemies within"? These issues are discussed next.

PROTEIN PRODUCTS OF ONCOGENES

Oncogenes encode proteins called *oncoproteins*, which resemble the normal products of protooncogenes with the exception that oncoproteins are devoid of important regula-tory elements, and their production in the transformed cells is not dependent on growth factors or other external signals. To aid in the understanding of the nature and functions of on-coproteins, it is necessary to briefly review the sequence of events that characterize normal cell proliferation; these were discussed earlier in Chapter 3. Under physiologic conditions, cell proliferation can be readily resolved into the following steps:

■ The binding of a growth factor to its specific receptor on the cell membrane
■ Transient and limited activation of the growth factor re-ceptor, which in turn activates several signal-transducing proteins on the inner leaflet of the plasma membrane
■ Transmission of the transduced signal across the cytosol to the nucleus via second messengers

■ Induction and activation of nuclear regulatory factors that initiate DNA transcription
■ Entry and progression of the cell into the cell cycle, re-sulting ultimately in cell division

With this background, we can readily identify oncogenes and oncoproteins as altered versions of their normal counter-parts and group them on the basis of their role in the signal transduction cascade and cell cycle regulation (Table 6–5).

Growth Factors. Beginning outside the cell, mutations of genes that encode growth factors can render them oncogenic. Such is the case with the protooncogene for platelet-derived growth factor (PDGF), which was initially discovered in the guise of the viral oncogene contained in the simian sarcoma virus (v-*sis*). Subsequently, several human tumor cell lines have been found to transcribe c-*sis*. Furthermore, it appears that several of the same tumors also possess receptors for PDGF and are hence subject to *autocrine stimulation*. Such an autocrine loop is not an uncommon characteristic of trans-formed cells. In many instances the growth factor gene itself is not altered or mutated, but the products of other oncogenes such as *ras* cause overexpression of growth factor genes, thus forcing the cell to secrete large amounts of growth factors such as transforming growth factor-α (TGF-α). This growth factor, you may recall, is related to the epidermal growth factor (EGF) and induces cell proliferation by binding to the EGF receptor.

In addition to c-*sis*, a group of related oncogenes that en-code homologs of fibroblast growth factors (e.g., *hst*-1 and *int*-2) has also been detected in several gastrointestinal and breast tumors.

■

Table 6–5. SELECTED ONCOGENES, THEIR MODE OF ACTIVATION, AND ASSOCIATED HUMAN TUMORS

Category	Protooncogenes	Mechanism of Activation	Associated Human Tumor
Growth factors			
PDGF-β chain	*sis*	Overexpression	Astrocytoma
Fibroblast growth factors	*hst*-1	Overexpression	Osteosarcoma
	int-2		Stomach cancer
			Bladder cancer
			Breast cancer
Growth factor receptors			
EGF receptor	*erb B*-1	Overexpression	Gliomas
family	*neu* (*erb B*-2)	Amplification	Breast, ovarian, and stomach cancers
	ret*	Point mutation	Medullary carcinoma of thyroid
Proteins involved in signal transduction			
GTP binding	*ras*	Point mutations	A variety of human cancers, including lung, colon, pancreas, and many leukemias
Tyrosine kinase	*abl*	Translocation	Chronic myeloid leukemia
			Acute lymphoblastic leukemia
Nuclear regulatory proteins			
Transcriptional activators	*myc*	Translocation	Burkitt's lymphoma
	N-*myc*	Amplification	Neuroblastoma
			Small cell carcinoma of lung
	L-*myc*	Amplification	Small cell carcinoma of lung
Cyclins	Cyclin D	Amplification	Breast cancer, esophageal cancer, lymphomas

* *ret* is a growth factor receptor with unknown ligand.
EGF, epidermal growth factor; GTP, guanosine triphosphate; PDGF, platelet-derived growth factor.

Growth Factor Receptors. The next group in the sequence of signal transduction involves growth factor receptors, and several oncogenes that encode growth factor receptors have been found. Both mutations and pathologic overexpression of normal forms of growth factor receptors have been detected in several tumors. Mutant receptor proteins deliver continuous mitogenic signals to cells, even in the absence of the growth factor in the environment. More common than mutations is overexpression of growth factor receptors. The best documented examples of overexpression involve the EGF receptor family. c-*erb B*-1, the EGF receptor, is overexpressed in up to 80% of squamous cell carcinomas of the lung. A related receptor, called c-*erb B*-2 (or c-*neu*), is amplified in 15% to 30% of breast cancers and adenocarcinomas of the lung, ovary, and salivary glands. These tumors are exquisitely sensitive to the mitogenic effects of very small amounts of growth factors, and not surprisingly, a high level of c-*erb B*-2 protein on breast cancer cells is a harbinger of poor prognosis.

Signal-Transducing Proteins. Several examples of oncoproteins that mimic the functions of normal cytoplasmic signal-transducing proteins have been found. Many such proteins are associated with the inner leaflet of the plasma membrane, where they receive signals from activated growth factor receptors and transmit them to the nucleus. Two important members in this category are c-*ras* and c-*abl*. Each of these will be discussed briefly.

Approximately 30% of all human tumors contain mutated versions of the *ras* gene. In some tumors, such as colon cancers, the incidence of *ras* mutations is even higher. Indeed, mutation of the *ras* gene is the single most common oncogene abnormality in human tumors. The *ras* family of proteins binds guanosine nucleotides (guanosine triphosphate [GTP] and guanosine diphosphate [GDP]), as do the well-known G proteins. Normal *ras* proteins flip back and forth between an excited signal-transmitting state and a quiescent state. In the inactive state, *ras* proteins bind GDP; when cells are stimulated by growth factors, inactive *ras* becomes activated by exchanging GDP for GTP (Fig. 6–17). The activated *ras* in turn activates downstream regulators of proliferation, including several cytoplasmic kinases, which flood the nucleus with signals for cell proliferation. However, the excited signal-emitting stage of the normal *ras* protein is short lived, because its intrinsic guanosine triphosphatase (GTPase) activity hydrolyzes GTP to GDP, thereby releasing a phosphate group

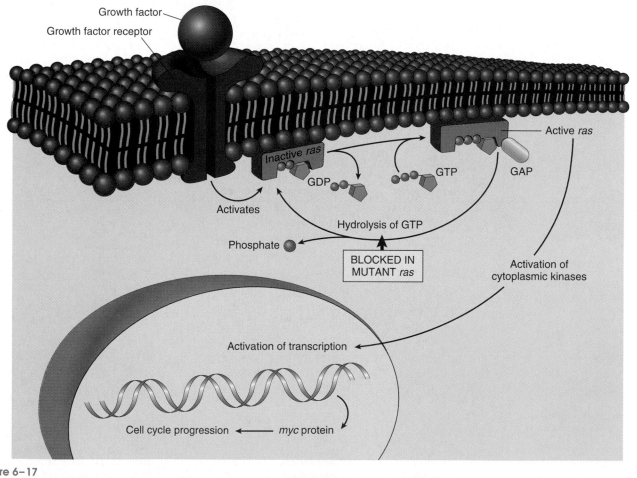

Figure 6–17

Model for action of *ras* genes. When a normal cell is stimulated through a growth factor receptor, inactive (GDP-bound) *ras* is activated to a GTP-bound state. Activated *ras* sends growth signals to the nucleus through cytoplasmic kinases. The mutant *ras* protein is permanently activated because of its inability to hydrolyze GTP, leading to continual stimulation of cell without any external trigger. GAP, GTP-ase activating protein.

and returning the protein to its quiescent ground state. The GTPase activity of the activated *ras* protein is dramatically magnified by a family of GTPase-activating proteins (GAPs). Thus, GAPs act as molecular "brakes" that prevent uncontrolled *ras* activation by favoring hydrolysis of GTP to GDP. Mutant *ras* proteins can bind GAPs, but their GTPase activity fails to be augmented. Hence the mutant proteins are "trapped" in their activated GTP-bound form, and the cell is led to believe that it must continue to proliferate. It follows from this scenario that the consequences of mutations in the *ras* protein would be mimicked by mutations in the GAPs that fail to restrain normal *ras* proteins. Indeed, a disabling mutation of neurofibromin 1 (NF-1), a GTPase-activating protein, is also associated with neoplasia (see "Cancer Suppressor Genes").

The c-*abl* protooncogene also encodes a plasma membrane–associated signal transducer protein that links external growth-promoting signals to cell proliferation. In its normal locale, on chromosome 9, the functions of c-*abl* are regulated, but when it is translocated to chromosome 22, as occurs in chronic myeloid leukemia, the normal regulatory elements are lost, and a hybrid gene composed of c-*abl* and some sequences from the break point cluster (*bcr*) region of chromosome 22 is formed. The *bcr*-c-*abl* gene encodes a potent tyrosine kinase that showers growth-promoting signals on the nucleus.

Nuclear Transcription Factors. Ultimately, all signal transduction pathways enter the nucleus and impact on a large bank of responder genes that orchestrate the cells' orderly advance through the mitotic cycle. Not surprisingly, therefore, mutations affecting genes that regulate transcription of DNA are associated with malignant transformation. A whole host of oncoproteins, including products of the *myc, myb, jun, fos,*

and *rel* oncogenes, have been localized to the nucleus. Of these, the *myc* gene is most commonly involved in human tumors. The c-*myc* protooncogene is expressed in virtually all cells, and the *myc* protein is rapidly induced when quiescent cells receive a signal to divide. The *myc* gene binds to the DNA, causing transcriptional activation of several growth-related genes, including cyclin D1, a gene whose product drives cells into the cell cycle (discussed later). In normal cells, *myc* levels decline to near basal level once the cell cycle begins. In contrast, oncogenic versions of the *myc* gene are associated with persistent expression or overexpression, thus contributing to sustained proliferation. Dysregulation of the *myc* gene occurs in Burkitt's lymphoma, a B-cell tumor; the related N-*myc* and L-*myc* genes are amplified in neuroblastomas and small cell cancers of lung, respectively.

Cyclins and Cyclin-Dependent Kinases. The ultimate outcome of all growth-promoting stimuli is the entry of quiescent cells into the cell cycle. As alluded to earlier (Chapter 3), the orderly progression of cells through the various phases of the cell cycle is orchestrated by cyclin-dependent kinases (CDKs) after they are activated by binding with another family of proteins called *cyclins*. The CDKs phosphorylate critical target proteins and are expressed constitutively during the cell cycle but in an inactive form. By contrast, various cyclins are synthesized during specific phases of the cell cycle, and their function is to activate the CDKs by binding to them. Upon completion of this task, cyclin levels decline rapidly. It is because of the cyclic nature of their production and degradation that these proteins have been termed *cyclins*. The cell cycle may thus be seen as a relay race in which each lap is regulated by a distinct set of cyclins, and as one set of cyclins leaves the track, the next set takes over (Fig. 6–18). Although each

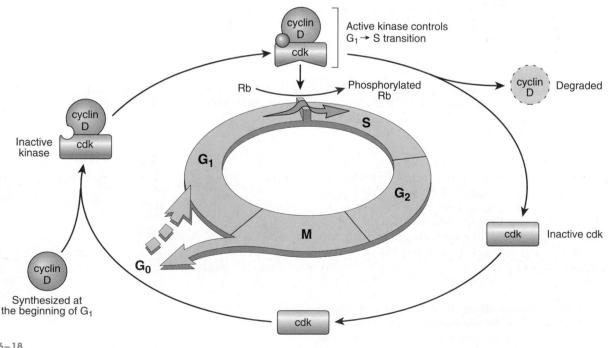

Figure 6–18   ■

Schematic illustrating the role of cyclins and cyclin-dependent kinases (CDK) in regulating the cell cycle. In the depicted example, inactive CDK is constitutively expressed; it is activated by binding to cyclin D that is synthesized in G_1. The activated CDK allows the cell to cross the $G_1 \rightarrow S$ checkpoint by phosphorylating retinoblastoma (Rb) protein. After the cell enters S phase, cyclin D is degraded, returning CDK to the inactive state.

phase of the circuitry is carefully monitored, the transition from G_1 to S is believed to be an extremely important checkpoint in the cell cycle clock. When a cell encounters growth-promoting signal, levels of the D family of cyclins go up, and the appropriate CDKs are activated. This checkpoint, as we shall see later, is guarded by the product of the retinoblastoma protein (pRB). Phosphorylation of pRB brought about by CDKs overcomes the $G_1 \rightarrow S$ hurdle and allows entry of cells into the DNA synthetic phase. Not surprisingly, therefore, mutations that dysregulate the expression of D cyclins allow the cells to move with abandon into the S phase. Such a mishap seems to be a common event in neoplastic transformation. The cyclin D genes are amplified and overexpressed in many esophageal, breast, and squamous cell carcinomas and in lymphomas. With this background it is not difficult to imagine that amplification of CDK4, the catalytic component of the D/CDK complex, may lead to a similar outcome. Indeed, this occurs in many glial tumors. Similarly, derangements affecting expression of other members of the cyclin/CDK families have been noted in tumors arising in the colon, parathyroids, and lymphoid tissues.

Activation of Oncogenes

In the preceding section we discussed how mutant forms of protooncogenes may provide gratuitous growth-stimulating signals. Next we focus on mechanisms by which protooncogenes are transformed into oncogenes. This is brought about by two broad categories of changes:

■ Changes in the structure of the gene, resulting in the synthesis of an abnormal gene product (oncoprotein) having an aberrant function
■ Changes in regulation of gene expression, resulting in enhanced or inappropriate production of the structurally normal growth-promoting protein

We can now discuss the specific lesions that lead to structural and regulatory changes that affect protooncogenes.

Point Mutations. The *ras* oncogene represents the best example of activation by point mutation. Several distinct mutations have been identified, all of which affect a domain critical to the GAP-induced hydrolysis of GTP; hence, mutant *ras* proteins have a reduced ability to hydrolyze GTP.

A very large number of human tumors carry *ras* mutations. The frequency of such mutations varies with different tumors, but in some types it is very high. For example, 90% of pancreatic adenocarcinomas contain a *ras* point mutation, as do about 50% of colon and thyroid cancers and 30% of lung adenocarcinomas and myeloid leukemias. Interestingly, *ras* mutations are very infrequent or even nonexistent in certain other cancers, particularly those arising in the ovary or breast, lending truth to the old adage that there is more than one way to skin a cat.

Chromosomal Translocations. Rearrangement of genetic material brought about by chromosomal translocation usually results in overexpression of protooncogenes, but in some cases the gene may incur structural changes as well. Translocation-induced overexpression of a protooncogene is best exemplified by Burkitt's lymphoma. All such tumors carry one of three translocations, each involving chromosome 8q24,

where the c-*myc* gene has been mapped. At its normal locus the expression of the *myc* gene is tightly controlled and is expressed only during certain stages of the cell cycle (Chapter 3). In Burkitt's lymphoma the most common form of translocation results in juxtaposition of the c-*myc*–containing segment of chromosome 8 to chromosome 14q band 32 (Fig. 6–19). This places c-*myc* close to the immunoglobulin heavy chain (Cμ) gene, a region with hectic transcriptional activity. Detached from its normal regulatory elements, the c-*myc* gene responds to relentless stimulation by its excitable and evidently seductive neighbor, and hence its product is expressed at a high level. Overexpression of the *bcl*-2 gene occurs in an analogous fashion. In virtually all follicular B-cell lymphomas, the *bcl*-2 gene, mapped on 18q21, is shifted to chromosome 14 near the immunoglobulin heavy chain gene.

The Philadelphia chromosome, characteristic of chronic myeloid leukemia, provides an example of genetic damage

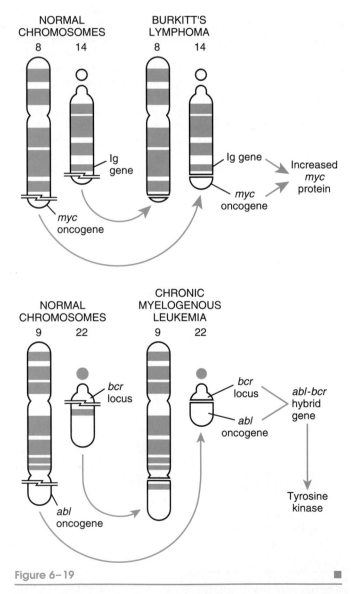

Figure 6–19 ■

The chromosomal translocations and associated oncogenes in Burkitt's lymphoma and chronic myelogenous leukemia.

wrought by translocation. In this case a reciprocal translocation between chromosomes 9 and 22 relocates a truncated portion of the protooncogene c-*abl* (from chromosome 9) to the breakpoint cluster (*bcr*) locus on chromosome 22. The hybrid c-*abl-bcr* gene encodes a chimeric protein that, like several other oncoproteins, has potent tyrosine kinase activity.

Gene Amplification. Activation of protooncogenes resulting from overexpression of their products may result from reduplication and manifold amplification of their DNA sequences. Such amplification may produce several hundred copies of the protooncogene in the tumor cell. Amplified genes can be detected by molecular studies or identified cytogenetically in the form of double minutes and homogeneous staining regions (Fig. 6–20). Increased expression of the oncoprotein can also be demonstrated by immunohistochemistry. The most interesting cases of amplification involve N-*myc* (a member of the *myc* family of genes) in neuroblastoma and c-*erb B*-2 in breast cancers. These genes are amplified in 30% to 40% of these two tumors, and in both settings this amplification is associated with poor prognosis. Similarly, amplification of L-*myc* and N-*myc* correlates strongly with disease progression in small cell cancer of the lung.

Cancer Suppressor Genes

You may recall that the eminent physicist Isaac Newton predicted that every action has an equal and opposite reaction. Although Newton was not a cancer biologist, his formulation holds true for cell growth. Whereas protooncogenes encode proteins that promote cell growth, the products of tumor suppressor genes apply brakes to cell proliferation. In this section we describe cancer suppressor genes, their products, and possible mechanisms by which loss of their function contributes to neoplastic transformation.

We begin our discussion with the retinoblastoma (*Rb*) gene, the first and prototypic cancer suppressor gene to be discovered. Like many advances in medicine, the discovery of cancer suppressor genes was accomplished by the study of a rare disease, in this case retinoblastoma, an uncommon childhood tumor. Approximately 60% of retinoblastomas are sporadic, and the remaining ones are familial, the predisposition to tumor being transmitted as an autosomal dominant trait. To account for the sporadic and familial occurrence of an identical tumor, Knudson, in 1974, proposed his now famous two-hit hypothesis, which in molecular terms can be stated as follows:

■ Two mutations ("hits") are required to produce retinoblastoma. These involve the *Rb* gene, located on chromosome 13q14. Both of the normal alleles of the *Rb* locus must be inactivated (two hits) for the development of retinoblastoma (Fig. 6–21).

■ In familial cases, children inherit one defective copy of the *Rb* gene in the germ line; the other copy is normal. Retinoblastoma develops when the normal *Rb* gene is lost in the retinoblasts as a result of somatic mutation. Because in retinoblastoma families only a single somatic mutation is required for expression of the disease, the familial transmission follows an autosomal dominant inheritance pattern.

■ In sporadic cases, both normal *Rb* alleles are lost by somatic mutation in one of the retinoblasts. The end result is the same: a retinal cell that has lost both of the normal copies of the *Rb* gene becomes cancerous.

Although the loss of normal *Rb* genes was discovered initially in retinoblastomas, it is now evident that homozygous loss of this gene is a fairly common event in several tumors, including osteosarcomas, breast cancer, small cell cancer of the lung, and some brain tumors.

At this point we should clarify some terminology. It follows from our discussion that a cell heterozygous at the *Rb* locus is normal. Cancer develops when the cell becomes *homozygous* for the mutant allele or, in other words, *loses heterozygosity* of the normal *Rb* gene. Because neoplastic transformation is associated with loss of both of the normal copies of the *Rb* gene, this and other cancer suppressor genes are also often called "recessive cancer genes."

The genetic damage that results in loss of the normal *Rb* gene may be a point mutation detected only by molecular analysis or a deletion of 13q14 (readily identified by cytogenetic studies). Indeed, detection of consistent nonrandom deletions of chromosomes, with associated loss of heterozygosity, has provided important clues to the locations of other cancer suppressor genes.

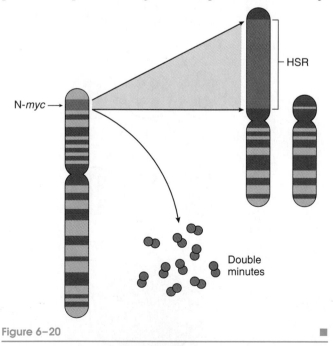

Figure 6–20   ■

Amplification of the N-*myc* gene in human neuroblastomas. N-*myc* gene, present normally on chromosome 2p, becomes amplified and is seen either as extra chromosomal double minutes or as a chromosomally integrated homogeneous-staining region (HSR). The integration involves other autosomes such as 4, 9, or 13. (Modified from Brodeur GM, et al: Clinical implication of oncogene activation in human neuroblastomas. Cancer 58:541, 1986. Copyright © 1986 American Cancer Society. Reprinted by permission of Wiley-Liss, Inc, a subsidiary of John Wiley & Sons, Inc.)

PROTEIN PRODUCTS OF TUMOR SUPPRESSOR GENES

The signals and signal-transducing pathways for growth inhibition are much less well understood than those for growth promotion. Nevertheless, it is reasonable to assume that, like mitogenic signals, growth inhibitory signals may originate outside the cell and utilize receptors, signal transducers, and nuclear transcription regulators to accomplish their effects. The tumor suppressor genes seem to encode various components of this growth inhibitory pathway.

Growth Inhibitory Factors. It is logical to expect that mutations in genes that encode soluble factors that bind to the cell membrane and transmit growth inhibitory signals may favor uncontrolled cell growth. One candidate tumor suppres-

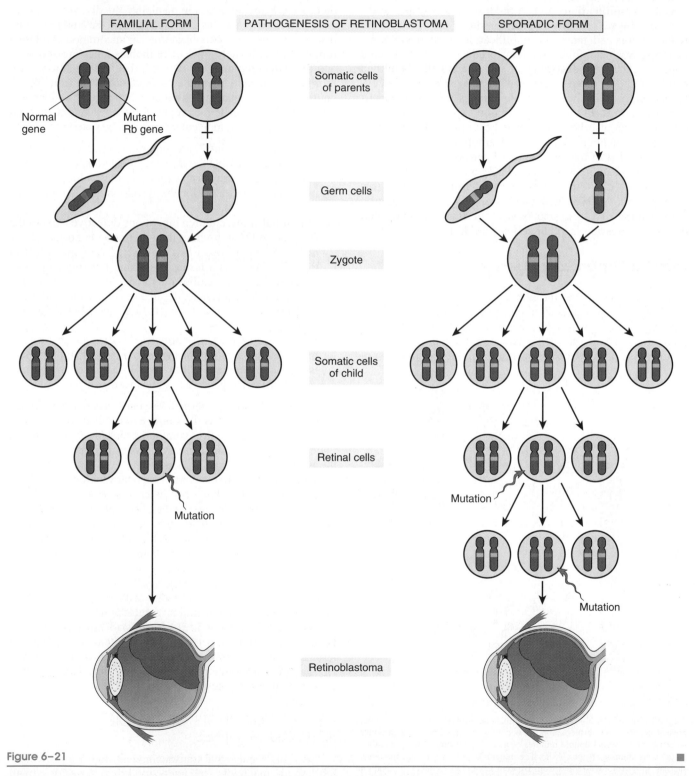

Figure 6–21

Pathogenesis of retinoblastoma. Two mutations of the Rb locus on Chromosome 13q14 lead to neoplastic proliferation of the retinal cells. In the familial form, all somatic cells inherit one mutant Rb gene from a carrier parent. The second mutation affects the Rb locus in one of the retinal cells after birth. In the sporadic form, on the other hand, both mutations at the Rb locus are acquired by the retinal cells after birth.

sor gene, breast cancer-1 (BRCA-1), has been tentatively assigned this role. It is speculated that the BRCA-1 protein is secreted from breast epithelium and that its normal function is to inhibit cell growth after binding to surface receptors. Patients with germ line mutations of BCRA-1 have greatly increased risk of breast and ovarian cancers. Approximately 5% to 10% of all breast cancers are familial, and it appears that mutations in BRCA-1 and another candidate tumor suppressor gene, BRCA-2 (of unknown function), account for these familial cases.

Molecules That Regulate Cell Adhesion. Several tumor suppressor genes encode molecules that are present on the cell surface or closely connected to them. One such gene, called *deleted in colon carcinoma (DCC),* is inactivated not only in most colon cancers, but also in carcinomas of the breast, prostate, pancreas, and endometrium. The structure of the DCC protein resembles cell surface molecules that are involved in cell-to-cell or cell-to-matrix interaction. Presumably, loss of the DCC gene products interferes with normal communication between cells and their environment and thus contributes to altered differentiation or proliferation. The gene encoding E-cadherin, a protein involved in the formation of intercellular junctions, is frequently mutated in invasive gastric carcinomas. Loss of E-cadherin reduces intercellular adhesiveness and may thus favor detachment and invasion.

Another well-known tumor suppressor gene, adenomatous polyposis coli (APC) also seems to be involved in regulating cellular adhesion. The APC protein is located in the cytoplasm but is linked to E-cadherin present on the cell surface. As with *Rb* and p53, mutations of APC may be inherited or acquired. Patients born with one mutant allele of APC invariably develop numerous adenomas of the colon. In virtually every case, a proportion of these adenomas progress to become malignant. Thus, individuals who inherit a mutant APC allele are at extremely high risk of developing a "second hit" at the APC locus and thus merit very careful follow-up.

Molecules That Regulate Signal Transduction. Downregulation of growth-promoting signals is another potential site at which products of tumor suppressor genes may be operative. The product of the NF-1 gene falls in this category. The NF-1 gene behaves very much like the APC gene. Individuals who inherit a mutant allele develop numerous benign neurofibromas, some of which progress to neurofibrosarcomas. The function of the NF-1 protein (neurofibromin) is intimately related to signal transduction via the *ras* proteins. Recall that the *ras* protein, involved in transmission of growth-promoting signals, flips back and forth between active and inactive states. The normal NF-1 gene encodes a GTPase-activating protein (GAP) that facilitates the conversion of active *ras* to inactive *ras*. With a loss of NF-1, *ras* may be trapped in its active, signal-emitting state.

Molecules That Regulate Nuclear Transcription and Cell Cycle. Ultimately, all positive and negative signals converge on the nucleus, where decisions to divide or not to divide are made. Not surprisingly, therefore, products of several tumor suppressor genes (*Rb,* WT-1, and p53) are localized to the nucleus.

Much is known about the *Rb* gene because this was the first tumor suppressor gene discovered. The *Rb* gene product (pRb) is a DNA-binding protein that is a key player in the regulation of cell cycle. It is expressed in every cell type examined, where it *exists in an active unphosphorylated and an inactive phosphorylated state.* Quiescent cells (in G_0 or early G_1) contain the active unphosphorylated pRb that prevents DNA synthesis by binding to and sequestering transcription factors that initiate cell replication. When the cells in G_1 are stimulated by growth factors, the concentration of D cyclins goes up, and the resultant activation of the cyclin D/CDKs leads to phosphorylation of pRb. *This is a critical event because phosphorylation of pRb sets free the transcripton factors, which then trigger DNA synthesis* (Fig. 6–22). It is obvious, therefore, that if the *Rb* protein is absent, or its ability to sequester transcription factors is derailed by mutations, the molecular brakes on the cell cycle are released, and the cells move blithely into the S phase. The central role of pRb in regulating the cell cycle is attested to by the discovery of a variety of growth-promoting and growth-inhibiting pathways, all of which converge on pRb.

■ It was mentioned earlier that cyclins and CDK regulate cell proliferation by facilitating pRb phosphorylation. Inhibitors of CDKs, of which there are several, exert growth suppressing effects, because by dampening cyclin/CDK actions they inhibit pRb phosphorylation. It can be surmised, therefore, that cyclins or CDKs may be converted into oncogenes by mutations that activate their functions; conversely, inhibitors of CDKs may act as tumor suppressor genes whose loss would prime the cell cycle by allowing unregulated activation of cyclins/CDKs. Indeed, inactivation of p16, a potent inhibitor of CDKs, has been noted in several tumors, including melanomas.

■ Transforming growth factor-β (TGF-β), a well-known inhibitor of proliferation of several (but not all) cell types, acts by inducing the synthesis of a CDK inhibitor whose downstream target is none other than pRb.

■ p53, a well-known tumor suppressor gene, described next, exerts its growth-inhibiting effect at least in part by acting on pRb.

■ The transforming proteins of human papillomaviruses (HPVs), believed to play a role in the causation of carcinoma of the uterine cervix, seem to act in part by neutralizing the growth inhibitory activities of pRb. These viral proteins bind to hypophosphorylated pRb at sites that normally sequester the transcription factors. Thus, the Rb protein is functionally deleted and the transcription factors are free to cause cell division.

p53, the other well-studied tumor suppressor gene, is located on chromosome 17p13.1, and is the single most common target for genetic alteration in human tumors. *Homozygous loss of the p53 gene is found in virtually every type of cancer,* including carcinomas of the lung, breast, and colon—the three leading causes of cancer deaths. In most instances, mutations that inactivate both copies of the p53 gene are acquired in somatic cells. Less commonly, some individuals inherit a mutant p53 allele. As with the *Rb* gene, inheritance of one mutant p53 allele predisposes individuals to develop malignant tumors, because only one more "hit" is needed to inactivate the second, normal, allele. Such individuals, said to have the *Li-Fraumeni syndrome,* are at a high risk of developing a wide variety of tumors, including carcinomas, sarcomas, lymphomas, and brain tumors.

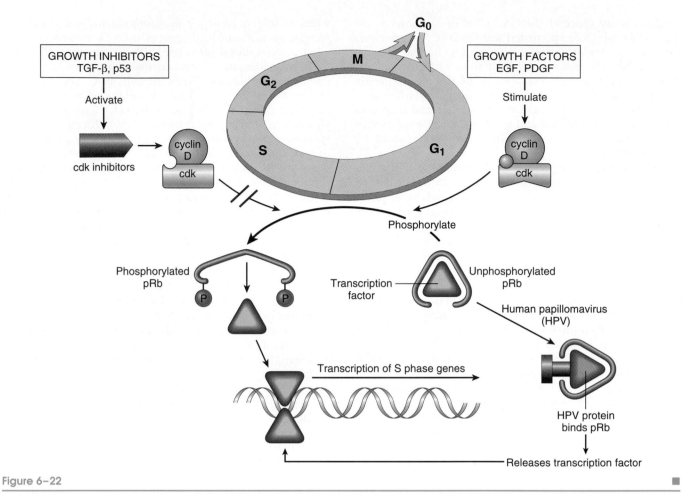

Figure 6–22

The central role of pRb in regulating the cell cycle. Several growth-promoting and growth-inhibitory pathways influence cellular proliferation by activating or inactivating the phosphorylation of pRb. DNA viruses like human papillomavirus (HPV) produce proteins that bind to pRb and cripple its ability to exert growth restraint by rendering it unable to sequester transcription factors.

Like the *Rb* gene, p53 also acts in the nucleus and has the ability to inhibit the cell cycle. However, unlike the *Rb* gene, p53 does not seem to police the normal cell but is called in to apply emergency brakes when the DNA is damaged by exposure to mutagenic chemicals or ionizing radiation (Fig. 6–23). With such an assault on genetic material, the normal p53 protein rapidly accumulates in the nucleus and causes the cells to arrest in G_1 phase. This task is accomplished by inducing the transcription of an inhibitor of cyclin-dependent kinase called p21. This, as we discussed earlier, inhibits the cyclin/CDK complexes and thus prevents the phosphorylation of pRb necessary for cells to enter the S phase. A pause in the cell cycle brought about by the action of p53 is welcome because it allows the cells time to repair DNA damage inflicted by mutagens. Indeed, p53 also helps this process directly by inducing transcription of some DNA repair enzymes. If the damaged DNA is repaired, the cell is allowed to complete the cycle. However, if for some reason the repair mechanisms fail, normal p53 stops the mutant cell from dividing and, as a last ditch effort, activates the cell-suicide genes. Thus, *a cell with damaged DNA that cannot be repaired is directed by the p53 gene to undergo apoptosis.* In view of these activities, p53 has been rightfully called a "guardian of the genome." With homozygous loss of p53, DNA damage goes unrepaired, mutations become fixed in dividing cells, and the cell reluctantly turns onto a one-way street that leads to malignant transformation. As with retinoblastoma protein, normal p53 can also be rendered nonfunctional by certain DNA viruses. Proteins encoded by oncogenic HPVs, hepatitis B virus, and possibly Epstein-Barr virus can bind to normal p53 proteins and nullify their protective functions. Thus, DNA viruses can subvert two of the best understood tumor suppressor genes, *Rb* and p53. A listing of the other tumor suppressor genes is provided in Table 6–6.

Genes That Regulate Apoptosis

Accumulation of neoplastic cells may result not only from activation of growth-promoting oncogenes or inactivation of growth-suppressing tumor suppressor genes, but also by mutations in the genes that regulate apoptosis. Just as cell growth is regulated by growth-promoting and growth-inhibiting genes, cell survival is conditioned by genes that promote and inhibit apoptosis. A large family of genes that regulate apop-

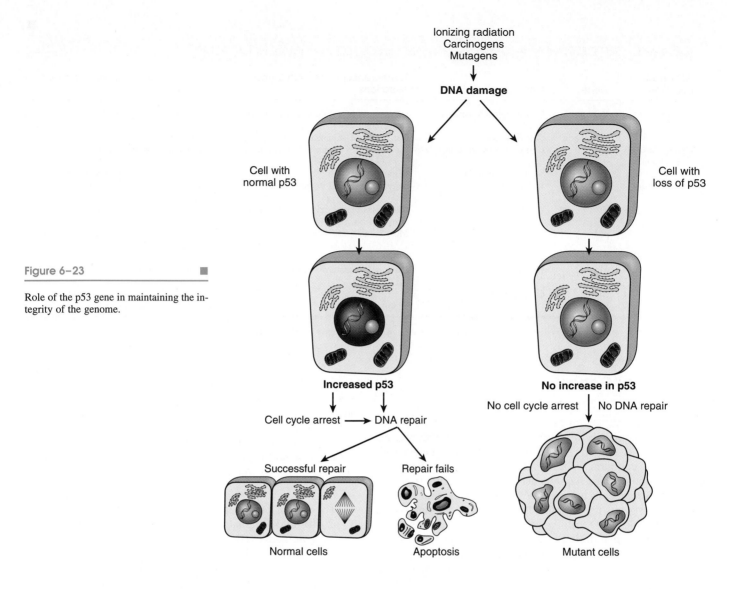

Figure 6–23   ■

Role of the p53 gene in maintaining the integrity of the genome.

tosis has been identified. Mercifully for students (and nonexperts), these genes can be remembered as a series of three-letter words beginning with a "b." Examples include *bcl*-2, *bcl*-x, *bax, bag, bad*, and, we are told, many more yet to come. *bcl*-2 is the prototypic anti-apoptosis gene. Located on chromosome 18, it is activated by translocation to the immunoglobulin (Ig) heavy chain locus on chromosome 14 in more than 80% of the B-cell tumors designated as follicular lymphomas (Chapter 12). The overexpressed *bcl*-2 protects lymphocytes from apoptosis and allows them to survive for prolonged periods; thus, there is a steady accumulation of lymphocytes, resulting in lymphadenopathy and marrow infiltration. Because these *bcl*-2 overexpressing lymphomas arise in large part from reduced cell death rather than excessive proliferation, they tend to be indolent (slow growing) compared with most other lymphomas. The mechanisms by which *bcl*-2 prevents apoptosis are not yet clear. However, it is well known that *bcl*-2 is not the only player in the apoptosis pathway. A related gene, *bax*, opposes *bcl*-2 action and hence accelerates cell death. The relative levels of these two genes

seem to regulate cell survival (Fig. 6–24). The other "b" genes listed above modify the actions of *bcl*-2 and *bax* in complex ways.

It was mentioned earlier that one of the functions of the normal p53 gene is to trigger apoptosis if the cells that are exposed to mutagenic agents cannot repair DNA damage. Thus, p53 may also be considered an apoptosis-inducing gene; it seems that p53 exerts this effect by increasing the transcription of *bax*.

The genetic regulation of apoptosis is of more than academic interest, because the *effectiveness of many chemotherapeutic agents depends on their ability to induce apoptosis in tumor cells*. It may be inferred from this discussion that tumors in which p53 is mutated are likely to be less sensitive to the action of chemotherapeutic agents that induce apoptosis. Such a correlation has indeed been noted in clinical studies. Thus, loss of normal p53 contributes to neoplastic transformation by allowing cells with DNA damage to proliferate and at the same time reduces the efficacy of anticancer therapy by inhibiting apoptosis, truly a "double whammy."

Table 6–6. SELECTED TUMOR SUPPRESSOR GENES INVOLVED IN HUMAN NEOPLASMS

Subcellular Location	Gene	Function	Tumors Associated With Somatic Mutations	Tumors Associated With Inherited Mutations
Cell surface	DCC	Cell-to-cell interactions	Carcinomas of colon, stomach, pancreas, prostate	Unknown
	E-cadherin	Cell adhesion	Carcinoma of stomach	Unknown
Under plasma membrane	APC	Cell-to-cell interactions (?)	Carcinomas of stomach, colon, pancreas	Familial adenomatosis polyposis coli; colon cancer
	NF-1	Signal transduction	Schwannomas	Neurofibromatosis type I and sarcomas
Cytoskeleton	NF-2	Unknown	Schwannomas and meningomas	Neurofibromatosis type II; acoustic schwannomas and meningiomas
Nucleus	*Rb*	Regulation of cell cycle	Retinoblastoma; osteosarcoma; carcinomas of breast, colon, lung	Retinoblastomas; osteosarcoma
	p53	Regulation of cell cycle and apoptosis	Most human cancers	Li Fraumeni syndrome; multiple carcinomas and sarcomas
	WT-1	Nuclear transcription	Wilms' tumor	Wilms' tumor
	p16	Regulation of cell cycle	Pancreatic, esophageal cancers	Malignant melanoma
Unknown	BRCA-1*	Growth inhibitor	?	Carcinomas of female breast and ovary
Unknown	BRCA-2	?	?	Carcinomas of male and female breast

* BRCA-1 is suspected to be a secreted growth inhibitory factor; but its exact subcellular localization and functions are under investigation.

DNA Repair Genes

Humans literally swim in a sea of environmental carcinogens. While exposure to naturally occurring DNA-damaging agents, such as ionizing radiation, sunlight, and dietary carcinogens, is common, cancer is a relatively rare outcome of such encounters. This happy state of affairs results from the ability of normal cells to repair DNA damage and thus prevent mutations in genes that regulate cell growth and apoptosis. In addition to possible DNA damage from environmental agents, the DNA of normal dividing cells is also susceptible to alterations resulting from errors that occur spontaneously during DNA replication. Such mistakes, if not repaired promptly, can

also push the cells further along the slippery slope of neoplastic transformation. The importance of DNA repair in maintaining the integrity of the genome is highlighted by several inherited disorders in which genes that encode proteins involved in DNA repair are defective. *Those born with such inherited mutations of DNA repair proteins are at a greatly increased risk of developing cancer.* Several examples are cited below:

■ The role of DNA repair genes in predisposition to cancer is illustrated dramatically by *h*ereditary *n*onpolyposis *co*lon *c*arcinoma (HNPCC) syndrome. This disorder, characterized by familial carcinomas of the colon affecting predominantly the cecum and proximal colon (Chapter 15),

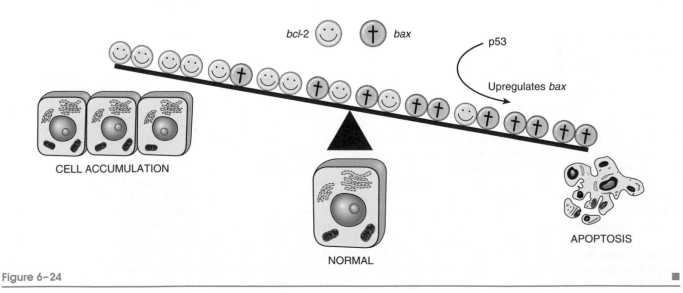

Figure 6–24

Regulation of cell death by *bcl-2*, *bax,* and p53. *bcl-2* dimers favor cell accumulation by inhibiting apoptosis; *bax* dimers favor apoptosis. The apoptosis-inducing affect of normal p53 genes is mediated in part by increasing the synthesis of *bax* protein.

results from defects in genes involved in DNA mismatch repair. When a strand of DNA is being repaired, these genes act as "spell checkers." Thus, for example, if there is an erroneous pairing of G with T rather than the normal A with T, the mismatch repair genes correct the defect. Without these "proofreaders," errors slowly accumulate in several genes, including protooncogenes and cancer suppressor genes. Mutations in at least four mismatch repair genes have been found to underlie HNPCC (Chapter 15). One such gene, called *human Msh-2*, maps to chromosome 2. Some patients are born with a defective copy of Msh-2 or another related DNA mismatch repair gene and acquire the "second hit" in the colonic epithelial cells. Thus, DNA repair genes behave like cancer suppressor genes in their mode of inheritance but are distinguished from tumor suppressor genes because they do not affect cell growth directly. While mismatch errors in DNA replication can occur in any dividing cell, carcinomas occur mainly in the proximal colon in those with HNPCC. In some families there is also an associated increase in endometrial cancers, but quite mysteriously, most tissues are spared.

■ Patients with another inherited disorder, xeroderma pigmentosum, are at increased risk for the development of cancers of the skin exposed to the ultraviolet light contained in sun rays. The basis of this disorder is also defective DNA repair. Ultraviolet light causes cross-linking of pyrimidine residues, thus preventing normal DNA replication. Such DNA damage is repaired by the nucleotide excision repair system. Several proteins and genes are involved in nucleotide excision repair, and an inherited loss of any one can give rise to xeroderma pigmentosum.

■ In addition to the examples mentioned earlier, a group of autosomal recessive disorders comprising Bloom's syndrome, ataxia telangiectasia, and Fanconi's anemia are characterized by hypersensitivity to other DNA-damaging agents such as ionizing radiation (Bloom's syndrome and ataxia telangiectasia) or DNA cross-linking agents, such as nitrogen mustard (Fanconi's anemia). Their phenotype is complex and includes, in addition to predisposition to cancer, other features such as neural symptoms (ataxia telangiectasia), anemia (Fanconi's anemia), and developmental defects (Bloom's syndrome). The ataxia telangiectasia gene seems to control several processes, including the normal functioning of the p53 gene, as well as genes that regulate growth factor functions. There is much current interest in this gene, because it is estimated that approximately 1% of the population is heterozygous and hence a carrier. While heterozygotes do not develop cancers, they are presumed to be at an increased risk for radiation-induced DNA damage, and therefore may be at risk of developing common cancers after exposure to doses of irradiation used in common radiologic procedures such as mammography.

Molecular Basis of Multistep Carcinogenesis

The notion that malignant tumors arise from a protracted sequence of events is supported by epidemiologic, experi-

mental, and molecular studies. Even before the discovery of oncogenes and cancer suppressor genes, cancer epidemiologists suggested that the age-associated increase in cancers could best be explained by postulating that five or six independent steps are required for tumorigenesis. More recently, the study of genetic changes in tumor cells has provided a firm molecular footing for the concept of multistep carcinogenesis:

■ DNA transfection experiments reveal that no single oncogene (e.g., *myc, ras*) can fully transform cells in vitro but that together *ras* and *myc* can transform fibroblasts.

■ Every human cancer that has been analyzed reveals multiple genetic alterations involving activation of several oncogenes and the loss of two or more cancer suppressor genes. Each of these alterations represents crucial steps in the progression from a normal cell to a malignant tumor. A dramatic example of incremental acquisition of the malignant phenotype is documented by the study of colon carcinoma. These lesions are believed to evolve through a series of morphologically identifiable stages: colon epithelial hyperplasia followed by formation of adenomas that progressively enlarge and ultimately undergo malignant transformation (Chapter 15). The proposed molecular correlates of this adenoma-carcinoma sequence are illustrated in Figure 6–25. According to this scheme, inactivation of the APC tumor suppressor gene occurs first, followed by activation of *ras* and, ultimately, loss of DCC and p53 genes. Although Figure 6–25 suggests a temporal sequence of mutations in specific genes, it should be noted that the order of mutations is considered less important than their total accumulation. Thus, in some cases loss of APC genes precedes *ras* mutation; in others, the sequence is reversed.

Figure 6–26 summarizes the possible functions and subcellular location of genes that may be altered in malignant tumors.

Karyotypic Changes in Tumors

The genetic damage that activates oncogenes or inactivates tumor suppressor genes may be subtle (e.g., point mutations) or large enough to be detected in a karyotype. In certain neoplasms, karyotypic abnormalities are nonrandom and common. Specific abnormalities have been identified in most leukemias and lymphomas and in an increasing number of nonhematopoietic tumors. The common types of nonrandom structural abnormalities in tumor cells are (1) balanced translocations, (2) deletions, and (3) cytogenetic manifestations of gene amplification. In addition, whole chromosomes may be gained or lost.

Balanced Translocations. Balanced translocations are extremely common, especially in hematopoietic neoplasms. Most notable is the Philadelphia (Ph[1]) chromosome in chronic myelogenous leukemia (CML), comprising a reciprocal and balanced translocation between chromosomes 22 and, usually, 9. As a consequence, chromosome 22 appears somewhat abbreviated. *This cytogenetic change, seen in more than 90% of cases of CML, is a reliable marker of the disease. The few Philadelphia chromosome negative cases of CML show mo-*

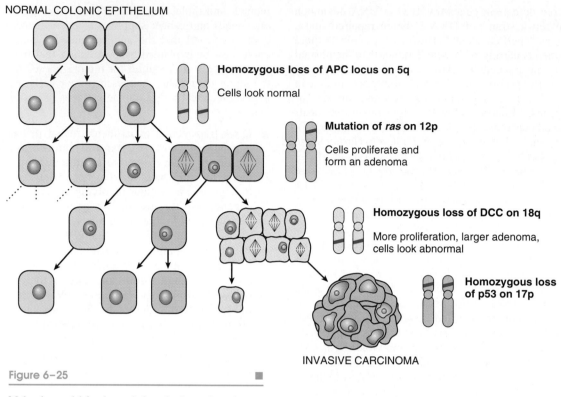

Figure 6–25 ■

Molecular model for the evolution of colorectal carcinoma.

lecular evidence of the bcr-c-abl rearrangement, the critical consequence of Ph[1] translocation. As another example, in more than 90% of cases of Burkitt's lymphoma, the cells have a translocation, usually between chromosomes 8 and 14. In follicular B-cell lymphomas, a reciprocal translocation between chromosomes 14 and 18 is extremely common.

Deletions. Chromosome deletions are the second most prevalent structural abnormality in tumor cells. *As compared with translocations, deletions are more common in nonhematopoietic solid tumors.* As discussed, deletions of chromosome 13q band 14 are associated with retinoblastoma. Deletions of 17p, 5q, and 18q, all noted in colorectal cancers, harbor three tumor suppressor genes. Deletion of 3p, noted in several tumors, is extremely common in small cell lung carcinomas, raising the suspicion that cancer suppressor genes will be found at this locale.

Gene Amplifications. There are two karyotypic manifestations of gene amplification: homogeneously staining regions (HSRs) on single chromosomes and double minutes (see Fig. 6–20), which are seen as very small paired fragments of chromatin. Neuroblastomas and breast cancers are the best studied examples of gene amplification involving the N-*myc* and c-*erb B*-2 genes, respectively.

BIOLOGY OF TUMOR GROWTH

The natural history of a typical malignant tumor can be resolved into several steps: neoplastic transformation of a cell, clonal expansion of the transformed cell, local invasion, and ultimately distant spread. In this sequence, the molecular basis of transformation has already been considered. Next we discuss the factors that affect growth of transformed cells, and last the biochemical and molecular basis of invasion and metastasis.

The formation of a tumor mass by the clonal descendants of a transformed cell is a complex process that is influenced by many factors. Some, such as doubling time of tumor cells, are intrinsic to the transformed cells, whereas others, such as angiogenesis, represent host responses elicited by tumor cells or their products. The multiple factors that influence tumor growth are considered under three headings: (1) kinetics of tumor cell growth, (2) tumor angiogenesis, and (3) tumor progression and heterogeneity.

KINETICS OF TUMOR CELL GROWTH

One can begin the consideration of tumor cell kinetics by asking the question, "How long does it take for the single transformed cell to produce a clinically overt mass?" This depends on three variables:

■ *The doubling time of tumor cells.* Because cell cycle controls exerted by the *Rb*, p53, and cyclins are deranged in many tumors, cells can be triggered into cycle more readily and without the usual restraints. However, the dividing cells do not complete the cell cycle more rapidly than do normal cells. In reality the total cell cycle time for many tumors is equal to or longer than that of corresponding normal cells.

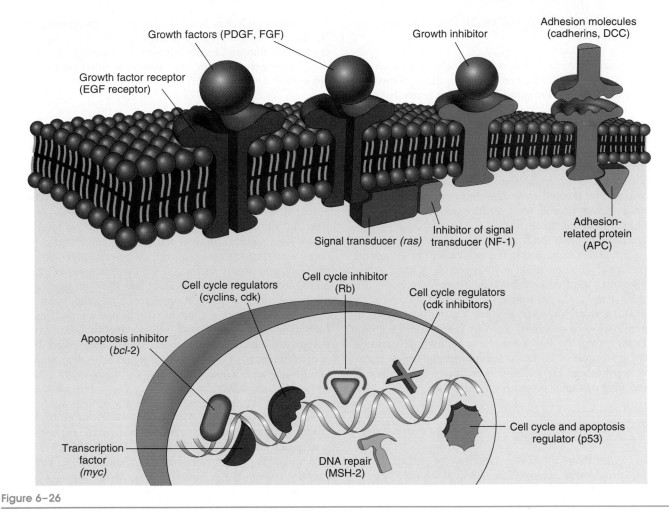

Figure 6–26   ■

Subcellular localization and functions of major classes of cancer-associated genes. The protooncogenes are colored red, the cancer suppressor genes blue, DNA repair genes green, and genes that regulate apoptosis purple.

■ *Growth fraction.* The growth fraction is the proportion of cells within the tumor cell population that are in the replicative pool. Clinical and experimental studies suggest that during the early, submicroscopic phase of tumor growth, most transformed cells are in the proliferative pool (Fig. 6–27). As tumors continue to grow, cells leave the replicative pool in ever-increasing numbers owing to shedding or lack of nutrients, by differentiating, and by reversion to G_0. Indeed, most cells within cancers remain in the G_0 phase. Thus, by the time a tumor is clinically detectable, most cells are not in the replicative pool. Even in some rapidly growing tumors, the growth fraction is approximately 20%.

■ *Cell production and loss.* Ultimately, the progressive growth of tumors and the rate at which they grow is determined by how much cell production exceeds cell loss. In some tumors, especially those with a relatively high growth fraction, the imbalance is large, resulting in more rapid growth than in those in which cell production exceeds cell loss by only a small margin.

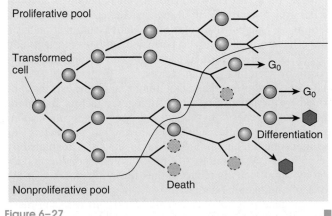

Figure 6–27   ■

Schematic representation of tumor growth. As the cell population expands, a progressively higher percentage of tumor cells leaves the replicative pool by reversion to G_0, differentiation, and death.

An understanding of tumor cell kinetics has important clinical implications:

■ *Cancer chemotherapy.* Almost all antineoplastic agents in current use are most effective on cycling cells. Hence, tumors with high growth fractions (e.g., high-grade lymphomas) are very susceptible to anticancer agents. In contrast, common solid tumors, such as colon cancer, that have low growth fractions are relatively resistant. In such cases the treatment strategy is to first shift tumor cells from G_0 into the cell cycle. This can be accomplished by debulking the tumor by surgery or radiation. The surviving tumor cells tend to reenter the cell cycle and thus become susceptible to drug therapy. Such considerations form the basis of combined-modality treatment.

■ *Latent period of tumors.* If all descendants of an originally transformed cell remained in the replicative pool, most tumors would become clinically detectable within a few months after the first cell division; however, most tumor cells leave the replicative pool, therefore the accumulation of cells is a relatively slow process. This in turn results in a latent period of several months to years before a tumor becomes clinically detectable. Nevertheless, several cell doublings occur in the latent period, during which mutations accumulate. These changes are pertinent to the understanding of tumor progression, described later.

TUMOR ANGIOGENESIS

Factors other than cell kinetics modify the growth of tumors. Most important among these is blood supply. Tumors cannot enlarge beyond 1 or 2 mm in diameter or thickness unless they are vascularized. Furthermore, *angiogenesis is a necessary biologic correlate of malignancy,* because without access to the vasculature, the tumor would fail to metastasize. How do growing tumors develop a blood supply? Several studies indicate that tumor angiogenesis is effected by secreted factors. Tumor-associated angiogenic factors are produced by tumor cells themselves and by inflammatory cells (e.g., macrophages) that infiltrate tumors. Of the dozen or so tumor-associated angiogenic factors, the two most important are basic fibroblast growth factor (bFGF) and vascular endothelial growth factor (VEGF). Others, such as TNF-α derived from macrophages, also contribute. Neovascularization has a dual effect on tumor growth: perfusion supplies nutrients and oxygen, and newly formed endothelial cells stimulate tumor growth by secreting growth factors.

Recent studies suggest that tumor angiogenesis is controlled by the balance between angiogenic factors and inhibitors of angiogenesis. In the latter category are thrombospondin and angiostatin. Quite interestingly, production of thrombospondin, an inhibitor of angiogenesis, is regulated by the p53 gene. With the loss of p53, thrombospondin production by tumor cells is reduced, thus tilting the balance in the favor of angiogenic factors.

Angiogenesis is not only essential for the growth of primary tumors, but also facilitates metastases. Highly vascular tumors are more prone to metastasize because of ready access to the vasculature. Indeed, in cancers of the breast, intratumor mi-crovessel density has been found to be a prognostic factor. Because of the critical role of angiogenesis in the growth and spread of tumors, much interest is focused on the use of angiogenesis inhibitors as adjuncts to other forms of therapy.

TUMOR PROGRESSION AND HETEROGENEITY

It is well established that over a period of time, many tumors become more aggressive and acquire greater malignant potential. This phenomenon is referred to as *tumor progression* and must be clearly distinguished from an increase in tumor size. Careful clinical and experimental studies reveal that increasing malignancy (e.g., accelerated growth, invasiveness, and ability to form distant metastases) is often acquired in an incremental fashion. This biologic phenomenon is related to the sequential appearance of subpopulations of cells that differ with respect to several phenotypic attributes, such as invasiveness, rate of growth, metastatic ability, karyotype, hormonal responsiveness, and susceptibility to antineoplastic drugs. Thus, *despite the fact that most malignant tumors are monoclonal in origin, by the time they become clinically evident, their constituent cells are extremely heterogeneous.* At the molecular level, tumor progression and associated heterogeneity most likely result from multiple mutations that accumulate independently in different cells, thus generating subclones with different characteristics.

What predisposes the original transformed cell to additional genetic damage is not entirely clear. Most investigators believe that transformed cells are genetically unstable. Such instability may result, for example, from the loss of p53, the so-called "guardian of the genome." As mentioned earlier, inherited or acquired mutations in DNA repair genes may also contribute to genomic instability. These and other unidentified factors render tumor cells susceptible to a high rate of random, spontaneous mutations during clonal expansion (Fig. 6–28). Some of these mutations may be lethal; others may spur cell growth by affecting other protooncogenes or cancer suppressor genes. The subclones so generated are subjected to immune and nonimmune selection pressures. For example, cells that are highly antigenic are destroyed by host defenses, whereas those with reduced growth factor requirements are positively selected. A growing tumor, therefore, tends to be enriched for those subclones that "beat the odds" and are adept at survival, growth, invasion, and metastases. Although progression is most obvious after a tumor is diagnosed, it is important to remember that during the latent period many cell doublings occur, and hence generation of heterogeneity begins well before the tumor is clinically evident.

The rate at which mutant subclones are generated is quite variable. In some tumors, such as osteosarcomas, metastatic subclones are already present when the patient walks into the physician's office. In others, typified by mixed salivary gland tumors, aggressive subclones develop late and infrequently. Knowledge of such biologic differences is of obvious importance to the clinical potential of cancers and to the management of cancer patients.

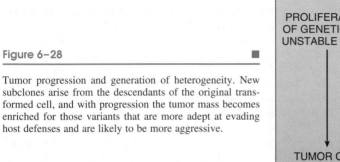

Figure 6-28 ■

Tumor progression and generation of heterogeneity. New subclones arise from the descendants of the original transformed cell, and with progression the tumor mass becomes enriched for those variants that are more adept at evading host defenses and are likely to be more aggressive.

Mechanisms of Local and Distant Spread

In an earlier part of this chapter it was emphasized that invasion and metastasis are biologic hallmarks of malignancy. Here we will concentrate on the mechanisms by which tumors infiltrate locally and are transported to distant sites.

The spread of tumors is a complex process involving a series of sequential steps, diagrammed in Figure 6–29. Quite predictably, this sequence of steps may be interrupted at any stage by either host or tumor-related factors. As mentioned earlier, cells within a tumor are heterogeneous with respect to metastatic potential. Only certain subclones possess the right combination of gene products to complete all the steps outlined in Figure 6–26. For the purpose of discussion, the metastatic cascade can be subdivided into two phases: invasion of extracellular matrix, and vascular dissemination and homing of tumor cells.

INVASION OF EXTRACELLULAR MATRIX

As is well known, human tissues are organized into a series of compartments separated from each other by two types of extracellular matrix (ECM): basement membranes and interstitial connective tissue. Although organized differently, each of these components of ECM is made up of collagens, glycoproteins, and proteoglycans. A review of Figure 6–26 will reveal that tumor cells must interact with the ECM at several stages in the metastatic cascade. A carcinoma must first breach the underlying basement membrane, then traverse the interstitial connective tissue, and ultimately gain access to the circulation by penetrating the vascular basement membrane. This cycle is repeated when tumor cell emboli extravasate at a distant site. Invasion of the ECM is an active process that can be resolved into four steps (Fig. 6–30):

■ Detachment of tumor cells from each other
■ Attachment of tumor cells to matrix components
■ Degradation of ECM
■ Migration of tumor cells

The first step in the metastatic cascade is a "loosening up" of tumor cells. As mentioned earlier, E-cadherins act as intercellular glues, and loss of E-cadherins increases the metastatic potential of carcinoma cells. Reduced surface expression of certain integrins is associated with an increase in the metastatic potential of melanomas.

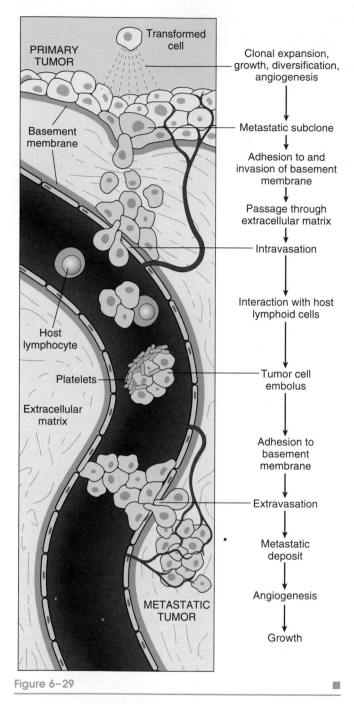

Figure 6–29 ■

The metastatic cascade. Schematic illustration of the sequential steps involved in the hematogenous spread of a tumor.

The next step, attachment of tumor cells to ECM proteins such as laminin and fibronectin, is important for invasion and metastasis. Normal epithelial cells have receptors for basement membrane laminin that are polarized at their basal surface. In contrast, carcinoma cells have many more receptors, and these are distributed all around the cell membrane. Furthermore, there is a correlation between the density of laminin receptors on breast carcinoma cells and lymph node metastases. A similar correlation exists between the ability to bind

fibronectin, the major glycoprotein of interstitial tissues, and invasiveness.

The third step in invasion is local degradation of the basement membrane and interstitial connective tissue. Tumor cells secrete proteolytic enzymes themselves or induce the host cells (e.g., fibroblasts) to elaborate proteases. Several matrix-degrading enzymes termed *metalloproteinases*, including gelatinases, collagenases, and stromelysins, are involved. Type IV collagenase is a gelatinase that cleaves type IV collagen of the epithelial and vascular basement membranes. Benign tumors of the breast, colon, and stomach show very little type IV collagenase activity, whereas their malignant counterparts overexpress this enzyme. Concurrently, the levels of metalloproteinase inhibitors are reduced, so the balance is tilted greatly toward tissue degradation. Similar correlations have been noted with other proteases, including cathepsin D. Overexpression of cathepsin D occurs in invasive breast cancers. Because of these observations, attempts are being made to use protease inhibitors as therapeutic agents.

Locomotion is the final step of invasion, propelling tumor cells through the degraded basement membranes and zones of matrix proteolysis. Migration seems to be mediated by tumor cell–derived cytokines such as autocrine motility factors. In addition, cleavage products of matrix components (e.g., collagen, laminin) and some growth factors (e.g., insulin-like growth factors I and II) have chemotactic activity for tumor cells. The latter could play a role in organ-selective homing of tumor cells.

VASCULAR DISSEMINATION AND HOMING OF TUMOR CELLS

Once in the circulation, tumor cells are vulnerable to destruction by the host immune cells, a topic discussed later in this chapter. In the bloodstream, some tumor cells form emboli by aggregating and adhering to circulating leukocytes, particularly platelets; aggregated tumor cells are afforded some protection from the antitumor host effector cells. However, most tumor cells circulate as single cells. Extravasation of free tumor cells or tumor emboli involves adhesion to the vascular endothelium, followed by egress through the basement membrane by mechanisms similar to those involved in invasion.

The site of extravasation, and hence the organ distribution of metastases, can generally be predicted by the location of the primary tumor and its vascular or lymphatic drainage. However, in many cases the natural pathways of drainage do not readily explain the distribution of metastases. As pointed out earlier, some tumors (e.g., lung cancers) tend to involve the adrenals with some regularity but almost never spread to skeletal muscle. Such organ tropism may be related to the expression of adhesion molecules by tumor cells whose ligands are expressed preferentially on the endothelium of target organs. Alternatively, some of the potential target organs may have an unfavorable environment and are therefore spared from metastases. They have poor soil, so to speak, for the growth of tumor seedlings. For example, the presence of high concentrations of protease inhibitors could prevent the establishment of a tumor colony.

However, despite the foregoing considerations, the precise

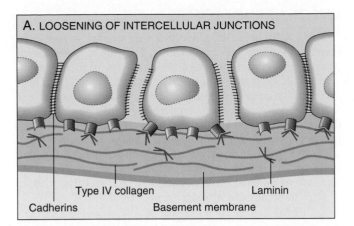

A. LOOSENING OF INTERCELLULAR JUNCTIONS

Cadherins
Type IV collagen
Basement membrane
Laminin

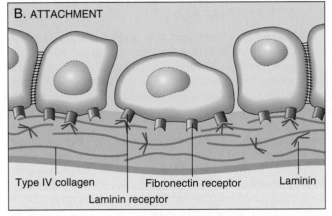

B. ATTACHMENT

Type IV collagen
Laminin receptor
Fibronectin receptor
Laminin

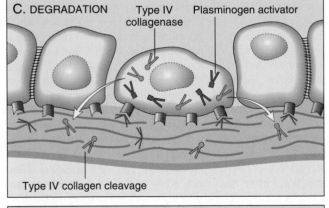

C. DEGRADATION
Type IV collagenase
Plasminogen activator
Type IV collagen cleavage

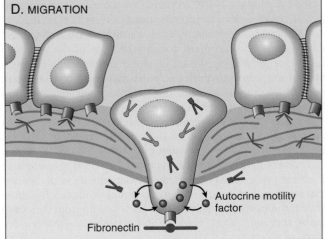

D. MIGRATION

Fibronectin
Autocrine motility factor

localization of metastases cannot be predicted with any form of cancer. Evidently many tumors have not read pathology textbooks!

MOLECULAR GENETICS OF METASTASES

It can be asked, "Are there oncogenes or tumor suppressor genes that elicit metastases as their principal or sole contribution to tumorigenesis?" This question is of more than academic interest, because if altered forms of certain genes promote or suppress the metastatic phenotype, their detection in a primary tumor may have prognostic as well as therapeutic implications. At present no single "metastasis gene" has been found. Indeed, since metastatic cells must acquire multiple properties (e.g., expression of adhesion receptors, production of collagenases, and motility factors), no single genetic alteration is likely to render a cell metastasis prone. Thus, it might be expected that mutations in the E-cadherin gene or genes that encode inhibitors of metalloproteinases would facilitate metastases by making the cells more invasive. Reduced expression of a gene called nm23 seems to be associated with metastatic potential in carcinomas of the breast, liver, ovary, and stomach. The function of nm23 in the metastatic cascade is unknown.

ETIOLOGY OF CANCER: CARCINOGENIC AGENTS

Genetic damage lies at the heart of carcinogenesis. What agents inflict such damage? Three classes of carcinogenic agents can be identified: chemicals, radiant energy, and oncogenic viruses. Chemicals and radiant energy are documented causes of cancer in humans, and oncogenic viruses are involved in the pathogenesis of tumors in several animals and at least some human tumors. In the following discussion each class of agents is considered separately, but it is important to note that several may act in concert or sequentially to produce the multiple genetic abnormalities characteristic of neoplastic cells.

Chemical Carcinogens

It has been about 200 years since the London surgeon Sir Percival Pott correctly attributed scrotal skin cancer in chimney sweeps to chronic exposure to soot. A few years later, based on this observation, the Danish Chimney Sweeps Guild

Figure 6–30 ■

Schematic illustration of the sequence of events in the invasion of epithelial basement membranes by tumor cells (A–D). Tumor cells detach from each other because of reduced adhesiveness, and then cells attach to the basement membrane via the laminin receptors and secrete proteolytic enzymes, including type IV collagenase and plasminogen activator. Degradation of the basement membrane and tumor cell migration follow.

ruled that its members must bathe daily. No public health measure since that time has achieved so much in the control of a form of cancer! Since that time, hundreds of chemicals have been shown to be carcinogenic in animals.

The following pertinent observations have emerged from the study of chemical carcinogens:

■ They are of extremely diverse structure and include both natural and synthetic products.

■ Some are direct-reacting and require no chemical transformation to induce carcinogenicity, but most are indirect-reacting and become active only after metabolic conversion. Such agents are referred to as *procarcinogens*, and their active end products are called *ultimate carcinogens.*

■ All chemical carcinogens, both the direct-reacting and the ultimate carcinogens, are highly reactive electrophiles (i.e., have electron-deficient atoms) that react with the electron-rich atoms in RNA, cellular proteins, and, mainly, DNA.

■ The carcinogenicity of some chemicals is augmented by agents that by themselves have little, if any, cancerous activity. Such augmenting agents have traditionally been called *promoters*; however, many carcinogens have no requirement for promoting agents.

■ Several chemical carcinogens may act in concert or with other types of carcinogenic influences (e.g., viruses or radiation) to induce neoplasia.

Some of the major agents are presented in Table 6–7. Only a few comments are offered on some.

■

Table 6–7. MAJOR CHEMICAL CARCINOGENS

Direct-acting carcinogens
Alkylating agents
    Anticancer drugs (cyclophosphamide, chlorambucil, nitrosou-
    reas, and others)
Acylating agents
    1-Acetyl-imidazole
    Dimethylcarbamyl chloride

Procarcinogens that require metabolic activation
Polycyclic and heterocyclic aromatic hydrocarbons
    Benz[a]anthracene
    Benzo[a]pyrene
    Dibenz[a,h]anthracene
    3-Methylcholanthrene
    7,12-Dimethylbenz[a]anthracene

Aromatic amines, amides, azo dyes
    2-Naphthylamine (β-naphthylamine)
    2-Acetylaminofluorene
    Dimethylaminoazobenzene (butter yellow)

Natural plant and microbial products
    Aflatoxin B_1
    Griseofulvin
    Betel nuts

Others
    Nitrosamine and amides
    Vinyl chloride, nickel, chromium
    Insecticides, fungicides
    Polychlorinated biphenyls (PCBs)
    Arsenic
    Asbestos

DIRECT-ACTING AGENTS

These substances, as already noted, require no metabolic conversion to become carcinogenic. They are in general weak carcinogens but are important because some of them are cancer chemotherapeutic drugs (e.g., alkylating agents) that have successfully cured, controlled, or delayed recurrence of certain types of cancer (e.g., leukemia, lymphoma, Hodgkin's disease, and ovarian carcinoma), only to later evoke a second form of cancer, usually leukemia. This is even more tragic when their initial use has been for non-neoplastic disorders such as rheumatoid arthritis or Wegener's granulomatosis. The risk of induced cancer is low, but the fact that it exists dictates judicious use of such agents.

INDIRECT-ACTING AGENTS

This designation indicates that these chemicals require metabolic conversion before they become active. Some of the most potent indirect chemical carcinogens—the polycyclic hydrocarbons—are present in fossil fuels. Benz[a]anthracene produces cancer wherever it is applied: when painted on the skin, it induces skin cancers; injected subcutaneously, it induces fibrosarcomas. Polycyclic agents are also produced in the combustion of organic substances. For example, benzo[a]pyrene and other carcinogens are formed in the high-temperature combustion of tobacco in cigarette smoking. *These products are implicated in the causation of lung cancer in cigarette smokers.* Polycyclic hydrocarbons may also be produced from animal fats during the process of broiling meats and are present in smoked meats and fish. The principal active products in many hydrocarbons are epoxides, which form covalent adducts (addition products) with molecules in the cell, principally DNA, but also with RNA and proteins.

Another class of indirect agents are the aromatic amines and azo dyes. Beta-naphthylamine was responsible, before its carcinogenicity was recognized, for a 50-fold increased incidence of bladder cancers in heavily exposed workers in the aniline dye and rubber industries. Many other occupational carcinogens are listed in Table 6–3. Some of the azo dyes were developed to color food (e.g., butter yellow to make margarine more enticing and scarlet red for maraschino cherries). What price aesthetics? Most of the aromatic amines and azo dyes are converted into ultimate carcinogens in the liver by the cytochrome P-450 oxygenase system and therefore induce hepatocellular carcinomas in experimental animals.

A few other agents merit brief mention. Nitrosamines and amides have aroused great concern because of the evidence that they can be formed endogenously in the acidic environment of the stomach. Various amines derived from food may undergo nitrosation with nitrites that have been added to food as preservatives or derived from nitrates by bacterial action. Repeatedly the question has been raised as to whether nitroso compounds could account for the increased incidence of gastric carcinoma in some populations. Nitroso compounds are also present in tobacco smoke and after absorption could lead to cancers in a variety of organs. Aflatoxin B_1 is of interest because it is a naturally occurring agent produced by some strains of *Aspergillus,* a mold that grows on improperly stored grains and nuts. There is a *strong correlation between the dietary level of this food contaminant and the incidence of hepatocellular carcinoma in some parts of Africa and the Far East.* However, there is an even stronger correlation between the prevalence of infection with hepatitis B virus and hepatocellular carcinoma. Thus, aflatoxin and hepatitis B virus may act in concert to produce hepatic cancers (Chapter 16). Saccharin and cyclamates have been incriminated as carcinogens in experimental animals, but because induction of cancer with these artificial sweeteners requires extremely large doses, their role in human carcinogenesis remains in doubt. Finally, attention should be called to vinyl chloride, arsenic, nickel, chromium, insecticides, fungicides, and polychlorinated biphenyls (PCBs) as potential carcinogens in the workplace and about the house.

MECHANISMS OF ACTION OF CHEMICAL CARCINOGENS

Because malignant transformation results from mutations that affect oncogenes and cancer suppressor genes, it will come as no surprise that most chemical carcinogens are mutagenic. Although any gene may be the target of chemical carcinogens, *ras* gene mutations are particularly common in several chemically induced cancers in rodents.

It was mentioned earlier that carcinogenicity of some chemicals is augmented by subsequent administration of "promoters" (such as phorbol esters, hormones, phenols, and drugs) that by themselves are nontumorigenic. To be effective, repeated or sustained exposure to the promoter must *follow* the application of the mutagenic chemical, or "initiator." The initiation-promotion sequence of chemical carcinogenesis raises an important question: Since promoters are not mutagenic, how do they contribute to tumorigenesis? Although the effects of tumor promoters are pleiotropic, *induction of cell proliferation is a sine qua non of tumor promotion.* Tetra-decanoylphorbol-acetate (TPA), a phorbol ester and the best-studied tumor promoter, is a powerful activator of protein kinase C, an enzyme that is a critical component of several signal transduction pathways, including those activated by growth factors. TPA also causes growth factor secretion by some cells. It seems most likely, therefore, that while the application of an initiator may cause the mutational activation of an oncogene such as *ras,* subsequent application of promoters leads to clonal expansion of initiated (mutated) cells. Such cells (especially after *ras* activation) have reduced growth factor requirements and may also be less responsive to growth inhibitory signals in their extracellular milieu. Forced to proliferate, the initiated clone of cells suffers additional mutations, developing eventually into a malignant tumor. The concept that sustained cell proliferation increases the risk of mutagenesis, and hence neoplastic transformation, is also applicable to human carcinogenesis. For example, pathologic hyperplasia of the endometrium (Chapter 19) and increased regenerative activity that accompanies chronic liver cell injury are associated with the development of cancer in these organs.

Before we leave the topic of chemical carcinogenesis, it must be emphasized that carcinogen-induced damage to DNA does not necessarily lead to initiation of cancer. Several forms of DNA damage (incurred spontaneously or through the action of carcinogens) can be repaired by cellular enzymes. Were this not the case, the incidence of environmentally induced cancer would in all likelihood be much higher. This is best exemplified by the rare hereditary disorders of DNA repair, including xeroderma pigmentosum, which is associated with defective DNA repair and a greatly increased risk of cancers induced by ultraviolet light and certain chemicals.

Radiation Carcinogenesis

Radiation, whatever its source—ultraviolet rays of sunlight, x-rays, nuclear fission, radionuclides—is an established carcinogen. The evidence is so voluminous that only a few examples will suffice. Many of the pioneers in the development of roentgen rays developed skin cancers. Miners of radioactive elements have suffered a tenfold increased incidence of lung cancers. Follow-up of survivors of the atomic bombs dropped on Hiroshima and Nagasaki has disclosed a markedly increased incidence of leukemia—principally acute and chronic myelocytic leukemia—after an average latent period of about 7 years. Decades later, the leukemia risk for those heavily exposed is still above the level for control populations, as is the mortality rate from thyroid, breast, colon, and pulmonary carcinoma and others. The nuclear power accident at Chernobyl in the former Soviet Union continues to exact its toll in the form of high cancer incidence in the surrounding areas. Even therapeutic irradiation has been documented to be carcinogenic. Thyroid cancers have developed in approximately 9% of those exposed during infancy and childhood to head and neck irradiation (Chapter 20). Thus, it is abundantly clear that radiation is strongly oncogenic. This effect of ionizing radiations is related to its mutagenic effects; it causes chromosome breakage, translocations, and point mutations. Because the latent period of irradiation-associated cancers is extremely long, it appears that cancer emerges only after the progeny of initially damaged cells accumulate additional mutations, induced possibly by other environmental factors.

The oncogenic effect of ultraviolet (UV) rays merits special mention because it highlights the importance of DNA repair in carcinogenesis. Natural UV radiation derived from the sun can cause skin cancers (melanomas, squamous cell carcinomas, and basal cell carcinomas). At greatest risk are fair-skinned people who live in locales that receive a great deal of sunlight. Thus, cancers of the exposed skin are particularly common in Australia and New Zealand. UV light has several biologic effects on cells. Of particular relevance to carcinogenesis is the ability to damage DNA by forming pyrimidine dimers. In normal persons, the altered DNA can usually be repaired by a series of repair enzymes, but in *individuals with xeroderma pigmentosum, the nucleotide excision repair mechanism is defective or deficient,* and hence there is a greatly increased predisposition to skin cancers. Three other disorders of DNA repair and genomic instability—ataxia telangiectasia, Fanconi's anemia, and Bloom's syndrome—are also characterized by an increased risk of cancer, related to some inability to repair environmentally induced DNA damage. They were discussed earlier (p 157).

Viral Oncogenesis

A large number of DNA and RNA viruses have proved to be oncogenic in animals as disparate as frogs and primates. However, despite intense scrutiny, only a few viruses have been linked with human cancer. Our discussion is limited predominantly to human oncogenic viruses.

RNA ONCOGENIC VIRUSES

The study of oncogenic retroviruses in animals has provided spectacular insights into the genetic basis of cancer. Animal retroviruses transform cells by two mechanisms. Some, called *acute transforming viruses*, contain a transforming viral oncogene such as *src, abl,* or *myb.* You may recall that v-*onc*s are transduced human protooncogenes. Others, called *slow transforming viruses* (e.g., mouse mammary tumor virus) do not contain a v-*onc,* but the proviral DNA is always found to be inserted near a protooncogene. Under the influence of a strong retroviral promoter, the adjacent normal or mutated protooncogene is overexpressed. This mechanism of transformation is called *insertional mutagenesis.* With this brief summary of retroviral oncogenesis in animals, we can turn to the only known human retrovirus that is associated with cancer.

Human T-Cell Leukemia Virus Type I. Human T-cell leukemia virus-I (HTLV-I) is associated with a form of T-cell leukemia/lymphoma that is endemic in certain parts of Japan and the Caribbean basin but is found sporadically elsewhere, including the United States. Like the acquired immunodeficiency syndrome (AIDS) virus, HTLV-I has tropism for CD4+ T cells, and hence this subset of T cells is the major target for neoplastic transformation. Human infection requires transmission of infected T cells via sexual intercourse, blood products, or breast feeding. Leukemia develops in only about 1% of infected individuals after a long latent period of 20 to 30 years.

There is little doubt that HTLV-I infection of T lymphocytes is necessary for leukemogenesis, but the molecular mechanisms of transformation are not entirely clear. Unlike acute transforming retroviruses, HTLV-I does not contain a v-*onc,* and unlike slow transforming retroviruses, no consistent integration next to a protooncogene has been discovered. The genomic structure of HTLV-I reveals the *gag, pol, env,* and long terminal repeat (LTR) regions typical of other retroviruses, but unlike other leukemia viruses, it contains another region, referred to as *tax.* It seems that the secrets of its transforming activity are locked in the *tax* gene. The product of this gene is essential for viral replication. The *tax* protein can also activate the transcription of several host cell genes, including genes encoding the cytokine interleukin 2 (IL-2) and its receptor, and the gene for the granulocyte-macrophage colony-stimulating factor (GM-CSF). From these and other observations the following scenario is emerging (Fig. 6–31): HTLV-I infection stimulates proliferation of T cells. This is brought about by the *tax* gene, which turns on genes that encode a T-cell growth factor, IL-2, and the IL-2 receptor, setting up an autocrine system for proliferation. At the same time, a paracrine pathway is activated by the increased production of GM-CSF. This myeloid growth factor, by acting on neigh-

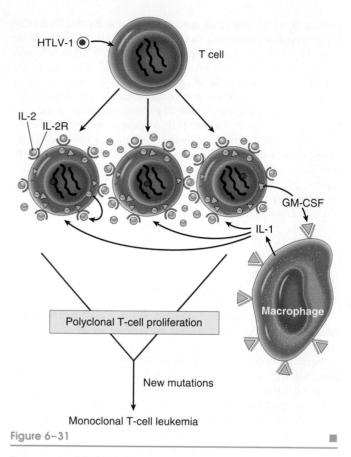

Figure 6–31 ■

Pathogenesis of HTLV-1–induced T-cell leukemia/lymphoma. HTLV-1 infects many T cells and initially causes polyclonal proliferation by autocrine and paracrine pathways. Ultimately, a monoclonal T-cell leukemia/lymphoma results when one proliferating T cell suffers additional mutations.

boring macrophages, induces increased secretion of other T-cell mitogens such as interleukin 1 (IL-1). Initially the T-cell proliferation is polyclonal, because the virus infects many cells. The proliferating T cells are at increased risk of secondary transforming events (mutations), which lead ultimately to the outgrowth of a monoclonal neoplastic T-cell population.

DNA ONCOGENIC VIRUSES

As with RNA viruses, several oncogenic DNA viruses that cause tumors in animals have been identified. Three DNA viruses—papillomavirus, Epstein-Barr virus (EBV), and hepatitis B virus (HBV)—are of special interest because they have been suspected of causing human cancer. Before we discuss the role of these viruses in carcinogenesis, a few general comments relating to transformation by DNA viruses are offered:

■ Transforming DNA viruses form stable associations with the host cell genome. The integrated virus is unable to complete its replicative cycle because the viral genes essential for completion of replication are interrupted during integration of viral DNA.

■ Those viral genes that are transcribed early (early genes) in the viral life cycle are important for transformation. They are expressed in transformed cells.

Human Papillomavirus. Approximately 50 genetically distinct types of HPV have been identified. Some types (e.g., 1, 2, 4, and 7) definitely cause benign squamous papillomas (warts) in humans (Chapters 19 and 22). HPVs have also been implicated in the genesis of several cancers, particularly squamous cell carcinoma of the cervix and anogenital region. Epidemiologic studies suggest that carcinoma of the cervix is caused by a sexually transmitted agent, and HPV is a prime suspect. DNA sequences of HPV types 16 and 18 are found in 75% to 100% of invasive squamous cell cancers and their presumed precursors (i.e., severe dysplasias and carcinoma in situ). In contrast with cervical cancers, genital warts with low malignant potential are associated with distinct HPV types, predominantly HPV-6 and HPV-11. The oncogenic potential of HPV can be related to products of two early viral genes, E6 and E7. The E7 protein binds to the retinoblastoma protein and displaces the transcription factors that are normally sequestered by *Rb*; the E6 protein binds to and inactivates the product of p53. Quite remarkably, the affinity of such interactions differs depending on the oncogenic potential of HPV. E6 and E7 proteins derived from high-risk HPVs (types 16, 18, and 31) bind to *Rb* and p53 with high affinity, whereas the E6 and E7 gene products of low-risk HPVs (types 6 and 11) bind with low affinity. Thus, *infection with high-risk HPV types simulates the loss of two important tumor suppressor genes that regulate the cell cycle.* However, infection with HPV itself is not sufficient for carcinogenesis. For example, when human keratinocytes are transfected with DNA from HPV 16, 18, or 31 in vitro, they are immortalized, but they do not form tumors in experimental animals. Co-transfection with a mutated *ras* gene results in full malignant transformation. These data strongly suggest that HPV in all likelihood acts in concert with other environmental factors (Chapter 19).

Epstein-Barr Virus. EBV has been implicated in the pathogenesis of four human tumors, Burkitt's lymphoma, B-cell lymphomas in immunosuppressed individuals (including those with AIDS), Hodgkin's disease, and nasopharyngeal cancer.

Burkitt's lymphoma is a tumor of B lymphocytes that is endemic in certain parts of Africa and sporadic elsewhere. In endemic areas, tumor cells in virtually all patients carry the EBV genome. EBV exhibits strong tropism for B cells and infects many B cells, causing them to proliferate. In vitro, such infection leads to immortalization of B cells, producing lymphoblastoid cell lines. These cell lines express several EBV-encoded antigens. In immunologically normal individuals, EBV-driven polyclonal B-cell proliferation in vivo is readily controlled, and the individual either remains asymptomatic or develops a self-limited episode of infectious mononucleosis (Chapter 12). In regions of the world where Burkitt's lymphoma is endemic, concomitant (endemic) malaria (or other infections) impairs immune competence, allowing sustained B-cell proliferation. In addition, the B cells do not express cell surface antigens that can be recognized by host T cells. Relieved from immunoregulation, such B cells are at increased risk of acquiring mutations such as the t(8,14) translocation, which activates the *myc* oncogene and is a consistent feature

of this tumor. The activation of c-*myc* causes further loss of growth control, and the stage is set for additional gene damage, which ultimately leads to the emergence of a monoclonal neoplasm. It should be noted that in nonendemic areas, 80% of tumors do not harbor the EBV genome, but all tumors possess the specific translocation. This suggests that B cells triggered by other mechanisms may also suffer similar mutations and give rise to non-African Burkitt's lymphoma.

In immunosuppressed patients, including those with HIV disease and organ transplant recipients, EBV-infected B cells undergo polyclonal expansion, producing in vivo counterparts of lymphoblastoid cell lines. Unlike tumor B cells in Burkitt's lymphoma, the B lymphoblasts in immunosuppressed patients do express cell surface antigens recognized by T cells. Hence, these potentially lethal proliferations can be subdued if the immunologic status of the host improves, as may occur with withdrawal of immunosuppressive drugs in transplant recipients.

Nasopharyngeal carcinoma is endemic in Southern China and some other locales, and the EBV genome is found in all tumors. As in Burkitt's lymphoma, EBV acts in concert with other unidentified factors.

Hepatitis B Virus. Although the epidemiologic evidence linking chronic HBV infection with hepatocellular carcinoma is strong (Chapter 16), the role of the virus in tumor production is unclear. The HBV genome does not encode any transforming proteins, and there is no consistent pattern of integration in liver cells. The oncogenic effect of HBV appears to be multifactorial. First, by causing chronic liver cell injury and accompanying regeneration, HBV predisposes the cells to mutations, caused possibly by environmental agents (such as dietary toxins). Mutational inactivation of p53 has been noted in liver cancers that occur in areas of the world where HBV and exposure to aflatoxins is endemic. Second, an HBV-encoded regulatory element called *x-protein* disrupts normal growth control of infected liver cells by transcriptional activation of several host cell protooncogenes (recall *tax* proteins of HTLV-I). This sequence is supported by the development of hepatocellular carcinomas in mice that are transgenic for the region of HBV DNA that encodes the x-protein. Third, in some patients viral integration seems to cause secondary rearrangements of chromosomes and possibly homozygous inactivation of the p53 gene. In addition, it has been reported that, like other DNA viruses, HBV x-protein may bind to and inactivate p53. Thus, it seems that virus-induced gene damage in regenerating liver cells may set the stage for multistep carcinogenesis.

HOST DEFENSE AGAINST TUMORS: TUMOR IMMUNITY

Malignant transformation, as has been discussed, is associated with complex genetic alterations, some of which may result in the expression of proteins that are seen as non-self by the immune system. The idea that tumors are not entirely self was conceived by Ehrlich, who proposed that immune-mediated recognition of autologous tumor cells may be a "positive mechanism" capable of eliminating transformed cells. Subsequently, Lewis Thomas and McFarlane Burnet formalized this concept by coining the term *immune surveillance* to refer to recognition and destruction of non-self tumor cells on their appearance. The very fact that cancers occur suggests that immune surveillance is imperfect; however, because some tumors escape such policing does not preclude the possibility that others may have been aborted. It is necessary therefore to explore certain questions about tumor immunity: What is the nature of tumor antigens? What host effector systems may recognize tumor cells? Is tumor immunity effective against spontaneous neoplasms? Can immune reactions against tumors be exploited for immunotherapy?

Tumor Antigens

Antigens that elicit an immune response have been demonstrated in many experimentally induced tumors and in some human cancers. They can be broadly classified into two categories: tumor-specific antigens (TSAs), which are present only on tumor cells and not on any normal cells, and tumor-associated antigens (TAAs), which are present on tumor cells and also on some normal cells.

Tumor-Specific Antigens. TSAs were initially demonstrated in chemically induced tumors of rodents. It was found that many chemically induced tumors express "private" or "unique" antigens not shared by other (histologically identical) tumors induced by the same chemical, even in the same animal. These antigens were recognized by cytotoxic T cells. Previously it was assumed that spontaneously arising human tumors are nonantigenic. However, more recent studies have led to the discovery of several tumor antigens that, while not unique to a given tumor, are generally not expressed on normal tissues. Hence they can serve as targets for tumor-specific cytotoxic T cells. As with all antigens recognized by cytotoxic T cells, TSAs expressed on human tumors are composed of a peptide that is bound to and presented to T cells by class I major histocompatibility complex (MHC) molecules. One such antigen, called *melanoma-associated antigen-1 (MAGE-1)*, initially thought to be restricted to melanomas, is expressed on 40% of melanomas, 20% of breast carcinomas, and 35% of non–small cell lung cancers. Of significance, this antigen is not expressed on any normal tissues except the testis. It is believed that the peptide forming the MAGE-1 antigen is derived from an embryonal protein that is not expressed on any normal cells (except testis) and whose expression is de-repressed in tumor cells. Similar antigens, called *BAGE* and *GAGE*, have also been detected in several human tumors. (Note how investigators have chosen the suffix "-age" for TSAs.)

In some pancreatic and breast carcinomas, peptides derived from abnormally glycosylated mucus can be recognized by cytotoxic T cells. These mucins differ from their normal counterparts, and hence tumor-specific T cells do not kill normal breast or pancreatic cells. CD8+ cytotoxic T lymphocytes that can specifically recognize such TSAs can be found among tumor-infiltrating lymphocytes and can be expanded in vitro for possible therapeutic use.

Tumor-Associated Antigens. Some human tumor antigens are not unique to the tumors; rather, they are shared by normal untransformed cells from which the tumor arose. These are called *differentiation-specific antigens*. They are peculiar to the differentiation state at which cancer cells are arrested. For example, CD10 (CALLA antigen), an antigen expressed in early B lymphocytes, is expressed in B-cell leukemias and lymphomas. Similarly, prostate-specific antigen (PSA) is expressed on normal as well as cancerous prostatic epithelium. Both serve as useful differentiation markers in the diagnosis of lymphoid and prostatic cancers. Melanomas and normal melanocytes, on the other hand, express a peptide derived from tyrosinase, an enzyme in the melanin biosynthetic pathway. The tyrosinase-derived antigen expressed on such cells can be recognized by cytotoxic T cells.

Antitumor Effector Mechanisms

Both cell-mediated and humoral immunity can have antitumor activity. The cellular effectors that mediate immunity were described in Chapter 5, so it is necessary here only to characterize them briefly (Fig. 6–32):

■ *Cytotoxic T lymphocytes.* The role of specifically sensitized cytotoxic T cells in experimentally induced tumors is well established. In humans they seem to play a protective role, chiefly against virus-associated neoplasms (e.g., EBV-induced Burkitt's lymphoma and HPV-induced tumors). The presence of MHC-restricted CD8+ cells that can kill autologous tumor cells within human tumors sug-

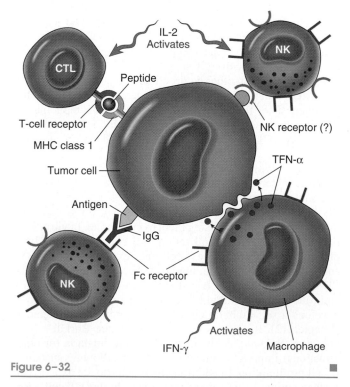

Figure 6–32 ■

Cellular effectors of antitumor immunity and some cytokines that modulate antitumor activities. The nature of antigen recognized by T cells is depicted in Figure 5–4.

gests that the role of T cells in immunity against human tumors may be broader than previously suspected.

■ *Natural killer cells.* Natural killer (NK) cells are lymphocytes that are capable of destroying tumor cells without prior sensitization; hence they may provide the first line of defense against tumors. After activation with IL-2, NK cells can lyse a wide range of human tumors, including many that appear to be nonimmunogenic for T cells. T cells and NK cells seem to provide complementary antitumor mechanisms. Tumors that fail to express MHC class I antigens cannot be recognized by T cells, but these tumors may trigger NK cells, because the latter are inhibited by recognition of normal autologous class I molecules (see Fig. 5–2). The nature of triggering receptors on NK cells is not known. In addition to direct lysis of tumor cells, NK cells can also participate in antibody-dependent cellular cytotoxicity (ADCC), as described in Chapter 5.

■ *Macrophages.* Activated macrophages exhibit somewhat selective cytotoxicity against tumor cells in vitro. T cells, NK cells, and macrophages may collaborate in antitumor reactivity, since interferon-γ (IFN-γ), a cytokine secreted by T cells and NK cells, is a potent activator of macrophages. These cells may kill tumors by mechanisms similar to those used to kill microbes (e.g., production of reactive oxygen metabolites; Chapter 1) or by secretion of tumor necrosis factor α (TNF-α). In addition to its many other effects, this cytokine is lytic for several tumor cells.

■ *Humoral mechanisms.* These may participate in tumor cell destruction by two mechanisms: activation of complement and induction of ADCC by NK cells.

Immunosurveillance

Given the host of possible and potential antitumor mechanisms, is there any evidence that they operate in vivo to prevent the emergence of neoplasms? The *strongest argument for the existence of immunosurveillance is the increased frequency of cancers in immunodeficient hosts.* About 5% of persons with congenital immunodeficiencies develop cancers, a rate that is about 200 times that for persons without such immunodeficiencies. Analogously, immunosuppressed transplant recipients and patients with AIDS have increased numbers of malignancies. It should be noted that most (but not all) of these neoplasms are lymphomas, often lymphomas of activated B cells. Particularly illustrative is the X-linked lymphoproliferative disorder (XLP). When affected boys develop an EBV infection, such infection does not take the usual self-limited form of infectious mononucleosis but instead evolves into a chronic or sometimes fatal form of infectious mononucleosis or, even worse, malignant lymphoma.

Most cancers occur in persons who do not suffer from any overt immunodeficiency. If immunosurveillance exists, how do cancers evade the immune system in immunocompetent hosts? To explain this, several escape mechanisms have been proposed:

■ *Selective outgrowth of antigen-negative variants.* During tumor progression, strongly immunogenic subclones may be eliminated.

■ *Loss or reduced expression of histocompatibility antigens.* Tumor cells may fail to express normal levels of human leukocyte antigen (HLA) class I, thereby escaping attack by cytotoxic T cells. Such cells, however, may trigger NK cells.

■ It may be recalled that sensitization of T cells requires two signals, one by foreign peptide presented by MHC, and the other by costimulatory molecules (Chapter 5); while tumor cells may express peptide antigens with class I molecules, they often do not express costimulatory molecules. This not only prevents sensitization, it may also render T cells anergic or, worse, cause them to undergo apoptosis.

■ *Immunosuppression.* Many oncogenic agents (e.g., chemicals and ionizing radiation) suppress host immune responses. Tumors or tumor products may also be immunosuppressive. For example, transforming growth factor β (TGF-β), secreted in large quantities by many tumors, is a potent immunosuppressant. In some cases the immune response induced by the tumor (e.g., activation of suppressor T cells) may itself inhibit tumor immunity.

While the increased occurrence of tumors in immunodeficient hosts supports the existence of immunosurveillance, *the strongest argument against the concept of immunosurveillance also derives from the study of immunosuppressed patients.* The most common forms of cancers in immunosuppressed and immunodeficient patients are lymphomas, notably immunoblastic B-cell lymphomas, which could be the consequence of abnormal immunoproliferative responses to microbial infections such as EBV or to the various therapeutic agents so often administered to these patients. Significantly, an increased incidence of the most common forms of cancer—lung, breast, and gastrointestinal tract—and multiple neoplasms might be anticipated in those who are immunodeficient, but these do not occur.

Immunotherapy of Human Tumors

Even if immune surveillance exists, for the patient who develops cancer, this protective mechanism has clearly failed. Can something be done to shore up defenses? The premise of immunotherapy is to either replace the suppressed components of the immune system or stimulate endogenous responses. Three general approaches are being tested in humans: adoptive cellular therapy, cytokine therapy, and antibody-based therapy.

Adoptive Cellular Therapy. Because incubation of peripheral blood lymphocytes with IL-2 generates lymphokine-activated killer (LAK) cells with potent antitumor activity in vitro, such cells can be utilized for adoptive immunotherapy. The patient's blood lymphocytes are cultured with IL-2 in vitro, and the LAK cells (generated principally from expansion of blood NK cells) are reinfused along with additional IL-2.

On the basis of the assumption that tumor-specific cytotoxic T cells are likely to be enriched among tumor-infiltrating lymphocytes (TILs), expanded and activated populations of TILs can be used for immunotherapy. Lymphocytes harvested from surgically resected tumor masses are cultured in IL-2 and then reinfused into the patient. To enhance the antitumor effects of TILs, the expanded cells can be transfected with cytokine genes, so that the tumor is attacked not only by cytotoxic T cells, but also by local release of antitumor cytokines. The efficacy of both of these modalities of cell-based therapy is still being evaluated.

Cytokine Therapy. Because cytokines can activate specific and nonspecific (inflammatory) host defenses, several cytokines, alone or in combination with other forms of treatment, are being evaluated for antitumor therapy. The use of IL-2 was mentioned earlier. In addition, interferon-α (IFN-α) and IFN-γ, TNF-α, and hematopoietic growth factors GM-CSF and granulocyte colony-stimulating factor (G-CSF) are also being tested in cancer patients. IFN-α has already shown considerable promise. It activates NK cells, increases expression of MHC molecules on tumor cells, and is also directly cytostatic. The most impressive results with IFN-α have been obtained in the treatment of hairy cell leukemia (Chapter 12).

Antibody-Based Therapy. Although antibodies against tumor-associated antigens have not proven to be efficacious, current interest lies in using antibodies as targeting agents for delivery of cell toxins. In one approach, monoclonal antibodies against certain B-cell lymphomas are conjugated with ricin (a potent toxin), and the resulting "immunotoxin" is infused into patients. The efficacy of such "magic bullets" in the treatment of leukemias and lymphomas is under investigation.

CLINICAL FEATURES OF NEOPLASIA

Ultimately the importance of neoplasms lies in their effects on people. Any tumor, even a benign one, may cause morbidity and mortality. Moreover, every new growth requires careful appraisal as to whether it is cancerous. This differentiation comes into sharpest focus with "lumps" in the female breast. Both cancers and many benign disorders of the female breast present as palpable masses. In fact, benign lesions are more common than cancers. Although clinical evaluation may suggest one or the other, "the only unequivocally benign breast mass is the excised and anatomically diagnosed one." This is equally true of all neoplasms. There are, however, instances when adherence to this dictum must be tempered by clinical judgment. Subcutaneous lipomas, for example, are quite common and readily recognized by their soft, yielding consistency. Unless they are uncomfortable, subject to trauma, or aesthetically disturbing, small lesions are often merely observed for significant increase in size. A few other examples might be cited, but it suffices to say that *with a few exceptions, all masses require anatomic evaluation.* In addition to the concern malignant neoplasms arouse, even benign lesions may have many adverse effects. The sections that follow consider (1) the effects of a tumor on the host, (2) the grading and clinical staging of cancer, and (3) the laboratory diagnosis of neoplasms.

Effects of Tumor on Host

Obviously, cancers are far more threatening to the host than are benign tumors. Nonetheless, both types of neoplasia may cause problems because of location and impingement on adjacent structures, effects on functional activity such as hormone synthesis, and the production of bleeding and secondary infections when the lesion ulcerates through adjacent natural surfaces. Any metastasis has the same potential. Cancers may also be responsible for cachexia (wasting) or paraneoplastic syndromes.

Location is of critical importance in both benign and malignant tumors. A small (1 cm) pituitary adenoma can compress and destroy the surrounding normal gland and give rise to hypopituitarism; a 0.5-cm leiomyoma in the wall of the renal artery may lead to renal ischemia and serious hypertension. A comparably small carcinoma within the common bile duct may induce fatal biliary tract obstruction.

Hormone production is seen with both benign and malignant neoplasms arising in endocrine glands. Adenomas and carcinomas arising in the β cells of the islets of the pancreas often produce hyperinsulinism, sometimes fatal. Analogously, some adenomas and carcinomas of the adrenal cortex elaborate corticosteroids that affect the patient (e.g., aldosterone, which induces sodium retention, hypertension, and hypokalemia). Such hormonal activity is more likely with a well-differentiated benign tumor than with a corresponding carcinoma.

Ulceration through a surface with consequent bleeding or secondary infection needs no further comment, but a few less obvious ramifications might be mentioned. The neoplasm, benign or malignant, that protrudes into the gut lumen may get caught in the peristaltic pull to telescope the neoplasm and its site of origin into the downstream segment of gut—intussusception (Chapter 15)—leading to ulceration of the mucosa or, even worse, intestinal obstruction or infarction.

It is evident that tumors create many problems, not only because of their local effects, but also in many other ways.

CANCER CACHEXIA

Many cancer patients suffer progressive loss of body fat and lean body mass, accompanied by profound weakness, anorexia, and anemia. This wasting syndrome is referred to as cachexia. Usually, an intercurrent infection brings a blessed end to the slow deterioration. There is in general some correlation between the size and extent of spread of the cancer and the severity of the cachexia. Small, localized cancers therefore are generally silent and produce no cachexia, but there are many exceptions.

The origins of cancer cachexia are multifactorial. Anorexia is a common problem in patients who have cancer, even those who do not have tumors of the gastrointestinal tract. Reduced food intake has been related to abnormalities in taste and in the central control of appetite, but reduced calorie intake is not sufficient to explain the cachexia of malignancy. In patients with cancer, calorie expenditure remains high, and basal metabolic rate is increased, despite reduced food intake. This is in contrast to the lower metabolic rate that occurs as an adaptational response in starvation. The basis of these metabolic abnormalities is not fully understood. Perhaps circulating factors such as TNF-α and IL-1, released from activated macrophages, are involved. TNF-α suppresses appetite and inhibits the action of lipoprotein lipase, thereby inhibiting the release of free fatty acids from lipoproteins. Recently, a novel proteoglycan that causes breakdown of skeletal muscle proteins has been detected in the urine of cancer patients. In healthy animals injection of this material causes acute weight loss without causing anorexia. There is no satisfactory treatment for cancer cachexia other than removal of the underlying cause, the tumor.

PARANEOPLASTIC SYNDROMES

Symptom complexes other than cachexia that appear in patients with cancer and that cannot be readily explained either by the local or distant spread of the tumor or by the elaboration of hormones indigenous to the tissue of origin of the tumor are referred to as paraneoplastic syndromes. They appear in 10% to 15% of patients with cancer, and it is important to recognize them for several reasons:

■ They may represent the earliest manifestation of an occult neoplasm.
■ In affected patients they may represent significant clinical problems and may even be lethal.
■ They may mimic metastatic disease and so confound treatment.

The paraneoplastic syndromes are diverse and are associated with many different tumors (Table 6–8). The most common syndromes are hypercalcemia, Cushing's syndrome, and nonbacterial thrombotic endocarditis; the neoplasms most often associated with these and other syndromes are bronchogenic and breast cancers and hematologic malignancies. Cushing's syndrome as a paraneoplastic phenomenon is usually related to ectopic production by the cancer of adrenocorticotropic hormone (ACTH) or ACTH-like polypeptides. The mediation of hypercalcemia, another common paraneoplastic syndrome, is multifactorial. Perhaps the most important factor is the synthesis of a parathyroid hormone–related protein (PTHrP) by tumor cells, especially squamous-cell carcinomas of the lung. (Although structurally PTHrP resembles parathyroid hormone, it can be distinguished from it by specific radioimmunoassays.) Also implicated are other tumor-derived factors such as TGF-α, a polypeptide factor that activates osteoclasts, and the active form of vitamin D. Another possible mechanism for hypercalcemia is widespread osteolytic metastatic disease of bone, but *it should be noted that hypercalcemia owing to skeletal metastases is not a paraneoplastic syndrome.* Sometimes one tumor induces several syndromes concurrently. Radioimmunoassays document, for example, that bronchogenic carcinomas may elaborate products identical to or having the effects of ACTH, antidiuretic hormone (ADH), parathyroid hormone, serotonin, and human chorionic gonadotropin, as well as other bioactive substances.

Paraneoplastic syndromes may take many other forms, such as hypercoagulability leading to venous thrombosis and nonbacterial thrombotic endocarditis (Chapter 11) or the development of clubbing of the fingers and hypertrophic osteoarthropathy in patients with lung carcinomas (Chapter 13). Still others will be encountered in the consideration of the cancers of the various organs of the body.

Grading and Staging of Cancer

Methods to quantify the probable clinical aggressiveness of a given neoplasm and, further, to express its apparent extent and spread in the individual patient are necessary for comparisons of end results of various forms of treatment. The results of treating extremely small, highly differentiated thyroid adenocarcinomas that are localized to the thyroid gland are likely to be different from those obtained from treating highly anaplastic thyroid cancers that have invaded the neck organs.

The *grading* of a cancer attempts to establish some estimate of its aggressiveness or level of malignancy based on the cytologic differentiation of tumor cells and the number of mitoses within the tumor. The cancer may be classified as grade I, II, III, or IV, in order of increasing anaplasia. Criteria for the individual grades vary with each form of neoplasia and so are not detailed here. Moreover, difficulties in establishing clear-cut criteria have led in some instances to descriptive characterizations (e.g., "well-differentiated adenocarcinoma with no evidence of vascular or lymphatic invasion" or "highly anaplastic sarcoma with extensive vascular invasion," and so forth).

Staging of cancers is based on the size of the primary lesion, its extent of spread to regional lymph nodes, and the presence or absence of metastases. This assessment is usually based on clinical and radiographic examination (CT, MRI) and in some cases surgical exploration. Two methods of staging are currently in use: the TNM system ("T" for primary tumor, "N" for regional lymph node involvement, and "M" for metastases) and the AJC (American Joint Committee) system. In the TNM system, T1, T2, T3, and T4, respectively, describe increasing size of the primary lesion; N0, N1, N2, and N3 indicate progressively advancing node involvement; and M0 and M1 reflect the absence or presence, respectively, of distant metastases. In the AJC method, the cancers are divided into stages 0 to IV, incorporating the size of primary lesions as well as the presence of nodal spread and of distant metastases. Examples of the application of these two staging systems are cited in subsequent chapters. It is worth noting that *when compared with grading, staging has proved to be of greater clinical value.*

Laboratory Diagnosis of Cancer

MORPHOLOGIC AND MOLECULAR METHODS

In most instances the laboratory diagnosis of cancer is not difficult. The two ends of the benign-malignant spectrum pose no problems; however, in the middle lies a "no-man's-land" where the wise tread cautiously. This issue was aptly emphasized earlier in this chapter; here the focus is on the roles of

Table 6-8. SOME PARANEOPLASTIC SYNDROMES

Clinical Syndromes	Major Forms of Underlying Cancer	Causal Mechanisms
Endocrinopathies		
Cushing's syndrome	Small cell cancer of the lung	ACTH or ACTH-like substance
	Pancreatic carcinoma	
	Neural tumors	
Syndrome of inappropriate ADH secretion	Small cell carcinoma of lung	ADH or atrial natriuretic factor
	Intracranial neoplasms	
Hypercalcemia	Squamous cell carcinoma of lung	Parathyroid hormone–related
	Breast carcinoma	protein (PTHrP), TGF-α,
	Renal carcinoma	vitamin D
Carcinoid syndrome	Bronchial carcinoid	Serotonin, bradykinin, ?hista-
	Pancreatic carcinoma	mine
	Gastric carcinoma	
Polycythemia	Renal carcinoma	Erythropoietin
	Cerebellar hemangioma	
	Hepatocellular carcinoma	
Nerve and muscle syndromes		
Disorders of the central and peripheral nervous systems	Small cell carcinoma of lung	?Immunologic, ?toxic
	Breast carcinoma	
Myasthenia gravis	Thymoma	?Immunologic
Osseous, articular, and soft tissue changes		
Hypertrophic osteoarthropathy and clubbing of the fingers	Carcinoma of lung	Unknown
Vascular and hematologic changes		
Venous thrombosis (Trousseau's phenomenon)	Pancreatic carcinoma	Hypercoagulability
	Lung carcinoma	
	Other cancers	
Nonbacterial thrombotic endocarditis	Advanced cancers	Hypercoagulability

ACTH, adrenocorticotropic hormone; ADH, antidiuretic hormone; TGF-α, transforming growth factor α.

the clinician (often a surgeon) and the pathologist in arriving at the correct diagnosis.

Clinicians tend to underestimate the contributions they make to the diagnosis of a neoplasm. Clinical data are invaluable for optimal pathologic diagnosis. Radiation-induced changes in the skin or mucosa can be similar to those of cancer. Sections taken from a healing fracture can mimic an osteosarcoma remarkably. Moreover, the laboratory evaluation of a lesion can be only as good as the specimen submitted for examination. The specimen must be adequate, representative, and properly preserved. Several sampling approaches are available, including excision or biopsy, fine-needle aspiration, and cytologic smears. When excision of a lesion is not possible, selection of an appropriate site for biopsy of a large mass requires awareness that the margins may not be representative, and the center may be largely necrotic. Analogously with disseminated lymphoma (i.e., involving many nodes), nodes in the inguinal region that drain large areas of the body often undergo reactive changes that may mask neoplastic involvement. The need for appropriate preservation of the specimen is obvious, yet it involves such issues as prompt immersion in a usual fixative (e.g., formalin solution), preservation of a portion in a special fixative (e.g., glutaraldehyde) for electron microscopy, or prompt refrigeration to permit optimal hormone or receptor analysis. Requesting "quick-frozen section" diagnosis is sometimes desirable, as, for example, in determining the nature of a breast lesion or in evaluating the margins of an excised cancer to ascertain that the entire neoplasm has been removed. This method, in which

a sample is quick-frozen and sectioned, permits histologic evaluation within minutes. It is then possible with, for example, a breast biopsy to determine whether the lesion is malignant and may require wider excision or sampling of axillary nodes for possible spread. The patient is thereby spared the expense and trauma of a subsequent operation. In experienced, competent hands, frozen-section diagnosis is very accurate, but there are particular instances when the better histologic detail provided by the more time-consuming routine methods is needed—as, for example, when extremely radical surgery, such as the amputation of an extremity, may be indicated. It is better to wait a few days, despite the drawbacks, than to perform inadequate or unnecessary surgery.

Fine-needle aspiration of tumors is another approach that is growing in popularity. It involves aspiration of cells from a mass, followed by cytologic examination of the smear. This procedure is most commonly employed with readily palpable lesions affecting the breast, thyroid, lymph nodes, and salivary glands. Modern imaging techniques enable the method to be extended to deeper structures such as the liver, pancreas, and pelvic lymph nodes. It obviates surgery and its attendant risks. Although it entails some difficulties, such as small sample size and sampling errors, in experienced hands it can be extremely reliable, rapid, and useful.

Cytologic (Papanicolaou) smears provide yet another method for the detection of cancer. This approach is widely used for the discovery of carcinoma of the cervix, often at an in situ stage, but it is also used with many other forms of suspected malignancy, such as endometrial carcinoma, bronchogenic carcinoma, bladder and prostate tumors, and gastric carcinomas; for the identification of tumor cells in abdominal, pleural, joint, and cerebrospinal fluids; and, less commonly, with other forms of neoplasia. Neoplastic cells are less cohesive than others and so are shed into fluids or secretions (Fig. 6–33). The shed cells are evaluated for features of anaplasia indicative of their origin in cancer.

Cytologic interpretation requires a great deal of expertise but can yield, with cervical smears, nearly 100% true-positive diagnosis (i.e., false-positive results are rare). However, there is a significant fraction of false-negative results, owing largely to sampling errors. It should be emphasized that *all positive findings are best confirmed by biopsy and histologic examination before therapy is instituted.* A negative report does not exclude the presence of a malignancy. The gratifying control of cervical cancer is the best testament to the value of the cytologic method.

It is well beyond the scope of this chapter to delve into the technical details of the anatomic diagnosis of cancer. Only a brief "state-of-the-art" summary will be made. Until relatively recently, the diagnosis of cancer was in some part science and in large part art, depending much on subjective judgments of histologic appearance. Involved was, and to some extent still is, the solomonic judgment of when the level of cytologic atypia is sufficient to demand the diagnosis of cancer. Innovations in immunocytochemistry, flow cytometry, and DNA probe analyses have proven to be helpful diagnostic aids and have added considerable objectivity to the laboratory diagnosis of cancer. These techniques can be applied to exfoliated cancer cells, tissue aspirates, or biopsy specimens. A few examples are illustrative. Monoclonal antibodies directed against intermediate filaments have proved to be valuable in the classification of otherwise poorly differentiated tumors. For example, detection of cytokeratin by immunoperoxidase staining allows distinction between poorly differentiated carcinoma and a large cell lymphoma. Detection of p53 by immunohistochemistry in tumor cell nuclei is usually indicative of a p53 mutation, because mutant but not normal p53 accumulates in the nuclei. T- and B-cell neoplasms can be identified on the basis of clonal rearrangement of their antigen receptor genes by employing Southern blot analysis. Leukemias and lymphomas can be classified by flow cytometric detection of differentiation-specific antigens (Chapter 12). Flow cytometry is also useful in assessing the DNA content of tumor cells. A relationship between DNA content (ploidy) and prognosis is becoming apparent for a variety of malignancies. Amplification of the N-*myc* oncogene, detected by cytogenetic or molecular methods, has proven to be of prognostic value in neuroblastomas. Detection of c-*abl-bcr* transcripts by polymerase chain reaction (PCR) can confirm the diagnosis of chronic myeloid leukemia in the small fraction that is Philadelphia chromosome–negative. Thus, molecular biology has moved from the laboratory to the bedside, and the diagnosis of malignant neoplasia has progressed from the level of "eyeballing" to the precision offered by molecular genetics.

BIOCHEMICAL ASSAYS

Biochemical assays for tumor-associated enzymes, hormones, and other tumor markers in the blood cannot be construed as modalities for the diagnosis of cancer; however, they contribute to finding cases and in some instances are useful in determining the effectiveness of therapy. The application of these assays will be considered with many of the specific forms of neoplasia discussed in other chapters, so only a few examples suffice here. Prostatic carcinoma can be suspected when elevated levels of PSA are found in the blood. Regrettably, the levels may also be elevated in benign prostatic hyperplasia, and hence elevations in PSA are not diagnostic of an underlying cancer (Chapter 18).

Radioimmunoassays for circulating hormones may point to the presence of tumors in the endocrine system and in some instances to the ectopic production of hormones by nonendocrine tumors.

A host of circulating tumor markers have been described, and new ones are identified every year. Only a few have stood the test of time and proved to be clinically useful. The two best-established are carcinoembryonic antigen (CEA) and α-fetoprotein. CEA, normally produced in embryonic tissue of the gut, pancreas, and liver, is a complex glycoprotein that is

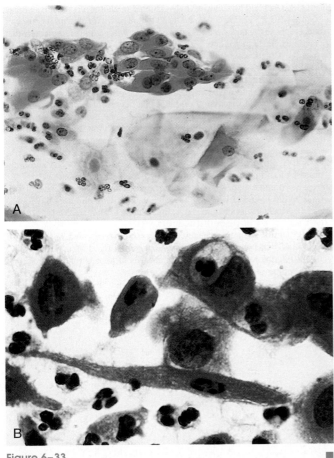

Figure 6–33

A, Normal cervicovaginal smear shows large flattened squamous cells and groups of metaplastic cells; interspersed are some neutrophils. There are no malignant cells. *B,* Abnormal cervicovaginal smear shows numerous malignant cells that have pleomorphic, hyperchromatic nuclei; interspersed are some normal polymorphonuclear leukocytes. (Courtesy of Dr. P.K. Gupta, Department of Pathology and Laboratory Medicine, University of Pennsylvania Medical Center, Philadelphia.)

elaborated by many different neoplasms. Depending on the serum level adopted as representative of a significant elevation, CEA is variously reported to be positive in 60% to 90% of colorectal carcinomas, 50% to 80% of pancreatic, and 25% to 50% of gastric and breast tumors. Much less consistently, elevated CEA levels have been described in other forms of cancer. In almost all types of neoplasia, the level of elevation is correlated with the body burden of tumor, so highest levels are found in those with advanced metastatic disease. However, CEA elevations have also been reported in many benign disorders, such as alcoholic cirrhosis, hepatitis, ulcerative colitis, Crohn's disease, and others. Occasionally levels of this antigen are elevated in apparently healthy smokers. *Thus, CEA assays lack both specificity and the sensitivity required for the detection of early cancers.* However, they are still useful in providing presumptive evidence of the possibility of colorectal carcinoma, because this tumor yields the highest CEA levels; these assays are particularly useful in the detection of recurrences after excision. With successful resection of the tumor, CEA disappears from the serum; its reappearance almost always spells the beginning of the end (Chapter 15).

The other well-established tumor marker is α-fetoprotein. Elevated circulating levels are encountered in adults with cancers arising principally in the liver and from yolk sac remnants in the gonads. Less regularly, it is elevated in teratocarcinomas and embryonal cell carcinomas of the testis, ovary, and extragonadal sites and occasionally in cancers of the stomach and pancreas. As with CEA, benign conditions, including cirrhosis, hepatitis, and pregnancy (especially with fetal distress or death), may cause modest elevations of α-fetoprotein. There is then a problem with both specificity and sensitivity, but the marker may still provide presumptive evidence of, for example, a hepatocellular carcinoma and is of value in the follow-up of therapeutic interventions. More details are found in Chapter 16. This cursory overview suffices to indicate the many laboratory approaches in use for the detection and diagnosis of tumors.

BIBLIOGRAPHY

Agarwala SS: Paraneoplastic syndromes. Med Clin North Am 80:173, 1996. (A recent overview of paraneoplastic syndromes.)

Birchmeier W: E-cadherin as a tumor (invasion) suppressor gene. BioEssays 17:97, 1995. (A short discussion of the role of E-cadherin in invasion.)

Chang F, et al: Implications of the p53 tumor-suppressor gene in clinical oncology. J Clin Oncol 13:1009, 1995. (A succinct review of the functions of p53 gene and clinical implications of the knowledge about p53 functions.)

Chung D, Rustgi AK: DNA mismatch repair and cancer. Gastroenterology 109:1685, 1995. (A topical discussion of the role of DNA mismatch repair genes in the origins of cancer.)

Cordon-Cardo C: Mutation of cell cycle regulators. Biological and clinical implications for human neoplasia. Am J Pathol 147:545, 1995. (A detailed discussion of cyclins and their dysregulation in human cancers.)

Cox LS, Lane DP: Tumor suppressors, kinases and clamps: how p53 regulates the cell cycle in response to DNA damage. BioEssays 17:501, 1995. (A detailed discussion of the role of p53 in the regulation of cell cycle.)

Folkman J: Clinical applications of research on angiogenesis. N Engl J Med 333:1757, 1995. (A concise discussion of the basic and clinical aspects of tumor angiogenesis.)

Herrington CS: Human papillomaviruses and cervical neoplasia. I. Classification virology, pathology, and epidemiology. J Clin Pathol 47:1066, 1994. (An excellent overview of the biology of human papilloma viruses and their role in carcinogenesis.)

Jiang WG, et al: Molecular and cellular basis of cancer invasion and metastasis: implications for treatment. Br J Surg 81:1576, 1994. (An excellent review of the multiple steps in the metastatic cascade.)

Karp JE, Broder S: Molecular foundations of cancer: new targets for intervention. Nature Med 1:309, 1995. (An excellent discussion of recent discoveries in the genetic alteration in cancer, with focus on cyclins, DNA repair genes and tumor suppressor genes.)

Klein G: Epstein-Barr virus strategy in normal and neoplastic B cells. Cell 77:791, 1994. (A concise review of the molecular basis of EBV-induced tumors.)

Nabel GR, Grunfeld C: Calories lost—another mediator of cancer cachexia? Nature Med 2:397, 1996. (An editorial that reviews the potential causes of cancer cachexia and describes the discovery of a novel molecule that causes cachexia in patients with cancer.)

Pamies RJ, Crawford DR: Tumor markers. An update. Med Clin North Am 80:185, 1996. (A discussion of tumor markers, and their utility in diagnosis and management of cancers.)

Ponta H, et al: Recent advances in the genetics of metastasis. Eur J Cancer 13:1995, 1994. (A discussion of genes that play a role in metastasis.)

Rennie J, Rusting R: Making headway against cancer. Sci Am 215:56, 1996. (An introduction to a series of excellent articles in the same issue written by leading authorities on the causation, spread, and developing therapies against cancer.)

Ruoslahti E: How cancer spreads. Sci Am 275:72, 1996. (A brief and lucid discussion of the mechanisms of tissue invasion and metastases.)

Steeg PS: Granin expectations in breast cancer? Nature Genet 12:223, 1996. (A brief discussion of BRCA-1 as a candidate growth inhibitory molecule.)

Steller H: Mechanisms and genes of cellular suicide. Science 257:1445, 1995. (A basic review of genes that control apoptosis.)

Tabor E: Tumor suppressor genes, growth factor genes, and oncogenes in hepatitis B virus-associated hepatocellular carcinoma. J Med Virol 42:357, 1994. (A good review of the molecular basis of hepatocellular carcinoma in the setting of hepatitis B virus infection.)

Van den Eynde B, Brichard VG: New tumor antigens recognized by T cells. Curr Opin Immunol 7:674, 1995. (A modern view of human tumor antigens.)

Weinberg RA: How cancer arises. Sci Am 275:62, 1996. (An excellent review on the molecular basis of cancer.)

7

Cl⁻   Na⁺

Genetic and Pediatric Diseases

Genetic Diseases

Traditionally, human diseases have been classified into three categories: (1) those that are genetically determined, (2) those that are almost entirely environmentally determined, and (3) those to which both nature and nurture contribute. However, progress in understanding the molecular basis of many so-called environmental disorders has tended to blur these distinctions. At one time microbial infections were cited as examples of disorders arising wholly from environmental influences, but it is now clear that to a considerable extent, an individual's genetic makeup influences his or her immune response and susceptibility to microbiologic infections. Despite the complexities of this nature-nurture interplay, there is little doubt that nature (i.e., the genetic component) plays a major, if not the determining, role in the occurrence and severity of many human diseases. Such disorders are far more frequent than is commonly appreciated.

Surveys indicate that as many as 20% of the pediatric inpatients in university hospital populations suffer from disorders of genetic origin. These data describe only the tip of the iceberg. Chromosome aberrations have been identified in up to 50% of spontaneous abortuses during the first trimester, and many more abortuses likely had gene mutations. Only those mutations compatible with independent existence constitute the reservoir of genetic disease in the population at large.

Because several pediatric disorders are of genetic origin, we will discuss developmental and pediatric diseases along with genetic diseases in this chapter. However, it must be borne in mind that all genetic disorders do not present in infancy and childhood, and conversely, many pediatric diseases are not of genetic origin. To the latter category belong diseases resulting from immaturity of organ systems. In this context it is helpful to clarify three commonly used terms: hereditary, familial, and congenital. *Hereditary disorders,* by definition, are derived from one's parents, are transmitted in the gametes through the generations, and therefore are *familial.* The term *congenital* simply implies "present at birth." It should be noted that some congenital diseases are not genetic (e.g., congenital syphilis). On the other hand, not all genetic diseases are congenital; Huntington disease, for example, begins to be expressed only after the third or fourth decade of life.

It is beyond the scope of this book to review normal human genetics, but it is beneficial to recall some fundamental concepts that have a bearing on the understanding of genetic diseases.

MUTATIONS

As is well known, the term *mutation* refers to permanent changes in the DNA. Those that affect germ cells are transmitted to the progeny and may give rise to inherited diseases. Mutations in somatic cells are not transmitted to the progeny but are important in the causation of cancers and some congenital malformations.

Details of specific mutations and their effects are discussed along with the relevant disorders throughout this text. Here we will cite only some common examples of gene mutations and their effects.

Point mutations result from the substitution of a single nucleotide base by a different base, resulting in the replacement of one amino acid by another in the protein product. The mutation giving rise to sickle cell anemia is an excellent example of a point mutation that alters the meaning of the genetic code (Fig. 7–1). Such mutations are sometimes called *missense mutations.*

In contrast, certain point mutations may change an amino acid codon to a chain termination, or *stop codon.* Such "nonsense" mutations interrupt translation, and the resultant truncated proteins are rapidly degraded. The effect of a nonsense mutation in the messenger RNA (m-RNA) of β-globin is illustrated in Figure 7–2.

Frameshift mutations occur when the insertion or deletion of one or two base pairs alters the reading frame of the DNA

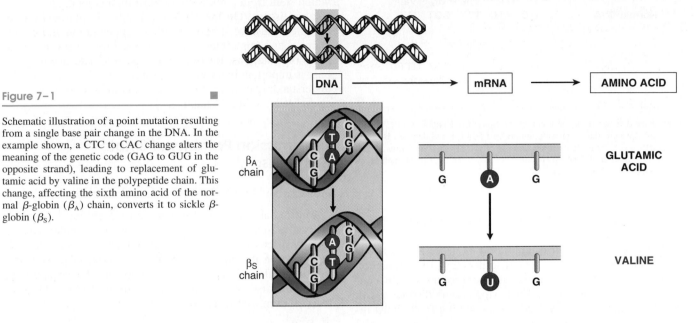

Figure 7–1 ■

Schematic illustration of a point mutation resulting from a single base pair change in the DNA. In the example shown, a CTC to CAC change alters the meaning of the genetic code (GAG to GUG in the opposite strand), leading to replacement of glutamic acid by valine in the polypeptide chain. This change, affecting the sixth amino acid of the normal β-globin (β_A) chain, converts it to sickle β-globin (β_S).

strand (Fig. 7–3). If the number of base pairs involved in a deletion is three or a multiple of three, frameshift does not occur; instead, a protein missing one or more amino acids is synthesized (Fig. 7–4).

Trinucleotide repeat mutations belong to a special category because these mutations are characterized by amplification of a sequence of three nucleotides. Although the specific nucleotide sequence that undergoes amplification differs in various disorders, all affected sequences share the nucleotides guanine (G) and cytosine (C). For example, in fragile X syndrome, prototypical of this category of disorders, there are 250 to 4000 tandem repeats of the sequence CGG within a gene called *FMR-1*. In normal populations the number of repeats is small, averaging 29. It is believed that expansions of the trinucleotide sequences prevent normal expression of the FMR-1 gene, thus giving rise to mental retardation. Another distinguishing feature of trinucleotide repeat mutations is that they are dynamic (i.e., the degree of ampli-

fication increases during gametogenesis). These features, discussed in greater detail later in this chapter, influence the pattern of inheritance and the phenotypic manifestations of the diseases caused by this class of mutations.

With this brief review of the nature of mutations, we can turn our attention to the three major categories of genetic disorders: (1) those related to mutant genes of large effect, (2) diseases with multifactorial (polygenic) inheritance, and (3) those arising from chromosomal aberrations. The first category, sometimes referred to as *mendelian disorders,* includes many uncommon conditions, such as the storage diseases and inborn errors of metabolism, all resulting from single-gene mutations of large effect. Most of these conditions are hereditary and familial. The second category includes some of the most common disorders of humans, such as hypertension and diabetes mellitus. Multifactorial, or polygenic, inheritance implies that both genetic and environmental influences condition the expression of a phenotypic characteristic or disease. The third category includes disorders that have been shown to be

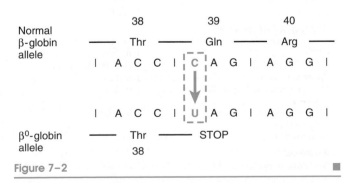

Figure 7–2 ■

Point mutation leading to premature chain termination. Partial mRNA sequence of the β-globin chain of hemoglobin showing codons for amino acids 38 to 40. A point mutation (C → U) in codon 39 changes glutamine (Gln) codon to a stop codon, and hence protein synthesis stops at the 38th amino acid.

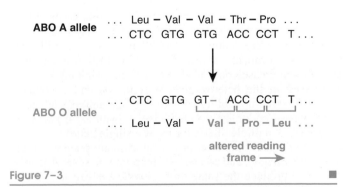

Figure 7–3 ■

Single-base deletion at the ABO (glycosyltransferase) locus, leading to a frameshift mutation responsible for the O allele. (From Thompson MW, et al: Thompson and Thompson Genetics in Medicine, 5th ed. Philadelphia, WB Saunders, 1991, p 134.)

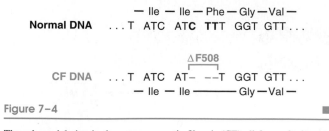

Normal DNA ...T ATC ATC TTT GGT GTT...
— Ile — Ile — Phe — Gly — Val —

ΔF508

CF DNA ...T ATC AT— ——T GGT GTT...
— Ile — Ile ———— Gly — Val —

Figure 7–4

Three-base deletion in the common cystic fibrosis (CF) allele results in synthesis of a protein that is missing amino acid 508 (phenylalanine). Because the deletion is a multiple of three this is not a frameshift mutation. (From Thompson MW, et al: Thompson and Thompson Genetics in Medicine, 5th ed. Philadelphia, WB Saunders, 1991, p 135.)

the consequence of numerical or structural abnormalities in the chromosomes.

To these well-known categories it is necessary to add a heterogeneous group of genetic disorders that, like mendelian disorders, involve single genes but do not follow simple mendelian rules of inheritance. These single-gene disorders with nonclassic inheritance include those resulting from triplet repeat mutations, those arising from mutations in mitochondrial DNA, and those in which the transmission is influenced by an epigenetic phenomenon called *genomic imprinting*.

Each of these four categories will be discussed separately.

MENDELIAN DISORDERS (DISEASES CAUSED BY SINGLE-GENE DEFECTS)

Single-gene defects (mutations) follow the well-known mendelian patterns of inheritance. Thus, the conditions they produce are often called *mendelian disorders*. The number of known mendelian disorders has grown to more than 5000. Although individually each is rare, altogether they account for approximately 1% of all adult admissions to hospitals and about 6% to 8% of all pediatric hospital admissions. Table 7–1 lists some of the more common mendelian disorders and their prevalence. Many of these are discussed in this chapter; most of the remaining ones are described elsewhere in the text.

Mutations involving single genes follow one of three patterns of inheritance: autosomal dominant, autosomal recessive, or X-linked. Although gene expression is usually described as dominant or recessive, it should be remembered that in some cases both alleles of a gene pair may be fully expressed in the heterozygote, a condition called *codominance*. Histocompatibility and blood group antigens are good examples of codominant inheritance, as well as of *polymorphism* (i.e., multiple allelic forms of a single gene).

A single-gene mutation may lead to many phenotypic effects (*pleiotropy*), and conversely, mutations at several genetic loci may produce the same trait (*genetic heterogeneity*). For example, Marfan syndrome, which results from a basic defect in connective tissue, is associated with widespread effects involving the skeleton, eye, and cardiovascular system, all of which stem from a mutation in fibrillin, a component of connective tissues. On the other hand, retinitis pigmentosa, an inherited cause of abnormal retinal pigmentation and consequent visual impairment, can be caused by several different types of mutations. Recognition of genetic heterogeneity not only is important in genetic counseling, but also facilitates the understanding of the pathogenesis of common disorders such as diabetes mellitus (Chapter 17).

Transmission Patterns of Single-Gene Disorders

AUTOSOMAL DOMINANT DISORDERS

Autosomal dominant disorders are manifested in the heterozygous state, so at least one parent of an index case is usually affected; both males and females are affected, and both can transmit the condition. When an affected person marries an unaffected one, every child has one chance in two of having the disease. The following features also pertain to autosomal dominant diseases:

■ With every autosomal dominant disorder, some patients do not have affected parents. Such patients owe their disorder to new mutations involving either the egg or the sperm from which they were derived. Their siblings are neither affected nor at increased risk of developing the disease.

■ Clinical features can be modified by reduced penetrance and variable expressivity. Some individuals inherit the mutant gene but are phenotypically normal. This is referred

Table 7–1. PREVALENCE OF SELECTED MONOGENIC DISORDERS AMONG LIVEBORN INFANTS

Disorder	Estimated Prevalence
Autosomal Dominant	
Familial hypercholesterolemia	1 in 500
Polycystic kidney disease	1 in 1250
Huntington disease	1 in 2500
Hereditary spherocytosis	1 in 5000
Marfan syndrome	1 in 20,000
Autosomal Recessive	
Sickle cell anemia	1 in 625 (US blacks)
Cystic fibrosis	1 in 2000 (Caucasians)
Tay-Sachs disease	1 in 3000 (US Jews)
Phenylketonuria	1 in 12,000
Mucopolysaccharidoses (all types)	1 in 25,000
Glycogen storage diseases (all types)	1 in 50,000
Galactosemia	1 in 57,000
X-Linked	
Duchenne muscular dystrophy	1 in 7000
Hemophilia	1 in 10,000

* From Wyngaarden JB, et al: Cecil Textbook of Medicine, 19th ed. Philadelphia, WB Saunders, 1992, p 121.

to as *reduced penetrance*. The factors that affect penetrance are not clearly understood. In contrast to penetrance, if a trait is seen in all individuals carrying the mutant gene but is expressed differently among individuals, the phenomenon is called *variable expressivity*. For example, polydactyly may be expressed in toes or in fingers as one or more extra digits.

■ In many conditions, the age at onset is delayed: symptoms and signs do not appear until adulthood (as in Huntington disease).

■ In autosomal dominant disorders, a 50% reduction in the normal gene product is associated with clinical symptoms. Because a 50% loss of enzyme activity can usually be compensated for, involved genes usually do not encode for enzyme proteins. Two major categories of nonenzyme proteins are usually affected in autosomal dominant disorders: (1) those involved in regulation of complex metabolic pathways, often subject to feedback control (examples are membrane receptors and transport proteins); and (2) key structural proteins, such as collagen and cytoskeletal components of the red cell membrane (e.g., spectrin). The biochemical mechanisms by which a 50% reduction in the levels of such proteins results in an abnormal phenotype are not fully understood. In some cases, especially when the gene encodes one subunit of a multimeric protein, the product of the mutant allele can interfere with the assembly of a functionally normal multimer. For example, the collagen molecule is a trimer in which the three collagen chains are arranged in a helical configuration. Each of the three collagen chains in the helix must be normal for the assembly and stability of the collagen molecule. Even with a single mutant collagen chain, normal collagen trimers cannot be formed, and hence there is a marked deficiency of collagen. In this instance, the mutant allele is called *dominant negative* because it impairs the function of a normal allele. This effect is illustrated by some forms of osteogenesis imperfecta (Chapter 21). Table 7–2 lists the more common autosomal dominant disorders. Most are discussed elsewhere in the text. Selected prototypical diseases are described later in this chapter.

AUTOSOMAL RECESSIVE DISORDERS

Autosomal recessive diseases make up the largest group of mendelian disorders. They occur when both of the alleles at a given gene locus are mutants; therefore, such disorders are characterized by the following features: (1) the trait does not usually affect the parents, but siblings may show the disease; (2) siblings have one chance in four of being affected (i.e., the recurrence risk is 25% for each birth); and (3) if the mutant gene occurs with a low frequency in the population, there is a strong likelihood that the proband is the product of a consanguineous marriage. In contrast to the features of autosomal dominant diseases, the following features generally apply to most autosomal recessive disorders:

■ The expression of the defect tends to be more uniform than in autosomal dominant disorders.
■ Complete penetrance is common.
■ Onset is frequently early in life.

Table 7–2. AUTOSOMAL DOMINANT DISORDERS

System	Disorder
Nervous	Huntington disease
	Neurofibromatosis
	Myotonic dystrophy
	Tuberous sclerosis
Urinary	Polycystic kidney disease
Gastrointestinal	Familial polyposis coli
Hematopoietic	Hereditary spherocytosis
	von Willebrand disease
Skeletal	Marfan syndrome*
	Ehlers-Danlos syndrome (some variants)*
	Osteogenesis imperfecta
	Achondroplasia
Metabolic	Familial hypercholesterolemia*
	Acute intermittent porphyria

* Discussed in this chapter. Other disorders listed are discussed in appropriate chapters of this book.

■ Although new mutations for recessive disorders do occur, they are rarely detected clinically. Because the affected individual is an asymptomatic heterozygote, several generations may pass before the descendants of such a person mate with other heterozygotes and produce affected offspring.

■ In many cases enzyme proteins are affected by the mutation. In heterozygotes, equal amounts of normal and defective enzyme are synthesized. Usually the natural "margin of safety" ensures that cells with half of their usual complement of the enzyme function normally.

To illustrate possible mechanisms by which an enzyme deficiency may give rise to an autosomal recessive disorder, Figure 7–5 provides an example of an enzyme reaction in which the substrate is converted by intracellular enzymes through intermediates into an end product. In this example, the final product exerts feedback control on enzyme 1. A minor pathway producing small quantities of M1 and M2 also exists. The biochemical consequences of an enzyme defect in such a reaction have two major implications:

1. Depending on the site of the block, accumulation of the substrate may be accompanied by build-up of one or both intermediates. Moreover, an increased concentration of intermediate 2 may stimulate the minor pathway and thus lead to an excess of M1 and M2. Under these conditions, tissue injury may result if the precursor, the intermediates, or the products of the minor pathways are toxic in high concentrations. For example, in galactosemia, a deficiency of galactose-1-phosphate uridylyltransferase leads to the accumulation of galactose and to consequent tissue damage. Similarly, a deficiency of phenylalanine hydroxylase results in the accumulation of phenylalanine. Excessive accumulation of complex substrates within the lysosomes as a result of a deficiency of degradative enzymes is responsible for a group of diseases generally referred to as *lysosomal storage diseases* (p 185).

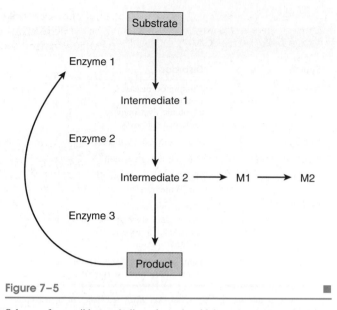

Figure 7–5 ■

Scheme of a possible metabolic pathway in which a substrate is converted to an end product by a series of enzyme reactions. M1, M2, products of a minor pathway.

2. The enzyme defect can lead to a metabolic block and a decreased amount of an end product that may be necessary for normal function. For example, a deficiency of melanin may result from lack of tyrosinase, which is necessary for the biosynthesis of melanin from its precursor, tyrosine. This results in a clinical condition called *albinism.* If the end product is a feedback inhibitor of the enzymes involved in the early reactions (for example, in Fig. 7–5 it is shown that the final product inhibits enzyme 1), the deficiency of the end product may permit overproduction of intermediates and their catabolic products, some of which may be injurious at high concentrations. A prime example of a disease with such an underlying mechanism is the Lesch-Nyhan syndrome (Chapter 21).

Enzyme deficiencies may act in other ways as well. For example, α_1-antitrypsin is a protease inhibitor whose chief function is to inactivate neutrophil elastase. In patients with α_1-antitrypsin deficiency, the elastic tissue in the walls of pulmonary alveoli falls prey to the unopposed destructive activity of neutrophil elastase, leading eventually to emphysema (Chapter 13).

Table 7–3 provides a list of the more common examples of autosomal recessive disorders. Some of these are discussed in this chapter, but most are described elsewhere, along with other diseases of the affected organ system.

X-LINKED DISORDERS

All sex-linked disorders are X-linked. To date, no Y-linked diseases are known. Save for determinants that dictate male differentiation, the only characteristic that may be located on the Y chromosome is the not altogether devastating attribute of hairy ears. Most X-linked disorders are X-linked recessive and are characterized by the following features:

■ They are transmitted by heterozygous female carriers virtually only to sons, who of course are hemizygous for the X chromosome.

■ Heterozygous females rarely express the full phenotypic change, owing to the presence of the paired normal allele; however, because of the inactivation of one of the X chromosomes in females (discussed later), it is remotely possible for the normal allele to be inactivated in most cells, permitting full expression of the disease in heterozygous females.

■ An affected male does not transmit the disorder to sons, but all daughters are carriers. Sons of heterozygous women have, of course, one chance in two of receiving the mutant gene.

There are a very few X-linked dominant diseases. Their inheritance pattern is characterized by transmission of the disease to 50% of the sons and daughters of an affected heterozygous female. An affected male cannot transmit the disease to his sons, but all daughters are affected. One example of such a disease is vitamin D–resistant rickets.

X-linked recessive disorders are much less common than disorders arising from autosomal mutations. Some of the more important conditions having this mode of transmission are listed in Table 7–4.

Although mendelian disorders are often grouped according to their patterns of transmission, it is perhaps more appropriate to categorize them on the basis of the nature of protein that is affected, because in large part the type of protein affected-determines the pattern of inheritance. Hence, in Table 7–5, selected single-gene disorders are classified into broad groupings on the basis of the protein abnormality. This classification is used to describe selected genetic diseases that are not covered elsewhere in the text.

■

Table 7–3. AUTOSOMAL RECESSIVE DISORDERS	
System	**Disorder**
Metabolic*	Cystic fibrosis*
	Phenylketonuria*
	Galactosemia*
	Homocystinuria
	Lysosomal storage diseases*
	α_1-Antitrypsin deficiency
	Wilson disease
	Hemochromatosis
	Glycogen storage diseases*
Hematopoietic	Sickle cell anemia
	Thalassemias
Endocrine	Congenital adrenal hyperplasia
Skeletal	Ehlers-Danlos syndrome (some variants)*
	Alkaptonuria
Nervous	Neurogenic muscular atrophies
	Friedreich ataxia
	Spinal muscular atrophy

* Discussed in this chapter. Many others are discussed throughout the text.

■

Table 7–4. X-LINKED RECESSIVE DISORDERS

System	Disease
Musculoskeletal	Duchenne muscular dystrophy
Blood	Hemophilia A and B Chronic granulomatous disease Glucose-6-phosphate dehydrogenase deficiency
Immune	Agammaglobulinemia Wiskott-Aldrich syndrome
Metabolic	Diabetes insipidus Lesch-Nyhan syndrome
Nervous	Fragile X syndrome*

* Discussed in this chapter.

Diseases Caused by Mutations in Structural Proteins

MARFAN SYNDROME

In this autosomal dominant disorder of connective tissues, the basic biochemical abnormality affects *fibrillin*. This glycoprotein, secreted by fibroblasts, forms microfibrillar aggregates in the extracellular matrix. These serve as scaffolding for the deposition of elastin and are considered integral components of elastic fibers. Both qualitative and quantitative defects in fibrillin have been noted in Marfan syndrome patients.

One of the fibrillin genes (FBN1) and the Marfan syndrome locus have both been mapped to chromosome 15q21.1. Furthermore, mutations in the fibrillin gene have been found in patients with Marfan syndrome.

Although connective tissue throughout the body is affected, the principal clinical manifestations relate to three systems: the skeleton, the eyes, and the cardiovascular system.

Skeletal abnormalities are the most obvious feature of Marfan syndrome. Patients have a slender, elongated habitus with abnormally long legs, arms, and fingers (arachnodactyly); a high, arched palate; and hyperextensibility of joints. A variety of spinal deformities, such as severe kyphoscoliosis, may appear. The chest is classically deformed, presenting either pectus excavatum (i.e., deeply depressed sternum) or a pigeon-breast deformity. President Lincoln is thought to have had features suggestive of Marfan syndrome. The most characteristic **ocular change** is bilateral dislocation, or subluxation, of the lens owing to weakness of its suspensory ligaments. It should be noted that the ciliary zonules that support the lens are devoid of elastin and are made up exclusively of fibrillin. Most serious, however, is the involvement of the **cardiovascular system.** Fragmentation of the elastic fibers in the tunica media of the aorta predisposes to aneurysmal dilation and aortic dissection (Chapter 10). Loss of medial support causes dilation of the aortic valve ring, giving rise to aortic incompetence. The car-

■

Table 7–5. BIOCHEMICAL BASIS AND INHERITANCE PATTERN OF SOME MENDELIAN DISORDERS

Protein Type/Function	Example	Pattern of Inheritance	Disease
Enzyme	Phenylalanine hydroxylase Hexosaminidase Adenosine deaminase	Autosomal recessive	Phenylketonuria Tay-Sachs disease Severe combined immuno-deficiency
Enzyme Inhibitor	α_1-Antitrypsin	Autosomal recessive	Emphysema and liver disease
Receptor	Low-density lipoprotein receptor	Autosomal dominant	Familial hypercholesterolemia
Transport Oxygen	Hemoglobin	Autosomal codominant*	α-Thalassemia β-Thalassemia Sickle cell anemia
Ions	Cystic fibrosis transmembrane conductance regulator	Autosomal recessive	Cystic fibrosis
Structural Extracellular	Collagen	Autosomal dominant	Osteogenesis imperfecta; Ehlers-Danlos syndromes†
	Fibrillin	Autosomal dominant	Marfan syndrome
Cell membrane	Dystrophin	X-linked recessive	Duchenne/Becker muscular dystrophy
	Spectrin, ankyrin, or protein 4.1	Autosomal dominant	Hereditary spherocytosis
Hemostasis	Factor VIII	X-linked recessive	Hemophilia A
Growth Regulation	Rb protein NF-1 protein	Autosomal dominant Autosomal dominant	Hereditary retinoblastoma Neurofibromatosis type 1

* Heterozygotes are either asymptomatic or have mild disease.
† Some variants of Ehlers-Danlos syndrome are autosomal recessive or X-linked recessive.

diac valves, especially the mitral and, less commonly, the tricuspid valve, may be excessively distensible and regurgitant (floppy valve syndrome), giving rise to congestive cardiac failure (Chapter 11). Death from aortic rupture may occur at any age. Such a calamity is the cause of death in 30% to 45% of affected individuals.

Although the lesions described above are typical of Marfan syndrome, they are not seen in all cases. There is much variation in clinical expression, and some patients may exhibit predominantly cardiovascular lesions with minimal skeletal and ocular changes. The variable expressivity is believed to be related to different allelic mutations in the fibrillin gene. Because of such variations, it is not feasible to develop a simple screening test that can detect all mutations that underlie Marfan syndrome.

EHLERS-DANLOS SYNDROMES

Ehlers-Danlos syndromes (EDSs) are characterized by defects in collagen synthesis or structure. As such, they belong to the same general category as Marfan syndrome. All are single-gene disorders, but the mode of inheritance encompasses all three of the mendelian patterns. This should not be surprising, because biosynthesis of collagen is a complex process that may be disturbed by genetic errors affecting any one of the numerous structural collagen genes or the genes that code for the enzymes necessary for post-transcriptional events, such as cross-linking of collagen fibers. It should be recalled that there are at least 12 distinct types of collagen, and all of them have characteristic tissue distributions and are the products of different genes. To some extent, the clinical heterogeneity of EDS can be explained on the basis of mutations in different collagen genes.

At least 10 clinical and genetic variants of EDS are recognized. Because defective collagen is present in all the variants, certain clinical features are common to all.

As might be expected, tissues rich in collagen, such as skin, ligaments, and joints, are frequently involved in most variants of EDS. Because the abnormal collagen fibers lack adequate tensile strength, *skin is hyperextensible and joints are hypermobile.* These features permit grotesque contortions, such as bending the thumb backward to touch the forearm and bending the knee forward to create almost a right angle. Indeed, it is believed that most contortionists have one of the EDSs; however, a predisposition to joint dislocation is one of the prices paid for this virtuosity. The skin is extraordinarily stretchable, extremely fragile, and vulnerable to trauma. Minor injuries produce gaping defects, and surgical repair or any surgical intervention is accomplished only with great difficulty because of the lack of normal tensile strength. The basic defect in connective tissue may lead to serious internal complications, including rupture of the colon and large arteries (EDS type IV); ocular fragility, with rupture of the cornea and retinal detachment (EDS type VI); and diaphragmatic hernias (EDS type I), among others.

The molecular bases of EDS are varied and include the following:

■ *Deficiency of the enzyme lysyl hydroxylase.* Decreased hydroxylation of lysyl residues in types I and III collagen interferes with the normal cross-links among collagen molecules. As might be expected, this variant (type VI), resulting from an enzyme deficiency, is inherited as an autosomal recessive disorder.

■ *Deficient synthesis of type III collagen owing to mutations in the pro-α_1 (III) gene.* This variant (type IV) is inherited as an autosomal dominant disorder and is characterized by weakness of tissues rich in type III collagen (e.g., blood vessels, bowel wall).

■ Defective conversion of procollagen type I to collagen, resulting from a mutation in the type I collagen gene in EDS type VII.

Diseases Caused by Mutations in Receptor Proteins

FAMILIAL HYPERCHOLESTEROLEMIA

Familial hypercholesterolemia is perhaps the most common of all mendelian disorders; the frequency of heterozygotes is 1 in 500 in the general population. It is caused by a mutation in the gene that specifies the receptor for low-density lipoprotein (LDL), the form in which 70% of total plasma cholesterol is transported. As you know, cholesterol may be derived from the diet or from endogenous synthesis. Dietary triglycerides and cholesterol are incorporated into chylomicrons in the intestinal mucosa, which drain via the gut lymphatics into the blood. These chylomicrons are hydrolyzed by an endothelial lipoprotein lipase in the capillaries of muscle and fat. The chylomicron remnants, rich in cholesterol, are then delivered to the liver. Some of the cholesterol enters the metabolic pool (to be described), and some is excreted as free cholesterol or bile acids into the biliary tract. The endogenous synthesis of cholesterol and LDL begins in the liver (Fig. 7–6). The first step in the synthesis of LDL is the secretion of triglyceride-rich very-low-density lipoprotein (VLDL) by the liver into the blood. In the capillaries of adipose tissue and muscle, the VLDL particle undergoes lipolysis and is converted to intermediate-density lipoprotein (IDL). Compared with VLDL, the content of triglyceride is reduced and that of cholesteryl esters enriched in IDL, but IDL retains on its surface two of the three VLDL-associated apoproteins, B-100 and E. Further metabolism of IDL occurs along two pathways: most of the IDL particles are taken up by the liver through the LDL receptor described below; others are converted to cholesterol-rich LDL by a further loss of triglycerides and apoprotein E. Two thirds of the resultant LDL are metabolized by the LDL receptor pathway and the rest by an LDL receptor–independent pathway, to be described later. The LDL receptor binds to apoproteins B-100 and E and hence is involved in the transport of both LDL and IDL. Although the LDL receptors are widely distributed, approximately 75% are located on hepatocytes, so liver plays an extremely important role in LDL metabolism.

The first step in the receptor-mediated transport of LDL involves binding to the cell surface receptor, followed by endocytotic internalization (Fig. 7–7). Within the cell, the en-

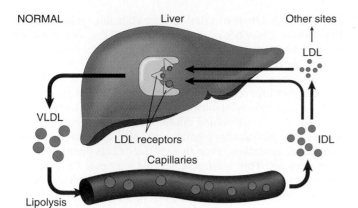

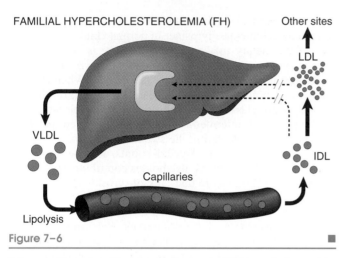

Figure 7-6   ■

Schematic illustration of low-density lipoprotein (LDL) metabolism and the role of the liver in its synthesis and catabolism, in normal persons and those with familial hypercholesterolemia. VLDL, very-low-density lipoprotein; IDL, intermediate-density lipoprotein.

docytic vesicles fuse with the lysosomes, and the LDL molecule is enzymically degraded, resulting ultimately in the release of free cholesterol into the cytoplasm. The cholesterol not only is utilized by the cell for membrane synthesis, but also takes part in intracellular cholesterol homeostasis by a sophisticated system of feedback control:

- It suppresses cholesterol synthesis by inhibiting the activity of the enzyme 3-hydroxy-3-methylglutaryl (3-HMG) coenzyme A reductase, which is the rate-limiting enzyme in the synthetic pathway.
- It activates the enzyme acyl-CoA:cholesterol acyltransferase (ACAT), which favors esterification and storage of excess cholesterol.
- It down-regulates the synthesis of cell surface LDL receptors, thus protecting cells from excessive accumulation of cholesterol.

The transport of LDL that does not involve LDL receptors, alluded to earlier, appears to take place in cells of the mononuclear-phagocyte system and possibly in other cells as well. Monocytes and macrophages have receptors for chemically modified (e.g., acetylated or oxidized) LDL. The amount catabolized by this "scavenger receptor" pathway is directly related to the plasma cholesterol level.

In familial hypercholesterolemia, mutations in the LDL receptor gene impair the intracellular transport and catabolism of LDL, resulting in accumulation of LDL cholesterol in the plasma. In addition, the absence of LDL receptors on liver cells also impairs the transport of IDL into the liver, and hence a greater proportion of plasma IDL is converted into LDL. Thus, patients with familial hypercholesterolemia develop excessive levels of serum cholesterol owing to the combined effects of reduced catabolism and excessive biosynthesis (see Fig. 7-6).

Familial hypercholesterolemia is an autosomal dominant disease. Heterozygotes have a two- to threefold elevation of plasma cholesterol levels, whereas homozygotes may have in excess of a fivefold elevation. Although their cholesterol lev-

Figure 7-7   ■

Sequential steps in the LDL pathway in cultured mammalian cells. LDL, low-density lipoprotein; HMG CoA reductase, 3-hydroxy-3-methylglutaryl coenzyme A reductase; ACAT, acyl-CoA:cholesterol acyltransferase. (From Goldstein JL, Brown MS: The LDL receptor defect in familial hypercholesterolemia. Implications for pathogenesis and therapy. Med Clin North Am 66:335, 1982.)

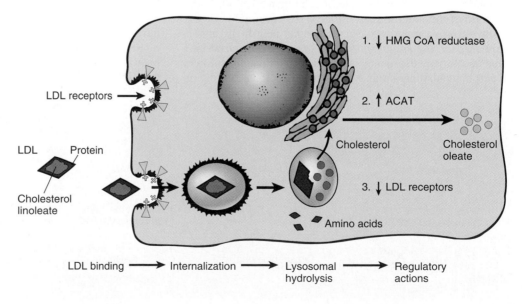

els are elevated from birth, heterozygotes remain asymptomatic until adult life, when they develop cholesterol deposits (xanthomas) along tendon sheaths and premature atherosclerosis resulting in coronary artery disease. Homozygous persons are much more severely affected, developing cutaneous xanthomas in childhood and often dying of myocardial infarction by the age of 15 years.

Analysis of the cloned LDL receptor gene has revealed that at least 35 different mutations can give rise to familial hypercholesterolemia. These can be grouped in four categories. Class I mutations, the most prevalent form, are associated with loss of receptor synthesis; with class II mutations, the receptor protein is synthesized, but its transport from the endoplasmic reticulum to the Golgi apparatus is impaired; class III mutations produce receptors that are transported to the cell surface but fail to bind LDL normally; class IV mutations, the rarest of all, give rise to receptors that fail to internalize after binding to LDL.

It should be emphasized that familial hypercholesterolemia is only one of several forms of hyperlipoproteinemia, most of which are not genetically determined.

Diseases Caused by Mutations in Enzyme Proteins

PHENYLKETONURIA

There are several variants of this inborn error of metabolism. The most common form, referred to as *classic phenylketonuria* (PKU), is quite common in persons of Scandinavian descent and is distinctly uncommon in blacks and Jews.

Homozygotes with this autosomal recessive disorder classically have a severe lack of phenylalanine hydroxylase, leading to hyperphenylalaninemia and PKU. Affected infants are normal at birth but within a few weeks develop a rising plasma phenylalanine level, which in some way impairs brain development. Usually by 6 months of life *severe mental retardation* becomes all too evident; fewer than 4% of untreated phenylketonuric children have IQ values greater than 50 or 60. About one third of these unfortunate children are never able to walk, and two thirds cannot talk. Seizures, other neurologic abnormalities, *decreased pigmentation of hair and skin,* and eczema often accompany the mental retardation in untreated children. Hyperphenylalaninemia and the resultant mental retardation

can be avoided by restriction of phenylalanine intake early in life. Hence, a number of screening procedures, including the Guthrie test, are routinely performed to detect PKU in the immediate postnatal period.

Many clinically normal female PKU patients, treated with diet early in life, reach childbearing age. Most of them have marked hyperphenylalaninemia because dietary treatment is discontinued after reaching adulthood. Children born to such women are profoundly mentally retarded and have multiple congenital anomalies, even though the infants themselves are heterozygotes. This syndrome, termed *maternal PKU,* results from the teratogenic effects of phenylalanine that crosses the placenta and affects the developing fetus. Hence, *it is imperative that maternal phenylalanine levels be lowered by dietary means before conception.*

The biochemical abnormality in PKU is an inability to convert phenylalanine into tyrosine. In normal children, less than 50% of the dietary intake of phenylalanine is necessary for protein synthesis. The rest is converted to tyrosine by the phenylalanine hydroxylase system (Fig. 7–8). When phenylalanine metabolism is blocked because of a lack of phenylalanine hydroxylase, minor shunt pathways come into play, yielding several intermediates that are excreted in large amounts in the urine and in the sweat. These impart a *strong musty or mousy odor* to affected infants. It is believed that excess phenylalanine or its metabolites contribute to the brain damage in PKU. Concomitant lack of tyrosine (Fig. 7–8), a precursor of melanin, is responsible for the light color of hair and skin.

At the molecular level, several mutant alleles of the phenylalanine hydroxylase gene have been identified, only some of which cause a severe deficiency of the enzyme and thus result in classic PKU. In those with a partial deficiency of phenylalanine hydroxylase, only modest elevations of phenylalanine levels occur, and there is no neurologic damage. This condition, referred to as *benign hyperphenylalaninemia,* is important to recognize, because affected individuals may well test positive in the widely utilized Guthrie screening test but will not develop the stigmata of classic PKU. Measurement of serum phenylalanine levels is necessary to differentiate benign hyperphenylalaninemia from PKU.

As alluded to earlier, a number of variant forms of PKU have been identified. These account for 3% to 10% of all cases of PKU and result from deficiencies of enzymes other than phenylalanine hydroxylase, such as dihydropteridine reductase (DHPR) (Fig. 7–8). *It is clinically important to recognize*

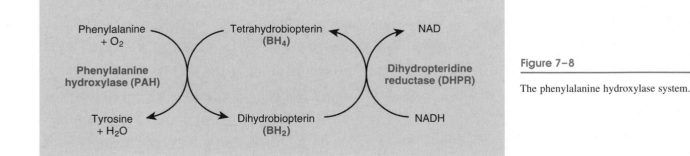

Figure 7–8 ■

The phenylalanine hydroxylase system.

these variant forms of PKU, because they cannot be treated by dietary restriction of phenylalanine.

GALACTOSEMIA

Galactosemia is an autosomal recessive disorder of galactose metabolism. Normally lactose, the major carbohydrate of mammalian milk, is split into glucose and galactose in the intestinal microvilli by lactase. Galactose is then converted to glucose in several steps, in one of which the enzyme galactose-1-phosphate uridyl transferase is required. Lack of this enzyme is responsible for galactosemia. As a result of this lack of transferase, galactose-1-phosphate and other metabolites, including galactitol, accumulate in many locations, including the liver, spleen, lens of the eye, kidney, and cerebral cortex.

The liver, eyes, and brain bear the brunt of the damage. The early-developing hepatomegaly is due largely to fatty change, but in time widespread scarring that closely resembles the cirrhosis of alcohol abuse may supervene (Chapter 16). Opacification of the lens (cataracts) develops, probably because the lens absorbs water and swells as galactitol, produced by alternative metabolic pathways, accumulates and increases its tonicity. Nonspecific alterations appear in the central nervous system, including loss of nerve cells, gliosis, and edema. There is still no clear understanding of the mechanism of injury to the liver and brain.

Almost from birth these infants fail to thrive. *Vomiting and diarrhea* appear within a few days of milk ingestion. *Jaundice and hepatomegaly* usually become evident during the first week of life. *Cataracts* develop within a few weeks, and within the first 6 to 12 months of life *mental retardation* may be detected. Accumulation of galactose and galactose-1-phosphate in the kidney impairs amino acid transport, resulting in aminoaciduria. There is an increased frequency of fulminant *Escherichia coli* septicemia.

Most of the clinical and morphologic changes can be prevented by early removal of galactose from the diet for at least the first 2 years of life. The diagnosis can be suspected by the presence in the urine of a reducing sugar other than glucose, but tests that directly identify the deficiency of the transferase in leukocytes and erythrocytes are more reliable. Antenatal diagnosis is possible in cultured fibroblasts from amniotic fluid.

LYSOSOMAL STORAGE DISEASES

Lysosomes, as is well known, contain a variety of hydrolytic enzymes that are involved in the breakdown of complex substrates, such as sphingolipids and mucopolysaccharides, into soluble end products. These large molecules may be derived from the turnover of intracellular organelles that enter the lysosomes by autophagocytosis, or they may be acquired from outside the cells by phagocytosis. With an inherited lack of a lysosomal enzyme, catabolism of its substrate remains incomplete, leading to accumulation of the partially degraded insoluble metabolites within the lysosomes (Fig. 7-9). As might be expected, these missing-enzyme syndromes are inherited as autosomal recessive disorders, and the storage of insoluble intermediates occurs mainly in cells of the mononuclear phagocyte system, because they ingest and degrade senescent red cells, leukocytes, and other tissue breakdown products.

The numerous lysosomal storage diseases can be divided into broad categories based on the biochemical nature of the substrates and the accumulated metabolites (Table 7-6). Within each group are several entities, each resulting from the deficiency of a specific enzyme. Fortunately for both medical students and the potential victims of the diseases, most of these conditions are very rare, and their detailed description is better relegated to specialized texts and reviews. Only a few of the more common conditions (Table 7-6) are considered

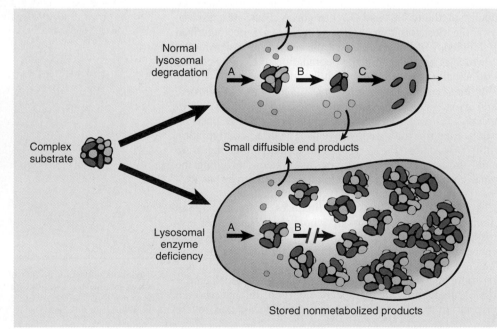

Figure 7-9   ■

Schematic diagram illustrating the pathogenesis of lysosomal storage diseases. In the example illustrated, a complex substrate is normally degraded by a series of lysosomal enzymes (A, B, and C) into soluble end products. If there is a deficiency or malfunction of one of the enzymes (e.g., B), catabolism is incomplete, and insoluble intermediates accumulate in the lysosomes.

Table 7–6. LYSOSOMAL STORAGE DISORDERS

Disease	Enzyme Deficiency	Major Accumulating Metabolite
Glycogenoses		
Type II (Pompe disease)	Lysosomal glucosidase	Glycogen
Sphingolipidoses		
G_{M1} (gangliosidoses)	G_{M1} ganglioside β-galactosidase	G_{M1} ganglioside, galactose-containing oligosaccharides
G_{M2} (gangliosidoses)		
Tay-Sachs disease	Hexosaminidase A	G_{M2} ganglioside
Gaucher disease	Glucocerebrosidase	Glucocerebroside
Neimann-Pick disease	Sphingomyelinase	Sphingomyelin
Mucopolysaccharidoses		
MPS I H (Hurler)	α-L-Iduronidase	Heparan sulfate Dermatan sulfate
MPS II (Hunter) (X-linked recessive)	L-Iduronosulfate sulfatase	Heparan sulfate Dermatan sulfate
Glycoproteinoses	Enzymes involved in degradation of oligosaccharide side chains of glycoproteins (several)	Several, depending on specific enzyme

here. Type II glycogen storage disease (Pompe disease), also a lysosomal disorder, is discussed later.

Tay-Sachs Disease (G_{M2} Gangliosidosis: Hexosaminidase α-Subunit Deficiency). Gangliosidoses are characterized by accumulation of gangliosides, principally in the brain, as a result of a deficiency of a catabolic lysosomal enzyme. Depending on the ganglioside involved, these disorders are subclassified into G_{M1} and G_{M2} categories. Tay-Sachs disease, by far the most common of all gangliosidoses, is characterized by deficiency of the α subunit of the enzyme hexosaminidase A, which is necessary for the degradation of G_{M2}. The brain is principally affected, because it is most involved in ganglioside metabolism. *The storage of G_{M2} occurs within neurons, axon cylinders of nerves, and glial cells throughout the central nervous system.* Affected cells appear swollen, possibly foamy. Electron microscopy reveals a whorled configuration within lysosomes (Fig. 7–10). These anatomic changes are found throughout the central nervous system (including the spinal cord), peripheral nerves, and autonomic nervous system. The retina is usually involved as well.

Tay-Sachs disease, like other lipidoses, is most common among Ashkenazi Jews, among whom the frequency of heterozygous carriers is estimated to be 1 in 30. Heterozygotes can be reliably detected by estimating the level of hexosaminidase in the serum. Antenatal diagnosis is possible, and detection of Tay-Sachs disease in the fetus is considered a possible indication for therapeutic abortion. Infants who are born suffer from mental retardation, blindness, and severe

neurologic dysfunctions that lead to certain death within 2 or 3 years.

Niemann-Pick Disease. This designation refers to a group of disorders that are clinically, biochemically, and genetically heterogeneous. The unifying feature of the Niemann-Pick group of diseases is the *lysosomal accumulation of sphingomyelin and cholesterol.* Biochemically, two major groups can be distinguished: patients with a deficiency of the sphingomyelin-cleaving enzyme sphingomyelinase (types A and B), and others in which this enzyme activity is normal or nearly so (types C and D). In the latter types, there is a primary defect in intracellular cholesterol esterification and transport. All types are rare, so remarks will be confined to the sphingomyelinase-deficient (type A) variant, which accounts for 75% to 80% of all cases. With a deficiency of sphingomyelinase, the breakdown of sphingomyelin into ceramide and phosphorylcholine is impaired, and excess sphingomyelin accumulates in all phagocytic cells and in the neurons. The phagocytic cells become stuffed with droplets or particles of the complex lipid, imparting a fine vacuolation or foaminess to the cytoplasm (Fig. 7–11). Because of their high content of phagocytic cells, *the organs most severely affected are the spleen, liver, bone marrow, lymph nodes, and lungs.* The splenic enlargement may be striking. In addition, the entire central nervous system, including the spinal cord and ganglia, is involved in this tragic, inexorable process. The affected

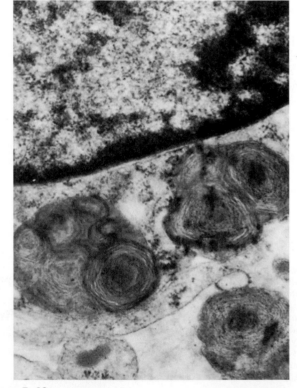

Figure 7–10 ■

Tay-Sachs disease. A portion of a neuron under the electron microscope shows prominent lysosomes with whorled configurations. Part of the nucleus is shown above. (Courtesy of Dr. Joe Rutledge, University of Texas Southwestern Medical School, Dallas, TX.)

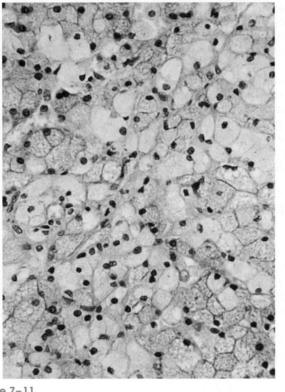

Figure 7-11   ■

Niemann-Pick disease. The foamy vacuolation of the cells in the spleen results from accumulations of sphingomyelin.

neurons are enlarged and vacuolated owing to the storage of lipids. This variant manifests itself in infancy with *massive visceromegaly and severe neurologic deterioration.* Death usually occurs within the first 5 years of life. Estimation of sphingomyelinase activity in the leukocytes or cultured fibroblasts can be used for diagnosis of suspected cases, as well as for detection of carriers. Antenatal diagnosis is possible by the use of cultured fibroblasts obtained by amniocentesis.

Gaucher Disease. There are three autosomal recessive variants of Gaucher disease. Common to all three is variably deficient activity of a glucocerebrosidase that normally cleaves the glucose residue from ceramide. This leads to an accumulation of glucocerebrosides in the reticuloendothelial cells and the formation of so-called Gaucher cells. Normally the glycolipids derived from the breakdown of senescent blood cells, particularly erythrocytes, are sequentially degraded. In Gaucher disease, the degradation stops at the level of glucocerebrosides, which, in transit through the blood as macromolecules, are engulfed by the phagocytic cells of the body, especially those in the liver, spleen, and bone marrow. These phagocytes (Gaucher cells) become enlarged, sometimes up to 100 μm, because of the accumulation of distended lysosomes, and develop a pathognomonic cytoplasmic appearance characterized as "wrinkled tissue paper" (Fig. 7–12). No distinct vacuolation is present.

One variant, type 1, also called the *chronic non-neuronopathic form,* accounts for 99% of cases of Gaucher disease. It is characterized by hepatosplenomegaly and the absence of

central nervous system involvement. The spleen often enlarges massively, filling the entire abdomen. Gaucher cells are found in the liver, spleen, lymph nodes, and bone marrow. Marrow replacement and cortical erosion may produce radiographically visible skeletal lesions, as well as a reduction in the formed elements of blood. Hypersplenism (Chapter 12) also contributes to the anemia and leukopenia. Type 1 has a predilection for Ashkenazi Jews and, unlike other variants, is compatible with long life. The type 2 variant is highly lethal, affects children by 6 months of age, and is characterized by severe central nervous system involvement. Although the liver and spleen are also involved, the clinical features are dominated by neurologic disturbances.

The type 3 (juvenile) variant involves the brain as well as viscera, but the course is intermediate between type 1 and 2. The three variants result from distinct mutations that affect the glucocerebrosidase gene.

The level of glucocerebrosidase in leukocytes or cultured fibroblasts is helpful in diagnosis and in the detection of heterozygotes. Current therapy is aimed at enzyme replacement by infusion of purified glucocerebrosidase. On the horizon is somatic gene therapy involving infusion of autologous hematopoietic stem cells transfected with the normal glucocerebrosidase gene in vitro.

Mucopolysaccharidoses. Mucopolysaccharidoses (MPSs) are characterized by defective degradation (and therefore storage) of mucopolysaccharides in various tissues. Recall that mucopolysaccharides form a part of ground substance and are

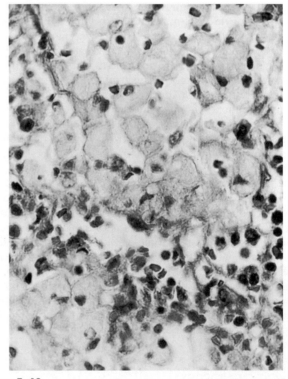

Figure 7-12   ■

The spleen in Gaucher disease. The large vacuolated cells have a ground-glass appearance and contain some faint wavy lines, creating some resemblance to wrinkled tissue paper.

synthesized in the connective tissues by fibroblasts. Most of the mucopolysaccharide is secreted into the ground substance, but a certain fraction is degraded within lysosomes. Several enzymes are involved in this catabolic pathway; it is the lack of these enzymes that leads to accumulation of mucopolysaccharides within the lysosomes. Several clinical variants of MPS, classified numerically from MPS I to MPS VII, have been described, each resulting from the deficiency of one specific enzyme. The mucopolysaccharides that accumulate within the tissues include dermatan sulfate, heparan sulfate, keratan sulfate, and (in some cases) chondroitin sulfate.

In general, the MPSs are progressive disorders characterized by involvement of multiple organs, including the liver, spleen, heart, and blood vessels. Most are associated with *coarse facial features, clouding of the cornea, joint stiffness, and mental retardation.* Urinary excretion of the accumulated mucopolysaccharides is often increased. All of these disorders except one are inherited as autosomal recessive conditions; the exception, Hunter syndrome, is an X-linked recessive disease. Of the seven recognized variants, only two well-characterized syndromes are discussed briefly here.

Hurler syndrome, also called *MPS I H,* results from a deficiency of *a*-L-iduronidase. Affected children have a life expectancy of 6 to 10 years. Like patients with most other forms of MPS, they develop coarse facial features associated with skeletal deformities, which creates an appearance referred to as *gargoylism.* Death is often due to cardiac complications resulting from the formation of raised endothelial and endocardial lesions by the deposition of mucopolysaccharides in the coronary arteries and heart valves. Accumulation of dermatan sulfate and heparan sulfate is seen in cells of the mononuclear phagocyte system, in fibroblasts, and within endothelium and smooth muscle cells of the vascular wall. The affected cells are swollen and have clear cytoplasm, resulting from the accumulation of periodic acid–Schiff (PAS)–positive material within engorged, vacuolated lysosomes. Lysosomal inclusions are also found in neurons, accounting for the mental retardation. Although most of the clinical features can be explained on the basis of excessive storage of mucopolysaccharides, joint stiffness, for example, probably results from disturbances in collagen synthesis, which occur secondary to the derangement in the ground substance.

The other variant of MPS, called *Hunter syndrome,* differs from Hurler syndrome in its mode of inheritance (X-linked), the absence of corneal clouding, and often its milder clinical course. As in Hurler syndrome, the accumulated mucopolysaccharides in Hunter syndrome are heparan sulfate and dermatan sulfate, but this results from a deficiency of L-iduronate sulfatase. Despite the difference in enzyme deficiency, an accumulation of identical substrates occurs because breakdown of heparan sulfate and dermatan sulfate requires both L-iduronidase and the sulfatase; if either one is missing, further degradation is blocked.

GLYCOGEN STORAGE DISORDERS (GLYCOGENOSES)

An inherited deficiency of any one of the enzymes involved in glycogen synthesis or degradation can result in excessive accumulation of glycogen or some abnormal form of glycogen in various tissues. The type of glycogen stored, its intracellular location, and the tissue distribution of the affected cells vary depending on the specific enzyme deficiency. Regardless of the tissue or cells affected, the glycogen is most often stored within the cytoplasm, or sometimes within nuclei. One variant, Pompe disease, is a form of lysosomal storage disease, because the missing enzyme is localized to lysosomes. Most glycogenoses are inherited as autosomal recessive diseases, as is common with "missing enzyme" syndromes.

Approximately a dozen forms of glycogenoses have been described on the basis of specific enzyme deficiencies. On the basis of pathophysiology they can be grouped into three categories:

■ *Hepatic forms.* Liver contains several enzymes that synthesize glycogen for storage and also break it down into free glucose. Hence, a deficiency of the hepatic enzymes involved in glycogen metabolism is associated with two major clinical effects: *enlargement of the liver owing to storage of glycogen and hypoglycemia owing to a failure of glucose production* (Fig. 7–13). von Gierke disease (type I glycogenosis), resulting from a lack of glucose-6-phosphatase, is the most important example of the hepatic form of glycogenoses (Table 7–7).

■ *Myopathic forms.* In striated muscle, glycogen, derived by the glycolytic pathway, is an important source of energy.

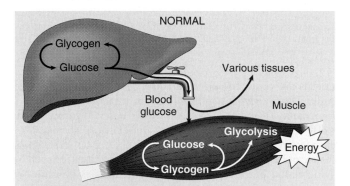

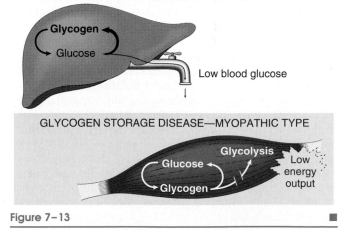

Figure 7–13 ■

Top, A simplified scheme of normal glycogen metabolism in the liver and skeletal muscles. *Middle,* The effects of an inherited deficiency of hepatic enzymes involved in glycogen metabolism. *Bottom,* The consequences of a genetic deficiency in the enzymes that metabolize glycogen in skeletal muscles.

Table 7–7.   PRINCIPAL SUBGROUPS OF GLYCOGENOSES

Clinicopathologic Category	Specific Type	Enzyme Deficiency	Morphologic Changes	Clinical Features
Hepatic type	Hepatorenal (von Gierke disease, type I)	Glucose-6-phosphatase	Hepatomegaly: intracytoplasmic accumulations of glycogen and small amounts of lipid, intranuclear glycogen. Renomegaly: intracytoplasmic accumulations of glycogen in cortical tubular epithelial cells	Failure to thrive, stunted growth, hepatomegaly, and renomegaly. Hypoglycemia due to failure of glucose mobilization, often leading to convulsions. Hyperlipidemia and hyperuricemia resulting from deranged glucose metabolism; many patients develop gout and skin xanthomas. Bleeding tendency due to platelet dysfunction. Mortality approximately 50%
Myopathic type	McArdle syndrome (type V)	Muscle phosphorylase	Skeletal muscle only—accumulations of glycogen predominant in subsarcolemmal location	Painful cramps associated with strenuous exercise. Myoglobinuria occurs in 50% of cases. Onset in adulthood (>20 yr). Muscular exercise fails to raise lactate level in venous blood. Compatible with normal longevity
Miscellaneous types	Generalized glycogenosis (Pompe disease, type II)	Lysosomal glucosidase (acid maltase)	Mild hepatomegaly: ballooning of lysosomes with glycogen creating lacy cytoplasmic pattern. Cardiomegaly: glycogen within sarcoplasm as well as membrane-bound. Skeletal muscle: similar to heart (see "cardiomegaly")	Massive cardiomegaly, muscle hypotonia, and cardiorespiratory failure within 2 yr. A milder adult form with only skeletal muscle involvement presents with chronic myopathy

When enzymes that are involved in glycolysis are deficient, glycogen storage occurs in muscles, and there is an associated muscle weakness due to impaired energy production. Typically, *the myopathic forms of glycogen storage diseases are marked by muscle cramps after exercise and failure of exercise to induce an elevation in blood lactate levels owing to a block in glycolysis.* McArdle disease (type V glycogenosis), resulting from a deficiency of muscle phosphorylase, is the prototype of myopathic glycogenoses.

■ Two other forms of glycogenosis do not fit into either of the two categories described above. Type II glycogenosis *(Pompe disease)* is caused by a deficiency of lysosomal acid maltase and so is associated with deposition of glycogen in virtually every organ, but cardiomegaly is most prominent. Brancher glycogenosis (type IV) is caused by deposition of an abnormal form of glycogen, with detrimental effects on the liver, heart, and muscles.

The principal subgroups of glycogen storage diseases are summarized in Table 7–7.

Diseases Caused by Mutations in Proteins That Regulate Cell Growth

As detailed in Chapter 6, two classes of genes, protooncogenes and cancer suppressor genes, regulate normal cell growth and differentiation. Mutations affecting these genes, most often in the somatic cells, are involved in the pathogenesis of tumors. In approximately 5% of all cancers, however, mutations affecting certain tumor suppressor genes are present in all cells of the body, including germ cells, and hence can be transmitted to the offspring. These mutant genes predispose the offspring to hereditary tumors, a topic discussed in greater detail in Chapter 6. Here, two prototypic familial tumors resulting from inherited mutations in growth-regulating genes are described.

NEUROFIBROMATOSIS: TYPES 1 AND 2

The neurofibromatoses consist of at least two autosomal dominant disorders affecting approximately 100,000 persons in the United States. They are referred to as *neurofibromatosis type 1* (previously known as *von Recklinghausen disease*) and *neurofibromatosis type 2* (previously called *bilateral acoustic neurofibromatosis*). Although the occurrence of neurogenic tumors is common to both, the two entities are clinically and genetically distinct. Neurofibromatosis type 1, which accounts for more than 90% of cases, has three major features:

1. Multiple neurofibromas develop, usually in the form of pedunculated nodules protruding from the skin. The neurofibromas are discrete, generally unencapsulated, soft nodules. In some cases, the tumors form large, multilobar, pendulous masses (plexiform neurofibromas). Although derived from Schwann cells, they contain a tangled array of all of the elements found in peripheral nerves (i.e.,

Schwann cells, neurites, and fibroblasts). Similar tumors, ranging from microscopic to monstrous masses, may occur in every conceivable site (e.g., along nerve trunks, the cauda equina, cranial nerves, in the retroperitoneum, orbit, tongue, and gastrointestinal tract).

2. Pigmented skin lesions known as "café-au-lait spots" sometimes overlie a neurofibroma. Infrequently, patients with neurofibromatosis type 1 (NF-1) have only the café-au-lait spots, an example of variable expressivity of a genetic defect.

3. Pigmented iris hamartomas, called *Lisch nodules*, do not present any clinical problem but are helpful in establishing the diagnosis.

In addition to being a disfiguring condition, neurofibromatosis may be extremely serious, either by virtue of the location of a lesion (e.g., within the spinal canal) or because one or more of the benign neurofibromas becomes transformed into a malignant neoplasm (in approximately 3% of patients). Usually the neurogenic sarcomas arise in the plexiform tumors attached to large nerve trunks of the neck or extremities. These patients also are at greater risk of developing other tumors, particularly optic gliomas, meningiomas, and pheochromocytomas. In addition, approximately 30% to 50% of patients have a wide variety of associated skeletal lesions. These include scoliosis, erosive bone defects, and bone cysts.

The NF-1 gene has been mapped to chromosome 17, and it encodes a protein that acts as a negative regulator of the *ras* oncoprotein. As detailed in Chapter 6, overactivity of the *ras* protein can contribute to tumorigenesis.

Type 2 neurofibromatosis is much rarer than is type 1. Although most patients have peripheral neurofibromas and café-au-lait spots, the defining feature of this variant is the presence of bilateral acoustic neuromas. The gene for type 2 neurofibromatosis has been mapped to chromosome 22 and is believed to be a tumor suppressor gene, but its function is not fully defined.

DISORDERS WITH MULTIFACTORIAL INHERITANCE

Multifactorial (also called *polygenic*) inheritance is involved in many of the physiologic characteristics of humans (e.g., height, weight, blood pressure, hair color). A multifactorial physiologic or pathologic trait may be defined as one governed by the additive effect of two or more genes of small effect but conditioned by environmental, nongenetic influences. Even monozygous twins reared separately may achieve different heights because of nutritional or other environmental influences. When surveyed in a large population, phenotypic attributes governed by multifactorial inheritance fall on a continuous Gaussian distribution (Fig. 7–14). Presumably there is some threshold effect, so that a disorder becomes manifest only when a certain number of effector genes, as well as conditioning environmental influences, are involved. The threshold effect also explains why parents of a child with a polygenic disorder may themselves be normal. Once the threshold value is exceeded, the severity of the disease is directly pro-

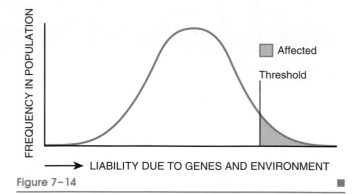

Figure 7–14 ■

Multifactorial inheritance. The continuous distribution of the liability to develop a multifactorial disease is determined by many genes and the environment. A threshold of liability indicates the limit beyond which disease is expressed. (From Elsas LJ II, Priest JH: Medical genetics. In Sodeman WA, Sodeman TM (eds): Pathologic Physiology: Mechanisms of Disease, 7th ed. Philadelphia, WB Saunders, 1985, p 59.)

portional to the number and the degree of influence of the pathologic genes.

The following features characterize multifactorial inheritance. These have been established for the multifactorial inheritance of congenital malformations and, in all likelihood, obtain for other multifactorial diseases.

■ The risk of expressing a multifactorial disorder is conditioned by the number of mutant genes inherited. Thus, the risk is greater in siblings of patients having severe expressions of the disorder.

■ The rate of recurrence of the disorder (in the range of 2% to 7%) is the same for all first-degree relatives (i.e., parents, siblings, and offspring) of the affected individual. Thus, if parents have had one affected child, the risk that the next child will be affected is between 2% and 7%. Similarly, there is the same chance that one of the parents will be affected.

■ The likelihood that both identical twins will be affected is significantly less than 100% but is much greater than the chance that both nonidentical twins will be affected. Experience has proved, for example, that the frequency of concordance for identical twins is in the range of 20% to 40%.

■ The risk of recurrence of the phenotypic abnormality in subsequent pregnancies depends on the outcome in previous pregnancies. When one child is affected, there is up to a 7% chance that the next child will be affected, but after two affected siblings, the risk rises to about 9%.

This form of inheritance is believed to underlie such common diseases as diabetes mellitus, hypertension, gout, schizophrenia, manic depression, and certain forms of congenital heart disease, as well as some skeletal abnormalities. Hypertension provides an excellent example of multifactorial inheritance. There is good evidence that the level of blood pressure of an individual, at least in some part, is under genetic control, apparently governed by multiple genes of small effect. The pressure levels of the population at large fall along a continuous Gaussian curve of distribution. At some arbitrary level of blood pressure, hypertension is said to exist, because pressures above this level are associated with a significant disadvantage to the individual. (Hypertension is described in Chapter 10.)

CYTOGENETIC DISORDERS

Before we embark on a discussion of chromosomal aberrations, it should be recalled that karyotyping is the basic tool of the cytogeneticist. A karyotype is a photographic representation of a stained metaphase spread in which the chromosomes are arranged in order of decreasing length. A variety of techniques for staining of chromosomes have been developed. With the widely used Giemsa stain (G-banding) technique, each chromosome set can be seen to possess a distinctive pattern of alternating light and dark bands of variable widths (Fig. 7–15). The use of banding techniques allows certain identification of each chromosome, as well as precise localization of structural changes in the chromosomes (to be described later).

Chromosomal abnormalities are much more frequent than is generally appreciated. It is estimated that approximately 1 of 200 newborn infants has some form of chromosomal abnormality. The figure is much higher in fetuses that do not survive to term. It is estimated that in 50% of first-trimester abortions, the fetus has a chromosomal abnormality. Cytogenetic disorders may result from alterations in the number or structure of chromosomes and may affect autosomes or sex chromosomes.

Numerical Abnormalities. In humans, the normal chromosome count is 46 (i.e., $2n = 46$). Any exact multiple of the haploid number (n) is called "euploid." Chromosome numbers such as $3n$ and $4n$ are called "polyploid." Polyploidy generally results in a spontaneous abortion. Any number that is not an exact multiple of n is called *aneuploid*. The chief cause of aneuploidy is nondisjunction of a homologous pair of chromosomes at the first meiotic division or a failure of sister chromatids to separate during the second meiotic division. The latter may also occur during somatic cell division, leading to the production of two aneuploid cells. Failure of pairing of homologous chromosomes followed by random assortment (anaphase lag) can also lead to aneuploidy. When nondisjunction occurs at the time of meiosis, the gametes formed have either an extra chromosome $(n + 1)$ or one less chromosome $(n - 1)$. Fertilization of such gametes by normal gametes would result in two types of zygotes: trisomic, with an extra chromosome $(2n + 1)$, or monosomic $(2n - 1)$. Monosomy involving an autosome is incompatible with life, whereas trisomies of certain autosomes and monosomy involving sex chromosomes are compatible with life. These, as we shall see, are usually associated with variable degrees of phenotypic abnormalities. *Mosaicism* is a term used to describe the presence of two or more populations of cells in the same individual. In the context of chromosome numbers, postzygotic mitotic nondisjunction would result in the pro-

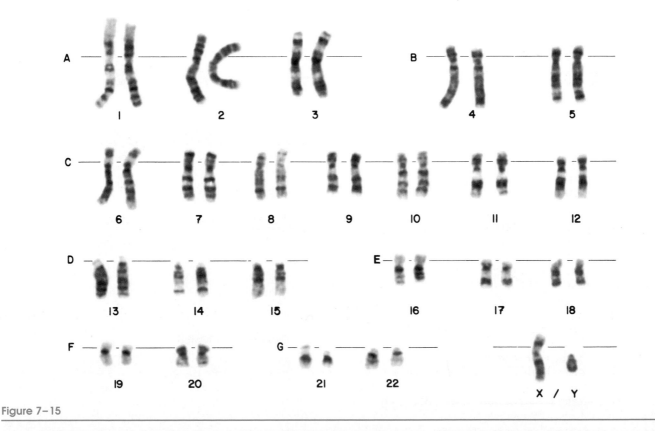

Figure 7–15

A normal male karyotype with G banding. (Courtesy of Dr. Patricia Howard-Peebles, Department of Pathology, University of Texas Southwestern Medical School, Dallas, TX.)

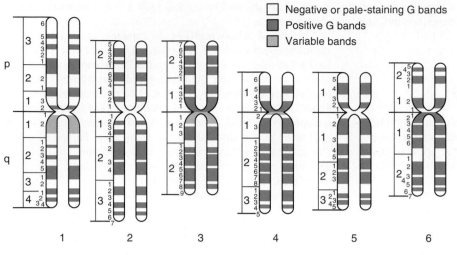

□ Negative or pale-staining G bands
■ Positive G bands
▨ Variable bands

Figure 7–16 ■

Diagrammatic representation of midmetaphase chromosome bands to indicate the nomenclature of arms, regions, and bands. (After Yunis JJ, Chandler MS: The chromosomes of man—clinical and biologic significance. A review. Am J Pathol 8: 466, 1977.)

duction of a trisomic and a monosomic daughter cell; the descendants of these cells would then produce a mosaic. As discussed later, mosaicism affecting sex chromosomes is common, whereas autosomal mosaicism is not.

Structural Abnormalities. Structural changes in the chromosomes usually result from chromosome breakage followed by loss or rearrangement of material. Such changes are usually designated using a cytogenetic shorthand in which "p" (petit) denotes the short arm of a chromosome, and "q," the long arm. Each arm is then divided into numbered regions (1, 2, 3, and so on) from centromere outward, and within each region the bands are numerically ordered (Fig. 7–16). Thus, 2q34 indicates chromosome 2, long arm, region 3, band 4. Loss and gain of material are denoted by minus and plus signs, respectively. The patterns of chromosomal rearrangement after breakage (diagrammed in Fig. 7–17) are as follows:

■ *Translocation* implies transfer of a part of one chromosome to another chromosome. The process is usually reciprocal (i.e., fragments are exchanged between two chro-

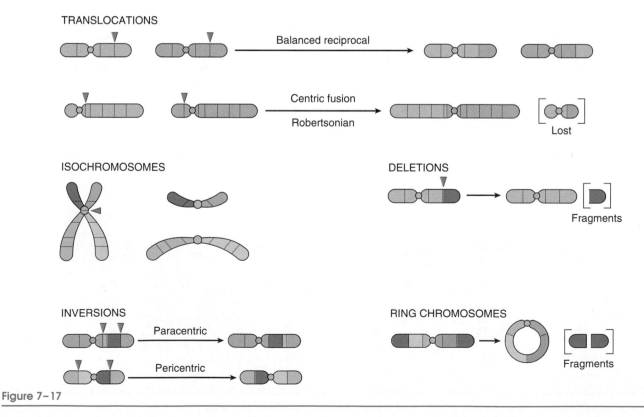

TRANSLOCATIONS

Balanced reciprocal

Centric fusion
Robertsonian

Lost

ISOCHROMOSOMES

DELETIONS

Fragments

INVERSIONS

Paracentric

Pericentric

RING CHROMOSOMES

Fragments

Figure 7–17 ■

Types of chromosomal rearrangements.

mosomes). In genetic shorthand, translocations are indicated by "t" followed by the involved chromosomes in numeric order, for example, 46,XX,t(2;5)(q31;p14). This would indicate a reciprocal translocation involving the long arm (q) of chromosome 2 at region 3, band 1, and the short arm of chromosome 5, region 1, band 4. When the entire broken fragments are exchanged, the resulting balanced reciprocal translocation (Fig. 7–17) is not harmful to the carrier, who has the normal number of chromosomes and the full complement of genetic material. However, during gametogenesis, abnormal (unbalanced) gametes will be formed, resulting in abnormal zygotes. A special pattern of translocation involving two acrocentric chromosomes is called *centric fusion-type,* or *Robertsonian,* translocation. Typically, the breaks occur close to the centromere, affecting the short arms of both the chromosomes. Transfer of the segments leads to one very large chromosome and one extremely small one (Fig. 7–17). The short fragments are lost, and the carrier has 45 chromosomes. Because the short arms of all acrocentric chromosomes have multiple copies of genes for ribosomal RNA, such loss is compatible with survival. However, difficulties arise during gametogenesis, resulting in the formation of unbalanced gametes that could lead to abnormal offspring.

■ *Isochromosomes* result when the centromere divides horizontally rather than vertically. One of the two arms of the chromosome is then lost, and the remaining arm is duplicated, resulting in a chromosome with two short arms only or two long arms only. The most common isochromosome present in live births involves the long arm of the X chromosome and is designated i(Xq). When fertilized by a gamete that contains a normal X chromosome, there is monosomy for genes on Xp and trisomy for genes on Xq.

■ *Deletion* involves loss of a portion of a chromosome. A single break may delete a terminal segment. Two interstitial breaks, with reunion of the proximal and distal segments, may result in loss of an intermediate segment. The isolated fragment, which lacks a centromere, almost never survives, and thus many genes are lost.

■ *Inversions* occur when there are two interstitial breaks in a chromosome, and the segment reunites after a complete turnaround.

■ A *ring chromosome* is a variant of a deletion. After loss of segments from each end of the chromosome, the arms unite to form a ring.

Against this background, we can turn first to some general features of chromosomal disorders, followed by some specific examples of diseases involving changes in the karyotype.

■ Chromosomal disorders may be associated with absence (deletion, monosomy), excess (trisomy), or abnormal rearrangements (translocations) of chromosomes.

■ In general, loss of chromosomal material produces more severe defects than does gain of chromosomal material.

■ Excess chromosomal material may result from a complete chromosome (trisomy) or part of a chromosome (Robertsonian translocation).

■ Imbalances of sex chromosomes (excess or loss) are tol-

erated much better than are similar imbalances of autosomes.

■ Sex chromosomal disorders often produce subtle abnormalities, sometimes not detected at birth. Infertility, a common manifestation, cannot be diagnosed until adolescence.

■ In most cases, chromosomal disorders result from de novo changes (i.e., parents are normal, and risk of recurrence in siblings is low). An uncommon but important exception to this principle is exhibited by the translocation form of Down syndrome.

Cytogenetic Disorders Involving Autosomes

Three autosomal trisomies (21, 18, and 13) and one deletion syndrome (cri du chat), which results from partial deletion of the short arm of chromosome 5, were the first chromosomal abnormalities identified. More recently, several additional trisomies and deletion syndromes have been described. Most of these disorders are quite uncommon, and all are characterized by clinical features that should permit ready recognition. Some of the features of the three most common entities are presented in Figure 7–18.

Only trisomy 21 occurs with sufficient frequency to merit further consideration.

TRISOMY 21 (DOWN SYNDROME)

Down syndrome is the most common of the chromosomal disorders. About 92% to 95% of affected persons have trisomy 21, so their chromosome count is 47. As mentioned earlier, the most common cause of trisomy, and therefore of Down syndrome, is meiotic nondisjunction. The parents of such children have a normal karyotype and are normal in all respects. *Maternal age has a strong influence on the incidence of Down syndrome.* It occurs in 1 in 1550 live births in women younger than 20 years, in contrast to 1 in 25 live births in women older than 45 years. The correlation with maternal age suggests that in most cases the meiotic nondisjunction of chromosome 21 occurs in the ovum. Indeed, in 95% of cases the extra chromosome is of maternal origin. The reason for the increased susceptibility of the ovum to nondisjunction is not fully understood. No effect of paternal age has been found in those cases where the extra chromosome is derived from the father.

In about 4% of all patients with trisomy 21, the extra chromosomal material is present not as an extra chromosome, but as a translocation of the long arm of chromosome 21 to chromosome 22 or 14. Such cases are usually familial, and the translocated chromosome is inherited from one of the parents, who is most frequently a carrier of a Robertsonian translocation. The consequences of the mating of a 14-21 translocation carrier (who may be phenotypically normal, with a chromosome count of 45) and a normal individual are depicted in Figure 7–19. Although theoretically the carrier has one chance in three of bearing a live child with Down syndrome, the observed frequency of affected children in such cases is much lower. The reasons for this discrepancy are not well understood. Approximately 1% of trisomy 21 patients are mosaics, usually having a mixture of 46- and 47- chro-

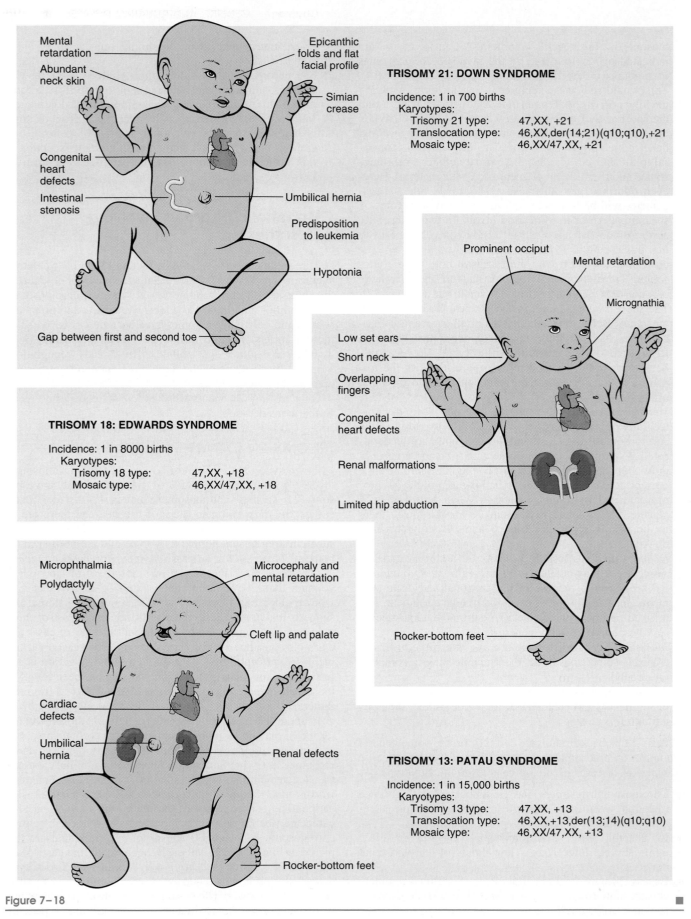

Mental retardation

Abundant neck skin

Epicanthic folds and flat facial profile

Simian crease

Congenital heart defects

Intestinal stenosis

Umbilical hernia

Predisposition to leukemia

Hypotonia

Gap between first and second toe

TRISOMY 21: DOWN SYNDROME

Incidence: 1 in 700 births
Karyotypes:
    Trisomy 21 type: 47,XX, +21
    Translocation type: 46,XX,der(14;21)(q10;q10),+21
    Mosaic type: 46,XX/47,XX, +21

TRISOMY 18: EDWARDS SYNDROME

Incidence: 1 in 8000 births
Karyotypes:
    Trisomy 18 type: 47,XX, +18
    Mosaic type: 46,XX/47,XX, +18

Prominent occiput

Mental retardation

Micrognathia

Low set ears

Short neck

Overlapping fingers

Congenital heart defects

Renal malformations

Limited hip abduction

Rocker-bottom feet

Microphthalmia

Polydactyly

Microcephaly and mental retardation

Cleft lip and palate

Cardiac defects

Umbilical hernia

Renal defects

TRISOMY 13: PATAU SYNDROME

Incidence: 1 in 15,000 births
Karyotypes:
    Trisomy 13 type: 47,XX, +13
    Translocation type: 46,XX,+13,der(13;14)(q10;q10)
    Mosaic type: 46,XX/47,XX, +13

Rocker-bottom feet

Figure 7–18

Clinical features and karyotypes of selected autosomal trisomies.

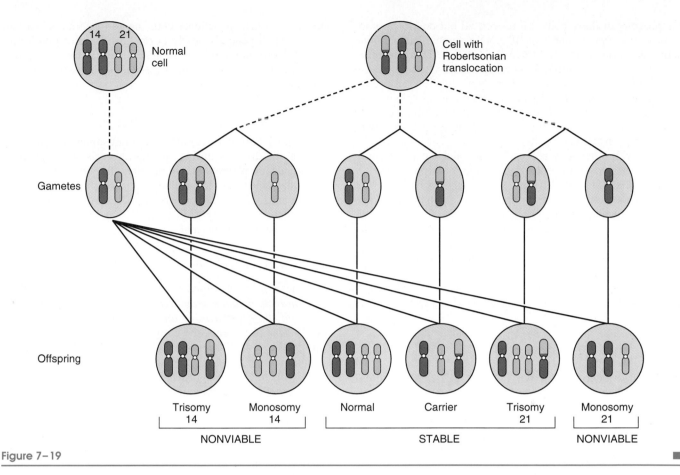

Figure 7–19   ■

Consequences of Robertsonian translocation (14-21) on gametogenesis and production of Down syndrome.

mosome cells. These result from mitotic nondisjunction of chromosome 21 during an early stage of embryogenesis. Symptoms in such cases are variable and milder, depending on the proportion of abnormal cells.

The clinical features of Down syndrome are illustrated in Figure 7–18. The combination of *epicanthic folds* and *flat facial profile* is quite characteristic. Trisomy 21 is a leading cause of *mental retardation.* The degree of mental retardation is severe: IQ varies from 25 to 50. Congenital malformations are common and quite disabling. Approximately 40% of patients with trisomy 21 are afflicted with *cardiac malformations,* which are responsible for most of the deaths in early childhood. *Serious infections* are another important cause of morbidity and mortality. As with most other clinical features, the basis of increased susceptibility to infection is not clearly understood. The chromosomal imbalance, in some undefined manner, also *increases the risk of developing acute leukemias.*

The overall prognosis for individuals with Down syndrome has improved remarkably in the recent past owing to better control of infections. Currently it is estimated that approximately 80% of those without congenital heart disease can expect to survive 30 years. The outlook is less favorable for those with cardiac malformations. Most of those who survive into middle age develop histologic, metabolic, and neurochemical changes of Alzheimer's disease (Chapter 23). Many develop frank dementia. The basis of this association is being actively investigated, with the hope of finding clues to the pathogenesis of Alzheimer's disease.

Cytogenetic Disorders Involving Sex Chromosomes

A number of abnormal karyotypes involving the sex chromosomes, ranging from 45,X to 49,XXXXY, are compatible with life. Indeed, males who are phenotypically normal have been identified as having two and even three Y chromosomes. Such extreme karyotypic deviations are not encountered with the autosomes. In large part this latitude relates to two factors: (1) lyonization of X chromosomes and (2) the scant amount of genetic information carried by the Y chromosome. The consideration of lyonization must begin with the Barr body, or sex chromatin, a prominent clump of chromatin attached to the nuclear membrane in the interphase nuclei of all somatic cells of females. In 1962, Mary Lyon proposed that the X, or *Barr, body represents one genetically inactivated X chromosome.* This inactivation occurs early in fetal life, about 16 days after conception, and randomly inactivates either the paternal or the maternal X chromosome in each of the primitive cells representing the developing embryo. Once inactivated, the same X chromosome remains genetically neutralized in all of the progeny of these cells. Moreover, all but one X chromosome is inactivated, and so a 48,XXXX female has only one active X chromosome and three Barr bodies. This phenomenon explains why normal females do not have a double dose (as compared with males) of phenotypic attributes coded by the X chromosome. The Lyon hypothesis also explains why normal females are in reality mosaics, containing two cell populations—one with an active maternal X, the other with an active paternal X.

Extra Y chromosomes are readily tolerated because the only information known to be carried on the Y chromosome appears to relate to male differentiation. It should be noted that whatever the number of X chromosomes, the presence of a Y invariably dictates the male phenotype. The Y body appears as a small, brightly fluorescent spot in interphase nuclei stained with fluorescent dyes and examined with the ultraviolet microscope. The genes for male differentiation are located on the short arm of the Y.

Three disorders—Klinefelter syndrome, XYY males, and Turner syndrome–arising in aberrations of sex chromosomes are described briefly.

KLINEFELTER SYNDROME

This syndrome is best defined as male hypogonadism that develops when there are at least two X chromosomes and one or more Y chromosomes. Most patients are 47,XXY. This karyotype results from nondisjunction of sex chromosomes during meiosis. The extra X chromosome may be of either maternal or paternal origin. Advanced maternal age and a history of irradiation of either parent may contribute to the meiotic error resulting in this condition. Approximately 15% of patients show mosaic patterns, including 46,XY/47,XXY, 47,XXY/48,XXXY, and variations on this theme. The presence of a 46,XY line in mosaics is usually associated with a milder clinical condition.

Although the following description applies to most patients, it should be noted that Klinefelter syndrome is associated with a wide range of clinical manifestations. In some it may be expressed only as hypogonadism, but most patients have a distinctive body habitus with an *increase in length between the soles and the pubic bone,* which creates the appearance of an elongated body. *Reduced facial and body hair* and *gynecomastia* are also frequently noted. The testes are markedly reduced in size, sometimes to only 2 cm in greatest dimension. Along with the *testicular atrophy,* the serum testosterone levels are lower than normal, and urinary gonadotropin levels are elevated.

The principal clinical effect of this syndrome is sterility. Only rarely are patients fertile, and these are presumably mosaics with a large proportion of 46,XY cells. The sterility is due to impaired spermatogenesis, sometimes to the extent of total azoospermia. Histologically, there is hyalinization of tubules, which appear as ghostlike structures in tissue section. By contrast, Leydig cells are prominent, owing to either hyperplasia or an apparent increase related to loss of tubules. Although Klinefelter syndrome may be associated with mental retardation, the degree of intellectual impairment is typically mild and in some cases is undetectable. The reduction in intelligence is correlated with the number of extra X chromosomes. Thus, in patients with the most common variant (XXY), intelligence is nearly normal, but in those with rare variant forms involving additional X chromosomes, significantly subnormal levels of intelligence, as well as more severe physical abnormalities, are found.

XYY MALES

The XYY karyotype results from nondisjunction at the second meiotic division during spermatogenesis. Most of these individuals are phenotypically normal, although they may be somewhat taller than usual, but they have been reported to display antisocial behavior. This remains a controversial issue; recent studies suggest that only 1% to 2% of XYY males exhibit behavioral abnormalities.

TURNER SYNDROME

Turner syndrome, *characterized by primary hypogonadism in phenotypic females, results from partial or complete monosomy of the short arm of the X chromosome.* In approximately 57% of patients, the entire X chromosome is missing, resulting in a 45,X karyotype. These patients are the most severely affected, and the diagnosis can often be made at birth or early in childhood. Typical clinical features associated with 45,X Turner syndrome include significant growth retardation, leading to abnormally short stature (below third percentile); webbing of the neck; low posterior hairline; cubitus valgus (an increase in the carrying angle of the arms); shieldlike chest with widely spaced nipples; high, arched palate; lymphedema of the hands and feet; and a variety of congenital malformations such as horseshoe kidney and coarctation of the aorta (Fig. 7–20). Affected girls fail to develop normal secondary sex characteristics, the genitalia remain infantile, breast development is inadequate, and little pubic hair appears. Most have primary amenorrhea, and morphologic examination reveals transformation of the ovaries into white streaks of fibrous stroma devoid of follicles. Ovarian estrogen levels are low, and the loss of feedback inhibition leads to elevated levels of pituitary gonadotropin. In adult patients, a combination of short stature and primary amenorrhea should prompt strong suspicion of Turner syndrome. The diagnosis is established by karyotyping.

Approximately 43% of patients with Turner syndrome are either mosaics (one of the cell lines being 45,X) or have structural abnormalities of the X chromosome. These are depicted in Figure 7–20. The most common is deletion of the small arm, resulting in the formation of an isochromosome of the long arm, 46,X,i(X)(q10). Combinations of deletions and mosaicism are reported. It is important to appreciate the karyotypic heterogeneity associated with Turner syndrome because it is responsible for significant variations in the phenotype. In contrast to the patients with monosomy X described above, those that are *mosaics or deletion variants may have an almost normal appearance and may present only with primary amenorrhea.*

It is pertinent to recall the Lyon hypothesis in the context of Turner syndrome. If only one active X chromosome were necessary for the development of normal females (as proposed in the Lyon hypothesis), patients with partial or complete loss

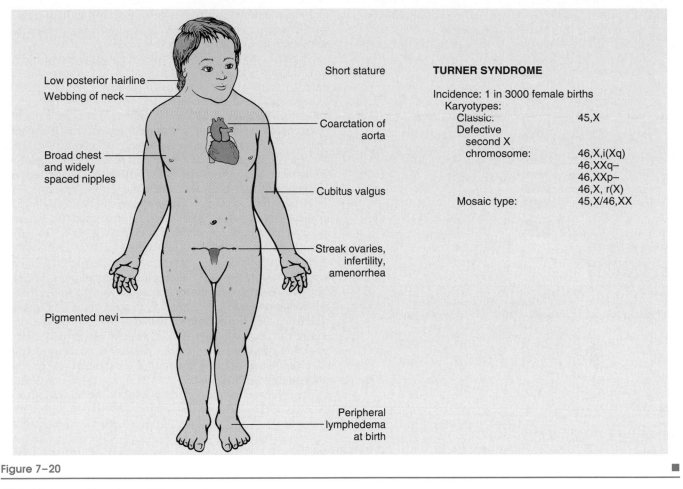

Figure 7–20   ■

Clinical features and karyotypes of Turner syndrome.

of one X chromosome would not be expected to display the stigmata of Turner syndrome. In view of this inconsistency and other recent observations, the Lyon hypothesis has been modified. It is currently believed that although one X chromosome is inactivated in all cells during embryogenesis, it is selectively reactivated in germ cells prior to first meiotic division. Furthermore, it seems that certain X chromosome genes remain active on both X chromosomes in many somatic cells of normal females. Thus, it seems that two copies of some X-linked genes are essential for normal gametogenesis and female development.

SINGLE-GENE DISORDERS WITH ATYPICAL PATTERNS OF INHERITANCE

Three groups of diseases resulting from mutations affecting single genes do not follow the mendelian rules of inheritance:

■ Diseases caused by triplet repeat mutations
■ Diseases caused by mutations in mitochondrial genes

■ Diseases associated with genomic imprinting

TRIPLET REPEAT MUTATIONS: FRAGILE X SYNDROME

Fragile X syndrome is the prototype of diseases in which the mutation is characterized by a long repeating sequence of three nucleotides. Other examples of diseases associated with trinucleotide repeat mutations include Huntington disease and myotonic dystrophy. In each of these conditions, *amplification of specific sets of three nucleotides within the gene disrupts its function.* Certain unique features of trinucleotide repeat mutations, to be described later, are responsible for the atypical pattern of inheritance of the associated diseases.

Fragile X syndrome is characterized by mental retardation and an abnormality in the X chromosome (Fig. 7–21). It is one of the most common causes of familial mental retardation. The cytogenetic alteration is induced by certain culture conditions and is seen as a *discontinuity of staining or constriction in the long arm of the X chromosome.* Clinically affected males have moderate to severe mental retardation. Although a variety of physical abnormalities have been reported, they are inconstant and not readily apparent. The only distinctive

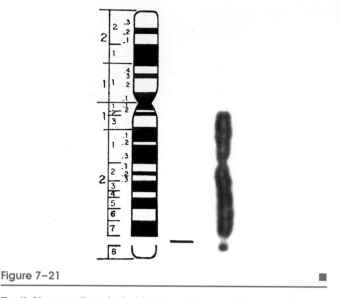

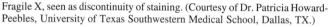

Figure 7-21 ■

Fragile X, seen as discontinuity of staining. (Courtesy of Dr. Patricia Howard-Peebles, University of Texas Southwestern Medical School, Dallas, TX.)

physical abnormality that can be detected in at least 80% of postpubertal males with fragile X syndrome is *macroorchidism* (enlargement of the testes).

Fragile X syndrome results from a mutation in the FMR-1 gene that maps to Xq27.3. As with all X-linked recessive disorders, this disease affects males. However, unlike other X-linked recessive disorders, approximately 20% of males who are known to carry the fragile X mutation are clinically and cytogenetically normal. These "carrier males" can transmit the disease to their grandsons through their phenotypically normal daughters. Another peculiarity is the presence of mental retardation in 50% of carrier females. These unusual features have been related to the dynamic nature of the mutation (Fig. 7-22). In the normal population the number of CGG repeats in the FMR-1 gene is small, averaging around 29, whereas affected individuals have 250 to 4000 repeats. These so-called full mutations are believed to arise through an intermediate stage of "premutations" characterized by 52 to 200 CGG repeats. Carrier males and females have premutations. It seems that during oogenesis the premutations can be converted to full mutations by further amplification of the CGG repeats, which can then be transmitted to both the sons and the daughters of the carrier female. These observations provide an explanation for why some carrier males are unaffected (they have premutations) and certain carrier females are affected (they inherit full mutations).

The presence of full mutations inhibits the transcription of

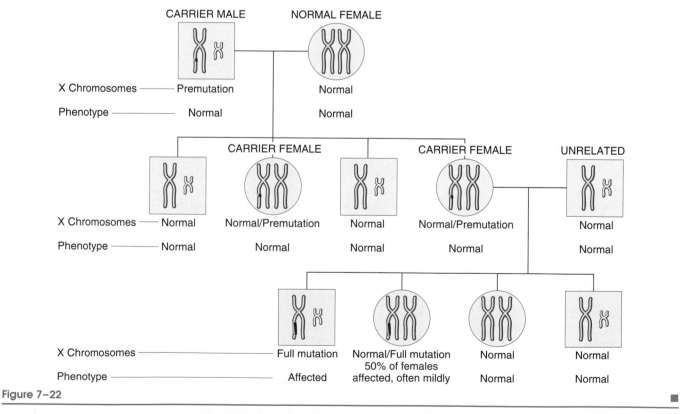

Figure 7-22 ■

Fragile X pedigree. Note that in the first generation all sons are normal and all females are carriers. During oogenesis in the carrier female, premutation expands to full mutation; hence in the next generation all males who inherit the X with full mutation are affected. However, only 50% of females who inherit the full mutation are affected, and often only mildly. (Original sketch courtesy of Dr. Nancy Schneider, Department of Pathology, University of Texas Southwestern Medical School, Dallas, TX.)

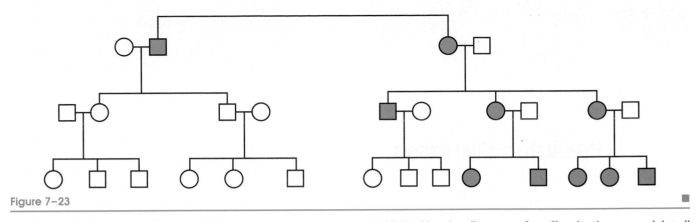

Figure 7–23

Pedigree of Leber's optic neuropathy, a disorder caused by mutation in mitochondrial DNA. Note that all progeny of an affected male are normal, but all children, male and female, of the affected female manifest disease.

the FMR-1 gene, which in turn leads to phenotypic abnormalities by mechanisms not fully understood. The diagnosis of this condition can be made by cytogenetic demonstration of the fragile site or, more reliably, by DNA probe analysis. With the molecular methods, the distinction between premutation and mutation can be made (p 216).

DISEASES CAUSED BY MUTATIONS IN MITOCHONDRIAL GENES

Mitochondria contain several genes that encode enzymes involved in oxidative phosphorylation. Inheritance of mitochondrial DNA differs from that of nuclear DNA in that the former is associated with *maternal inheritance.* This peculiarity results from the fact that ova contain mitochondria within their abundant cytoplasm, whereas spermatozoa contain few, if any, mitochondria. Hence, the mitochondrial DNA complement of the zygote is derived entirely from the ovum. Thus, mothers transmit mitochondrial genes to all of their offspring, both male and female; however, daughters but not sons transmit the DNA further to their progeny (Fig. 7–23).

Diseases caused by mutations in mitochondrial genes are rare. Leber's hereditary optic neuropathy is the prototypical disorder in this group. This neurodegenerative disease manifests itself as progressive bilateral loss of central vision that leads in due course to blindness.

GENOMIC IMPRINTING: PRADER-WILLI AND ANGELMAN SYNDROMES

As is well known, all humans inherit two copies of each gene, carried on homologous maternal and paternal chromosomes. It has usually been assumed that there is no difference between normal homologous genes derived from the mother or father. Indeed, this is true for many genes. However, it has now been established that with respect to some genes, functional differences exist between the paternal and maternal

genes. These differences arise from an epigenetic process called *genomic imprinting,* whereby certain genes are differentially "marked" during paternal and maternal gametogenesis, resulting in differential expression of these genes in the individual.

Genomic imprinting is best illustrated by considering two uncommon genetic disorders: Prader-Willi syndrome and Angelman syndrome.

Prader-Willi syndrome is characterized by mental retardation, short stature, hypotonia, obesity, small hands and feet, and hypogonadism. In 50% to 60% of cases, an interstitial deletion of band q12 in the long arm of chromosome 15 [i.e., del(15)(q11;q13)] can be detected. In many patients without a detectable cytogenetic abnormality, DNA probe analysis reveals smaller deletions within the same region. *It is striking that in all cases the deletion affects the paternally derived chromosome 15.* In contrast with Prader-Willi syndrome, patients with the phenotypically distinct *Angelman syndrome* are born with a deletion of the same chromosomal region derived from their mothers. Patients with Angelman syndrome are also mentally retarded, but in addition they present with ataxic gait, seizures, and inappropriate laughter. Because of the laughter and ataxia, this syndrome is also called the *happy puppet syndrome.* A comparison of these two syndromes clearly demonstrates the "parent-of-origin" effects on gene function. If all the paternal and maternal genes contained within chromosome 15 were expressed in an identical fashion, clinical features resulting from these deletions would be expected to be identical regardless of the parental origin of chromosome 15.

The molecular basis of imprinting is not clear. However, it is established that imprinting is an epigenetic process that most likely occurs during gametogenesis. Because DNA methylation affects gene expression, it is strongly suspected that imprinting is associated with differential DNA methylation of paternal and maternal genes. In addition to the two rare chromosomal disorders described above, it should be noted that parent-of-origin effects have been documented in a variety of single-gene disorders, including Huntington disease, myotonic dystrophy, and neurofibromatosis.

Pediatric Diseases

As mentioned earlier and illustrated by several examples, many diseases of infancy and childhood are of genetic origin. Others, although not genetic, are either unique to children or take distinctive forms in this stage of life and so merit the designation *pediatric diseases.*

During each stage of development, infants and children are prey to a somewhat different group of diseases (Table 7–8). Clearly, diseases of infancy (i.e., the first year of life) pose the highest risk of mortality. During this phase, the neonatal period (the first 4 weeks of life) is unquestionably the most hazardous time.

Once the infant survives the first year of life, the outlook brightens considerably. However, it is sobering to note that between 1 year and 15 years of age, injuries resulting from accidents are the leading cause of death. Not all conditions listed in Table 7–8 are described in this chapter, but only a select few that are more common. Although general principles of neoplastic disease and specific tumors are discussed in other chapters, a few tumors of children are described to highlight the differences between pediatric and adult neoplasms.

CONGENITAL MALFORMATIONS

Congenital malformations can be defined as structural defects that are present at birth, but some, such as cardiac defects and renal anomalies, may not become clinically apparent until years later. As will be evident from the ensuing discussion, the term *congenital* does not imply or exclude a genetic basis for malformations. It is estimated that about 3% of newborns have a major malformation, defined as a malformation having either cosmetic or functional significance. As indicated in Table 7–8, such malformations are a leading cause of infant mortality. Moreover, they continue to be a significant cause of illness, disability, and death throughout the early years of life.

Before describing the etiology and pathogenesis of congenital malformations, it is essential to define some of the terms used to describe errors in morphogenesis.

■ *Malformations* represent primary errors of morphogenesis. They may present in several patterns. Some, such as congenital heart diseases, involve single body systems, whereas in other cases multiple malformations involving many organs and tissues may coexist.
■ *Deformations*, in contrast to malformations, arise later in fetal life and represent alterations in form or structure resulting from mechanical factors. We will consider deformations later in this chapter.
■ *Disruptions*, the third main error in morphogenesis, result from secondary destruction of an organ or body region that was previously normal in development. *Amniotic bands*, denoting rupture of amnion with resultant formation of "bands" that encircle, compress, or attach to parts of the developing fetus, are the classic example of a disruption. Vascular insults may also cause disruptions. Understandably, disruptions are not heritable and hence are not associated with risk of recurrence in subsequent pregnancies.
■ *Sequence* refers to multiple congenital anomalies that re-

Table 7–8. CAUSES OF DEATH AND AGE

Causes	Rate*
Under 1 yr: All Causes	692
Perinatal conditions	
Intrauterine growth retardation/low birth weight	
Respiratory distress syndrome	
Intrauterine hypoxia/birth asphyxia	
Birth trauma	
Others	
Congenital anomalies	
Sudden infant death syndrome	
Pneumonia	
Gastrointestinal disorders	
1–4: All Causes	43.3
Injuries	
Congenital anomalies	
Malignant neoplasms	
Homicide	
Diseases of the heart	
5–9 yr: All Causes	18.5
Injuries	
Malignant neoplasms	
Congenital anomalies	
Homicide	
Diseases of the heart	
10–14 yr: All Causes	18.5
Injuries	
Malignant neoplasms	
Suicide	
Homicide	
Congenital anomalies	

* Number of deaths per 100,000 population.

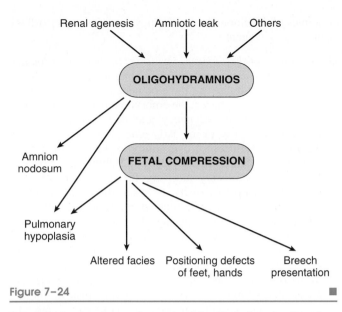

Renal agenesis   Amniotic leak   Others

OLIGOHYDRAMNIOS

Amnion
nodosum

FETAL COMPRESSION

Pulmonary
hypoplasia

Altered facies   Positioning defects   Breech
of feet, hands   presentation

Figure 7–24   ■

Schematic diagram of the pathogenesis of the oligohydramnios (Potter) sequence.

sult from secondary effects of a single localized aberration in organogenesis. The initiating event may be a malformation, deformation, or a disruption. An excellent example is the oligohydramnios (or Potter) sequence (Figs. 7–24 and 7–25). Oligohydramnios, denoting decreased amniotic fluid, may be caused by a variety of unrelated maternal, placental, or fetal abnormalities. Chronic leakage of amniotic fluid owing to rupture of the amnion, uteroplacental insufficiency resulting from maternal hypertension or severe toxemia, and renal agenesis in the fetus (as fetal urine is a major constituent of amniotic fluid) all are causes of oligohydramnios. The fetal compression associated with significant oligohydramnios in turn results in a classic phenotype in the newborn infant, including flattened facies and positional abnormalities of the hands and feet (Fig. 7–25). The hips may be dislocated. Growth of the chest wall and the contained lungs is also compromised, sometimes to such an extent that survival is not possible.

■ *Malformation syndrome* refers to the presence of several defects that cannot be explained on the basis of a single localizing initiating error in morphogenesis. Syndromes are most often caused by a single causative factor (e.g., viral infection or a specific chromosomal abnormality) that simultaneously affects several tissues.

■ In addition to the global definitions listed above, some general terms are applied to organ-specific malformations. *Agenesis* refers to complete absence of an organ or its analage; *atresia* describes the absence of an opening, usually of a hollow visceral organ or duct such as intestines and bile ducts; *aplasia* and *hypoplasia* are used to indicate incomplete development or underdevelopment of an organ. Unlike agenesis, the organ is present but underdeveloped.

Etiology. Known causes of human malformations can be grouped into two major categories: genetic and environmental (Table 7–9). Almost half have no recognized cause.

Genetic causes of malformations include all the previously

discussed mechanisms of genetic disease. Virtually all chromosomal syndromes are associated with congenital malformations. Examples include Down syndrome and other trisomies, Turner syndrome, and Klinefelter syndrome. Most chromosomal disorders arise during gametogenesis and hence are not familial. Single-gene mutations, characterized by mendelian inheritance, may underlie major malformations. On the whole, these are less common than those resulting from chromosomal aberrations, and they are exemplified by rare disorders such as polydactyly and syndactyly. Much more commonly, congenital malformations are suspected to result from multifactorial inheritance, a term that implies the interaction of two or more genes of small effect with environmental factors. Included in this category are some relatively common malformations such as cleft lip and palate. The recurrence risks and mode of transmission of multifactorial disorders have been described earlier in this chapter (p 190).

Environmental influences such as viral infections, drugs, and irradiation to which the mother was exposed during pregnancy may cause fetal malformations. Among the viral infections listed in Table 7–9, the effects of rubella and cytomegalovirus have been studied most extensively. Although maternal rubella and the resultant rubella syndrome have been virtually eliminated as a result of immunization with rubella vaccine, this viral infection serves as an important model of environmental teratogenesis and hence will be discussed briefly.

As with all environmental teratogens, the *gestational age at which fetal exposure* to rubella occurs is critically important. The at-risk period for untoward results of rubella infection extends from shortly before conception to the 16th week of gestation, the hazard being greater in the first 8 weeks than

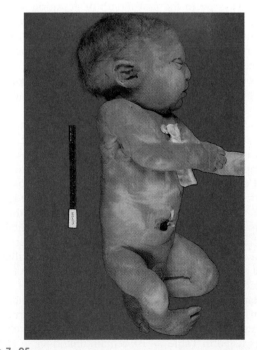

Figure 7–25   ■

Infant with oligohydramnios/Potter sequence. Note flattened facial features and deformed foot (talipes equinovarus).

Table 7-9. CAUSES OF CONGENITAL MALFORMATIONS IN HUMANS

Cause	Malformed Live Births (%)
Genetic	
Chromosomal aberrations	10–15
Mendelian inheritance	2–10
Multifactorial	20–25
Environmental	
Maternal/placental infections	2–3
Rubella	
Toxoplasmosis	
Syphilis	
Cytomegalovirus	
Human immunodeficiency virus	
Maternal disease states	6–8
Diabetes	
Phenylketonuria	
Endocrinopathies	
Drugs and chemicals	~1
Alcohol	
Folic acid antagonists	
Androgens	
Phenytoin	
Thalidomide	
Warfarin	
13-*cis*-Retinoic acid	
Others	
Irradiation	~1
Unknown	40–60

Adapted from Stevenson RE, et al (ed): Human Malformations and Related Anomalies. New York, Oxford University Press, 1993, p 115.

in the second 8 weeks. The incidence of malformations is reduced from 50% in the first month of gestation to 20% or 7% if infection occurs in the second or third month, respectively. The triad of congenital heart defects, cataracts, and deafness represents the classic manifestations of the rubella syndrome.

A variety of drugs and chemicals have been suspected to be teratogenic, but perhaps less than 1% of congenital malformations are caused by these agents. The list includes thalidomide; folate antagonists; androgenic hormones; alcohol; anticonvulsants; warfarin (oral anticoagulant); and 13-*cis*-retinoic acid, which is used in the treatment of severe acne. For example, *thalidomide,* once used as a tranquilizer in Europe and currently being considered for its immunosuppressive properties, caused an extremely high incidence (50% to 80%) of limb malformations. *Alcohol,* perhaps the most widely used agent today, is an important environmental teratogen. Affected infants show growth retardation, microcephaly, atrial septal defect, short palpebral fissures, maxillary hypoplasia, and several other minor anomalies. These together are labeled the *fetal alcohol syndrome.*

The genetic and environmental factors discussed above account for no more than 50% of all congenital malformations. The causes of most birth defects, including the relatively common ones listed in Table 7–10, remain unknown.

Pathogenesis. The pathogenesis of congenital malformations is complex and still poorly understood. Certain general

principles of developmental pathology are relevant regardless of the etiologic agent:

■ *The timing of the prenatal insult has an important impact on both the occurrence and the type of malformation produced.* The intrauterine development of humans can be divided into two phases: the embryonic period, occupying the first 9 weeks of pregnancy, and the fetal period, which terminates at birth. In the early embryonic period (first 3 weeks after fertilization), an injurious agent damages either enough cells to cause death and abortion, or only a few cells, presumably allowing the embryo to recover without developing defects. Between the third and ninth weeks the embryo is extremely susceptible to teratogenesis; the peak sensitivity during this period is between the fourth and fifth weeks. It is during this period that organs are being created out of the germ cell layers. The fetal period that follows organogenesis is marked chiefly by further growth and maturation of the organs, with greatly reduced susceptibility to teratogenic agents. Instead, the fetus is susceptible to growth retardation or injury to already formed organs. For example, in the first trimester, viral infections such as rubella produce malformations by disrupting the developmental program, but later during pregnancy the result of virus infections is usually tissue injury accompanied by inflammation (e.g., congenital encephalitis). Timing of the teratogenic insult is also important with respect to the specific malformation produced. It is therefore possible for a given agent to produce different malformations if exposure occurs at different times of gestation. In general, malformations resulting from incomplete morphogenesis usually have their origin when the development of the organ in question is not yet completed. For example, a ventricular septal defect may occur from exposure to a teratogen before 6 weeks of gestation, because the ventricular septum closes at this time.

Table 7-10. APPROXIMATE FREQUENCY OF THE MORE COMMON CONGENITAL MALFORMATIONS IN THE UNITED STATES

Malformation	Frequency per 10,000 Total Births
Hypospadias	28.23
Clubfoot without neural defects	25.61
Ventricular septal defect	15.23
Cleft lip with or without cleft palate	9.05
Congenital dislocation of hip without neural defects	8.92
Patent ductus arteriosus	7.50
Spina bifida without anencephaly	4.78
Anencephaly	3.14
Atrial septal defect	1.70

Adapted from Edmonds LD, James LM: Temporal trends in the incidence of malformations in the United States: selected years, 1970–71, 1982–83. MMWR (CDC Surveillance Summaries). 34(255): 155, 355, 1985.

■ *Genes that regulate morphogenesis may be the target of teratogens.* Because many congenital malformations result from errors in morphogenesis, genes that control developmental events are likely to be affected by teratogens. Once such class of genes, called *Hox* genes, regulates transcription of several other genes, and in experimental animals, agents that alter *Hox* gene expression are known to produce malformations. In humans, retinoic acid is known to regulate some *Hox* genes during normal development. Infants born to mothers treated with retinoic acid for severe acne develop *retinoic acid embryopathy.* This is characterized by defects in the central nervous system, heart, and face.

DEFORMATIONS

Deformations are common problems, affecting approximately 2% of newborn infants to varying degrees. Fundamental to the pathogenesis of deformations is localized or generalized compression of the growing fetus by abnormal biomechanical forces, leading eventually to a variety of structural abnormalities. In contrast to malformations, there is no intrinsic defect in morphogenesis, although fetal malformations may initiate a sequence of changes that ultimately lead to deformations. The most common underlying factor responsible for deformations is uterine constraint. Between the 35th and 38th weeks of gestation, rapid increase in the size of the fetus outpaces the growth of the uterus, and the relative amount of amniotic fluid (which normally acts as a cushion) also decreases. Thus, even the normal fetus is subjected to some form of uterine constraint. However, several factors increase the likelihood of excessive compression of the fetus, including maternal conditions such as first pregnancy, small uterus, malformed (bicornuate) uterus, and leiomyomas. Factors relating to the fetus, such as multiple fetuses, oligohydramnios, and abnormal fetal presentation, may also be involved.

PERINATAL INFECTIONS

Infections of the fetus and neonate may be acquired transcervically (ascending infections) or transplacentally (hematologic infections).

Transcervical, or *ascending, infections* involve spread of infection from the cervicovaginal canal and may be acquired in utero or during birth. Most bacterial infections (e.g., *β*-hemolytic *Streptococcus*) and a few viral infections (e.g., herpes simplex) are acquired in this manner. In general, the fetus acquires the infection by "inhaling" infected amniotic fluid into the lungs or by passing through an infected birth canal during delivery. Fetal infection is usually associated with inflammation of the placental membranes (chorioamnionitis) and inflammation of the umbilical cord (funisitis). This mode of spread usually gives rise to pneumonia and, in severe cases, to sepsis and meningitis.

Transplacental infections are usually caused by viruses, parasites, and some bacteria (e.g., *Treponema pallidum*). The infecting microbes gain access to the fetal bloodstream through chorionic villi. Unlike ascending infections, the effects of transplacental infection are more widespread. The most important transplacental infections can be conveniently remembered by the acronym "TORCH". The TORCH complex may be caused by any of the following: *Toxoplasma* (T), rubella (R), cytomegalovirus (C), herpes virus (H), or a number of other (O) microbes such as *T. pallidum*. These agents are grouped together because they may evoke similar clinical and pathologic manifestations, including fever, encephalitis, chorioretinitis, hepatosplenomegaly, pneumonia, myocarditis, and hemolytic anemia. Congenital CMV infection and syphilis are described in Chapters 13 and 18, respectively.

PREMATURITY AND INTRAUTERINE GROWTH RETARDATION

It is well established that children born before completion of the full period of gestation have higher morbidity and mortality rates than full-term infants. The immaturity of organ systems in preterm infants (i.e., those born before 37 or 38 weeks) makes them especially vulnerable to conditions such as respiratory distress syndrome. As might be expected, those born before completion of gestation also weigh less than normal (<2500 gm). However, it should be noted that up to one third of infants who weigh less than 2500 gm are born at term and are therefore undergrown rather than immature. These *small-for-gestational-age (SGA) infants suffer from intrauterine growth retardation (IUGR).* Although in many cases the specific cause is unknown, IUGR may result from fetal, maternal, or placental abnormalities.

■ Among fetal causes are those that impair growth despite an adequate uteroplacental axis. These include chromosomal disorders, congenital malformations, and congenital infections. When caused by factors intrinsic to the fetus, growth retardation is symmetric (i.e., affects all organ systems equally).
■ Placental causes include any factor that compromises the uteroplacental supply line. This may result from placenta previa, placental abruption, placental thrombosis, or infections. With placental (and maternal) causes of IUGR, the growth retardation is asymmetric (i.e., the brain is spared relative to visceral organs such as the liver).

Maternal factors are by far the most common cause of SGA infants. These include vascular diseases such as toxemia and chronic hypertension. In addition, maternal narcotic abuse, alcoholism, and heavy cigarette smoking adversely affect fetal growth.

The SGA infant is handicapped not only in the perinatal period, but also in childhood and adult life. These individuals are at increased risk for cerebral dysfunction, learning disabilities, and sensory (i.e., visual, hearing) impairment.

RESPIRATORY DISTRESS SYNDROME OF THE NEWBORN

There are many causes of respiratory distress in the newborn, including excessive sedation of the mother, fetal head injury during delivery, aspiration of blood or amniotic fluid, and intrauterine hypoxia brought about by coiling of the umbilical cord about the neck. However, the most common cause is respiratory distress syndrome (RDS), also known as *hyaline membrane disease* because of the formation of "membranes" in the peripheral airspaces of infants who succumb to this condition. Approximately 60,000 cases of RDS are reported each year in the United States, with annual deaths totaling 5000.

Pathogenesis. *RDS is basically a disease of premature infants.* It affects 15% to 20% of those born between 32 and 36 weeks' gestation, and the prevalence increases to 60% for infants delivered before 28 weeks. Other contributing influences are diabetes in the mother, cesarean section before the onset of labor, and prenatal asphyxia. Males are at greater risk than females.

The fundamental defect in RDS is the inability of the immature lung to synthesize sufficient surfactant. Surfactant is a complex of surface-active lipids, principally (dipalmitoyl)phosphatidylcholine (lecithin) and at least two proteins thought to be essential to the normal function and metabolism of the lipid. It is synthesized by type II pneumocytes and, with the healthy newborn's first breath, rapidly coats the surface of alveoli, reducing surface tension and thus decreasing the pressure required to keep alveoli open. In a lung deficient in surfactant, alveoli tend to collapse, and a relatively greater inspiratory effort is required with each breath to open the alveoli. The infant rapidly tires of breathing, and generalized atelectasis sets in. The resulting hypoxia sets into motion a sequence of events that lead to epithelial and endothelial damage and eventually to the formation of hyaline membranes (Fig. 7–26).

Surfactant synthesis is regulated by hormones. Corticosteroids stimulate the formation of surfactant lipids and associated apoproteins. Thyroxine acts synergistically with corticosteroids, but insulin antagonizes this effect. Uncontrolled diabetes in a pregnant woman gives rise to compensatory hyperinsulinism in the fetus, which in turn can suppress surfactant synthesis. This may explain the higher risk of RDS in infants born to diabetic mothers. Labor is known to increase surfactant synthesis, hence the association with cesarean section.

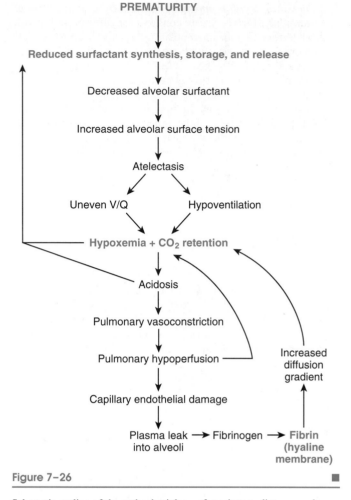

PREMATURITY

Reduced surfactant synthesis, storage, and release

↓

Decreased alveolar surfactant

↓

Increased alveolar surface tension

↓

Atelectasis

↙ ↘

Uneven V/Q   Hypoventilation

↘ ↙

Hypoxemia + CO₂ retention

↓

Acidosis

↓

Pulmonary vasoconstriction

↓

Pulmonary hypoperfusion

↓

Capillary endothelial damage

↓

Plasma leak → Fibrinogen → Fibrin
into alveoli   (hyaline membrane)

Increased diffusion gradient

Figure 7–26 ■

Schematic outline of the pathophysiology of respiratory distress syndrome. V/Q, ventilation-perfusion ratio. (From Oh W, Stern L: Respiratory diseases of the newborn. In Stern L, Vert P (eds): Neonatal Medicine. New York, Masson Publishing USA, 1987, p 396.)

(Fig. 7–27). These "membranes," produced by increased capillary permeability, consist mainly of fibrinogen and fibrin admixed with necrotic epithelial cells. In addition to the formation of membranes, there is intense vascular congestion. If the infant dies after several days, evidence of reparative changes, including proliferation of alveolar lining cells and interstitial fibrosis, is seen.

MORPHOLOGY. The lungs in RDS infants are of normal size but are heavy and relatively airless. They have a mottled purple color, and microscopically the tissue appears solid, with poorly developed, generally collapsed (atelectatic) alveoli. If the infant dies within the first several hours of life, only necrotic cellular debris is present in the terminal bronchioles and alveolar ducts. Later in the course, hyaline membranes line the respiratory bronchioles, alveolar ducts, and random alveoli

Clinical Features. Although with other causes of respiratory distress the newborn may be apneic or hypoxic from the moment of birth, infants with RDS usually appear normal at birth but within minutes to a few hours develop a labored, grunting respiration that progressively worsens and, unless controlled by therapy, causes death. Indeed, RDS is the major cause of death in the neonatal period.

Treatment is designed to support ventilation until the infant is able to breathe on its own, which in milder cases can be expected by the third or fourth day of life. Therapy with aerosolized natural or recombinant surfactant is widely utilized for

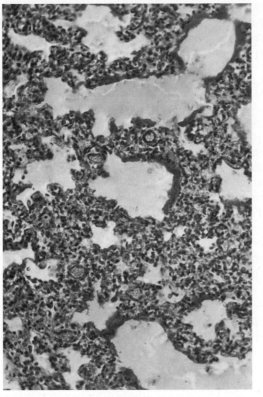

Figure 7-27

Hyaline membrane disease. There is atelectasis of the alveoli and dilation of the alveolar ducts, which are filled with fluid and lined by thick hyaline membranes.

both prophylaxis and treatment of RDS. The greater the birth weight and gestational age, the better the outlook. Death and morbidity may result not only from hypoxemia, but also from (1) intraventricular hemorrhage, to which the immature brain is particularly vulnerable during hypoxemia; (2) heart failure secondary to patent ductus arteriosus; and (3) necrotizing enterocolitis.

A minority of infants who survive suffer long-term sequelae related to neurodevelopmental defects and chronic lung disease. The neurologic abnormalities result from the effects of hypoxia on neurons or from intracerebral hemorrhage. The chronic lung disease, manifested as *bronchopulmonary dysplasia,* is multifactorial. It results from the primary anoxic injury, as well as from exposure to the high concentrations of oxygen and positive-pressure ventilation required for the treatment of this disease. Pathologic findings in bronchopulmonary dysplasia include hyperplasia and squamous metaplasia of bronchial epithelium, peribronchial fibrosis, fibrotic obliteration of bronchioles, and overdistended alveoli.

The most effective method of reducing the morbidity and mortality from RDS is prevention—notably, prevention of premature delivery until the maturing lung is capable of adequate surfactant synthesis. Reasonably reliable estimates of fetal pulmonary maturity can be achieved by measuring the concentration of surfactant phospholipids (e.g., lecithin) in amniotic fluid obtained by amniocentesis. Other noninvasive measurements of fetal maturity (e.g., ultrasound) are commonly employed. When the test indicates pulmonary imma-

turity, efforts are made to delay delivery until the lung matures. If early delivery is unavoidable, administration of corticosteroids to the mother may decrease the risk of RDS by increasing surfactant synthesis.

SUDDEN INFANT DEATH SYNDROME

The current definition of sudden infant death syndrome (SIDS) is "the sudden and unexpected death of an infant less than 1 year of age whose death remains unexplained after the performance of a complete autopsy, examination of the scene of death, and review of the case history." SIDS is sometimes referred to as *crib death* or *cot death,* because most infants succumb during sleep.

SIDS accounts for approximately 8000 deaths in the United States annually. In 90% of cases the infant is under 6 months of age; most are between the ages of 2 and 4 months. Usually death occurs during sleep and without any apparent struggle. Although the cause of SIDS is unknown, several factors related to both the mother and the infant are associated with an increased risk of SIDS (Table 7-11). For reasons not quite clear, there is an increased risk of SIDS in infants who sleep in a prone position, prompting the American Academy of Pediatrics to recommend placing infants in the supine position when laying them down to sleep.

Anatomic studies of victims have yielded a variety of findings, although these are usually subtle, of uncertain significance, and not present in all cases. By definition an overt cause of death, such as bronchopneumonia or a lethal malformation, is lacking. In some cases microscopic alterations have been identified in the structures that control respiratory and cardiac rhythm (brain stem, carotid bodies, vagus nerves) and in tissues sensitive to chronic hypoxemia (brain, lungs, periadrenal brown fat). These changes could well lead to or be secondary to chronic hypoxia, so the possibility exists that they are not, of themselves, the basic defects.

Most authorities believe that SIDS is not a single entity but a disorder with multiple origins. In some infants it may be a manifestation of an inborn error of fatty acid metabolism, such as a deficiency of medium-chain acyl coenzyme A (acyl-CoA) dehydrogenase. In others it may result from a neural developmental delay that may manifest as a respiratory dysfunction. In still others it may be an unusual manifestation of a microbial infection. The litany of hypotheses could be contin-

Table 7-11. FACTORS ASSOCIATED WITH SIDS

Maternal	Infant
Youth (<20 yr of age)	Prematurity
Unmarried	Low birth weight
Short intergestational intervals	Male sex
Low socioeconomic group	Product of a multiple birth
Smoking	Not the first sibling
Drug abuse	SIDS in a prior sibling
Black race (? socioeconomic)	

ued, but suffice it to say that none of these theories, alone or in combination, can at present explain these tragic deaths.

ERYTHROBLASTOSIS FETALIS (HEMOLYTIC DISEASES OF THE NEWBORN)

Erythroblastosis fetalis may be defined as an antibody-induced hemolytic disease in the newborn that is caused by blood group incompatibility between mother and fetus. Such an incompatibility occurs only when the fetus inherits red cell antigenic determinants from the father that are foreign to the mother. Important in this respect are the ABO and Rh blood group antigens. The incidence of hemolytic disease owing to Rh incompatibility has declined remarkably in recent years as a result of successful prophylaxis of this disorder, resulting from increased understanding of its pathogenesis.

Etiology and Pathogenesis. The underlying basis of erythroblastosis fetalis is the immunization of the mother by blood group antigens on fetal red cells and the free passage of antibodies from the mother through the placenta to the fetus. Fetal red cells may reach the maternal circulation during the last trimester of pregnancy, when the cytotrophoblast is no longer present as a barrier, or during childbirth itself. The mother thus becomes sensitized to the foreign antigen.

Of the numerous antigens included in the Rh system, only the D antigen is the major cause of Rh incompatibility. Several factors influence the immune response to Rh-positive fetal red cells that reach the maternal circulation.

■ Concurrent ABO incompatibility protects the mother against Rh immunization because the fetal red cells are promptly coated by isohemagglutinins and removed from the maternal circulation.

■ The antibody response depends on the dose of immunizing antigen; hence, hemolytic disease develops only when the mother has experienced a significant transplacental bleed (more than 1 ml Rh-positive red cells).

■ The isotype of the antibody is important because immunoglobulin G (IgG) (but not immunoglobulin M [IgM]) antibodies can cross the placenta. The initial exposure to Rh antigen evokes the formation of IgM antibodies, so Rh disease is very uncommon with the first pregnancy. Subsequent exposure during the second or third pregnancy generally leads to a brisk IgG antibody response.

Appreciation of the role of prior sensitization in the pathogenesis of Rh erythroblastosis has led to its remarkable control in recent years. Currently, Rh-negative mothers are administered anti-D globulin soon after the delivery of an Rh-positive baby. The anti-D antibodies mask the antigenic sites on the fetal red cells that may have leaked into the maternal circulation during childbirth, thus preventing long-lasting sensitization to Rh antigens.

Owing to the remarkable success achieved in prevention of Rh hemolytic disease, fetomaternal ABO incompatibility is currently the most common hemolytic disease of newborns. *Although ABO incompatibility occurs in approximately 20%* to 25% of pregnancies, only a small fraction of infants subsequently born develop hemolytic disease, and in general the disease is much milder than is Rh hemolytic disease.* ABO hemolytic disease occurs almost exclusively in infants of group A or B who are born of group O mothers. The normal anti-A and anti-B isohemagglutinins in group O mothers are usually of the IgM type and so do not cross the placenta. However, for reasons not well understood, certain group O women possess IgG antibodies directed against group A or B antigens (or both) even without prior sensitization. Therefore, the first-born may be affected. Fortunately, even with transplacentally acquired antibodies, lysis of the infant's red cells is minimal. Two factors seem to be responsible for this happy circumstance: (1) neonatal red cells express group A and B antigens poorly and (2) the widespread presence of these antigens on other tissue cells serves to "soak up" some of the transferred antibodies. There is no effective method of preventing hemolytic disease resulting from ABO incompatibility.

MORPHOLOGY. The anatomic findings in erythroblastosis fetalis vary with the severity of the hemolytic process. Infants may be stillborn, die within the first few days, or recover completely. In its mildest form, the anemia may be only slight, and the child may survive without further complication. More severe hemolysis gives rise to jaundice and other features associated with hemolytic anemias (Chapter 12). In very severe cases, hypoxic injury to the heart and liver may lead to circulatory and hepatic failure, with resultant generalized edema. This pattern is known as **hydrops fetalis.** In most cases the liver and spleen are enlarged, with the degree depending on the severity of the hemolytic process and the compensatory extramedullary erythropoiesis. In all forms, the bone marrow shows hyperplasia of erythroid precursors, and extramedullary hematopoiesis is present in the liver, spleen, and possibly other tissues such as the kidneys, lungs, and even the heart. The increased hematopoietic activity accounts for the presence in the peripheral circulation of large numbers of immature red cells, including reticulocytes, normoblasts, and erythroblasts (hence the name erythroblastosis fetalis).

When hyperbilirubinemia is marked (usually above 20 mg/dl in full-term infants, often less in premature infants), the central nervous system may be damaged (**kernicterus**). The circulating unconjugated bilirubin is taken up by the brain tissue, on which it apparently exerts a toxic effect. It is interesting that adults are protected from this effect of hyperbilirubinemia by the blood-brain barrier.

Clinical Course. The clinical patterns of erythroblastosis fetalis vary from fetal hydrops fetalis to extremely mild degrees of anemia in otherwise healthy infants. Kernicterus may manifest itself by apathy and poor feeding and later by mental retardation, cerebral irritability, extrapyramidal signs, and cranial nerve palsies.

Because severe erythroblastosis fetalis can be treated, early recognition of the disorder is imperative. That which results from Rh incompatibility may be more or less accurately predicted, because it correlates well with rapidly rising Rh antibody titers in the mother during pregnancy. Amniotic fluid obtained by amniocentesis may show high levels of bilirubin. The human antiglobulin test (Coombs' test, Chapter 12) is positive on fetal cord blood if the red cells have been coated by maternal antibody. Exchange transfusion of the infant is an effective form of therapy. Postnatally, phototherapy is helpful because visible light converts bilirubin to readily excreted dipyrroles. As already discussed, in an overwhelming majority of cases, administration of anti-D globulins to the mother can prevent the occurrence of Rh erythroblastosis.

Group ABO erythroblastosis fetalis is more difficult to predict but is readily monitored by awareness of the blood incompatibility between mother and father and by hemoglobin and bilirubin determinations in the vulnerable newborn infant.

CYSTIC FIBROSIS

With an incidence of 1 in 2000 live births, cystic fibrosis (CF) is the most common lethal genetic disease that affects white populations. It is distinctly uncommon among Asians and blacks. CF is associated with a widespread defect in the secretory process of all exocrine glands. Indeed, abnormally viscid mucous secretions that block the airways and the pancreatic ducts are responsible for the two most important clinical manifestations: recurrent and chronic pulmonary infections and pancreatic insufficiency. In addition, although the exocrine sweat glands are structurally normal (and remain so throughout the course of this disease), *a high level of sodium chloride in the sweat is a consistent and characteristic biochemical abnormality in CF.*

Pathogenesis. Although a large number of abnormalities have been described in CF, *the primary defect is in the transport of chloride (Cl⁻) ions across epithelia.* The changes in mucus are considered secondary to the disturbance in transport of Cl⁻ ions. In normal epithelia, the transport of Cl⁻ ions across the cell membrane occurs through transmembrane proteins that form chloride channels. These channels are like gates through which Cl⁻ ions enter or leave the cell. There are two types of Cl⁻ channels: those that are opened by a cyclic adenosine monophosphate (cAMP)–dependent pathway, and others that are regulated by Ca⁺⁺ ions. In CF, the cAMP-dependent Cl⁻ channels, also called the *cystic fibrosis transmembrane conductance regulator (CFTR),* are defective. Mutations in the CFTR gene render the epithelial membranes relatively impermeable to Cl⁻ ions (Fig. 7–28). However, the impact of this defect on transport function is tissue specific. In sweat glands, for example, the concentrations of Na+ and Cl⁻ secreted into the gland lumen are normal, but the epithelium that lines the sweat ducts is impermeable to Cl⁻. Hence, as the sweat moves toward the surface, the normal reabsorp-

tion of Cl⁻ through CFTR, and the accompanying cation Na+, fails to occur. This is responsible for the high concentration of NaCl in the sweat of CF patients. In the respiratory tract, the flow of Cl⁻ ions and the consequences of CFTR mutation are quite different. In the normal airway epithelium, Cl⁻ is secreted into the airways through cAMP-dependent chloride channels. The impaired transport of Cl⁻ from the epithelium into the lumen of the airways causes a series of secondary effects, which lead ultimately to increased absorption of Na+ and water from the airspace to the blood. This lowers the water content of the mucus blanket coating the respiratory epithelium. The resulting dehydration of the mucus layer leads to defective mucociliary action and the accumulation of viscid secretions that obstruct the air passages and predispose to recurrent pulmonary infections (Fig. 7–29).

The CF gene is located on chromosome 7 (7q31-32), and to date more than 300 mutations have been identified in this gene. Approximately 70% of patients have a common mutation characterized by a three base pair deletion leading to the deletion of phenylalanine at amino acid position 508 (ΔF508). The remaining 30% of cases have a variety of other genetic lesions, including frameshifts, missense, and nonsense mutations. To some extent, the severity of clinical manifestations and the organ systems involved are related to the nature of the mutation. The ΔF508 mutation, the most common form, leads to a virtual absence of CFTR in the cell membrane and hence extreme impermeability to Cl⁻ ions. These patients have severe disease with early pancreatic insufficiency and variable degrees of respiratory disease. By contrast, some of the other, much less common, mutations give rise to Cl⁻ channels that allow relatively normal chloride transport; patients with such mutations may have male sterility (owing to obstruction of vas deferens) as the only manifestation of the disease.

MORPHOLOGY. The anatomic changes in CF are highly variable and depend on the type of mutation and hence the severity of expression of this genetic disorder. **Pancreatic abnormalities** are present in approximately 85% of patients. These abnormalities may consist only of accumulations of mucus, leading to dilation of ducts; in more advanced cases the ducts may become totally plugged, causing atrophy of the exocrine glands (Fig. 7–30); the islets of Langerhans are usually, but not always, spared. The ducts may be converted into cysts separated only by islets of Langerhans and an abundant fibrous stroma, a picture that gave rise to the designation *fibrocystic disease of the pancreas.* Loss of pancreatic secretion may lead to severe malabsorption, particularly of fats. A resultant lack of vitamin A, a fat-soluble vitamin, may then contribute to squamous metaplasia of the linings of the ducts. Changes similar to those in the pancreas may develop in the salivary glands. **Pulmonary lesions** are seen in almost every case and, with adequate treatment of the pancreatic problems, are the most serious aspect of this dis-

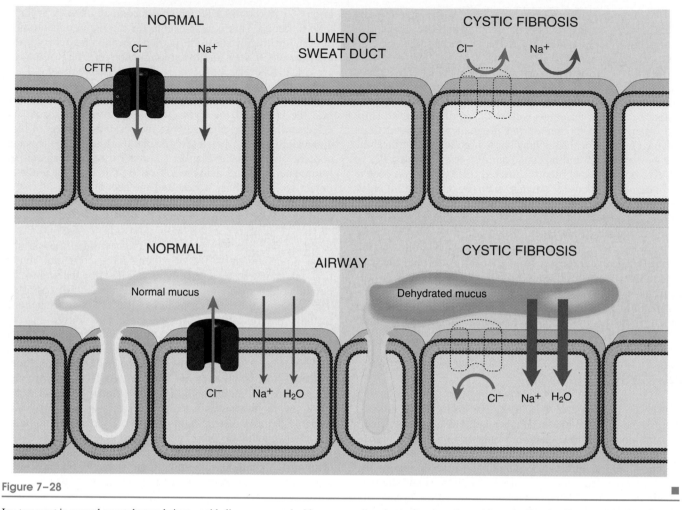

Figure 7–28 ■

Ion transport in normal sweat duct and airway epithelium, compared with corresponding tissues from a patient with cystic fibrosis. Absence of the Cl⁻ channel, cystic fibrosis transmembrane conductance regulator (CFTR), prevents reabsorption of Cl⁻ and therefore Na⁺ in the sweat duct, thus accounting for the high salt content of sweat. In the airways, failure of Cl⁻ secretion from the cells to the airspaces indirectly causes increased reabsorption of Na⁺ ions and water, rendering the mucus dehydrated.

ease. Retention of abnormally viscid mucin within the small airways leads to dilation of bronchioles and bronchi with secondary infection, so that severe chronic bronchitis, bronchiectasis, and lung abscesses (Chapter 13) are frequent sequelae. *Staphylococcus aureus* and *Pseudomonas aeruginosa* are the two pathogens most commonly isolated in CF patients. For reasons not clear, the mucoid form of *P. aeruginosa,* rarely found in persons who do not have CF, is found in more than 50% of those who have the disease. There is increasing frequency of infections with another microbe, *Burkholderia cepacia,* an opportunistic bacterium that is particularly difficult to eradicate. The subtended pulmonary parenchyma may undergo emphysema or atelectasis (Chapter 13). Obstruction of the small bowel secondary to impacted viscid mucin **(meconium ileus)** is not an uncommon complication in newborns. In approximately 25% of patients, inspissation of mucin within

the bile ducts impairs excretion of bile, adding to the malabsorption problems. In time, **biliary cirrhosis** (Chapter 16) may develop, but in only about 2% of patients. The ducts and glands of the male reproductive tract are commonly affected; obstruction of vas deferens, epididymis, and seminal vesicles results in azoospermia and sterility in more than 95% of CF males.

Clinical Features. The clinical manifestations of this condition are extremely varied and range from mild to severe and from onset at birth to onset years later. Approximately 5% to 10% of cases come to clinical attention at birth or soon after because of an attack of *meconium ileus.* More commonly, manifestations of *malabsorption* (e.g., large, foul stools; abdominal distention; and poor weight gain) appear during the first year of life. The faulty fat absorption may induce deficiency of the fat-soluble vitamins, resulting in manifestations

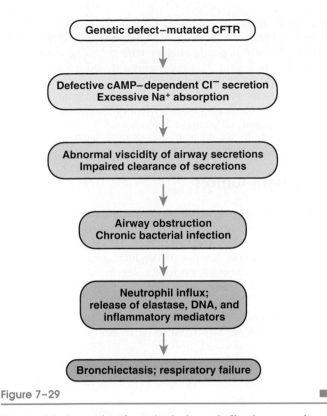

```
Genetic defect–mutated CFTR
            ↓
Defective cAMP–dependent Cl⁻ secretion
Excessive Na⁺ absorption
            ↓
Abnormal viscidity of airway secretions
Impaired clearance of secretions
            ↓
Airway obstruction
Chronic bacterial infection
            ↓
Neutrophil influx;
release of elastase, DNA, and
inflammatory mediators
            ↓
Bronchiectasis; respiratory failure
```

Figure 7–29 ■

Pathophysiologic sequelae of mutation in the cystic fibrosis transmembrane regulator (CFTR) gene, leading to bronchiectasis and respiratory failure. (Modified from Knowles MR, et al: Pharmacologic modulation of salt and water in the airway epithelium of cystic fibrosis. Am J Respir Crit Care Med 151 (Suppl 3):S65, 1995.)

of avitaminosis A, D, or K. If the child survives these hazards, *pulmonary problems* such as chronic cough, persistent lung infections, obstructive pulmonary disease, and cor pulmonale may make their appearance. Persistent pulmonary infections are responsible for 80% to 90% of the deaths. With improved control of infections, more patients are currently surviving to adulthood; median life expectancy is approximately 26 years.

The diagnosis of CF is based on clinical findings and the biochemical abnormalities in sweat. A properly administered and interpreted sweat test is crucial to the diagnosis. An increase in sweat electrolytes (often the mother makes the diagnosis because her infant tastes salty), along with one or more major clinical features, is necessary for diagnosis. Until recently there has been no reliable test for detection of heterozygotes or for antenatal diagnosis; however, because the CF gene has been cloned and more than two thirds of patients owe their disease to a single mutation, detection of carriers with the most common mutation is now possible. The number of mutations that can give rise to CF is very large, however, and therefore population-based screening studies are not feasible.

The treatment of CF is largely symptomatic, but gene therapy is on the horizon. Transfer of the CFTR gene into cells of CF patients corrects the Cl⁻ transport defect in vitro, and with suitable vectors it may be possible to devise effective strategies for transferring the gene in vivo.

TUMORS AND TUMOR-LIKE LESIONS OF INFANCY AND CHILDHOOD

Malignant neoplasms are the second most common cause of death in children between the ages of 4 and 14 years; only accidents exact a higher toll. Benign tumors are even more common than are cancers.

It is difficult to segregate, on morphologic grounds, true tumors from tumor-like lesions in the infant and child. In this context, two special categories of tumor-like lesions should be recognized.

■ *Heterotopia* and *choristoma* refer to microscopically normal cells or tissues that are present in abnormal locations. Examples of heterotopias include a rest of pancreatic tissue found in the wall of the stomach or small intestine, or a small mass of adrenal cells found in the kidney, lungs, ovaries, or elsewhere. Heterotopic rests are usually of little significance, but they can be confused clinically with neoplasms.

■ *Hamartoma* refers to an excessive but focal overgrowth of cells and tissues native to the organ in which it occurs. Although the cellular elements are mature and identical to those found in the remainder of the organ, they do not reproduce the normal architecture of the surrounding tissue. Hamartomas can be thought of as the linkage between

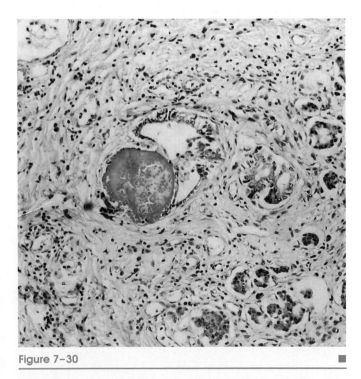

Figure 7–30 ■

Cystic fibrosis of the pancreas. A dilated duct plugged with inspissated mucin is seen in center field. The atrophic acini are completely replaced by fibrous tissue that contains several surviving islets of Langerhans. (Courtesy of Dr. Dennis Burns, Department of Pathology, University of Texas Southwestern Medical School, Dallas, TX.)

malformations and neoplasms. The line of demarcation between a hamartoma and a benign neoplasm is frequently tenuous and is variously interpreted. Hemangiomas, lymphangiomas, rhabdomyomas of the heart, and adenomas of the liver are considered by some to be hamartomas and by others to be true neoplasms.

Benign Tumors

Virtually any tumor may be encountered in the pediatric age group, but three—hemangiomas, lymphangiomas, and sacrococcygeal teratomas—deserve special mention here because they occur commonly in childhood.

Hemangiomas are the most common tumors of infancy. Architecturally, they do not differ from those encountered in adults (Chapter 10). In children, most are located in the skin, particularly on the face and scalp, where they produce flat to elevated, irregular, red-blue masses; some of the flat, larger lesions are referred to as *port wine stains*. Hemangiomas may enlarge along with the growth of the child, but in many instances they spontaneously regress (Fig. 7–31). In addition to their cosmetic significance, they can represent one facet of the hereditary disorder von Hippel–Lindau disease (Chapter 5).

Lymphangiomas represent the lymphatic counterpart of hemangiomas. They are characterized by cystic and cavernous spaces lined by endothelial cells and filled with pale fluid. They may occur on the skin but, more importantly, are also encountered in the deeper regions of the neck, axilla, mediastinum, and retroperitoneum. Although histologically benign, they tend to increase in size after birth and may encroach on mediastinal structures or nerve trunks in axilla.

Sacrococcygeal teratomas occur more frequently in females than in males (Fig. 7–32). In view of the overlap in the mechanisms underlying teratogenesis and oncogenesis, it is interesting that approximately 10% of sacrococcygeal teratomas are associated with congenital anomalies, primarily defects of the hindgut and cloacal region and other midline defects (e.g., meningocele, spina bifida) not believed to result from local effects of the tumor. Approximately 75% of these tumors are histologically mature with a benign course, and about 12% are unmistakably malignant and lethal (Chapter 18). The remainder are designated as immature teratomas, and their malignant potential correlates with the amount of immature tissue elements present. Most of the benign teratomas are encountered in younger infants (<4 months), whereas children with malignant lesions tend to be somewhat older.

Malignant Tumors

The organ systems involved most commonly by malignant neoplasms in infancy and childhood include the hematopoietic system, neural tissue, and soft tissues. This is in sharp contrast to adults, in whom tumors of the lung, heart, prostate, and colon are the most common forms. The most common malignant tumors of infancy and childhood are listed in Table 7–12.

Malignant tumors of infancy and childhood differ biologically and histologically from those in adults. The main differences are as follows:

- Relatively frequent demonstration of a close relationship between abnormal development (teratogenesis) and tumor induction (oncogenesis)
- Prevalence of underlying genetic aberrations
- Tendency of fetal and neonatal malignancies to spontaneously regress or cytodifferentiate
- Improved survival or cure of many childhood tumors, so that more attention is now being paid to minimizing the adverse delayed effects of chemotherapy and radiotherapy in survivors, including the development of second malignancies

Histologically, many malignant pediatric neoplasms are unique. In general, they tend to have a primitive (embryonal) rather than pleomorphic-anaplastic microscopic appearance, and frequently they exhibit features of organogenesis specific

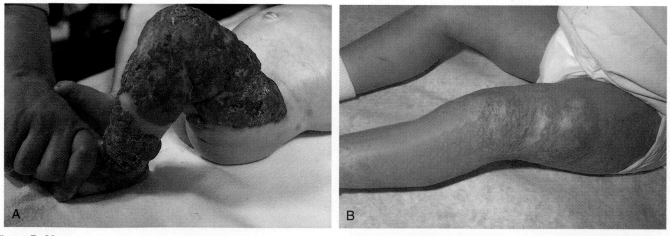

Figure 7–31

Congenital capillary hemangioma at birth (*A*) and at 2 years of age (*B*) after the lesion had undergone spontaneous regression. (Courtesy of Dr. Eduardo Yunis, Children's Hospital of Pittsburgh.)

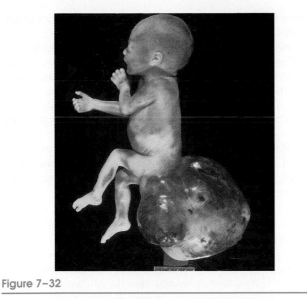

Figure 7–32   ■

Sacrococcygeal teratoma. Note the size of the lesion compared with that of the infant.

to the site of tumor origin. Because of their primitive histologic appearance, many childhood tumors have been collectively referred to as *small, round, blue cell tumors*. These are characterized by sheets of cells with small, round nuclei. The list of tumors in this category includes neuroblastoma, lymphoma, rhabdomyosarcoma, Ewing's sarcoma (peripheral neuroectodermal tumor), and occasionally Wilms' tumor. Rendering a definitive diagnosis is usually possible on the basis of histologic examination alone, but when necessary, clinical and radiographic findings, combined with ancillary studies (e.g., chromosome analysis, immunoperoxidase stains, and electron microscopy) are used. Three common tumors—neuroblastoma, retinoblastoma, and Wilms' tumor—are described here to highlight the differences between pediatric tumors and those in adults.

NEUROBLASTOMA

This neoplasm is one of the most common extracranial childhood solid tumors; it accounts for about 15% of all childhood cancer deaths. Most (80% to 90%) are found in children younger than 5 years, many in the first year of life.

Of neural crest origin, *neuroblastomas may arise anywhere in the sympathetic nervous system* from the head to the pelvis. About 75% arise within the abdomen: about half in the adrenal glands and the other half in the abdominal paravertebral autonomic ganglia. Similar neoplasms rarely arise in the brain. Most occur sporadically, but a few are familial with autosomal dominant transmission, and in such cases the neoplasms may involve both of the adrenals or multiple primary autonomic sites.

MORPHOLOGY. These tumors range from microscopic nodules (usually in infants) to masses that virtually fill the abdomen. Smaller tumors may appear to be circumscribed or even encapsulated,

but larger masses often grow into nearby organs (kidney, liver, pancreas). Advanced disease frequently invades the renal vein, often extending into the inferior vena cava. On cross-section they are gray-white, soft, and friable, and larger tumors often have areas of hemorrhage, necrosis, cystic degeneration, and calcification.

Histologically, the cells, growing in solid sheets, are round to ovoid and primitive looking with large, hyperchromatic nuclei surrounded by scant cytoplasm. It is evident that such total lack of differentiation makes it difficult to distinguish these neoplasms from other small, round, blue cell tumors. However, more characteristic features can often be identified in neuroblastomas: for example, rosettes (Homer Wright pseudorosettes), in which the tumor cells are arranged about the periphery of a central space filled with fibrillar extensions of the cells. Other helpful features are immunochemical reactions for neuron-specific enolase and small, membrane-bound, catecholamine-containing cytoplasmic secretory granules.

Some neoplasms show signs of differentiation. Clusters or scattered larger cells having more abundant cytoplasm with large vesicular nuclei, and a prominent nucleolus may be found in tumors composed largely of primitive neuroblasts. Even better differentiated lesions may contain many more large cells resembling neurons; such neoplasms merit the designation **ganglioneuroma.** Some tumors metastasize widely through the hematogenous and lymphatic systems, particularly to liver, lungs, and bones.

Staging of neuroblastomas (Table 7–13) assumes great importance in establishing a prognosis. Special note should be taken of stage IV-S, because, as will be seen, the outlook for these patients is excellent, despite the spread of disease.

Table 7–12.   COMMON MALIGNANT NEOPLASMS OF INFANCY AND CHILDHOOD

0–4 yr	5–9 yr	10–14 yr
Leukemia	Leukemia	
Retinoblastoma	Retinoblastoma	
Neuroblastoma	Neuroblastoma	
Wilms' tumor		
Hepatoblastoma	Hepatocarcinoma	Hepatocarcinoma
Soft tissue sarcoma (especially rhabdomyosarcoma)	Soft tissue sarcoma	Soft tissue sarcoma
Teratomas		
Central nervous system tumors	Central nervous system tumors	
	Ewing's tumor	
	Lymphoma	Osteogenic sarcoma
		Thyroid carcinoma
		Hodgkin's disease

Table 7–13. STAGING OF NEUROBLASTOMAS

Stage	
I	Tumor confined to organ of origin.
II	Tumor extends in continuity beyond organ of origin but does not cross midline. Ipsilateral lymph nodes may or may not be involved.
III	Tumor extends in continuity beyond the midline. Ipsilateral lymph nodes may or may not be involved.
IV	Metastatic disease to viscera, distant lymph nodes, soft tissue, and skeleton.
IV-S	Patients who would be stage I or II but who have distant disease of liver, skin, or bone marrow (without evidence of bone involvement).

From Silverman ML, Lee AK: Anatomy and pathology of the adrenal glands. Urol Clin North Am 16:417, 1989.

Clinical Course. In young children less than 2 years of age, neuroblastomas generally present with protuberant abdomen owing to an abdominal mass, fever, and weight loss. In older children they may remain unnoticed until metastases cause hepatomegaly, ascites, and bone pain. About 90% of neuroblastomas, regardless of location, produce catecholamines (similar to the catecholamines associated with pheochromocytomas), which are an important diagnostic feature (i.e., elevated blood levels of catecholamines and elevated urine levels of metabolites, vanillylmandelic acid [VMA], and homovanillic acid [HVA]). Despite the elaboration of catecholamines, hypertension is much less frequent with these neoplasms than with pheochromocytomas.

Many factors influence prognosis, but the most important are the stage of the tumor and the age of the patient. Children under 1 year of age have a much more favorable outlook than do older children at a comparable stage of disease. Most often in this age group the neoplasms are stage I or II. Stage IV-S is indeed special. As noted in Table 7–13, these patients would be classified as being in stage I or II but for the presence of metastases, which are limited to liver, skin, and bone marrow. Such infants have an excellent prognosis with minimal therapy. The biologic basis of this welcome behavior is not clear.

Molecular and genetic analysis of these tumors also provides prognostic information. Deletion of the short arm of chromosome 1 (1p32), resulting possibly in the loss of a tumor suppresser gene, is usually associated with aggressive disease. Amplification of the N-*myc* oncogene is also a harbinger of poor prognosis.

RETINOBLASTOMA

Retinoblastoma is the most common malignant eye tumor of childhood. From a pathologic as well as a clinical standpoint, retinoblastoma is unusual in several aspects when compared with most other solid tumors. Retinoblastoma can be multifocal and bilateral, it undergoes spontaneous regression, patients have a high incidence of second primary tumors, and it frequently occurs as a congenital tumor. The incidence decreases with age, most cases being diagnosed before the age of 4 years.

Retinoblastomas occur in both familial and sporadic patterns. *Familial cases typically develop multiple tumors that are bilateral,* although they may be unifocal and unilateral. Of the sporadic nonheritable tumors, all are unilateral and unifocal. Patients with familial retinoblastoma are also at increased risk for developing *osteosarcoma* and other soft tissue tumors.

As detailed in Chapter 6, retinoblastoma serves as a prototype of a diverse group of human cancers associated with recessive, loss-of-function mutations at distinct genetic loci harboring cancer suppressor genes.

MORPHOLOGY. Retinoblastoma is believed to arise from a cell of neuroepithelial origin, usually in the posterior retina. The tumors tend to be nodular masses, often with satellite seedings. On light microscopic examination, undifferentiated areas of these tumors are composed of small, round cells with large hyperchromatic nuclei and scant cytoplasm, resembling undifferentiated retinoblasts.

Differentiated structures are found within many retinoblastomas, the most characteristic of these being the rosettes described by Flexner and Wintersteiner (**Flexner-Wintersteiner rosettes,** Fig. 7–33). These structures consist of clusters of cuboidal or short columnar cells arranged around a central lumen. The nuclei are displaced away from the lumen, which by light microscopy appears to have a limiting membrane resembling the external limiting membrane of the retina.

Tumor cells may disseminate beyond the eye through the optic nerve or subarachnoid space. The most common sites of distant metastases are the central nervous system, skull, distal bones, and lymph nodes.

Clinical Features. The tumor may be present at birth, but most commonly it presents at 2 years of age. The presenting findings include poor vision, strabismus, a whitish hue to the pupil, and pain and tenderness in the eye. Approximately 60% to 70% of the tumors are associated with a germ-line mutation in the *Rb* gene and are hence heritable. The remaining 30% to 40% of the tumors develop sporadically. Untreated the tumors are usually fatal, but after early treatment with enucleation, chemotherapy, and radiotherapy, survival is the rule. As noted earlier, some tumors spontaneously regress, and patients with retinoblastoma are at increased risk for developing osteosarcoma and other soft tissue tumors.

WILMS' TUMOR

Wilms' tumor is the most common primary tumor of the kidney in children. Most cases occur between 2 and 5 years of age. This tumor illustrates several important concepts of childhood tumors: the relationship between congenital malformation and increased risk of tumors, the histologic simi-

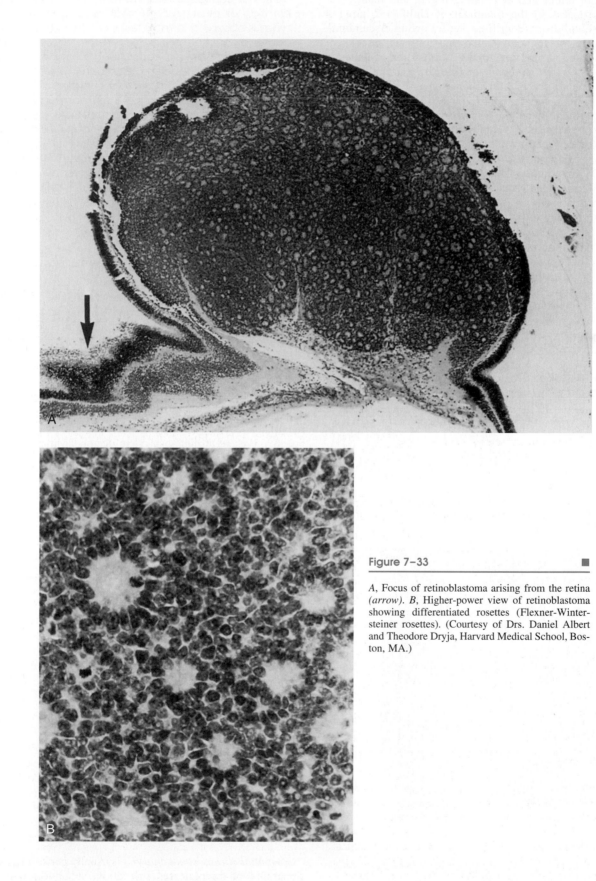

A, Focus of retinoblastoma arising from the retina *(arrow)*. *B*, Higher-power view of retinoblastoma showing differentiated rosettes (Flexner-Wintersteiner rosettes). (Courtesy of Drs. Daniel Albert and Theodore Dryja, Harvard Medical School, Boston, MA.)

larity between tumor and developing organ, and finally the remarkable success in the treatment of childhood tumors. Each of these will be evident from the following discussion.

Three groups of congenital malformations are associated with an increased risk of developing Wilms' tumor. Patients with the *WAGR syndrome*, characterized by *a*niridia, *g*enital abnormalities, and mental *r*etardation, have a 33% chance of developing Wilms' tumor. Both of these conditions are associated with loss of genetic material on chromosome 11p13, where the putative cancer suppressor gene WT-1 has been mapped. Another group of patients, those with the so-called *Denys-Drash syndrome*, also have an extremely high risk of developing Wilms' tumor. This syndrome is characterized by gonadal dysgenesis and renal abnormalities. The genetic abnormality in this group of patients has also been mapped to 11p13. A third group of patients, those afflicted by the *Beck-with-Wiedmann syndrome*, also has an increased risk of developing Wilms' tumor. These patients have enlargement of body organs, hemihypertrophy, renal cysts, and enlargement of adrenal cortical cells. The genetic locus involved in these patients is also on chromosome 11, but at 11p15.5. These associations suggest that in some cases congenital malformation and tumorigenesis represent related manifestations of genetic damage affecting a single gene or closely linked genes.

MORPHOLOGY. Grossly, Wilms' tumor tends to present as a large, solitary, well-circumscribed mass, although 10% are either bilateral or multicentric at the time of diagnosis. On cut section the tumor is soft, homogeneous, and tan to gray, with occasional foci of hemorrhage, cyst formation, and necrosis (Fig. 7–34).

Microscopically, Wilms' tumors are characterized by recognizable attempts to recapitulate different stages of nephrogenesis. The classic triphasic combination of blastemal, stromal, and epithelial cell types is observed in most lesions, although the percentage of each component is variable (Fig. 7–35). Epithelial "differentiation" is usually in the form of abortive tubules or glomeruli. Stromal cells are usually fibrocytic or myxoid in nature, although skeletal muscle "differentiation" is not uncommon. Rarely, other heterologous elements are identified, including squamous or mucinous epithelium, smooth muscle, adipose tissue, cartilage, and osteoid and neurogenic tissue. Approximately 5% of tumors contain foci of anaplasia (cells with large, hyperchromatic, pleomorphic nuclei and abnormal mitoses), the only histologic feature correlating with prognosis.

Clinical Course. Patients' complaints are usually referable to the tumor's enormous size. Commonly there is a readily palpable abdominal mass, which may extend across the midline and down into the pelvis. Less often, the patient presents with fever and abdominal pain, with hematuria or, occasionally, intestinal obstruction as a result of pressure from the tumor. The outlook for patients with Wilms' tumor is generally very good. Excellent results are obtained with a combination of radiotherapy, nephrectomy, and chemotherapy. Two-year survival rates are as high as 90%, and survival for 2 years usually implies a cure. These results are all the more remarkable because in many of these patients pulmonary metastases, present at diagnosis, may disappear after institution of the therapeutic regimen.

DIAGNOSIS OF GENETIC DISEASES

Diagnosis of genetic diseases requires examination of genetic material (i.e., chromosomes and genes). Hence, two general methods are employed: cytogenetic analysis and molecular analysis. Cytogenetic analysis requires karyotyping.

Prenatal chromosome analysis should be offered to all patients who are at risk of cytogenetically abnormal progeny. It can be performed on cells obtained by amniocentesis, on chorionic villus biopsy, or on umbilical cord blood. Some important indications are the following:

■ Advanced maternal age (>34 years) because of greater risk of trisomies
■ A parent who is a carrier of a balanced reciprocal translocation, robertsonian translocation, or inversion (in these cases the gametes may be unbalanced, and hence the progeny would be at risk for chromosomal disorders)
■ A previous child with a chromosomal abnormality
■ A parent who is a carrier of an X-linked genetic disorder (to determine fetal sex)

Postnatal chromosome analysis is usually performed on peripheral blood lymphocytes. Indications are as follows:

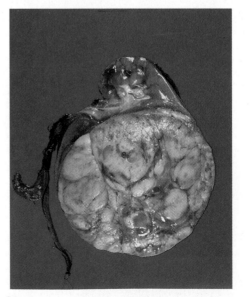

Figure 7–34

Wilms' tumor in the lower pole of the kidney with the characteristic tan-to-gray color and well-circumscribed margins.

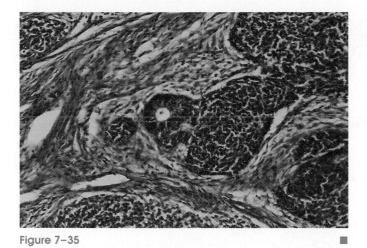

Figure 7-35   ■

Triphasic histology of Wilms' tumor with a stromal, less cellular area on the left, spindle-shaped cells, and epithelial (one clear tubule in the center) and blastemal (tightly packed blue cells) elements. (Courtesy of Dr. Charles Timmons, Department of Pathology, University of Texas Southwestern Medical School, Dallas, TX.)

■ Multiple congenital anomalies
■ Unexplained mental retardation and/or developmental delay
■ Suspected aneuploidy (e.g., features of Down syndrome)
■ Suspected unbalanced autosome (e.g., Prader-Willi syndrome)
■ Suspected sex chromosomal abnormality (e.g., Turner syndrome)
■ Suspected fragile X syndrome
■ Infertility (to rule out sex chromosomal abnormality)
■ Multiple spontaneous abortions (to rule out the parents as carriers of balanced translocation; both partners should be evaluated)

Many genetic diseases are caused by subtle changes in individual genes that cannot be detected by karyotyping. Traditionally, the diagnosis of single-gene disorders has depended on the identification of abnormal gene products (e.g., mutant hemoglobin or enzymes) or their clinical effects, such as anemia or mental retardation (e.g., phenylketonuria). Now it is possible to identify mutations at the level of DNA and offer gene diagnosis for several mendelian disorders. The use of recombinant DNA technology for the diagnosis of inherited diseases has several distinct advantages over other techniques:

■ It is remarkably sensitive. The amount of DNA required for diagnosis by molecular hybridization techniques can be readily obtained from 100,000 cells. Furthermore, the use of polymerase chain reaction (PCR) allows several million–fold amplification of DNA or RNA, making it possible to utilize as few as 1 or 100 cells for analysis. Tiny amounts of whole blood or even dried blood can supply sufficient DNA for PCR amplification.
■ DNA-based tests are not dependent on a gene product that may be produced only in certain specialized cells (e.g., brain) or expression of a gene that may occur late in life. Because virtually all normal cells of the body contain the same DNA in inherited genetic disorders, each postzygotic cell carries the mutant gene.

These two features have profound implications for the prenatal diagnosis of genetic diseases, because a sufficient number of cells can be obtained from a few milliliters of amniotic fluid or from a biopsy of chorionic villus that can be performed as early as the first trimester.

There are two distinct approaches to the diagnosis of single-gene diseases by recombinant DNA technology: direct detection of mutations, and indirect detection based on linkage of the disease gene with a harmless "marker gene." These two methods are described below.

Direct Gene Diagnosis

Victor McKusick, an eminent geneticist, has appropriately called direct gene diagnosis the *diagnostic biopsy of the human genome*. Such diagnosis depends on the detection of an important qualitative change in the DNA. There are two variations of direct gene diagnosis.

One technique relies on the fact that some mutations alter or destroy certain restriction sites on the normal DNA. For example, in the normal β-globin gene (HbA) there are three sites that are recognized by the restriction enzyme Mst II (Fig. 7-36). The sickle mutation responsible for sickle cell anemia (Chapter 12) involves a single base pair change (A $\rightarrow$ T) that abolishes one of the three MST II sites. When DNA from a normal individual is digested with Mst II and hybridized with the radioactive complementary DNA (cDNA) probe specific for the β-globin gene, a single 1.15-kb band that reacts with the probe is detected on Southern blot analysis (such a band results from the formation of identical 1.15-kb fragments from each of the two normal chromosomes). On the other hand, a similar analysis of DNA from the cells of a patient homozygous for the sickle cell hemoglobin (HbS) gene leads to the formation of a single larger (1.35-kb) fragment, owing to the loss of the Mst II sites from both chromosomes. In heterozygotes, the normal chromosome yields a 1.15-kb band, whereas the chromosome carrying the mutation gives rise to the 1.35-kb band. Thus, Southern blot analysis reveals two different-sized bands, allowing detection of a heterozygote carrier.

If the mutation does not alter any known restriction site, an alternative approach based on the use of allele-specific oligonucleotides can be utilized (Fig. 7-37). For example, many cases of α_1-antitrypsin (α_1-AT) deficiency are due to a single G $\rightarrow$ A change in the α_1-AT gene, producing the so-called Z allele (Chapter 13). Two oligonucleotides, having at their center the single base by which the normal and mutant gene differ, are synthesized. Such allele-specific oligonucleotides can then be used as radiolabeled probes in a Southern blot analysis. The oligonucleotide containing the sequence of the normal gene hybridizes with both the normal and the mutant DNA, but hybridization to the mutant DNA is unstable, owing to the single base pair mismatch. Thus, under stringent conditions of hybridization, the labeled normal probe produces a strong autoradiographic signal with DNA from a normal individual, no signal in the DNA extracted from a patient homozygous for the mutant gene, and a faint signal with DNA from a heterozygote. With the probe containing the mutant sequence, the pattern of hybridization is reversed. Of course,

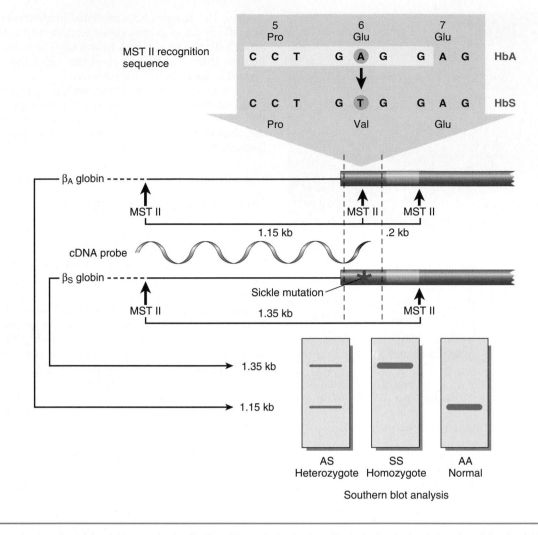

Figure 7–36 ■

Direct gene diagnosis: detection of the sickle mutation by Southern blot analysis. An A → T substitution in the sixth codon of the β_A globin gene yields the β_S allele. This substitution eliminates an Mst II recognition site in the β-globin DNA. Thus, when digested with Mst II and probed with an appropriate cDNA, the β_S allele generates a 1.35-kb fragment rather than the normal 1.15-kb fragment.

heterozygotes react with both probes because they carry one normal and one mutant gene.

PCR Analysis. This method, whereby a DNA sequence can be greatly amplified, is now widely used in molecular diagnosis. If RNA is used as the starting material, it is first reverse transcribed (RT) to obtain cDNA and then amplified by PCR. This method is often abbreviated as RT-PCR.

As with the other methods of direct gene diagnosis, the sequence of the normal gene must be known. To detect the mutant gene, two primers that bind to the 3′ and 5′ ends of the normal sequence are designed. By utilizing appropriate DNA polymerases and thermal cycling, the target DNA is greatly amplified, producing millions of copies of the DNA sequence between the two primer sites. If the specific mutation is known to affect a restriction site, then the amplified DNA can be digested. Because the mutation affects a restriction site, the mutant and normal alleles will give rise to products of different sizes. These would appear as different bands on agarose gel electrophoresis. If, on the other hand, the sequence

of the normal gene is known but that of the mutant allele is unknown, the vastly amplified DNA obtained from the patient can be sequenced by conventional methods. By comparison with the sequence of the normal gene, the disease-causing mutation can be pinpointed.

PCR analysis is also very useful when a mutation is associated with deletions or expansions. As discussed earlier, several diseases, such as the fragile X syndrome, are associated with trinucleotide repeats. Figure 7–38 reveals how PCR analysis can be used to detect this mutation. Two primers that bind to a sequence at the 5′ end of the FMR-1 gene, which is affected by trinucleotide repeats, are used to amplify the intervening sequences. Because there are large differences in the number of repeats, the size of the PCR products obtained from the DNA of normal individuals, or those with premutation, is quite different. These size differences are revealed by differential migration of the amplified DNA products on a gel. Currently the full mutation cannot be detected by PCR analysis because the affected segment of

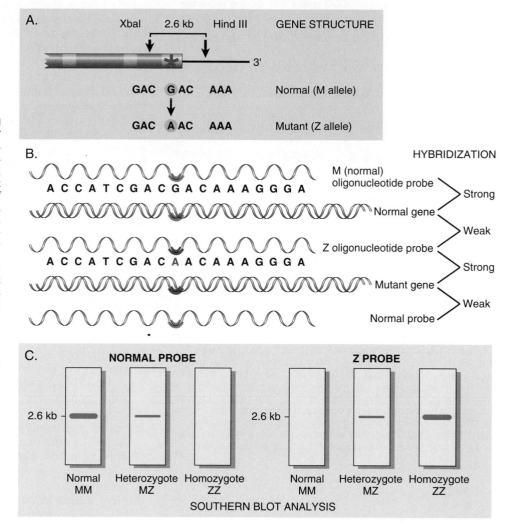

Figure 7-37 ■

Direct gene diagnosis by using an oligonucleotide probe, and Southern blot analysis. *A,* A G → A change converts a normal α₁-antitrypsin allele (allele M) to a mutant Z allele. This change involves exon V of the α₁-antitrypsin gene, which lies between restriction sites for the enzymes Xba I and Hind III. *B,* The principle of oligonucleotide probe analysis. Two synthetic oligonucleotide probes, one corresponding in sequence to the normal allele (M allele probe) and the other corresponding to the mutant allele (Z allele probe), are lined up against normal and mutant genes, and the expected pattern of hybridization with different combinations is indicated on the right. *C,* The results of Southern blot analysis when DNA from normal individuals or those heterozygous or homozygous for the mutant Z allele is digested (with Xba I and Hind III) and probed with the normal (M) or Z oligonucleotide probe.

DNA is too large for conventional PCR. In such cases, a Southern blot analysis of genomic DNA has to be performed (Fig. 7–38).

Linkage Analysis

Direct gene diagnosis is possible only if the mutant gene and its normal counterpart have been identified and cloned and their nucleotide sequences are known. In a large number of genetic diseases, including some that are relatively common, information about the gene sequence is lacking. Therefore, alternative strategies must be employed to track the mutant gene on the basis of its linkage to detectable genetic markers. In essence, one has to determine whether a given fetus or family member has inherited the same relevant chromosomal region(s) as a previously affected family member. It follows, therefore, that the success of such a strategy depends on the ability to distinguish the chromosome that carries the mutation from its normal homologous counterpart. This is accomplished by exploiting naturally occurring variations in DNA sequences that give rise to so-called restriction fragment length polymorphisms (RFLPs). Because RFLPs form the backbone of indirect DNA diagnosis, they will be discussed briefly.

Examination of DNA from any two persons will reveal variations in the DNA sequences involving approximately one nucleotide in every 200 to 500 base pair stretch. Most of these variations occur in noncoding regions of the DNA and are hence phenotypically silent; however, these single–base pair changes may abolish or create recognition sites for restriction enzymes, thereby altering the length of DNA fragments produced after digestion with certain restriction enzymes. Using appropriate DNA probes that hybridize with sequences in the vicinity of the polymorphic sites, it is possible to detect the DNA fragments of different lengths by Southern blot analysis. To summarize, the term *restriction fragment length polymorphism* refers to variation in fragment length between individuals that results from DNA sequence polymorphisms.

With this background, we can discuss how RFLPs can be used in gene tracking. Figure 7–39 illustrates the principle of RFLP analysis. In this example of an autosomal recessive disease, both of the parents are heterozygote carriers and the children are normal, are carriers, or are affected. In the illus-

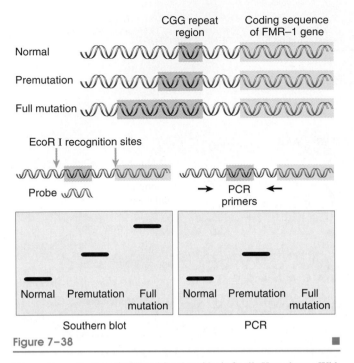

Figure 7–38 ■

Diagnostic application of PCR and Southern blot in fragile X syndrome. With PCR, the differences in the size of CGG repeat between normal and pre-mutation give rise to products of different sizes and mobility. With a full mutation, the region between the primers is too large to be amplified by conventional PCR. In Southern blot analysis the DNA is cut by enzymes that flank the CGG repeat region and is then probed with a complementary DNA that binds to the affected part of the gene. A single small band is seen in normal males, a higher-molecular-weight band in males with premutation, and a very large (usually diffuse) band in those with the full mutation.

trated example, the normal chromosome (A) has two restriction sites, 7.6-kb apart, whereas chromosome B, which carries the mutant gene, has a DNA sequence polymorphism resulting in the creation of an additional (third) restriction site for the same enzyme. Note that the additional restriction site has not resulted from the mutation. When DNA from such an individual is digested with the appropriate restriction enzyme and probed with a cloned DNA fragment that hybridizes with a stretch of sequences between the restriction sites, the normal chromosome yields a 7.6-kb band, whereas the other chromosome (carrying the mutant gene) produces a smaller, 6.8-kb, band. Thus, on Southern blot analysis two bands are noted. It is possible by this technique to distinguish family members who have inherited both normal chromosomes from those who are heterozygous or homozygous for the mutant gene.

To summarize, RFLP analysis makes it possible to track the transmission of a single chromosome region through a family and to see if a particular single-gene disease is co-inherited with a polymorphic site. It is therefore possible to utilize this method for antenatal diagnosis by examining fetal DNA. However, because the probe does not identify the disease gene itself, certain limitations become apparent:

■ First, for prenatal diagnosis several relevant family members must be available for testing. A DNA sample from a previously affected child is necessary to determine the RFLP pattern that is associated with the homozygous genotype.
■ Second, key family members must be heterozygous for an RFLP (i.e., the two homologous chromosomes must be distinguishable). This may require the use of multiple restriction enzymes and several different probes for closely linked genes.
■ Third, normal exchange of chromosomal material between homologous chromosomes (recombination) during game-

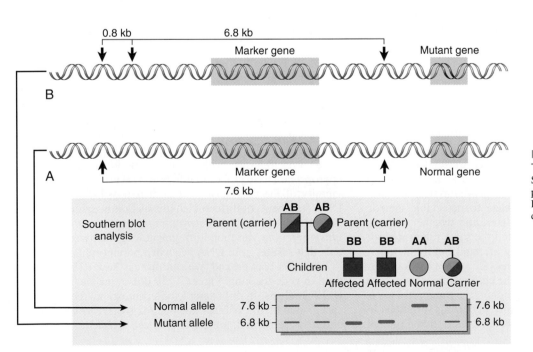

Figure 7–39 ■

Schematic illustration of the principles underlying restriction fragment length polymorphism analysis in the diagnosis of genetic diseases.

togenesis may lead to "separation" of the mutant gene from the polymorphism pattern with which it had been previously coinherited. This may lead to an erroneous genetic prediction in a subsequent pregnancy. Obviously, the closer the linkage, the smaller is the likelihood of recombination and thus of a false result. Such errors can also be reduced by utilizing probes on both (3′ and 5′) sides of the mutation.

RFLPs have been useful in the antenatal diagnosis of CF, Huntington disease, and adult polycystic kidney disease, among others. It is obvious that when a disease gene is identified and cloned, direct gene diagnosis becomes the preferred method.

BIBLIOGRAPHY

Barlow DP: Gametic imprinting in mammals. Science 270:1610, 1995. (A discussion of the process of imprinting and its consequences.)

Francke U, Furthmayr H: Marfan syndrome and other disorders of fibrillin. N Engl J Med 330:1384, 1994. (A short editorial on the molecular basis of Marfan syndrome.)

Green DM, et al: Wilms' tumor. CA Cancer J Clin 46:46, 1996. (An excellent review that covers epidemiology, genetics, clinical features, and treatment of Wilms' tumor.)

Jennings C: How trinucleotide repeats may function. Nature 378:127, 1995. (A short commentary on the mechanisms by which trinucleotide repeat mutations may cause disease, with a focus on Huntington disease.)

Johns DR: Mitochondrial DNA and disease. N Engl J Med 333:638, 1995. (An excellent review of diseases caused by inheritance of mitochondrial DNA.)

Knowles MR, et al: Pharmacologic modulation of salt and water in the airway epithelium in cystic fibrosis. Am J Respir Crit Care Med 151 (Suppl 3): S65, 1995. (This entire supplement covers the genetics, molecular basis, and gene therapy of CF.)

Korf B: Molecular diagnosis (in two parts). N Engl J Med 332:1218, 1995, and 332:1499, 1995. (An easy-to-understand primer of modern methods of molecular diagnosis.)

Laxova R: Fragile X syndrome. Adv Pediatr 41:305, 1994. (A detailed review of the cytogenetic, molecular, and clinical features of fragile X syndrome.)

Lazoff M, Kauffman F: Sudden infant death syndrome—part I: general features. Acad Emerg Med 2:926, 1995. (A comprehensive and well-written discussion of SIDS.)

Matthay KK: Neuroblastoma: a clinical challenge and biologic puzzle. CA Cancer J Clin 45:179, 1995. (An easy-to-read and up-to-date discussion of neuroblastomas.)

Nicholls RD: New insights reveal complex mechanisms involved in genomic imprinting. Am J Hum Genet 54:733, 1994. (A scholarly and detailed article on the mechanisms of genomic imprinting for the advanced reader.)

Singer RH: Triplet repeats and human disease. Molecular Medicine Today 2:65, 1996. (An excellent and brief review of the pathogenesis of triplet repeat mutations in human disease.)

Verma RP: Respiratory distress syndrome of the newborn infant. Obstet Gynecol Surv 50:542, 1995. (An excellent review of the pathogenesis and clinical features of RDS in the newborn.)

Warren ST: The expanding world of trinucleotide repeats. Science 271:1374, 1996. (A broad list of human diseases caused by trinucleotide repeat mutations and the general features of such expansions.)

Welsh MJ, Smith AE: Cystic fibrosis. Sci Am 273:52, 1995. (A clearly written article on the molecular basis and symptomatology of cystic fibrosis.)

8

Environmental Diseases

The contributions made by Dr. Mary F. Lipscomb to the Environmental
Diseases chapter in the previous edition of this book are gratefully acknowledged.

Environmental pathology theoretically could encompass the study of all diseases that are not entirely genetic. Furthermore, even the expression of inherited disorders can be influenced by environmental factors. Recognizing, however, that very few diseases are purely environmental or genetic, we will limit our discussion to some general concepts and illustrative diseases that develop from (1) pollution of the environment, particularly of air; (2) use and abuse of drugs and physical agents, including radiation; and (3) over- or undernutrition. The discussion begins with an overview of environmental pollution and then turns to air pollution and its impact on the lungs.

ENVIRONMENTAL POLLUTION

Microorganisms contaminating food and water have long been a major cause of morbidity and mortality in third world countries; in recent years, concerns about contamination of food and water by pesticides and industrial waste are increasing worldwide. Air is polluted in many communities by industrial waste or the products of automobile exhausts.

A *pollutant* is an agent in the environment that can cause disease in those who are exposed. Thus, agents that are "naturally" present but in abnormal quantities, such as ozone, may be considered pollutants just as well as those that are not naturally present, such as polychlorinated biphenyls (PCBs). Pollutants produce disease by several mechanisms. Acute toxicity may be produced directly, when an agent induces inflammation or necrosis, or indirectly, when an immune response causes a hypersensitivity reaction. These acute reactions are referred to as *proximal effects* of the pollutant. More difficult to study, and therefore to evaluate, are the distal effects of pollutants. These may take such forms as subclinical chronic inflammation and fibrosis, resulting from ongoing toxic effects and/or hypersensitivity reactions, or degenerative changes that lead to organ malfunction, as might occur in the central nervous system of children with chronic lead toxicity. The effects of a number of chemicals that may contaminate food and water are discussed with nontherapeutic agents later in this chapter. A discussion of the health consequences of air pollution follows.

Air Pollution

Air pollution has been a continuing problem in industrialized areas. Smog, the visible accumulation of air pollutants, is particularly heavy in cities where coal combustion is a source of energy and in certain communities where automobile exhaust fumes accumulate. Coal combustion results in release into the air of sulfur oxides and particulates (a so-called reducing smog). This form of smog is common in the northeastern United States and in some European cities. In the past, high levels of sulfur oxides and particulates have been clearly linked to increased morbidity and mortality, especially among persons with preexisting lung disease. "Photochemical oxidant smog" results when incompletely burned hydrocarbons release carbon monoxide (CO), carbon dioxide (CO_2), and nitrogen oxides. The action of sunlight on these primary pollutants leads to the release of secondary pollutants, including ozone and free radicals with oxidizing properties. This type of pollution occurs in cities such as Los Angeles, California. The effects of such pollution on morbidity and mortality are difficult to document. It seems, however, that *small decrements in pulmonary function occur in persons who inhabit areas where this form of pollution is heavy.*

Although air pollutants can affect many organ systems (e.g., lead absorbed through the respiratory tract can produce extrapulmonary disease, discussed later), the lung itself usually bears the brunt and is particularly vulnerable when there is underlying lung disease, especially chronic obstructive lung disease (Chapter 13).

The pulmonary changes seen with various air pollutants range from minor irritation to the initiation of debilitating fibrotic disease to the induction of cancer (Table 8–1). Except for the pneumoconioses, which will be discussed in this chapter, and some general comments on smoking, all pollutant-caused lung diseases are discussed in Chapter 13.

The following factors determine whether an air pollutant causes lung injury and what form the injury takes:

■ *Solubility in water.* A water-soluble molecule such as sulfur dioxide (SO_2) is dissolved readily in secretions in the upper air passages. This effect is referred to as the *scrubbing* action of the upper air passages and results in protection of the lower air passages.

■ *Particle size and airway anatomy.* Particles greater than 5 or 10 μm are unlikely to reach distal airways, whereas particulates smaller than 0.5 μm tend to act like gases and move in and out of the alveoli, often without substantial deposition or injury. Particles that are 1 to 5 μm are the most dangerous, because they impact at bifurcations of the distal airways.

■ *Concentration and chemical reactivity.* Low concentrations of SO_2 (< 0.1 ppm) produce only eye irritation. Concentrations in the range of 2 to 5 ppm (found in smog under some conditions) overcome the scrubbing action of the nose and cause increased airway resistance. Very high levels (> 20 ppm), achieved under experimental conditions, result in decreased mucociliary clearance and even pulmonary edema.

■

Table 8–1. PATTERNS OF LUNG INJURY RELATED TO AIR POLLUTION

Lung Response	Pathogenic Mechanisms
Acute or chronic inflammation (e.g., chronic bronchitis)	Direct cell injury
Emphysema	Enhanced proteolysis
Asthma	Allergic or irritant effect
Hypersensitivity pneumonitis	Immunologic injury
Pneumoconiosis	Fibrotic reactions caused by cytokines released from macrophages and other recruited leukocytes
Neoplasia	Mutagenic and promoting effects

■ *Duration of exposure.* The longer the period of exposure to a pollutant continuously present in air, the greater the accumulation in the lungs. This is an important factor in occupational exposures that result in pneumoconiosis. Because even those who work outside the home spend more than 50% of their time in their homes, the pollution of the air inside the home can be an important problem. The list of indoor air pollutants is long. Some examples include formaldehyde derived from formaldehyde foam insulation (a possible cause of allergic reactions); radon and radon daughters (as risk factors for lung cancer); nitric oxide (NO), nitrous oxide (NO_2), and CO derived from gas ranges and their pilot lights (possible causes of respiratory irritation and CO poisoning); and asbestos used in building insulation (possible cause of lung fibrosis and cancer).

■ *Host clearance mechanisms.* The decreased capacity to clear inhaled particles that occurs in lung diseases such as emphysema, chronic bronchitis, and cystic fibrosis leads to higher accumulations of potentially toxic substances in the lungs.

Table 8–2. EFFECTS OF SELECTED TOBACCO SMOKE CONSTITUENTS

Substance	Effect
Tar	Carcinogenesis
Polycyclic aromatic hydrocarbons	Carcinogenesis
Nicotine	Ganglionic stimulation and depression, tumor promotion
Phenol	Tumor promotion and irritation
Benzopyrene	Carcinogenesis
Carbon monoxide	Impaired oxygen transport and utilization
Formaldehyde	Toxicity to cilia and irritation
Oxides of nitrogen	Toxicity to cilia and irritation
Nitrosamine	Carcinogenesis

Tobacco Smoke

Of all air pollutants, tobacco smoke is the one associated with the highest prevalence of disease. On the basis of a large 40-year study of male physicians in Great Britain, it is estimated that about 50% of all regular cigarette smokers will die of smoking-related diseases. For more than 30 years, the U.S. Surgeon General has identified tobacco smoking as the single most common cause of preventable mortality. Happily, during this time the percentage of adults who smoke has decreased from 43% to 30%. Nevertheless, the number of smokers remains large, and it appears that the smoke inhaled by nonsmoking bystanders also has adverse health effects. The following discussion summarizes the detrimental effects of cigarette smoking, the reversal of these effects with cessation of smoking, and the evidence that passive smoke inhalation is also injurious to health. It should be noted that even though cigarette smoking is the prime culprit, pipe and cigar smoking, albeit less hazardous, are not without risk.

The number of potentially noxious chemicals in tobacco smoke is extraordinary. Table 8–2 provides only a partial list and includes the likely mechanism by which each of these agents produces injury. This injury translates into a number of important diseases (Fig. 8–1), all of which are discussed in detail in later chapters. However, we should point out here the mechanisms for the most important diseases caused by cigarette smoke.

Emphysema, chronic bronchitis, and lung cancer are common lung diseases, and cigarette smoking is by far the most common cause of these disorders. Agents in smoke have a direct irritant effect on the tracheobronchial mucosa, producing inflammation and increased mucus production (bronchitis). Cigarette smoke also results in the recruitment of leukocytes to the lung and increased local elastase production, with subsequent injury to lung tissue and emphysema. Components of cigarette smoke, particularly tars, are potent mutagens and cancer promoters, so that 85% of cancers in the lung arising from the bronchial epithelium (bronchogenic carcinoma) are related to cigarette smoking. The risk for development of these three diseases is related to the dose of exposure, frequently expressed in terms of "pack years" (e.g., one pack daily for 20 years equals 20 pack years).

In addition to lung disease, *atherosclerosis and its major complication, myocardial infarction, have also been strongly linked to cigarette smoking;* causal mechanisms likely relate to several factors, including increased platelet aggregation, decreased myocardial oxygen supply (because of significant lung disease) accompanied by an increased oxygen demand, and a decreased threshold for ventricular fibrillation.

As might be expected, cessation of smoking leads to substantial benefits. The 1990 U.S. Surgeon General's report summarized the data on this issue. The overall risk of dying in individuals of all ages is increased if the individuals smoke but is reduced somewhat within a year after quitting. The risk continues to decrease for at least 15 years, which is the extent of time for which data are currently available. Not shown in Figure 8–1 is the effect of smoking on the unborn fetus. Maternal smoking increases the risk of spontaneous abortions and still births and results in intrauterine growth retardation (Chapter 7); birth weights of infants born to mothers who stopped smoking before pregnancy are normal.

Breathing sidestream smoke *(passive smoke inhalation)* is also associated with some of the same detrimental effects that result from active smoking. It is estimated that the relative risk of lung cancer in nonsmokers exposed to environmental smoke is about 1.5 times that of nonsmokers who are not exposed to smoke. While this increase in risk may appear small, it translates into a significant health hazard. The U.S. Environmental Protection Agency estimates that in the United States, approximately 3000 lung cancer deaths in nonsmokers over the age of 35 years can be attributed each year to environmental tobacco smoke. Even more striking is the increased risk of coronary atherosclerosis and fatal myocardial infarction. Recent studies estimate that every year 30,000 to 60,000 cardiac deaths in the United States are associated with exposure to passive smoke. Children living in households with an adult who smokes show an increased incidence of respiratory illnesses and asthma.

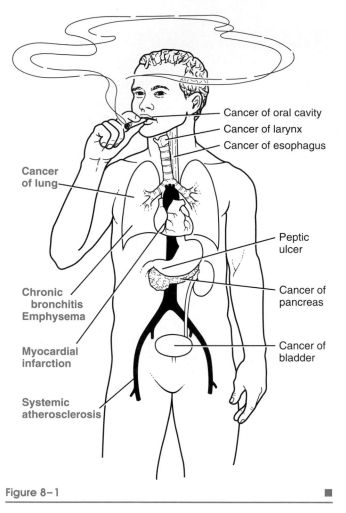

Cancer of oral cavity
Cancer of larynx
Cancer of esophagus

Cancer of lung

Peptic ulcer

Chronic bronchitis Emphysema

Cancer of pancreas

Myocardial infarction

Cancer of bladder

Systemic atherosclerosis

Figure 8–1 ■

Adverse effects of smoking: the more common on the left and the somewhat less common on the right.

Pneumoconioses

Pneumoconiosis is a term originally coined to describe the non-neoplastic lung reaction to inhalation of mineral dusts. The term has been broadened to include diseases induced by organic as well as inorganic particulates, and some experts also regard chemical fume- and vapor-induced non-neoplastic lung diseases as pneumoconioses.

The mineral dust pneumoconioses—the four most common result from exposure to coal dust, silica, asbestos, and beryllium—nearly always result from exposure in the workplace. However, the increased risk of cancer as a result of asbestos exposure extends to family members of asbestos workers and to other individuals exposed to asbestos outside the workplace. Table 8–3 indicates the pathologic conditions associated with each mineral dust and the major industries in which the dust exposure is sufficient to produce disease.

Pathogenesis. The reaction of the lung to mineral dusts depends on factors previously discussed, including size, shape, solubility, and reactivity of the particles. Coal dust is relatively inert, and large amounts must be deposited in the lungs before lung disease is clinically detectable. Silica, asbestos, and beryllium are more reactive than coal dust, resulting in fibrotic reactions at lower concentrations. A unifying concept for the development of lesions in all pneumoconioses is depicted in Figure 8–2. Most inhaled dust is removed by entrapment in the mucous blanket and rapid removal from the lung by ciliary movement. However, some of the particles become impacted at alveolar duct bifurcations, where macrophages accumulate and endocytose the impacted particulates. The more reactive particulates trigger the macrophage to release a number of products that are toxic to the lung, mediating an inflammatory response and initiating fibroblast proliferation and collagen deposition. Important macrophage mediators for tissue damage, inflammatory cell recruitment, and fibroblast growth stimulation include (1) oxygen radicals and proteases; (2) leukotriene B_4 (LTB_4) and the cytokines interleukin 8 (IL-8), MIP-1α, tumor necrosis factor α (TNF-α), and interleukin 6 (IL-6), which recruit and activate inflammatory cells; and (3) the cytokines IL-1, TNF-α, fibronectin, platelet-derived growth factor (PDGF), and insulin-like growth factor 1 (IGF-1), which induce fibrogenesis. Some of the particles may be taken up by epithelial cells or cross the epithelial cell lining and interact directly with fibroblasts and interstitial macrophages. Some may reach the lymphatics either by direct drainage or within migrating macrophages and thereby initiate an immune response to components of the particulates and/or to self proteins, modified by the particles. This then leads to an amplification and

■

Table 8–3. MINERAL DUST–INDUCED LUNG DISEASE

Agent	Disease	Exposure
Coal dust	Simple coal workers' pneumoconiosis: macules and nodules	Coal mining
	Complicated coal workers' pneumoconiosis: PMF, Caplan's syndrome	
Silica	Acute silicosis, chronic silicosis, PMF, Caplan's syndrome	Sandblasting, quarrying, mining, stone cutting, foundry work, ceramics
Asbestos	Asbestosis, Caplan's syndrome, pleural effusions, pleural plaques, or diffuse fibrosis, mesothelioma, carcinoma of the lung, larynx, stomach, colon	Mining, milling, and fabrication of ores and materials; installation and removal of insulation
Beryllium	Acute berylliosis, beryllium granulomatosis	Nuclear energy and aircraft industries

PMF, progressive massive fibrosis.

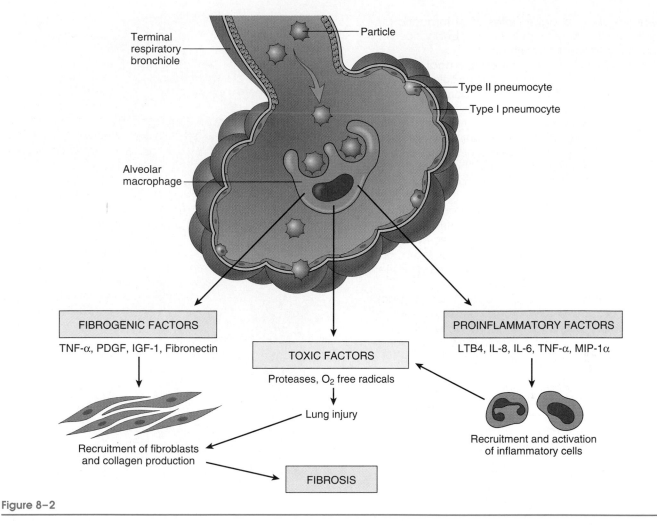

Figure 8–2   ■

Pathogenesis of pneumoconiosis. Inhaled particulates usually impact at the bifurcations of terminal respiratory bronchioles, where they are engulfed by alveolar macrophages, which are then stimulated to secrete (1) various fibrogenic factors that recruit fibroblasts and induce collagen synthesis, (2) toxic factors that initiate lung injury directly, and (3) proinflammatory factors that recruit additional inflammatory cells.

extension of the local reaction. Tobacco smoking worsens the effects of all inhaled mineral dusts, and more so with asbestos than with any other particle.

COAL WORKERS' PNEUMOCONIOSIS

A number of British novels, including D. H. Lawrence's *Sons and Lovers,* poignantly describe the tragedy of the coal miners at the turn of the century who toiled lifelong underground, only to die of "black lung" complicated by tuberculosis. Dust reduction in the coal mines has drastically reduced the incidence of coal dust–induced disease. The spectrum of lung findings in coal workers is wide, ranging from *asymptomatic anthracosis,* in which pigment accumulates without a perceptible cellular reaction, to *simple coal workers' pneumoconiosis* (CWP), in which cellular accumulations of macrophages occur with little to no pulmonary dysfunction, and *complicated CWP* or *progressive massive fibrosis* (PMF), in which fibrosis is extensive and lung function is compromised (Table 8–3). Although statistics vary, it appears that fewer than 10% of cases of simple CWP progress to PMF. It should

be noted that PMF is a generic term that applies to a confluent fibrosing reaction in the lung; this can be a complication of any one of the four pneumoconioses discussed here.

The pathogenesis of both simple and complicated CWP is incompletely understood. In particular, it is not clear what causes the lesions of simple CWP to progress to PMF. Contaminating silica in coal mine dust has been suggested to favor progressive disease; recent evidence suggests, however, that complex interactions of different compounds in coal mine dust, rather than silica alone, are responsible for PMF.

MORPHOLOGY. Pulmonary anthracosis is the most innocuous coal-induced pulmonary lesion in coal miners and is also commonly seen in all urban dwellers and tobacco smokers. Inhaled carbon pigment is engulfed by alveolar or interstitial macrophages, which then accumulate in the connective tissue along the lymphatics, including the pleural lymphatics, or in organized lymphoid tissue along the bronchi or in the lung hilus. At autopsy, linear streaks and aggregates of anthracotic pigment readily identify pulmonary lymphatics and mark the pulmonary lymph nodes.

Simple CWP is characterized by **coal macules** and the somewhat larger **coal nodule.** The coal macule consists of dust-laden macrophages; the nodule in addition contains small amounts of a delicate network of collagen fibers. Although these lesions are scattered throughout the lung, the upper lobes and upper zones of the lower lobes are more heavily involved. They are primarily located adjacent to respiratory bronchioles, the site of initial coal dust accumulation. In due course, dilation of adjacent alveoli occurs, a condition sometimes referred to as **centrilobular emphysema.** However, by definition emphysema is associated with destruction of alveolar septa, and whether this occurs in primary CWP has not been clearly demonstrated.

Complicated CWP (PMF) occurs on a background of simple CWP and generally requires many years to develop. It is characterized by intensely blackened scars larger than 2 cm, sometimes up to 10 cm in greatest diameter. They are usually multiple (Fig. 8–3). Microscopically the lesions consist of dense collagen and pigment. The center of the lesion is often necrotic, resulting most likely from ischemia.

Caplan's syndrome is defined as the coexistence of rheumatoid arthritis with a pneumoconiosis, leading to the development of distinctive nodular pulmonary lesions that develop fairly rapidly. Like rheumatoid nodules (Chapter 5), the nodular lesions in Caplan's syndrome exhibit central necrosis surrounded by fibroblasts, macrophages, and collagen. This syndrome also occurs in asbestosis and silicosis.

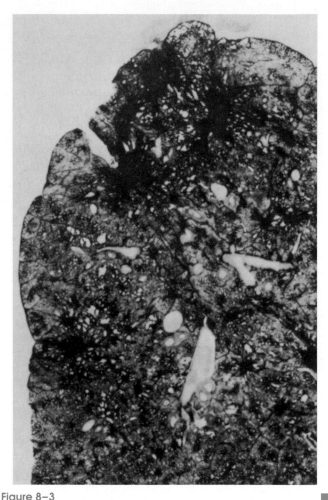

Figure 8–3 ■

Progressive massive fibrosis superimposed on coal workers' pneumoconiosis. The large blackened scars are principally in the upper lobe. Note the extensions of scars into surrounding parenchyma and retraction of adjacent pleura. (Courtesy of Dr. Werner Laquer, Dr. Jerome Kleinerman, and the National Institute of Occupational Safety and Health.)

Clinical Course. CWP is usually a benign disease that produces little decrement in lung function. Even mild forms of complicated CWP fail to demonstrate abnormalities of lung function. However, in a minority of cases PMF develops, leading to increasing pulmonary dysfunction, pulmonary hypertension, and cor pulmonale. Once PMF develops, it may progress, even if further exposure to dust is prevented. The incidence of clinical tuberculosis is increased in persons with CWP, but whether this reflects a greater vulnerability to infection or, instead, socioeconomic factors inherent in the life of miners is unclear. There is also some evidence that exposure to coal dust increases the incidence of chronic bronchitis and emphysema independent of smoking, thus complicating the management of the patient with CWP. However, to date there is no compelling evidence that CWP in the absence of smoking predisposes an individual to cancer.

SILICOSIS

Silicosis is a lung disease caused by inhalation of crystalline silicon dioxide (silica). Currently the most prevalent chronic occupational disease in the world, silicosis usually presents, after decades of exposure, as a slowly progressing, nodular, fibrosing pneumoconiosis. As shown in Table 8–3, workers in a large number of occupations are at risk, especially sandblasters and many mine workers. Less commonly, very heavy exposure over months to a few years can result in acute silicosis, a lesion characterized by the generalized accumulation of a lipoproteinaceous material within alveoli.

Silica occurs in both crystalline and amorphous forms, but crystalline forms (including quartz, crystobalite, and tridymite) are biologically the most active. Of these, quartz is most commonly implicated in silicosis. Talc, vermiculite, and mica are examples of noncrystalline silicates that are less common causes of pneumoconioses.

After inhalation, particles of quartz smaller than 5 μm may reach the terminal airways, and those approximately 1 μm are particularly apt to be retained and to cause fibrosis. Animals exposed to silica demonstrate a steady increase in macrophages and lymphocytes in the alveolus and interstitium. As discussed earlier, the recruited macrophages play a pivotal role by secreting factors that lead to fibroblast proliferation and collagen production. As with CWP, the initial lesions tend to localize in the upper lung zones, although the reasons for this distribution are obscure. *In contrast with CWP, however, early lesions of silicosis are more fibrotic and less cellular.* It seems likely that factors secreted by macrophages that ingest coal dust have less potent fibroblast-stimulating capability than do those secreted by macrophages that ingest silica.

> **MORPHOLOGY. Silicosis** is characterized grossly in its early stages by tiny, barely palpable, discrete, pale-to-blackened (if coal dust is also present) nodules in the upper zones of the lungs. As the disease progresses, these nodules may coalesce into hard, collagenous scars (Fig. 8–4). Some nodules may undergo central softening and cavitation as a result of superimposed tuberculosis or ischemia. The intervening lung parenchyma may be compressed or overexpanded, and a honeycomb pattern may develop. Fibrotic lesions may also occur in the hilar lymph nodes and pleura. Sometimes thin sheets of calcification occur in the lymph nodes and are appreciated radiographically as "eggshell" calcification (e.g., calcium surrounding a zone lacking calcification). If the disease continues to progress, expansion and coalescence of lesions produces PMF. Histologically, the nodular lesions consist of concentric layers of hyalinized collagen surrounded by a dense capsule of more condensed collagen (Fig. 8–5). Examination of the nodules by polarized microscopy reveals birefringent silica particles.

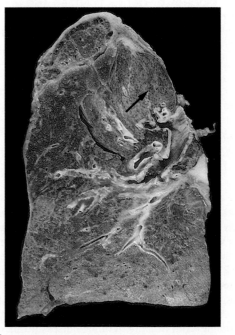

Figure 8–4 ■

Advanced silicosis seen on transection of lung. Scarring has contracted the upper lobe into a small dark mass *(arrow)*. Note the dense pleural thickening. (Courtesy of Dr. John Godleski, Brigham and Women's Hospital, Boston.)

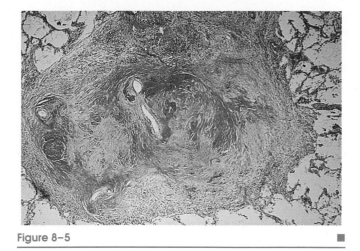

Figure 8–5 ■

Several coalescent collagenous silicotic nodules. (Courtesy of Dr. John Godleski, Brigham and Women's Hospital, Boston.)

Clinical Course. The disease is usually detected in routine chest radiographs performed on asymptomatic workers. The radiographs typically show a fine nodularity in the upper zones of the lung, but pulmonary function is either normal or only moderately affected. Most patients do not develop shortness of breath until late in the course, after PMF is present. At this time the disease may be progressive, even if the patient is no longer exposed. The disease is slow to kill, but impaired pulmonary function may severely limit activity. As with CWP, susceptibility to tuberculosis is increased, but there is no evidence that silicosis predisposes individuals to the development of bronchogenic carcinoma.

ASBESTOSIS AND ASBESTOS-RELATED DISEASES

Asbestos is a family of crystalline hydrated silicates with a fibrous geometry. On the basis of epidemiologic studies, occupational exposure to asbestos is linked to (1) parenchymal interstitial fibrosis (asbestosis); (2) bronchogenic carcinoma; (3) pleural effusions; (4) localized fibrous plaques or, rarely, diffuse pleural fibrosis; (5) mesotheliomas; and (6) laryngeal and perhaps other extrapulmonary neoplasms, including colon carcinomas. An increased incidence of asbestos-related cancer in family members of asbestos workers has alerted the general public to the potential hazards of asbestos in the environment. For instance, asbestos is widely present in insulation and is detectable in water and air.

Pathogenesis. Concentration, size, shape, and solubility of the different forms of asbestos dictate whether disease will occur. There are two distinct forms of asbestos: *serpentine* (in which the fiber is curly and flexible) and *amphibole* (in which the fiber is straight, stiff, and brittle). There are several subtypes of curly and straight asbestos fibers. The serpentine *chrysotile* accounts for most of the asbestos used in industry. It is important to make the distinction between various forms of amphiboles and serpentines, because amphiboles, even though less prevalent, are more pathogenic than the serpentine chrysotile, particularly with respect to induction of malignant pleural tumors (mesotheliomas). Indeed, some studies of mesotheliomas have shown the link is almost invariably to amphibole exposure. The greater pathogenicity of straight and stiff amphiboles is apparently related to several factors:

■ The serpentine chrysotiles, with their more flexible, curled structure, are likely to become impacted in the upper respiratory passages and removed by the mucociliary elevator. Those that are trapped in the lungs are gradually leached from the tissues because they are more soluble than amphiboles.
■ The straight, stiff amphiboles align themselves in the airstream and are hence delivered deeper into the lungs, where they may penetrate epithelial cells and reach the interstitium.

Despite these differences, both asbestos forms are fibrogenic, and increasing doses are associated with a higher incidence of all asbestos-related diseases except mesothelioma. In contrast to other inorganic dusts that induce cellular and fibrotic lung reactions, asbestos can also act as both a tumor initiator and a promoter, at least in experimental animals. However, potentially toxic chemicals adsorbed onto the asbestos fibers undoubtedly contribute to the pathogenicity of the fibers. For example, *the adsorption of carcinogens in tobacco smoke onto asbestos fibers may well be important to the remarkable synergy between tobacco smoking and the development of bronchogenic carcinoma in asbestos workers.*

Asbestosis, like other pneumoconioses, causes fibrosis by interacting with lung macrophages. It is not completely understood, however, why some inorganic dusts, exemplified by silicosis, cause nodular fibrosis, whereas others, such as asbestos, cause diffuse interstitial fibrosis. The more diffuse distribution may be related to the ability of asbestos to reach alveoli more consistently, its ability to penetrate epithelial cells, or both.

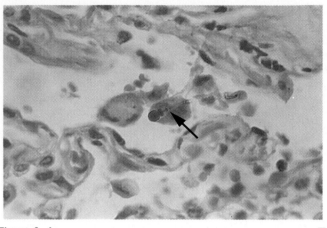

Figure 8–6 ■

High-power detail of an asbestos body, revealing the typical beading and knobbed ends *(arrow).*

MORPHOLOGY. **Asbestosis** is marked by diffuse pulmonary interstitial fibrosis. These changes are indistinguishable from those resulting from other causes of diffuse interstitial fibrosis (Chapter 13), except for the presence of asbestos bodies, which are seen as **golden brown, fusiform or beaded rods with a translucent center. They consist of asbestos fibers coated with an iron-containing proteinaceous material** (Fig. 8–6). Asbestos bodies apparently arise when macrophages attempt to phagocytose asbestos fibers; the iron is presumably derived from phagocyte ferritin. It should be noted that asbestos bodies can sometimes be found in the lungs of normal persons, but usually in much lower concentrations and without an accompanying interstitial fibrosis.

Asbestosis begins as fibrosis around respiratory bronchioles and alveolar ducts and extends to involve adjacent alveolar sacs and alveoli. Contraction of the fibrous tissue distorts the native architecture, creating enlarged airspaces enclosed within thick fibrous walls. In this way the affected regions become honeycombed. In contrast to CWP and silicosis, asbestosis begins in the lower lobes and subpleurally, but the middle and upper lobes of the lungs become affected as fibrosis progresses. Simultaneously, the visceral pleura undergoes fibrous thickening and sometimes binds the lungs to the chest wall. Large parenchymal nodules typical of Caplan's syndrome may appear in a few patients who have concurrent rheumatoid arthritis. The scarring may trap and narrow pulmonary arteries and arterioles, causing pulmonary hypertension and cor pulmonale (Chapter 11).

Pleural plaques are the most common manifestation of asbestos exposure and are well-circumscribed plaques of dense collagen (Fig. 8–7), often containing calcium. They develop most frequently on the anterior and posterolateral aspects of the **parietal** pleura and over the domes of the diaphragm. They do not contain asbestos bodies, and only rarely do they occur in persons who have no history or evidence of asbestos exposure. Uncommonly, asbestos exposure induces pleural effusions, which are usually serous but may be bloody. Rarely, diffuse visceral pleural fibrosis may occur and, in advanced cases, bind the lung to the thoracic cavity wall.

Both bronchogenic carcinomas and mesotheliomas develop in workers exposed to asbestos. The risk of bronchogenic carcinoma is increased about fivefold for asbestos workers; the relative risk for mesotheliomas, normally a very rare tumor (two to 17 cases per 1 million persons), is more than 1000-fold greater. Concomitant cigarette smoking greatly increases the risk of bronchogenic carcinoma but not that of mesothelioma. These asbestos-related tumors are morphologically indistinguishable from cancers of other causes and are described in Chapter 13.

Clinical Course. The clinical findings in asbestosis are indistinguishable from those of any other diffuse interstitial lung disease (Chapter 13). Typically, progressively worsening

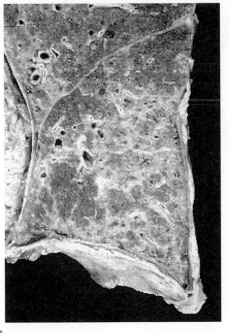

Figure 8-7 ■

Asbestosis. Markedly thickened visceral pleura covers the lateral and dia-phragmatic surface of lung. Note also severe interstitial fibrosis diffusely affecting the lower lobe of the lung.

dyspnea appears 10 to 20 years after exposure. The dyspnea is usually accompanied by a cough associated with production of sputum. The disease may remain static or progress to congestive heart failure, cor pulmonale (Chapter 11), and death. The development of Caplan's syndrome may accelerate the clinical course. Pleural plaques are usually asymptomatic and are detected on radiographs as circumscribed densities. Asbestosis complicated by lung or pleural cancer is associated with a particularly grim prognosis.

BERYLLIOSIS

Heavy exposure to airborne dusts or to fumes of metallic beryllium or its oxides, alloys, or salts may induce *acute pneumonitis; more protracted low-dose exposure may cause pulmonary and systemic granulomatous lesions that closely mimic sarcoidosis* (Chapter 13). In recent years, limitations on worker exposure to beryllium have resulted in the disappearance of acute berylliosis and a marked reduction in the incidence of chronic disease. Currently, workers in the nuclear and aerospace industries who work with beryllium alloys are at highest risk for exposure.

Chronic berylliosis is caused by induction of T cell–mediated immunity in genetically susceptible individuals. Indeed, linkage to specific alleles of major histocompatibility complex (MHC) class II genes has been demonstrated. It appears that beryllium acts as a hapten that binds to proteins and renders them immunogenic for CD4+ helper T cells. The resultant delayed hypersensitivity leads to the formation of non-caseating granulomas in the lungs and hilar nodes or, less commonly, in spleen, liver, kidneys, adrenals, and distant lymph nodes. The pulmonary granulomas become progres-sively fibrotic, giving rise to irregular, fine nodular densities detected on chest radiographs. Hilar adenopathy is present in about half of the cases.

Chronic berylliosis may not result in clinical manifestations until many years after exposure, when the patient presents with dyspnea, cough, weight loss, and arthralgias. Some cases stabilize, others remit and relapse, and still others progress to pulmonary failure. Epidemiologic evidence links heavy be-ryllium exposure to an increased incidence of cancer.

■ INJURY BY CHEMICAL AGENTS

There is a nearly endless list of chemical and biologic agents that can be injurious when inhaled, ingested, injected, or absorbed through the skin. Some may produce injury in the course of therapy for another disease (therapeutic agents); others (nontherapeutic agents) are introduced accidentally or intentionally into the body. Some of the latter agents (e.g., alcohol and other drugs of abuse) are used principally because of their psychotropic or mind-altering effects.

A perspective on the magnitude of the problem of chemical injury is gained by examining poison control center data. In 1989, about 2.1 million poison exposures resulted in calls to poison control centers. Of these exposures, 91% were in the home, 73% involved oral intake, and 61% of victims were children younger than 6 years. As might be expected, the most frequent offending agents were substances commonly available in the home, such as cleaning agents, analgesics, cosmetics, plants, or cold preparations. In 88% of cases, the episode resulted in either minor or no toxic effects. The remaining patients suffered significant toxicity, and at least 590 died.

The following principles are important in understanding the mechanisms of chemical injury:

■ *Dose.* In general, the higher the dose, the greater the toxicity, although small doses may cause serious sequelae, particularly over a protracted period. An example is impairment of mental development in children chronically exposed to low levels of lead.
■ *Requirement for metabolic conversion.* Some agents (e.g., certain alkaline cleaning materials) are directly toxic to cells and hence injure the mucosa of the oral cavity, esophagus, and stomach when swallowed. In contrast, many drugs, including alcohol, are converted in the liver to compounds that are more toxic than the parent compound. Thus, there may be little or no injury at the site of entry, and the liver may bear the brunt of injury.
■ *Sites of absorption, accumulation, or excretion.* For chemicals that are direct cell toxins, the site of entry is obviously important in determining the type of injury. The site of accumulation is also important. The aminoglycoside antibiotics, for instance, are particularly prone to accumulate in the endolymph and perilymph of the ear and in the renal cortex, thus explaining the propensity of these drugs (e.g., tetracycline) to cause ototoxicity and nephrotoxicity.
■ *Individual variation.* An important determinant of the rate of drug metabolism is inherited polymorphisms in the enzymes that metabolize the drugs. For example, the rate of

acetylation of the antihypertensive drug hydralazine is genetically determined. Individuals who are slow acetylators are more likely to develop drug-induced lupus (Chapter 5) than are rapid acetylators, possibly because prolonged elevation of the plasma level of native drug enhances its capacity to initiate an immune response.

■ *The capacity of the chemical to induce an immune response.* Many chemicals are not directly toxic but inflict injury by inducing an immune response. For example, penicillin may induce an immunoglobulin E (IgE)–mediated anaphylactic response or an immunoglobulin G (IgG)–mediated hemolytic anemia in those who are genetically prone to develop type I or type II hypersensitivity reactions to this drug (Chapter 5).

Injury by Therapeutic Agents (Adverse Drug Reactions)

Adverse drug reactions refer to untoward effects of drugs that are given in conventional therapeutic settings. These reactions are extremely common in the practice of medicine. Several examples were given in the discussion of general principles above; Table 8–4 lists common pathologic findings in adverse drug reactions and the drugs most frequently involved. Because they are widely used, estrogens and oral contraceptives (OCs) will be discussed in more detail. In addition, because acetaminophen and aspirin, commonly used as nonprescription drugs, are important causes of accidental or intentional overdose, they also merit additional comment. Sedatives and hypnotic and anxiolytic agents are also important causes of drug injury, but injury associated with their use is usually in the context of abuse.

EXOGENOUS ESTROGENS AND ORAL CONTRACEPTIVES

Estrogens and OCs are discussed separately because (1) estrogens for postmenopausal syndrome may be given alone and are usually natural estrogens, and (2) OCs contain synthetic estrogens, always with progesterone.

Exogenous Estrogens. Estrogen therapy, once used primarily for the distressing symptoms of menopause, is currently also used widely in postmenopausal women, with or without added progesterones, to prevent or slow the progression of osteoporosis (Chapter 21). Given the fact that endogenous hyperestrinism increases the risk of developing endometrial carcinoma and, likely, breast carcinoma, there is understandable concern about the use of exogenous estrogens as therapeutic agents. Current data support the following adverse effects of estrogen therapy:

■ *Endometrial carcinoma.* Unopposed estrogen therapy increases the risk of endometrial carcinoma three- to sixfold after 5 years of use and more than 10-fold after 10 years, when compared with the risk in women who had not used hormones. This risk is drastically reduced or even eliminated when progestins are added to the therapeutic regimen.

■ *Breast carcinoma.* Although some studies continue to point to an increased risk of this form of cancer with the

Table 8–4.	SOME COMMON ADVERSE DRUG REACTIONS AND THEIR AGENTS
Reaction	**Major Offenders**
Blood Dyscrasias (feature of almost half of all drug-related deaths)	
Granulocytopenia, aplastic anemia, pancytopenia	Antineoplastic agents, immunosuppressives, and chloramphenicol
Hemolytic anemia, thrombocytopenia	Penicillin, methyldopa, quinidine
Cutaneous	
Urticaria, macules, papules, vesicles, petechiae, exfoliative dermatitis, fixed drug eruptions	Antineoplastic agents, sulfonamides, hydantoins, many others
Cardiac	
Arrhythmias	Theophylline, hydantoins
Cardiomyopathy	Doxorubicin, daunorubicin
Renal	
Glomerulonephritis	Penicillamine
Acute tubular necrosis	Aminoglycoside antibiotics, cyclosporin, amphotericin B
Tubulointerstitial disease with papillary necrosis	Phenacetin, salicylates
Pulmonary	
Asthma	Salicylates
Acute pneumonitis	Nitrofurantoin
Interstitial fibrosis	Busulfan, nitrofurantoin, bleomycin
Hepatic	
Fatty change	Tetracycline
Diffuse hepatocellular damage	Halothane, isoniazid, acetominophen
Cholestasis	Chlorpromazine, estrogens, contraceptive agents
Systemic	
Anaphylaxis	Penicillin
Lupus erythematosus syndrome (drug-induced lupus)	Hydralazine, procainamide
Central Nervous System	
Tinnitus and dizziness	Salicylates
Acute dystonic reactions and parkinsonian syndrome	Phenothiazine antipsychotics
Respiratory depression	Sedatives

use of unopposed estrogen (i.e., for postmenopausal replacement), the weight of the evidence suggests that the increased risk is very small, if any, and is not influenced by the addition of progestins to the formulation (Chapter 19).

■ *Thromboembolism.* Although estrogen therapy might be expected to increase the risk of this complication because synthetic estrogens stimulate the production of coagulation factors by the liver, statistics have not borne this out. This happy outcome is perhaps related to the more frequent use of natural estrogens, which appear to be less thrombogenic than synthetic estrogens.

■ *Cardiovascular disease.* Myocardial infarction and stroke are among the leading causes of death in postmenopausal women, and hence there is considerable interest in the effects of estrogens on the incidence of cardiovascular disease. Estrogens tend to elevate the level of high-density lipoprotein (HDL) and reduce the level of low-density lipoprotein (LDL). This lipid profile is protective against the development of atherosclerosis. Progestins, on the other hand, tend to lower HDL and elevate LDL, which counters the estrogen effect. Recent epidemiologic studies of the role of estrogens have shown a 40% to 50% decrease in the risk of ischemic heart disease in women who received postmenopausal estrogen therapy, compared with those who did not receive estrogens. The general consensus seems to be that unopposed estrogens are likely to be beneficial. The addition of sequential progestins does not alter the benefit of estrogen regimens. The risk of strokes seems unaltered by estrogen therapy.

Oral Contraceptives. Although OCs have been in use for over 30 years, and despite innumerable analyses of their effects, experts continue to disagree about their safety and adverse effects. These drugs nearly always contain a synthetic estradiol and variable amounts of a progestin (combined OCs), but a few preparations contain only progestins. Currently, prescribed OCs contain smaller amounts of estrogens (< 50 μg per day) and are clearly associated with fewer side effects than were earlier formulations. Hence, the results of epidemiologic studies must be interpreted in the context of the dosage. Nevertheless, there is reasonable evidence to support the following conclusions about the effects of these drugs:

■ *Breast carcinoma.* The issue of breast cancer risk is controversial. Despite the disagreements, the prevailing opinion is that there is a slight increase in breast cancer risk when combined OCs are used by women under the age of 45 years, particularly nulliparous women younger than 25 years. For women over the age of 45 years, the risk, if any, is negligible.
■ *Endometrial cancer.* There is no increased risk, and very likely OCs exert a protective effect.
■ *Cervical cancer.* OCs carry some increased risk, which is correlated with duration of use. More recent studies suggest that the increased risk may be more strongly correlated with life style than with the drug (Chapter 19).
■ *Ovarian cancer.* OCs protect against ovarian cancer; the longer they are used, the greater the protection, and this protection persists for some time after OC use stops.
■ *Thromboembolism.* The OCs used in the past (> 50-μg estrogens) were clearly associated with an increased risk of venous thrombosis and pulmonary thromboembolism because of increased hepatic synthesis of coagulation factors and reduced levels of antithrombin III. Data with the newer (second-generation) formulations (< 50-μg estrogens) suggest that the overall risk is much less, especially in women less than 35 years old who do not smoke and do not have other predisposing influences such as diabetes. More recently, third-generation OCs, which combine low-dose estrogens with synthetic progestins, have been introduced because the synthetic progestins affect LDL and HDL levels to a lesser extent than natural progestins, and hence the risk of acute myocardial infarction is reduced. However, quite unexpectedly, the third-generation OCs confer a higher risk of venous thrombosis than do second-generation OCs. Furthermore, there is an even greater risk of venous thrombosis in users who are carriers of a mu-

tation in factor V. As stated earlier (Chapter 4), the carrier rate of the factor V mutation is fairly high (2% to 15%) in whites. With all of these potential complications, the risks and benefits of these newest OCs are under careful scrutiny.
■ *Hypertension.* Even the newer, low-estrogen formulations of OCs cause a slight increase in blood pressure. The effect is more marked in older women with a family history of hypertension.
■ *Cardiovascular disease.* As discussed, estrogens and progestins have opposing effects on HDL and LDL levels. The overall effect on the levels of these lipoproteins seems to depend on the preparations used, particularly the dose of progestin in the formulation. There is considerable uncertainty regarding the risk of atherosclerosis and myocardial infarction in users of OCs. This stems from the fact that several variables (e.g., the estrogen content of the formulation; the age of the women studied; and the presence or absence of other risk factors for atherosclerosis, especially smoking) can influence the outcome of epidemiologic studies. Recent evidence seems to absolve OCs: it appears that nonsmoking, healthy women younger than 45 years who use the newer, low-estrogen formulations do not incur an increased risk of ischemic heart disease. Conversely, young women smokers who use the pill are 10 times more likely to suffer myocardial infarction than are users who do not smoke.
■ *Hepatic adenoma.* There is a well-defined association between the use of OCs and this rare benign hepatic tumor, especially in older women who have used OCs for prolonged periods.
■ *Gallbladder disease.* The slightly increased risk found with older formulations is not seen with the newer ones.

Obviously, the pros and cons of OC use must be viewed in the context of their wide applicability and acceptance as a form of contraception that protects against unwanted pregnancies with their attendant hazards.

ACETAMINOPHEN

When taken in very large doses, this widely used nonprescription analgesic and antipyretic causes *hepatic necrosis.* The window between the usual therapeutic dose (0.5 gm) and the toxic dose (15 to 25 gm) is large, however, and the drug is ordinarily very safe. Toxicity begins with nausea, vomiting, diarrhea, and sometimes shock, followed in a few days by evidence of jaundice; with serious overdosage, liver failure ensues, with centrilobular necrosis that may extend to the entire lobule. Some patients show evidence of concurrent renal and myocardial damage.

ASPIRIN (ACETYLSALICYLIC ACID)

Overdose may result from accidental ingestion by young children; in adults, overdose is frequently suicidal. The major untoward consequences are metabolic with few morphologic changes. At first respiratory alkalosis develops, followed by metabolic acidosis that often proves fatal before anatomic changes can appear. Ingestion of as little as 2 to 4 gm by children or 10 to 30 gm by adults may be fatal, but survival has been reported after doses five times larger.

Chronic aspirin toxicity (salicylism) may develop in persons who take 3 gm or more daily, the dose required to treat chronic inflammatory conditions. Chronic salicylism is manifested by headache, dizziness, ringing in the ears (tinnitus), difficulty hearing, mental confusion, drowsiness, nausea, vomiting, and diarrhea. The central nervous system changes may progress to convulsions and coma. The morphologic consequences of chronic salicylism are varied. Most often there is an acute erosive gastritis (Chapter 15), which may produce overt or covert gastrointestinal bleeding and lead to gastric ulceration. A bleeding tendency may appear concurrently with chronic toxicity, because aspirin acetylates platelet cyclooxygenase and blocks the ability to make thromboxane A$_2$, an activator of platelet aggregation. Petechial hemorrhages may appear in the skin and internal viscera, and bleeding from gastric ulcerations may be exaggerated.

Proprietary analgesic mixtures of aspirin and phenacetin or its active metabolite, acetaminophen, when taken over a span of years, have caused renal papillary necrosis, referred to as *analgesic nephropathy* (Chapter 14).

Injury by Nontherapeutic Toxic Agents

Table 8–5 lists some of the more common agents involved in acute poisoning, along with their major pathologic effects. The purpose of this list is to emphasize both the diversity of agents that may cause injury and the variety of responses that toxins can produce. A more detailed discussion of two common environmental pollutants, lead and CO, follows. Inhalation is the route of entry for CO and an important route for lead, but both manifest injury in extrapulmonary organs.

LEAD

Acute lead poisoning may occur under unusual circumstances (e.g., battery burning). More commonly, lead compounds accumulate slowly until they reach toxic levels. Adults usually present with *colicky abdominal pain, fatigue,* and perhaps *headache,* but in infants and children, lead poisoning may remain unsuspected until it erupts in a *catastrophic encephalopathic crisis.* Lead poisoning has proved to be one of the most difficult environmental health problems to control, and part of this difficulty stems from the lack of distinctive early manifestations.

There are innumerable sources of lead in the environment (Fig. 8–8). Indeed, it is hard to avoid exposure to lead. Environmental lead is absorbed either through the gastrointestinal tract or through the lungs. Identification of the principal environmental sources of lead is a controversial issue, but most experts agree that urban air, dirt, and food are the major conduits. Some years ago, automotive engines and industries polluted the air with about 450,000 tons of lead per year. With the use of unleaded gasoline, the lead content of urban air has been significantly reduced. Volatilized lead is particularly hazardous, because most is absorbed in the lungs. By contrast, only a fraction of ingested lead is absorbed. Urban adults have a daily intake of 100 to 150 μg of lead in water and food,

Table 8–5. SOME COMMON NONTHERAPEUTIC TOXIC AGENTS AND THE MAJOR ASSOCIATED PATHOLOGIC EFFECTS

Agent	Pathologic Effects
Carbon monoxide	Binds with hemoglobin with high affinity, causing systemic hypoxia
Cleaning compounds	
Bleach (sodium hypochlorite)	Local irritant, unlikely to scar
Caustic (acid or basic) agents	Local erosions with scarring
Chloroform, carbon tetrachloride	CNS depression, liver necrosis
Cyanide	Blocking of cytochrome oxidase activity, resulting in rapid death owing to severe hypoxia
Ethylene glycol (antifreeze)	CNS depression, metabolic acidosis, acute tubular necrosis
Insecticides	
Chlorinated hydrocarbon (e.g., DDT)	CNS stimulant, accumulates in fat stores for long periods. ? carcinogenic
Organophosphates	Acetylcholinesterase inhibition (muscle weakness, cardiac arrhythmias, respiratory depression)
Isopropanol (rubbing alcohol)	Similar to those of ethanol (gastritis, CNS depression)
Mercurials	
High-dose mercury vapors	Pneumonitis
Low-dose exposure	Intention tremors, memory loss, gingivitis, skin rashes, nephrotic syndrome
Methanol (Sterno, antifreeze)	CNS depression, acidosis, blindness
Mushrooms	
Amanita muscaria	Parasympathomimetic symptoms, including bradycardia, hypotension
Amanita phalloides	Gastrointestinal symptoms with shock, convulsions, coma
Petroleum distillates (kerosene, benzene, gasoline)	Respiratory depression, gastrointestinal inflammation, severe pneumonitis
Polychlorinated biphenyls (PCBs)	Insidious development of chloracne, visual loss, impotence

only about 10% of which is absorbed. Although children have, on average, a lower intake, they unfortunately absorb about 50%. Flaking lead paint in older houses and soil contamination pose major hazards to youngsters, and ingestion of up to 200 μg per day may occur.

Most of the absorbed lead (80% to 85%) is taken up by bone, the blood accumulates about 5% to 10%, and the remainder is distributed throughout the soft tissues. In children, excess lead interferes with the normal remodeling of calcified cartilage and primary bone trabeculae in the epiphyses, leading to increased bone density, which is detected as radiodense "lead lines" on radiographs (Fig. 8–9). Lead lines of a different sort may also occur in the gums, where excess lead stimulates hyperpigmentation of the gum tissue adjacent to the teeth. Excretion of lead occurs via the kidneys, thereby exposing these organs to potential damage.

Lead causes injury by binding to disulfide groups in pro-

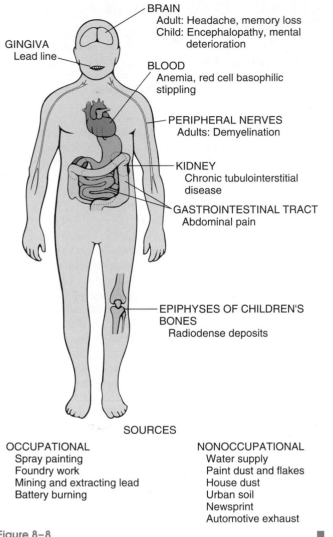

BRAIN
Adult: Headache, memory loss
Child: Encephalopathy, mental
deterioration

GINGIVA
Lead line

BLOOD
Anemia, red cell basophilic
stippling

PERIPHERAL NERVES
Adults: Demyelination

KIDNEY
Chronic tubulointerstitial
disease

GASTROINTESTINAL TRACT
Abdominal pain

EPIPHYSES OF CHILDREN'S
BONES
Radiodense deposits

SOURCES

OCCUPATIONAL
Spray painting
Foundry work
Mining and extracting lead
Battery burning

NONOCCUPATIONAL
Water supply
Paint dust and flakes
House dust
Urban soil
Newsprint
Automotive exhaust

Figure 8–8   ■

Clinical and pathologic features of lead poisoning.

Brain damage is prone to occur in children. It may be very subtle, producing mild dysfunction, or it may be massive and lethal. In young children, sensory, motor, intellectual, and psychologic impairments have been described, including reduced IQ; learning disabilities; retarded psychomotor development; blindness; and, in more severe cases, psychoses, seizures, and coma. The anatomic changes underlying the more subtle functional deficits are ill defined, but there is concern that some of the defects may be permanent. At the more severe end of the spectrum are marked brain edema, demyelination of the cerebral and cerebellar white matter, and necrosis of cortical neurons accompanied by diffuse astrocytic proliferation. In adults, the central nervous system is less often affected, but frequently a peripheral **demyelinating neuropathy** appears, typically involving the motor innervation of the most commonly used muscles. Thus, the extensor muscles of the wrist and fingers are often the first to be affected, followed by paralysis of the peroneal muscles.

The **gastrointestinal tract** is also a major source of clinical manifestations. Lead "colic," characterized by extremely severe, poorly localized abdominal pain, is often associated with sufficient spasm and rigidity of the abdominal wall to create the impression of an acute "surgical abdomen." Other findings are shown in Figure 8–8.

teins, including enzymes, altering their tertiary structure. The major anatomic targets of lead toxicity are the blood, nervous system, gastrointestinal tract, and kidneys (see Fig. 8–8).

Blood changes resulting from lead accumulation occur fairly early and are characteristic. Lead interferes with normal heme biosynthesis by inhibiting the enzymes aminolevulinic acid dehydratase (ALA-D) and ferroketolase (which is involved in incorporation of iron into the protoporphyrin molecule to form heme). As a consequence of this latter enzyme defect, zinc-protoporphyrin is formed instead of heme. Thus, the elevated blood level of zinc-protoporphyrin or its product, free erythrocyte protoporphyrin, is an important indicator of lead poisoning. Typically, a **microcytic, hypochromic, mild hemolytic anemia and**—even more distinctive—**punctate basophilic stippling of the erythrocytes** appear.

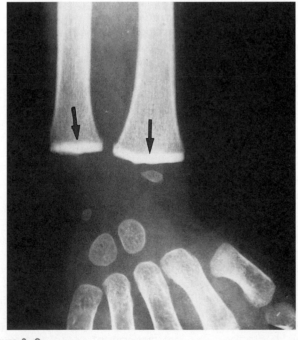

Figure 8–9   ■

Lead poisoning. Impaired remodeling of calcified cartilage in the epiphyses *(arrows)* of the wrist has caused a marked increase in their radiodensity, so that they are as radiopaque as the cortical bone. (Courtesy of Dr. G. W. Dietz, Department of Radiology, University of Texas Southwestern Medical School, Dallas, TX.)

The diagnosis of lead poisoning requires constant awareness of its prevalence. The diagnosis may be suspected on the basis of neurologic changes in children or unexplained anemia with basophilic stippling in red cells. Elevated blood lead and free erythrocyte protoporphyrin levels (above 50 μg/dl) or, alternatively, zinc-protoporphyrin levels are required for definitive diagnosis.

CARBON MONOXIDE

This nonirritating, colorless, tasteless, odorless gas produced by the imperfect oxidation of carbonaceous materials continues to be a cause of accidental and suicidal death. Its sources include automotive engines, industrial processes using fossil fuels, home heating with fossil fuels (not natural gas), and cigarette smoke. The exhaust of automotive engines is about 5% CO; in a small, closed garage the average car exhaust can induce lethal coma within 5 minutes. CO kills by inducing central nervous system depression, which appears so insidiously that victims may not be aware of their plight and indeed may be unable to help themselves.

CO acts as a systemic asphyxiant. *Hemoglobin has a 200-fold greater affinity for CO than for oxygen.* The resultant carboxyhemoglobin is incapable of carrying oxygen and furthermore interferes with the release of oxygen from oxyhemoglobin. Systemic hypoxia appears when the hemoglobin is 20% to 30% saturated with CO, and unconsciousness and death are likely with 60% to 70% saturation. Depending on the rate of conversion to carboxyhemoglobin and the ultimate severity, one of two clinical patterns can be recognized.

Acute poisoning is marked by a characteristic **generalized cherry-red color of the skin and mucous membranes, resulting from the carboxyhemoglobin.** If death occurs, depending on the rapidity of onset, morphologic changes may not be present; with longer survival the brain may be slightly edematous, with punctate hemorrhages and hypoxia-induced neuronal changes. The morphologic changes are not specific for CO; they simply imply systemic hypoxia. When exposure has not been prolonged and only moderate hypoxia has occurred, complete recovery is possible. However, sometimes impairments of memory, vision, hearing, and speech remain.

Chronic poisoning may appear because the carboxyhemoglobin, once formed, is remarkably stable and, with low-level persistent exposure, may accumulate to a life-threatening concentration in the blood. The slowly developing hypoxia can insidiously evoke widespread changes in the central nervous system; these are particularly marked in the basal ganglia and lenticular nuclei. With cessation of exposure to CO, the victim usually recovers, but often there are permanent neurologic sequelae. The diagnosis of CO poisoning is critically dependent on the identification of significant levels of carboxyhemoglobin in the blood.

ALCOHOL AND OTHER DRUGS OF ABUSE

Drug abuse may be defined as the use of a mind-altering substance in a way that differs from generally approved medical or social practices. Ethanol is imbibed, at least partly, for its mood-altering properties but when used in moderation is socially acceptable and not injurious. When excessive amounts are used, alcohol can cause marked physical and psychologic damage. Table 8–6 provides a classification of drugs that are abused, with examples of each. Our purpose here is to describe the pathology directly associated with the abuse of alcohol, therapeutic agents, and illicit drugs.

Ethanol. In many populations 80% to 90% of adults consume ethanol. Unfortunately, consumption is excessive in 5% to 10% of adult males and about 5% of adult females in most Western societies. It is estimated that in the United States there are more than 10 million chronic alcoholics and an additional 7 million who drink enough to suffer adverse effects.

The major effects of acute alcohol intake are exerted on the central nervous system, but with chronic use other organs are also affected. After ingestion, ethanol is absorbed unaltered in the stomach and small intestine. It is then distributed to all the tissues and fluids of the body in direct proportion to the blood level. Less than 10% of absorbed alcohol is excreted unchanged in the urine, sweat, and breath. The amount exhaled is proportional to the blood level and forms the basis of the breath test employed by law enforcement agencies.

Most of the alcohol in the blood is biotransformed to acetaldehyde in the liver through two major pathways (Fig. 8–10). Acetaldehyde formed by either pathway is further metabolized by acetaldehyde dehydrogenase. With relatively low levels of alcohol intake, this conversion is mediated primarily by alcohol dehydrogenase. At higher levels, the microsomal P-450 system becomes more important. Indeed, high blood levels of alcohol enhance the activity of this system. A man

■

Table 8–6. CLASSIFICATION OF DRUGS OF ABUSE

Class	Examples
Sedatives and hypnotics	Alcohol, barbiturates, benzodiazepines
CNS sympathomimetics or stimulants	Cocaine, amphetamines, methylphenidate (Ritalin), weight loss products
Opioids	Heroin, morphine, methadone, and almost all prescription analgesics
Cannabinols	Marijuana, hashish
Hallucinogens or psychedelics	Lysergic acid diethylamide (LSD), mescaline, psilocybin, phencyclidine (PCP)
Inhalants	Aerosol sprays, glues, toluene, gasoline, paint thinner, amyl nitrite, nitrous oxide
Nonprescription drugs	Ingredients: Atropine, scopolamine, weak stimulants, antihistamines, weak analgesics

Modified from Schuckit MA (ed): Drug and Alcohol Abuse: A Clinical Guide to Diagnosis and Treatment, 3rd ed. New York, Plenum Press, 1989.

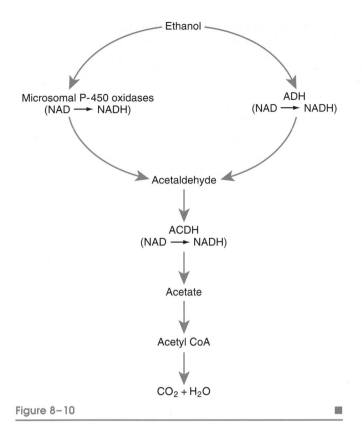

Ethanol

Microsomal P-450 oxidases
(NAD → NADH)

ADH
(NAD → NADH)

Acetaldehyde

ACDH
(NAD → NADH)

Acetate

Acetyl CoA

$CO_2 + H_2O$

Figure 8–10   ■

Metabolism of alcohol. With occasional intake the major pathway is via hepatic alcohol dehydrogenase (ADH). In chronic alcoholism the P-450 system is induced and plays a more important role. ACDH, hepatic acetaldehyde dehydrogenase; NAD, nicotinamide adenine dinucleotide; NADH, reduced NAD.

of average size and weight metabolizes about 9 gm of alcohol (about ¾ ounce of whiskey) per hour regardless of the blood level. However, genetic polymorphisms of liver alcohol and acetaldehyde dehydrogenases have been identified, some associated with more rapid metabolism of substrate than others. Moreover, chronic alcoholics develop a measure of tolerance as a result of enzyme induction (particularly of the microsomal P-450 system), leading to an increased rate of metabolism. Thus, there is some individual variability in the ability to handle alcohol, but the variations are confined to a narrow range.

Acute alcoholism exerts its effects mainly on the central nervous system, but it may induce hepatic and gastric changes that are reversible in the absence of continued alcohol consumption. The hepatic changes are described in Chapter 16. The gastric changes constitute acute gastritis and ulceration (Chapter 15). In the central nervous system, alcohol is a depressant, first affecting subcortical structures (probably the high brain stem reticular formation) that modulate cerebral cortical activity. Consequently, there is stimulation and disordered cortical, motor, and intellectual behavior. At progressively higher blood levels, cortical neurons and then lower medullary centers are depressed, including those that regulate respiration. Respiratory arrest may follow.

Blood alcohol levels and the degree of impairment of central nervous system function in nonhabituated drinkers are closely correlated. In individuals of average size, consumption of 180 ml (6 ounces) of distilled spirits in a relatively brief time results in a blood alcohol level of approximately 100 mg/dl. This level induces obvious ataxia and is usually considered the legal upper limit of sobriety. Drowsiness occurs at about 200 mg/dl, stupor at 300 mg/dl, and profound anesthesia, if not death, at 400 to 500 mg/dl. Fortunately, fatal levels are rarely encountered because stupor or vomiting of gastric contents intervenes.

Chronic alcoholism is responsible for morphologic alterations in virtually all organs and tissues in the body, particularly the liver and stomach. Only the gastric lesions that appear immediately after exposure can be related to the direct effects of ethanol on the mucosal vasculature. The origin of the other chronic changes is less clear. Acetaldehyde, a major oxidative metabolite of ethanol, is a very reactive compound and has been proposed as the mediator of the widespread tissue and organ damage. Although the catabolism of acetaldehyde is more rapid than that of alcohol, chronic ethanol consumption reduces the oxidative capacity of the liver, raising the blood level of acetaldehyde, which is augmented by the increased rate of ethanol metabolism in the habituated drinker. Other suggested mechanisms of injury include increased free radical activity and, possibly, immune reactions against hepatic neoantigens generated by acetaldehyde or free radical–induced alteration of proteins. Dependence on alcohol seems to be genetically regulated. This is supported by studies in twins; the concordance rate for chronic alcoholism is significantly more common in monozygotic twins than in dizygotic twins. Family studies also support this notion. It is believed that multiple genes contribute to the genetic vulnerability. This is an area of active investigation.

Whatever the basis, chronic alcoholics suffer significant morbidity and a shortened life span related principally to damage to the liver, gastrointestinal tract, central nervous system, cardiovascular system, and pancreas.

■ *Liver.* Alcohol, the most common cause of hepatic injury, may lead to cirrhosis (Chapter 16). Cirrhosis of the liver is the ninth leading cause of death in the United States.

■ *Gastrointestinal tract.* Massive bleeding from gastritis, gastric ulcer, or esophageal varices (associated with cirrhosis) may prove fatal.

■ *Central nervous system.* A deficiency of thiamine is common in chronic alcoholics; the principal lesions of this deficiency are peripheral neuropathies and the Wernicke-Korsakoff syndrome (discussed later in this chapter and in Chapter 23). Cerebral atrophy, cerebellar degeneration, and optic neuropathy may also occur, possibly directly related to alcohol or its products.

■ *Cardiovascular system.* Direct injury to the myocardium may produce dilated congestive cardiomyopathy (Chapter 11). Although moderate amounts of alcohol have been shown to increase levels of HDL and decrease the incidence of coronary heart disease, heavy consumption, with attendant liver injury, results in a decrease in levels of HDL, accompanied by an increase in the likelihood of coronary heart disease. Chronic alcoholism is associated with an increased incidence of hypertension.

■ *Pancreas.* Excess alcohol intake increases the risk of acute and chronic pancreatitis (Chapter 17).

■ *Other.* The heavy use of ethanol during pregnancy can cause fetal alcohol syndrome (i.e., growth retardation and some reduction in mental function in the child).

Cocaine. In the past decade cocaine, along with its derivative "crack," has become a major substance of abuse; there are an estimated 2 to 6 million cocaine abusers in the United States. Cocaine, an alkaloid extracted from the leaves of the coca plant, is usually prepared in the form of a water-soluble powder, cocaine hydrochloride, but when sold on the street, it is liberally diluted with talcum powder, lactose, or other look-alikes. Crystallization of the pure alkaloid from cocaine hydrochloride yields nuggets of crack (so called because of the cracking or popping sound it makes when heated). The pharmacologic actions of cocaine and crack are identical, but the latter is far more potent. Both forms of the drug are absorbed from all sites and so can be snorted, smoked after mixing with tobacco, ingested, or injected subcutaneously or intravenously.

Cocaine produces an intense euphoria with so-called reinforcing qualities, making it one of the most addicting of all drugs. Experimental animals will press a lever more than 1000 times and forgo food and drink to obtain the drug. In the cocaine abuser, although physical dependence appears not to occur, the psychologic withdrawal is profound and can be extremely difficult to treat. Recurrent intense cravings to re-experience drug-associated "highs" are particularly severe in the first several months after abstinence, but they can recur for years.

The most serious physical side effects of cocaine use relate to its acute toxic effects on the cardiovascular system and can be most readily understood by considering the sympathicomimetic action of the drug (Fig. 8–11). Cocaine *acts to facilitate neurotransmission both in the central nervous system, where it blocks the reuptake of dopamine, and at adrenergic nerve endings, where it blocks the reuptake of both epinephrine and norepinephrine* while stimulating the presynaptic release of norepinephrine. The net effect is the accumulation of these two neurotransmitters at adrenergic nerve endings, resulting in excess stimulation, manifested by tachycardia and hypertension. These effects are compounded because cocaine also induces myocardial ischemia, the basis for which is multifactorial. Cocaine causes *coronary artery vasoconstriction, promotes thrombus formation* by facilitating platelet aggregation, and induces premature atherosclerosis in long-term users. Cocaine-induced coronary vasospasm is potentiated by cigarette smoking—a common habit among cocaine users. Thus, on the one hand, cocaine induces increased myocardial oxygen demand by its sympathicomimetic action. On the other hand, it reduces coronary blood flow, thus setting the

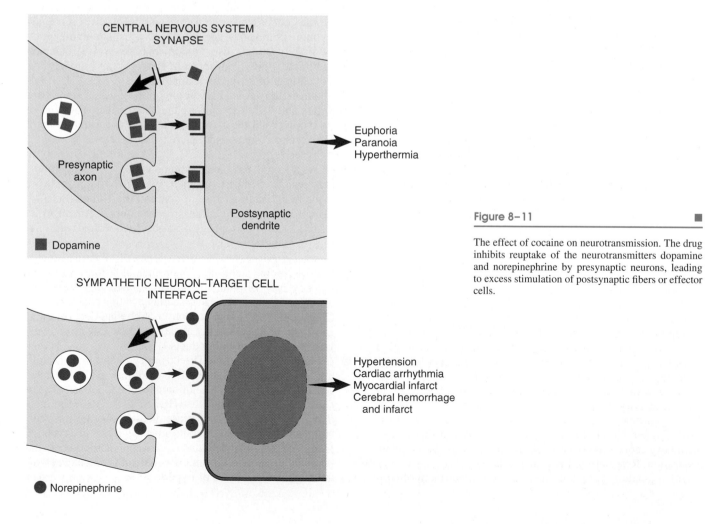

Figure 8–11 ■

The effect of cocaine on neurotransmission. The drug inhibits reuptake of the neurotransmitters dopamine and norepinephrine by presynaptic neurons, leading to excess stimulation of postsynaptic fibers or effector cells.

stage for myocardial ischemia that may lead to myocardial infarction. In addition to its detrimental effects on myocardial oxygenation, cocaine can also precipitate *lethal arrhythmias* by enhanced sympathetic activity, as well as by disrupting normal ion (K+, Ca+, Na+) transport in the myocardium. These toxic effects are not necessarily dose related, and a lethal event may occur in a first-time abuser with what is a typical mood-altering dose. The following are some manifestations of acute cocaine toxicity:

■ Sympathetic nervous system stimulation, resulting in dilated pupils, vasoconstriction, an increase in arterial blood pressure, and tachycardia.
■ Lethal arrhythmias and myocardial infarction.
■ Cerebral infarction and intracranial hemorrhage, the latter in persons who have preexisting vascular malformations and probably related to the sudden acute elevations in blood pressure. The most common central nervous system findings are hyperpyrexia (thought to be caused by aberrations of the dopaminergic pathways that control body temperature) and seizures.
■ Rhabdomyolysis, sometimes accompanied by renal failure; the mechanism is not understood but may relate to intense vasoconstriction together with a direct effect of the drug on muscle.

In contrast to acute toxicity, chronic cocaine use may result in (1) perforation of the nasal septum in cocaine snorters; (2) decreased lung diffusing capacity in those who inhale the smoke from cocaine; and (3) rarely, the development of dilated cardiomyopathy.

The hazards of cocaine abuse extend to pregnancy and the fetus. These include abruptio placentae, premature labor, intrauterine growth retardation, and possible teratogenesis.

Heroin. Heroin, although not as widely used as cocaine, is even more hazardous. It is an addicting opioid, closely related to morphine, derived from the poppy plant. It is sold on the street cut (diluted) with an agent, often talc or quinine; in this setting, the size of the dose not only is variable but also is usually unknown to the buyer. The heroin, along with any contaminating substances, is usually self-administered intravenously or subcutaneously. Effects are varied and include euphoria, hallucinations, somnolence, and sedation. Heroin has a wide range of adverse physical effects related to (1) the pharmacologic action of the agent, (2) reactions to the cutting agents or contaminants, (3) hypersensitivity reactions to the drug or its adulterants (quinine itself has neurologic, renal, and auditory toxicity), and (4) diseases contracted incident to the use of the needle.

■ Sudden death, usually related to overdose, is an ever-present risk because drug purity is generally unknown and may range from 2% to 90%. Sudden death can also occur if tolerance for the drug, built up over time, is lost (as during a period of incarceration). The mechanisms of death include profound respiratory depression, arrhythmia and cardiac arrest, and severe pulmonary edema.
■ Pulmonary complications include moderate to severe edema, septic embolism, lung abscess, opportunistic infections, and foreign body granulomas from talc and other adulterants. Although granulomas occur principally in the lung, they are sometimes found in the mononuclear-phag-

ocyte system, particularly in the spleen, liver, and lymph nodes that drain the upper extremities. Examination under polarized light often highlights trapped talc crystals, sometimes enclosed within foreign body giant cells.
■ Infectious complications are common. The four sites most commonly affected are the skin and subcutaneous tissue, heart valves, liver, and lungs. In a series of addicts admitted to the hospital, more than 10% had endocarditis, which often takes a distinctive form involving right-sided heart valves, particularly the tricuspid. Most cases are caused by *Staphylococcus aureus,* but fungi and a multitude of other organisms have also been implicated. Viral hepatitis is the most common infection among addicts and is acquired by the casual sharing of dirty needles. In the United States this practice has also led to a very high incidence of acquired immunodeficiency syndrome (AIDS) in drug addicts, an incidence second only to that in homosexual men.
■ Cutaneous lesions are probably the most frequent telltale sign of heroin addiction. Acute changes include abscesses, cellulitis, and ulcerations owing to subcutaneous injections. Scarring at injection sites, hyperpigmentation over commonly used veins, and thrombosed veins are the usual sequelae of repeated intravenous inoculations.
■ Kidney disease is a relatively common hazard. The two forms most frequently encountered are amyloidosis and focal glomerulosclerosis, and both induce heavy proteinuria and the nephrotic syndrome. Amyloidosis is secondary to chronic skin infections (Chapter 5).

Marijuana. Marijuana, or "pot," is the most widely used illegal drug. It is made from the leaves of the *Cannabis sativa* plant, which contain the psychoactive substance Δ^9-tetrahydrocannabinol (THC). When it is smoked, about 50% of the THC is absorbed; when ingested, only about 5% to 10% is absorbed. Despite numerous studies, the central question of whether the drug has persistent adverse physical and functional effects remain unresolved. Some of the untoward anecdotal effects may be allergic or idiosyncratic reactions or may possibly be related to contaminants in the preparations rather than to marijuana's pharmacologic effects. On the other hand, two beneficial effects of THC are its capacity to decrease intraocular pressure in glaucoma and to combat intractable nausea secondary to cancer chemotherapy.

■ The functional and organic central nervous system consequences of marijuana have received greatest scrutiny. Clearly, the use of pot distorts sensory perception and impairs motor coordination, but these acute effects generally clear in 4 to 5 hours. With continued use, these changes may progress to cognitive and psychomotor impairment, such as inability to judge time, speed, and distance. Among adolescents, such changes often lead to automobile accidents.
■ Not unexpectedly, the lungs are affected by chronic pot smoking; laryngitis, pharyngitis, bronchitis, cough and hoarseness, and asthma-like symptoms have all been described, along with mild but significant airway obstruction. Smoking a marijuana cigarette, compared with a tobacco cigarette, is associated with a threefold increase in the amount of tar inhaled and retained in the lungs. Presumably, the larger puff volume, deeper inhalation, and longer breath holding are responsible. Concern continues that

long-term smokers of marijuana may also be at increased risk for lung cancer.
■ Marijuana increases the heart rate and sometimes blood pressure, and in a person with a fixed coronary artery, narrowing may cause angina.
■ Marijuana may induce chromosome damage in somatic and germ cells, but the evidence is not incontrovertible. A large study involving many thousands of female marijuana users revealed lower infant birth weights, shorter gestation periods, and an increased number of malformations among the offspring. Because the peak use of marijuana is among teenagers and young adults, these provocative findings require further study.

Inhalants. These agents of abuse have achieved great popularity among very young persons. Favorites among the inhalants are glue, paint thinner, nail polish remover, and many substances in aerosol cans such as hair spray and room deodorizers. As a group, the solvents and aerosolizers act as powerful central nervous system depressants; because they repress inhibitory pathways, they produce a transient "high" much like that of acute alcoholism. For the most part, the neurologic and psychologic effects (impairment in judgment, disorientation, and manic euphoria) are transitory, but deaths from heart failure have been reported, possibly because the solvents and fluorocarbons in aerosol cans intensify the effects of epinephrine on the heart.

INJURY BY PHYSICAL AGENTS

Injury induced by physical agents is divided into the following categories: mechanical trauma, thermal injury, electrical injury, and injury produced by ionizing radiation. Understanding the pathology of these forms of injury is clearly important to the physician who undertakes therapy and also, when death is the outcome, to the forensic pathologist, who may be required to determine the proximate cause of death and the medicolegal ramifications.

Mechanical Trauma

Mechanical forces may inflict damage in several ways. The impact of the body with a moving or stationary object can result in compression, stretching, torsion, or penetration of tissues. The type of injury depends on the type of object, the amount of energy discharged at impact, and the tissues or organs that bear the impact. With regard to particular tissues injured, bone and head injuries result in unique damage and are discussed elsewhere (Chapter 23). All soft tissues react similarly to mechanical forces, and the patterns of injury can be summarized in five terms: abrasion, contusion, laceration, incised wound, and puncture wound.

ABRASION. An abrasion is a wound produced by scraping or rubbing, resulting in removal of the superficial layer. Skin abrasions may remove only the epidermal layer.

CONTUSION. A contusion, or bruise, is a wound usually produced by a blunt object and characterized by damage to blood vessels and extravasation of blood into tissues.

LACERATION. A laceration is a tear or disruptive stretching of tissue caused by the application of force by a blunt object. In contrast to an incision, most lacerations have jagged, irregular edges.

INCISED WOUND. An incised wound is one inflicted by a sharp instrument.

PUNCTURE WOUND. A puncture wound is caused by a long narrow instrument and is termed **penetrating** when the instrument pierces the tissue and **perforating** when it traverses a tissue to also create an exit wound. Gunshot wounds are special forms of puncture wounds that demonstrate distinctive features important to the forensic pathologist. For example, a wound from a bullet fired at close range leaves powder burns, whereas one fired from more than 4 or 5 feet away does not.

One of the most common causes of mechanical injury is vehicular accidents; injuries sustained typically result from the driver or passenger (1) hitting a part of the interior of the vehicle or being hit by an object that enters the passenger compartment during the crash, such as the motor; (2) being thrown from the vehicle; or (3) being trapped in a burning vehicle. The pattern of injury relates to whether one or all three of these mechanisms are operative. For example, in a head-on collision, a common pattern of injury sustained by a driver who is not wearing a seat belt includes trauma to the head (windshield impact), chest (steering column impact), and knees (dashboard impact). Under these conditions, common chest injuries include sternal and rib fractures, heart contusions, aortic lacerations (Fig. 8–12), and (less commonly) lacerations of the spleen and liver. Thus, in caring for an automobile injury victim, it is essential to remember that *superficial abrasions, contusions, and lacerations are often accompanied by similar internal wounds. Indeed, in many cases external evidence of serious internal damage is completely absent.*

Thermal Injury

Both excess heat and excess cold are important causes of injury. Burns are all too common and are discussed first; a brief discussion of hyperthermia and hypothermia follows.

THERMAL BURNS

In the United States, burns cause 5000 deaths per year and result in the hospitalization of more than 10 times that many persons. Many victims are children, who are often scalded by hot liquids. Fortunately, marked decreases have been seen in both mortality rates and length of hospitalizations since the 1970s. This improved prognosis results from a better understanding of the systemic effects of massive burns and discov-

Despite continuous improvement in therapy, any burn exceeding 50% of the total body surface, whether superficial or deep, is grave and potentially fatal. With burns of more than 20% of the body surface, there is a rapid shift of body fluids into the interstitial compartments, both at the burn site and systemically, which can result in hypovolemic shock (Chapter 4). The mechanisms include an increase in local interstitial osmotic pressure (from release of osmotically active constituents of dying cells) and both neurogenic and mediator-induced increases in vascular permeability. Because protein from the blood is lost into interstitial tissue, generalized edema, including pulmonary edema, may become severe if fluids used for volume replacement are not osmotically active.

Another important consideration in patients with burns is the degree of *injury to the airways and lungs.* Inhalation injury is frequent in persons trapped in burning buildings and may result from the direct effect of heat on the mouth, nose, and upper airways or from the inhalation of toxic components in smoke. Water-soluble gases such as chlorine, sulfur oxides, and ammonia may react with water to form acids or alkalis, particularly in the upper airways, and to produce inflammation and swelling, which may lead to partial or complete airway obstruction. Lipid-soluble gases such as nitrous oxide and products of burning plastics are more likely to reach deeper airways, producing pneumonitis. Unlike shock, which develops within hours, pulmonary manifestations may not develop for 24 to 48 hours. Thus, the initial absence of respiratory symptoms does not necessarily imply that there has been no respiratory injury.

Secondary *burn infection* is an important complication in all burn patients who have lost epidermis. Organ system failure resulting from burn sepsis continues to be the leading cause of death in burned patients. The burn site is ideal for growth of microorganisms; the serum and debris provide nutrients, and the burn injury compromises blood flow, blocking effective inflammatory responses. The most common offender is the opportunist *Pseudomonas aeruginosa,* but antibiotic-resistant strains of other common hospital-acquired bacteria, such as *S. aureus,* and fungi, particularly *Candida* species, may also be involved. Furthermore, cellular and humoral defenses against infections are compromised, and both lymphocyte and phagocyte functions are impaired. Direct bacteremic spread and release of toxic substances such as endotoxin from the local site exert dire consequences. Pneumonia or septic shock with renal failure and/or the acute respiratory distress syndrome (ARDS) (Chapter 13) are the most common serious sequelae. Aggressive, early debridement of burn wounds is designed not only to provide a clean, vascular surface on which wound repair can proceed, but also to provide phagocytes ready access to infecting microorganisms. Topical antibiotics may help, but burn infection continues to be an important problem.

Another very important pathophysiologic effect of burns is

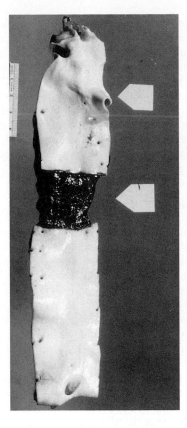

Figure 8–12 ■

Transverse rupture of the descending thoracic aorta incurred in an automobile accident. (Courtesy of Dr. Charles Petty, Department of Pathology and Forensic Medicine, University of Texas Southwestern Medical School, Dallas, TX.)

eries of better ways to prevent wound infection and facilitate healing of skin surfaces.

The clinical significance of burns depends on the following important factors:

■ Depth of the burn
■ Percentage of body surface involved
■ Possible presence of internal injuries from inhalation of hot and toxic fumes
■ Promptness and efficacy of therapy, especially fluid and electrolyte management and prevention or control of wound infections

A *full-thickness burn* involves total destruction of the epidermis and dermis, with loss of the dermal appendages that would have provided cells for epithelial regeneration. Both *third-* and *fourth-degree burns* are in this category. In *partial-thickness burns,* at least the deeper portions of the dermal appendages are spared. Partial-thickness burns include *first-degree burns* (epithelial involvement only) and *second-degree burns* (both epidermis and superficial dermis).

the *development of a hypermetabolic state* with excess heat loss and an increased need for nutritional support. It is estimated that when more than 40% of the body surface is burned, the resting metabolic rate may approach twice normal. The consequence is breakdown of tissue, which may result in loss of essential protein stores, reaching lethal proportions comparable to starvation within several weeks. Thus, it is essential to keep the patient's room temperature elevated to reduce body heat loss and to implement appropriate nutritional supplementation.

HYPERTHERMIA

Prolonged exposure to elevated ambient temperatures can result in heat cramps, heat exhaustion, and heat stroke.

■ *Heat cramps* result from loss of electrolytes via sweating. Cramping of voluntary muscles, usually in association with vigorous exercise, is the hallmark. Heat-dissipating mechanisms are able to maintain normal core body temperature.

■ *Heat exhaustion* is probably the most common heat syndrome. Its onset is sudden, with prostration and collapse, and it results from a failure of the cardiovascular system to compensate for hypovolemia, secondary to water depletion. After a period of collapse, which is usually brief, equilibrium is spontaneously re-established.

■ *Heat stroke* is associated with high ambient temperatures and high humidity. Thermoregulatory mechanisms fail, sweating ceases, and core body temperature rises. Body temperatures of 112° to 113°F have been recorded in some terminal cases. Clinically, a rectal temperature of 106°F or higher is considered a grave prognostic sign, and the mortality rate for such patients exceeds 50%. The underlying mechanism is marked generalized peripheral vasodilation with peripheral pooling of blood and a decreased effective circulating blood volume. Necrosis of the muscles and myocardium may occur. Arrhythmias, disseminated intravascular coagulation, and other systemic effects are common. Elderly persons, individuals undergoing intense physical stress (including young athletes and military recruits), and persons with cardiovascular disease are prime candidates for heat stroke.

HYPOTHERMIA

Prolonged exposure to low ambient temperature leads to hypothermia, a condition seen all too frequently in homeless persons. Lowering of body temperature is hastened by high humidity in cold, wet clothing and dilation of superficial blood vessels as a result of the ingestion of alcohol. At about 90°F, loss of consciousness occurs, followed by bradycardia and atrial fibrillation at lower core temperatures.

Local Reactions. Chilling or freezing of cells and tissues causes injury in two ways:

1. Direct effects are probably mediated by physical dislocations within cells and high salt concentrations incident to the crystallization of the intra- and extracellular water.
2. Indirect effects are exerted by circulatory changes. Depending on the rate at which the temperature drops and the duration of the drop, slowly developing chilling may induce vasoconstriction and increased permeability, leading

to edematous changes. Such changes are typical of "trench foot." Atrophy and fibrosis may follow. Alternatively, with sudden sharp drops in temperature that are persistent, the vasoconstriction and increased viscosity of the blood in the local area may cause ischemic injury and degenerative changes in peripheral nerves. In this situation, only after the temperature begins to return toward normal do the vascular injury and increased permeability with exudation become evident. However, during the period of ischemia, hypoxic changes and infarction of the affected tissues may develop (e.g., gangrene of toes or feet).

Electrical Injury

Electrical injuries, which may result in death, can arise from low-voltage currents (i.e., in the home and workplace), high-voltage currents from high-power lines, or lightning. Injuries are of two types: (1) burns and (2) ventricular fibrillation or cardiac and respiratory center standstill resulting from disruption of normal electrical impulses. The type of injury and the severity and extent of burning depend on the amperage and path of the electric current within the body.

It is important to remember that current flow (amperes) equals voltage (volts) divided by resistance (ohms). Obviously, current flow, and therefore injury, is less if voltage is low or resistance is high. Unfortunately, voltage in the household and workplace (120 or 220 V) is high enough so that with low resistance at the site of contact (as when the skin is wet; resistance is higher when the skin is dry), sufficient current can pass through the body to ground to cause serious injury, including ventricular fibrillation. If current flow continues long enough, it generates sufficient heat to produce burns at the site of entry and exit as well as in internal organs. An important characteristic of alternating current, the type available in most homes, is that it induces tetanic muscle spasm, so that if an energized object is grasped, irreversible clutching is likely to occur, prolonging the period of current flow. This results in a greater likelihood of developing extensive electrical burns and, in some cases, spasm of the chest wall muscles, producing death from asphyxia. Currents generated from high-voltage sources cause similar damage; however, because of the large current flows generated, these are more likely to produce paralysis of medullary centers and extensive burns. Lightning also produces high-voltage electrical injury.

Before leaving the subject of electrical injury, a word about the health risk of exposure to electromagnetic fields (EMFs) is in order. Some epidemiologic studies have linked exposure to EMFs among electrical workers (especially those who work on high-power lines) and children living near high-power lines to an increased risk for cancer, particularly leukemias, lymphomas, and cancers in the nervous system. However, after an analysis of all available data, a panel of U.S. experts has concluded that EMFs do not pose a human health hazard.

Injury Produced by Ionizing Radiation

Ionizing radiation is a double-edged sword: it provides an invaluable means of clinical diagnosis and for some tumors a curative mode of therapy, but at the same time it is a potent mutagen and destroyer of cells. Cosmic radiation and emissions from naturally occurring terrestrial radionuclides (radon gas) are omnipresent; diagnostic x-ray procedures are common occurrences, as is radiotherapy for cancers. Public concern about the location of nuclear waste disposal sites and the safety of nuclear reactors reflects a widespread awareness of the potential dangers of ionizing radiation.

Ionizing radiation occurs in two forms: (1) electromagnetic waves (x-rays and gamma rays) and (2) high-energy neutrons and charged particles (alpha and beta particles and protons). All forms of ionizing radiation exert their effects on cells by displacing electrons from molecules and atoms with which they collide, causing ionization and inducing a cascade of events that may alter the cell transiently or permanently. The most important target molecule in living cells is DNA. Ionizing radiation may directly damage DNA (direct target theory), but more often it indirectly damages DNA by inducing the formation of free radicals, particularly those that form from the radiolysis of water (indirect target theory). Other cell molecules that may also be direct or indirect targets of radiant injury include lipids in cell membranes and proteins that function as critical enzymes. The transfer of energy to a target atom or molecule from the incident source of radiant energy occurs within microfractions of a second, yet its biologic effect may not become apparent for minutes or, if the effect is on DNA, even decades.

The following terms are used to express radiation dose:

■ *Roentgen* (R) is a unit of x- or gamma irradiation defined by the quantity of induced ionization in air. Thus, it is a measure of exposure.
■ *Radiation absorbed dose* (rad) and *grays* (Gy) are units that express the energy absorbed by target tissue from gamma and x-rays. A rad or its equivalent, the centigray (cGy), is the dose that results in absorption of 100 ergs of energy per gram of tissue.
■ *Curie* (Ci) defines the disintegrations per second of a spontaneously disintegrating radionuclide (radioisotope). One Ci is equal to 3.7×10^{10} disintegrations per second.

These three measurements do not directly quantify energy transferred per unit of tissue and therefore do not predict the biologic effects of radiation. The following terms provide a better approximation of such information:

■ *Linear energy transfer* (LET) expresses energy loss per unit of distance traveled as electron volts per micrometer. This value depends on the type of ionizing radiation. LET is very high for alpha particles, less so for beta particles, and even less for gamma rays and x-rays. Thus, alpha and beta particles penetrate short distances and interact with many molecules within that short distance. Gamma rays and x-rays penetrate deeply but interact with relatively few molecules per unit distance. It should be evident that if equivalent amounts of energy entered the body in the form of alpha and gamma radiation, the alpha particles would induce heavy damage in a restricted area, whereas gamma rays would dissipate energy over a longer course and produce considerably less damage per unit of tissue.
■ *Relative biologic effectiveness* (RBE) is simply a ratio that represents the relationship of the LETs of various forms

of irradiation to cobalt gamma rays and megavolt x-rays, both of which have an RBE of unity (1).

Effects of Ionizing Radiation on Cells and Tissues. The primary target of ionizing radiation is DNA. Except at extremely high doses that impair DNA transcription, DNA damage is compatible with survival if the cell remains in the intermitotic phase; however, during mitosis, cells that have incurred irreparable DNA damage die, because chromosome abnormalities prevent normal division. Understandably, therefore, *tissues with a high rate of cell turnover, such as bone marrow and the mucosa of the gastrointestinal tract, are extremely vulnerable to radiation,* and the injury is manifest early after exposure. Tissues with slower turnover rates, such as liver and endothelium, are not affected immediately after irradiation but are depopulated slowly, because dividing cells cannot be replaced. Tissues with nondividing cells, such as brain and myocardium, do not demonstrate radiation effects except at doses that are so high that DNA transcription or some other molecule vital to the normal functioning of the cell is affected. In summary, within days of exposure to radiant energy, tissues containing many rapidly dividing cells show evidence of radiation injury, while tissues that contain few dividing cells show little injury.

Because tissues are made up of many cell types, the effects of radiation are complex. For example, vascular injury can result in changes that interfere with repair, and therefore parenchymal cells may reveal manifestations of radiation injury months to years later. Endothelial cells, which are moderately sensitive to irradiation, may be damaged, and the resultant narrowing or occlusion of the blood vessels may lead to impaired healing of parenchymal cells or chronic ischemic atrophy. Vascular changes in the central nervous system after irradiation can lead to late manifestations of radiation damage, although nerve cells were not directly affected by the ionizing radiation.

In addition to the number of replicating cells in a tissue, several other important parameters determine whether injury will occur in irradiated tissue. These include (1) the rate of the dose delivered, (2) the capacity of the cells to repair themselves, and (3) the effect of oxygen. An important practical application of this knowledge is in designing strategies for radiation treatment of cancer.

The rate of delivery significantly modifies the biologic effect. Although the effect of radiant energy is cumulative, delivery in divided doses may allow cells to repair some of the damage in the intervals. Thus, fractional doses of radiant energy have a cumulative effect only to the extent that repair during the intervals is incomplete. Radiotherapy of tumors exploits the fact that, in general, normal cells are capable of more rapid repair and recovery and so do not sustain as much cumulative radiation injury as do tumor cells. Oxygenation amplifies radiation damage to cells and tissues. Radiant energy may interact with molecular oxygen to induce free radicals, such as superoxide, which can then interact with atoms and molecules to compound the cellular injury. The oxygen effect is significant in the radiotherapy of neoplasms. The center of rapidly growing tumors may be poorly vascularized and therefore somewhat hypoxic, making radiotherapy less effective. A summary of the biologic effects of ionizing radiation is provided in Figure 8–13.

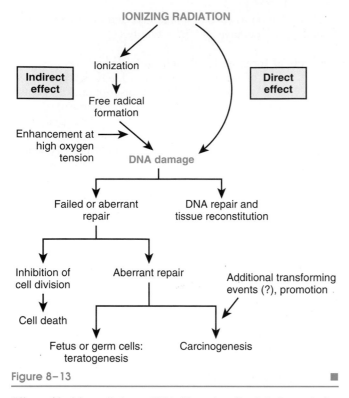

Figure 8–13

Effects of ionizing radiation on DNA. The major effect is indirect, via free radical formation.

MORPHOLOGY. At the **molecular level,** the DNA sustains a variety of alterations. These include the formation of pyrimidine dimers, cross-links, single-strand or double-strand breaks, and various rearrangements. Most single-strand breaks are rapidly repaired, often within minutes; double-strand breaks are more often irreparable. These alterations lead to a wide range of structural changes in chromosomes, including deletions, breaks, translocations, and fragmentation. The mitotic spindle often becomes disorderly, and polyploidy and aneuploidy may be encountered. At the **cellular level,** nuclear swelling and condensation and clumping of chromatin may appear; sometimes the nuclear membrane breaks. All forms of abnormal nuclear morphology may be produced. Giant cells with pleomorphic nuclei or more than one nucleus may appear and persist for years after exposure. At extremely high dose levels of radiant energy, nuclear pyknosis or lysis appears quickly as a marker of cell death.

In addition to affecting DNA and nuclei, radiant energy may induce a variety of **cytoplasmic changes,** including cytoplasmic swelling, mitochondrial distortion, and degeneration of the endoplasmic reticulum. Plasma membrane breaks and focal defects may appear. The histologic constellation of cellular pleomorphism, giant cell formation, conformational changes in nuclei, and

mitotic figures creates a more than passing similarity between radiation-injured cells and cancer cells, a problem that plagues the pathologist evaluating postirradiation tissues for the possible persistence of tumor cells.

At the light microscopic level, vascular changes are prominent in irradiated tissues. During the immediate postirradiation period, vessels may show only dilation. Later, or with higher doses, a variety of degenerative changes appear, including endothelial cell swelling and vacuolation, or even dissolution with total necrosis of the walls of small vessels such as capillaries and venules. Affected vessels may rupture or thrombose. Still later, endothelial cell proliferation and collagenous hyalinization with thickening of the media are seen in irradiated vessels, resulting in marked narrowing or even obliteration of the vascular lumina.

Effects on Organ Systems. Figure 8–14 depicts the organs that are particularly radiosensitive, together with common early and late manifestations.

The *hematopoietic and lymphoid systems are extremely susceptible to radiant injury* and deserve special mention here. With high dose levels and large exposure fields, severe lymphopenia may appear within hours of radiation, along with shrinkage of the lymph nodes and spleen. Radiation directly destroys lymphocytes, both in the circulating blood and in tissues (nodes, spleen, thymus, gut). With sublethal doses of irradiation, regeneration from viable precursors is prompt, leading to restoration of a normal lymphocyte count in the blood within weeks to months. The circulating granulocyte count may first rise but begins to fall toward the end of the first week. Levels near zero may be reached during the second week. If the patient survives, recovery of the normal granulocyte count may require 2 to 3 months. Platelets are similarly affected, with the nadir of the count occurring somewhat later than that of granulocytes; recovery is similarly delayed. Hematopoietic cells in the bone marrow, including red cell precursors, are also quite sensitive to radiant energy. Erythrocytes are radioresistant, but anemia may nonetheless appear after 2 to 3 weeks and persist for months because of marrow damage.

Another effect of irradiation on organ systems that deserves special mention relates to *malignant transformation* (see Fig. 8–13 and Chapter 6). Any cell capable of division that has sustained a mutation has the potential to become cancerous. Thus, an increased incidence of neoplasms may occur in any organ after radiation. The level of radiation required to increase the risk of cancer development is difficult if not impossible to determine. Radiation in very large doses kills cells and therefore is not associated with occurrence of tumors. Sublethal but relatively high doses are clearly associated with an increased risk. This is documented by the increased incidence of neoplasms in survivors of the atomic bombing of Hiroshima and Nagasaki, in radiologists of bygone years, and in miners of uranium ores. Exposure to low-dose irradiation has its risks as well, as will be evident from the following discussion of the relationship of radon to bronchogenic carcinoma.

Radon is a ubiquitous alpha particle–emitting product of

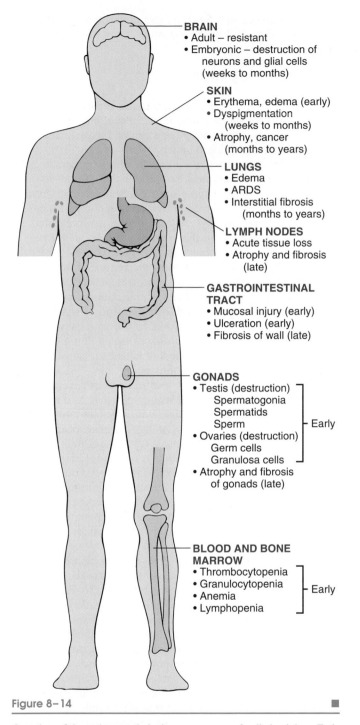

BRAIN
• Adult – resistant
• Embryonic – destruction of
  neurons and glial cells
  (weeks to months)

SKIN
• Erythema, edema (early)
• Dyspigmentation
  (weeks to months)
• Atrophy, cancer
  (months to years)

LUNGS
• Edema
• ARDS
• Interstitial fibrosis
  (months to years)

LYMPH NODES
• Acute tissue loss
• Atrophy and fibrosis
  (late)

**GASTROINTESTINAL
TRACT**
• Mucosal injury (early)
• Ulceration (early)
• Fibrosis of wall (late)

GONADS
• Testis (destruction)
  Spermatogonia
  Spermatids
  Sperm   ⎤ Early
• Ovaries (destruction)
  Germ cells
  Granulosa cells   ⎦
• Atrophy and fibrosis
  of gonads (late)

**BLOOD AND BONE
MARROW**
• Thrombocytopenia
• Granulocytopenia   ⎤ Early
• Anemia
• Lymphopenia   ⎦

Figure 8–14

Overview of the major morphologic consequences of radiation injury. Early changes occur in hours to weeks; late changes occur in months to years. ARDS, adult respiratory distress syndrome.

the spontaneous decay of uranium. Because radon is a gas, it moves freely in and out of the lungs and generally does not accumulate in tissues, nor does it cause damage because, as previously discussed, alpha emitters penetrate tissues very poorly. In contrast, two radon decay by-products (or radon "daughters") are alpha particle–emitting particulates. These particulates are more readily deposited in lung tissue and can accumulate, producing short-range DNA damage. Over a pe-

Table 8–7. SYNDROMES ASSOCIATED WITH VARIOUS LEVELS OF TOTAL BODY IRRADIATION

Syndrome	Dose (rad)	Clinical Manifestations
Hematopoietic	200–500	Nausea and vomiting, lympho-penia, thrombocytopenia, neutropenia, later anemia
Gastrointestinal	500–1000	Severe gastrointestinal symptoms, including diarrhea, hemorrhage, emaciation; at higher doses, death within days; at lower doses, hematopoietic system manifestations
Cerebral	>5000	Listlessness and drowsiness, followed by convulsions, coma, and death within hours

riod of time, cells that suffer sufficient unrepaired DNA damage may become neoplastic and give rise to lung carcinomas. It is not currently known what levels of radon might be safe, but the question is of considerable importance, because radon is ubiquitous and may accumulate in buildings, particularly where ventilation is poor. Fortunately, the levels of radon currently thought to be safe are only uncommonly exceeded, except in those regions of the United States where uranium is closer to the surface and home construction practices facilitate leakage and entrapment of gases from the soil in basements.

Total Body Radiation. Exposure of large areas of the body to even very small doses of radiation may have devastating effects. Although 10 to 50 rad of gamma or x-ray exposure may exert no discernible effects, 50 to 100 rad may cause as many as 10% of exposed individuals to manifest nausea and vomiting, fatigue, and transient decreases in lymphocytes and granulocytes. As little as 100 to 300 rad of radiant energy in total body exposure delivered in one dose may induce an "acute radiation syndrome." To place this radiation level in context, it must be appreciated that doses of 4000 rad or more are often used in carefully shielded patients for radiotherapy of tumors. The lethal range in humans for total body radiation begins at about 200 rad, and at 700 rad, death is certain without medical intervention. Three often fatal acute radiation syndromes have been identified: (1) hematopoietic, (2) gastrointestinal, and (3) cerebral (Table 8–7).

NUTRITIONAL DISEASES

Adequate nutrition continues to be one of the most important concerns of humankind. In third world countries, undernutrition or protein-energy malnutrition (PEM) continues to be common, and in industrialized societies the most frequent diseases (atherosclerosis, cancer, diabetes, and hypertension) have all been linked to some form of dietary impropriety.

An adequate diet should provide (1) energy, in the form of carbohydrates, fats, and proteins; (2) essential (as well as nonessential) amino acids and fatty acids to be utilized as building blocks for synthesis of structural and functional proteins and lipids; and (3) vitamins and minerals, which function as co-enzymes or hormones in vital metabolic pathways or, as in the case of calcium and phosphate, as important structural components. In *primary malnutrition,* one or all of these components is missing from the diet. By contrast, in *secondary,* or *conditional, malnutrition*, the supply of nutrients is adequate, but malnutrition may result from nutrient malabsorption, impaired nutrient utilization or storage, excess nutrient losses, or increased need for nutrients.

In developing nations, the incidence of overt hunger is high, and the incidence of more subtle forms of undernutrition is even higher. Vitamin A deficiencies are rampant in certain parts of Africa, iodine deficiencies occur in regions where iodized salt is not available, and iron deficiency is often seen in infants fed exclusively milk diets. Thus, ignorance about the nutritional value of foods also plays an important role in malnutrition. In the United States, the National Research Council recommends daily allowances for protein, vitamins, and minerals for healthy adults, specifying ranges for both men and women. These standards represent the scientifically based general consensus of the safe (not minimal) amounts of each nutrient necessary to maintain good health. Debates continue as to optimal levels of fat and fiber to prevent cardiovascular disease and cancer, and this subject will be briefly discussed later.

It must be emphasized that affluent societies are not immune to a significant incidence of undernutrition. The following listing of common causes in the United States highlights this point:

■ *Ignorance and poverty.* Homeless persons, aged individuals, and children of the poor demonstrate effects of PEM as well as trace nutrient deficiencies. Even the affluent may fail to recognize that infants, adolescents, and pregnant women have increased nutritional needs.

■ *Chronic alcoholism.* Alcoholics may sometimes suffer PEM but are more frequently deficient in several vitamins, especially thiamine, pyridoxine, folate, and vitamin A, owing to a combination of dietary deficiency, defective gastrointestinal absorption, abnormal nutrient utilization and storage, increased metabolic needs, and an increased rate of loss. A failure to recognize the likelihood of thiamine deficiency in chronic alcoholics may result in irreversible brain damage (e.g., Korsakoff's psychosis, discussed later).

■ *Acute and chronic illnesses.* The basal metabolic rate (BMR) becomes accelerated in many illnesses (in patients with extensive burns, it may double), resulting in an increased daily requirement for all nutrients. Failure to appreciate this fact can compromise recovery.

■ *Self-imposed dietary restriction.* Anorexia nervosa, bulimia nervosa, and less overt eating disorders affect a large population who are concerned about body image or suffer from an unreasonable fear of cardiovascular disease.

Other, less common causes of malnutrition include the malabsorption syndromes, genetic diseases, specific drug therapies (which block uptake or utilization of particular nutrients), and total parenteral nutrition (TPN).

In the sections that follow, we will barely skim the surface of nutritional disorders. Included in the discussion are PEM, deficiencies of most of the vitamins and trace minerals, obesity, and a brief overview of the relationships of diet to ath-erosclerosis and cancer. Several other nutrients and nutritional issues are discussed in the context of specific disorders throughout the text.

Protein-Energy Malnutrition

Severe PEM is a disastrous disease. It is far too common in third world countries, where up to 25% of children may be affected; in these countries it is a major factor in the high death rates among children under 5 years of age.

PEM refers to a *range of clinical syndromes* characterized by an inadequate dietary intake of protein and calories to meet the body's needs. It is important to remember that, from a functional standpoint, there are two protein compartments in the body: the *somatic protein compartment*, represented by the skeletal muscles, and the *visceral protein compartment*, represented by protein stores in the visceral organs, primarily the liver. These two compartments are regulated differently, and as we shall see, the somatic compartment is affected more severely in marasmus, and the visceral compartment is depleted more severely in kwashiorkor. Before discussing the clinical presentations of the two polar forms of severe malnutrition (marasmus and kwashiorkor), some comments will be made on the clinical assessment of undernutrition and some of its general metabolic characteristics.

The diagnosis of PEM is obvious in its most severe forms; in mild to moderate forms, the usual approach is to compare the body weight for a given height with standard tables; other parameters are also helpful, including evaluation of fat stores, muscle mass, and serum proteins. With a loss of fat, the major storage form of energy, the thickness of skinfolds (which includes skin and subcutaneous tissue) is reduced. If the somatic protein compartment is catabolized, the resultant reduction in muscle mass is reflected by reduced circumference of the midarm. Measurement of serum proteins (albumin, transferrin, and others) provides a measure of the adequacy of the visceral protein compartment.

The most common victims of PEM worldwide are children. A child whose weight falls to less than 80% of normal is considered malnourished. When the level falls to 60% of normal weight for sex and age, the child is considered to have *marasmus.* A marasmic child suffers growth retardation and loss of muscle. The loss of muscle mass results from catabolism and depletion of the somatic protein compartment. This seems to be an adaptational response that serves to provide the body with amino acids as a source of energy. Interestingly, the visceral protein compartment, which is presumably more precious and critical for survival, is depleted only marginally, and hence *serum albumin levels are either normal or only slightly reduced.* In addition to muscle proteins, subcutaneous fat is also mobilized and used as a fuel. With such losses of muscle and subcutaneous fat, the *extremities are emaciated;* by comparison, the head appears too large for the body. Anemia and manifestations of multivitamin deficiencies are present, and there is evidence of *immune deficiency,* particularly of T cell–mediated immunity. Hence, concurrent infections are usually present, and they impose an additional stress on an already weakened body.

Kwashiorkor occurs when protein deprivation is relatively greater than the reduction in total calories. This is the most common form seen in African children who have been weaned

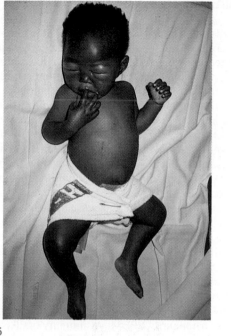

Figure 8-15   ■

Kwashiorkor. The infant shows generalized edema, seen in the form of puffiness of the face, arms, and legs.

(often too early, owing to the arrival of another child) and are subsequently fed an exclusively carbohydrate diet. The prevalence of kwashiorkor is also high in impoverished countries of Southeast Asia. Less severe forms may occur worldwide in persons with chronic diarrheal states in which protein is not absorbed or in those with conditions in which chronic protein loss occurs (e.g., protein-losing enteropathies, the nephrotic syndrome, or after extensive burns).

Kwashiorkor is a more severe form of malnutrition than marasmus. Unlike marasmus, marked protein deprivation is associated with severe loss of the visceral protein compartment, and the resultant hypoalbuminemia gives rise to generalized or dependent edema (Fig. 8-15). The weight of children with severe kwashiorkor is typically 60% to 80% of normal. However, the true loss of weight is masked by the increased fluid retention (edema). In further contrast to ma-

rasmus, there is relative sparing of subcutaneous fat and muscle mass. The modest loss of these compartments may also be masked by edema. Children with kwashiorkor have characteristic *skin lesions,* with alternating zones of hyperpigmentation, areas of desquamation, and hypopigmentation, giving a "flaky paint" appearance. *Hair changes* include overall loss of color or alternating bands of pale and darker hair; straightening, fine texture; and loss of firm attachment to the scalp. Other features that differentiate kwashiorkor from marasmus include an enlarged, *fatty liver* (resulting from reduced synthesis of carrier proteins) and a tendency to develop very early apathy, listlessness, and loss of appetite. As in marasmus, other vitamin deficiencies are likely to be present, as are *defects in immunity* and *secondary infections.* The latter add to the catabolic state, thus setting up a vicious cycle. It should be emphasized that marasmus and kwashiorkor are two ends of a spectrum, and considerable overlap exists.

Secondary PEM is not uncommon in chronically ill or hospitalized patients within the United States. Both marasmus-like and kwashiorkor-like syndromes (with intermediate forms) may develop. Table 8-8 summarizes the secondary forms of these two syndromes.

The central anatomic changes in PEM are (1) growth failure; (2) peripheral edema in kwashiorkor; and (3) loss of body fat and atrophy of muscle, more marked in marasmus.

The **liver** in kwashiorkor, but not in marasmus, is enlarged and fatty; superimposed cirrhosis is rare.

In kwashiorkor (rarely in marasmus) the **small bowel** shows a decrease in the mitotic index in the crypts of the glands, associated with mucosal atrophy and loss of villi and microvilli. In such cases, concurrent loss of small intestinal enzymes occurs, most often manifested as disaccharidase deficiency. Hence, infants with kwashiorkor initially may not respond well to a full-strength, milk-based diet. With treatment, the mucosal changes are reversible.

The **bone marrow** in both kwashiorkor and marasmus may be hypoplastic, owing mainly to decreased numbers of red cell precursors. How

Table 8-8. COMPARISON OF SEVERE MARASMUS-LIKE AND KWASHIORKOR-LIKE SECONDARY PROTEIN–ENERGY MALNUTRITION (PEM)

Syndrome	Clinical Setting	Time Course	Clinical Features	Laboratory Findings	Prognosis
Marasmus-like PEM	Chronic illness (e.g., chronic obstructive lung disease, cancer)	Months	History of weight loss Muscle wasting Absent subcutaneous fat	Normal or mildly reduced serum proteins	Variable; depends on underlying disease
Kwashiorkor-like PEM	Acute, catabolic illness (e.g., severe trauma, burns, sepsis)	Weeks	Normal fat and muscle Edema Easily pluckable hair	Serum albumin <2.8 gm/dl	Poor

Modified from Bennett JC, Plum F (eds): Cecil Textbook of Medicine, 20th ed. Philadelphia, WB Saunders, 1996, p 1156.
Original table adapted from Weinsier RL, et al: Handbook of Clinical Nutrition, 2nd ed. St. Louis, CV Mosby, 1989.

much of this derangement is due to a deficiency of protein and folates or to reduced synthesis of transferrin and ceruloplasmin is uncertain. Thus, anemia is usually present, most often hypochromic microcytic anemia, but a concurrent deficiency of folates may lead to a mixed microcytic-macrocytic anemia.

The **brain** in infants who are born to malnourished mothers and who suffer PEM during the first 1 or 2 years of life has been reported by some observers to show cerebral atrophy, a reduced number of neurons, and impaired myelinization of the white matter, but there is no universal agreement on the validity of these findings.

Many **other changes** may be present, including (1) thymic and lymphoid atrophy (more marked in kwashiorkor than in marasmus), (2) anatomic alterations induced by intercurrent infections, particularly with all manner of endemic worms and other parasites, and (3) deficiencies of other required nutrients such as iodine and vitamins.

Anorexia Nervosa and Bulimia

Anorexia nervosa is self-induced starvation, resulting in marked weight loss; bulimia is a condition in which the patient binges on food and then induces vomiting. These eating disorders occur primarily in previously healthy young women who have developed an obsession with attaining thinness.

The clinical findings in anorexia nervosa are generally similar to those in severe PEM. In addition, effects on the endocrine system are prominent. *Amenorrhea,* resulting from decreased secretion of gonadotropin-releasing hormone (Gn-RH) (and subsequent decreased secretion of luteinizing hormone [LH] and follicle-stimulating hormone [FSH]), is so common that its presence is a diagnostic feature for the disorder. Other common findings, related to decreased thyroid hormone release, include cold intolerance, bradycardia, constipation, and changes in the skin and hair. The skin becomes dry and scaly and may be yellow owing to excess carotene in the blood. Body hair may be increased but is usually fine and pale (lanugo). Bone density is decreased, most likely owing to low estrogen levels, which mimic the postmenopausal acceleration of osteoporosis. As expected with severe PEM, anemia, lymphopenia, and hypoalbuminemia may be present. A major complication of anorexia nervosa is an increased susceptibility to cardiac arrhythmia and sudden death, resulting in all likelihood from hypokalemia.

In bulimia, binge eating is the norm. Huge amounts of food, principally carbohydrates, are ingested, only to be followed by induced vomiting. Although menstrual irregularities are common, amenorrhea occurs in fewer than 50% of bulimia patients, probably because weight and gonadotropin levels are maintained near normal. The major medical complications relate to continual induced vomiting and include (1) electrolyte imbalances (hypokalemia), which predispose the patient to cardiac arrhythmias; (2) pulmonary aspiration of gastric contents; and (3) esophageal and cardiac rupture.

Vitamin Deficiencies

Thirteen vitamins are necessary for health; four—A, D, E, and K—are fat soluble, and the remainder are water soluble. The distinction between fat- and water-soluble vitamins is important, because although fat-soluble vitamins are more readily stored in the body, they are likely to be poorly absorbed in gastrointestinal disorders of fat malabsorption (Chapter 15). Small amounts of some vitamins can be synthesized endogenously—vitamin D from precursor steroids, vitamin K and biotin by the intestinal microflora, and niacin from tryptophan, an essential amino acid—but the rest must be supplied in the diet. A deficiency of vitamins may be primary (dietary in origin) or secondary (because of disturbances in intestinal absorption, transport in the blood, tissue storage, or metabolic conversion). In the following sections, the major vitamins, together with their well-defined deficiency states, are discussed individually (with the exception of B_{12} and folate, which are discussed in Chapter 12), beginning with the fat-soluble vitamins. However, it should be emphasized that deficiencies of a single vitamin are uncommon, and the expression of a deficiency of a combination of vitamins may be submerged in concurrent PEM. A summary of all the essential vitamins, along with their functions and deficiency syndromes, are presented in Table 8–9.

VITAMIN A

Vitamin A is actually a group of related natural and synthetic chemicals that exert a hormone-like activity or function. The relationship of some important members of this group is presented in Figure 8–16. *Retinol,* perhaps the most important form of vitamin A, is the transport form and, as the retinol ester, also the storage form. It is oxidized in vivo to the aldehyde *retinal* (the form used in visual pigment) and the acid *retinoic acid.* Important dietary sources of vitamin A are animal derived (e.g., liver, fish, eggs, milk, butter). Yellow and leafy green vegetables such as carrots, squash, and spinach supply large amounts of carotenoids, many of which are provitamins that can be metabolized to active vitamin A in vivo; the most important of these is beta-carotene. A widely used term, *retinoids,* refers to both natural and synthetic chemicals that are structurally related to vitamin A but do not necessarily have vitamin A activity.

As with all fats, the digestion and absorption of carotenes and retinoids require bile, pancreatic enzymes, and some level of antioxidant activity in the food. *Retinol,* whether derived from ingested esters or from beta-carotene (through an intermediate oxidation step involving retinal), is transported in chylomicrons to the liver for esterification and storage. More than 90% of the body's vitamin A reserves are stored in the liver, predominantly in the perisinusoidal stellate (Ito) cells. In normal persons who consume an adequate diet, these reserves are sufficient for at least 6 months' deprivation. *Retinoic acid,* on the other hand, can be absorbed unchanged; it represents a small fraction of vitamin A in the blood and is active in epithelial differentiation and growth but not in the maintenance of vision.

When dietary intake of vitamin A is inadequate, the retinol esters in the liver are mobilized, and released retinol is then bound to a specific retinol-binding protein (RBP), synthesized

Table 8–9.   VITAMINS: MAJOR FUNCTIONS AND DEFICIENCY SYNDROMES

Nutrient	Function	Deficiency Syndromes
Fat-Soluble Vitamins		
Vitamin A	Visual protein; hormonal regulation of cell growth	Night blindness, xerophthalmia, keratomalacia, metaplasia of columnar epithelium, immune deficiency
Vitamin D	Facilitates Ca and PO_4 absorption from intestine; helps maintain plasma Ca and PO_4 levels	Rickets in children, osteomalacia in adults, hypocalcemic tetany
Vitamin E	Antioxidant; maintenance of nervous system	Spinocerebellar syndrome
Vitamin K	Cofactor for hepatic carboxylation of prothrombin; factors VII, IX, and X; and proteins C and S	Bleeding diathesis
Water-Soluble Vitamins		
Thiamine (B_1)	As thiamine pyrophosphate functions as a coenzyme essential for maintaining nervous system	Wet and dry beriberi; Wernicke-Korsakoff syndrome
Riboflavin (B_2)	Cofactor in several enzymes, including FMN and FAD	Ariboflavinosis: cheilosis, glossitis, dermatitis, keratitis
Niacin	Component of coenzymes NAD and NADP	Pellagra: dementia, diarrhea, dermatitis
Pyridoxine (B_6)	Forms pyridoxal-5-phosphate, a coenzyme in many reactions	Cheilosis, glossitis, dermatitis, peripheral neuropathy
Pantothenic acid	Component of coenzyme A and acyl carrier protein	Recognized only under experimental conditions: constitutional and gastrointestinal symptoms, paresthesias, cramps, impaired coordination
Biotin	Cofactor in several carboxylation reactions	Deficiencies extremely rare: lassitude, anorexia, dermatitis, atrophic glossitis, myalgia, ECG changes, hypothermia, mild anemia
Folate	Coenzyme in transfer and utilization of 1-carbon units; essential step in nucleic acid synthesis	Megaloblastic anemia
Cyanocobalamin (B_{12})	Role in utilization of folate in nucleic acid synthesis, also essential for maintenance of nervous system	Megaloblastic anemia, subacute combined degeneration
Vitamin C	Cofactor in hydroxylation and amidation reactions	Scurvy

FMN, flavin mononucleotide; FAD, flavin adenine dinucleotide; NAD, nicotinamide adenine dinucleotide; NADP, nicotinamide adenine dinucleotide phosphate; ECG, electrocardiogram.

in liver. The uptake of retinol by the various cells of the body is dependent on surface receptors specific for RBP, rather than receptors specific for the retinol. Retinol is transported across the cell membrane, where it binds to a cellular retinol-binding protein and the RBP is released back into the blood.

Function. In humans the best-defined functions of vitamin A are as follows:

■ Maintaining normal vision in reduced light
■ Potentiating the differentiation of specialized epithelial cells, mainly mucus-secreting cells
■ Enhancement of immunity to infections, particularly in children

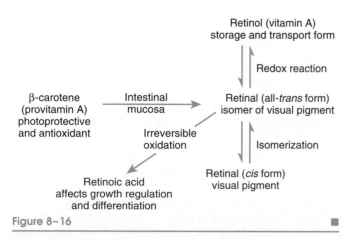

Figure 8–16   ■

Interrelationships of retinoids and their major functions.

In addition, the retinoids, beta-carotene, and some related carotenoids have been shown to function as photoprotective and antioxidant agents.

The *visual process* involves four forms of vitamin A–containing pigments: rhodopsin in the rods, the most light-sensitive pigment and therefore important in reduced light, and three iodopsins in cone cells, each responsive to specific colors in bright light. The synthesis of rhodopsin from retinol involves (1) oxidation to all-*trans*-retinal, (2) isomerization to 11-*cis*-retinal, and (3) interaction with the rod protein, opsin, to form rhodopsin. When a photon of light impinges on the dark-adapted retina, rhodopsin undergoes a sequence of configurational changes to ultimately yield all-*trans*-retinal and opsin. In the process, a nerve impulse is generated (by changes in membrane potential) that is transmitted via neurons from the retina to the brain. During dark adaptation some of the all-*trans*-retinal is reconverted to 11-*cis*-retinal, but most is reduced to retinol and lost to the retina, dictating the need for continuous input of retinol.

Vitamin A plays an important role in the orderly *differentiation of mucus-secreting epithelium;* when a deficiency state exists, the epithelium undergoes squamous metaplasia and differentiation to a keratinizing epithelium. The mechanism is not precisely understood, but in cell culture systems, retinoic acid (retinol is much less potent) regulates the gene expression of a number of cell receptors and secreted proteins, including receptors for growth factors.

Vitamin A plays some role in *host resistance to infections.* This beneficial effect of vitamin A seems to derive in part from its ability to stimulate the immune system, possibly through the formation of a recently discovered metabolite called *14-hydroxy retinol.* In addition, it appears that during infections, the bioavailability of vitamin A is reduced. The acute-phase response that accompanies many infections reduces the formation of retinol-binding protein in the liver, resulting in depression of circulating retinol levels, which in turn leads to reduced tissue availability of vitamin A. In keeping with this, supplements of the vitamin during the course of infections such as measles dramatically improves the clinical outcome.

It has been suspected that vitamin A and the carotenoids may play a role in preventing cancer. The following three mechanisms have been proposed:

1. The regulatory effect of retinoic acid on growth and differentiation has an anticarcinogenic effect.
2. The immunity-enhancing function of vitamin A has a protective effect.
3. The antioxidant function of the carotenoids prevents oxidant-induced mutagenic effects.

Despite these potential mechanisms, two recently completed studies have dashed any hopes of cancer prevention by dietary supplementation of beta-carotene and vitamin A. There was no reduction of cancer incidence, even in those at high risk for lung cancer as a result of cigarette smoking and asbestos exposure. In contrast, the structurally related retinoids are of benefit in the treatment of acute promyelocytic leukemia (Chapter 12), and some synthetic retinoids are reported to prevent recurrence of hepatocellular carcinomas following surgical resection. In addition, certain non-neoplastic skin diseases, including severe acne and psoriasis, are often controlled and cured by some synthetic retinoids devoid of vitamin A activity.

Deficiency State. Vitamin A deficiency occurs worldwide either on the basis of general undernutrition or as a conditioned deficiency among individuals having some cause for malabsorption of fats. One of the earliest manifestations of vitamin A deficiency is impaired vision, particularly in reduced light (night blindness). Because vitamin A and retinoids are involved in maintaining the differentiation of epithelial cells, persistent deficiency gives rise to a series of changes, the most devastating of which occur in the eyes. Collectively, the ocular changes are referred to as *xerophthalmia* (dry eye). First, there is dryness of the conjunctivae (xerosis) as the normal lachrymal and mucus-secreting epithelium is replaced by keratinized epithelium. This is followed by the buildup of keratin debris in small opaque plaques (Bitot's spots) and, eventually, erosion of the roughened corneal surface with softening and destruction of the cornea (keratomalacia) and total blindness.

In addition to the ocular epithelium, the epithelium lining the upper respiratory passages and urinary tract is replaced by keratinizing squamous cells (squamous metaplasia). Loss of the mucociliary epithelium of the airways predisposes to secondary pulmonary infections, and desquamation of keratin debris in the urinary tract predisposes to renal and urinary bladder stones. Hyperplasia and hyperkeratinization of the epidermis with plugging of the ducts of the adnexal glands may produce follicular or papular dermatosis. The pathologic

effects of vitamin A deficiency are summarized in Figure 8–17.

Another very serious consequence of avitaminosis A is immune deficiency. This impairment of immunity leads to higher mortality rates from common infections such as measles, pneumonia, and infectious diarrhea. In parts of the world where vitamin A deficiency is endemic, dietary supplements reduce mortality by 20% to 30%.

Vitamin A Toxicity. Both short- and long-term excess of vitamin A may produce toxic manifestations, a point of some concern because of the megadoses being popularized by certain health food stores. The clinical consequences of acute hypervitaminosis A include headache, vomiting, stupor, and papilledema, symptoms also suggestive of brain tumor. Chronic toxicity is associated with weight loss, nausea, and vomiting; dryness of the mucosa of the lips; bone and joint pain; hyperostosis; and hepatomegaly with parenchymal damage and fibrosis. Although synthetic retinoids used for the treatment of acne are not associated with the complications listed above, their use in pregnancy should be avoided owing to a well-established increase in the incidence of congenital malformations.

VITAMIN D

The major function of vitamin D is the *maintenance of normal plasma levels of calcium and phosphorus.* In this capacity, it is required for the prevention of bone diseases (rickets in growing children whose epiphyses have not already closed and osteomalacia in adults) and of hypocalcemic tetany. With respect to tetany, vitamin D maintains the correct concentration of ionized calcium in the extracellular fluid compartment required for normal neural excitation and relaxation of muscle. Insufficient ionized calcium in the extracellular fluid results in continuous excitation of muscle, leading to the convulsive state, hypocalcemic tetany. Our attention here will be focused on the function of vitamin D in the regulation of serum calcium levels.

Metabolism of Vitamin D. Humans have two possible sources of vitamin D: endogenous synthesis in the skin, and diet. There are large amounts of the precursor 7-dehydrocholesterol in the skin; ultraviolet (UV) light in sunlight converts it to vitamin D_3. Depending on the skin's level of melanin pigmentation, which absorbs UV light, and the amount of exposure to sunlight, about 80% of the vitamin D needed can be endogenously derived. The remainder must be obtained from dietary sources such as deep-sea fish, plants, and grains. In plant sources, vitamin D is present in its precursor form (ergosterol), which is converted to vitamin D_2 in the body. In many countries, various foods are fortified with vitamin D_2. Since D_3 and D_2 undergo identical metabolic transformations and have identical functions, both will hereafter be referred to as vitamin D.

The metabolism of vitamin D can be outlined as follows:

1. Absorption of vitamin D in the gut or synthesis from precursors in the skin.
2. Binding to a plasma α_1-globulin (D-binding protein [DBP]) and transport to liver.
3. Conversion to 25-hydroxyvitamin D (25-OH-D) by 25-hydroxylase in the liver.

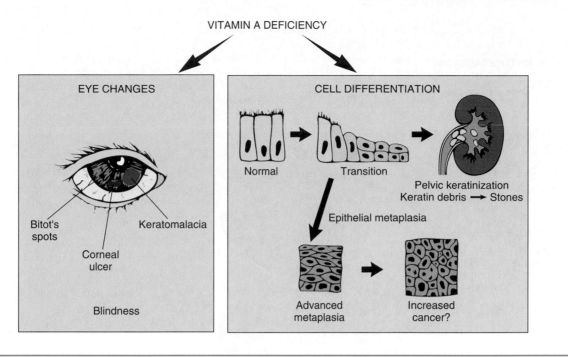

Figure 8–17   ■

Vitamin A deficiency. Its major consequences in the eye, in the production of keratinizing metaplasia of specialized epithelial surfaces, and its possible role in potentiating neoplasia.

4. Conversion of 25-OH-D to 1,25-$(OH)_2$-D by α_1-hydroxylase in the kidney; *biologically this is the most active form of vitamin D.*

The production of 1,25-$(OH)_2$-D by the kidney is regulated by three mechanisms:

1. In a feedback loop, increased levels of 1,25-$(OH)_2$-D down-regulate synthesis of this metabolite by inhibiting the action of α_1-hydroxylase, and decreased levels have the opposite effect.
2. Hypocalcemia stimulates secretion of parathyroid hormone, which in turn augments the conversion of 25-OH-D to 1,25-$(OH)_2$-D by activating α_1-hydroxylase.
3. Hypophosphatemia directly activates α_1-hydroxylase and thus increases formation of 1,25-$(OH)_2$-D.

Functions of Vitamin D. 1,25-$(OH)_2$-D, the biologically active form of vitamin D, is best regarded as a steroid hormone. Like other steroid hormones, it acts by binding to a high-affinity receptor that is widely distributed. However, the essential functions of vitamin D — the maintenance of normal plasma levels of calcium and phosphorus — involve actions on the intestines, bones, and kidneys. The active form of vitamin D

■ Stimulates intestinal absorption of calcium and phosphorus
■ Collaborates with parathyroid hormone in the mobilization of calcium from bone
■ Stimulates the parathyroid hormone (PTH)–dependent reabsorption of calcium in the distal renal tubules

How 1,25-$(OH)_2$-D stimulates intestinal absorption of calcium and phosphorus is still somewhat unclear. The weight of evidence favors the view that it binds to epithelial receptors, activating the synthesis of calcium transport proteins. The increased absorption of phosphorus is independent of the effects on calcium transport.

The effects of vitamin D on bone depend on the plasma levels of calcium. On the one hand, with hypocalcemia, 1,25-$(OH)_2$-D collaborates with PTH in the resorption of calcium and phosphorus from bone to support blood levels. On the other hand, vitamin D is required for normal mineralization of epiphyseal cartilage and osteoid matrix. It is still not clear how the resorptive function is mediated, but direct activation of osteoclasts is ruled out. It is more likely that vitamin D favors differentiation of osteoclasts from their precursors (monocytes). The precise details of mineralization of bone when vitamin D levels are adequate are also uncertain. It is widely believed that the main function of vitamin D is to maintain calcium and phosphorus at supersaturated levels in the plasma. However, vitamin D–mediated increases in the synthesis of the calcium-binding proteins, osteocalcin and osteonectin, in the osteoid matrix may also play a role.

Equally unclear is the role of vitamin D in renal reabsorption of calcium. PTH is clearly necessary, but it is believed that vitamin D is also. There is no substantial evidence that vitamin D participates in renal reabsorption of phosphorus. An overview of the normal metabolism of vitamin D and the consequences of a deficiency are depicted in Figure 8–18.

Deficiency States. Rickets in growing children and osteomalacia in adults are worldwide skeletal diseases, but in developed countries they rarely occur as a result of dietary deficiencies. Both forms of skeletal disease may result from deranged vitamin D absorption or metabolism or, less commonly, from disorders that affect the function of vitamin D or disturb calcium or phosphorus homeostasis. A summary of the causes of rickets and osteomalacia is given in Table 8–

NORMAL VITAMIN D METABOLISM

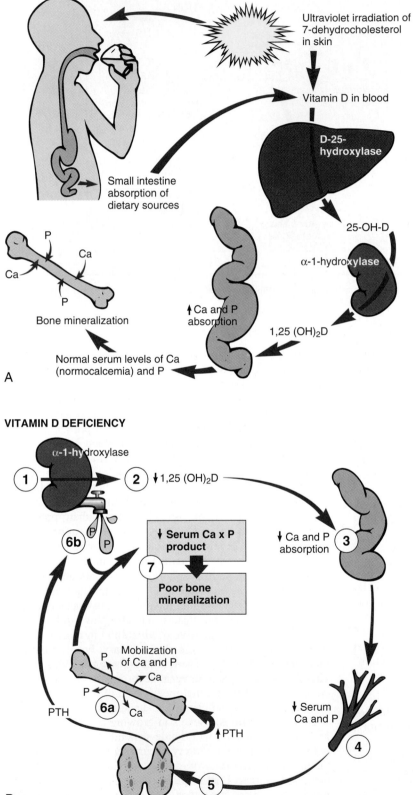

VITAMIN D DEFICIENCY

Figure 8–18 ■

A, Schema of normal vitamin D metabolism. *B,* Vitamin D deficiency. There is inadequate substrate for the renal hydroxylase (1), yielding a deficiency of $1,25(OH)_2D$ (2), and deficient absorption of calcium and phosphorus from the gut (3), with consequent depressed serum levels of both (4). The hypocalcemia activates the parathyroid glands (5), causing mobilization of calcium and phosphorus from bone (6a). Simultaneously, the parathyroid hormone (PTH) induces wasting of phosphate in the urine (6b) and calcium retention. Consequently, the serum levels of calcium are normal or nearly normal but the phosphate is low; hence, mineralization is impaired (7).

Table 8–10. CAUSES OF RICKETS OR OSTEOMALACIA

1. Decreased endogenous synthesis of vitamin D
   a. Inadequate exposure to sunlight
   b. Heavy melanin pigmentation of skin (blacks)

2. Decreased absorption of fat-soluble vitamin D in the intestine
   a. Dietary lack
   b. Biliary tract, pancreatic, or intestinal dysfunction

3. Enhanced degradation of vitamin D and 25(OH)-D
   a. Phenytoin, phenobarbital, rifampin induction of cytochrome P-450 enzymes

4. Impaired synthesis of 25(OH)-D
   a. Diffuse liver diseases

5. Decreased synthesis of $1,25(OH)_2$-D
   a. Advanced renal disease with failure
   b. Vitamin D–dependent rickets type I (inherited deficiency of renal α_1-hydroxylase)

6. Target organ resistance to $1,25(OH)_2$-D
   a. Vitamin D–dependent rickets type II (congenital lack of or defective receptors for active metabolite)

7. Phosphate depletion
   a. Poor absorption—long-term use of antacids, which bind phosphates and render them insoluble
   b. Renal tubular disorders, acquired or genetic, causing increased excretion

10. Whatever the basis, a deficiency of vitamin D tends to cause hypocalcemia. When hypocalcemia occurs, PTH production is increased, which (1) activates renal α_1-hydroxylase, thus increasing the amount of active vitamin D and calcium absorption; (2) mobilizes calcium from bone; (3) decreases renal calcium excretion; and (4) increases renal excretion of phosphate. Thus, the serum level of calcium is restored to near normal, but hypophosphatemia persists, and so mineralization of bone is impaired.

An understanding of the morphologic changes in rickets and osteomalacia is facilitated by a brief summary of normal bone development and maintenance. The development of flat bones in the skeleton involves intramembranous ossification, while the formation of long tubular bones reflects endochondral ossification. With intramembranous bone formation, mesenchymal cells differentiate directly into osteoblasts, which synthesize the collagenous osteoid matrix on which calcium is deposited. In contrast, with endochondral ossification, growing cartilage at the epiphyseal plates is provisionally mineralized and then progressively resorbed and replaced by osteoid matrix, which undergoes mineralization to create bone (Fig. 8–19B).

MORPHOLOGY. The basic derangement in both rickets and osteomalacia is an excess of unmineralized matrix. The changes that occur in the growing bones of children with rickets, however, are complicated by inadequate provisional calcification of epiphyseal cartilage deranging endochondral bone growth. The following sequence ensues in rickets:

- Overgrowth of epiphyseal cartilage due to inadequate provisional calcification and failure of the cartilage cells to mature and disintegrate
- Persistence of distorted, irregular masses of cartilage, many of which project into the marrow cavity (Fig. 8–19A)
- Deposition of osteoid matrix on inadequately mineralized cartilaginous remnants (Fig. 8–19A)
- Disruption of the orderly replacement of cartilage by osteoid matrix, with enlargement and lateral expansion of the osteochondral junction (Fig. 8–19A)
- Abnormal overgrowth of capillaries and fibroblasts in the disorganized zone because of microfractures and stresses on the inadequately mineralized, weak, poorly formed bone
- Deformation of the skeleton due to the loss of structural rigidity of the developing bones

The conformation of the gross skeletal changes depends on the severity of the rachitic process; its duration; and, in particular, the stresses to which individual bones are subjected. During the nonambulatory stage of infancy, the head and chest sustain the greatest stresses. The softened occipital bones may become flattened, and the parietal bones can be buckled inward by pressure; with the release of the pressure, elastic recoil snaps the bones back into their original positions **(craniotabes).** An excess of osteoid produces **frontal bossing** and a **squared appearance to the head.** Deformation of the chest results from overgrowth of cartilage or osteoid tissue at the costochondral junction, producing the **"rachitic rosary."** The weakened metaphyseal areas of the ribs are subject to the pull of the respiratory muscles and thus bend inward, creating anterior protrusion of the sternum **(pigeon breast deformity).** The inward pull at the margin of the diaphragm creates **Harrison's groove,** girdling the thoracic cavity at the lower margin of the rib cage. The pelvis may become deformed. When an ambulating child develops rickets, deformities are likely to affect the spine, pelvis, and long bones (e.g., tibia), causing, most notably, **lumbar lordosis** and **bowing of the legs** (Fig. 8–20).

In adults the lack of vitamin D deranges the normal bone remodeling that occurs throughout life. The newly formed osteoid matrix laid down by osteoblasts is inadequately mineralized, thus producing the excess of persistent osteoid characteristic of **osteomalacia.** Although the contours of the bone are not affected, the bone is weak and vulnerable to gross fractures or microfractures, which are most likely to affect vertebral bodies and femoral necks.

Histologically, the unmineralized osteoid can be visualized as a thickened layer of matrix (which stains pink in hematoxylin and eosin preparations) arranged about the more basophilic, normally mineralized trabeculae.

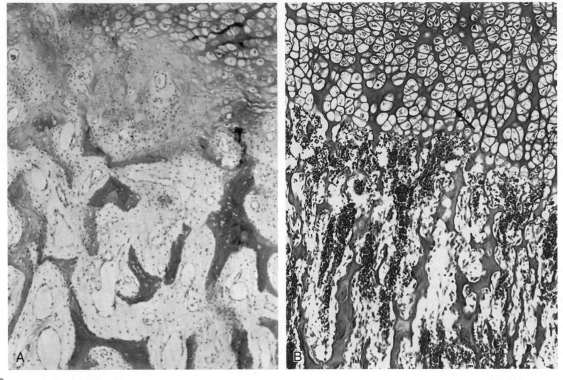

Figure 8-19 ■

A, Detail of a rachitic costochondral junction. The palisade of cartilage is lost. Some of the trabeculae are old, well-formed bone, but the paler ones consist of uncalcified osteoid. B, For comparison, normal costochondral function from a young child demonstrates the orderly transition from cartilage to new bone formation.

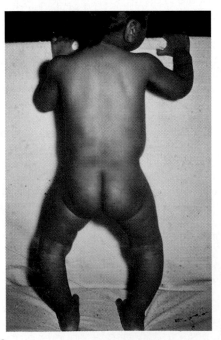

Figure 8-20 ■

Rickets. The bowing of legs in a toddler due to the formation of poorly mineralized bones is evident.

Persistent failure of mineralization in adults leads eventually to loss of skeletal mass, referred to as *osteopenia*. It is then difficult to differentiate osteomalacia from other osteopenias such as osteoporosis (Chapter 21). Osteoporosis, unlike osteomalacia, results from reduced production of osteoid, the protein matrix of the bone. Recent studies suggest that vitamin D may also be essential for preventing demineralization of bones. In certain familial forms of osteoporosis, the defect has been localized to the vitamin D receptor. It appears that certain genetically determined variants of the vitamin D receptor are associated with an accelerated loss of bone minerals with aging.

VITAMIN E

A group of eight closely related fat-soluble compounds—four tocopherols and four tocotrienols—all exhibit vitamin E biologic activity, but α-tocopherol is the most active and the most widely available. Vitamin E is abundant in so many foods—vegetables, grains, nuts and their oils, dairy products, fish, and meat—that a diet sufficient to sustain life is unlikely to be insufficient in vitamin E. The absorption of tocopherols, as of all fat-soluble vitamins, requires normal biliary tract and pancreatic function. After absorption, vitamin E is transported in the blood in the form of chylomicrons, which rapidly equilibrate with the plasma lipoproteins, mainly LDLs. Unlike vitamin A, which is stored predominantly in the liver, vitamin

E accumulates throughout the body, mostly in fat depots but also in liver and muscle.

This essential nutrient is one of a group of *antioxidants that serve to scavenge free radicals formed in redox reactions throughout the body* (Chapter 1). It plays a role in termination of free radical–generated lipid peroxidation chain reactions, particularly in cellular and subcellular membranes that are rich in polyunsaturated lipids. This action complements that of selenium, which, as a constituent of glutathione peroxidase, also metabolizes peroxides before they cause membrane damage. For reasons that are not clear, the nervous system is a particular target of vitamin E deficiency. Although the basis for this affinity is not entirely clear, it is speculated that neurons with long axons are particularly vulnerable because of their large membrane surface area. Mature red cells may also be vulnerable to vitamin E deficiency because they are at risk for oxidative injury imposed by the generation of superoxide radicals during oxygenation of hemoglobin.

Hypovitaminosis E resulting from a deficient diet is uncommon in the Western world and occurs almost exclusively in association with (1) fat malabsorption that accompanies cholestasis, cystic fibrosis, and primary small intestinal disease; (2) infant low birth weight with immature liver and gastrointestinal tract; and (3) abetalipoproteinemia, a rare autosomal recessive disorder in which transport of vitamin E is abnormal because the apoprotein B component of chylomicrons, LDLs, and very-low-density lipoproteins (VLDLs) is not synthesized.

MORPHOLOGY. The anatomic changes found in the nervous system depend on the duration and severity of the deficiency state. Most consistent is **degeneration of the axons in the posterior columns of the spinal cord, with focal accumulation of lipopigment and loss of nerve cells in the dorsal root ganglia, attributed to a dying-back type of axonopathy.** Myelin degeneration in sensory axons of peripheral nerves may also be present, and in more marked cases, degenerative changes in the spinocerebellar tracts may occur as well. In occasional cases, features of both primary and denervation muscle disease have been observed in skeletal muscle.

Vitamin E–deficient erythrocytes are more susceptible to oxidative stress and have a shorter half-life in the circulating blood.

The neurologic manifestations of vitamin E deficiency are depressed or, more often, absent tendon reflexes; ataxia; dysarthria; loss of position and vibration sense; and loss of pain sensation. Muscle weakness is also common. In addition, there may be impaired vision and disorders of eye movement, sometimes progressing to total ophthalmoplegia. Anemia is not a feature of the deficiency state in adults but is often found in premature infants and is probably multifactorial in origin.

In closing, attention should be drawn to the ongoing interest in the possible protective effects of vitamin E against atherosclerosis and cancer, the two most common causes of death in the United States. In the case of atherosclerosis, it is sug-gested that vitamin E may inhibit atheroma formation by reducing the oxidation of LDL (Chapter 10); in the context of cancer, the antioxidant effect is postulated to reduce mutagenesis. However, to date, epidemiologic studies designed to assess the protective role of vitamin E in these two conditions remain inconclusive.

VITAMIN K

Vitamin K is a required cofactor for a liver microsomal carboxylase that is necessary to convert glutamyl residues in certain protein precursors to γ-carboxyglutamates. *Clotting factors VII, IX, and X and prothrombin all require carboxylation of glutamate residues for functional activity.* Carboxylation provides calcium-binding sites and thus allows calcium-dependent interaction of these clotting factors with a phospholipid surface involved in the generation of thrombin (Chapter 4). In addition, activation of anticoagulant proteins C and S also requires glutamate carboxylation. In recent years, a diverse group of proteins with no connection to coagulation have also been found to be vitamin K dependent. Such proteins have been found in a wide variety of tissues, including kidney, bone, placenta, and lung. As with the proteins involved in coagulation, vitamin K serves to facilitate carboxylation of glutamyl residues in these other proteins as well. Of particular interest is osteocalcin, a noncollagenous protein secreted by osteoblasts; as with the coagulation proteins, γ-carboxylation of osteocalcin facilitates binding to calcium. Thus, *it appears that vitamin K may favor calcification of bone proteins.* Hence, much interest is focused on delineating the role of vitamin K in bone metabolism.

In the course of the reaction of vitamin K with its substrate proteins, its active (reduced) form is oxidized to an epoxide but then is promptly reduced back by a liver epoxide reductase (Fig. 8–21). Thus, in a healthy liver vitamin K is efficiently recycled, and the daily dietary requirement is low. Furthermore, endogenous intestinal bacterial flora readily synthesize the vitamin. Nevertheless, there is a small but definite need for exogenous vitamin, which fortunately is widely available in the usual Western diet. Deficiency usually occurs (1) in fat malabsorption syndromes, particularly with biliary tract dis-

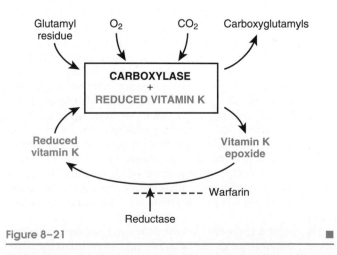

Figure 8–21

The biochemical events in the carboxylation of vitamin K-dependent proteins.

ease, as with the other fat-soluble vitamins; (2) after destruction of the endogenous vitamin K–synthesizing flora, particularly with ingestion of broad-spectrum antibiotics; (3) in the neonatal period, when liver reserves are small, the bacterial flora is not yet developed, and the level of vitamin K in breast milk is low; and (4) in diffuse liver disease, even in the presence of normal vitamin K stores, because hepatocyte dysfunction interferes with the synthesis of the vitamin K–dependent coagulation factors. In patients with thromboembolic disease, therapeutically desirable vitamin K deficiency is induced by coumarin anticoagulants (e.g., warfarin). These agents block the activity of liver epoxide reductase and thereby prevent regeneration of reduced vitamin K (Fig. 8–21).

The major consequence of vitamin K deficiency (or of inefficient utilization of vitamin K by the liver) is the development of a *bleeding diathesis*. In neonates, it causes hemorrhagic disease of the newborn. Its most serious manifestation is intracranial hemorrhage, but bleeding may occur at any site, including skin, umbilicus, and viscera. The estimated 3% prevalence of vitamin K–dependent bleeding diathesis among neonates warrants routine prophylactic vitamin K therapy for all newborns. However, in normal full-term infants, by 1 week of age, endogenous flora provide sufficient vitamin K to correct any lingering deficit. In adults suffering from vitamin K deficiency or decreased synthesis of vitamin K–dependent factors, a bleeding diathesis may occur, characterized by *hematomas, hematuria, melena, ecchymoses,* and *bleeding from the gums.*

THIAMINE

Thiamine is widely available in the diet, although refined foods such as polished rice, white flour, and white sugar contain very little. During absorption from the gut, thiamine undergoes phosphorylation to produce thiamine pyrophosphate (TPP), the functionally active coenzyme form of the vitamin. TPP has three major functions: (1) it regulates oxidative decarboxylation of alpha-ketoacids, leading to the synthesis of adenosine triphosphate (ATP); (2) it acts as a cofactor for transketolase in the pentose phosphate pathway; and (3) in a little-understood manner, it maintains neural membranes and normal nerve conduction (chiefly of peripheral nerves).

In underdeveloped countries where a large part of the scant diet consists of polished rice, as occurs in many areas of Southeast Asia, thiamine deficiency sometimes develops. In developed countries, clinically evident thiamine deficiency, although uncommon on a strictly dietary basis, *affects as many as one fourth of chronic alcoholics admitted to general hospitals.* A thiamine deficiency state may also result from the pernicious vomiting of pregnancy or from debilitating illnesses that impair the appetite, predispose to vomiting, or cause protracted diarrhea. Because a subclinical deficiency state may be converted to overt disease by extended intravenous glucose therapy or refeeding of chronically malnourished persons (particularly alcoholics), care must be taken that adequate amounts of thiamine are administered concurrently.

The major targets of thiamine deficiency are the peripheral nerves, the heart, and the brain, so persistent thiamine deficiency gives rise to three distinctive syndromes:

■ A polyneuropathy (dry beriberi)
■ A cardiovascular syndrome (wet beriberi)
■ Wernicke-Korsakoff syndrome

Typically, these three syndromes appear in this sequence, but on occasion the deficiency manifests as only one of them. The *polyneuropathy is usually symmetric and takes the form of a nonspecific peripheral neuropathy with myelin degeneration* and disruption of axons involving motor, sensory, and reflex arcs. It usually first appears in the legs, but it may also extend to the arms, so classically these patients present with toe-, foot-, and wristdrop. The progressive sensory loss is accompanied by muscle weakness and hypo- or areflexia.

Beriberi heart disease (wet beriberi) is associated with peripheral vasodilation, leading to more rapid arteriovenous shunting of blood, high-output cardiac failure, and eventually peripheral edema. The heart may be normal, have subtle changes, or be markedly enlarged and globular (owing to four-chamber dilation), with pale, flabby myocardium. The dilation thins the ventricular walls. Mural thrombi are often present, particularly in the dilated atria.

In protracted severe deficiency states, most often encountered in chronic alcoholics in the Western world, Wernicke-Korsakoff syndrome may appear. It usually develops against a background of peripheral neuropathy and cardiac insufficiency, but in some instances it is the only manifestation of thiamine deficiency. The details of this syndrome are presented in Chapter 23. Briefly, Wernicke's encephalopathy is marked by ophthalmoplegia; nystagmus; ataxia of gait and stance; and derangement of mental function, characterized by global confusion, apathy, listlessness, and disorientation. Korsakoff's psychosis takes the form of serious impairment of remote recall (retrograde amnesia), inability to acquire new information, and confabulation. Wernicke's encephalopathy and Korsakoff's psychosis are not distinct syndromes but rather are successive stages of a single central nervous system disease that have the same pathophysiologic substrate.

The central nervous system lesions affect *the mamillary bodies, the periventricular regions of the thalamus, the floor of the fourth ventricle, and the anterior region of the cerebellum.* There are hemorrhages and degenerative changes in the neurons (Chapter 23). The three major syndromes of thiamine deficiency are summarized in Figure 8–22.

RIBOFLAVIN

Riboflavin is a critical component of the coenzymes flavin mononucleotide (FMN) and flavin adenine dinucleotide (FAD), which participate in a wide range of oxidation–reduction reactions. In addition, flavin in covalent linkage is incorporated into succinic dehydrogenase and monoamine oxidase as well as into other mitochondrial enzymes. It is widely distributed in meat, dairy products, and vegetables as free riboflavin or riboflavin phosphate and is absorbed in the upper gastrointestinal tract.

Ariboflavinosis still occurs as a primary deficiency state among persons in economically deprived and developing countries. Under such circumstances, it is frequently accompanied by deficiencies of other vitamins and proteins. In industrialized nations, a deficiency is most likely to be encoun-

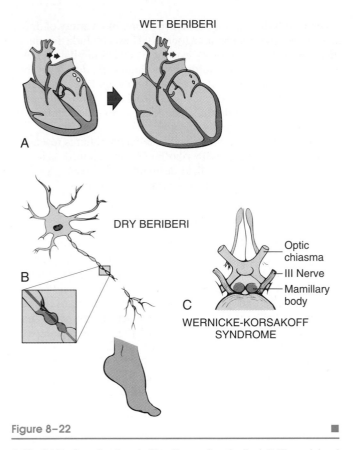

WET BERIBERI

A

DRY BERIBERI

B

C

Optic
chiasma
III Nerve
Mamillary
body

WERNICKE-KORSAKOFF
SYNDROME

Figure 8–22   ■

A, The flabby, four-chambered, dilated heart of wet beriberi. *B,* The peripheral neuropathy with myelin degeneration leading to footdrop, wristdrop, and sensory changes in dry beriberi. *C,* Hemorrhages into the mamillary bodies in the Wernicke-Korsakoff syndrome.

tered in alcoholics and in persons who have chronic infections, advanced cancer, or other debilitating diseases.

MORPHOLOGY. Ariboflavinosis is associated with changes at the angles of the mouth (known as cheilosis or cheilitis), glossitis, and ocular and skin changes.

Cheilosis is usually the first and most characteristic sign of this deficiency state. It begins as areas of pallor at the angles of the mouth. Later cracks or fissures may appear, radiating from the corners of the mouth, which tend to become secondarily infected.

With **glossitis** the **tongue** becomes atrophic, taking on a magenta hue strongly resembling the red-blue coloration of cyanosis (Fig. 8–23).

The **eye change** is a superficial interstitial keratitis. In the earlier stages the superficial layers of the cornea are invaded by capillaries. Interstitial inflammatory infiltration and exudation follow, producing opacities and sometimes ulcerations of the corneal surface.

A greasy, scaling **dermatitis** over the nasolabial folds may extend into a butterfly distribution to involve the cheeks and skin about the ears. Scrotal and vulvar lesions are common. In well-defined cases, atrophy of the skin may also develop. Erythroid hypoplasia in the **bone marrow** is typically present but is usually not marked.

NIACIN

Niacin is the generic designation for nicotinic acid and its functionally active derivatives (e.g., nicotinamide). In the form of nicotinamide, it is an essential component of two coenzymes, nicotinamide adenine dinucleotide (NAD) and nicotinamide adenine dinucleotide phosphate (NADP), both of which play central roles in cellular intermediary metabolism. NAD functions as a coenzyme for a variety of dehydrogenases involved in the metabolism of fat, carbohydrate, and amino acids. NADP participates in a variety of dehydrogenation reactions, particularly in the hexose-monophosphate shunt of glucose metabolism.

Niacin can be derived from the diet or may be synthesized endogenously. It is widely available in grains, legumes, and seed oils and in much smaller quantities in meats. In some grains it is present in bound form and therefore not absorbable; the niacin in maize (corn), in particular, is bound, so the niacin deficiency syndrome, *pellagra,* has appeared with unexpected frequency among native populations that subsist largely on maize. Niacin can also be synthesized endogenously from tryptophan. Thus, pellagra may result from either a niacin or a tryptophan deficiency. *In industrialized countries pellagra is encountered sporadically (usually in combination with other vitamin deficiencies), principally among alcoholics and persons suffering from chronic debilitating illnesses.* It may also occur with protracted diarrheal states, with diets that are grossly deficient in protein, and with long-term administration of drugs such as isoniazid and 6-mercaptopurine.

In pharmacologic doses, nicotinic acid lowers plasma LDL levels by reducing hepatic synthesis of VLDL, and hence it is used in the treatment of hypercholesterolemia.

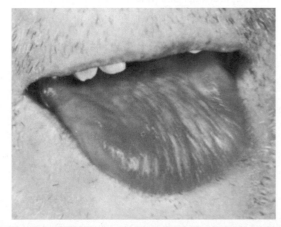

Figure 8–23   ■

The glazed, shiny, atrophic tongue of riboflavin deficiency.

MORPHOLOGY. The term **pellagra,** strictly speaking, refers to rough skin. The clinical syndrome, however, is classically identified by most clinicians by the "three Ds": dermatitis, diarrhea, and dementia.

Dermatitis is usually bilaterally symmetric and is found mainly on exposed areas of the body. The changes at first comprise redness, thickening, and roughening of the skin, which may be followed by extensive scaling and desquamation, producing fissures and chronic inflammation (Fig. 8–24). Similar lesions may occur in the mucous membranes of the mouth and vagina.

Diarrhea is caused by atrophy of the columnar epithelium of the gastrointestinal tract mucosa, followed by submucosal inflammation. Atrophy may be followed by ulceration.

Dementia results from degeneration of the neurons in the brain, accompanied by degeneration of the corresponding tracts in the spinal cord. The spinal cord lesions bear a close resemblance to the posterior column alterations observed in pernicious anemia.

PYRIDOXINE (VITAMIN B₆)

A primary, clinically overt deficiency of vitamin B_6 is rare in humans, but subclinical conditioned deficiency states, paradoxically, are thought to be quite common. Three naturally occurring substances—pyridoxine, pyridoxal, and pyridoxamine—together with the phosphate forms of each, possess vitamin B_6 activity and are generically referred to as *pyridoxine*. All are equally active metabolically, and all are converted in the tissues to the coenzyme form, pyridoxal 5-phosphate. This coenzyme participates as a cofactor for a large number of enzymes involved in transaminations, carboxylations, and deaminations in the metabolism of lipids and amino acids and in the immune response.

Vitamin B_6 is present in virtually all foods; however, food processing may destroy pyridoxine and in the past was responsible for severe deficiency in infants fed poorly controlled dried milk preparations. Secondary hypovitaminosis B_6 is pro-

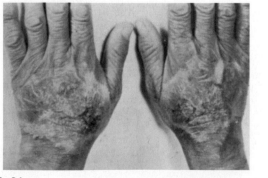

Figure 8–24 ■

The sharply demarcated, characteristic scaling dermatitis of pellagra.

duced most often by long-term use of any of a variety of drugs that act as pyridoxine antagonists. These include isoniazid (used to treat tuberculosis), estrogens, and penicillamine. Alcoholics are also prone to develop vitamin B_6 deficiency because acetaldehyde, an alcohol metabolite, enhances pyridoxine degradation. Pregnancy is associated with increased demand. Thus, pyridoxine supplementation is required in these conditions.

Clinical findings in vitamin B_6–deficient patients resemble those seen in patients with riboflavin and niacin deficiency. Patients may have seborrheic dermatitis, cheilosis, glossitis, peripheral neuropathy, and sometimes convulsions.

VITAMIN C (ASCORBIC ACID)

A deficiency of vitamin C leads to the development of scurvy, characterized principally by bone disease in growing children and hemorrhages and healing defects in both children and adults. Unlike some other vitamins, ascorbic acid cannot be synthesized endogenously, and therefore humans are dependent on intake with food. Ascorbic acid is present in milk and some animal products (liver, fish) and is abundant in a variety of fruits and vegetables. All but the most restricted diets provide adequate amounts of vitamin C.

With the abundance of ascorbic acid in many foods, scurvy has ceased to be a global problem, although it is sometimes encountered even in affluent populations as a conditioned deficiency, particularly among elderly individuals, persons who live alone, and alcoholics—all groups that often have erratic and inadequate eating patterns. Occasionally scurvy appears in patients undergoing peritoneal dialysis and hemodialysis and among food faddists. Tragically, the condition sometimes appears in infants who are maintained on formulas of processed milk without supplementation.

Ascorbic acid functions in a variety of biosynthetic pathways by accelerating hydroxylation and amidation reactions. The most clearly established *function of vitamin C is the activation of prolyl and lysyl hydroxylases from inactive precursors, providing for hydroxylation of procollagen.* Inadequately hydroxylated precursors cannot acquire a stable helical configuration and cannot be adequately cross-linked, so they are poorly secreted from the fibroblast. Those that are secreted lack tensile strength, are more soluble, and are more vulnerable to enzymatic degradation. Collagen, which normally has the highest content of hydroxyproline, is most affected, particularly in blood vessels, accounting for the predisposition to hemorrhages in scurvy. In addition, it appears that a deficiency of vitamin C leads to *suppression of the rate of synthesis of collagen peptides,* independent of an effect on proline hydroxylation.

While the role of vitamin C in collagen synthesis has been known for many decades, it is only in relatively recent years that its antioxidant properties have been recognized. Vitamin C can scavenge free radicals directly in aqueous phases of the cell and can act indirectly by regenerating the antioxidant form of vitamin E. Thus, vitamins E and C act in concert. It is because of these synergistic actions that both of these vitamins have attracted interest as agents that may retard atherosclerosis by reducing the oxidation of LDL (Chapter 10).

Scurvy in a growing child is far more dramatic than in an adult. **Hemorrhages** constitute one of the most striking features. Because the defect in collagen synthesis results in inadequate support of the walls of capillaries and venules, purpura and ecchymoses often appear in the skin and in the gingival mucosa. Furthermore, the loose attachment of the periosteum to bone, together with the vascular wall defects, leads to extensive **subperiosteal hematomas** and **bleeding into joint spaces** after minimal trauma. Retrobulbar, subarachnoid, and intracerebral hemorrhages may prove fatal.

Skeletal changes may also develop in infants and children. The primary disturbance is in the formation of osteoid matrix, rather than in mineralization or calcification, such as occurs in rickets. In scurvy, the palisade of cartilage cells is formed as usual and is provisionally calcified. However, there is insufficient production of osteoid matrix by osteoblasts. Resorption of the cartilaginous matrix then fails or slows, and as a consequence there is cartilaginous overgrowth, with long spicules and plates projecting into the metaphyseal region of the marrow cavity, and sometimes widening of the epiphysis (Fig. 8–25). The scorbutic bone yields to the stresses of weight bearing and muscle tension, with bowing of the long bones of the lower legs and abnormal depression of the sternum with outward projection of the ends of the ribs. The bone changes in adults are similar to those in children, with decreased formation of osteoid matrix, but deformation does not occur.

In severely scorbutic children and adults, **gingival swelling, hemorrhages,** and **secondary bacterial periodontal infection** are common. A distinctive **perifollicular, hyperkeratotic, papular rash** that may be ringed by hemorrhage often appears. **Wound healing and localization of focal infections are impaired** because of the derangement in collagen synthesis. Anemia is common, resulting from bleeding and from a secondary decrease in iron absorption (Chapter 12). The major features of scurvy are summarized in Figure 8–26.

Trace Elements

A number of minerals are essential for health. Calcium and phosphorus are required in large amounts and were considered in the discussion of vitamin D. Trace elements are metals that

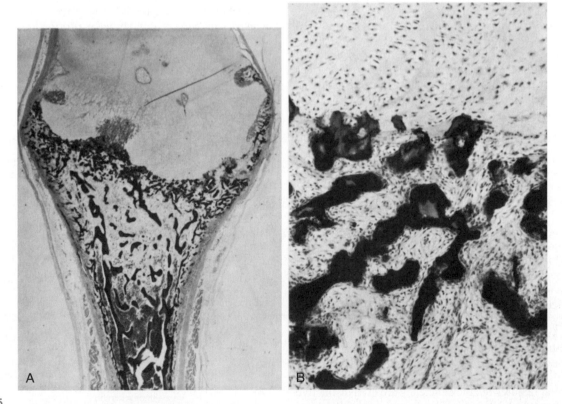

Figure 8–25

A, Longitudinal section of a scorbutic costochondral junction with widening of the epiphyseal cartilage and projection of masses of cartilage into the adjacent bone. *B,* Detail of a scorbutic costochondral junction. The orderly palisade is totally destroyed. There is dense mineralization of the spicules but no evidence of newly formed osteoid.

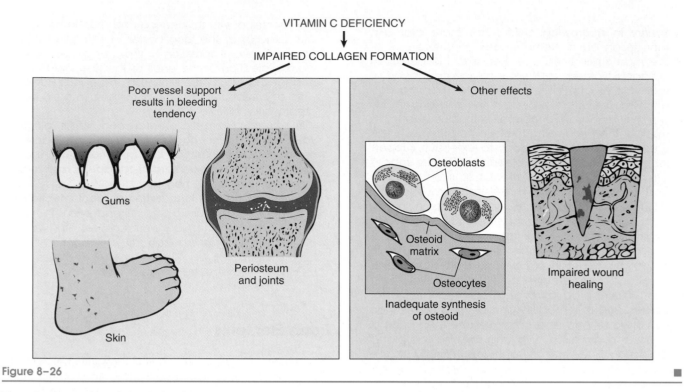

Figure 8–26 ■

The major consequences of vitamin C deficiency.

occur at concentrations smaller than 1 μg per gram of wet tissue. *Of the various trace elements found in the body, only five — iron, zinc, copper, selenium, and iodine — have been associated with well-characterized deficiency states.* In theory, a deficiency of a trace element might occur for many of the same reasons as a vitamin deficiency, but three influences are particularly relevant: (1) inadequate supplementation in preparations used for total parenteral nutrition, (2) interference with absorption by dietary constituents, and (3) inborn errors of metabolism leading to abnormalities of trace metal absorption. Dietary interference as a mechanism was first noted among inhabitants of Egypt and Iran who subsisted largely on unrefined cereals; sufficient phytic acid and fiber were present in the diet to bind and block zinc absorption. Genetic malabsorption syndromes involving a trace element are very rare. In one, failure to synthesize metallothionein (a metal-binding protein) in intestinal mucosal cells blocks absorption of both copper and zinc.

Table 8–11 provides brief comments on the role of several trace elements in health and disease. Additional comments are offered only for zinc and selenium deficiency.

Zinc Deficiency. A lack of zinc is very unusual because it is reasonably abundant in meats, fish, shellfish, whole-grain cereals, and legumes. Most cases of zinc deficiency have been related to either total parenteral nutrition unsupplemented by zinc or the aforementioned rare genetic syndrome that interferes with absorption.

The essential features of zinc deficiency are (1) a distinctive rash, most often around the eyes, nose, mouth, anus, and distal parts, called *acrodermatitis enteropathica* (Fig. 8–27); (2) anorexia, often accompanied by diarrhea; (3) growth retardation in children; (4) impaired wound healing; (5) hypogonadism with diminished reproductive capacity; (6) altered immune function; (7) impaired night vision related to altered vitamin A metabolism; (8) depressed mental function; and (9) an increased incidence of congenital malformations in infants of zinc-deficient mothers. Zinc deficiency should be suspected

Table 8–11.	FUNCTIONS OF TRACE METALS AND DEFICIENCY SYNDROMES	
Nutrient	**Function**	**Deficiency Syndromes**
Iron	Essential component of hemoglobin, as well as a number of iron-containing metalloenzymes	Hypochromic, microcytic anemia
Zinc	Component of enzymes, principally oxidases	Acrodermatitis enteropathica, growth retardation, infertility
Iodine	Component of thyroid hormone	Goiter and hypothyroidism
Selenium	Component of glutathione peroxidase	Myopathy, rarely cardiomyopathy
Copper	Component of cytochrome C oxidase, dopamine β-hydroxylase, tyrosinase, lysyloxidase, and unknown enzyme involved in cross-linking keratin	Muscle weakness, neurologic defects, hypopigmentation, abnormal collagen cross-linking
Manganese	Component of metalloenzymes, including oxidoreductases, hydrolases, and lipases	No well-defined deficiency syndrome
Fluoride	Mechanism unknown	Dental caries

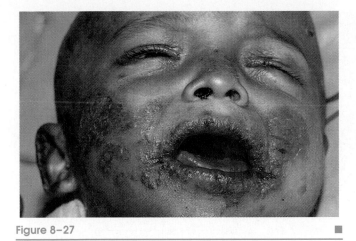

Figure 8–27   ■

Zinc deficiency with hemorrhagic dermatitis around the mouth and eyes.

in any case of obscure growth retardation or infertility associated with a distinctive rash (acrodermatitis enteropathica). Oral zinc supplementation is promptly curative.

Selenium Deficiency. Selenium, like vitamin E, protects against oxidative damage of membrane lipids. The deficiency of this element is well known in China as *Keshan disease*, which presents as a congestive cardiomyopathy, mainly in children and young women. It results from a markedly low level of the metal in soil, water, and food.

Obesity

Obesity is epidemic in the United States. Approximately 20% to 30% of men and 30% to 40% of women in the United States are obese. Because it is highly correlated with an increased incidence of several diseases, it is important to define and recognize it, to understand its causes, and to be able to initiate appropriate measures to prevent it or to treat it.

How does one measure fat accumulation? There are several highly technical ways to approximate the measurement, but for practical considerations the following ones are commonly used:

- Some expression of weight in relation to height, especially the measurement referred to as the *body mass index* (BMI)
- Skinfold measurements
- Various body circumferences, particularly the ratio of the waist-to-hip circumference

The BMI, expressed in kilograms per square meter, is closely correlated to body fat. A BMI of approximately 25 kg/m^2 is considered normal. It is generally agreed that a 20% excess in body weight (BMI greater than 27 kg/m^2) imparts a health risk. This is illustrated in Figure 8–28. Note that in this figure, a BMI below 20 kg/m^2 is also associated with an increased mortality rate. This may be related to smoking and its attendant risks, because smoking is known to decrease appetite and, subsequently, the BMI.

The untoward effects of obesity are related not only to the total body weight but also to the distribution of the stored fat. Central or visceral obesity, in which fat accumulates in the

trunk and in the abdominal cavity (in the mesentery and around viscera), is associated with a much higher risk for several diseases than is excess accumulation of fat diffusely in subcutaneous tissue.

The etiology of obesity is complex and incompletely understood. However, simply put, *obesity is a disorder of energy balance. When food-derived energy chronically exceeds energy expenditure, the excess calories are stored as triglycerides in adipose tissue.* The two sides of the energy equation, intake and expenditure, are finely regulated by neural and hormonal mechanisms. In most individuals, when food intake increases, so does the consumption of calories, and vice versa. Hence, body weight is maintained within a narrow range for many years. Apparently, this fine balance is maintained by an internal setpoint, or "lipostat," that can sense the quantity of the energy stores (adipose tissue) and appropriately regulate the food intake as well as the energy expenditure. The molecular nature of the lipostat remained obscure for many years, but starting in 1994, a series of breathtaking discoveries changed the picture. The current understanding of the neurohumoral mechanisms involved in weight control is illustrated in Figure 8–29 and described briefly here. It is now established that adipocytes communicate with the satiety centers in the brain by secreting a polypeptide hormone called *leptin.* By mechanisms not fully understood, output of leptin is regulated by the adequacy of the fat stores. With abundant fat stores, leptin secretion is stimulated, and the hormone travels to the hypothalamus, where it binds to leptin receptors. This interaction has multiple effects: a marked decrease in the production of *neuropeptide Y* (NPY), a powerful stimulator of appetite, and increased synthesis of a counter-regulatory hormone called *glucagon-like peptide 1* (GLP-1), which inhibits the appetite. Furthermore, in experimental animals, stimulation of the leptin receptor also increases energy expenditure, physical activity, and production of heat. Thermogenesis seems to be controlled by leptin receptor–mediated hypothalamic signals that increase the release of norepinephrine from sympathetic nerve endings in adipose tis-

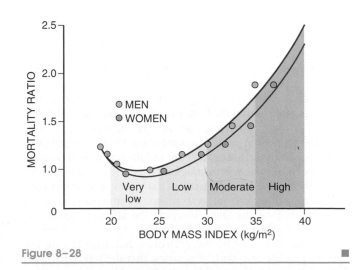

Figure 8–28   ■

Mortality ratios for men and women at different levels of body mass index. (Data from Lew EA, Garfinkel L: Variations in mortality by weight among 750,000 men and women. J Chronic Dis 32:563–576, 1979.)

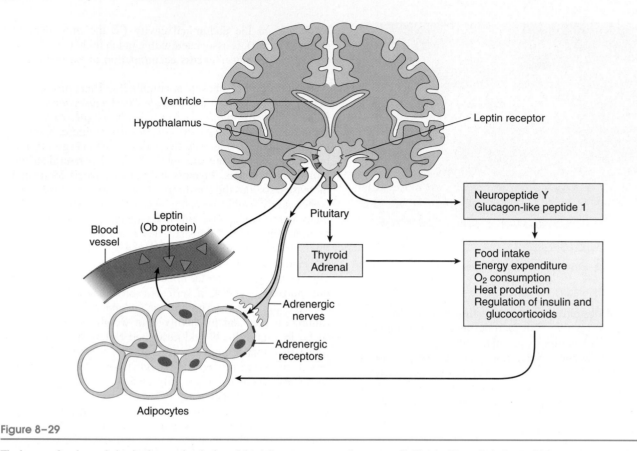

Figure 8-29

The hormonal and neural circuits that regulate body weight. Adipocytes secrete a hormone called leptin (also called *ob* protein) in response to nutritional status (available fat stores) and hormones such as insulin and glucocorticoids. Leptin is transported to the hypothalamus via the circulation, where it binds to the leptin receptor. This interaction regulates energy balance by affecting satiety (food intake) and energy expenditure. Leptin decreases the synthesis and secretion of the appetite stimulant neurotransmitter neuropeptide Y, and increases the synthesis of the counterregulatory neurotransmitter glucagon-like peptide 1. In addition, through neuronal pathways, the activation of leptin receptor in the hypothalamus increases the release of norepinephrine from sympathetic nerve terminals that innervate adipose tissue. Norepinephrine binds to the β_3-adrenergic receptors on fat cells and leads to increased metabolism of fatty acids and dissipation of the energy as heat. (Modified from Scott J: New chapter for the fat controller. Nature 379:113, 1996. Reprinted with permission from *Nature*. Copyright 1996 Macmillan Magazines Limited.)

sue. The fat cells express β_3-adrenergic receptors that, when stimulated by norepinephrine, cause fatty acid hydrolysis and also uncouple energy production from storage. Thus, the fats are literally burned, and the energy so produced is dissipated as heat. There are other catabolic effects mediated by leptin, all transduced through its hypothalamic receptor, which in turn communicates with other endocrine glands via the hypothalamic pituitary axis.

This schema is buttressed by the observation that in rodents, mutations that disable the leptin gene or its receptor give rise to massive obesity. (Indeed, because of the massive obesity of leptin-deficient mice, leptin is sometimes called *ob* protein.) Such mice continue to eat and gain weight because the leptin–leptin receptor system is uncoupled. Mice with a mutant leptin gene fail to sense the adequacy of fat stores, and hence they behave as if they are undernourished. Conversely, in mice with mutations of the leptin receptor, the afferent signals impinging on the hypothalamus fail to affect appetite and energy expenditure. Preliminary studies in obese humans indicate that leptin levels are elevated, suggesting that the leptin receptor may not be responsive to increased leptin levels.

While it is too soon to tell whether human obesity is caused by dysfunctions of the leptin system, there is little doubt that genetic influences play an important role in weight control. Support comes from a study in which identical twins, reared apart, had a remarkable concordance in the degree of obesity. However, as with all complex traits, obesity is not merely a genetic disease. There are definite environmental factors; the prevalence of obesity in Asians who immigrate to the United States is much higher than in those who remain in their native land. These changes in all likelihood result from changes in the type and amount of dietary intake. After all, even with bad genes, obesity would not occur without intake of food!

Obesity, particularly *central obesity, increases the risk for a number of conditions,* including diabetes, hypertension, hypertriglyceridemia, low HDL cholesterol (Chapter 10), and possibly coronary artery disease. The mechanisms underlying these associations are complex and likely to be interrelated. Obesity, for instance, is associated with *insulin resistance* and hyperinsulinemia, important features of non–insulin-dependent, or type II, diabetes, and weight loss is associated with improvement (Chapter 17). It has been speculated that excess insulin, in turn, may play a role in the retention of sodium, expansion of blood volume, production of excess norepinephrine, and smooth muscle proliferation that are the hallmarks of hypertension. Regardless of whether these pathogenic mechanisms are actually operative, *the risk of developing hypertension among previously normotensive persons increases proportionately with weight.*

Obese persons are likely to have hypertriglyceridemia and a low HDL cholesterol value, and these factors may increase the risk of *coronary artery disease* in the *very* obese. It should be emphasized that the association between obesity and heart disease is not straightforward, and such linkage as there may be relates more to the associated diabetes and hypertension than to weight per se.

Cholelithiasis (gallstones) is six times more common in obese than in lean subjects. The mechanism is mainly an increase in total body cholesterol, increased cholesterol turnover, and augmented biliary excretion of cholesterol in the bile, which in turn predisposes to the formation of cholesterol-rich gallstones (Chapter 16).

Hypoventilation syndrome is a constellation of respiratory abnormalities in very obese persons. It has been called the *pickwickian syndrome,* after the fat lad who was constantly falling asleep in Charles Dickens' *Pickwick Papers.* Hypersomnolence, both at night and during the day, is characteristic and is often associated with apneic pauses during sleep, polycythemia, and eventual right-sided heart failure.

Marked adiposity predisposes to the development of degenerative joint disease *(osteoarthritis).* This form of arthritis, which typically appears in older persons, is attributed in large part to the cumulative effects of wear and tear on joints. It is reasonable to assume that the greater the body burden of fat, the greater the trauma to joints with passage of time.

The relationship between *obesity and stroke* is unclear, and opposing views can be found in the literature. According to some, the true relationship is between stroke and hypertension, not between stroke and obesity per se (i.e., obese patients who are not hypertensive are not at higher risk for stroke).

Equally controversial is the relationship between *obesity and cancer,* particularly cancers arising in the endometrium and breast. Here the problem is complicated by the role of particular foods, such as animal fats, which may be independently associated with cancer and obesity. Nevertheless, it seems that obese women are at a higher risk of developing endometrial cancer than are lean women in the same age group. This relationship may be indirect; high estrogen levels are associated with increased risk of endometrial cancer (Chapter 19), and obesity is known to raise estrogen levels. With breast cancer, the data are controversial. It seems that in postmenopausal women who live in countries with a moderate or low risk of breast cancer (e.g., Japan), central obesity is associated with an increased risk of breast cancer. Again, the role of sex hormones is a confounding factor.

DIET AND SYSTEMIC DISEASES

The problems of under- and overnutrition, as well as specific nutrient deficiencies, have been discussed; however, the composition of the diet, even in the absence of any of these problems, may make a significant contribution to the causation and progression of a number of diseases. A few examples suffice here.

Currently one of the most important and controversial issues is the contribution of diet to atherogenesis. The central question is, "Can dietary modification—specifically, reduc-tion in the consumption of cholesterol and saturated animal fats (e.g., eggs, butter, beef)—reduce serum cholesterol levels and prevent or retard the development of atherosclerosis (most importantly, coronary heart disease)?" The average adult in the United States consumes an inordinate amount of fat and cholesterol daily, with a ratio of saturated fatty acids to poly-unsaturated fatty acids of about 3:1. Lowering the level of saturates to the level of the polyunsaturates effects a 10% to 15% reduction in serum cholesterol level within a few weeks. Vegetable oils (e.g., corn and safflower oils) and fish oils contain polyunsaturated fatty acids and are good sources of such cholesterol-lowering lipids. Fish oil fatty acids belonging to the omega-3, or n-3, family have more double bonds than do the omega-6, or n-6, fatty acids found in vegetable oils. Substitution of a portion of the saturated fat with a fish oil for a 4-week period has been shown to effect a substantial reduction in serum levels of triglycerides and VLDLs but can result in increased LDL cholesterol levels. A study of Dutch men whose usual daily diet contained 30 gm of fish revealed a substantially lower frequency of death from coronary heart disease than that among comparable controls. Thus, although dietary modification can affect heart disease, currently there are insufficient data to suggest that long-term supplementation of food with omega-3 fatty acids is of benefit in reducing coronary artery disease.

There are other examples of the effect of diet on disease:

■ Hypertension is beneficially affected by restricting sodium intake.
■ Dietary fiber, or roughage, resulting in increased fecal bulk, has a preventive effect against diverticulosis of the colon.
■ Caloric restriction has been convincingly demonstrated to increase life span in experimental animals. The basis of this striking observation is not clear. It seems, however, that in such animals, the age-related decline in immuno-logic functions is modest, and the animals are more resistant to experimental carcinogenesis.
■ Even lowly garlic has been touted to protect against heart disease (and also, alas, kisses), although research has yet to prove unequivocally this effect.

DIET AND CANCER

With respect to carcinogenesis, three aspects of the diet are of concern: (1) the possible content of exogenous carcinogens, (2) the potential that carcinogens might be endogenously synthesized from dietary components, and (3) a possible lack of protective factors. Relative to exogenous carcinogens, aflatoxins are clearly carcinogenic. There is increasing debate about the carcinogenicity of food additives, artificial sweeteners, and contaminating pesticides. Artificial sweeteners (cyclamates and saccharine) have been implicated in bladder cancers, but convincing evidence is lacking.

The concern about endogenous synthesis of carcinogens or promoters from components of the diet relates principally to gastric carcinomas. With gastric carcinoma, nitrosamines and nitrosamides are believed by some to be carcinogens because they have been clearly shown to induce gastric cancer in animals. These compounds can be formed in the body from nitrites and amines or amides derived from digested proteins.

Sources of nitrites include sodium nitrite, added to foods as a preservative, and nitrates, present in common vegetables, which are reduced in the gut by bacterial flora. There is, then, the potential for endogenous production of carcinogenic agents from dietary components, which might well have an effect on the stomach exposed to high concentrations.

High animal fat intake combined with low fiber intake has been implicated in the causation of colon cancer. The most convincing explanation of these associations is as follows: high fat intake increases the level of bile acids in the gut, which in turn modifies intestinal flora, favoring the growth of microaerophilic bacteria. The bile acids or bile acid metabolites produced by these bacteria might serve as carcinogens or promoters. The protective effect of a high-fiber diet might relate to (1) increased stool bulk and decreased transit time, which decrease the exposure of mucosa to putative offenders, and (2) the capacity of certain fibers to bind carcinogens and thereby protect the mucosa. Attempts to document these theories in clinical and experimental studies have, on the whole, led to contradictory results.

Finally, some dietary components have been considered anticarcinogenic. As mentioned earlier, vitamins C and E, beta-carotenes, and selenium could be protective because of their antioxidant properties. Oxidants can cause mutations, the first step in carcinogenesis. However, to date there is no convincing evidence that these antioxidant vitamins are effective chemopreventive agents.

Thus, we must conclude that despite many tantalizing trends and proclamations by "diet gurus," to date there is no definite proof that diet can cause or protect against cancer. Nonetheless, concern persists that carcinogens lurk in things as pleasurable as a juicy steak and rich ice cream.

BIBLIOGRAPHY

Bagshaw S: The combined oral contraceptive. Risks and adverse effects in perspective. Drug Safety 12:91, 1995. (A short, modern perspective on the adverse effects of oral contraceptives.)

Becklake MR: Fiber burden and asbestos-related lung disease: determinants of dose-response relationships. Am J Respir Crit Care Med 150:1488, 1994. (A detailed discussion of the factors associated with the development of asbestosis.)

Doll R, et al: Mortality in relation to smoking: 40 years' observations on male British doctors. Br Med J 309:901, 1994. (An excellent, detailed prospective study of mortality related to cigarette smoking.)

Flier JS: The adipocyte: storage depot or node on the energy information superhighway? Cell 80:15, 1995. (An excellent discussion of the role of adipocytes in the neurohormonal circuitry that regulates body weight.)

Glantz SA, Parmley WW: Passive smoking and heart disease. JAMA 273: 1047, 1995. (A review of studies that implicate passive smoking in the causation of ischemic heart disease; also includes a good discussion of the mechanisms by which cigarette smoke affects myocardial function and atherogenesis.)

Greenberg ER, Sporn MB: Antioxidant vitamins, cancer, and cardiovascular disease. N Engl J Med 334:1189, 1996. (An editorial summarizing the results of two large clinical trials designed to test the cancer-preventive effects of beta-carotene and vitamin A. The role of vitamin E in protecting against cardiovascular disease is also discussed.)

Kaiser J: Power lines and health. Panel finds EMFs pose no threat. Science 274:910, 1996. (A short commentary on the conclusions arrived at by a panel of the National Research Council.)

Lewis MA, et al: Third generation oral contraceptives and risk of myocardial infarction: an international case-control study. Br Med J 312:88, 1996. (An international study that demonstrated reduced risk of myocardial infarction in users of third-generation oral contraceptives.)

Lupulescu A: Estrogen use and cancer incidence: a review. Cancer Invest 13: 287, 1995. (A balanced review of the evidence relating to cancer risk in women who use estrogen.)

Meyer KC: Beryllium and lung disease. Chest 106:942, 1994. (A short discussion of an occupational lung disease that is mediated by induction of cell-mediated immunity.)

Muto Y, et al: Prevention of second primary tumors by an acyclic retinoid, polyprenoic acid, in patients with hepatocellular carcinoma. N Engl J Med 334:1561, 1996. (A study that describes the chemopreventive action of a synthetic retinoid in patients with liver cancer.)

Rump AFE, et al: The pathophysiology of cocaine cardiotoxicity. Forensic Sci Int 71:103, 1995. (A review of the adverse cardiac effects of cocaine.)

Samsioe Göran: Coagulation and anticoagulation effects of contraceptive steroids. Am J Obstet Gynecol 170:1523, 1994. (A concise review of the effects of oral contraceptives on the coagulation system.)

Scott J: New chapter for the fat controller. Nature 379:113, 1996. (Editorial summarizing breakthroughs in the understanding of leptin and its receptor system.)

Vanhèe D, et al: Cytokines and cytokine network in silicosis and coal workers' pneumoconiosis. Eur Respir J 8:834, 1995. (An excellent discussion of the pathogenesis of pneumoconiosis.)

Weiss N: Third-generation oral contraceptives: how risky? Lancet 346:1570, 1995. (An editorial on the risk of venous thrombosis in patients who use third-generation oral contraceptives, including those who are carriers of factor V mutations.)

9

General Pathology of Infectious Diseases

JOHN SAMUELSON, MD, PhD

The contributions of Dr. Arlene Sharpe to the chapter "The Response to Infection" in the previous edition of this text are gratefully acknowledged.

Modern industrial societies have made great progress in preventing and treating infectious diseases. Thanks to safe, uncontaminated water supplies, improved living conditions, widespread vaccination, and availability of effective antibiotics, death from infectious disease now occurs mainly in patients who are severely debilitated by other chronic diseases, are infected with the human immunodeficiency virus (HIV), or are being treated with immunosuppressive drugs. Instead, noninfectious diseases such as atherosclerosis, cancer, and dementia are the most frequent causes of morbidity and mortality. By contrast, in developing countries, where malnutrition and poor hygiene are widespread, infectious diseases kill tens of millions each year. Most deaths occur among children and are a result of respiratory and gastrointestinal infections caused by common viruses and bacteria rather than by "exotic" tropical diseases.

Table 9–1 presents in chronologic sequence 10 major breakthroughs in our understanding of infectious diseases and their causes, selected with the intent of providing an historical perspective for the concepts of microbial pathogenesis to be discussed here. Jenner's discovery in 1798 that milkmaids working with cows were resistant to smallpox paved the way to an understanding of cross-reactive immunity. Vaccinia virus (cowpox) induces immune reactions that neutralize subsequent infection with the much more virulent variola virus of smallpox. Because of an heroic vaccination campaign by the World Health Organization and others, smallpox is the first and only disease of humans that has been eradicated from the earth. Metchnikoff's discovery in 1884 of the process of phagocytosis, whereby leukocytes ingest foreign particles, initiated the study of white cells and cell-mediated immunity in the protection against infection.

Koch established the criteria for linking a specific microorganism to a specific disease: (1) the organism is regularly found in the lesions of the disease, (2) the organism can be isolated as single colonies on solid medium, (3) inoculation of this culture causes disease in an experimental animal, and (4) the organism can be recovered from lesions in the animal. To this end, bacterial surface antigens defined by Lancefield's serotypes have been used to link particular bacterial strains with particular diseases (e.g., group A *Streptococcus* with scarlet fever, rheumatic heart disease, and glomerulonephritis). Avery identified DNA as the genetic material that encoded the pneumococcal capsule, an important virulence factor. The successful culture of polioviruses by Enders and Weller led to the development of a formalin-killed and attenuated live vaccines to prevent crippling infections by polio.

The goal of this chapter is to discuss mechanisms by which infectious organisms cause disease. In discussing these mechanisms, two separate but interrelated aspects must be considered: (1) the specific properties of the organisms causing the infection, and (2) the host response to infectious agents. Only a few of the many human infections will be used to illustrate the concepts of microbial pathogenesis; greater coverage of particular organisms is found in the chapters that describe diseases by organ system (e.g., hepatitis B virus [HBV] in Chapter 16 and *Mycobacterium tuberculosis* in Chapter 13). In addition, the role of the immune system and immunodeficiencies (including acquired immunodeficiency syndrome [AIDS]) in microbial infection are discussed in Chapter 5.

CATEGORIES OF INFECTIOUS AGENTS

Organisms that cause infectious diseases range in size from the 20-nm poliovirus to the 10-m tapeworm *Taenia saginata* (Table 9–2).

Viruses. Animal viruses are obligate intracellular agents that depend on the host metabolic machinery for their replication. Viruses are classified by the type of nucleic acid they contain—either DNA or RNA, but not both—and by the shape of their protein coat or capsid. Viral pathogens account for a major share of all human infections, many of which cause acute illness (e.g., colds or influenza epidemics). Other viruses are not eliminated from the body but persist for years, continuing to multiply and remaining demonstrable (chronic infection) or surviving in some latent noninfectious form with the potential to be reactivated later. For example, the herpes zoster virus, the cause of chickenpox, may persist in the dorsal root ganglia and be periodically activated to cause the painful skin condition called *shingles*. Different species of viruses can produce the same pathologic features (e.g., upper respiratory tract infections), and a single virus (e.g., cytomegalovirus [CMV]) can produce different clinical manifestations depending on the host's resistance and age (Chapter 13).

Because viruses are only 20 to 300 nm in size, individual viruses are best visualized with the electron microscope, where they may appear spherical if capsid proteins form an icosahedron or cylindrical if they form a helix. Some viral particles aggregate within the cells they infect and form characteristic *inclusion bodies*, which may be diagnostic with the light microscope. For example, CMV-infected cells are enlarged and show a large eosinophilic nuclear inclusion and smaller basophilic cytoplasmic inclusions (Fig. 9–1); herpesviruses form a large nuclear inclusion surrounded by a clear

Table 9–1. TEN MAJOR DISCOVERIES IN MICROBIAL PATHOGENESIS

Year	Investigator	Discovery
1796	Jenner	Vaccination against smallpox
1865	Pasteur	Proof of germ theory and the beginning of modern biology
1882	Koch	Criteria for proof of causality in infectious disease
1884	Metchnikoff	Description of phagocytosis by macrophages
1902	Ross	Identification of mosquito vector for *Plasmodium falciparum* malaria
1906	Ehrlich	Description of chemotherapeutic agents
1908	Ellerman and Bang	Viral oncogenesis in chickens
1933	Lancefield	Serotyping of organisms and association of bacterial clones with disease
1945	Avery	Identification of DNA as genetic material and the start of the molecular biology revolution
1949	Enders	Culture of viruses and production of the polio vaccine

Table 9–2. CLASSES OF HUMAN MICROBIAL PATHOGENS

Taxonomic Class	Size	Site of Propagation	Sample Species and Related Disease	
Viruses	20–30 nm	Obligate intracellular	Poliovirus	Poliomyelitis
Chlamydiae	200–1000 nm	Obligate intracellular	*Chlamydia trachomatis*	Trachoma
Rickettsiae	300–1200 nm	Obligate intracellular	*Rickettsia prowazekii*	Typhus fever
Mycoplasmas	125–350 nm	Extracellular	*Mycoplasma pneumoniae*	Atypical pneumonia
Bacteria, spirochetes, mycobacteria	0.8–15 μm	Cutaneous Mucosal Extracellular Facultative intracellular	*Staphylococcus epidermidis* *Vibrio cholerae* *Streptococcus pneumoniae* *Mycobacterium tuberculosis*	Wound infection Cholera Pneumonia Tuberculosis
Fungi imperfecti	2–200 μm	Cutaneous Mucosal Extracellular Facultative intracellular	*Trichophyton* sp. *Candida albicans* *Sporothrix schenckii* *Histoplasma capsulatum*	Tinea pedis ("athlete's foot") Thrush Sporotrichosis Histoplasmosis
Protozoa	1–50 mm	Mucosal Extracellular Facultative intracellular Obligate intracellular	*Giardia lamblia* *Trypanosoma gambiense* *Trypanosoma cruzi* *Leishmania donovani*	Giardiasis Sleeping sickness Chagas' disease Kala-azar
Helminths	3 mm–10 m	Mucosal Extracellular Intracellular	*Enterobius vermicularis* *Wuchereria bancrofti* *Trichinella spiralis*	Pinworm Filariasis Trichinosis

halo; smallpox and rabies viruses both form characteristic cytoplasmic inclusions. Often viral inclusions are difficult to find (e.g., HBV), and many viruses do not give rise to inclusions (e.g., HIV, Epstein-Barr virus [EBV]).

Bacteriophages, Plasmids, and Transposons. Bacteriophages, plasmids, and transposons are mobile genetic elements that infect bacteria and indirectly cause human diseases by encoding bacterial virulence factors, including adhesins, toxins, and enzymes that confer drug resistance. The addition of a bacteriophage or plasmid converts nonpathogenic bacteria into virulent ones, and plasmids encoding antibiotic resistance frequently make therapy difficult and expensive (e.g., vancomycin-resistant enterococci and methacillin-resistant staphylococci, both of which are endemic in many hospitals).

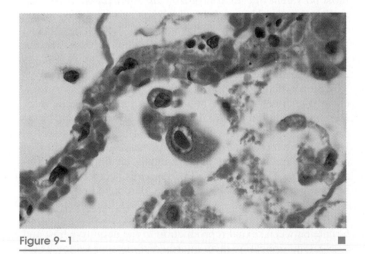

Cytomegalovirus. Distinct nuclear and ill-defined cytoplasmic inclusions in the lung.

Bacteria. Bacterial cells are prokaryotes, which lack nuclei and endoplasmic reticulum. Recently the double-stranded DNA genome of one bacterium (*Haemophilus influenzae*) has been sequenced in its entirety. Bacteria have cell walls composed of two phospholipid bilayer membranes separated by a peptidoglycan layer (gram-negative organisms) or an inner membrane surrounded by a peptidoglycan layer (gram-positive organisms) (see Fig. 9–9).

A normal healthy person is colonized by as many as 10^{12} bacteria on the skin, 10^{10} bacteria in the mouth, and 10^{14} bacteria in the alimentary tract. Bacteria colonizing the skin include *Staphylococcus epidermidis*, *Corynebacterium* spp., and *Propionibacterium acnes* (the cause of acne among adolescents). Aerobic and anaerobic bacteria, particularly *Streptococcus mutans,* contribute to a dense microbial mass called *dental plaque,* a major cause of tooth decay. In the colon, more than 99.9% of bacteria are anaerobic, including *Bacteroides* spp. Many bacteria remain extracellular when they invade the body, whereas *facultative intracellular bacteria* (e.g., *Mycobacterium* spp.) can survive and replicate either outside of host cells or within host cells.

Chlamydia,* Rickettsiae, and *Mycoplasma. These infectious agents are grouped together because they are similar to bacteria (they divide by binary fusion and are susceptible to antibiotics) but lack certain structures (e.g., *Mycoplasma* organisms do not have a rigid cell wall) or metabolic capabilities (e.g., *Chlamydia* spp. cannot synthesize ATP). Chlamydiae and rickettsiae are obligate intracellular agents that replicate in phagosomes of epithelial cells and in the cytoplasm of endothelial cells, respectively. *Chlamydia trachomatis* is the leading infectious cause of female sterility (by scarring and narrowing the fallopian tubes) and blindness (by trachoma, a chronic inflammation of the conjunctiva that eventually scars and opacifies the cornea).

Rickettsiae are transmitted by arthropod vectors, including lice (epidemic typhus), ticks (Q fever, Rocky Mountain spotted fever [RMSF]), and mites (scrub typhus). By injuring the endothelial cells, rickettsiae cause a hemorrhagic vasculitis that is often visible as a skin rash (Fig. 9–2), but they may also cause a transient pneumonia or hepatitis (Q fever) or injure the central nervous system and cause death (RMSF and epidemic typhus).

Mycoplasma organisms and the closely related *Ureaplasma* organisms are the tiniest free-living organisms known (125 to 300 nm). *Mycoplasma* infections spread from person to person in aerosols. The organisms bind to the surface of epithelial cells in the airways, and cause an atypical pneumonia characterized by peribronchiolar infiltrates of lymphocytes and plasma cells (Chapter 13). *Ureaplasma* infections are transmitted venereally and may cause nongonococcal urethritis (NGU) (Chapter 18).

Fungi. Fungi possess thick, ergosterol-containing cell walls and grow as perfect, sexually reproducing forms in vitro and as imperfect forms in vivo; the latter include budding yeast cells and slender tubes (hyphae). Some yeast forms produce spores, which are resistant to extreme environmental conditions, while hyphae may produce fruiting bodies called *conidia*. Some fungal species (e.g., those of the *Tinea* group, which cause "athlete's foot") are confined to the superficial layers of the human skin; other "dermatophytes" preferentially damage the hair shafts or nails. Certain fungal species invade the subcutaneous tissue, causing abscesses or granulomas, as happens in sporotrichosis and in tropical mycoses.

Deep fungal infections can spread systemically to destroy vital organs in immunocompromised hosts, but heal spontaneously or remain latent in otherwise normal hosts. Some deep fungal species are limited to a particular geographic region (e.g., *Coccidioides, Histoplasma,* and *Blastomyces*). Opportunistic fungi (e.g., *Candida, Aspergillus, Mucor,* and *Cryptococcus*; Fig. 9–3), by contrast, are ubiquitous contaminants colonizing the normal human skin or gut without causing illness. Only in immunosuppressed individuals do opportunistic fungi give rise to life-threatening infections, characterized by tissue necrosis, hemorrhage, and vascular occlusion, with

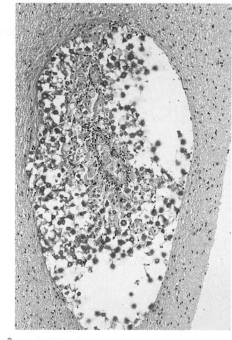

Figure 9–3 ■

Mucicarmine stain of cryptococci in a Virchow-Robin perivascular space of the brain (soap-bubble lesion).

minimal or no inflammatory response. In addition, AIDS patients, late in their course, are frequent victims of the opportunistic fungus-like organism *Pneumocystis carinii.*

Protozoan Parasites. Parasitic protozoa are motile, single-celled eukaryotes that are among the foremost causes of disease and death in developing countries (e.g., 1 million deaths per year caused by *Plasmodium falciparum* malaria). In industrialized countries, protozoa are widely prevalent but are less often lethal (e.g., *Trichomonas, Giardia, Entamoeba,* and *Toxoplasma*). The simplest protozoan parasite is *Trichomonas,* which has a single flagellated form, is sexually transmitted, and colonizes the vagina and the male urethra. The most prevalent intestinal protozoa are *Entamoeba histolytica* and *Giardia lamblia,* each of which has two forms: (1) motile trophozoites that attach to the intestinal epithelial wall and may invade *(E. histolytica)*, and (2) immobile cysts that are infectious when eaten because they have a chitin wall that is resistant to stomach acids.

Protozoa that reside in plasma (e.g., *Trypanosoma brucei,* cause of African sleeping sickness), in red blood cells (e.g., *Plasmodia*), and in macrophages (e.g., *Leishmania*) are transmitted by insect vectors, in which they replicate extracellularly and are motile. *Toxoplasma,* an intracellular parasite that causes severe infections in individuals lacking cellular immunity (e.g., fetuses or AIDS patients), is acquired when humans ingest intramuscular cysts in undercooked meat.

Helminths. Parasitic worms are highly differentiated multicellular organisms. Their life cycles are complex; most alternate between sexual reproduction in the definitive host and asexual multiplication in an intermediary host or vector. Thus, depending on parasite species, humans may harbor adult worms (e.g., *Ascaris*), immature forms (e.g., *Toxocara canis*),

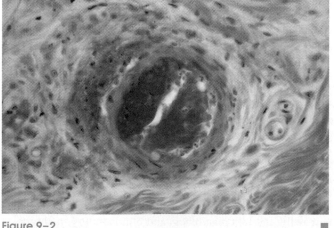

Figure 9–2 ■

Rocky Mountain spotted fever with thrombosed vessel and vasculitis.

or asexual larval forms (e.g., *Echinococcus*). Adult worms, once resident in humans, do not multiply in number but generate eggs or larvae destined for the next phase of the cycle. An exception is *Strongyloides*, the larvae of which can become infective inside the gut and cause overwhelming auto-infection in immunosuppressed persons. There are two important consequences of the lack of replication of adult worms: (1) disease is often caused by inflammatory responses to the eggs rather than to the adults (e.g., schistosomiasis; Fig. 9–4), and (2) the severity of disease is proportional to the number of organisms that have infected the host (e.g., 10 hookworms have little effect, whereas 1000 hookworms cause severe anemia by consuming 100 ml of blood per day).

There are three major classes of helminths: roundworms, flatworms, and flukes. These are briefly described as follows:

1. Roundworms (nematodes) are characterized by a collagenous tegument and a nonsegmented structure. These include *Ascaris*, hookworms, and *Strongyloides* among the intestinal worms and the filariae and *Trichinella* among the tissue invaders.
2. Flatworms (cestodes) are gutless worms, whose head (scolex) sprouts a ribbon of flat segments (proglottids) covered by absorptive tegument. In this class are pork, beef, and fish tapeworms and cystic tapeworm larvae (cysticerci and hydatid cysts).
3. Flukes (trematodes), which are primitive leaf-like worms with a syncytial tegument, include the oriental liver and lung flukes and the blood-dwelling schistosomes. All human parasitic helminths are extracellular except for the larvae of *Trichinella spiralis,* which encyst for a very long time in skeletal muscles.

Ectoparasites. Ectoparasites are insects (lice, bedbugs, fleas) or arachnids (mites, ticks) that attach and live on or in the skin. These arthropods may cause itching and excoriations (e.g., pediculosis caused by lice attached to hair shafts, or scabies caused by mites burrowing into the stratum corneum). At the site of the bite, mouth parts may be found in association with a mixed infiltrate of lymphocytes, macrophages, and eosinophils. In addition, attached arthropods can be vectors for other pathogens that produce characteristic skin lesions (e.g., the expanding erythematous plaque caused by the Lyme disease spirochete *Borrelia burgdorferi,* which is transmitted by deer ticks).

We will now discuss the pathogenesis of infection, beginning with the normal host defenses against the entry and establishment of infectious agents and how these defenses can be overwhelmed.

HOST BARRIERS TO INFECTION AND HOW THEY BREAK DOWN

Host barriers to infection prevent access of microbes to the body and their subsequent spread throughout the tissues. The first barriers are intact skin and mucosal surfaces and the secretions that these surfaces produce (e.g., lysozyme in tears degrades the peptidoglycan wall of bacteria). These are formidable defenses against most infections. Only four of every 10 exposures to gonococci result in gonorrhea, and it takes 10^{11} vibrios to produce cholera in human volunteers with normal gastric juices. Still, some infectious agents are able to overcome these barriers, so that as few as 100 *Shigella* organisms, *Giardia* cysts, or *M. tuberculosis* organisms, are sufficient to cause illness. In general, respiratory, gastrointestinal, and genitourinary tract infections occur in healthy persons and are caused by relatively virulent organisms that are able to damage intact epithelial barriers. In contrast, most skin infections are caused by less virulent organisms entering the skin through cuts or insect bites.

Skin

The human skin is normally inhabited by a variety of bacterial and fungal species, including some potential opportunists such as *S. epidermidis* and *Candida albicans*. This rich cutaneous flora maintains itself in metabolic equilibrium and thus inhibits overgrowth of any single resident species or virulent newcomer pathogen. In addition, the dense, keratinized outer skin layer bearing resident microbes is constantly shed and renewed. The low pH of the skin (about 5.5) and the presence of fatty acids also inhibit microbial growth, but wet skin is more permeable to microorganisms. Human papillomavirus (HPV), the cause of venereal warts, and *Treponema pallidum,* the agent of syphilis, both penetrate warm, moist skin during sexual intercourse. Superficial infections of the stratum corneum of the epidermis by *Staphylococcus aureus* (impetigo) or by cutaneous fungi are all aggravated by heat and humidity. Schistosome larvae released from fresh water snails penetrate swimmers' skin by releasing collagenase, elastase, and other enzymes that dissolve the extracellular matrix. Most other microorganisms penetrate through lesions in skin, including superficial pricks (fungal infections), deep wounds (staphylococci), burns *(Pseudomonas aeruginosa),* and diabetic and pressure-related foot sores (multibacterial infections). Intravenous catheters in hospitalized patients frequently cause bacteremia with *Staphylococcus* spp. or gram-

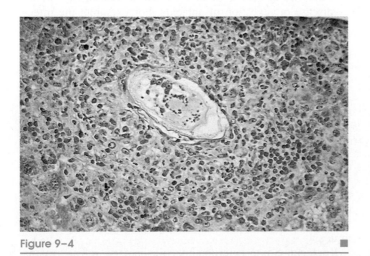

Figure 9–4

Schistosoma mansoni granuloma with a miracidium-containing egg *(center)* and numerous scattered eosinophils.

negative organisms. Needle sticks, whether intentional (by drug abusers) or unintentional (by health care workers), expose the recipient to potentially infected blood and may transmit HBV, HIV, and hepatitis C virus (HCV).

Bites by fleas, ticks, mosquitoes, mites, and lice break the skin and transmit diverse infectious organisms, including arboviruses (causes of yellow fever and encephalitis), rickettsiae, bacteria (plague, Lyme disease), protozoa (malaria, leishmaniasis), and helminths (filariasis). The protozoans and helminths undergo important developmental changes in their insect vectors, and their infectivity may be much enhanced by the release from the insects of potent anticoagulants or vasodilators. For example, the infectivity of *Leishmania* in mice is increased 1000-fold by coinjection with saliva from the sandfly vector. Finally, animal bites may cause infections with anaerobic bacteria or with the deadly rabies virus.

Urogenital Tract

Even though urine can support the growth of many bacteria, the urinary tract is normally sterile because it is flushed many times per day. Women have more than 10 times as many urinary tract infections (UTIs) as men, because the distance between the urinary bladder and the bacteria-laden skin (i.e., the length of the urethra) is 5 cm in women, as compared with 20 cm in men. In addition, girls and boys with obstruction of urinary flow and/or reflux of urine into the ureters are much more susceptible to UTIs. When UTI spreads retrograde from the bladder to the kidney, it causes acute and chronic pyelonephritis (discussed in Chapter 14), which is the major preventable cause of renal failure. The pathogens that infect the urinary tract (mostly bacteria from the perianal area or from an infected sexual partner [e.g., with *Gonococcus*]) are those that adhere best to the epithelium of the urinary tract. Most acute UTIs are caused by a few strains of *Escherichia coli* that have adherent fimbria, while chronic infections are caused by *Proteus, Pseudomonas, Klebsiella,* or *Enterococcus* spp. that are often drug resistant.

During the reproductive years, the vagina has a unique defense against colonization by pathogenic organisms. Under the control of estrogen, the epithelial cells of the vagina produce glycogen, which is broken down to lactic acid by hyperinfection with Döderlein's lactobacilli. The acid pH suppresses many other organisms, except for those causing sexually transmitted diseases.

Respiratory Tract

Some 10,000 microorganisms, including viruses, bacteria, and fungi, are inhaled daily by every city inhabitant. The distance these microorganisms travel into the respiratory system is inversely proportional to their size. Large microbes are trapped in the mucociliary blanket that lines the nose and the upper respiratory tract. Microorganisms are trapped in the mucus secreted by goblet cells and are then transported by ciliary action to the back of the throat, where they are swallowed and cleared. Organisms smaller than 5 μm travel directly to the alveoli, where they are phagocytosed by alveolar macrophages or by neutrophils recruited to the lung by cytokines.

Damage to the mucociliary defense results from repeated insults in smokers and in patients with cystic fibrosis, while acute injury occurs in intubated patients and in those who aspirate gastric acid. Virulent respiratory pathogens escape the intact mucociliary defense by attaching via hemagglutinins to carbohydrates on epithelial cells in the lower respiratory tract and pharynx (e.g., influenza virus). Furthermore, influenza, parainfluenza, and mumps viruses use viral neuraminidase to lower the viscosity of mucus and free themselves from entrapment. Certain organisms (e.g., *H. influenzae*) release factors that inhibit ciliary motion. Secondary respiratory infections with *Streptococcus pneumoniae* or *Staphylococcus* spp., which lack specific adherence factors, occur after viral damage to epithelial cells. *M. tuberculosis* causes respiratory infection because it is able to escape phagocytotic killing by the macrophage. Finally, opportunistic fungi infect the lungs when cellular immunity is depressed and leukocytes are deficient in number (e.g., *P. carinii* in AIDS patients and *Aspergillus* spp. in patients receiving chemotherapy).

Intestinal Tract

Most gastrointestinal pathogens are transmitted by food or drink contaminated with human feces, and therefore exposure can be reduced by frequent handwashing, use of clean water, and proper cooking methods. Defenses against microbial invasion through the gastrointestinal tract include (1) the mucus covering of epithelial cells, (2) acid in gastric juices, (3) pancreatic enzymes, (4) the detergent bile salts, and (5) secreted antibodies (immunoglobulin A [IgA]). In addition, pathogenic organisms must compete for nutrients with nonpathogenic bacteria already growing within the intestinal lumen (mostly anaerobes), and all organisms are passed from the body each day in the stool.

Like many respiratory infections, most gastrointestinal infections occur in healthy persons who are exposed to relatively virulent organisms that can escape the normal host defenses. Several conditions interfere with these gastrointestinal defenses:

■ *Decrease of gastric acid.* This can be caused by chronic disease or ingestion of antacids. For example, the infectious dose of cholera bacteria is reduced from 10^{11} organisms to 10^4 if gastric pH is increased.

■ *Treatment with antibiotics.* Antibiotics alter the normal flora so that it is overrun by pathogenic bacteria (e.g., *Clostridium difficile,* an important cause of pseudomembranous enterocolitis [Chapter 15]).

■ *Interference with normal bowel motion or outright obstruction* (e.g., blind loop syndrome).

Viruses. Most enveloped viruses are killed by secretions and so cannot enter via the gut, but nonenveloped enteropathic viruses, such as hepatitis A virus, are resistant to stomach acids, intestinal proteases, and bile. Rotaviruses infect and damage intestinal epithelia; reoviruses pass through mucosal M cells into the blood without causing any detectable local injury.

Bacteria. Some enteropathogenic bacteria release toxins that can damage the host without invading or multiplying in the gut wall (e.g., food poisoning by *Staphylococcus* spp., and

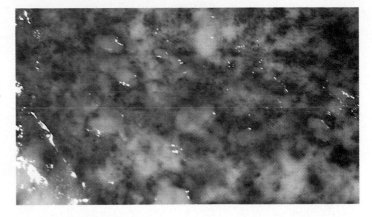

Figure 9–5   ■

Close-up of colonic mucosa in *Shigella* colitis with erythema, ulceration, and pseudomembrane formation (white plaques).

Clostridium botulinum). Other bacteria (e.g., *Vibrio cholerae* and toxigenic *E. coli*) use their flagellae to move along a chemotactic gradient through the mucus layer covering colonic epithelial cells, and attach via specific adhesins to sugars in the brush border of epithelial cells. There the bacteria multiply and release toxins that cause epithelial cells to secrete large volumes of fluid into the lumen. The result is a watery diarrhea by which the physiology of the intestinal epithelium and of the host is dramatically affected, although histopathologic changes are relatively slight. In contrast, other bacteria (e.g., *Shigella, Salmonella,* and *Campylobacter* spp.) invade and disrupt the intestinal epithelium and so cause ulcerations, inflammation, and hemorrhage, which present clinically as dysentery (Fig. 9–5). Finally, some bacteria (e.g., *Salmonella typhi* and *Yersinia* spp.) pass through the epithelium and enter Peyer's patches, where they multiply and cause pathologic changes.

Parasites. Intestinal parasites break the protective barriers by a number of different mechanisms. The cyst forms of protozoan parasites *E. histolytica* and *G. lamblia* are infectious because they are resistant to stomach acids, while the motile trophozoite forms cause injury by attaching via parasite lectins to sugars on the intestinal epithelium cells. *Giardia* and *Cryptosporidium* spp. damage the epithelium without stromal invasion, while *Entamoeba* organisms cause contact-mediated cytolysis by releasing a channel-forming pore protein (similar to that of cytotoxic lymphocytes) that inserts into the target epithelial cell plasma membrane and depolarizes it (Fig. 9–6). Some helminth parasites can damage the host by remaining in the intestinal lumen and consuming essential nutrients (e.g., the fish tapeworm, which depletes the host of vitamin B_{12}) or by mechanically obstructing the bile duct (e.g., *Ascaris*). Ancylostomas (hookworms) suck the blood from the intestinal vessels and so may cause severe iron-deficiency anemia. Finally, some helminth larvae pass innocuously through the intestines and then encyst in muscle (e.g., *Trichinella*) or the central nervous system (e.g., cysticerci).

Spread of Microbes Throughout the Body

Microbes spread rapidly along the wet epithelial surfaces of the intestines, lungs, and genitourinary tract and, slowly, if

at all, on the dry surface of the skin (Fig. 9–7). Many microbes do not travel beyond the epithelium because they proliferate only in superficial layers of epithelia (e.g., HPV organisms), but others are able to penetrate (e.g., streptococci and staphylococci, which secrete hyaluronidase, which in turn degrades the extracellular matrix between host cells). The routes of microbial spread initially follow tissue planes of least resistance and the regional lymphatic and vascular anatomy. For example, staphylococci cause a locally expanding skin abscess (furuncle), followed by a regional lymphadenitis that sometimes leads to bacteremia (blood-borne infection) and colonization of distant organs deep to the body's surfaces (heart, liver, brain, spleen, bones). Once in the blood, organisms are transported by a variety of means. HBV and polioviruses, most bacteria and fungi, occasional protozoan parasites (e.g., African trypanosomes), and all helminths are transported free in the plasma. Herpesviruses, HIV, CMV, *Mycobacterium, Leishmania,* and *Toxoplasma* are carried by leukocytes. Certain viruses (e.g., Colorado tick fever virus) and parasites (e.g., plasmodia, babesia) are carried by red cells.

Dissemination of pathogens in the blood can lead to systemic signs of infection, including fever, which is caused by host cytokines released in response to bacterial endotoxin

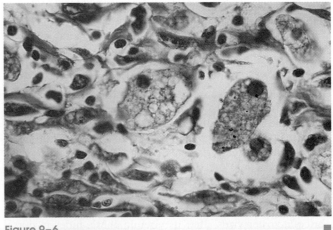

Figure 9–6   ■

Amebiasis of the colon with three *Entamoeba histolytica* trophozoites.

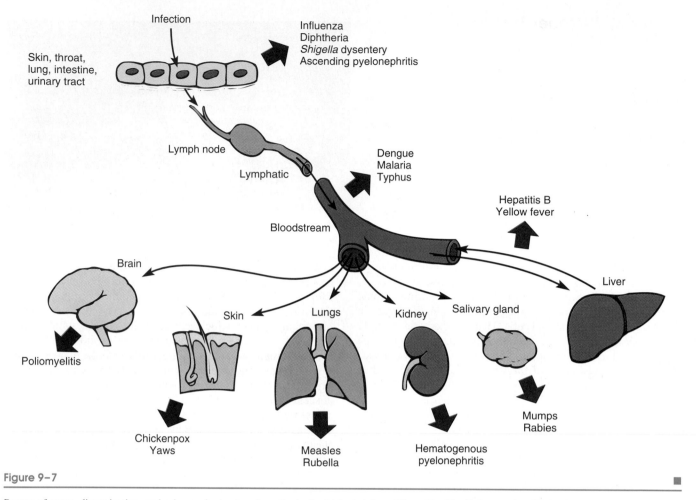

Figure 9–7

Routes of entry, dissemination, and release of microbes from the body. (Adapted from Mims CA: The Pathogenesis of Infectious Disease. Orlando, FL, Academic Press, 1987.)

(Chapter 2). Massive sustained bloodstream invasion by pyogenic bacteria and certain parasites (e.g., malaria) may be fatal. Infectious foci disseminated by blood are called *secondary foci* and usually have a widespread distribution, either in a single organ (e.g., miliary, or seedlike, distribution of progressive tuberculosis within the lung) or through many tissues (e.g., microabscesses throughout the kidneys, intestines, and skin caused by septic emboli shed from a staphylococcal aortic valve infection). Invasive microbes quickly spread within fluid-lined cavities such as pleura, peritoneum, and meninges.

Frequently organisms cause major disease manifestations at sites distant from the point of entry. For example, the chickenpox virus enters through the lungs but causes rashes in the skin; polioviruses enter through the intestine but selectively cause damage to motor neurons; and *Schistosoma mansoni* penetrate the skin but eventually localize in blood vessels of the portal system and the mesentery, causing damage to the liver and intestines. Rabies viruses track to the brain in a retrograde fashion along nerves, while the varicella-zoster virus, after its viremic phase, hides in dorsal root ganglia, whence it may travel along the nerves and cause shingles.

Severe damage to the developing fetus occurs when infectious organisms circulate in the mother's blood or reach the uterus from the vagina to infect the placenta and the fetus. Placental or fetal infections with bacteria frequently cause premature birth or stillbirth, while viral infections can also cause maldevelopment of the fetus, depending on the time of infection (Chapter 7). Rubella infection in the first trimester may cause congenital heart disease, mental retardation, cataracts, or deafness in the infant, whereas little damage is caused by rubella infection in the third trimester. In contrast, transmission of treponemes gives rise to syphilis only when the organisms invade the fetus late in the second trimester, but then they cause a severe fetal osteochondritis and periostitis that leads to multiple bony lesions (Chapter 18).

Because the fetus receives antibodies but not cell-mediated immunity from the mother, opportunistic pathogens common to AIDS patients (e.g., CMV, herpesviruses, and *Toxoplasma*) may cause severe damage to the fetus. During the birth process, infants can also become infected with the mother's viruses and bacteria, which may subsequently cause acquired immunodeficiency (HIV), chronic hepatitis or liver cancer (HBV), blindness (chlamydia), and multisystem organ failure (herpesviruses).

Release of Microbes From the Body

For transmission of disease, the exit of infectious agents from the host's body is as important as their entry into it. Many of the mechanisms by which infectious organisms are cleared from the infected individual are responsible for their spread from one person to another, including skin shedding, coughing, sneezing, urination, and defecation. Stool pathogens that are resistant to drying (e.g., bacterial spores, protozoan cysts, nematode eggs) survive in the environment for a long time, whereas certain viruses must be quickly passed from person to person, often by direct contact. Stool-contaminated food and water are important vehicles for spread of epidemic and endemic pathogens. Viruses that infect the salivary glands (e.g., herpesvirus, mumps virus) are released during talking, singing, spitting, and kissing. All classes of organisms are transmitted by intimate mucosal or venereal contact, including viruses (e.g., herpesvirus, HPV, HBV, HIV), chlamydia, bacteria (*T. pallidum* and *Neisseria gonorrhoeae*), fungi *(Candida),* protozoa *(Trichomonas),* and arthropods *(Phthiris pubis,* or crab lice). Microorganisms transmitted by blood-sucking arthropods must be in the blood to infect the next insect that feeds, even when the major lesions caused by them are in the brain (viral encephalitis), liver, spleen *(Leishmania donovani),* or heart *(Trypanosoma cruzi* in Chagas' disease).

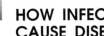

HOW INFECTIOUS AGENTS CAUSE DISEASE

Having reviewed the manner by which infectious agents break host barriers, we will examine how they injure cells and cause tissue damage. There are three general mechanisms:

1. Infectious agents can contact or enter host cells and directly cause cell death.
2. Pathogens can release endotoxins or exotoxins that kill cells at a distance, release enzymes that degrade tissue components, or damage blood vessels and cause ischemic injury.
3. Pathogens can induce host cell responses that may cause additional tissue damage, usually by immune-mediated mechanisms.

Immune-mediated injury is discussed in Chapter 5. Here we describe some of the specific mechanisms whereby viruses and certain bacteria cause cell and tissue injury.

Mechanisms of Virus-Induced Injury

Viruses damage host cells by entering the cell and replicating at the host's expense. They have specific surface viral proteins (ligands) that bind to particular host proteins (receptors), many of which have known functions. For example,

HIV binds to CD4 involved in T-cell activation and to chemokine receptors, EBV binds to the complement receptor CD21 on B cells, and rhinoviruses bind to intercellular adhesion molecule 1 (ICAM-1) on mucosal cells. For several viruses, x-ray crystallographic studies have identified the specific part of the viral attachment protein that binds to a particular segment of the host cell receptor.

The presence or absence of host cell proteins that allow the virus to attach is one reason for *viral tropism,* or the tendency of certain viruses to infect specific cells but not others. Similarly, some paramyxoviruses are not infectious until their envelope glycoproteins undergo proteolytic cleavage by tissue proteases to reveal the cryptic viral attachment sites that bind to host cells. A second major cause of viral tropism is the ability of the virus to replicate inside some cells but not in others. Viral enhancer or promoter sequences determine this specificity. For example, the JC papovavirus infection of the brain is restricted to oligodendroglia in the central nervous system (Chapter 23). Studies of foreign DNA expression in cultured cells show that the JC virus promoter and enhancer DNA sequences upstream from the viral genes are active in cultured glial cells but not in other cell types. Similarly, when JC virus genes are injected into transgenic mice, oligodendroglial dysfunction is dependent on the presence of particular JC virus promoter and enhancer sequences that are recognized by glial cell–specific proteins involved in messenger RNA (mRNA) synthesis.

Once attached, the entire virion, or a portion containing the genome and essential polymerases, penetrates the cell cytoplasm by (1) translocation of the entire virus across the plasma membrane, (2) fusion of the viral envelope with the cell membrane, or (3) receptor-mediated endocytosis and fusion with endosomal membranes. Within the cell the virus uncoats, separating its genome from its structural components and loses its infectivity. Viruses then replicate, using enzymes that are distinct for each virus family. For example, RNA polymerase is used by negative-sense RNA viruses to generate positive-sense mRNA, while reverse transcriptase is used by retroviruses to generate DNA from their RNA template. These virus-specific enzymes provide points at which drugs may be used to inhibit viral replication. Viruses also use host enzymes for viral synthesis, and such enzymes may be present in some but not all of the tissues. Newly synthesized viral genomes and capsid proteins are assembled into progeny virions in the nucleus or cytoplasm and are either released directly (unencapsulated viruses) or bud through the plasma membrane (encapsulated viruses).

Viruses kill host cells and cause tissue damage in a number of ways (Fig. 9–8):

■ Viruses may inhibit host cell DNA, RNA, or protein synthesis. For example, the poliovirus inactivates "cap-binding protein," a protein essential for translation of host cell mRNAs, but leaves translation of poliovirus mRNAs unaffected.
■ Viral proteins may insert into the host cell's plasma membrane and directly damage its integrity or promote cell fusion (HIV, measles, and herpesviruses).
■ Viruses replicate efficiently and lyse host cells. For example, respiratory epithelial cells are killed by explosive rhinovirus or influenza virus multiplication, liver cells by

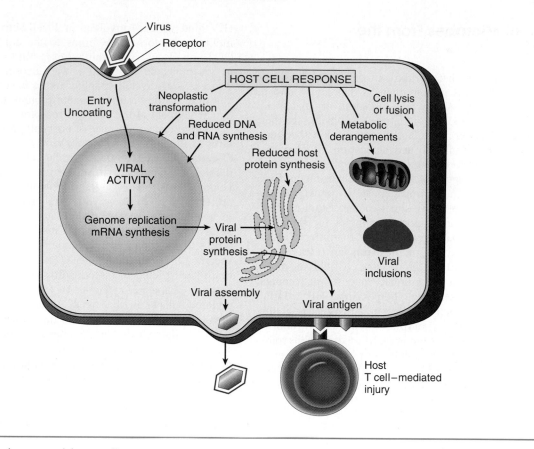

Figure 9–8

Mechanisms by which viruses cause injury to cells.

yellow fever virus, and neurons by poliovirus or rabies viruses.

■ Virus proteins on the surface of the host cells may be recognized by the immune system, and the host lymphocytes attack the virus-infected cells (e.g., liver cells infected with HBV).

■ Viruses may also damage cells involved in host antimicrobial defense, leading to secondary infections. For example, viral damage to respiratory epithelium predisposes to the subsequent development of pneumonia caused by pneumococci or *Haemophilus* organisms, while HIV depletes CD4+ helper lymphocytes and opens the floodgates for many opportunistic infections.

■ Viral killing of cells of one type may cause damage to other cells that are dependent on their integrity. Denervation by the attack of poliovirus on motor neurons causes atrophy, and sometimes death, of distal skeletal muscle cells.

■ Slow virus infections (e.g., subacute sclerosing panencephalitis caused by measles virus) culminate in severe progressive disease after a long latency period.

In addition to all the potential mechanisms of killing cells, viruses (e.g., EBV, HPV, HBV, and human T-cell lymphotropic virus I [HTLV-I]) can cause cell proliferation and transformation, resulting in the formation of cancer (Chapter 6).

Mechanisms of Bacteria-Induced Injury: Bacterial Adhesins and Toxins

Bacterial damage to host tissues depends on their ability to adhere to and enter host cells or to deliver toxins. *The coordination of bacterial adherence and toxin delivery is so important to bacterial virulence that the genes encoding adherence proteins and toxins are frequently regulated together by specific environmental signals.* For example, changes in temperature, osmolarity, or pH trigger the synthesis by *Bordetella pertussis* of some 20 different proteins, including the filamentous hemagglutinin, fimbrial proteins, and pertussis toxin. Similarly, the virulence of enterotoxic *E. coli* depends on the expression of adherence proteins that allow the bacteria to bind to the intestinal epithelial cells and coordinate synthesis and release of heat-labile or heat-stable toxins that cause intestinal cells to secrete isotonic fluids.

Bacterial Adhesins. Bacterial adhesins are molecules that bind bacteria to host cells. They are limited in type but have a broad range of host cell specificity. The surface of gram-positive cocci such as streptococci is covered with two molecules that may mediate adherence of the bacteria to host cells (Fig. 9–9). First, *lipotechoic acids* are hydrophobic molecules that bind to the surface of all eukaryotic cells but have a higher affinity to particular receptors on blood cells and oral epithelial cells. Second, a nonfibrillar adhesin called *protein F* binds

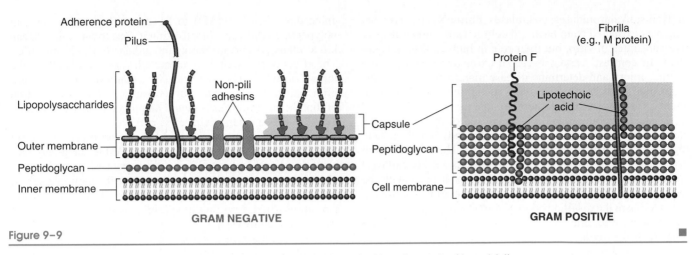

Figure 9–9   ■

Some molecules on the surface of gram-negative and gram-positive bacteria involved in pathogenesis of bacterial diseases.

to fibronectin, an extracellular matrix protein also found on most host cells. M proteins, which form fibrillae on the surface of gram-positive bacteria, as well as a carbohydrate capsule, prevent phagocytosis by host macrophages.

Fimbriae or *pili* on the surface of gram-negative rods and cocci are nonflagellar filamentous structures composed of repeating subunits. While sex pili are used to exchange genes carried on plasmids or transposons from one bacterium to another, most pili mediate adherence of bacteria to host cells. The base of the subunit that anchors the pilus to the bacterial cell wall is similar for widely divergent bacteria (e.g., *Mycobacterium, Pseudomonas, Neisseria*). At the tips of the pili are minor protein components that determine to which host cells the microbes will attach (bacterial tropism). In *E. coli* these minor proteins are antigenically distinct and are associated with particular infections (e.g., type I bind mannose and cause lower urinary tract infections, type P bind galactose and cause pyelonephritis, type S bind sialic acid and cause meningitis). A single bacterium can express more than one type of pilus, as well as adhesins not located in pili (e.g., proteins I and II of gonococci). Other molecules on the surface of gram-negative bacteria important for virulence are lipopolysaccharides and a carbohydrate capsule (discussed later).

Unlike viruses, which infect a broad range of host cells, facultative intracellular bacteria are more restricted and infect epithelial cells (*Shigella* and enteroinvasive *E. coli*), macrophages *(M. tuberculosis, Mycobacterium leprae),* or both *(S. typhi).* Most of these bacteria attach to host cell integrins, plasma membrane proteins that bind complement, or extracellular matrix proteins, including fibronectin, laminin, and collagen (Chapter 3). For example, *Legionella* organisms, *M. tuberculosis,* and the protozoan *Leishmania* all bind to CR3, the cell receptor for complement C3bi. In contrast to rickettsiae, the facultative intracellular bacteria are unable to directly penetrate the host cells but are endocytosed by the epithelial cells or phagocytosed by the macrophages. *Shigella* and enteroinvasive *E. coli* use a plasmid-encoded hemolysin to escape from the endocytic vacuole into the cytoplasm. Once in the cytoplasm, *Shigella* and *E. coli* inhibit host protein synthesis, rapidly replicate, and within 6 hours lyse the host cells.

In contrast, *Salmonella* and *Yersinia* organisms replicate within the phagolysosome of the macrophage, while *Mycobacterium* and *Legionella* organisms inhibit the acidification that normally occurs after endosome fusion with the lysosome. In the absence of a host cellular immune response, many replicating organisms persist within the macrophages (e.g., lepromatous leprosy, *Mycobacterium avium* infection in AIDS patients), but activated macrophages can kill these organisms or limit their growth.

Bacterial Endotoxin. Bacterial endotoxin is a lipopolysaccharide (LPS) that is a structural component of the outer cell wall of gram-negative bacteria. LPS is composed of a long-chain fatty acid anchor (lipid A) connected to a core sugar chain, both of which are the same in all gram-negative bacteria. Attached to the core sugar is a variable carbohydrate chain (O antigen), which is used to serotype and distinguish different bacteria. The many biologic activities of endotoxins are discussed elsewhere in this book and include induction of fever (Chapter 2), septic shock (Chapter 4), disseminated intravascular coagulation (Chapter 12), the acute respiratory distress syndrome (Chapter 13), and a variety of effects on cells of the immune system. All the biologic activities of endotoxin come from lipid A and the core sugars. They are mediated both by direct effects of endotoxin and by the induction of host cytokines such as interleukin 1 (IL-1), tumor necrosis factor (TNF), and others.

Bacterial superantigens (e.g., *Staphylococcus* enterotoxins and toxic shock syndrome toxin [TSST]) cause fever, shock, and multisystem organ failure by a mechanism distinct from that of endotoxin. Bacterial superantigens bind to the major histocompatibility complex (MHC) class II molecules on the surface of many antigen-presenting cells (APCs), without the usual internal processing or discrimination. These superantigen-containing APCs then indiscriminately stimulate numerous T cells to secrete excess interleukin 2 (IL-2), which in turn causes overproduction of TNF and other cytokines responsible for the systemic disturbances.

Bacterial Exotoxins. Many potentially harmful products are secreted by bacteria, yet relatively few have been proved to have defined deleterious effects in vivo. Leukocidins, hemolysins, hyaluronidases, coagulases, fibrinolysins, and other enzymes extracted from bacterial cultures act on their respective substrates in vitro, but their role in human disease is unclear. In contrast, certain bacterial exotoxins directly cause cellular injury and determine disease manifestations, and the molecular mechanisms underlying such injury have been well studied. The effects of diphtheria toxins, for example, are well established. Diphtheria toxin is composed of fragment B (the carboxyl end) and fragment A (the amino end), which are held together by a disulfide bridge (Fig. 9–10). The toxin binds to glycoproteins on the surface of target cells via its carboxyl end and enters the acidic endosome, where it fuses with the endosomal membrane and enters the cell cytoplasm. Within the cytoplasm the disulfide bond of diphtheria toxin is reduced and broken, releasing the enzymatically active amino fragment A of the toxin, which catalyzes the covalent transfer of adenosine diphosphate (ADP)–ribose from nicotinamide-ad-

enine dinucleotide (NAD) to EF-2 (an elongation factor in polypeptide synthesis), inactivating it. One toxin molecule can kill a cell by ADP-ribosylating more than 10^6 EF-2 molecules. The effect of the toxin is to create a layer of dead cells in the throat, on which *Corynebacterium diphtheriae* bacteria outgrow competing bacteria. Subsequently, wide dissemination of diphtheria toxin causes neural and myocardial dysfunction. The heat-labile enterotoxins of *V. cholerae* and of *E. coli* also have an A-B structure and are ADP-ribosyl transferases, but these enzymes catalyze transfer from NAD to the guanyl nucleotide–dependent regulatory component of adenylate cyclase. This generates excess cyclic adenosine monophosphate (cAMP), which causes intestinal epithelial cells to secrete isoosmotic fluid, resulting in voluminous diarrhea and loss of water and electrolytes.

The gram-positive anaerobic *Clostridium perfringens,* the agent of gas gangrene, literally digests host tissues, including the relatively resistant collagens. Its α-toxin is a lecithinase that disrupts plasma membranes, including those of red and white blood cells. *Clostridium tetani,* a wound contaminant, secretes an exotoxin called *tetanoplasmin* that interferes with release of inhibitory transmitter substances such as γ-aminobutyric acid from presynaptic terminals of the spinal interneurons. This results in violent muscle contractions that characterize tetanic spasm. *C. botulinum* toxins block the release of cholinergic neurotransmitters, particularly at the neuromuscular junctions, resulting in progressive paralysis of the limbs, respiratory muscles, and cranial motor nerves. Remarkably, both botulinum and tetanus toxins are endopeptidases that cleave synaptobrevins, which are proteins involved in synaptic vesicle formation.

IMMUNE EVASION BY MICROBES

Humoral and cellular immune responses that protect the host from most infections and the mechanisms of immune-mediated damage to host tissues induced by microbes (e.g., anaphylactic reactions, immune complex reactions) were discussed in Chapter 5. Here we will focus on the ways in which microorganisms escape the host immune system by (1) remaining inaccessible; (2) cleaving antibody, resisting complement-mediated lysis, or surviving in phagocytotic cells; (3) varying or shedding antigens; and (4) causing specific or nonspecific immunosuppression.

Microbes that propagate in the lumen of the intestine (e.g., toxin-producing *C. difficile*) or gallbladder (e.g., *S. typhi*) are inaccessible to the host immune defenses, including secretory IgA. Viruses shed from the luminal surface of epithelial cells (e.g., CMV in urine or milk and poliovirus in stool) or those that infect the keratinized epithelium (poxviruses that cause molluscum contagiosum) are also inaccessible to the host humoral immune system. Some organisms establish infections by rapidly invading host cells before the host humoral response becomes effective (e.g., malaria sporozoites entering liver cells; *Trichinella* and *Trypanosoma cruzi* entering skeletal and cardiac muscles, respectively). Some larger parasites (e.g., the larvae of tapeworms) form cysts in host tissues that

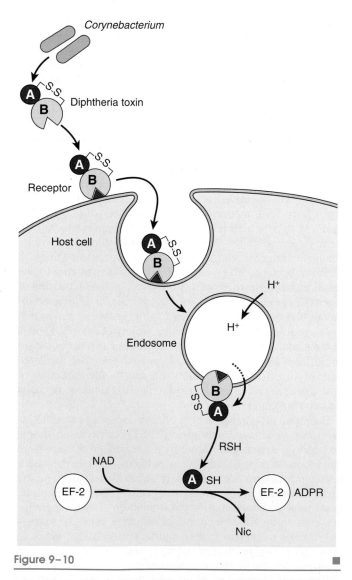

Figure 9–10 ■

Inhibition of cellular protein synthesis by diphtheria toxin. See text for abbreviations. (Adapted from Collier RJ: Corynebacteria. In Davis BD, et al (eds): Microbiology. New York, Harper & Row, 1990.)

are covered by a dense fibrous capsule that walls them off from host immune responses.

The carbohydrate capsule on the surface of all the major pathogens that cause pneumonia or meningitis (*Pneumococcus, Meningococcus, Haemophilus, Klebsiella,* and *E. coli*) makes them more virulent by covering bacterial antigens and preventing phagocytosis of the organisms by neutrophils. *Pseudomonas* bacteria secrete a leukotoxin that kills neutrophils. Some *E. coli* have K antigens that prevent activation of complement by the alternative pathway and lysis of the cells. Conversely, some gram-negative bacteria have very long polysaccharide O antigens, which bind host antibody and activate complement at such distance from the bacterial cells that the organisms fail to lyse. Staphylococci are covered by protein A molecules that bind the Fc portion of the antibody and so inhibit phagocytosis. *Neisseria, Haemophilus,* and *Streptococcus* all secrete proteases that degrade antibodies.

Viral infection evokes neutralizing antibodies, which prevent viral attachment, penetration, or uncoating. This highly specific immunity is the basis of antiviral vaccination, but it cannot protect against viruses with many antigenic variants (e.g., rhinoviruses or influenza viruses). Pneumococci are capable of more than 80 permutations of their capsular polysaccharides, so that in repeated infections the host is unlikely to recognize the new serotype. *Neisseria gonorrhoeae* have pilar (attachment) proteins composed of a constant region and a hypervariable region. The latter allows *Neisseria* to change its antigens during infection and prevent immune clearance. Similarly, the spirochete *Borrelia recurrentis* causes a relapsing fever by repeatedly switching its surface antigens before each successive clone is exterminated by the host. Successive clones of African trypanosomes also vary their major surface antigen to escape host antibody responses. Cercariae of *S. mansoni* shed parasite antigens, which are recognized by host antibodies or activate complement by the alternative pathway, within minutes of penetrating the skin. Finally, viruses that infect lymphocytes (HIV and EBV) directly damage the host immune system and cause opportunistic infections (e.g., AIDS).

SPECIAL TECHNIQUES FOR DIAGNOSIS OF INFECTIOUS AGENTS

Some infectious agents or their products can be directly observed in H and E–stained sections (e.g., the inclusion bodies formed by CMV and herpesvirus; bacterial clumps, which usually stain blue; *Candida* and *Mucor,* among the fungi; most protozoans; and all helminths). However, many infectious agents are best visualized after staining with special stains that identify organisms based on particular characteristics of their cell walls or coat (Gram, acid-fast, silver, mucicarmine, and Giemsa stains) or after labeling with specific antibody probes (Table 9–3). Regardless of the staining technique, organisms are usually best visualized at the advancing edge of a lesion rather than at its center, particularly if there is necrosis. Because these morphologic techniques cannot speciate organisms, determine drug sensitivity, or identify virulence char-

Table 9–3. SPECIAL TECHNIQUES FOR DIAGNOSIS OF INFECTIOUS AGENTS

Technique	Agent(s) Detected
Gram stain	Most bacteria
Acid-fast stain	*Mycobacteria, Nocardia* (modified)
Silver stains	Fungi, *Legionella, Pneumocystis*
Periodic acid–Schiff	Fungi, amebae
Mucicarmine	Cryptococci
Giemsa	Campylobacteria, *Leishmania,* malaria
Antibody probes	Viruses, rickettsiae
Culture	All classes
DNA probes	Viruses, bacteria, protozoa

acteristics, cultures of lesional tissue must be performed. PCR-based methods are used to identify microbes that grow slowly in culture (*Mycobacteria* or CMV organisms) or cannot be cultured at all (HBV and HCV). In addition, DNA sequence analysis has been used to classify bacteria that have never been cultured, including those that cause Whipple's disease (a gram-positive actinobacteria related to *Actinomyces* and *Streptomyces*) and hepatic peliosis and bacillary angiomatosis (a rickettsia).

Regardless of the method of microbial identification, the final step in diagnosis of infectious pathogens is correlation of the suspect organism with the lesion caused and the signs and symptoms produced.

INFLAMMATORY RESPONSE TO INFECTIOUS AGENTS

This chapter concludes with a summary of the most common histologic patterns of host responses induced by infectious agents. In contrast to the vast molecular diversity of parasites, the patterns of inflammatory response to these agents are limited, as are the mediator mechanisms that direct these responses. At the microscopic level, therefore, many pathogens evoke identical reaction patterns, and few of the features are unique to or pathognomonic of each agent. Broadly speaking, there are five histologic patterns of tissue reaction: suppurative polymorphonuclear inflammation, mononuclear inflammation, cytopathic-cytoproliferative inflammation, necrotizing inflammation, and chronic inflammation and scarring.

Suppurative Polymorphonuclear Inflammation. This is the familiar reaction to acute tissue damage described in Chapter 2, marked by increased vascular permeability and neutrophilic exudation. The neutrophils are attracted to the site of infection by release of chemoattractants from *the rapidly dividing "pyogenic" bacteria that evoke this response, mostly extracellular gram-positive cocci and gram-negative rods.* The bacterial chemoattractants include secreted bacterial peptides, all of which contain *N*-formyl methionine residues at their amino terminals that are recognized by specific receptors on neutrophils. Alternatively, bacteria attract neutrophils

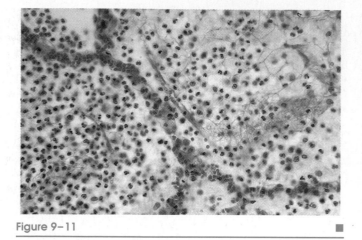

Figure 9-11 ■

Pneumococcus pneumonia. Note the intra-alveolar polymorphonuclear exudate and intact alveolar septa.

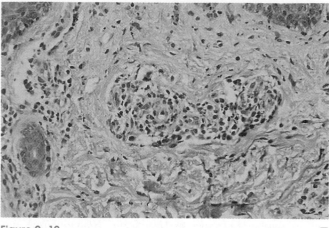

Figure 9-12 ■

Secondary syphilis in the dermis with perivascular lymphoplasmacytic infiltrate and endothelial proliferation.

indirectly by releasing endotoxin, which stimulates macrophages to secrete IL-1 or TNF, or by cleaving complement into the chemoattractant peptide C5a. Massing of neutrophils results in the formation of pus. The size of exudative lesions may vary tremendously, from tiny microabscesses formed in multiple organs during sepsis secondary to a colonized heart valve, to distended pus-filled fallopian tubes caused by *N. gonorrhoeae* (the gonococcus), diffuse involvement of the meninges during *H. influenzae* infection, or pneumonia in which multiple lobes of the lung are involved. How destructive the lesions are depends on their location and the organism involved. For example, pneumococci usually spare pulmonary alveolar walls and cause lobar pneumonia, permitting resolution (Fig. 9-11), while staphylococci and *Klebsiella* species destroy alveolar walls and form abscesses, which can only be followed by scarring (Chapter 13). Bacterial pharyngitis heals without sequelae, whereas untreated acute bacterial inflammation can destroy a joint in a matter of days.

Mononuclear Inflammation. Diffuse, predominantly mononuclear interstitial infiltrates are a common feature of all chronic inflammatory processes, but when they occur acutely, they are *often a response to viruses, intracellular bacteria, or intracellular parasites. In addition, spirochetes and helminths cause chronic inflammation.* Which mononuclear cell predominates within the inflammatory lesion depends on the host immune response to the organism. For example, many plasma cells are seen in the primary and secondary lesions of syphilis (Fig. 9-12), while lymphocytes predominate in HBV or in viral infections of the brain. These lymphocytes represent cell-mediated immunity against the pathogen or the pathogen-infected cells. At the other extreme, macrophages filled with *M. avium* are present in many tissues of AIDS patients, who have no helper T cells left and can mount no immune response to the organisms. In *M. leprae* infection and cutaneous leishmaniasis, some persons mount a strong immune response so that their lesions contain few organisms, few macrophages, and many lymphocytes; others with a weak immune response have lesions that contain many organisms, many macrophages, and few lymphocytes (Fig. 9-13). Granulomatous inflammation (described in detail in Chapter 2) is a distinctive

form of mononuclear inflammation usually evoked by relatively slow-dividing infectious agents (e.g., *M. tuberculosis*) and by agents of relatively large size (e.g., schistosome eggs). Granulomatous inflammation almost always reflects a cell-mediated immune reaction (Chapter 5).

Cytopathic-Cytoproliferative Inflammation. These reactions, usually produced by viruses, are characterized by damage to individual host cells, with little or no host inflammatory response. Some viruses replicate within cells and make viral aggregates that are visible as inclusion bodies (e.g., CMV, adenovirus) or induce cells to fuse and form polykaryons (e.g., measles, herpesviruses). Focal cell damage may cause epithelial cells to become discohesive and form blisters (e.g., chickenpox virus). Viruses can also cause epithelial cells to proliferate and take unusual forms (e.g., venereal warts by HPV or the umbilicated papules of molluscum contagiosum by pox viruses). Finally, viruses can cause dysplastic changes and cancers in epithelial cells and lymphocytes (Chapter 6).

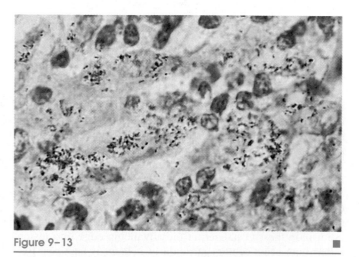

Figure 9-13 ■

Leprosy. High-power view of acid-fast bacilli proliferating in foamy macrophages.

Necrotizing Inflammation. *C. perfringens* and other organisms that secrete very strong toxins cause such rapid and severe tissue damage that cell death is the dominant feature. Because so few inflammatory cells are involved, these lesions resemble infarcts, with disruption or loss of basophilic nuclear staining and preservation of cellular outlines. Often clostridia are opportunistic pathogens introduced into muscle tissue by penetrating trauma or by infection of the bowel in a neutropenic host. Similarly, the parasite *E. histolytica* causes colonic ulcers and liver abscesses characterized by extensive tissue destruction with liquefactive necrosis in the absence of an inflammatory infiltrate. Occasionally viruses can cause necrotizing inflammation when host cell damage is particularly widespread and severe; for example, there may be total destruction of the temporal lobes of the brain by herpesvirus or of the liver by HBV.

Chronic Inflammation and Scarring. The final common pathway of many infections is chronic inflammation, which may lead to extensive scarring (e.g., chronic gonococcal salpingitis). Chronic HBV infection may cause cirrhosis of the liver, in which dense fibrous septae surround nodules of regenerating hepatocytes. For some organisms that are relatively inert, the exuberant host scarring response is the major cause of disease (e.g., the "pipestem" fibrosis of the liver caused by schistosome eggs or gummas of tertiary syphilis in the liver, CNS, and bones).

These patterns of tissue reaction are useful for analyzing the infective processes, but they frequently overlap. For example, a cutaneous lesion of leishmaniasis may contain two separate histopathologic regions: a central ulcerated area filled with neutrophils, and a peripheral region containing a mixed infiltrate of lymphocytes and mononuclear cells, where the leishmanial parasites are located. The lung of an AIDS patient may be infected with CMV, which causes cytolytic changes and *Pneumocystis,* which causes interstitial inflammation. Similar patterns of inflammation can also be seen in tissue responses to physical or chemical agents and in inflammatory diseases of unknown cause (e.g., sarcoidosis).

It is evident that many factors that relate to the invader and the host modify the development and nature of the microbe-induced disease and its outcome. This chapter has emphasized the structural and molecular mechanisms relevant to the interaction between microbe and host. However, it should also be remembered that, considering the multiplicity of potential invaders, most infectious diseases are caused by a relatively small number of agents that differ in geographic locales and are determined largely by environmental, socioeconomic, and public health factors.

BIBLIOGRAPHY

Binford CH, O'Connor DH: Pathology of Tropical and Extraordinary Diseases, Vols I and II. Washington, DC, Armed Forces Institute of Pathology, 1976. (To date, some of the best descriptions and illustrations of the histopathology of infectious diseases.)

Enders JF, et al: Cultivation of the Lansing strain of poliomyelitis virus in culture of various human embryonic tissues. Science 109:85, 1949. (Report of the Nobel prize–winning work that led to the polio vaccines.)

Finlay BB, Falkow S: Common themes in microbial pathogenicity. Microbial Rev 53:210, 1989. (An overview of bacterial pathogenesis.)

Fischetti VA: Streptococcal M protein. Sci Am 264:58, 1991.

Hultgren SJ, et al: Pilus and nonpilus bacterial adhesion: assembly and function in cell recognition. Cell 73:887, 1993.

Johnson HM, et al: Superantigens in human disease. Sci Am 266:92, 1992.

Mekalanos JJ: Environmental signals controlling expression of virulence gene determinants in bacteria. J Bacteriol 174:1, 1992. (A review of mechanisms of global regulation of pathogenicity of bacteria.)

Mims CA: The Pathogenesis of Infectious Disease. Orlando, FL, Academic Press, 1987. (An extensive discussion of the mechanisms of microbial pathogenesis.)

Sayers AA, Whitt DD: Bacterial Pathogenesis. A Molecular Approach. Washington, DC, ASM Press, 1994. (A well-selected set of examples of the molecular basis of bacterial diseases.)

Schiavo G, et al: Tetanus and botulinum-B neurotoxins block neurotransmitter release by proteolytic cleavage of synaptobrevin. Nature 359:832, 1992.

Spangler B: Structure and function of cholera toxin and the related *Escherichia coli* heat-labile enterotoxin. Microbiol Rev 56:622, 1992.

von Lichtenberg F: Pathology of Infectious Disease. New York, Raven Press, 1991. (An authoritative and concise presentation of the broad gamut of microbial diseases, with excellent coverage of the resultant morphologic lesions.)

Walsh J: Estimating the burden of illness in the tropics. In Warren KS, Mahmoud AAF (eds): Tropical and Geographical Medicine. New York, McGraw-Hill, 1990. (An overview of the epidemiology of infectious diseases in the developing world.)

Zhang QY: Gene conversion in *Neisseria gonorrhoeae*: evidence for its role in pilus antigenic variation. Proc Natl Acad Sci USA 89:5366, 1992.

Diseases of Organ Systems

10

Blood Vessels

Vascular disorders are responsible for more morbidity and mortality than any other category of human disease. Among them, arterial diseases are the most important. They achieve this unenviable preeminence by (1) narrowing vessels and thus producing ischemia of tissues perfused by such vessels; (2) damaging the endothelial lining and thus promoting intravascular thrombosis, a process that contributes to critical ischemia of vital organs such as the heart and brain; (3) weakening the walls of vessels, predisposing to dilation or possibly rupture; and (4) contributing to the pathogenesis of some of the most common diseases in humans, namely, atherosclerosis, hypertension, and diabetes. Although disorders of veins are by no means trivial, they are dwarfed in significance by the diseases of arteries, in particular atherosclerosis. In the following discussions, the various conditions are divided into those that affect the arteries, those that affect the veins, and those that affect the lymphatics; this is followed by a brief consideration of vascular tumors, because whatever their origin, they are quite similar clinically and anatomically.

Before we discuss the individual diseases, mention should be made of the general properties and reactions of the two cellular components of blood vessels—endothelium and vascular smooth muscle—that are involved in many of the disorders.

Endothelial Cells. Vascular endothelium is a versatile multifunctional tissue that has many synthetic and metabolic properties (Table 10–1). As a semipermeable membrane, endothelium controls the transfer of small and large molecules into the arterial wall and through the walls of capillaries and venules. In most regions the intercellular junctions are normally impermeable to such molecules, but the relatively labile junctions between endothelial cells (ECs) may widen under the influence of hemodynamic factors (e.g., high blood pressure) and vasoactive agents (e.g., histamine in inflammation) (Chapter 2). Moreover, ECs play a role in the maintenance of a nonthrombogenic blood–tissue interface (Chapter 4), the modulation of blood flow and vascular resistance, the metabolism of hormones, the regulation of immune and inflammatory reactions, and the growth regulation of other cell types, particularly smooth muscle cells (SMCs). Thus, the endothelium is an active participant in the interaction between blood and tissues. In addition to contributing to the formation of thrombi, endothelial injury may be responsible, at least in part, for the initiation of atherosclerosis and the vascular lesions of hypertension and other disorders.

With the several antithrombotic properties of ECs, it is not surprising that mechanical denudation of the endothelial lining with exposure of blood to subendothelial connective tissue initiates thrombosis. An important conceptual advance, however, is the realization that *structurally intact ECs can respond to various stimuli by adjusting some of the constitutive functions and by expressing some newly acquired (induced) properties.* The term *endothelial dysfunction* is often used to describe several types of potentially reversible changes in the functional state of ECs that occur as a response to environmental stimuli. In particular, ECs can be *activated* by a number of stimuli, principally cytokines, resulting in the induction of endothelial leukocyte adhesion molecules, growth factors, cytokines, and vasoactive mediators.

Vascular Smooth Muscle Cells. Vascular smooth muscle cells are capable of many functions, including vasoconstriction and dilation in response to normal or pharmacologic stimuli; synthesis of various types of collagen, elastin, and proteoglycans; elaboration of growth factors and cytokines; and migration and proliferation. Smooth muscle proliferation and production of extracellular matrix components contribute to atherosclerotic plaque.

The migratory and proliferative activity of SMCs is physiologically regulated by both growth promoters and inhibitors. Promoters include platelet-derived growth factor (PDGF), which is derived not only from platelets, but also from ECs and macrophages; basic fibroblast growth factor (bFGF); and interleukin 1 (IL-1). Inhibitors include heparan sulfates, nitric oxide (NO)/endothelium-derived relaxing factor (EDRF), interferon-gamma, and transforming growth factor β (TGF-β). Vascular injury stimulates SMC growth by disrupting the physiologic balance between SMC growth inhibition and growth stimulation.

Reconstitution of the damaged vascular wall, including endothelium, comprises a physiologic healing response with the formation of a *neointima*. Under certain circumstances, intimal thickening as a healing response becomes exaggerated, resulting in *intimal thickening/hyperplasia*, which can cause stenosis or occlusion of small and medium-sized blood vessels or vascular grafts. Such a scenario contributes to many important clinical disorders. The initial injurious stimulus in these disorders varies from predominantly mechanical (angioplasty restenosis) to predominantly immunologic (transplant arteriosclerosis) to multifactorial (atherosclerosis).

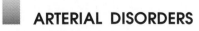

ARTERIAL DISORDERS

Arteriosclerosis

Arteriosclerosis is the generic term for three patterns of vascular disease, all of which cause thickening and inelasticity of arteries:

Table 10–1. ENDOTHELIAL CELL PROPERTIES AND FUNCTIONS

Maintenance of permeability barrier	Modulation of blood flow and vascular reactivity
Elaboration of anticoagulant and antithrombotic molecules	Vasoconstrictors: endothelin, ACE
Prostacyclin	Vasodilators: NO/EDRF, prostacyclin
Thrombomodulin	
Plasminogen activator	Regulation of inflammation and immunity
Heparin-like molecules	IL-1, IL-6, IL-8
Elaboration of prothrombotic molecules	Adhesion molecules
von Willebrand factor (factor VIII-vWF)	Histocompatibility antigens
	Regulation of cell growth
Tissue factor	Growth stimulators: PDGF, CSF, FGF
Plasminogen activator inhibitor	Growth inhibitors: heparin, TGF-β
Extracellular matrix production (collagen, proteoglycans)	Oxidation of LDL

ACE, angiotensin-converting enzyme (AI → AII); NO/EDRF, nitric oxide/endothelium-derived relaxing factor; IL, interleukin; PDGF, platelet-derived growth factor; CSF, colony-stimulating factor; FGF, fibroblast growth factor; TGF-β, transforming growth factor β; LDL, low-density lipoprotein.

■ The dominant pattern is atherosclerosis, characterized by the formation of intimal fibrofatty plaques that often have a central grumous core rich in lipid—hence the term "atherosclerosis," from the Greek stem *athera,* meaning "gruel or porridge."

■ The second morphologic form of arteriosclerosis is the rather trivial *Mönckeberg's medial calcific sclerosis,* characterized by calcifications in the media of muscular arteries. It is usually encountered in medium-sized muscular arteries in persons older than 50 years. The calcifications take the form of irregular medial plates or discrete transverse rings; they create a nodularity on palpation and are readily visualized radiographically. Occasionally the calcific deposits undergo ossification. Since these medial lesions do not encroach on the vessel lumen, medial calcific sclerosis is largely of anatomic interest alone; however, arteries so affected may also develop atherosclerosis.

■ Disease of small arteries and arterioles *(arteriolosclerosis)* is the third pattern. Small vessel sclerosis is most often associated with hypertension and diabetes mellitus. There are two anatomic variants, hyaline and hyperplastic, depending on the cause and rate of progression of disease. Both cause thickening of vessel walls with luminal narrowing and may in the aggregate induce ischemic injury to tissues or organs. Since the lesions are often associated with hypertension, they are described later in the chapter.

Here we will consider only atherosclerosis, which is so clearly the most important form that it is often loosely referred to as *arteriosclerosis.*

ATHEROSCLEROSIS

No disease in the United States (or other developed countries) is responsible for more deaths, has stimulated more research, and has engendered more controversy about how best to control it than atherosclerosis (AS). Basically it is characterized by intimal plaques called *atheromas* that protrude into the lumen, weaken the underlying media, and undergo a series of complications. AS alone accounts for more than half of all deaths in the Western world. Although any artery may be affected, the major targets are the aorta and the coronary and cerebral arteries. Coronary AS induces ischemic heart disease (IHD) and, when the arterial lesions are complicated by thrombosis, the most serious form of IHD, myocardial infarction (MI), which alone is responsible for 20% to 25% of all deaths in the United States.

Atherothrombotic disease of the cerebral vessels is the major cause of brain infarcts, or strokes, one of the most common forms of neurologic disease. In addition, AS often produces critical ischemia of the intestines and lower extremities and is a major cause of abdominal aortic aneurysms (abnormal dilations) that sometimes rupture to produce massive fatal hemorrhage. The disease begins in early childhood and progresses slowly over the decades. Thus, in some sense AS is a pediatric disease, and if its toll is to be reduced, measures must be instituted early before it rears its ugly head and provokes one of its unfortunate consequences.

Epidemiology. AS is virtually ubiquitous among the populations of North America, Europe, Australia, New Zealand, the Soviet Union, and other developed nations. In contrast, as judged by the number of deaths attributable to IHD (including MI), it is much less prevalent in Central and South America, Africa, Asia, and the Orient. For example, the mortality rate for IHD in the United States is six times higher than that in Japan. Indeed, in most developed nations, AS and its sequelae have assumed nearly epidemic proportions, but happily in the United States there is evidence that the epidemic has been brought under control. Between 1968 (the peak year) and 1984 there was a nearly 40% decrease in the death rate from IHD and a 53% decrease in death from strokes. The basis for this fortunate trend is not entirely clear but has reasonably been attributed to changes in living habits, including reduced cigarette smoking, altered dietary habits with reduced consumption of cholesterol and other saturated animal fats, better control of hypertension, and improved methods of treatment of nonfatal myocardial infarcts.

Risk Factors. The prevalence and severity of the disease, and therefore the age when it is likely to cause tissue or organ injury, are related to a number of factors, some constitutional and therefore immutable, but others acquired and potentially controllable. The constitutional factors include age, sex, and familial background.

■ *Age.* Age is a dominant influence. Although early lesions of AS appear in childhood, clinically significant disease, as judged by the death rates from IHD, rises with each decade, even into advanced age. For example, from age 40 to age 60 there is a greater than fivefold increase in the incidence of MI.

■ *Sex.* Other factors being equal, males are much more prone to AS than females. Females are more or less sheltered from advanced, disease-producing AS until menopause, so MI is uncommon in premenopausal women unless they are predisposed by diabetes or some unusual (possibly familial) form of hyperlipidemia or have severe hypertension. Between ages 35 and 55 years, the mortality rate from IHD for white women is one fifth that for white men. After menopause, protection slowly dwindles, until the frequency of MI becomes the same in both sexes by the seventh to eighth decade of life.

■ *Familial Predisposition.* There is a well-defined familial predisposition to AS and IHD. In some instances it relates to familial clustering of other risk factors, such as hypertension and diabetes. In other instances, it involves well-defined hereditary genetic derangements in lipoprotein metabolism that result in excessively high blood lipid levels. The prototype of these conditions is familial hypercholesterolemia, but in addition there are a growing number of familial dyslipoproteinemias, many of which result from mutations that yield defective apolipoproteins. Recall that these are proteins bound to the various blood lipid fractions, which have many functions, among them activating or inhibiting particular enzymes, facilitating transmembrane transport of certain lipoproteins, and serving as ligands to high-affinity cellular receptors that guide the lipoproteins to specific sites of catabolism.

There are four major acquired risk factors that are at least in some part amenable to control: (1) hyperlipidemia, (2) hypertension, (3) cigarette smoking, and (4) diabetes. In addition, there are a number of less important, "soft" risks.

Hyperlipidemia is virtually universally acknowledged to be a major risk factor for AS. Most of the evidence specifically implicates hypercholesterolemia, but hypertriglyceridemia may also play a role, although it is not as significant as hypercholesterolemia. Recall from an earlier discussion that the various classes of blood lipids are transported as lipoproteins complexed to specific apoproteins.

The major evidence implicating hypercholesterolemia in the genesis of AS includes the following:

■ High-cholesterol diets can produce atherosclerotic plaques in experimental animals, including nonhuman primates, that are nearly identical to those observed in human disease.

■ The major lipids in atheromas (plaques) are cholesterol and cholesteryl esters derived from the plasma.

■ Many large-scale epidemiologic analyses have demonstrated a significant correlation between the total plasma cholesterol or low-density lipoprotein (LDL) level and the severity of AS as judged by the mortality rate from IHD. The higher the total cholesterol level, the greater the risk of symptomatic and fatal atherosclerotic disease. No threshold clearly separates persons at risk from those free of risk, but in general, atherosclerotic events are very uncommon with total serum cholesterol levels below 150 mg/dl. Hypertriglyceridemia, as manifested by elevated very-low-density lipoprotein (VLDL) levels, is also associated with some increased risk.

■ Genetic or acquired disorders (e.g., familial hypercholesterolemia, diabetes mellitus, hypothyroidism) that cause hypercholesterolemia lead to premature and severe AS; an example is familial hypercholesterolemia, which in the homozygous state is often associated with MI before age 20 years (Chapter 7).

■ When levels of serum cholesterol are lowered by diet or drugs, there is evidence in animals that some atherosclerotic plaques regress, or fail to progress, within months, and that the risk of cardiovascular mortality in selected patients is reduced.

■ Genetic manipulations of lipid components in mice (e.g., apolipoprotein E deficiency) lead to abnormal lipid metabolism and atheromatous lesions in these animals.

It is important at this point to emphasize the inverse relationship between symptomatic AS and the high-density lipoprotein (HDL) level. HDL participates in reverse transport of cholesterol and is believed to mobilize this lipid from cells and presumably from atherosclerotic plaques and transport it to the liver for excretion in the bile. *The higher the levels of HDL, the lower is the risk of IHD.* Hence, there is great interest in dietary methods of lowering serum LDL and raising serum HDL. Nondietary influences may also affect the level of blood lipids. Exercise and moderate consumption of ethanol both raise the HDL level, whereas obesity and smoking lower it.

Hypertension is a major risk factor for AS at all ages and may well be more important than hypercholesterolemia after age 45. Men age 45 to 62 whose blood pressure exceeds 160/95 mm Hg have a more than fivefold greater risk of IHD than those with blood pressures of 140/90 mm Hg or lower. Both systolic and diastolic levels are important in increasing risk.

Smoking, another important risk factor, is thought to account for the relatively recent increase in the incidence and severity of AS in women. When one or more packs of cigarettes are smoked per day for several years, the death rate from IHD increases by up to 200%. Cessation of smoking reduces this increased risk in time.

Diabetes mellitus induces hypercholesterolemia and a markedly increased predisposition to AS. Other factors being equal, the incidence of MI is twice as high in diabetics as in nondiabetics. There is also an increased risk of strokes and, even more striking, perhaps a 100-fold increased risk of AS-induced gangrene of the lower extremities. Indeed, in the absence of diabetes, atherosclerotic gangrene of the lower extremities is uncommon.

Other Factors. These are sometimes referred to as minor, or "soft," risk factors because they are associated with a less pronounced and difficult-to-quantitate risk. These include (1) insufficient regular physical activity; (2) competitive, stressful life style with "type A" personality behavior (although this is controversial); (3) obesity; (4) the use of oral contraceptives; (5) hyperuricemia; (6) high carbohydrate intake; and (7) hyperhomocysteinemia. The last has recently received increased attention, and a role for hemocysteine as a deleterious agent in AS is currently being pursued.

In closing this discussion of risk factors, it is important to note that *multiple factors impose more than an additive effect.* When three risk factors are present (e.g., hyperlipidemia, hypertension, and smoking), the heart attack rate is seven times greater than when none are present. Two risk factors increase the risk fourfold. However, the converse is equally important: AS may develop in the absence of any apparent risk factors, so even those who live "the prudent life" and have no apparent genetic predispositions are not immune to this killer disease.

Pathogenesis. Understandably, the commanding importance of AS has stimulated enormous efforts to discover its cause, and a number of hypotheses for its pathogenesis have been proposed. The currently favored theory, and the one receiving the greatest attention is the response-to-injury hypothesis (Fig. 10–1). It best accommodates the various risk factors discussed. Central to this thesis are the following features:

1. The development of focal areas of chronic endothelial injury, usually subtle, with resulting increased endothelial permeability or other evidence of endothelial dysfunction.
2. Increased insudation of lipoproteins into the vessel wall, mainly LDL or modified LDL with its high cholesterol content, and also VLDL.
3. A series of cellular interactions in these foci of injury involving ECs, monocytes/macrophages, T lymphocytes, and SMCs of intimal or medial origin.
4. Proliferation of smooth muscle cells in the intima with formation of extracellular matrix by the SMCs (Fig. 10–1).

Each of these aspects of the atherogenic process will now be considered.

Endothelial Injury. Chronic or repeated endothelial injury is the cornerstone of the response-to-injury hypothesis. Although endothelial denuding injuries certainly initiate atherosclerotic changes in experimental animals, the naturally occurring disease of humans begins with some form of nondenuding, subtle injury. Circulating endotoxins, hypoxia, products derived from cigarette smoke, viruses, and specific endothelial toxins such as homocysteine (accounting for the premature and severe AS of homocystinurics) could be in-

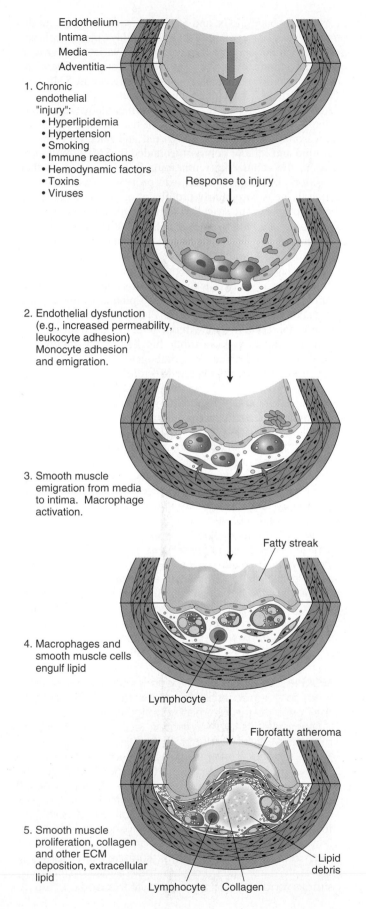

Endothelium
Intima
Media
Adventitia

1. Chronic
   endothelial
   "injury":
   • Hyperlipidemia
   • Hypertension
   • Smoking
   • Immune reactions
   • Hemodynamic factors
   • Toxins
   • Viruses

Response to injury

2. Endothelial dysfunction
   (e.g., increased permeability,
   leukocyte adhesion)
   Monocyte adhesion
   and emigration.

3. Smooth muscle
   emigration from media
   to intima. Macrophage
   activation.

Fatty streak

4. Macrophages and
   smooth muscle cells
   engulf lipid

Lymphocyte

Fibrofatty atheroma

5. Smooth muscle
   proliferation, collagen
   and other ECM
   deposition, extracellular
   lipid

Lipid
debris

Lymphocyte   Collagen

Figure 10–1   ■

The response-to-injury theory of atherogenesis. ECM, extracellular matrix.

volved, but thought to be much more likely are (1) hemodynamic disturbances (shear stress, turbulent flow) and (2) adverse effects of hypercholesterolemia, perhaps acting in concert.

Shear stress and turbulent flow cause increased endothelial permeability and cell turnover, enhanced receptor-mediated LDL endocytosis, and increased endothelial adhesivity to leukocytes. These alterations are associated with altered gene expression of important molecules, such as cytokines, adhesion molecules, and coagulation proteins. The complex geometry of the arterial system, with its twists and turns and branchings, could give rise to turbulent flow patterns with variable levels of shear stress capable of causing focal areas of such endothelial dysfunction. In support of this notion is a well-defined tendency for plaques to occur at mouths of exiting vessels, branch points, and along the posterior wall of the descending and abdominal aorta, which is caught between the "anvil" of the vertebral column and the "hammer" of the arterial pulse.

Hyperlipidemia contributes to atherogenesis in several ways:

■ Chronic hyperlipidemia, particularly hypercholesterolemia, may itself initiate endothelial dysfunction.
■ With chronic hyperlipidemia, lipoproteins accumulate within the intima at sites of endothelial injury or dysfunction.
■ Most important, it provides the opportunity for modification of lipid in the arterial wall, largely by oxidative mechanisms, yielding modified LDL. Oxidative modification of LDL is currently thought to be a significant aspect of the atherogenic process. It is proposed that LDL in the microenvironment of interadherent monocytes and endothelial cells is exposed to free radicals generated by these activated cells. Oxidized LDL contributes to atherogenesis in the following ways: (1) it is readily ingested by macrophages through the scavenger receptor that is distinct from the LDL receptor (Chapter 7); (2) it is chemotactic for circulating monocytes; (3) it increases monocyte adhesion; (4) it inhibits the motility of macrophages already in lesions, thus favoring the recruitment and retention of macrophages in the lesions; (5) it stimulates release of growth factors and cytokines; (6) it is cytotoxic to endothelial and SMCs; and (7) it is immunogenic. Indeed, it has been shown that it is possible to confer some protection against AS in animals by treating them with antioxidants. This has provoked much interest in the possible protective role of antioxidants such as vitamin E in human AS.

Cellular Events in Atherogenesis. A complex series of cellular events similar to those that occur in chronic inflammation (Chapter 2) are involved in the formation of atheromatous plaques. After some form of endothelial injury, monocytes adhere and migrate between ECs to localize subendothelially. There they become transformed into macrophages and avidly engulf lipoproteins, largely oxidized LDL, to become foam cells (Fig. 10–2). Recall that oxidized LDL is chemotactic to monocytes and immobilizes macrophages at sites where it ac-

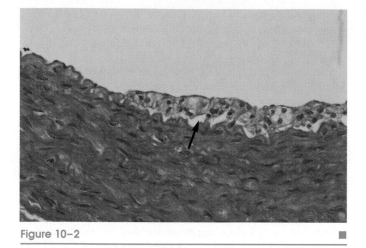

Figure 10-2

Photomicrograph of fatty streaks in an experimental hypercholesterolemic rabbit, demonstrating intimal macrophage-derived foam cells *(arrow)*.

cumulates. Macrophages also proliferate in the intima. If the injury is denuding, platelets also adhere to the endothelium. Early in the evolution of the lesion, SMCs, some of medial origin, migrate and gather in the intima, where they proliferate, and some take up lipids to also be transformed into foam cells. As long as the hypercholesterolemia persists, monocyte adhesion, subendothelial migration of SMCs, and accumulation of lipids within the macrophages and SMCs continue, eventually yielding aggregates of foam cells in the intima, which are apparent macroscopically as *fatty streaks.* These, many believe, are the forerunners of fully evolved atheromas. Should the hypercholesterolemia be ameliorated, these fatty streaks may regress, but if they persist, they continue to evolve.

In view of the large number of secretory products and biologic activities of macrophages, detailed in the discussion of inflammation (Chapter 2), it is likely that they play a role in the progression of atherosclerotic lesions. For example, macrophages produce IL-1 and tumor necrosis factor (TNF), which increase adhesion of leukocytes; several chemokines (e.g., monocyte chemoattractant protein 1 [MCP-1]) generated by macrophages may further recruit leukocytes into the plaque. Macrophages produce toxic oxygen species that also cause oxidation of the LDL in the lesions; recall that oxidized LDL is recognized by the scavenger receptor. Finally, growth stimulators and growth inhibitors elaborated by macrophages (see later) may modulate the proliferation of SMCs and the deposition of extracellular matrix in the lesions. T lymphocytes (both CD4 and CD8+) are also present in atheromas, but the precise stimuli for their recruitment and their roles in the evolution of atheromas are uncertain.

Proliferation of SMCs about the focus of foam cells converts the fatty streak into a mature fibrofatty atheroma. Arterial SMCs can synthesize collagen, elastin, and glycoproteins. A number of growth factors have been implicated in the proliferation of SMCs, most importantly PDGF, which is released from platelets adherent to the focus of endothelial injury but is also produced by macrophages, ECs, and SMCs. Additional candidate mitogens are FGF and transforming growth factor α. Indeed, the evolving atheroma has been likened to a chronic inflammatory reaction, with activated T cells, mono-

cytes/macrophages, ECs, and SMCs all expressing or contributing a variety of cytokines that could play roles in cell adhesion, locomotion, and replication. A variety of growth inhibitors modulate smooth muscle proliferation. These include heparin-like molecules, present in ECs and SMCs, or TGF-β, derived from ECs or macrophages.

At this stage in atherogenesis, the intimal plaque represents a central aggregation of foam cells of macrophage and SMC origin, some of which may have died and released extracellular lipid and cellular debris surrounded by SMCs. With progression, the cellular-fatty atheroma is modified by further deposition of collagen, elastin, and proteoglycans. This connective tissue is particularly prominent on the intimal aspect, where it produces the so-called *fibrous cap.* Thus evolves the fully mature *fibrofatty atheroma.* Some atheromas undergo considerable cellular proliferation and connective tissue formation to yield *fibrous plaques.* Others retain a central core of lipid-laden cells and fatty debris.

Thrombosis is a complication of late-stage AS, and organization of thrombi may contribute to plaque formation and their encroachment on the lumen. Platelets generally do not adhere to the arterial wall without prior severe injury or endothelial denudation; more subtle biochemical disruptions of a normal EC could render it thrombogenic.

Lipoprotein Lp(a) is an altered form of LDL that contains the apolipoprotein B-100 portion of the LDL linked to apolipoprotein A (apo A), itself a large glycoprotein molecule with a high degree of structural homology to plasminogen (a key protein in fibrinolysis). Lipoprotein Lp(a) could be atherogenic by various mechanisms, including interference with both LDL and plasminogen metabolism or promotion of SMC proliferation. Indeed, epidemiologic studies have shown a correlation between increased blood levels of lipoprotein Lp(a) and coronary and cerebral vascular disease, independent of the level of total cholesterol or LDL.

Figure 10–1 summarizes the major proposed mechanism of atherogenesis. This considers AS as a chronic inflammatory response of the vascular wall to a variety of initiating events that can occur early in life. Multiple mechanisms contribute to plaque formation and progression, including endothelial dysfunction, monocyte adhesion and infiltration, smooth muscle proliferation, extracellular matrix deposition, lipid accumulation, and thrombosis.

MORPHOLOGY. Atherosclerotic lesions evolve over time, so it is necessary to characterize them from their origin to their ultimate configuration.

Many experts believe that at least some atheromas arise as **fatty streaks** in the first years of life. These subendothelial lesions begin as 1-mm, soft, yellow, intimal discolorations **(fatty dots)** that progressively enlarge by becoming thicker and slightly elevated while they elongate in the long axis of the vessel to produce typical fatty streaks 1 to 3 mm wide and up to 1.5 cm long (Fig. 10–3). Some may not be elevated and so are better seen after staining the aortic surface with oil red O, a stain for lipid. Early in their evolution, fatty streaks tend to be in the region of the aortic valve

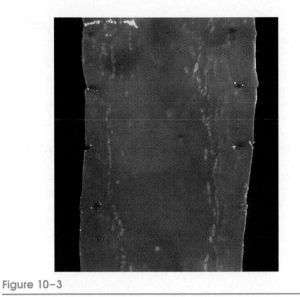

Figure 10–3   ■

Atherosclerosis. The barely elevated, lipid-laden fatty streaks are seen in two vertical rows near the ostia of vertebral branches of the aorta. (From the teaching collection of the Department of Pathology, University of Texas Southwestern Medical School, Dallas, TX.)

ring, in the posterior wall of the descending thoracic aorta, and adjacent to the orifices of the intercostal arteries in the thoracic aorta. With age they increase in number and at the same time progress down the aorta to involve the abdominal portion. When persons reach about 10 years of age, fatty streaks also appear in the coronary arteries, most abundantly in the proximal segment of the left coronary artery.

Histologically, fatty streaks are intimal aggregations of foam cells with vacuolated cytoplasm derived from both macrophages and SMCs (see Fig. 10–2). A few T lymphocytes may be present at the margins. In larger aggregates there may be some extracellular lipid debris derived from the death of foam cells, but there is little cellular proliferation in the margins. Although fatty streaks may be the forerunners of fully evolved atheromas, some undoubtedly regress, because many fatty streaks are located at sites in the aorta that typically are little involved in the fully developed disease (e.g., the arch of the aorta). Moreover, fatty streaks are equally prevalent in all children, regardless of race, geography, and predisposition to the later development of AS. It is now thought that the fatty streaks that progress are those that form over segments of thick intima, called **adaptive intimal thickening,** which are present in everyone from birth, particularly at bifurcations.

The atheromatous plaque is the hallmark of AS. It may have a rich lipid content, but more usually it is a fibrofatty lesion, and sometimes it is almost solidly cellular and fibrotic. Plaques range up to several centimeters in largest dimension and, depending on the content of lipid, may be bright yellow to gray intimal lesions raised several millimeters above the surface of the surrounding intima. Irregular in shape, they may coalesce to form maplike configurations. On transection there is usually a central core of yellow grumous debris enclosed within a firmer, poorly defined wall and covered by a tough, gray-white, fibrous cap. As noted earlier, in some plaques there is scant lipid and only a tough, elevated, gray-white lesion.

Plaques tend to be found in certain locations; in descending order of extent and severity of involvement, these locations are the lower abdominal aorta, coronary arteries, popliteal arteries, descending thoracic aorta, internal carotid arteries, and circle of Willis. Other medium-sized muscular arteries may also be affected, but the vessels of the upper extremities, mesenteric arteries, and renal arteries are largely spared, save for their ostia. The aortic arch also tends to be spared, except when the patient has underlying syphilitic aortitis. As the disease evolves, there is a tendency for more plaques to be formed, and in severe cases they may virtually coat the abdominal aorta. Similarly, they become more numerous in the coronary arteries but are usually most abundant in the first 6 cm. Although their protrusion into the lumen of the aorta does not significantly threaten the patency of this vessel, in smaller arteries, particularly the coronaries and those of the brain, AS may significantly impair blood flow, particularly when the lesions become complicated, as will soon be detailed.

Microscopically, **plaques have essentially three components: (1) cells, including vascular SMCs, blood-derived monocytes/macrophages, and a scattering of lymphocytes; (2) connective tissue fibers and matrix; and (3) lipids.** Some plaques contain relatively small amounts of lipid and are composed almost entirely of connective tissue cells together with collagen and elastin fibers and proteoglycans to create the so-called **fibrous plaque** (Fig. 10–4). In others, the cellular and matrix elements create an intimal "fibrous cap" overlying a center containing a variable mixture of proteoglycans; cellular debris; fibrin and other plasma proteins; and, most importantly, an **extracellular lipid core** composed of cholesterol (which may form needle-like crystals) and cholesteryl esters—the classic **fibrofatty atheroma** (Fig. 10–5). In the margins of this soft center are a few or many lipid-laden foam cells. As the plaques enlarge, they cause atrophy and fibrosis of the underlying media, impairing wall elasticity and strength; evoke a lymphocytic infiltrate in the contiguous adventitia; and develop new small blood vessels **(angiogenesis)** about their margins. Mural thrombi may form on plaques and become organized and incorporated into them; canalization of the organizing thrombi is an additional mechanism of vascularization of the plaques.

The typical atheroma may undergo one of four

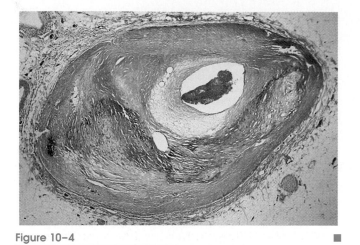

Figure 10-4 ■

An eccentric atheromatous plaque that has markedly narrowed the lumen of a coronary artery. Parts of the atheroma appear purple-blue owing to calcification. The lumen contains a fragment of postmortem clot. (Courtesy of Tom Rogers, MD, Department of Pathology, University of Texas Southwestern Medical School, Dallas, TX.)

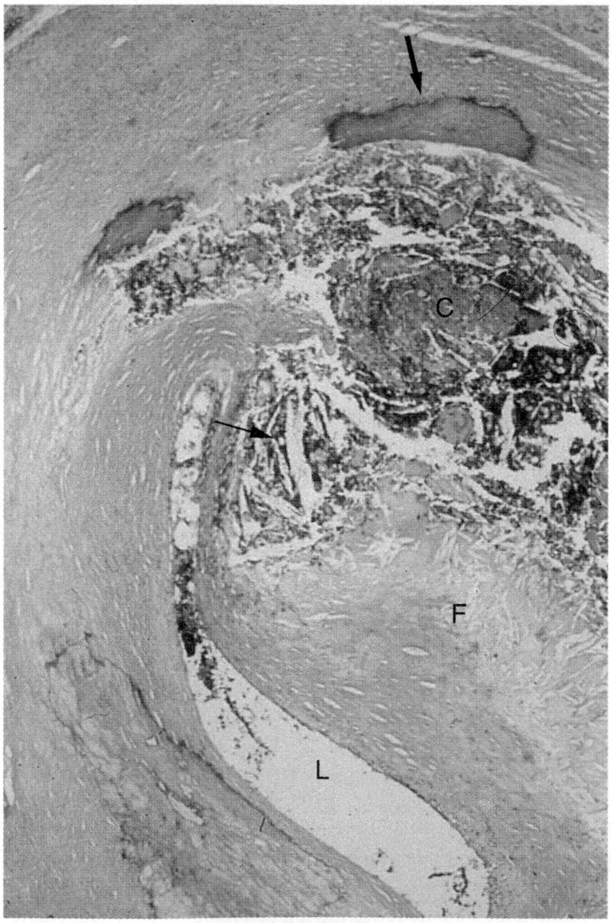

Figure 10-5 ■

High-power detail of an atherosclerotic plaque. Note the fibrous cap (F) projecting into the lumen (L) and the necrotic core (C). Areas of calcification *(thick arrow)* and cholesterol clefts *(thin arrow)* are also present. (Courtesy of Sid Murphree, MD, Department of Pathology, University of Texas Southwestern Medical School, Dallas, TX.)

changes, giving rise to so-called **complicated plaques:**

- In advanced disease, plaques frequently undergo patchy or massive **calcification,** and arteries may be converted to virtual pipestems.
- **Fissuring or ulceration of the luminal surface** with rupture of the plaque may discharge debris into the bloodstream **(cholesterol emboli).**
- Fissured or ulcerated lesions may develop **superimposed thrombosis** (Fig. 10-6).
- **Hemorrhage** into a plaque may result from loss of endothelial integrity (early ulceration), leading to progressive influx of blood from the vessel lumen, or the hemorrhage may arise from the periplaque capillaries described. The hemorrhage may balloon the plaque and lead to its rupture.

Plaques may develop the four complications in any combination. It is evident that **ulceration, thrombosis, and intraplaque hemorrhage have serious consequences in smaller vessels such as those of the heart and brain, because they may cause total vascular occlusion.** In larger vessels (e.g., the aorta), such complications have little effect on the luminal diameter, but damage to the underlying media may yield an **atherosclerotic aneurysm** (p 299) typically in the distal aorta below the renal arteries.

A recent American Heart Association committee classified atherosclerotic lesions into six types, beginning with the earliest fatty dots, through stages of fatty streaks, atheromas, and fibroatheromas, to the complicated lesions (Fig. 10-7).

Clinical Significance. The clinical implications and potential consequences of AS have already been amply emphasized. Understandably, then, intensive efforts are under way to devise means to reduce its toll. These involve primary prevention programs for persons who have never suffered an acute atherosclerotic event, aimed at preventing or delaying the formation of atheromatous plaques or possibly causing regression in persons who have never suffered an acute athero-

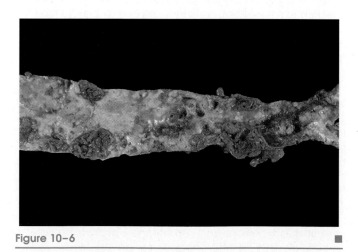

Figure 10-6 ■

Advanced atherosclerosis of the abdominal aorta showing multiple thrombi overlying several ulcerated plaques.

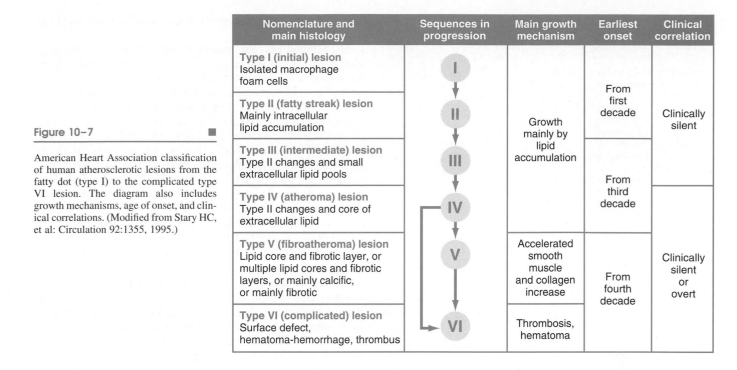

Nomenclature and main histology	Sequences in progression	Main growth mechanism	Earliest onset	Clinical correlation
Type I (initial) lesion Isolated macrophage foam cells	I	Growth mainly by lipid accumulation	From first decade	Clinically silent
Type II (fatty streak) lesion Mainly intracellular lipid accumulation	II			
Type III (intermediate) lesion Type II changes and small extracellular lipid pools	III		From third decade	
Type IV (atheroma) lesion Type II changes and core of extracellular lipid	IV			
Type V (fibroatheroma) lesion Lipid core and fibrotic layer, or multiple lipid cores and fibrotic layers, or mainly calcific, or mainly fibrotic	V	Accelerated smooth muscle and collagen increase	From fourth decade	Clinically silent or overt
Type VI (complicated) lesion Surface defect, hematoma-hemorrhage, thrombus	VI	Thrombosis, hematoma		

Figure 10–7 ■

American Heart Association classification of human atherosclerotic lesions from the fatty dot (type I) to the complicated type VI lesion. The diagram also includes growth mechanisms, age of onset, and clinical correlations. (Modified from Stary HC, et al: Circulation 92:1355, 1995.)

sclerotic event, and secondary prevention programs intended to prevent recurrence of acute atherosclerotic events such as MI. The media are filled with advice (some of it quite sound) on primary prevention: cessation of cigarette smoking; treatment of hypertension; weight reduction by control of total calorie intake coupled with increased exercise; moderation of alcohol consumption; and, most importantly, lowering blood cholesterol levels, particularly LDL and VLDL, while increasing HDL. Thus, the great current interest in replacing saturated fats (red meat, eggs, butter, and other fat-laden dairy products) with mono- or polyunsaturated fats, such as are in olive, corn, and safflower oils and the omega-3 fatty acids derived from fish. Such methods are not always successful in lowering high blood levels of cholesterol, and therefore there is growing interest in the use of lipid-lowering drugs, particularly in patients with genetic hyperlipidemias.

Although the controversy persists, most of the evidence indicates that treatment of hypercholesterolemia, whether by diet or drugs, reduces the mortality rate from IHD. Moreover, it is also hoped that lipid-lowering regimens will favor the regression of already developed atherosclerotic plaques, as has been documented in animals. In addition, several angiographic studies in humans suggest that lipid-lowering diets retard the progression of coronary artery narrowing and even reduce the size of plaques. Analogously, secondary prevention programs based on attempts to lower blood lipid levels and prevent thrombotic complications using antiplatelet drugs have successfully reduced the frequency of recurrent myocardial infarcts. Despite the encouraging results, a minority of investigators decry the preoccupation with blood lipids, pointing out that the pathogenesis of this disease is undoubtedly multifactorial. However, if we wait until all the pieces of the puzzle have been put together, thousands of possibly preventable deaths may have occurred.

Hypertension and Hypertensive Vascular Disease

Hypertension is associated with both functional and morphologic alterations in blood vessels. In this section we will discuss the pathogenesis of hypertension and the resulting morphologic changes of the vasculature.

HYPERTENSION

Elevated blood pressure is a common and staggering health problem. It is an important risk factor in both coronary heart disease and cerebrovascular accidents; it may also lead to congestive heart failure (hypertensive heart disease), aortic dissection, and renal failure. A sustained diastolic pressure greater than 90 mm Hg or a sustained systolic pressure in excess of 140 mm Hg are generally considered to constitute hypertension. Using these criteria, screening programs reveal that 25% of persons in the general population are hypertensive. The prevalence increases with age. Blacks are affected about twice as often as whites and seem more vulnerable to the complications of hypertension.

About 90% to 95% of hypertension is idiopathic and apparently primary (essential hypertension). Of the remaining 5% to 10%, most is secondary to renal disease or, less often, to narrowing of the renal artery, usually by an atheromatous plaque (renovascular hypertension). Infrequently, secondary hypertension is the result of adrenal disorders such as primary aldosteronism, Cushing's syndrome, and pheochromocytoma; neurologic diseases; and other disorders (Table 10–2).

Both essential and secondary hypertension may be either benign or malignant, according to the clinical course. In most cases hypertension remains at a modest level and fairly stable over years to decades and, unless an MI or cerebrovascular

Table 10–2. TYPES OF HYPERTENSION

Primary or Essential Hypertension
Secondary Hypertension
  Renal
      Acute glomerulonephritis
      Chronic renal disease
      Renal artery stenosis
      Renal vasculitis
      Renin-producing tumors
  Endocrine
      Adrenocortical hyperfunction (Cushing's syndrome)
      Oral contraceptives
      Pheochromocytoma
      Acromegaly
      Myxedema
      Thyrotoxicosis (systolic)
  Vascular
      Coarctation of aorta
      Polyarteritis nodosa
      Aortic insufficiency (systolic)
  Neurogenic
      Psychogenic
      Increased intracranial pressure
      Polyneuritis, bulbar poliomyelitis, others

accident supervenes, is compatible with long life. This form of the disorder is termed *benign hypertension.* About 5% of hypertensive persons show a rapidly rising blood pressure, which, if untreated, leads to death within 1 or 2 years. This is called *accelerated* or *malignant hypertension.* The full-blown clinical syndrome of malignant hypertension includes severe hypertension (diastolic pressure greater than 120 mm Hg); renal failure; and retinal hemorrhages and exudates, with or without papilledema. This form of hypertension may develop in previously normotensive persons but more often is superimposed on preexisting benign hypertension, either essential or secondary.

Pathogenesis of Essential Hypertension

Blood pressure is a complex trait that is determined by the interaction of multiple genetic and environmental factors. Therefore, it should not be surprising that the pathogenesis of essential hypertension is complex. Because the potential mechanisms of hypertension constitute aberrations of normal regulatory processes, the physiologic regulation of blood pressure is discussed next, followed by pathologic considerations.

Blood Pressure Regulation. The magnitude of the arterial pressure depends on two fundamental hemodynamic variables: cardiac output and total peripheral resistance (Fig. 10–8). Cardiac output is influenced by blood volume, which is greatly dependent on body sodium. Thus, sodium homeostasis is central to blood pressure regulation. For the most part, total peripheral resistance is accounted for by resistance of the arterioles, which is predominantly related to lumen size. The latter in turn is determined by the thickness of the arteriolar wall and the effects of neural and hormonal influences that either constrict or dilate these vessels. Vasoconstricting agents are angiotensin II, catecholamines, thromboxane, leukotrienes, and endothelin. Vasodilators include kinins, prostaglandins, and NO. Certain metabolic products (e.g., lactic acid,

hydrogen ions, and adenosine) and hypoxia are also local vasodilators.

The kidneys play an important role in blood pressure regulation by influencing both peripheral resistance and sodium homeostasis. Renin elaborated by the juxtaglomerular cells of the kidney transforms *plasma angiotensinogen to angiotensin I,* and the latter is converted to *angiotensin II* by angiotensin-converting enzyme (ACE) (Fig. 10–9). Angiotensin II alters blood pressure by increasing both peripheral resistance and blood volume. The former effect is achieved largely by its ability to cause vasoconstriction through direct action on vascular smooth muscle, the latter by stimulation of aldosterone secretion, which increases distal tubular reabsorption of sodium and thus of water. In addition, two other renal factors have an important bearing on sodium homeostasis: *the glomerular filtration rate (GFR) and GFR-independent natriuretic factors.* When blood volume is reduced, the GFR falls; this in turn leads to increased reabsorption of sodium by proximal tubules in an attempt to conserve sodium and expand blood volume. GFR-independent factors include atrial natriuretic factor (ANF), or atriopeptin, a group of peptides secreted by heart atria in response to volume expansion; these peptides inhibit sodium reabsorption in distal tubules and cause vasodilation. Abnormalities in these renal mechanisms are implicated in the pathogenesis of secondary hypertension in a variety of renal diseases but, as we shall see, they also play important roles in essential hypertension.

Mechanisms of Hypertension. *Arterial hypertension occurs when changes develop that alter the relationship between blood volume and total arterial resistance.* For many of the secondary forms of hypertension, these factors are reasonably well understood, as, for example, in so-called renovascular hypertension. In this condition, renal artery stenosis causes decreased glomerular flow and pressure in the afferent arteriole of the glomerulus and induces renin secretion by the juxtaglomerular cells; this initiates angiotensin II–induced vasoconstriction; increased peripheral resistance; and, through the aldosterone mechanism, increased sodium reabsorption and increased blood volume. Similarly, in pheochromocytoma, a tumor of the adrenal medulla, catecholamines produced by tumor cells cause episodic vasoconstriction and thus induce hypertension.

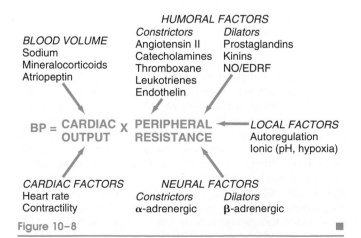

Figure 10–8

Blood pressure regulation. NO/EDRF, nitric oxide–endothelium-derived relaxing factor.

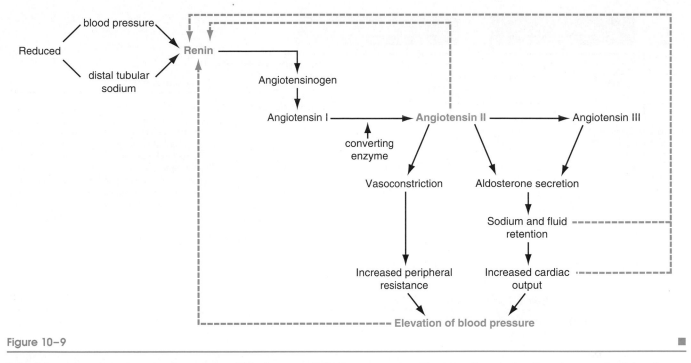

Figure 10–9   ■

Role of the renin-angiotensin system in regulation of blood pressure. Solid lines represent positive interactions; broken lines show negative interactions or feedback inhibition.

More controversial is the cause of essential hypertension. Indeed, if there is agreement at all, it is that a single cause or mechanism is unlikely to account for all cases of essential hypertension. Instead it is thought that a number of *genetic and environmental factors that affect cardiac output, peripheral resistance, or both, result in elevated blood pressure, and these factors may differ in both type and degree in different patients with hypertension.*

Genetic factors clearly play a role, as evidenced by studies comparing blood pressure in monozygotic and dizygotic twins, studies of familial aggregation of hypertension, and adoption studies. Hypertension has been induced in experimental animals by inbreeding, and some of the genes implicated in experimental hypertension have been defined. In humans, rare forms of severe hypertension caused by mutations in single genes have been identified. These include (1) gene defects in enzymes involved in aldosterone metabolism (aldosterone synthase, 11β-hydroxylase) that lead to an adaptive increase in secretion of aldosterone, increased salt and water resorption, plasma volume expansion, and ultimately hypertension; and (2) mutations in an epithelial sodium channel protein that lead to increased distal tubular sodium reabsorption induced by aldosterone, resulting in a moderately severe form of salt-sensitive hypertension called *Liddle's syndrome.*

Although it is clear that single gene defects are not involved in essential hypertension, inherited variations in blood pressure may depend on the cumulative effects of allelic forms of several genes that affect blood pressure. For example, genetic linkage analysis has shown that predisposition to essential hypertension is associated with specific molecular variants of the gene encoding angiotensinogen, the physiologic substrate of renin—a major regulator of the renin-angiotensin system.

The studies on the mendelian disorders and angiotensinogen genes discussed above have been interpreted to favor the primacy of defects in renal sodium homeostasis in hypertension. Such scenarios suggest the existence of genetic defects that result in reduced renal sodium excretion, in the presence of normal arterial pressure, as the initiating event in essential hypertension. Decreased sodium excretion leads to an increase in fluid volume and a high cardiac output. In the face of increasing cardiac output, peripheral vasoconstriction occurs (as a result of autoregulation) to prevent the overperfusion of tissues that would result from an unchecked increase in cardiac output. Such autoregulation, however, leads to increased peripheral resistance and, along with it, elevated blood pressure. At higher blood pressures, enough additional sodium can be excreted by the kidneys to equal intake and prevent fluid retention. Thus, an altered but steady state of sodium excretion is achieved (Fig. 10–10).

Other hypotheses, in contrast, postulate that increased peripheral resistance is the initiating event in hypertension. Such increased resistance may be caused either by factors that induce *functional* vasoconstriction, or by stimuli that induce *structural* changes in the vessel wall (i.e., hypertrophy, remodeling, and hyperplasia of SMCs), leading to a thickened wall, or by both effects. Vasoconstrictive influences may consist of (1) behavioral or neurogenic factors, as evidenced by the reduction in blood pressure achieved with meditation (the relaxation response); (2) increased release of vasoconstrictor agents such as angiotensin II or endothelin; or (3) a primary increased sensitivity of vascular smooth muscle, possibly caused by genetic defects in smooth muscle reactivity. Such vasoconstrictive influences, if exerted repeatedly, may themselves cause structural thickening of the resistance vessels, which in turn perpetuates increased blood pressure. Indeed, a number of vasoconstrictors, such as angiotensin II, also cause smooth muscle hypertrophy and hyperplasia; conversely, a number of growth factors, such as PDGF, are vasoconstric-

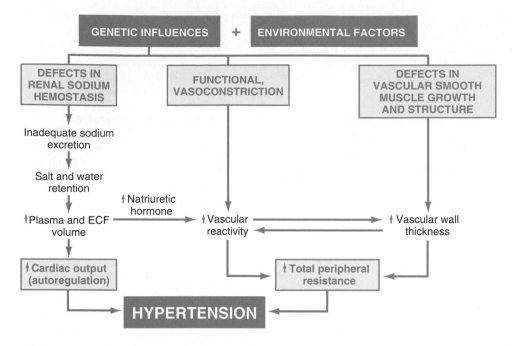

GENETIC INFLUENCES + ENVIRONMENTAL FACTORS

DEFECTS IN RENAL SODIUM HEMOSTASIS

FUNCTIONAL, VASOCONSTRICTION

DEFECTS IN VASCULAR SMOOTH MUSCLE GROWTH AND STRUCTURE

Inadequate sodium excretion

Salt and water retention

↑Natriuretic hormone

↑Plasma and ECF volume

↑Vascular reactivity

↑Vascular wall thickness

↑Cardiac output (autoregulation)

↑Total peripheral resistance

HYPERTENSION

Figure 10–10 ■

Hypothetical scheme for the pathogenesis of essential hypertension, implicating genetic defects in renal excretion of sodium, functional regulation of vascular tone, and structural regulation of vascular caliber. Environmental factors, especially increased salt intake, potentiate the effects of genetic factors. The resultant increase in cardiac output and peripheral resistance contributes to hypertension. ECF, extracellular fluid.

tors. More recent work, however, has suggested that the structural changes may indeed be early events in hypertension, preceding rather than being strictly secondary to the vasoconstriction. This has led to the hypothesis that genetic or environmentally induced defects, possibly in intracellular signaling, affect ion fluxes and cell cycle genes that modulate both smooth cell growth, causing wall thickening, and increased vascular tone, resulting in vasoconstriction.

Environmental factors are also involved in the expression of hypertension. The role of the environment is illustrated by the lower incidence of hypertension in Chinese people living in their native country, compared with persons of Chinese descent living in the United States. Such factors include stress, obesity, smoking, inactivity, and heavy consumption of salt. It must be stressed that in both of the major hypotheses of hypertension discussed—those that primarily involve sodium retention and those that emphasize primary increases in vascular resistance—heavy sodium intake augments the hypertension.

To summarize, essential hypertension is a complex disorder that almost certainly has more than one cause. It may be initiated by disturbances in any of the factors that control blood pressure (e.g., environmental stress, salt intake, estrogens) but act in the genetically predisposed individual. Although the susceptibility genes for hypertension are currently unknown, they may well include genes that govern responses to sodium load, levels of pressor substances, reactivity of vascular smooth muscle to pressor agents, or smooth muscle cell growth. In established hypertension, both increased blood volume and increased peripheral resistance contribute to the increased pressure (Fig. 10–10).

VASCULAR PATHOLOGY IN HYPERTENSION

The earliest changes in resistance vessels in human hypertension are not well known. In experimental animals, smooth

muscle hyperplasia, hypertrophy, and remodeling, as well as increased deposition of amorphous material in the vessel wall, are characteristic of early hypertensive vasculopathy. In well-established human disease, hypertension is associated with two forms of small blood vessel disease: *hyaline arteriolosclerosis and hyperplastic arteriolosclerosis.* Both lesions are clearly related to elevations in blood pressure and are most prominently seen in the kidneys; hence they are described in greater detail in Chapter 14. Hypertension also accelerates atherogenesis and causes changes in the structure of the walls of blood vessels that potentiate both aortic dissection and cerebrovascular hemorrhage.

HYALINE ARTERIOLOSCLEROSIS. This condition is encountered frequently in elderly patients, whether normotensive or hypertensive, but it is more generalized and more severe in patients with hypertension. The condition is also seen commonly in diabetes and forms part of the microangiography characteristic of diabetic disease. Whatever the clinical setting, the vascular lesion consists of a homogeneous, pink, hyaline thickening of the walls of arterioles, with loss of underlying structural detail and with narrowing of the lumen (Fig. 10–11).

The narrowing of the arteriolar lumina causes impairment of the blood supply to affected organs, particularly well exemplified in the kidneys. Thus, hyaline arteriolosclerosis is a major morphologic characteristic of benign nephrosclerosis, in which the arteriolar narrowing causes diffuse renal ischemia and symmetric contraction of the kidneys (Chapter 14).

HYPERPLASTIC ARTERIOLOSCLEROSIS. The hyperplastic type of arteriolosclerosis is generally related to more acute or severe elevations in blood pres-

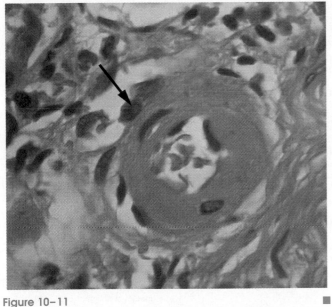

Figure 10-11 ■

Hyaline arteriosclerosis. An arteriole in the kidney shows hyaline thickening of the wall.

sure and is therefore characteristic of malignant hypertension (i.e., diastolic pressure greater than 120 mm Hg). This form of arteriolar disease can be identified with the light microscope by virtue of its onion-skin, concentric, laminated thickening of the walls of arterioles with progressive narrowing of the lumina (Fig. 14-19 in Chapter 14). There is hypertrophy and hyperplasia of the vascular SMCs and thickening and reduplication of the basement membrane. Frequently, but not invariably, these hyperplastic changes are accompanied by deposits of fibrinoid and acute necrosis of the vessel walls, referred to as **necrotizing arteriolitis**. The arterioles in all tissues throughout the body may be affected, with favored sites being the kidney, periadrenal fat, gallbladder, and peripancreatic and intestinal arterioles.

Vasculitis

The term vasculitis is applied to any inflammatory involvement of an artery, vein, or venule; when the aorta is affected, it is referred to as *aortitis*. One or a relatively few vessels may be affected, as, for example, in a localized area of infection, irradiation, or mechanical trauma, or in the Arthus reaction. In a number of clinicopathologic entities that are more or less distinctive conditions, the vasculitis is more widespread. These are termed *systemic necrotizing vasculitides*. Many of these entities have an immunologic basis; we will first discuss common pathogenetic mechanisms.

Immune Complexes. Many types of vasculitis are thought to be induced by immune complexes. This is supported by the following:

■ The vascular lesions resemble those found in experimental

immune complex–mediated conditions, such as the local Arthus phenomenon and serum sickness.

■ DNA–anti-DNA immune complexes and complement are present in the vascular lesions of systemic lupus erythematosus (SLE)–associated vasculitis.

■ In some patients, viruses and other antigens have been localized in the lesions, together with immunoglobulin and complement, and immune complexes are found in the circulation.

■ There is a high incidence of hepatitis B surface antigen (HBsAg) and HBsAg–anti-HBsAg immune complexes in the sera and, with complement, in the vascular lesions of some patients with vasculitis. In patients with chronic hepatitis C virus (HCV) infection and glomerulonephritis, HCV/RNA and cryoprecipitates containing immunoglobulin G (IgG) anti-HCV antibodies are detected.

Whether complexes accumulate in vessel walls by deposition from the circulation, by in situ formation, or by a combination of these mechanisms is unclear.

Antineutrophil Cytoplasmic Antibodies. Serum from many patients with vasculitis reacts in immunofluorescence and immunochemical assays with cytoplasmic antigens in neutrophils, indicating the presence of antineutrophil cytoplasmic autoantibodies (ANCAs). Two relatively distinct patterns of neutrophil immunofluorescence are observed: perinuclear (called *P-ANCA*) and cytoplasmic (called *C-ANCA*). P-ANCAs are directed largely toward myeloperoxidase in the primary granules of neutrophils. The major neutrophil antigen involved in C-ANCA is a neutral leukocyte protease (proteinase 3). There is some correlation between the type of ANCA and the specific vasculitis syndrome. The C-ANCA pattern is detected in most patients with active Wegener's granulomatosis and microscopic polyarteritis. In contrast, P-ANCA is observed frequently in patients with polyarteritis nodosa and primary glomerular disease.

ANCAs are proving to be useful diagnostic indicators in the study of vasculitis; their presence and titers usually correlate with disease activity. What triggers their induction, however, and the precise mechanism by which they cause disease are unclear. One postulated sequence is that these antibodies activate neutrophils, causing a respiratory burst and degranulation, thereby stimulating the release of toxic oxygen free radicals and lytic enzymes from neutrophils. This results in EC and tissue damage. Such neutrophil activation is potentiated by the cytokines associated with these diseases, possibly triggered by intercurrent infections. In addition, there is evidence that antibodies to proteinase 3 inhibit β_1-antitrypsin activity, thus potentiating tissue damage.

Classification. Most classifications of systemic vasculitis depend on the size of the involved blood vessels, the anatomic site, the histologic characteristics of the lesion, and the clinical manifestations. The nomenclature used here is that developed at the Chapel Hill Consensus Conference on the Nomenclature of Systemic Vasculitides (Table 10-3 and Fig. 10-12). We will now briefly review some types of vasculitis.

POLYARTERITIS NODOSA

Polyarteritis nodosa (PAN) is a disease of medium-sized to small arteries that is characterized by transmural acute nec-

Table 10–3. MAJOR VASCULITIS SYNDROMES

Syndrome	Vessels Involved	Distribution of Vascular Involvement	Principal Morphologic Features
Polyarteritis nodosa	Medium-sized and small arteries	GI tract, liver, kidney, pancreas, muscles, other sites	Panmural acute necrotizing arteritis with fibrinoid necrosis, neutrophil and eosinophil infiltration, and extension into adventitia
Wegener's granulomatosis	Small to medium-sized arteries	Upper and lower respiratory tracts; occasionally eye, skin, heart	Acute and chronic (sometimes granulomatous) angiitis with prominent eosinophils and occasional giant cells in association with extravascular granulomas
Microscopic polyangiitis (hypersensitivity vasculitis, microscopic polyarteritis)	Venules, capillaries, arterioles	Widespread, but particularly skin	Necrosis and neutrophilic infiltration of venules with leukocytoclasis
Temporal (cranial) arteritis	Elastic tissue–rich major arteries	Head, including ocular and intracranial vessels; uncommonly systemic	Chronic mononuclear inflammatory infiltration, mostly in inner half of the media, with giant cells and granuloma formation
Kawasaki's arteritis	Small and medium-sized arteries	Skin, ocular and oral mucosa, coronary arteries, but may be widespread	Acute and chronic infiltration, mainly with lymphocytes and macrophages, and with endothelial cell necrosis and immunoglobulin deposition
Thromboangiitis obliterans (Buerger's disease)	Medium-sized and small arteries and veins	Extremities	Acute and chronic inflammatory infiltration of arteries and veins, often with giant cells, granulomas, intravascular thrombi containing microabscesses, and later perivascular fibrosis trapping nerve trunks

rotizing inflammation of these vessels. The involvement is peculiarly focal, random, and episodic. It often produces irregular aneurysmal dilation, nodularity, and vascular obstruction and sometimes infarctions. Virtually any organ or tissue of the body may be affected, with the striking exception of the lungs and the aorta with its primary branches.

PAN appears most often in middle-aged adults, although individuals of any age may be affected, from infancy to the advanced years of life.

In the classic case, PAN involves **arteries of medium to small size in any organ,** with the possible exception of the lung. The distribution of lesions, in descending order of frequency, is kidneys, heart, liver, and gastrointestinal tract, followed by pancreas, testes, skeletal muscle, nervous system, and skin. Individual lesions are **sharply segmental** and indeed on microscopic evaluation may not involve the entire circumference of the vessel. They tend to be at branch points and bifurcations. Aneurysmal dilation and **nodularity** may appear in the area of involvement; however, sometimes the lesions are exclusively microscopic and produce no visible gross changes. Whatever the gross appearance, the vasculitis during the acute phase is characterized by **transmural inflammation of the arterial wall** with a heavy infiltrate of neutrophils, eosinophils, and mononuclear cells, frequently accompanied by fibrinoid necrosis of the inner half of the vessel wall (Fig. 10–13). Typically the inflammatory reaction permeates the adventitia. The lumen may become **thrombosed.** In some lesions only a portion of the circumference is affected, leaving segments of normal arterial wall juxtaposed to areas of vascular inflammation. At a later stage the acute inflammatory infiltrate begins to disappear and is replaced by fibrous thickening of the vessel wall accompanied by a mononuclear infiltrate. The fibroblastic proliferation may extend into the adventitia, contributing to the firm nodularity that sometimes marks the lesions. At a still later stage, all that remains is marked fibrotic thickening of the affected vessel, devoid of significant inflammatory infiltration. **Particularly characteristic of PAN is that all stages of activity may coexist in different vessels or even within the same vessel.** Thus, whatever the inflammatory insult, it is apparently recurrent and strangely haphazard.

The clinical signs and symptoms of this disease are as var-

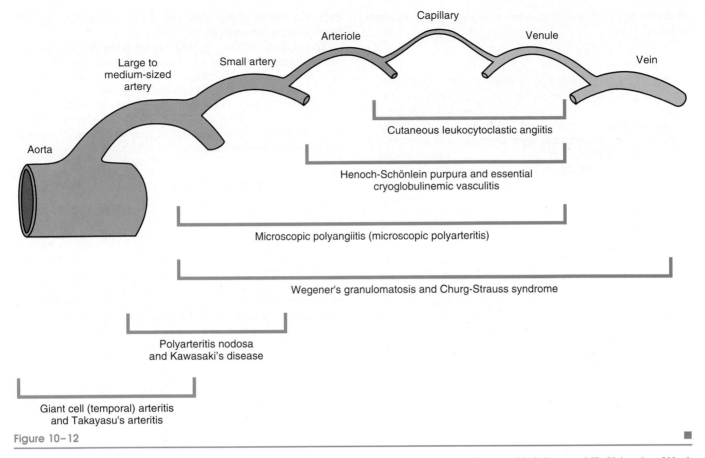

Capillary

Arteriole

Venule

Small artery

Vein

Large to
medium-sized
artery

Aorta

Cutaneous leukocytoclastic angiitis

Henoch-Schönlein purpura and essential
cryoglobulinemic vasculitis

Microscopic polyangiitis (microscopic polyarteritis)

Wegener's granulomatosis and Churg-Strauss syndrome

Polyarteritis nodosa
and Kawasaki's disease

Giant cell (temporal) arteritis
and Takayasu's arteritis

Figure 10–12   ■

Diagrammatic representation of the lesions of the vasculature involved by various forms of vasculitides. (Courtesy of J. C. Jennette, MD, University of North Carolina at Chapel Hill, NC.)

ied as the sites of vascular involvement. Malaise, fever, weakness, and weight loss may usher in the disease. Eventually organ damage appears. Renal involvement is one of the prominent manifestations of PAN and a major cause of death. Hypertension is common and may precede the apparent renal disease. Vascular lesions in the gastrointestinal tract produce a wide variety of symptoms, including abdominal pain, diarrhea, and melena. *About 30% of patients with PAN have hepatitis B antigen in their serum, and as mentioned earlier, P-ANCAs are often present in the serum and correlate with disease activity.*

The presentations are so diverse that clinical diagnosis often needs to be established by biopsy of suspected areas of involvement, with favored sites being kidney and skeletal muscle.

WEGENER'S GRANULOMATOSIS

Wegener's granulomatosis (WG) is classically characterized by the triad of (1) necrotizing granulomas of the upper respiratory tract (ear, nose, throat), the lower respiratory tract, or both; (2) necrotizing or granulomatous vasculitis of small arteries and veins, predominantly in the lungs but possibly elsewhere; and (3) necrotizing, often crescentic, glomerulonephritis. There are, however, instances of "limited WG," in which the kidneys are unaffected and the involvement is restricted to the respiratory tract, and, conversely, more widespread WG, with vasculitis involving the eye, skin, and (rarely) other organs, notably the heart. These systemic distributions may produce clinical syndromes very similar to PAN, save that the lungs are involved. Males are affected

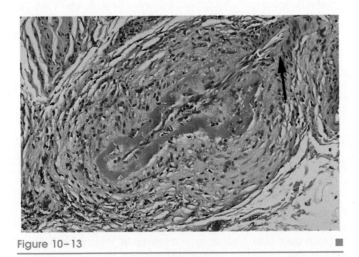

Figure 10–13   ■

Polyarteritis nodosa. Segmental fibrinoid necrosis *(central pink zone)* with marked inflammatory thickening of the vessel wall. Note in the upper right corner the remaining small, normal segment of artery wall *(arrow)*. (Courtesy of Sid Murphree, MD, Department of Pathology, University of Texas Southwestern Medical School, Dallas, TX.)

somewhat more often than females, at an average age of about 40 years.

Morphologically, the upper respiratory tract lesions range from inflammatory sinusitis resulting from the development of **mucosal granulomas** to **ulcerative lesions of the nose, palate, or pharynx, rimmed by necrotizing granulomas and accompanying vasculitis.** In the lungs, dispersed focal necrotizing granulomas may coalesce to produce radiographically visible nodules that may undergo cavitation. Microscopically, the granulomas reveal a geographic pattern of necrosis rimmed by lymphocytes, plasma cells, macrophages, and variable numbers of giant cells. In association with such lesions there is a **necrotizing or granulomatous vasculitis** of small, and sometimes larger, arteries and veins (Fig. 10–14). The necrotizing pattern produces a vasculitis that is indistinguishable from that in polyarteritis. Scattered eosinophils may be present in the inflammatory foci. With severe disease, involvement of the vessels extends down to the level of alveolar capillaries, sometimes producing large areas of alveolar hemorrhage. Focal segmental necrotizing or crescentic glomerulonephritis is present in most, but not all, cases (Chapter 14).

The precise pathogenesis of WG is unknown. C-ANCAs are present in the serum in more than 95% of these patients, and the dramatic response to immunosuppressive therapy clearly points to an immunologically mediated disease; however, the nature of the initiating agents and underlying immune defects are unclear.

The clinical features of WG can be deduced from the anatomic findings, so it remains only to point out that the course of untreated disease is progressive, with a 2-year mortality rate of more than 90%. When the diagnosis is established, appropriate therapy (i.e., immunosuppressive drugs, cyclophosphamide, possibly prednisone, and sometimes antibacterial drugs) produces a gratifying response in most patients, with only occasional relapses.

MICROSCOPIC POLYANGIITIS (MICROSCOPIC POLYARTERITIS, HYPERSENSITIVITY VASCULITIS)

This type of necrotizing vasculitis generally affects smaller vessels than PAN (arterioles, capillaries, and venules). Furthermore, unlike PAN, in a single patient, all lesions tend to be of the same age. It typically involves the skin, mucous membranes, lungs, brain, heart, gastrointestinal tract, kidneys, and muscle. Necrotizing glomerulonephritis and pulmonary capillaritis are particularly common. The major resultant clinical features are hemoptysis, hematuria, and proteinuria; bowel pain or bleeding; and muscle pain or weakness. Cutaneous vasculitis is manifested by palpable purpura. In many cases an immunologic reaction to an antigen, such as drugs (e.g., penicillin), microorganisms (e.g., streptococci), heterologous proteins, and tumor antigens, can be traced as the precipitating cause, but there are *few or no demonstrable immune deposits in this type of vasculitis.*

MORPHOLOGY. In contrast to PAN, muscular and large arteries are spared; thus, macroscopic infarcts similar to those seen in PAN are uncommon. Histologically, segmental fibrinoid necrosis of the media may be present, but in some lesions the change is limited to infiltration with neutrophils, which become fragmented as they follow the vessel wall **(leukocytoclasia).** The term **leukocytoclastic angiitis** is given to such lesions, most commonly found in postcapillary venules. Immunoglobulins and complement components are often present in the vascular lesions of the skin, especially if these are examined within 24 hours of development, but in general, there is a paucity of immunoglobulin demonstrable by immunofluorescence microscopy ("pauci-immune injury").

With the exception of those who develop widespread renal or brain involvement, most patients respond well simply to removal of the offending agent. P-ANCAs are present in 70% of patients. Disseminated vascular lesions of hypersensitivity angiitis may also appear in a number of relatively distinct syndromes, including Henoch-Schönlein purpura, essential mixed cryoglobulinemia, vasculitis associated with some of the connective tissue disorders, and vasculitis associated with malignancy. These are discussed with the specific entities elsewhere in this book.

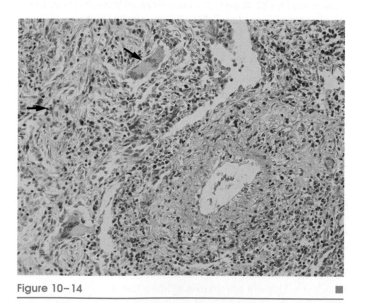

Figure 10–14 ■

Wegener's granulomatosis. There is inflammation (vasculitis) of a small artery, along with adjacent granulomatous inflammation, in which epithelioid cells and giant cells *(arrows)* can be seen. (Courtesy of Sid Murphree, MD, Department of Pathology, University of Texas Southwestern Medical School, Dallas, TX.)

TEMPORAL (GIANT CELL, CRANIAL) ARTERITIS

The most common of the arteritides, temporal arteritis, is characterized by segmental acute and chronic (most often granulomatous) vasculitis involving predominantly the larger arteries in the head, particularly the branches of the carotid artery. Favored locations are the temporal arteries and the terminal branches of the ophthalmic artery, involvements that may lead to unilateral (rarely bilateral) blindness. Other vessels may be affected, including the aorta and arteries to the brain and the breast, but almost never are heart and lungs involved. Temporal arteritis usually occurs in elders (after age 50) with a 2 : 1 or 3 : 1 female-to-male ratio. In about half of cases, the arteritis develops on a background of polymyalgia rheumatica, a flulike illness in elders, marked by pain and stiffness in the proximal muscles of the hip and shoulder girdles, neck, and buttocks, but in the remaining cases it arises de novo.

Characteristically, short segments of one or more affected arteries develop **nodular thickenings with reduction of the lumen**, possibly to a slitlike orifice, which may become thrombosed. Histologically, two patterns are seen. In the more common variant there is **granulomatous inflammation** of the inner half of the media centered on the internal elastic membrane marked by a mononuclear infiltrate, multinucleate giant cells of both foreign body and Langerhans type, and fragmentation of the internal elastic lamina (Fig. 10–15). In the other, less common pattern, granulomas are rare or absent, and there is only a nonspecific panarteritis with a mixed inflammatory infiltrate composed largely of lymphocytes and macrophages admixed with some neutrophils and eosinophils but no giant cells. Occasionally in this variant there is some fibrinoid necrosis. The later healed stage of both of these patterns reveals only collagenous thickening of the vessel wall; organization of the luminal thrombus sometimes transforms the artery into a fibrous cord.

The pathogenesis of temporal arteritis is unknown, but on the basis of the granulomatous nature of the inflammation, association with certain human leukocyte DR antigens (HLA-DR) and the response to corticosteroid therapy, T cell–mediated injury is suspected.

Clinically this condition may begin with only vague constitutional symptoms—fever, fatigue, weight loss—without localizing signs or symptoms, but in most instances there is facial pain or headache, which is severe, sometimes unilateral, and often most intense along the course of the superficial temporal artery. The vessel itself may be nodular and painful to palpation. More serious are ocular symptoms, which sometimes appear quite abruptly in about half of all patients and range from diplopia to transient or complete vision loss. Hence the urgency in establishing the diagnosis promptly, as treatment with steroids is remarkably effective. The diagnosis depends on biopsy and histologic confirmation, but because of the segmental nature of the involvement, adequate biopsy requires at least a 2- to 3-cm length of artery. Thus, a negative biopsy result does not rule out the condition.

TAKAYASU'S ARTERITIS (PULSELESS DISEASE)

Takayasu's arteritis (pulseless disease) is a *chronic vasculitis that affects principally the aorta and its main branches and sometimes the pulmonary arteries.* The aortic involvement may be restricted to the arch alone, may spare the arch and affect the rest of the aorta, or in some cases may involve the entire aorta. Uncommonly, the major branches of the aortic arch are more severely affected than the aorta. This condition occurs predominantly in persons younger than 40 years and shows a strong female preponderance. Although previously it was reported most often in Asians, Takayasu's arteritis is global in distribution. The cause and pathogenesis of this disease are unknown, although immune mechanisms are suspected.

Gross morphologic changes, when present, are thickening of the aortic wall with intimal wrinkling and narrowing of the orifices of the great vessels that arise from areas of involvement, accounting for the name **pulseless disease.** The origins of the coronary and renal arteries may be similarly affected. Sometimes the vasculitis extends some distance into the aortic branches, and in about half of cases it also involves the pulmonary arteries. The histologic changes evolve over time. In the earlier active stage, there is a prominent granulomatous arteritis with giant cells, principally restricted to the media and adventitia but sometimes extending throughout the thickness of the vessel wall with patchy destruction of the muscu-loelastic lamellae of the media. Later, or after

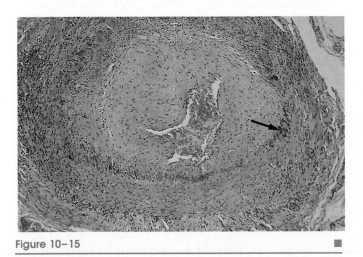

Figure 10–15   ■

Temporal (giant cell) arteritis. Circumferential giant cells mark the location of degenerated internal elastic membrane *(arrow).*

treatment with steroids, the inflammatory reaction is predominantly marked by collagenous fibrosis involving all layers of the vessel wall but particularly the intima, accompanied by lymphocytic infiltration. When the root of the aorta is affected, it may undergo dilation, producing aortic valve insufficiency. Narrowing of the coronary ostia may lead to MI.

Most patients (usually young women) have symptoms of vascular insufficiency of the extremities, mainly the upper extremities, with coldness or numbness of the fingers. Involvement of the more distal aorta may lead to claudication of the legs and of cranial vessels, leading to visual disturbances and neurologic manifestations. Involvement of pulmonary arteries may lead to pulmonary hypertension and manifestations of cor pulmonale. The course of the disease is variable. In some persons there is rapid progression, but in others a quiescent stage is reached in 1 or 2 years, permitting long-term survival, albeit sometimes with visual or neurologic deficits.

KAWASAKI'S DISEASE (MUCOCUTANEOUS LYMPH NODE SYNDROME)

An acute febrile illness of infancy and early childhood, Kawasaki's disease is self-limited in many instances, but in most cases vasculitis of the coronary arteries appears, sometimes leading to aneurysm formation and possibly superimposed thrombosis. From 0.5% to 1% of patients die of myocardial infarction.

The cause of the condition is unknown, but there is evidence that the vasculitis is based on an immunoregulatory defect characterized by T-cell and macrophage activation, secretion of cytokines, polyclonal B-cell hyperactivity, and the formation of autoantibodies to endothelial and smooth muscle cells, leading to acute vasculitis. The nature of the initiating antigen remains unknown, but it is currently speculated that in genetically susceptible persons, a variety of common infectious agents (most likely viral) may trigger the sequence of changes described.

The acute phase of disease begins with vasculitis and perivasculitis of small vessels (arterioles, venules, and capillaries). Small vessel changes resemble those of microscopic polyangiitis, save that the inflammation is maximal in the intima. Later, larger arteries in the body, including the coronary arteries, may be affected with changes similar to those of polyarteritis. At this time myocarditis, pericarditis, or valvulitis may appear. The acute phase eventually begins to subside spontaneously or in response to treatment, but it is during this subsiding phase that the acute vasculitis of the coronary arteries often leads to aneurysm formation and sometimes associated thrombosis with myocardial infarction.

The characteristic clinical features are fever, bilateral non-purulent conjunctivitis, and erythema of the palms of the hands and soles of the feet, accompanied by edema and, later, desquamation. This is followed by the development of a rash composed of erythematous plaques or even pustules. Lymphadenopathy, frequently present at this time, is usually limited to a single node in the neck. All of these manifestations are relatively unthreatening compared with the involvement of the heart, which leads to arrhythmias; cardiac dilation with mitral insufficiency; congestive heart failure; and, most ominously, myocardial infarction.

THROMBOANGIITIS OBLITERANS (BUERGER'S DISEASE)

Buerger's disease is a remitting, relapsing, inflammatory disorder that often leads to thrombosis of medium-sized vessels, principally the tibial and radial arteries, with secondary extension to the adjacent veins and nerves. It is mainly a disease of male cigarette smokers ages 25 to 50 years, and the relatively recent increase in incidence among females is attributed to changing smoking practices since the 1970s. Buerger's disease often leads to vascular insufficiency in the extremities and sometimes gangrene, and therefore it must be differentiated from other causes of peripheral vascular disease, such as AS and thromboembolism.

The cause and pathogenesis of Buerger's disease are unknown, but they are clearly related in some way to the *use of tobacco products.* Many patients show hypersensitivity to intradermally injected tobacco extracts. Conceivably, some derivative of tobacco or tobacco smoke might have direct endothelial toxicity or incite an immunologic reaction in predisposed persons. There is an increased prevalence of HLA-A9 and -B5 in these patients, and the condition is far more common in Israel, Japan, and India than in the United States and Europe, all of which hints at genetic influences.

Thromboangiitis is characterized by **sharply segmental acute and chronic vasculitis of medium-sized and small arteries** with secondary spread to contiguous veins and nerves. Often the vascular supply to the extremities, upper as well as lower, is affected. By contrast, AS affects predominantly the larger arteries, mostly those in the lower extremities. Microscopically, acute and chronic inflammation permeates the arterial walls, accompanied by thrombosis of the lumen, which may undergo organization and recanalization. Characteristically, the thrombus contains small microabscesses marked by a central focus of neutrophils surrounded by granulomatous inflammation (Fig. 10–16). The inflammatory process extends into and about the accompanying veins and nerves, and in time all three structures become encased in fibrous tissue.

Often clinically manifest Buerger's disease is preceded by Raynaud's phenomenon or recurrent episodes of migratory thrombophlebitis of superficial veins. *Raynaud's phenomenon*

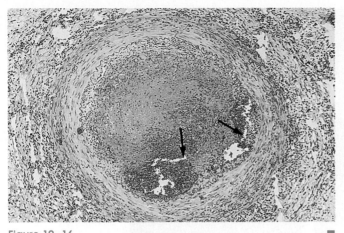

Figure 10–16 ■

Thromboangiitis obliterans (Buerger's disease). The lumen is occluded by a thrombus containing two abscesses *(arrows)*. The vessel wall is infiltrated with leukocytes.

refers to arterial insufficiency of the acral parts secondary to some other disorder that is responsible for arterial narrowing (e.g., SLE, systemic sclerosis, AS, or Buerger's disease). Indeed, Raynaud's phenomenon may be the first manifestation of any of these conditions. Eventually the classic manifestations of vascular insufficiency (claudication and color and temperature changes) appear. In contrast to the insufficiency caused by AS, in Buerger's disease the insufficiency tends to be accompanied by severe pain, even at rest, related undoubtedly to the neural involvement. Chronic ulcerations of the toes, feet, or fingers may appear, perhaps followed in time by frank gangrene. Abstinence from cigarette smoking in the early stages of the disease often brings dramatic relief from further attacks.

Aneurysms

Abnormal dilations of arteries or veins are called *aneurysms*. They are described here because they are much more frequent and important in arteries, especially the aorta. They develop wherever there is marked weakening of the wall of a vessel. Any vessel may be affected by a wide variety of disorders that weaken arterial walls, including congenital defects, local infections (mycotic aneurysms), trauma (traumatic aneurysms or arteriovenous aneurysms), or systemic diseases. The two principal causes of aortic aneurysms are AS and cystic medial necrosis. Syphilis can also cause aortic aneurysms. Congenital defects of the intracranial arteries, *saccular berry aneurysms,* are also fairly frequent; they represent an important cause of cerebrovascular accidents (CVAs) (Chapter 23). Much has been made in the past about the terms *saccular, fusiform, cylindroid,* and *berry-shaped* in relation to the gross appearance of an aneurysm. However, these shapes are not specific for any disease or clinical manifestations. Having made these comments, we can deal with the three major etiologic forms of aortic aneurysms.

ATHEROSCLEROTIC (ABDOMINAL) ANEURYSMS

AS is by far the most common cause of aortic aneurysms. They are most frequent in males (5:1 ratio) after the fifth decade of life. Any site in the aorta may be affected, including the thoracic aorta, but the *great preponderance occur in the abdominal aorta, usually below the renal arteries.* Although AS is a major etiologic factor in abdominal aortic aneurysms, it has recently been claimed that genetic defects in a connective tissue component responsible for the strength of blood vessels could provide a particularly susceptible substrate on which AS, hypertension, or both, could act to weaken the aortic wall.

Atherosclerotic aneurysms take the form of saccular (balloon-like), cylindroid, or fusiform swellings, sometimes up to 15 cm in greatest diameter and of variable length (up to 25 cm). As would be expected, at these sites there is severe complicated AS, which destroys the underlying tunica media and thus weakens the aortic wall. Mural thrombus frequently is found within the aneurysmal sac. In saccular forms, the thrombus may completely fill the outpouching up to the level of the surrounding aortic wall (Fig. 10–17). The elongated fusiform or cylindroid patterns more often have layers of mural thrombus that only partially fill the dilation.

The clinical consequences of these aneurysms depend principally on their location and size. Occlusion of the iliac, renal, or mesenteric arteries may result either from pressure by the aneurysmal sac or from propagation of the thrombus. The thrombus may embolize. As enlarging pulsatile masses, these aneurysms not only simulate tumors, but also progressively erode adjacent structures such as the vertebral bodies. They have been known to erode the wall of the gut or, when they occur in the thorax, the wall of the trachea or esophagus. Rupture is the most feared consequence and is related to the size of the dilation. In general, when they are smaller than 6 cm in diameter, these aneurysms rarely rupture, whereas up to 50% of patients with larger lesions die of rupture within 10 years of the diagnosis. Fortunately, since most such aneurysms occur below the level of the renal arteries, many can be replaced with prosthetic arterial channels with excellent results. The operative mortality rate before rupture is about 5%; after rupture, it rises sharply, to 50%.

SYPHILITIC AORTITIS AND ANEURYSM

The tertiary stage of syphilis shows a predilection for the cardiovascular and nervous systems. Fortunately, with better control and treatment of syphilis in its early stages, these involvements are becoming less common. The obliterative endarteritis characteristic of tertiary syphilis may involve small vessels in any part of the body, but it is clinically most devastating when it affects the vasa vasorum of the aorta. Such involvement gives rise to thoracic aortitis, which in turn leads

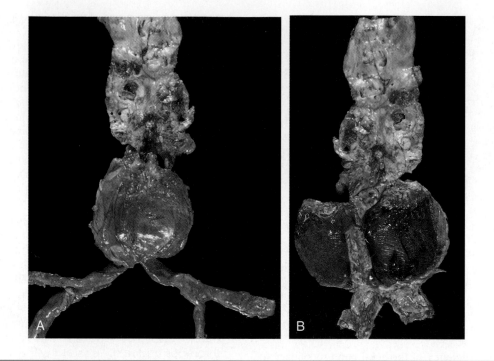

Figure 10-17

Atherosclerotic abdominal aneurysm above the iliac bifurcation. *A,* Unopened, external surface of aneurysm. *B,* Lumen of aneurysm filled completely with a thrombus.

to the aneurysmal dilation of the aorta and aortic valve ring characteristic of full-blown cardiovascular syphilis.

Syphilitic aortitis is almost always confined to the **thoracic aorta,** usually the ascending and transverse portions, and rarely extends below the diaphragm. **The obliterative endarteritis causes narrowing of the vasa vasorum that supply oxygen to the aortic media.** This leads to ischemic destruction of the elastic tissue and muscle of the media and to subsequent development of stellate fibrous scars in the media and fibrous thickening of the adventitia. With contraction of the irregular medial scars, longitudinal wrinkling, or "tree barking," of the intimal surface ensues. The scarring may envelop and narrow the ostia of vessels arising from the aorta, including those of the coronary arteries.

With destruction of the tunica media, the aorta loses its elastic support and tends to become dilated, producing a syphilitic aneurysm. Secondary atherosclerotic involvement of these damaged areas is almost invariable and may contribute to the weakening of the aortic wall. The end result is diffuse involvement by calcified atherosclerotic plaques, which obliterate the intimal "tree bark" pattern. **Even when these aneurysms are complicated by AS, their location in the thorax tends to distinguish them from typical atherosclerotic aneurysms, which rarely affect the aortic arch and never involve the root of the aorta.** When the aneurysmal dilation includes the aortic valve ring, the valvular commissures are widened, and the valve leaflets are stretched, so that their free margins tend to roll and become thickened. Incompetence of the valve leads to marked, sometimes extraordinary, hypertrophy and dilation of the left ventricle, with resultant heart weights of up to 1000 gm. Such a heart is known as cor bovinum.

Syphilitic aortitis with aneurysmal dilation may give rise to (1) respiratory difficulties as a result of encroachment on the lungs and airways; (2) difficulty in swallowing, owing to compression of the esophagus; (3) persistent brassy cough from pressure on the recurrent laryngeal nerve; (4) pain caused by erosion of bone (ribs and vertebral bodies); and (5) cardiac disease. As the aneurysm leads to dilation of the aortic root, signs of aortic valvular insufficiency develop. Most patients with syphilitic aneurysms die of heart failure as a result of aortic valvular incompetence.

AORTIC DISSECTION (DISSECTING HEMATOMA)

Aortic dissection is a catastrophic illness characterized by dissection of blood along the laminar planes of the media, along with formation of a blood-filled channel within the aortic wall. Such a channel often ruptures, causing massive hemorrhage. Aortic dissection is not usually associated with marked dilation of the aorta, and thus the older term *dissecting aneurysm* is no longer used. Aortic dissection occurs principally in two groups of patients: men 40 to 60 years of age, in whom hypertension is almost invariably an antecedent (more than 90% of cases of dissection); and patients with an abnormality of connective tissue that affects the aorta (e.g., Marfan syndrome, discussed later and in Chapter 7). Rarely, for unclear reasons, aortic dissection occurs during pregnancy. In contrast, dissection is unusual in the face of severe AS.

MORPHOLOGY. Dissections almost always originate with intimal tears, although in about 5% of cases none are found. While these tears may occur anywhere in the aorta, 90% are within 10 cm of the aortic valve. The next most common site of origin is in the descending thoracic aorta, just distal to the origin of the left subclavian artery.

The tear is usually longitudinal or oblique and 4 to 5 cm long. Blood entering this defect usually penetrates into the media and propagates in the medial laminar planes, typically between the outer and the middle third of the media. Concurrent AS is usually present, consonant with the patient's age and risk factors, but only infrequently does an ulcerated plaque constitute the site of origin of the intimal tear. The hemorrhage may dissect proximally toward the heart, sometimes into the coronary arteries, or it may rupture into the pericardial sac or pleural cavity. In other instances it dissects distally for some distance, sometimes into the iliac and femoral arteries. In long dissections, the hemorrhage may re-rupture back into the aortic lumen through a second distal intimal tear to produce a false lumen, or **double-barreled aorta,** through which blood may flow, thus protecting against rupture into one of the body cavities or periaortic structures. Over the course of years, the false lumen may become endothelialized and indeed develop AS. While the entire circumference of the aorta or other vessel may be involved, in some instances the hematoma is confined to one arc of the circumference,

sparing a portion. With dissection into the smaller branches of the aorta, the inner layers may collapse on themselves, causing significant vascular obstruction.

Histologically, in most cases there are few abnormal findings in the aortic walls save for the dissection and its content of blood, which may be unchanged if the victim dies abruptly; or it may have undergone more or less organization depending on how long the patient has survived. In about 20% of cases there are focal areas of medial degeneration producing so-called **cystic medial necrosis.** These ill-defined lesions constitute focal clefts or irregular defects created by loss of elastica and SMCs that are filled with amorphous basophilic extracellular matrix (Fig. 10–18). There is no accompanying inflammatory reaction, and the media separating these random lesions may be normal. **Such changes are present in most patients with Marfan syndrome, but in fewer than 20% of other dissections.**

The pathogenesis of aortic dissection in patients with Marfan syndrome, an autosomal dominant disease, has been traced to genetic defects in *fibrillin*, a connective tissue protein involved in elastic tissue formation (Chapter 7). This syndrome is characterized by cardiovascular, skeletal, and ocular manifestations, all attributable to the fibrillin mutations. The precise role of cystic medial necrosis is unclear. The fact that most non–Marfan syndrome patients have no cystic medial necrosis in the dissected aorta and that this lesion is sometimes encountered in elders as an incidental finding indicate that such medial lesions are neither sufficient nor critical to the development of dissection. Hypertension is present in most patients (70% to 90%) and conceivably could in some manner predispose patients to medial degeneration and to the propagation of the dissection.

Clinical Course. The risk and nature of serious complica-

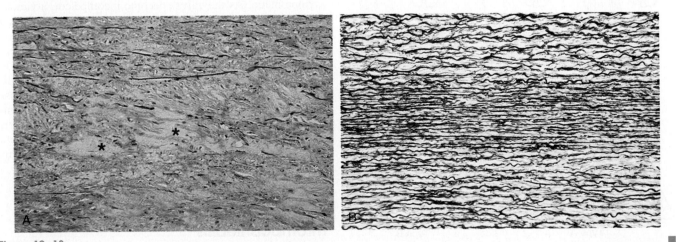

Figure 10–18

Cystic medial degeneration. *A,* Disruption and fragmentation of elastic lamellae of the aortic media, with formation of areas devoid of elastin (*) that resemble cystic spaces, from a patient with Marfan syndrome. *B,* Normal media for comparison showing the regular layered pattern of elastic tissue. Both photographs are of tissue stained with the elastic tissue stain, highlighting elastin as black.

tions of dissection depend on the level of the aorta affected. Aortic dissections are generally classified into two types: (1) the more common (and dangerous) proximal lesions, involving either the ascending portion only or both the ascending and the descending aorta (types I and II of DeBakey's classification, often collectively called type A), and (2) distal lesions not involving the ascending part and usually beginning distal to the subclavian artery (DeBakey type III, often called type B) (Fig. 10–19). The classic clinical symptoms of aortic dissection are the *sudden onset of excruciating pain,* usually beginning in the anterior chest, radiating to the back, and moving downward as the dissection progresses. This intense *pain can be readily confused with that of acute MI.* The antemortem diagnosis of aortic dissection and the differentiation of the various types are based largely on aortic angiography, but noninvasive techniques—two-dimensional cardiac ultrasound (especially transesophageal echocardiography), computed tomography (CT), and magnetic resonance imaging (MRI)—are increasingly useful.

At one time, aortic dissection was almost invariably fatal, but the prognosis has markedly improved. The development of surgical procedures involving plication of the aortic wall and early institution of intensive antihypertensive therapy permit salvage of 65% to 75% of patients with dissections.

VENOUS DISORDERS

Although none of the disorders of veins has the impressive frequency of AS, several, such as varicose veins and phlebothrombosis, are extremely common. Varicose veins induce a great deal of discomfort and morbidity but are rarely life

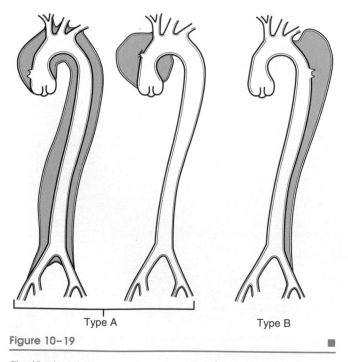

Figure 10–19 ■

Classification of dissection into types A and B. Type A (proximal) involves the ascending aorta; type B (distal) does *not* involve the ascending aorta.

Type A   Type B

threatening. On the other hand, phlebothrombosis, although somewhat less prevalent, may have lethal consequences. Discussions of these two venous disorders, as well as of the relatively rare involvements of the superior and inferior venae cavae, follow.

Varicose Veins

Varicose veins are abnormally dilated, tortuous veins; this condition is caused by increased intraluminal pressure and, to a lesser extent, by loss of support of the vessel wall. Although any vein in the body may be affected, *the superficial veins of the leg are by far the most frequently involved.* This predilection is due to high venous pressure in the legs when they are dependent, coupled with the relatively poor tissue support for the superficial, as opposed to the deep, veins. Even in otherwise normal persons, these factors produce a tendency toward the development of varices with advancing age. Indeed, this disorder is seen in approximately 50% of persons after age 50 years. There is a familial tendency to develop varicose veins relatively early in life. Because of the venous stasis in the lower legs caused by pregnancy, females are more often afflicted than males. In addition, any impediment to venous flow, such as an encroaching neoplasm or an encircling surgical dressing, promotes the development of varicosities in the legs or elsewhere.

Attention should be called to two special sites of varix formation. *Hemorrhoids* result from varicose dilation of the hemorrhoidal plexus of veins at the anorectal junction. The causative mechanism is presumed to be prolonged pelvic congestion resulting, for example, from repeated pregnancies or chronic constipation and straining at stools. The second and more important special site of varicosities is the esophagus, and this form is encountered virtually only in patients who have cirrhosis of the liver and its attendant portal hypertension (Chapter 16). Rupture of an *esophageal varix* may be more serious than the primary liver disease itself.

Clinical Course. Sometimes distention of the veins in the legs is painful, although most often early varicose veins are asymptomatic. As the valves become incompetent, a vicious circle is established, and the resultant venous stasis further increases intraluminal pressure. Marked venous congestion with edema may occur. Such edema impairs circulation, rendering the affected tissues extremely vulnerable to injury. In these severe cases, trophic changes, stasis dermatitis, cellulitis, and varicose ulcerations are common. Although varicose veins frequently thrombose, embolization to the lungs is uncommon from the superficial leg veins. Hemorrhoids, as is well known, not only are uncomfortable, but also may be a source of bleeding. Sometimes they thrombose, and in this distended state, they are prone to painful ulceration.

Phlebothrombosis and Thrombophlebitis

These two designations are synonyms for thrombus formation in veins. This condition was described in some detail in Chapter 4. Recall that the thrombi most often arise in the deep veins of the lower extremities. Frequently they are silent clinically but have the distressing potential of giving rise to emboli that lodge in the lungs to produce pulmonary embolism and infarction, which are extremely important causes of morbidity and mortality. Recall, too, that phlebothrombosis is most often associated with cardiac failure, prolonged bed rest or immobilization of an extremity, postoperative and postpartal states, neoplasia, and any form of severe trauma, particularly extensive burns. In patients with cancer, particularly primary carcinomas in the abdominal cavity, the venous thromboses have a tendency to appear spontaneously in one site, only to disappear and be followed by thromboses in other veins, giving rise to the entity referred to as *migratory thrombophlebitis (Trousseau's sign)*. Because of the clinical settings in which phlebothrombosis appears, pulmonary embolization often constitutes the final mortal blow to those already gravely ill.

Obstruction of Superior Vena Cava (Superior Vena Caval Syndrome)

This dramatic entity is usually caused by neoplasms that compress or invade the superior vena cava. Most commonly, a primary bronchogenic carcinoma or a mediastinal lymphoma is the underlying lesion. Occasionally other lesions, such as an aortic aneurysm, may impinge on the superior vena cava. Regardless of the cause, the consequent obstruction produces a distinctive clinical complex referred to as the superior vena caval syndrome. It is manifested by dusky cyanosis and marked dilation of the veins of the head, neck, and arms. Commonly the pulmonary vessels are also compressed, and consequently respiratory distress may develop.

Obstruction of Inferior Vena Cava (Inferior Vena Caval Syndrome)

This is analogous to the superior vena caval syndrome and may be caused by many of the same processes. Neoplasms may either compress or penetrate the walls of the inferior vena cava. In addition, one of the most common causes of inferior vena caval obstruction is upward propagation of a thrombus from the femoral or iliac vein. Certain neoplasms, particularly hepatocellular carcinoma and renal cell carcinoma, show a striking tendency to grow within the lumina of the veins, extending ultimately into the inferior vena cava.

As would be anticipated, obstruction to the inferior vena cava induces marked edema of the legs; distention of the superficial collateral veins of the lower abdomen; and, when the renal veins are involved, massive proteinuria.

■ LYMPHATIC DISORDERS

Disorders of the lymphatic channels fall into two categories: primary diseases, which are extremely uncommon, and secondary processes, which develop in association with inflammation (lymphangitis) or cancer. In both patterns there is frequently obstruction to the lymphatic channels, followed by lymphedema, entirely analogous to the edema that develops distal to venous obstructions.

Lymphangitis

Infections that spread into the lymphatics may either drain through these channels without causing any reaction or produce acute inflammatory involvement—a process known as lymphangitis. The most common causative agents of lymphangitis are the group A β-hemolytic streptococci, although any virulent pathogen may be responsible. The inflammation is marked by redness and dilation of the channels (red streaks), as well as local tenderness. An acute leukocytic exudate is found within the lumina. Almost inevitably the lymph nodes of drainage are involved with acute lymphadenitis. When these barriers to further spread are overwhelmed, infection may eventually drain into the venous system and initiate bacteremia or septicemia.

Lymphedema

Lymphedema is divided into primary and secondary forms. *Secondary lymphedema* may develop from (1) postinflammatory scarring of lymphatic channels, (2) spread of malignant neoplasms with obstruction of either the lymphatic channels or nodes of drainage, (3) radical surgical procedures with excision of regional lymph nodes (e.g., the removal of axillary nodes in radical mastectomy), (4) postradiation fibrosis, or (5) filariasis.

In contrast, *primary lymphedema* may occur as an isolated congenital defect (simple congenital lymphedema), or it may be familial, in which case it is known as *Milroy's disease* or *heredofamilial congenital lymphedema*. Both entities are presumed to be caused by faulty development of lymphatic channels, possibly with poor structural strength, permitting abnormal dilation and incompetence of the lymphatic valves. Classically, these disorders involve the lower extremities, although they may affect other areas, sometimes in a rather sharply limited, bizarre distribution. Both simple congenital lymphedema and Milroy's disease are present from birth. In contrast, a third form of primary lymphedema, known as *lymphedema praecox*, appears between the ages of 10 and 25 years, usually in females. The cause is unknown. This disorder begins in one or both feet, and the edema slowly accumulates throughout life so that the involved extremity may swell to many times its normal size; the process may extend upward to affect the trunk. The size of the limb may produce some disability, but more serious complications such as superimposed infection or chronic ulcerations may also occur.

With lymphedema from any cause, the morphologic changes in the lymphatics consist of dilation distal to the point of obstruction, accompanied by increases in interstitial fluid. Persistence of edema leads to interstitial fibrosis, which is most evident subcutaneously. The thickened skin assumes the texture of orange peel, a finding termed *peau d'orange;* often this is seen in the female breast when there is widespread lymphatic dissemination of a primary cancer. Enlargement of the affected part, brawny induration, infection (cellulitis), and chronic skin ulcers are common sequelae to persistent primary lymphedema.

VASCULAR TUMORS

Tumors of vessels (blood or lymphatic) run the gamut from benign lesions that usually produce vascular channels to borderline, more cellular tumors referred to as *hemangioendotheliomas* and overtly malignant neoplasms termed *hemangiosarcomas* or *angiosarcomas*. Although the well-differentiated benign tumor can be readily distinguished from the anaplastic cancer, the line in the middle of the spectrum dividing the benign from the malignant is poorly defined, but in general the following criteria apply:

■ Benign tumors produce readily recognized vascular channels filled with blood cells or, in the case of lymphatics, with transudate. The lining cells of the channels are identical to normal endothelial cells.
■ Malignant tumors are much more solidly cellular and form few or no vascular channels.
■ Solidly cellular neoplasms often have cytologic anaplasia, including mitotic figures.

The differentiation of solidly cellular angiosarcomas from other spindle cell neoplasms (e.g., fibrosarcoma or leiomyosarcoma) is at times difficult. Helpful in this regard is the finding of endothelial specific antigens, such as factor VIII–related antigens, by immunocytochemistry.

There are, in addition, a few vascular lesions that lie in the gray area between non-neoplastic and neoplastic. Most benign angiomas—capillary and cavernous—are present from birth and expand along with the growth of the child. Many regress spontaneously at or before puberty. Are these true neoplasms or merely hamartomatous congenital anomalies? Regardless, the common angiomatous birthmark that is quite distressing to mothers of infants may well disappear spontaneously at puberty. Other interface lesions are the *granuloma pyogenicum* and the *pregnancy tumor*. Granuloma pyogenicum usually is secondary to some chronic localized infection and is an exuberant overgrowth of granulation tissue rich in vascular channels. Pregnancy tumor is a granuloma pyogenicum occurring in the gingiva of pregnant women. Pregnancy tumors almost always regress spontaneously after delivery, but the granuloma pyogenicum may require excision or cauterization.

Another vascular lesion more clearly non-neoplastic is the *spider telangiectasia*. It is a more or less radial array of somewhat dilated subcutaneous arteries or arterioles about a central core. Because they have arteriolar or arterial connections, they may pulsate. They tend to be on the face, neck, or upper chest and are most frequent in pregnant women and in patients with liver cirrhosis. The hyperestrinism found in these two settings is believed in some way to play a role in the development of these telangiectases. However, in the autosomal dominant *Osler-Weber-Rendu disease,* these telangiectases are clearly genetic malformations present from birth. They are distributed widely over the skin and mucous membranes of the oral cavity; lips; respiratory, gastrointestinal, and urinary tracts; liver; brain; and spleen. Any one of these innumerable lesions may rupture to cause such problems as nosebleeds, hematuria, or bleeding into the gut, but only rarely are these bleeding episodes serious.

Now we turn to the undoubted vascular neoplasms.

Hemangiomas

Hemangiomas may be composed of masses of cavernous or capillary-like channels filled with either blood or lymph.

MORPHOLOGY. Cavernous hemangiomas may arise in blood vessels or in lymphatics. The cavernous hemangiomas often occur on the skin and mucosal surfaces of the body but may also arise in viscera, particularly in the liver, spleen, pancreas, and, rarely, the brain. In the rare autosomal dominant von Hippel-Lindau disease, these vascular tumors may occur within the cerebellum, brain stem, retina, and sometimes in the pancreas and liver, along with other visceral neoplasms. In infants, cavernous hemangiomas sometimes constitute large lesions of the skin of the face or scalp, the so-called port wine stains or birthmarks. Cavernous hemangiomas are generally red-blue, compressible, spongy lesions that are 2 to 3 cm in diameter, sharply defined at their margins, and composed of large cavernous spaces filled with fluid blood; they sometimes have partially thrombosed channels (Fig. 10–20). In most instances these cavernous lesions have little clinical significance, and in children they may regress. When picked up in internal organs by CT or MRI scans, they must be differentiated from more ominous lesions. Those in the brain are most threatening, since they may cause pressure symptoms or rupture.

A capillary hemangioma is an unencapsulated

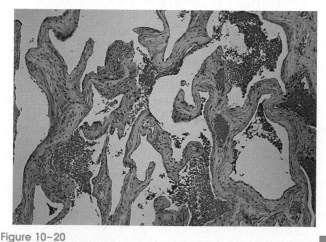

Figure 10–20 ■

Cavernous hemangioma with large, irregular, endothelium-lined spaces, some filled with blood. (Courtesy of Tom Rogers, MD, Department of Pathology, University of Texas Southwestern Medical School, Dallas, TX.)

tangle of closely packed capillaries separated by a scant connective tissue stroma. The channels are usually filled with fluid blood; however, thrombosis and fibrous organization within some of the component capillaries are common. The ECs of the lining appear normal. Although any organ or tissue may be involved, capillary hemangiomas usually occur in the skin, subcutaneous tissues, or mucous membranes of the oral cavity and lips. On gross inspection, they appear as bright red to blue lesions, ranging from a few millimeters to several centimeters in diameter. They may be level with the surface of the surrounding tissue, slightly elevated, or occasionally even pedunculated. Uncommonly, capillary hemangiomas take the form of large, flat, maplike discolorations that cover large areas of the face or upper parts of the body, producing port wine stains analogous to those caused by cavernous hemangiomas.

Capillary hemangiomas, because they are usually on the skin or mucous membranes, are significant only because they are vulnerable to traumatic ulceration and bleeding.

Glomangioma (Glomus Tumor)

This uncommon but curious benign lesion, which arises from the modified SMCs of a glomus body, is invariably small, red-blue, and exquisitely painful to the slightest pressure. It is most commonly encountered in the distal fingers and toes, especially under the nails. The tumors are small and on the order of 5 mm in diameter. When in the skin, they are slightly elevated, rounded, red-blue, firm nodules. Under the nail they appear as minute foci of fresh hemorrhage. Histologically, they are composed of branching vascular channels enclosed within a stroma bearing nests or larger aggregates of glomus cells, which are small; round to cuboidal; and regular in size and shape, with central dark nuclei. On electron microscopy they have features of modified SMCs. They are usually readily excised and cured.

Hemangioendothelioma and Angiosarcoma

Both of these neoplasms represent the malignant counterparts of the benign angiomatous lesions. The hemangioendothelioma constitutes an intermediate grade between the benign hemangiomas and the unmistakably malignant anaplastic angiosarcoma.

In the *hemangioendothelioma*, vascular channels are usually readily discernible within the masses of proliferating, reasonably well-differentiated endothelial cells. Occasionally the cells are plump and resemble epithelial cells (*epithelioid hemangioendothelioma*). In the *angiosarcoma*, vascular channels may be virtually inapparent. Thus, the angiosarcoma is composed of masses of anaplastic spindle cells with sparsely scattered, poorly formed vascular channels, themselves lined by tumorous endothelial cells (Fig. 10–21). Both patterns of tumors are found in the same locations as their benign counterparts and tend to be larger, more solid, less obviously vascular, and more unmistakably invasive. In some cases the tumor cells contain Weibel-Palade bodies and/or factor VIII–related antigens.

The angiosarcomas are of interest because they are associated with distinct carcinogens, including arsenic compounds, polyvinylchloride (used in plastics industries), or the radioactive agent Thorotrast (formerly used in radiography).

Kaposi's Sarcoma

At one time thought to be an uncommon neoplasm of elderly, mostly Jewish, men of European extraction, Kaposi's sarcoma (KS) has come into prominence because several variant forms have been identified. The form that affects elderly men is referred to as *classic KS.* Another pattern, called *African* or *endemic KS,* is endemic among black African young men and children. A third variant occurs in immunosuppressed transplantation patients, and yet another highly virulent variant, called *epidemic KS,* is particularly common in acquired immunodeficiency syndrome (AIDS) patients.

Classic KS is an indolent disease that typically begins with red-blue inflamed-looking lesions (one or more) on the distal lower extremities. Over the course of years, the lesions tend to become more numerous centripetally and more nodular, and they are sometimes complicated by involvement of the lymph nodes, gastrointestinal tract, lung, liver, and other viscera. Rarely the visceral lesions precede the cutaneous ones. Even with dissemination, the course of the disease is indolent and only occasionally fulminant, and 90% of the patients die

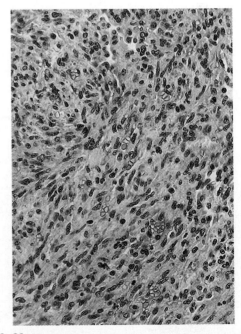

Figure 10–21 ■

Photomicrograph of angiosarcoma showing plump, atypical endothelial cells with occasional vascular channels.

of intercurrent disease. About one third have a history of or develop lymphoma.

Endemic KS, which is particularly prevalent among the Bantus of South Africa, has the same geographic distribution as Burkitt's lymphoma. Whites in this same locale have no increased prevalence of KS. Among young males the disease may be benign, resembling the classic pattern, or extremely aggressive. Occasionally the virulent form is largely restricted to lymph nodes, sparing the skin but occasionally involving the viscera. This "lymphadenopathic pattern" is particularly likely to occur in children with KS, often in the first years of life.

KS in immunosuppressed patients tends to be indolent but is sometimes aggressive and more or less resembles the classic pattern. The lesions sometimes regress when immunosuppressive therapy is discontinued.

Epidemic KS seen in AIDS may begin with a nodular skin or mucosal lesion but spreads rapidly to nodes and viscera. Despite the spread of the disease, most patients die of opportunistic infections (as do most patients with AIDS) or of an intercurrent lymphoma. For completely obscure reasons, 90% to 95% of all AIDS-associated KS occurs in homosexual men, far out of proportion to their representation in the AIDS population, but the incidence of KS among homosexual men has declined dramatically, from about 40% to about 20%, in recent years.

The pathogenesis of KS is sill unclear, as is the nature of the undifferentiated spindle-shaped tumor cells. Current theories suggest either primitive mesenchymal or endothelial cell derivation of tumor cells. For AIDS-associated KS, there is considerable evidence that locally produced growth factors, acting in a paracrine or autocrine fashion, cause unchecked growth of cells. Furthermore, as discussed in Chapter 5, both human immunodeficiency virus (HIV) products and human

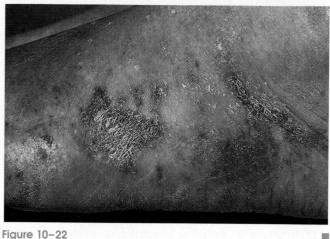

Figure 10–22 ■

Kaposi's sarcoma showing red-purple coalescent multiple macules and plaques.

herpesvirus type 8 may play a role in the etiology of these tumors.

MORPHOLOGY. In the relatively indolent, classic disease of older men, and sometimes in the other variants, three stages can be identified: patch, plaque, and nodule. The **patches** comprise pink to red to purple solitary or multiple macules that in the classic disease are usually confined to the distal lower extremities or feet (Fig. 10–22). Microscopic examination discloses only dilated, perhaps irregular and angulated blood vessels lined by

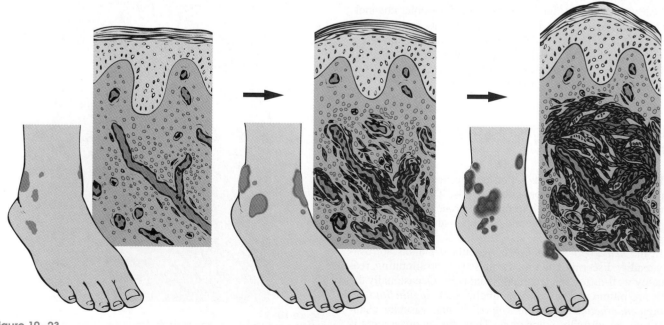

Figure 10–23 ■

Schematic representation of the progressive gross and microscopic stages of Kaposi's sarcoma.

normal-looking endothelial cells with an interspersed infiltrate of lymphocytes, plasma cells, and macrophages (sometimes containing hemosiderin). Such lesions are difficult to distinguish from granulation tissue. Over time, lesions in the classic disease spread proximally and usually convert into larger, violaceous, **raised plaques** that reveal dermal, dilated, jagged vascular channels lined by somewhat plump spindle cells accompanied by perivascular aggregates of similar spindled cells. Scattered between the vascular channels are red cells, hemosiderin-laden macrophages, lymphocytes, and plasma cells. Pink hyaline globules of uncertain nature may be found in the spindled cells and macrophages. Occasional mitotic figures may be present.

At a still later stage, the skin and mucous membrane lesions may become **nodular** and more distinctly neoplastic and may be composed of sheets of plump, proliferating spindle cells, mostly in the dermis or subcutaneous tissues (Fig. 10–23). Particularly characteristic in this cellular background are scattered small vessels and slitlike spaces that often contain rows of red cells characteristically arranged in a "boxcar" pattern. More marked hemorrhage, hemosiderin pigment, lymphocytes, and occasional macrophages may be admixed with this cellular background. Mitotic figures are common, as are the round, pink, cytoplasmic globules. At this stage the lesion comes to resemble an angiosarcoma or fibrosarcoma. The nodular stage is often accompanied by involvement of lymph nodes and of viscera, particularly in the African and AIDS-associated diseases.

Clinical Course. The presentation and natural course of KS vary widely and are significantly affected by the setting in which it occurs. Some of these details were presented earlier. Whereas the classic form at the outset is largely restricted to the surface of the body, in the endemic and epidemic subsets, the condition at presentation tends to be more widespread, particularly in persons who have AIDS. Visceral involvement is often present when the cutaneous manifestations appear. Whereas the classic disease is relatively indolent and compatible with long survival, both the endemic and epidemic patterns are much more aggressive and usually fatal within 2 to 5 years. Regrettably, no form of therapy has proved very effective.

BIBLIOGRAPHY

American Heart Association Committee on Vascular Lesions of the Council on Arteriosclerosis, Stary HC (chair): A definition of advanced types of atherosclerosis lesions and a histological classification of atherosclerosis. Circulation 92:1355, 1995.

Berk BC, Alexander RW: Biology of the vascular wall in hypertension. In Brenner BM (ed): Brenner and Rector's The Kidney, Vol II, 5th ed. Philadelphia, WB Saunders, 1996, pp 2049–2070. (An excellent review of the increasing evidence of primary role of vascular wall pathobiology in hypertension.)

Cotran RS, Briscoe DM: Endothelial cells in inflammation. In Kelly WN, et al (eds): Textbook of Rheumatology. Philadelphia, WB Saunders, 1997, pp 183–198. (A review of endothelial cells.)

Dajani AS, et al: Diagnosis and therapy of Kawasaki disease in children. Circulation 87:1776, 1993.

Davies PF: Shear stress and atherosclerosis. Physiol Rev 75:519, 1995.

Ernst CB: Abdominal aortic aneurysms. N Engl J Med 328:1167, 1993.

Fuster V, et al (eds): Atherosclerosis and Coronary Artery Disease. Philadelphia, Lippincott-Raven, 1996. (A comprehensive two-volume set with excellent chapters on the pathogenesis and pathology of atherosclerosis.)

Gimbrone MA Jr: Vascular endothelium in health and disease. In Haber E (ed): Molecular Cardiovascular Medicine. New York, Scientific American, 1995, pp 49–61.

Glasser SP, Selwyn AP, Ganz P: Atherosclerosis, risk factors and vascular endothelium. Am Heart J 1996 (in press).

Jennette JC, et al: Nomenclature of systemic vasculitides: the proposal of an international consensus conference. Arthritis Rheum 37:187, 1994.

Jennette JC, Falk RJ: Antineutrophil cytoplasmic autoantibodies: discovery, specificity, disease associations and pathogenic potential. Adv Pathol Lab Med 8:313, 1995. (A summary of recent advances in the role of ANCA in vasculitis.)

Kaplan NM: Systemic hypertension: mechanisms and diagnosis. In Braunwald ED (ed): Heart Disease, 5th ed. Philadelphia, WB Saunders, 1997.

Kurokawa K, et al (eds): Hypertension: causes and consequences of renal injury. Kidney Int 49:S1, 1996. (A compendium of articles on renal factors in hypertension.)

Lifton RP: Molecular genetics of human blood pressure variation. Science 272:676, 1996. (A review of known single gene defects leading to hypertension.)

Resnick N, Gimbrone M: Hemodynamic factors are regulators of endothelial gene expression. FASEB J 9:874, 1995.

Ross R: The pathogenesis of atherosclerosis: a perspective for the 1990s. Nature 362:801, 1993.

Schoen FV, Gimbrone MA Jr (eds.): Cardiovascular Pathology: Clinicopathologic Correlations and Pathogenetic Mechanisms. Baltimore, Williams & Wilkins, 1996. (Excellent chapters on atherogenesis, aortic aneurysms, and vasculitis.)

Somer T, Finegold SM: Vasculitides associated with infections, immunization and antimicrobial drugs. Clin Infect Dis 20:1010, 1995.

11

The Heart

DENNIS K. BURNS, MD
VINAY KUMAR, MD

In addition to serving as an unfailing source of inspiration to poets, the human heart also accomplishes the enormous task of propelling over 6000 liters of blood through the body daily during the lifetime of the individual. In most cases, it performs its duties quietly and efficiently, providing the tissues with a steady supply of vital nutrients and facilitating the excretion of waste products. As might be anticipated, cardiac dysfunction can be associated with devastating physiologic consequences. Heart disease remains the leading cause of death and disability in the industrialized nations of the world and currently accounts for nearly 40% of all deaths in the United States. The major categories of cardiac diseases considered in this chapter include coronary artery disease, hypertensive heart disease, heart disease caused by intrinsic pulmonary diseases (cor pulmonale), valvular heart diseases, primary myocardial diseases, and selected congenital heart diseases. A few comments about pericardial diseases and cardiac neoplasms are also offered. Before considering details of specific heart diseases, we will review salient features of congestive heart failure (CHF), the common end point of many different types of heart disease.

CONGESTIVE HEART FAILURE

Congestive heart failure (CHF) is a multisystem derangement that occurs, in most cases, when the heart is no longer able to eject the blood delivered to it by the venous system. Excluded from this definition are conditions in which inadequate cardiac output occurs because of blood loss or some other process that impairs the return of blood to the heart. In an additional minority of cases, heart failure may result because of greatly increased demands for blood by the tissues, a process sometimes referred to as *high output failure.* Inadequate cardiac output, also termed *forward failure,* is almost always accompanied by increased congestion of the venous circulation (*backward failure*). This occurs because the failing ventricle is unable to eject the normal volume of venous blood delivered to it during diastole. This results in an increase in the volume of blood in the ventricle at the end of diastole, an elevation in end-diastolic pressure within the heart, and, finally, elevated venous pressure. CHF may involve the left side of the heart, the right side, or all of the cardiac chambers.

The most common causes of left-sided cardiac failure are systemic hypertension, mitral or aortic valve disease, ischemic heart disease, and primary diseases of the myocardium. *The most common cause of right-sided heart failure is left ventricular failure,* with its associated pulmonary congestion and elevation in pulmonary arterial pressure. Right-sided failure may also occur in the absence of left heart failure in patients with intrinsic diseases of the lung (cor pulmonale), in patients with primary diseases of the pulmonary vasculature, and in patients with pulmonic or tricuspid valve disease. It sometimes follows congenital heart diseases in which there is a left-to-right shunt.

As the heart begins to fail, a number of local *compensatory mechanisms* are triggered in an attempt to maintain normal cardiac output. Initially there is an increase in the activity of the sympathetic nervous system. Catecholamines cause both a more forceful contraction of the heart muscle (a positive inotropic effect) and an increase in heart rate. Over time, the overburdened heart may respond to increased demands by undergoing hypertrophy, in much the same way as the skeletal muscles enlarge to accommodate increased loads. If the combination of sympathetic activity and hypertrophy proves insufficient to expel all the venous blood that drains into the heart, end-diastolic pressure and volume increase, causing the heart to dilate. This leads to elongation and stretching of individual cardiac muscle fibers. In accordance with the Frank-Starling relationship, these lengthened fibers initially contract more forcibly, thereby increasing cardiac output (Fig. 11–1). If the dilated ventricle is able to maintain cardiac output at a level that meets the needs of the body, the patient is said to be in *compensated heart failure.* Beyond a certain point, however, further dilation no longer results in increased contractility, but instead leads to a progressive decrease in myocardial contractility and a decline in cardiac output. When this point is passed, patients enter a phase termed *decompensated heart failure.*

Heart failure causes changes in other organs as well. As noted previously, cardiac failure inevitably includes an element of backward failure, the result of which is *congestion of the venous circulation.* In a patient with left-sided failure, this

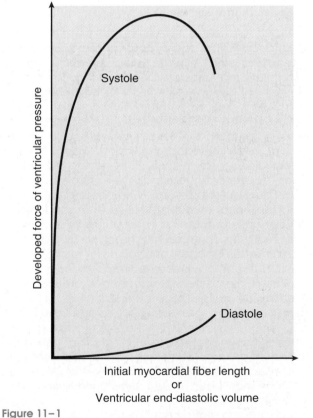

Figure 11–1   ■

Frank-Starling curve demonstrating the relationship between resting myocardial fiber length and force of myocardial contraction. During the initial phases of heart failure, ventricular dilation results in a more forceful myocardial contraction. With more severe degrees of dilation, however, myocardial contractility begins to decline, causing a decrease in cardiac output ("forward failure") and increased end-diastolic and venous pressures ("backward failure").

results in passive congestion of the pulmonary circulation. With increasing failure of the left heart, the hydrostatic pressure in the pulmonary vasculature increases sufficiently to cause leakage of fluid and, occasionally, erythrocytes into the interstitial tissue and airspaces of the lungs to *produce pulmonary edema.* Congestion of the pulmonary circulation also causes an increase in pulmonary vascular resistance and, with it, an increased workload on the right side of the heart. This increased burden, if sustained and severe, may ultimately cause the right heart to fail also. Failure of the right heart in turn contributes to the development of *systemic venous congestion and soft tissue edema* (Chapter 4).

As the heart fails, a number of *systemic alterations also occur as the body attempts to maintain cardiac output at near-normal levels.* Decompensated heart failure is associated with decreased perfusion of the kidneys, which in turn causes local activation of the renin-angiotensin system. Aldosterone is released in response to activation of the renin-angiotensin system and causes the renal tubules to resorb both sodium and water. This sequence of events, sometimes called secondary hyperaldosteronism, increases the total plasma volume of extracellular fluid. However, unless the performance of the cardiac pump improves, the failing heart is unable to pump the increased intravascular volume, which remains pooled in the veins, thereby adding further to systemic and pulmonary venous congestion. This ultimately contributes further to both pulmonary and soft tissue edema.

MORPHOLOGY. The failing **cardiac chambers are dilated,** and often hypertrophied as well. In **left-sided failure** the **lungs** are boggy and congested, and the cut surface exudes a frothy mixture of edema fluid and surfactant. Microscopically, the pulmonary alveolar capillaries are congested. There is transudation of fluid, initially limited to perivascular interstitial spaces, causing widening of the alveolar septa. In time, it overflows into the alveoli **(pulmonary edema).** The protein-poor edema fluid stains pale pink. With persistent elevation of pulmonary venous pressure, the capillaries may become tortuous, and may rupture to produce small hemorrhages into the alveolar spaces. Alveolar macrophages phagocytose red blood cells and eventually become filled with hemosiderin. These pigmented macrophages are called **heart failure cells.** Long persistence of septal edema often induces fibrosis within the alveolar walls, which, together with the accumulation of hemosiderin, is characteristic of **chronic venous congestion** of lungs. Such lungs are dark brown in color and firm in consistency, and hence this appearance has been called **brown induration of the lungs.**

Long-standing **right heart failure** is associated with congestion of the abdominal viscera, soft tissue edema, and (in some cases) fluid in the pleural, pericardial, and abdominal cavities. Changes in the **liver** include chronic passive congestion, characterized by atrophy of hepatocytes around the central veins that gives rise to a nutmeg-like appearance on the cut surface of the organ (see Fig. 4–3 in Chapter 4). Hemorrhagic necrosis of centrilobular hepatocytes is common in severe cases. With long-standing cardiac failure, the liver may become fibrotic and (in extreme cases) may develop diffuse fibrosis, sometimes called cardiac cirrhosis (Chapter 16).

Clinical Features. The most common manifestation of left ventricular failure is *dyspnea,* or a sense of breathlessness. This is caused predominantly by decreased lung compliance resulting from pulmonary edema and congestion, and by increased activity of autonomic stretch receptors within the lung. Dyspnea is most noticeable during periods of physical activity (*exertional dyspnea*). It is also prominent when the person is lying down (*orthopnea*), because of the increased amount of venous blood returned to the thorax from the lower extremities and because the diaphragm is elevated in this position. *Paroxysmal nocturnal dyspnea* is an especially dramatic form of dyspnea that awakens the patient with sudden, severe shortness of breath, accompanied by coughing, a choking sensation, and (in many cases) wheezing. Other manifestations of left ventricular failure include muscle fatigue, an enlarged heart, tachycardia, a third heart sound (S_3), and fine rales at the lung bases, produced by the flow of air through edematous pulmonary alveoli. With progressive ventricular dilation, the papillary muscles are displaced laterally, causing mitral regurgitation and a high-pitched systolic murmur. Chronic dilation of the left atrium may also occur, and it is often associated with the development of *atrial fibrillation,* manifested by an "irregularly irregular" heartbeat.

As stated earlier, right-sided heart failure is most often caused by left-sided failure. Its major consequences are *systemic venous congestion* and *soft tissue edema.* Systemic venous congestion is manifested clinically by distended neck veins and an enlarged, sometimes tender, liver. It is also associated with an increased frequency of deep venous thrombi and pulmonary embolism (Chapter 4). Edema causes weight gain and usually becomes apparent first in the dependent areas of the body, such as the feet and lower legs. With more severe degrees of ventricular failure, the edema may become generalized. Pleural effusions are common, particularly on the right side, and may be accompanied by pericardial effusions and ascites. Unlike inflammatory edema, the edema fluid in CHF has a low protein content.

As CHF progresses, patients may become frankly cyanotic and acidotic owing to decreased tissue perfusion. Ventricular arrhythmias caused by myocardial irritability and overactivity of the sympathetic nervous system are common and are an important cause of sudden death in this setting.

ISCHEMIC HEART DISEASE

Ischemic heart disease, also designated *coronary heart disease,* refers to a group of closely related syndromes caused by an imbalance between the myocardial oxygen demand and blood supply. The most common cause of ischemic heart disease is a reduction in coronary arterial blood supply due to atherosclerosis of the coronary arteries.

Ischemic heart disease is the single most common cause of death in economically developed countries of the world, including the United States and western Europe, where it is responsible for about one third of all deaths. Depending on the rate and severity of coronary artery narrowing and the myocardial response, one of four syndromes may develop: (1) various forms of *angina pectoris* (chest pain), (2) *acute myocardial infarction (MI)*, (3) *sudden cardiac death,* and (4) *chronic ischemic heart disease with congestive heart failure.* These syndromes are late manifestations of coronary atherosclerosis that probably begins during childhood.

Epidemiology. Clinical manifestations of coronary atherosclerosis may occur at any age, but they are most common in older adults, with a peak incidence after the age of 60 years in men and 70 years in women. Men are more commonly affected than women until the ninth decade, by which time the frequency of coronary artery disease is similar in both sexes. Factors that contribute to the development of coronary atherosclerosis are similar to those responsible for atherosclerosis in general, and include *hypertension, diabetes mellitus, smoking,* and *high levels of low-density lipoprotein (LDL) cholesterol* (Chapter 10). *Genetic factors* undoubtedly play an important role in the development of coronary atherosclerosis. In some families the genetic influences include inheritance of some of the previously mentioned risk factors (e.g., hypercholesterolemia, diabetes mellitus). In other cases of familial coronary artery disease the specific genetic abnormalities have not been defined.

Much attention has also been given to factors that might reduce the risk of coronary atherosclerosis. *Regular exercise,* by decreasing myocardial oxygen demand and increasing myocardial vascularity, appears to significantly reduce the risk of coronary artery disease and its sequelae. It appears that *moderate consumption of red wine* and perhaps other alcoholic beverages may also reduce the risk of coronary artery disease, possibly by increasing levels of high-density lipoprotein (HDL) cholesterol. Welcome though these associations may be to connoisseurs of fine wine and the sedentary individuals among us, the beneficial effects of moderate alcohol consumption are probably slight at best. More important, they do not compensate for the detrimental effects of smoking, an indiscriminate diet, or a lack of exercise.

Pathogenesis. Symptomatic ischemic heart disease is typically associated with a *critical stenosis, defined as a 75% or greater reduction in the lumen of one or more coronary arteries by atherosclerotic plaque.* With this level of *fixed obstruction,* the augmented coronary blood flow that may occur as a result of compensatory coronary vasodilation is insufficient to meet even moderate increases in myocardial oxygen demand. In addition to chronic, fixed atherosclerotic plaques, various superimposed lesions also play an important role in the development of myocardial ischemia. These include

■ Acute changes in plaque morphology
■ Platelet aggregation
■ Coronary artery thrombosis
■ Coronary artery vasospasm

Acute changes in the morphology of chronic atherosclerotic

plaques include fissuring, hemorrhage into the plaque, and overt plaque rupture with embolization of atheromatous debris into distal coronary vessels. In addition to causing enlargement of the plaque, local disruption of plaque increases the risk of platelet aggregation and thrombosis at that site.

Local platelet aggregation in the coronary arteries has been documented in patients with unstable angina pectoris (discussed below) and in patients who undergo sudden cardiac death. Both mechanical occlusion of small blood vessels by small platelet aggregates and coronary vasospasm induced by mediators released from the platelet aggregates may contribute to myocardial ischemia in such cases.

Coronary artery thrombosis is almost always associated with a severe atherosclerotic plaque. Local disruption of atheromatous plaques plays an important role in the development of thrombi by exposing thrombogenic, lipid-rich plaque debris to the blood (Fig. 11–2). Thrombi are identified most often in patients who have suffered a myocardial infarct involving the full thickness of the myocardium (transmural myocardial infarct), although they may also occur in patients with other clinical manifestations of cardiac ischemia, such as unstable angina pectoris.

Coronary artery spasm usually occurs in patients with at least some preexisting atherosclerosis. It has been associated with one particular type of angina pectoris, termed *Prinzmetal's (variant) angina.* The mechanism for coronary vasospasm is not entirely clear. At the site of plaque disruption, it may be induced by the release of vasospastic mediators such as thromboxane A_2 by platelet aggregates. Endothelial dysfunction may also precipitate vasospasm by reduced elaboration of endothelial cell–derived relaxing factors. Increased adrenergic activity and smoking have also been implicated.

Uncommonly, processes other than atherosclerosis or its complications may compromise blood flow through the coro-

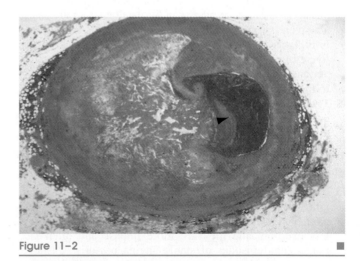

Figure 11–2   ■

Photomicrograph of an atherosclerotic coronary artery, with rupture of the atherosclerotic plaque and an overlying occlusive thrombus. The thrombus is deep red and crescentic in shape; it is completely filling the markedly narrowed coronary artery lumen. More than 80% of the lumen is filled by an atherosclerotic plaque, which shows a central soft area in which cholesterol, represented by clear spaces, is present. The left side of the deep red thrombus is hugging the area of plaque rupture *(arrow).* (Courtesy of Dr. Sid Murphree, Department of Pathology, University of Texas Southwestern Medical School, Dallas, TX.)

nary arteries. These include emboli originating from vegetations on the aortic or mitral valves, and coronary vasculitis. Severe systemic hypotension may also be associated with decreased coronary artery flow and myocardial ischemia, particularly in patients with preexisting coronary atherosclerosis. In addition to factors that compromise coronary blood flow, increased myocardial oxygen demand may also contribute to the development of myocardial ischemia. This may occur with left ventricular myocardial hypertrophy, as well as other conditions that place an increased demand on the heart, such as hypertension and diseases of the heart valves. With this overview of the pathogenesis of myocardial ischemia, we can turn our attention to the specific clinical presentations of ischemic heart disease and the morphologic changes associated with them.

Angina Pectoris

The term *angina pectoris* refers to the presence of *intermittent chest pain caused by reversible myocardial ischemia.* Three major variants of angina pectoris are recognized: typical (stable) angina pectoris, Prinzmetal's (variant) angina, and unstable angina pectoris. More than one pattern of angina may be present in a given patient.

■ *Typical angina pectoris* refers to episodic chest pain associated with exertion or some other form of stress. The pain is classically described as a crushing or squeezing substernal sensation, which may radiate down the left arm. Stable angina pectoris is often, but not invariably, associated with a *fixed degree of atherosclerotic narrowing* (usually 75% or greater) of one or more coronary arteries. With this degree of obstruction, the myocardial oxygen demand may be adequate under basal conditions but cannot be augmented sufficiently to meet the increased requirements imposed by exercise or other conditions that stress the heart. The pain is usually relieved by rest (reducing demand) or nitroglycerin. This vasodilator reduces venous blood delivered to the heart (and hence cardiac work) by effecting venous dilation, and in larger doses increases blood supply to the myocardium by coronary vasodilation.

■ *Prinzmetal's, or variant, angina* refers to angina that occurs at rest or, in some cases, awakens the patient from sleep. Angiographic studies have shown that Prinzmetal's angina is associated with coronary artery *spasm*, usually near an atherosclerotic plaque. It also responds to the administration of vasodilators.

■ *Unstable angina pectoris*, sometimes called *crescendo* angina, is characterized by the increased frequency of anginal pain. The attacks tend to be precipitated by progressively less exertion, and they are more intense and often last longer than episodes of stable angina pectoris. Unstable angina is a harbinger of more serious, potentially irreversible, myocardial ischemia and hence has sometimes been referred to as *preinfarction angina*. In most patients it is induced by acute plaque change with superimposed partial thrombosis, distal embolization of the thrombus, and/or vasospasm. The morphologic changes in the heart are essentially those of coronary atherosclerosis and its associated lesions.

Myocardial Infarction

The term *myocardial infarction* (MI) indicates the *development of a defined area of myocardial necrosis caused by local ischemia.* Acute MI is the single most common cause of death in industrialized nations. In the United States, an estimated 1.5 million people per year suffer an MI, with roughly 500,000 fatalities. Among fatal cases, nearly half of the patients die before reaching the hospital. The risk of acute MI increases progressively throughout life. Between the ages of 45 and 54, men are four to five times as likely to develop an MI as women. As with ischemic heart disease in general, however, the risk of disease becomes the same in both sexes after 80 years of age. The major risk factors for acute MI are the same as those discussed previously for coronary atherosclerosis (see also Chapter 10).

Pathogenesis. Although any of the forms of coronary artery disease discussed earlier may cause acute MI, angiographic studies indicate that *most acute MIs are caused by coronary artery thrombosis.* Preexisting atherosclerosis plays a very important role in the development of coronary thromboses, as noted previously. In most cases, careful histologic examination reveals a disruption of an underlying atherosclerotic plaque (e.g., fissure formation), which serves as the nidus for the generation of the thrombus. Vasospasm and platelet aggregation may contribute to coronary artery occlusion, but they are seldom, if ever, the sole cause of the occlusion. Sometimes, particularly in the case of infarcts limited to the subendocardial myocardium, thrombi may be absent. In such cases, hypoperfusion of coronary vessels already compromised by atherosclerosis is presumably sufficient to cause a subendocardial infarct.

Myocardial necrosis begins within approximately 20 to 30 minutes of the time of coronary artery occlusion. Under normal circumstances, the subendocardial region of the myocardium is the most poorly perfused region of the ventricular wall; not only is it the last area to receive blood from branches of the epicardial coronary arteries, but the relatively high intramural pressures that exist in this area further compromise inflow of blood. *Because of this increased vulnerability to ischemic injury, myocardial infarcts typically begin in the subendocardial region.* The zone of necrosis extends externally over the next several hours, to involve the mid- and subepicardial areas of the myocardium. The infarct usually reaches its full size within a period of 3 to 6 hours. During this period of evolution, lysis of the thrombus by the administration of thrombolytic agents (e.g., streptokinase or tissue plasminogen activator) may limit the size of the infarct. The progression of ischemic necrosis in the myocardium is summarized in Figure 11–3.

The location of an MI is determined by the site of the occlusion and by the anatomy of the coronary circulation. Occlusion of the left anterior descending coronary artery typically causes an infarct in the anterior and apical areas of the left ventricle and adjacent interventricular septum (anteroapical MI). Occlusion of the right coronary artery is responsible for most infarcts involving the posterior and basal portions of the left ventricle. The underlying anatomy of the coronary circulation also has a significant influence on the location of the infarct. For example, occlusion of the right coronary artery would have different consequences in an individual whose

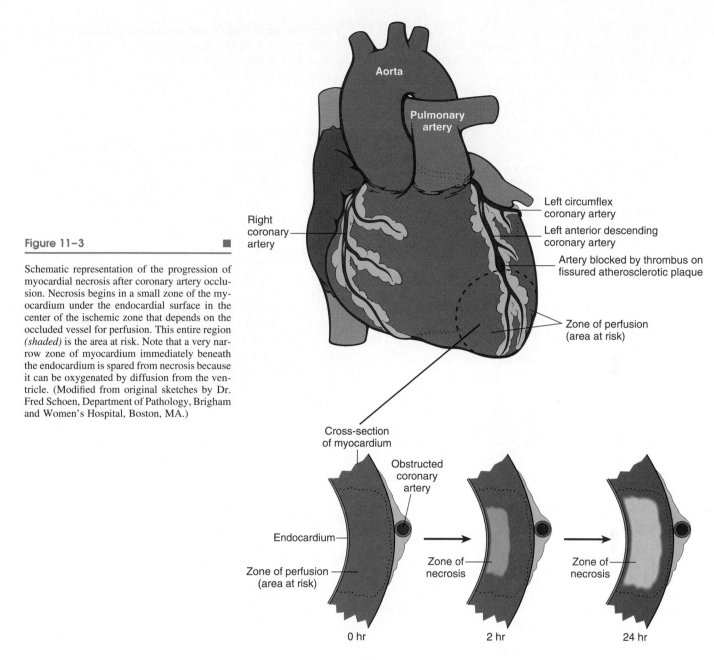

Figure 11–3 ■

Schematic representation of the progression of myocardial necrosis after coronary artery occlusion. Necrosis begins in a small zone of the myocardium under the endocardial surface in the center of the ischemic zone that depends on the occluded vessel for perfusion. This entire region *(shaded)* is the area at risk. Note that a very narrow zone of myocardium immediately beneath the endocardium is spared from necrosis because it can be oxygenated by diffusion from the ventricle. (Modified from original sketches by Dr. Fred Schoen, Department of Pathology, Brigham and Women's Hospital, Boston, MA.)

posterior ventricle was supplied by branches of the right coronary (right dominant circulation) than in a person whose posterior wall was supplied by branches of the circumflex coronary artery (left dominant circulation).

The size of the infarct is influenced by several factors. In general, occlusion of more proximal segments of the coronary arteries produces larger infarcts, involving the full thickness of the myocardium. Conversely, thrombi in more distal arterial branches tend to cause smaller infarcts. The extent of the infarct is also influenced by the degree of collateral circulation that exists at the time of the occlusion. In patients with longstanding coronary atherosclerosis, collateral circulation may develop over time in response to chronic ischemia. Such collateral vessels may limit the size of the infarct, particularly in the epicardial regions of the myocardium.

MORPHOLOGY. The appearance of a myocardial infarct is determined primarily by its age. The essential sequence of events, which are reviewed in more detail below, is that of **coagulation necrosis and inflammation,** followed by the **formation of granulation tissue, resorption of the necrotic myocardium,** and, finally, **organization of the granulation tissue to form a fibrous scar.** These events occur in a fairly predictable pattern, allowing one to estimate the age of a given infarct from its gross and microscopic appearance. It should be noted, however, that other factors may modify the appearance of an infarct. Because smaller infarcts tend to heal more rapidly than larger lesions, the morphology of a myocardial infarct is also influenced by its **size.** Other variables, such as **recurrent infarcts** in the same territory, and **reperfusion** of necrotic myocardium after fibrinolysis or surgical removal of the coronary thrombus, also affect the appearance of a myocardial infarct.

The frequencies of occlusion of various coronary arteries and the distribution of the resultant infarcts are as follows:

Left anterior descending coronary artery (40%–50%)	Anterior and apical left ventricle; anterior two thirds of the interventricular septum
Right coronary artery (30%–40%)	Posterior wall of the left ventricle; posterior one third of the interventricular septum (in persons with right-dominant coronary circulation)
Left circumflex coronary artery (15%–20%)	Lateral wall of left ventricle (may also involve the posterior wall in persons with left-dominant coronary circulation)

Myocardial infarcts may involve most of the thickness of the ventricular wall, in which case they are termed **transmural infarcts,** while those restricted to the inner one third of the myocardium are designated **subendocardial infarcts.** Virtually all transmural infarcts involve the left ventricle (including the interventricular septum). Sometimes those in the posterior wall and septum extend into the adjacent right ventricular wall. Isolated infarction of the right ventricle or the atria is rare.

The morphologic changes associated with MI are listed in Table 11–1. **For the first 12 hours,** no changes are evident on gross examination. Between 18 and 24 hours, a slight pallor may be noted. Microscopically, **coagulation necrosis** becomes apparent by about 12 to 18 hours, at which time the cytoplasm of the necrotic myocytes becomes increasingly eosinophilic, with a loss of cross-striations, while the nuclei begin to undergo fragmentation (karyorrhexis) or contraction (pyknosis). **Neutrophils** are attracted by the necrotic myocardium, and a neutrophilic infiltrate becomes apparent during the initial 18 to 24 hours. Neutrophils are present in all myocardial infarcts by 48 hours, reach a peak on days 5 to 6, and subsequently diminish. Some degree of hemorrhage may be present but is usually not extensive unless lysis or mechanical removal of the coronary thrombus has permitted reperfusion of the necrotic zone. At the periphery of the infarct, some myocytes may contain brightly eosinophilic, coarse, transverse bands termed **contraction**

Table 11–1. SEQUENCE OF CHANGES IN MYOCARDIAL INFARCTION

Time	Gross	Light Microscope	Electron Microscope	Other
0–30 min	No change	No change	*Reversible* changes (mitochondrial swelling, relaxation of myofibrils)	Loss of enzyme activity; glycogen loss
1–2 hr	No change	Few "wavy" fibers at margin of infarct	*Irreversible* changes (sarcolemmal disruption, electron-dense mitochondrial deposits)	
4–12 hr	No change	Early coagulation necrosis; edema; occasional neutrophils; minimal hemorrhage		
18–24 hr	Slight pallor	Continuing coagulation necrosis (nuclear pyknosis and disintegration; cytoplasmic eosinophilia); "contraction band" necrosis at periphery of infarct; neutrophilic infiltrate		
24–72 hr	Pallor	Complete coagulation necrosis of myofibers; heavy neutrophilic infiltrate with early fragmentation of neutrophil nuclei		
4–7 days	Central pallor with hyperemic border	Macrophages appear; early disintegration and phagocytosis of necrotic fibers; granulation tissue visible at edge of infarct		
10 days	Maximally yellow, soft, shrunken; purple border	Well-developed phagocytosis; prominent granulation tissue in peripheral areas of infarct		
7–8 wk	Firm, gray	Fibrosis		

bands. These structures, produced by hypercontraction of myofibrils in dying cells, are induced by the influx of calcium ions from the plasma into cells with damaged cell membranes (Fig. 11–4). Hence, contraction bands tend to be more prominent when there is early reperfusion of the ischemic area. A thin zone of residual viable myocytes is usually present immediately beneath the surface of the endocardium, where direct diffusion of nutrients from the ventricular cavity is sufficient to sustain the cells. However, cells in this immediate subendocardial area are not completely normal; they often assume a vacuolated appearance, termed **myocytolysis,** resulting from influx of water across injured cell membranes.

By days 4 to 5, the infarct appears grossly as a pale, firm, fairly well-defined region with a hyperemic border (Fig. 11–5). Macrophages, fibroblasts, and capillaries first appear at the margins of the infarct on about the fourth day, migrating progressively toward the center of the lesion over the next several weeks. During this period, macrophages begin to phagocytize the necrotic myocytes.

By day 10, the necrotic area is yellow, soft, and sunken; the granulation tissue is visible grossly at the edge of the infarct as a red-purple zone. Microscopically, the periphery of the infarct has been replaced by granulation tissue. Pigmented macrophages, laden with the remnants of necrotic myocytes, are present in large numbers. Early maturation of the granulation tissue is manifested by the appearance of collagen fibers at the periphery of the infarct.

Phagocytosis of necrotic myocytes and maturation of granulation tissue continue over the next

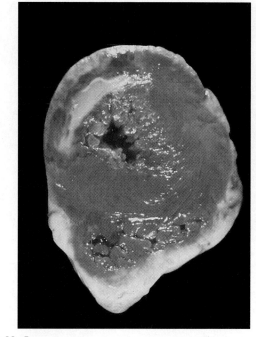

Figure 11–5   ■

Acute MI, 5 to 7 days old. The infarct is visible as a well-demarcated, pale yellow lesion in the posterolateral region of the left ventricle. The border of the infarct is accentuated by a dark red zone of acute inflammation.

several weeks. **By the end of the fourth week,** virtually all of the necrotic myocardium has been resorbed, with only a few residual islands visible microscopically. As the granulation tissue matures, its vascularity diminishes, while the amount of collagen increases. **By approximately the eighth week,** most infarcts have been replaced by dense scar tissue and can be considered healed. The ventricular wall is thinned, firm, and gray at the site of the healed infarct (Fig. 11–6).

Several important complications may be encountered in patients who have suffered myocardial infarcts, particularly if they are **transmural.** These occur at different times during the evolution of the infarct and can be summarized as follows:

■ **Papillary muscle dysfunction** occurs frequently in patients with MIs. In most cases, it is caused by local bulging of the injured left ventricular wall at the site of attachment of the papillary muscle, ischemia and impaired contractility of the papillary muscle, or generalized dilation of the left ventricle in the setting of heart failure. Less commonly (less than 1% of cases of MI), **an infarcted papillary muscle may rupture,** with resultant detachment of the chordae tendineae and severe mitral insufficiency. Papillary muscle rupture is most common about 3 days after the development of the infarct. It causes acute left ventricular failure and is associated with a high rate of mortality.

■ **External rupture of the infarct** occurs in up to 13%

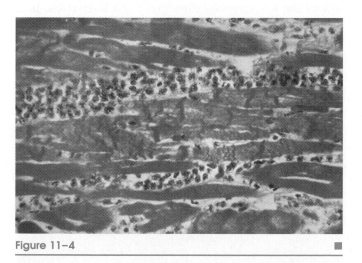

Figure 11–4   ■

Photomicrograph of a 48-hour-old myocardial infarct (MI). The cardiac muscle fibers are brightly eosinophilic owing to coagulative necrosis, and an infiltrate of neutrophils is seen in between the fibers. In addition, the myocardial fibers show contraction bands in the form of deeply stained transverse bands. (Courtesy of Dr. Sid Murphree, Department of Pathology, University of Texas Southwestern Medical School, Dallas, TX.)

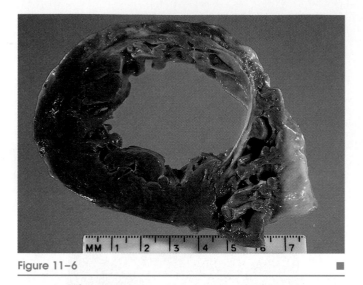

Figure 11–6 ■

Healed MI. By about 2 months, the necrotic myocardium has been completely replaced by dense scar tissue, visible here as a thinned gray area in the left ventricular myocardium.

of cases of MI. This catastrophic event may occur at any time during the first 2 weeks of the infarct, but it is most common between days 4 and 7, when extensive softening of the myocardium has occurred but granulation tissue and fibrosis are poorly developed. The rupture usually develops over the course of several days, during which time blood dissects progressively through the soft, necrotic myocardium (Fig. 11–7). Rupture through the epicardial surface causes massive hemopericardium, with resultant cardiac tamponade. Less commonly (1% to 3% of cases of MI), **rupture of the intraventricular septum** may occur. It causes an acute left-to-right shunt, with resultant CHF.

■ **Mural thrombi,** which may develop on the endocardial surface overlying an infarct, are potential sources for systemic emboli and their complications, such as brain infarcts. Such thrombi are particularly common in patients who develop a ventricular aneurysm (discussed below). Organization of mural thrombi typically produces an area of dense endocardial fibrosis.

■ Clinically apparent **acute pericarditis** occurs in up to 15% of patients with MI within 2 to 4 days after the development of a transmural infarct. It may cause a significant pericardial effusion.

■ **Ventricular aneurysms** are a late complication of large transmural MIs and are caused by the bulging of the noncontractile fibrous myocardium during systole. They are most common in the anteroapical region of the heart, where they appear as a thin-walled, fibrous outpouching of the ventricular wall (Fig. 11–8). A mural thrombus is often present. In addition to serving as a source of emboli, ventricular aneurysms may cause congestive heart failure, papillary muscle dysfunction, and recurrent arrhythmias. Surgical resection is beneficial in some cases.

Clinical Features. The onset of MI is usually accompanied by severe, crushing substernal chest pain, which may radiate to the neck, jaw, epigastrum, shoulder, or left arm. In about 50% of patients the MI is preceded by episodes of angina pectoris. In contrast to the pain of angina pectoris, however, the pain associated with an MI typically lasts several hours to days and is not significantly relieved by nitroglycerin. The pulse is generally rapid and weak, and patients are often diaphoretic. Dyspnea is common and is caused by impaired contractility of the ischemic myocardium, with resultant pulmonary congestion and edema. With massive MIs involving over 40% of the left ventricle, cardiogenic shock develops. In a

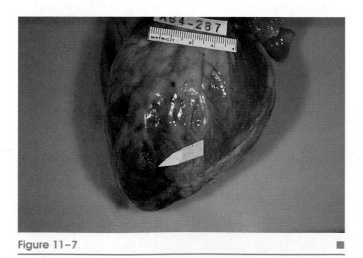

Figure 11–7 ■

Myocardial rupture 6 days after an MI. The patient developed a cardiac tamponade and died. (From the teaching collection of the Pathology Department, University of Texas Southwestern Medical School, Dallas, TX.)

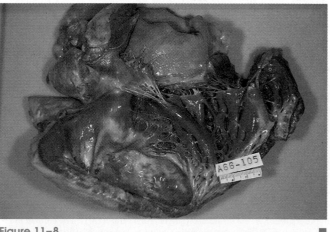

Figure 11–8 ■

Healed MI with a ventricular aneurysm. The aneurysm is visible as a thin-walled outpouching of the ventricular wall. Such aneurysms are often complicated by thrombosis, arrhythmias, and heart failure.

sizable minority of patients (20% to 30%) the MI does not cause chest pain. Such "silent" MIs are particularly common in patients with underlying diabetes mellitus and hypertension, and in elderly patients.

Electrocardiographic abnormalities are an important manifestation of MI. These include changes such as Q waves, ST-segment abnormalities, and T-wave inversion. Arrhythmias caused by electrical abnormalities of the ischemic myocardium and by conduction disturbances are common.

After the onset of an acute ischemic event, one of several pathways may be followed. Regrettably, one pathway is very brief: sudden coronary death caused by a ventricular arrhythmia (25% of patients). Of patients who reach the hospital, approximately 10% to 20% experience no complications. The remaining 80% to 90% develop one or more of the following:

- Cardiac arrhythmias (75% to 95%)
- Left ventricular failure with mild to severe pulmonary edema (60%)
- Cardiogenic shock (10%)
- Rupture of free wall, septum, papillary muscle (4% to 8%)
- Thromboembolism (15% to 49%)

Laboratory evaluation is an integral part of the clinical management of a suspected MI. A number of enzymes and other proteins are released into the circulation by dying myocardial cells. Measurement of the level of some of these molecules in the serum is helpful in the diagnosis of myocardial infarcts. The various myocardial markers used to monitor the evolution of MI, and their patterns of elevation, are summarized below:

- *Creatine kinase (CK)* is an enzyme that is highly concentrated in brain, myocardium, and skeletal muscle. The enzyme is composed of two dimers designated "M" and "B." CK-MM is derived predominantly from skeletal muscle and heart; CK-BB from brain, lung, and many other tissues; and CK-MB principally from myocardium, although variable amounts of the MB form are also present in skeletal muscle. *Total CK activity* begins to rise within 2 to 4 hours of an MI, peaks at 24, and returns to normal within approximately 72 hours. Although *total CK activity is one of the most sensitive determinants of acute myocardial necrosis, it is not specific,* because CK is also elevated in other conditions, such as skeletal muscle injury. The specificity for the detection of MI is enhanced by measurement of the CK-MB fraction. CK-MB rises within 2 to 4 hours of the onset of an MI, peaks at 18 hours, and usually disappears by 48 hours. Although minor elevations of CK-MB occur in patients with extensive skeletal muscle injury, the amount of CK-MB relative to total CK is much higher in MI than in any other condition in which the CK level is elevated. This is sometimes expressed as a CK index. *An absence of a change in the levels of CK and CK-MB during the first 2 days after the development of chest pain essentially excludes the diagnosis of MI.*
- *Lactate dehydrogenase (LD)* is another myocardial enzyme that has been used extensively in the past to evaluate suspected MIs. Total LD activity begins to rise within 24 hours of an MI, peaks at approximately 72 hours, and persists for about a week. LD is present in a large number of tissues in addition to myocardium, including skeletal muscle, erythrocytes, kidney, liver, and lung. Hence, the diagnostic value of total LD measurements is limited by lack of specificity. Like CK, LD exists in several different isoforms, and measurement of specific LD isoenzymes can enhance its specificity. Myocardium is particularly rich in the LD-1 isoenzyme, and thus the level of the LD-1 isoenzyme relative to the level of the LD-2 isoenzyme is more useful than assay of total LD levels alone. With the introduction of troponin assays, the measurement of LD levels for the diagnosis of MI is becoming obsolete.

- More recently, *determinations of serum levels of certain myocardial proteins* have shown great promise in the evaluation of suspected MI. *Troponins* are contractile proteins found in human skeletal and cardiac muscle. Different isoforms of these proteins exist in mature skeletal muscle and myocardium. By the use of sensitive immunologic assays, it has been possible to distinguish cardiac troponin T (cTnT) and troponin I (cTnI) from troponins of skeletal muscle origin. Cardiac troponin I is only found in heart muscle during adult life, and is thus more specific than CK-MB, which is also found in skeletal muscles in small proportion. Cardiac troponin I is not detected in serum after pure skeletal muscle injury, and is therefore a reliable marker of myocardial necrosis, even when confounding skeletal muscle injury exists. After an acute MI, both cTnT and cTnI levels rise at about the same time as CK-MB. The diagnostic sensitivity of cardiac troponin measurements is similar to that of CK-MB in the early stages of acute MI. However, troponin levels remain elevated for 4 to 7 days after the acute event, allowing the diagnosis of an acute MI long after CK-MB levels have returned to normal. Both cTnT and cTnI levels have also been shown to have prognostic value in patients with unstable angina, elevated levels correlating with the subsequent development of acute MI. *Of the two cardiac troponins, cTnI is more cardiospecific than cTnT.*

Chronic Ischemic Heart Disease

The term *chronic ischemic heart disease,* sometimes called *ischemic cardiomyopathy,* is used to describe the development of progressive congestive heart failure as a consequence of long-term ischemic myocardial injury. Many cases are associated with a history of angina pectoris and may be preceded by recognized infarcts. In other cases the condition may develop more insidiously.

MORPHOLOGY. The coronary arteries invariably contain areas of **moderate to severe atherosclerosis.** The heart is **enlarged,** sometimes to a striking degree, secondary to **dilation of all cardiac chambers.** Multiple areas of **myocardial fibrosis,** often including foci of transmural scarring, are usually present. A moderate degree of **hypertrophy** of the remaining myocardium is common. Despite the hypertrophy, however, wall thickness may be normal because of the concomitant dilation. The endocardium is thick and opaque, and thrombi in varying stages of organization may be adherent to the endocardial surface. Microscopy reveals extensive myocardial fibrosis, due to chronic ischemia. Among the remaining myocytes, both atrophic and hypertrophic fibers are present. Vacuolation of the sarcoplasm of some myofibers is common, particularly in the subendocardial areas.

Clinical Features. Chronic ischemic heart disease is characterized by the development of severe, progressive heart failure, sometimes punctuated by episodes of angina pectoris or MI. Arrhythmias are common and, along with congestive heart failure and intercurrent MI, account for many deaths. This form of ischemic heart disease may be difficult to distinguish clinically from dilated cardiomyopathy (p 330).

Sudden Cardiac Death

Sudden death has been defined in many different ways, ranging from instantaneous death to death occurring within 24 hours of the onset of symptoms. Excluded from most definitions of sudden death are events such as homicide, suicide, accidental trauma, and exposure to lethal toxins. Sudden death can be caused by a wide range of diseases, including heart disease, pulmonary embolism, ruptured aortic aneurysm, disorders of the central nervous system, and infections. *Most cases of sudden death in the Western world are caused by heart disease.* Sudden cardiac death accounts for approximately 300,000 deaths each year in the United States and for about 50% of all deaths caused by cardiovascular disease. The major forms of cardiac diseases associated with sudden death are listed in Table 11-2. *The most common cause of sudden cardiac death is ischemic heart disease.* Chronic ischemia predisposes the myocardium to the development of lethal ventricular arrhythmias, usually in the form of ventricular fibrillation, which is the most common cause of sudden death in these cases. In some cases, sudden death is preceded by other

■

Table 11-2. CARDIAC CAUSES OF SUDDEN DEATH

Coronary artery diseases
Coronary atherosclerosis
Developmental abnormalities (anomalous origin, hypoplasia)
Coronary artery embolism
Other (vasculitis, dissection)

Myocardial diseases
Cardiomyopathies
Myocarditis and other infiltrative processes
Right ventricular dysplasia

Valvular diseases
Mitral valve prolapse
Aortic stenosis and other forms of left ventricular outflow obstruction
Endocarditis

Conduction system abnormalities

Modified from Virmani R, Roberts WC: Sudden cardiac death. Hum Pathol 18: 485, 1987.

---

clinical manifestations of myocardial ischemia. Tragically, however, sudden death is the initial manifestation of ischemic heart disease in about 50% of patients with the disease.

MORPHOLOGY. The most common cardiac lesions in sudden death are those of coronary atherosclerosis and its complications. In most cases the degree of atherosclerosis is marked, with more than 75% reduction in the cross-sectional area of two or more vessels. The proximate cause of sudden cardiac death is not entirely clear in many cases. According to some studies, acute plaque rupture followed by coronary thrombosis and possibly vasospasm triggers fatal ventricular arrhythmias. However, according to other studies, occlusive thrombi are present in less than half of all patients and are uncommon in patients who collapse and die instantaneously. Other morphologic manifestations of ischemic heart disease, such as recent or remote myocardial infarcts, patchy myocardial fibrosis, wavy fiber change, or contraction band necrosis, are usually present. Other structural cardiac abnormalities have also been associated with sudden death and should be carefully sought in cases of sudden death associated with minimal atherosclerosis. These changes include various primary myocardial disorders (discussed later), conduction system abnormalities, and developmental abnormalities of the coronary arteries.

Summary of Ischemic Heart Disease. *Cardiac ischemia resulting from atherosclerosis of the coronary arteries may present with several well-defined but somewhat overlapping syndromes (Fig. 11-9). Typical angina results from an increased myocardial oxygen demand that cannot be met owing to fixed critical stenosis of the coronary arteries. The three acute coronary syndromes (unstable angina, acute MI, and, possibly, sudden cardiac death) seem to result from acute changes in fixed atherosclerotic lesions. In unstable angina, a small fissure or rupture of an atherosclerotic plaque triggers platelet aggregation, vasoconstriction, and formation of a mural thrombus that may not be occlusive; thus, there is severe but transient reduction in myocardial oxygenation. Acute MI occurs when complete thrombotic occlusion is superimposed on acute plaque disruption. Sometimes acute plaque rupture and the resultant thrombosis and vasospasm induce a rapidly fatal arrhythmia that causes sudden cardiac death. Finally, in some patients, chronic and progressive coronary atherosclerosis causes gradual loss of myocardium that eventuates in congestive heart failure. Such patients are diagnosed as having chronic ischemic heart disease.*

HYPERTENSIVE HEART DISEASE

As discussed in Chapter 10, chronic hypertension is a common disorder associated with considerable morbidity. Inadequately controlled hypertension has serious effects on many

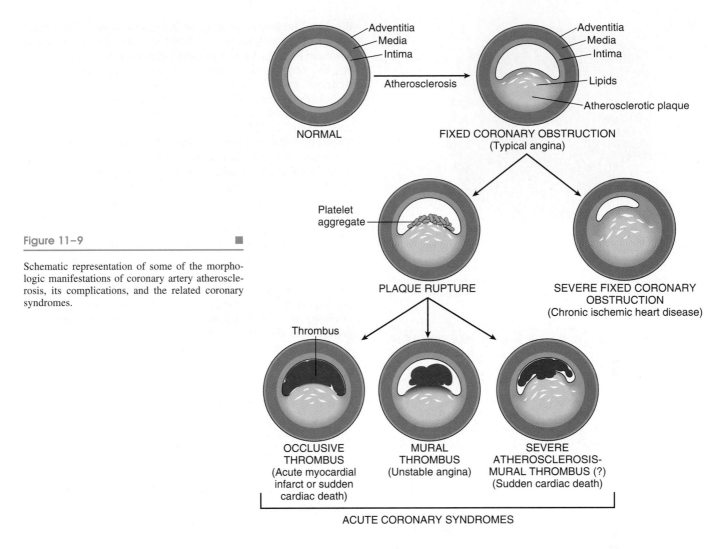

Figure 11–9 ■

Schematic representation of some of the morphologic manifestations of coronary artery atherosclerosis, its complications, and the related coronary syndromes.

organs, including the heart, brain, and kidneys. Our comments here will focus on the cardiac complications of this disorder. Other effects of hypertension are discussed elsewhere in the text, along with other diseases of specific organs.

The diagnosis of hypertensive heart disease is based on the presence of *left ventricular hypertrophy in an individual with a history of hypertension,* and in whom other causes of ventricular hypertrophy (e.g., aortic stenosis or primary hypertrophic cardiomyopathy) have been excluded. The stimulus to ventricular hypertrophy in patients with hypertension is a sustained pressure load on the left ventricular myocardium. The cellular events leading to myocardial hypertrophy are poorly understood but appear to involve both local mechanical effects and growth factors, which lead in turn to changes in the genes controlling the expression of myosin, actin, and other cellular constituents.

The *metabolic requirements* of hypertrophic myocardium, understandably, are greater than those of normal myocardium. With increasing hypertrophy, the metabolic requirements continue to increase but the ability of the heart to meet these demands decreases. This occurs because hypertrophy renders the myocardium stiff, and therefore ventricular compliance and stroke volume are decreased. At the same time, the dis-

tance over which oxygen and other nutrients delivered by the capillaries must diffuse is increased. To make matters worse, chronic hypertension also predisposes to atherosclerosis. In concert, these various changes predispose the hypertrophic myocardium to ischemic injury, eventually resulting in the development of congestive heart failure, myocardial infarcts, or arrhythmias.

MORPHOLOGY. The essential feature of hypertensive heart disease is **left ventricular hypertrophy.** The hypertrophy typically involves the wall in a symmetric, circumferential pattern termed **concentric hypertrophy** (Fig. 11–10). The weight of the heart usually exceeds 450 gm. On occasion, particularly in long-standing cases, hypertrophy may be more pronounced in the septal area, mimicking the appearance of hypertrophic cardiomyopathy (discussed later). The size of the chamber is normal in the early stages of hypertensive heart disease, but in long-standing cases some degree of dilation is common. As left ventricular failure

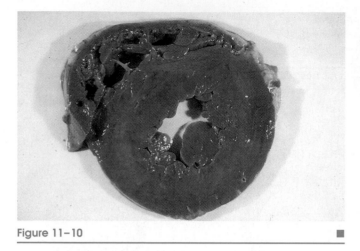

Figure 11-10 ■

Concentric left ventricular hypertrophy in a patient with longstanding hypertension. Any process, including systemic hypertension, that imposes a chronic pressure load on the left ventricle can cause similar changes.

progresses, right ventricular hypertrophy and dilation may also develop. Coronary artery disease is present in most cases, with its associated morphologic effects on the myocardium. Microscopically, the cardiac myocytes are enlarged and contain large, hyperchromatic, "boxcar"-shaped nuclei. The nuclear changes are caused by tetraploidy, presumably reflecting abortive attempts at cell replication. Superimposed ischemic changes, including interstitial fibrosis and recent or remote infarcts, are common.

Clinical Features. In its early stages, while the cardiac output is maintained at normal levels, hypertensive heart disease may cause no symptoms. In these patients, the diagnosis is usually based on the detection of left ventricular enlargement in chest radiographs or echocardiograms, or by electrocardiographic evidence of left ventricular hypertrophy. As the left ventricle begins to fail, the clinical manifestations of heart failure appear. Heart failure in the setting of hypertension is associated with a poor prognosis, with only 50% of patients surviving 5 years after diagnosis. Signs and symptoms of myocardial ischemia, such as angina pectoris, often punctuate the course of hypertensive cardiac disease. In addition, progressive renal damage or cerebrovascular accidents may occur. The risk of sudden cardiac death is also increased.

COR PULMONALE

The term *cor pulmonale,* or *pulmonary heart disease*, is used to describe disease of the right-sided cardiac chambers caused by pulmonary hypertension resulting from pulmonary parenchymal or pulmonary vascular disease. Excluded from this definition are cases of pulmonary hypertension caused by left ventricular failure or other primary diseases of the left heart, and pulmonary hypertension caused by congenital heart disease. The condition may be acute or chronic. The major causes of cor pulmonale are listed in Table 11–3, the more common being pulmonary emboli, chronic obstructive and restrictive lung diseases, and pulmonary vascular diseases.

Acute cor pulmonale is most often caused by pulmonary embolism. When emboli acutely obstruct more than 50% of the pulmonary vascular bed, the sudden increase in the burden on the right side of the heart causes right ventricular failure. The right ventricle is typically dilated but is not hypertrophied.

Chronic cor pulmonale can be caused by any of the diseases listed in Table 11–3, all of which cause pulmonary hypertension. Of these, the *most common cause is chronic obstructive lung disease* (Chapter 13). In chronic cor pulmonale, in contrast to acute cor pulmonale, sustained pulmonary hypertension allows sufficient time for the development of compensatory right ventricular hypertrophy. Over time, as in the case of left ventricular failure in patients with systemic hypertension, the right ventricle progressively dilates and is ultimately unable to maintain cardiac output at normal levels. When this occurs, symptoms and signs typical of congestive heart failure develop. Acute decompensation may occur at any point in a patient with chronic cor pulmonale.

MORPHOLOGY. In isolated **acute cor pulmonale**, the right ventricle is usually dilated. However, if sudden death occurs, for example, after massive pulmonary embolism, the heart may appear normal in size. **Chronic cor pulmonale** is characterized by right ventricular, and often right atrial, hypertrophy. In extreme cases, the thickness of the right ventricular wall may exceed that of the left ventricle. When ventricular failure develops, the right ventricle and atrium may also be dilated. Such dilation may mask right ventricular hypertro-

Table 11-3. DISORDERS THAT PREDISPOSE TO COR PULMONALE

Diseases of the lungs
Chronic obstructive lung disease
Diffuse pulmonary interstitial fibrosis
Extensive persistent atelectasis
Cystic fibrosis

Diseases of pulmonary vessels
Pulmonary embolism
Primary pulmonary vascular sclerosis
Extensive pulmonary arteritis (e.g., Wegener's granulomatosis)
Drug-, toxin-, or radiation-induced vascular sclerosis

Disorders affecting chest movement
Kyphoscoliosis
Marked obesity (pickwickian syndrome)
Neuromuscular diseases

Disorders inducing pulmonary arteriolar constriction
Metabolic acidosis
Hypoxemia
Chronic altitude sickness
Obstruction to major airways
Idiopathic alveolar hypoventilation

phy. However, the weight of the heart is increased. Because chronic cor pulmonale occurs in the setting of chronically elevated pulmonary arterial pressure, the pulmonary arteries often contain atheromatous plaques and other lesions of pulmonary hypertension (Chapter 13).

■ VALVULAR HEART DISEASES

Diseases of the heart valves include a diverse group of acquired and congenital lesions. Some of these occur in isolation and others in association with other heart diseases. In this section, we will devote our attention to primary valvular diseases. Valvular lesions that occur in association with congenital cardiac malformations will be considered later, along with other congenital heart diseases. Syphilis, an important cause of aortic valve disease, is discussed in Chapter 10 along with other disorders of the aorta.

Deformed cardiac valves may cause disease by two major mechanisms. First, *they impose a major hemodynamic burden on the cardiac chambers* by causing obstruction (stenosis) or regurgitation (incompetence), or sometimes a combination of the two. Second, the *abnormal valves are more susceptible to infection* and thus predispose patients to infective endocarditis and its many complications. The important forms of acquired valvular disease affecting the mitral and aortic valves are listed in Table 11–4. With the possible exception of infective endocarditis, lesions of the tricuspid and pulmonic valves are much less common; therefore, most of our discussion will focus on diseases of the aortic and mitral valves.

Rheumatic Fever and Heart Disease

Rheumatic fever is an acute, immunologically mediated, multisystem inflammatory disease that follows, after a few weeks, an episode of group A streptococcal pharyngitis. It is interesting to note that rheumatic fever does not follow infections by similar streptococci at other sites, such as the skin. The incidence and mortality rate of rheumatic fever have declined remarkably in many parts of the world over the past 30 years thanks to improved socioeconomic conditions, rapid diagnosis and treatment of streptococcal pharyngitis, and an unexplained decrease in the virulence of group A streptococci. Nevertheless, in third world countries, and in many crowded, economically depressed urban areas in the Western world, rheumatic fever remains an important public health problem. Rheumatic fever may cause heart disease during its acute phase (*acute rheumatic carditis*), or it may cause *chronic valvular deformities* that may not manifest themselves until many years after the acute disease. Fortunately, rheumatic fever occurs in only about 3% of patients with group A streptococcal pharyngitis. However, after an initial attack, there is increased vulnerability to reactivation of the disease with subsequent pharyngeal infections.

The pathogenesis of acute rheumatic fever and its chronic sequelae is not fully understood. It is strongly suspected that *acute rheumatic fever is a hypersensitivity reaction induced by group A streptococci.* It is proposed that antibodies directed against the M proteins of certain strains of streptococci cross-react with tissue glycoproteins in the heart, joints, and other tissues. The onset of symptoms 2 to 3 weeks after infection and the absence of streptococci from the lesions support the concept that rheumatic fever results from an immune response against the offending bacteria. Because the nature of cross-reacting antigens has been difficult to define, it has also been suggested that the streptococcal infection evokes an autoimmune response against self-antigens. The major aspects of the pathogenesis and morphology of rheumatic carditis are summarized in Figure 11–11.

Table 11–4.	MAJOR ETIOLOGIES OF ACQUIRED HEART VALVE DISEASE	

Mitral Valve Disease	Aortic Valve Disease
Mitral Stenosis	**Aortic Stenosis**
Postinflammatory scarring (rheumatic heart disease)	Postinflammatory scarring (rheumatic heart disease)
	Senile calcific aortic stenosis
	Calcification of congenitally deformed valve
Mitral Regurgitation	**Aortic Regurgitation**
Abnormalities of leaflets and commissures	Intrinsic valvular disease
Postinflammatory scarring	Postinflammatory scarring (rheumatic heart disease)
Infective endocarditis	Infective endocarditis
Mitral valve prolapse	Aortic disease
Abnormalities of tensor apparatus	Degenerative aortic dilation
Rupture of papillary muscle	Syphilitic aortitis
Papillary muscle dysfunction (fibrosis)	Ankylosing spondylitis
Rupture of chordae tendineae	Rheumatoid arthritis
Abnormalities of left ventricular cavity and/or annulus	Marfan syndrome
Left ventricular enlargement (myocarditis, congestive cardiomyopathy)	
Calcification of mitral ring	

Modified from Schoen FJ: Surgical pathology of removed natural and prosthetic valves. Hum Pathol 18:558, 1987.

MORPHOLOGY. In **acute rheumatic fever,** inflammatory infiltrates may occur in a wide range of sites, including synovium, joints, skin, and (most important) the heart. The initial tissue reaction is that of focal fibrinoid necrosis. This provokes a mixed inflammatory response, which may take the form of either a diffuse cellular infiltrate or a localized aggregation of cells that resembles a granuloma. Areas of fibrosis eventually develop at sites of inflammation. **Fibrosis is particularly common in cardiac tissues,** where it is responsible for the valvular deformities seen in chronic rheumatic heart disease.

Acute rheumatic carditis is characterized by inflammatory changes in all three layers of the

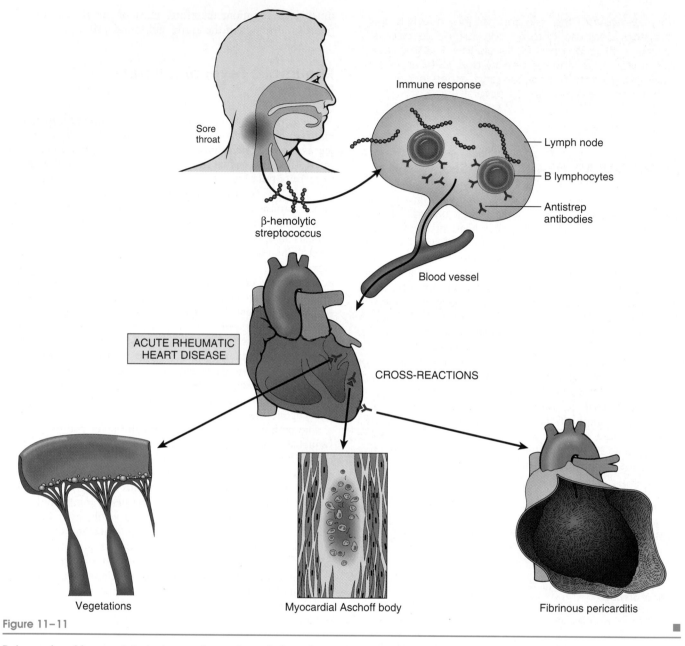

Sore throat

β-hemolytic streptococcus

Immune response

Lymph node

B lymphocytes

Antistrep antibodies

Blood vessel

ACUTE RHEUMATIC HEART DISEASE

CROSS-REACTIONS

Vegetations

Myocardial Aschoff body

Fibrinous pericarditis

Figure 11–11 ■

Pathogenesis and key morphologic changes of acute rheumatic heart disease. Acute rheumatic fever causes changes in the endocardium, myocardium, and epicardium. Chronic rheumatic heart disease is almost always caused by deformity of the heart valves, particularly the mitral and aortic valves.

heart, and thus is appropriately designated a pan-carditis. The hallmark of acute rheumatic carditis is the presence of multiple foci of inflammation within the connective tissues of the heart, termed **Aschoff bodies** (Fig. 11–12). They contain a central focus of fibrinoid necrosis, surrounded by a chronic mononuclear inflammatory infiltrate, and occasional large histiocytes with vesicular nuclei and abundant basophilic cytoplasm, termed **Anitschkow cells.** Aschoff bodies may be found anywhere in the connective tissues of the heart. In the myocardium, they often lie in close proximity to a small vessel and may encroach on its wall. In ad-

dition to Aschoff bodies, the myocardium may also contain diffuse interstitial inflammatory infiltrates. In severely affected cases, the myocarditis may result in generalized dilation of the cardiac chambers. **Pericardial involvement** is manifested grossly and microscopically by the presence of fibrinous pericarditis, sometimes associated with a serous or serosanguineous pericardial effusion. Involvement of the **endocardium** is common and may affect any valve. However, valvular inflammation tends to be most pronounced in the mitral and aortic valves. The affected valves are edematous and thickened and show foci of fibrinoid

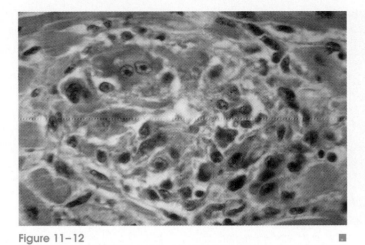

Figure 11-12

Aschoff body in a patient who died of acute rheumatic carditis. In the interstitium of the myocardium there is a circumscribed (granulomatous) collection of mononuclear inflammatory cells. There are some large histiocytes with prominent nucleoli, and a prominent binucleate histiocyte. The central necrosis seen within these lesions is not prominent in this field. (Courtesy of Sid Murphree, M.D. Department of Pathology, University of Texas Southwestern Medical School, Dallas, TX.)

necrosis, but Aschoff nodules are not common. The inflammation of the valve predisposes to the formation of small vegetations, seen as wartlike excrescences, particularly along the lines of valve closure (**verrucous endocarditis**) (Fig. 11-13). The acute changes may resolve without sequelae or may progress to cause significant scarring and chronic valvular deformities, described below. Changes encountered in other organs include nonspecific **arthritis of the large joints,** characterized by chronic inflammatory infiltrates and edema in the involved joints and periarticular soft tissues. In contrast to the cardiac lesions, the arthri-

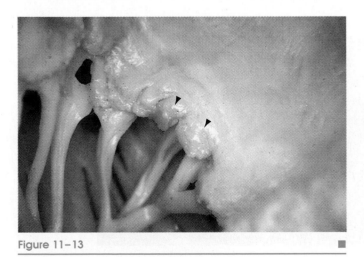

Figure 11-13

Acute rheumatic mitral valvulitis superimposed on chronic rheumatic heart disease. Small vegetations are visible along the line of closure of the mitral valve leaflet *(arrows).* Previous episodes of rheumatic valvulitis have caused fibrous thickening and fusion of the chordae tendineae.

tis is self-limited and does not cause chronic deformity. **Pulmonary involvement** is uncommon; it is manifested by chronic interstitial inflammatory infiltrates and fibrinous inflammation of the pleural surface. **Skin changes** take the form of **subcutaneous nodules** or **erythema marginatum.** Microscopically, the skin nodules reveal focal lesions that are essentially large Aschoff bodies. Erythema marginatum is seen as a maculopapular rash.

Chronic rheumatic heart disease is characterized by irreversible deformity of one or more cardiac valves, resulting from previous episodes of acute valvulitis. Valves on the left side of the heart are involved more frequently than those on the right side. Scarring of the valve leaflets may cause a reduction in the diameter of the valve orifice (**stenosis**), or it may prevent proper closure of the valve leaflets, resulting in **regurgitation** of blood during diastole. Sometimes stenosis and regurgitation coexist, although one hemodynamic defect usually predominates. Valvular stenosis and regurgitation increase the demands on the myocardium because of increased pressure load or volume load, or both, which, if severe enough, eventually causes **cardiac failure.** Damage to the valves also predisposes the patients to superimposed **infective endocarditis.**

Chronic rheumatic mitral valvulitis causes stenosis more often than regurgitation, and it is the most common cause of mitral stenosis. It occurs more frequently in females than in males, for reasons that remain unclear. In **mitral stenosis,** the valve leaflets and chordae tendineae are thick, rigid, and interadherent (Fig. 11-14A). The mitral orifice is narrowed to a slitlike channel, sometimes designated a "fish-mouth" deformity (Fig. 11-14B). The left atrium is dilated and hypertrophied, and the endocardial surface is often thickened, particularly above the posterior mitral leaflet. Mural thrombi may be present (Fig. 11-14B), representing a potential source of systemic emboli. The lungs are firm and heavy as a result of chronic passive congestion, and in long-standing cases the right ventricle and atrium are dilated and hypertrophied as well.

In cases of **mitral regurgitation,** the deformed mitral leaflets are retracted, and the added volume load on the left ventricle causes left ventricular dilation and hypertrophy.

Chronic aortic valvulitis is encountered more often in males than in females. Aortic disease is almost invariably associated with an element of mitral valvulitis. In patients with **aortic stenosis,** the valve cusps are thickened, firm, and adherent to each other, and the resultant aortic valve orifice is reduced to a rigid, triangular channel (Fig. 11-15B). Aortic stenosis places a pressure load on the left ventricle, which undergoes concentric hypertrophy. Subsequent left ventricular failure is associated with dilation of the chamber and other mor-

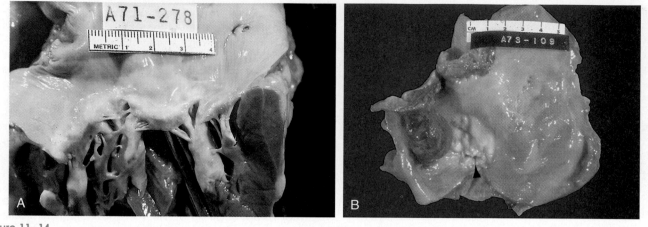

Figure 11–14

Chronic (healed) rheumatic myocarditis. *A,* The mitral valve leaflets are thickened, opaque, and fused at the commissures. The chordae tendineae are also thickened and shortened as a result of fibrosis. *B,* Seen from the left atrial side, the mitral valve appears markedly stenotic, appearing as a pinhole *(arrow).* The opened dilated left atrium contains a large thrombus resulting from stasis of blood in this chamber.

phologic sequelae of congestive heart failure. Fibrosis of the valve leaflets may also cause them to retract toward the aortic wall, resulting in **aortic regurgitation.**

Clinical Features. *Acute rheumatic fever* occurs anywhere from 10 days to 6 weeks after an episode of pharyngitis caused by group A streptococci. Because only a minority of infected patients develop rheumatic fever, genetic susceptibility that regulates the hypersensitivity reaction is suspected. The peak incidence is between the ages of 5 and 15, although younger children and adults may also develop the disease. Although pharyngeal cultures for streptococci are negative by the time the illness begins, antibodies to one or more streptococcal enzymes, such as streptolysin O and DNAse B, are present in the sera of most patients. Reliable assays, such as the Strep-

tozyme test, are widely available for the detection of these antibodies. The predominant clinical manifestations of acute rheumatic fever are those of arthritis and carditis. The *arthritis,* much more common in adults than in children, preferentially occurs in larger joints and tends to involve different joints sequentially (migratory polyarthritis). Clinical features related to *acute carditis* include pericardial friction rubs, weak heart sounds, tachycardia, and arrhythmias. The myocarditis may cause cardiac dilation that may give rise to functional mitral valve insufficiency, or even congestive heart failure. Less than 5% of patients with rheumatic fever succumb to the acute disease.

Chronic rheumatic carditis usually does not cause clinical manifestations for years or even decades after the initial episode of rheumatic fever. The signs and symptoms of valvular disease depend on which cardiac valve or valves are involved. In addition to various cardiac murmurs, cardiac hypertrophy and dilation, and congestive heart failure, patients with

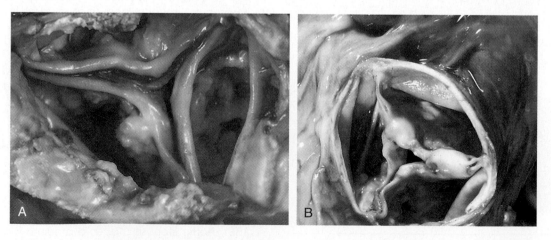

Figure 11–15

Degenerative calcific aortic stenosis. *A,* View from the aortic side of an unopened, markedly deformed tricuspid aortic valve. Calcific masses protrude into the sinuses of Valsalva. Note that the valve commissures are not fused. *B,* In contrast, healed rheumatic aortic valvulitis shows aortic stenosis due to fibrosis and fusion of the valves and the commissures.

chronic rheumatic heart disease may suffer from arrhythmias (particularly atrial fibrillation in the setting of mitral stenosis), thromboembolic complications, and infective endocarditis. Timely surgical replacement of diseased valves has greatly improved the outlook for patients with rheumatic heart disease.

Calcific Aortic Stenosis

Degenerative changes in the cardiac valves are an inevitable part of the aging process. Such changes can be thought of as the valvular counterparts of age-related arteriosclerosis, and they include fibrosis of the valve leaflets, usually accompanied by some degree of calcification. Valve sclerosis occurs most frequently in the aortic and mitral valves. In most cases, age-related valve sclerosis is asymptomatic and is discovered incidentally in chest radiographs or at the time of autopsy. In some patients, the sclerosis may be severe enough to cause clinically apparent disease. *Sclerosis and calcification of the aortic valve is the most common cause of isolated aortic stenosis in the United States.* This lesion, sometimes called *degenerative calcific aortic stenosis (DCAS)*, may occur in a congenitally bicuspid or unicuspid aortic valve, or it may develop in previously normal semilunar valve cusps. Calcification of the mitral valve is usually asymptomatic, but in some cases it may cause conduction disturbances.

> **MORPHOLOGY. In DCAS the aortic valve leaflets are rigid** and **deformed by irregular calcified masses.** The calcium deposits lie behind the valve cusps and extend into the sinus of Valsalva (Fig. 11–15*A*). Stigmata of rheumatic valvulitis, such as fusion of aortic valve commissures, are not present; these features help to distinguish DCAS from chronic rheumatic aortic valvulitis (Fig. 11–15*B*). Degenerative changes in the mitral valve are restricted to fibrosis and calcification along the lines of closure and within the valve annulus. Concentric hypertrophy of the left ventricle and ventricular dilation are commonly seen with long-standing disease.

Clinical Features. Like aortic stenosis in general, the cardinal manifestations of DCAS include angina pectoris, syncope, and (in later stages) congestive heart failure. DCAS arising in a previously normal valve is usually asymptomatic until the eighth or ninth decade. Calcific aortic stenosis may also occur in *congenitally bicuspid* aortic valves, and in these abnormal valves, greater wear and tear leads to earlier degenerative changes. Thus, these lesions become clinically manifest 10 to 20 years earlier than DCAS. Regardless of the cause of aortic stenosis, physical examination discloses a harsh crescendo-decrescendo systolic murmur and left ventricular hypertrophy. *Angina* occurs because of the increased oxygen requirements of the hypertrophied myocardium coupled with reduced aortic outflow and, in many patients, concomitant coronary artery disease. *Syncope* reflects poor perfusion of the

brain. Untreated aortic stenosis usually causes death within 3 to 4 years of the onset of symptoms, either from congestive heart failure or from a lethal arrhythmia. DCAS is an important indication for surgical valve replacement.

Mitral Valve Prolapse

As noted in the preceding sections (and in Table 11–4), mitral regurgitation may occur in patients with rheumatic heart disease, ischemic heart disease, or congestive heart failure of any origin. However, the most common cause of isolated mitral regurgitation is a disorder known as *mitral valve prolapse*, first recognized by Barlow in the 1960s. Mitral valve prolapse is one of the most common cardiac disorders, occurring in about 5% of the general adult population. Most cases are discovered between the ages of 20 and 40; the disease is more common in women than in men. It is characterized by an accumulation of loose ground substance within the leaflets and chordae of the mitral valve, which causes the valve to become "floppy" and incompetent during systole. Mitral valve prolapse may arise as a complication of Marfan syndrome or similar connective tissue disorders, but it occurs most often as an isolated, nonfamilial abnormality.

> **MORPHOLOGY. The mitral valve cusps, particularly the posterior cusp, are soft and enlarged, causing a characteristic ballooning of the valve leaflets** into the left atrium during systole (Fig. 11–16). The chordae tendineae, which are often elongated and fragile, may rupture in severe cases. The mitral annulus may be dilated. Histologic examination reveals excessive amounts of loose, edematous, faintly basophilic tissue within the valve

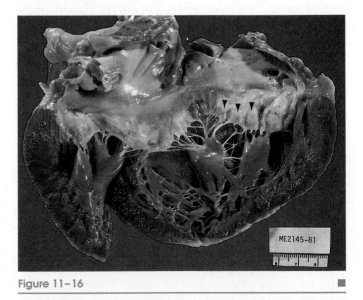

Figure 11–16   ■

Mitral valve prolapse. The opened mitral valve shows ballooning (*arrows*) of the valve leaflets into the left atrium. (From the teaching collection of the Pathology Department, University of Texas Southwestern Medical School, Dallas, TX.)

leaflets and chordae. Similar changes may be seen in the tricuspid and, less commonly, the pulmonic valve.

Clinical Features. Most patients with mitral valve prolapse are asymptomatic. In a minority of cases, however, patients may complain of palpitations, fatigue, or atypical chest pain. Auscultation of the chest discloses a sharp *midsystolic click, caused by abrupt tension on the redundant valve leaflets and chordae tendineae, followed by a late systolic murmur.* In severe cases there may be hemodynamically significant mitral regurgitation and congestive heart failure, particularly if the chordae or valve leaflets rupture. Patients with mitral valve prolapse are also at increased risk for the development of infective endocarditis, arrhythmias, and sudden death.

Nonbacterial Thrombotic Endocarditis

Nonbacterial thrombotic endocarditis (NBTE) is characterized by the deposition of small masses of fibrin, platelets, and other blood components on the leaflets of the cardiac valves. In contrast to the vegetations of infective endocarditis, discussed in the next section, *the valvular lesions of NBTE are sterile and do not contain microorganisms.* Valvular damage is not a prerequisite for NBTE. Indeed, the condition is usually found on previously normal valves. The pathogenesis of NBTE is incompletely understood; it is thought that subtle endothelial abnormalities and hypercoagulable states predispose to its development. Malignancies, particularly adenocarcinomas, have been identified in up to 50% of patients with NBTE. These patients also exhibit other features of hypercoagulability such as deep venous thrombosis. Although NBTE may occur in otherwise healthy individuals, a wide variety of diseases associated with general debility or wasting are associated with an increased risk of NBTE. The term *marantic endocarditis* has also been used to describe this entity, in recognition of the increased frequency of NBTE in cachectic patients.

Grossly, NBTE is characterized by groups of small nodules on the lines of valve closure, similar to the valvular lesions of acute rheumatic fever. The nodules usually measure less than 5 mm in diameter but may become fairly large and friable (Fig. 11–17). The valve leaflets appear normal on gross inspection. Although any valve may be affected, the aortic valve is the most common site, followed by the mitral valve. Microscopically, the nodules are composed of eosinophilic material (fibrin) and a delicate layer of aggregated platelets. The underlying valve is typically free of inflammation or fibrosis, in contrast to the valves in acute rheumatic fever. The lesions of NBTE often resolve spontaneously, leaving in their wake delicate strands of fibrous tissue, termed *Lambl's excrescences.*

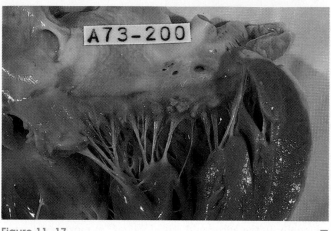

Figure 11–17 ■

Nonbacterial thrombotic endocarditis. Irregular yellow-tan vegetations are present on the mitral valve. Note that unlike the valves in chronic rheumatic carditis (Fig. 11–14), this valve shows normal thin leaflets, and the chordae tendineae are thin and glistening. (From the teaching collection of the Pathology Department, University of Texas Southwestern Medical School, Dallas, TX.)

Clinical Features. NBTE is usually asymptomatic. Sometimes, particularly in patients with larger lesions, fragments of the vegetations may embolize and cause infarcts in the brain and other organs. The lesions of NBTE also serve as a potential nidus for bacterial colonization and thus may be complicated by the development of infective endocarditis.

Infective Endocarditis

The term *infective endocarditis* designates infection of the cardiac valves or mural surface of the endocardium, resulting in the formation of an adherent mass of thrombotic debris and organisms, termed a *vegetation.* Virtually any type of microorganism is capable of causing endocarditis, although most cases are caused by bacteria.

Infective endocarditis has traditionally been subdivided into acute and subacute forms. Cases of *acute endocarditis* are classically associated with infection of the valves by organisms of high virulence, such as *Staphylococcus aureus.* Such organisms are capable of infecting even structurally normal valves and cause rapidly progressive infection, with little accompanying local host reaction. *Subacute endocarditis,* in contrast, is typically associated with infection of previously abnormal valves by organisms of lower virulence, such as α-hemolytic streptococci. The resultant infections tend to progress somewhat more slowly and are often accompanied by the development of a local inflammatory reaction and granulation tissue in the affected valve. In the era of antibiotics, however, therapy often modifies the morphology and clinical progression of disease, thus blurring the distinction between acute and subacute cases.

Etiology and Pathogenesis. Infection occurs when organisms are implanted on the endocardial surface during episodes of bacteremia. In some instances the cause of the hematogenous infection is obvious, as in the case of intravenous drug abusers who inject contaminated material directly into the bloodstream; an infection elsewhere or a previous dental, surgical, or other interventional procedure (e.g., catheterization) may also seed the bloodstream. In other cases, however, the source of bacteremia is occult, presumably related to trivial injuries to the skin or mucosal surfaces, as may be encountered, for example, during brushing of teeth.

Conditions that increase the risk of infective endocarditis can be segregated into three categories: (1) preexisting cardiac abnormalities, (2) prosthetic heart valves, and (3) intravenous drug abuse.

■ A number of cardiac abnormalities predispose individuals to infective endocarditis. The risk of endocarditis is increased by any condition that causes increased hemodynamic trauma to the endocardial surface, such as high pressure shunts within the heart (e.g., small ventricular septal defects) or chronic valvular diseases (e.g., chronic rheumatic heart disease, DCAS, mitral valve prolapse).

■ With an increasing number of patients undergoing valve replacement surgery, prosthetic valves now account for 10% to 20% of cases of infective endocarditis. There is no difference in the incidence of endocarditis between mechanical and bioprosthetic valves. The frequency of endocarditis is also increased, as might be expected, in individuals with indwelling intravascular catheters.

■ Intravenous drug abusers are at a high risk for development of infective endocarditis. In this setting, infective endocarditis usually occurs on previously normal valves.

The causative organisms differ somewhat in the three high-risk groups. Endocarditis of native (not prosthetic) valves is caused most commonly (50% to 60% of cases) by α-hemolytic (viridans) streptococci, which usually attack previously damaged valves. The more virulent *S. aureus* organisms attack healthy or deformed valves and are responsible for 10% to 20% of cases. The roster of the remaining bacteria includes enterococci and the so-called HACEK group (*Haemophilus*, *Actinobacillus*, *Cardiobacterium*, *Eikenella*, and *Kingella*), all commensals in the oral cavity. Prosthetic valve endocarditis is caused most commonly by coagulase-negative staphylococci (e.g., *S. epidermidis*). Other agents include gram-negative bacilli and fungi. In intravenous drug abusers, *S. aureus*, commonly found on the skin, is the major offender; other, less frequent, causes include streptococci, gram-negative rods, and fungi.

Infective endocarditis is a particularly difficult infection to eradicate because of the avascular nature of the heart valves. In view of the paucity of blood vessels, the inflammatory response to the infection is relatively scant, if present at all, and hence even avirulent organisms can proliferate in an uncontrolled fashion. Before effective antibiotics were available, infective endocarditis was almost always fatal.

MORPHOLOGY. The hallmark of infective endocarditis is the presence of valvular vegetations containing bacteria or other organisms. The **aortic** (Fig. 11–18A) and **mitral valves** are the most common sites of infection, although the valves of the **right heart** may also be involved, particularly in cases of endocarditis occurring in intravenous drug abusers (Fig. 11–18B). The vegetations may be single or multiple and may involve more than one valve. The appearance of the vegetations is influenced by the type of organism responsible for the infection, the degree of host reaction to the infection, and previous antibiotic therapy. **Fungal endocarditis,** for example, tends to cause larger vegetations than does bacterial infection. Although highly virulent organisms tend to cause acute endocarditis, treatment with antibiotics may curb the infection sufficiently to change the morphology of the vegetations to a more subacute form.

The vegetations in cases of classic **acute endocarditis** begin as small excrescences, which may be grossly indistinguishable from those of NBTE. As

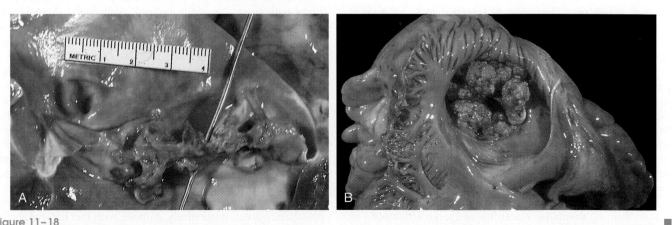

Figure 11–18

A, Acute bacterial endocarditis of the aortic valve. There are irregular vegetations attached to the valve, which has been severely damaged and perforated. The metal probe is traversing a hole in the valve leaflet. *B,* Opened right atrium shows large, irregular, friable vegetations causing virtual occlusion of the tricuspid valve. Such vegetations are often noted in intravenous drug abusers.

the organisms proliferate, the vegetations enlarge progressively and eventually form bulky, friable lesions that may obstruct the valve orifice (Fig. 11–18B). The vegetations cause rapid destruction of the valves, often resulting in rupture of the leaflets, chordae tendineae, or papillary muscles. The infection may eventually extend through the valve into the adjacent myocardium to produce abscesses in the perivalvular tissue, termed **ring abscesses.** Microscopic examination of the vegetations reveals large numbers of organisms admixed with fibrin and blood cells. When confined to the valve, the vegetations elicit virtually no inflammatory response. A brisk neutrophilic inflammatory response occurs once the infection extends beyond the avascular valves. **Systemic emboli** may occur at any time because of the friable nature of the vegetations, and they may cause infarcts in the brain, kidneys, myocardium, and other tissues. Because the embolic fragments contain large numbers of virulent organisms, **abscesses often develop at the sites of such infarcts.**

The vegetations of **subacute endocarditis** tend to be somewhat firmer and are associated with less valvular destruction than those of acute endocarditis, although the distinction between the two forms may be difficult. Subacute infections are less likely to erode into the myocardium, and perivalvular abscesses are uncommon. Microscopically, the vegetations of typical subacute infective endocarditis are distinguished from those of acute disease by the presence of **granulation tissue** at their bases. With the passage of time, fibrosis, calcification, and a chronic inflammatory infiltrate may develop. **Systemic emboli** may also develop in subacute endocarditis. In contrast to those of acute endocarditis, however, **the resultant infarcts are less likely to undergo suppuration** because of the less virulent nature of the offending organisms.

Clinical Features. The onset of infective endocarditis may be gradual or explosive, depending on the organism responsible for the infection. Low-grade *fever,* malaise, and weight loss are characteristic of cases caused by organisms of low virulence, while more acute cases, in contrast, typically present with high fevers, shaking chills, and other evidence of overt septicemia. *Cardiac murmurs* are almost always present, although they may be difficult to detect early in the course of acute endocarditis. The *spleen is often enlarged,* and clubbing of the digits may be seen, particularly in subacute cases. *Systemic emboli* are very common in all forms of infective endocarditis, manifesting as neurologic deficits, retinal abnormalities, necrosis of the digits, and infarcts of the myocardium and other viscera. Pulmonary emboli may occur in patients with right-sided endocarditis and large vegetations on the tricuspid or pulmonic valves. Entrapment of infected emboli in the walls of blood vessels may cause local infection and weakening of the vessel wall, with the formation of so-

called *mycotic* aneurysms. Petechiae (small hemorrhages) may be seen on the skin or mucosal surfaces. They may be caused by microemboli or deposition of immune complexes formed in response to chronic antigenemia. *Renal lesions* are common and include both renal infarcts and glomerulonephritis, the latter resulting from the trapping of immune complexes in the glomeruli. Over a period of days to months, progressive valvular destruction in untreated cases results in valvular regurgitation and congestive heart failure.

Repeated blood cultures are extremely important in the evaluation of patients with suspected infective endocarditis. Cultures for both aerobic and anaerobic organisms should be obtained the moment the possibility of endocarditis is considered. In a minority of cases of infective endocarditis blood cultures remain negative, because of either the fastidious nature of the organism or the effects of previous antibiotic therapy.

Prosthetic Cardiac Valves

The introduction of effective prosthetic heart valves has radically altered the prognosis of patients with many of the valvular diseases discussed above. Two types of prosthetic valves are used: those derived from animals (bioprosthetic valves) and man-made (mechanical) valves. Each type of valve has its advantages and disadvantages. Several complications are common to all prosthetic valves.

Mechanical deterioration is a particularly important complication of bioprosthetic valves. Virtually all biologic valve leaflets undergo some degree of stiffening after implantation. This loss of mobility may be sufficient to cause significant valvular stenosis. Calcification of the leaflets is also common and may contribute to the stenosis. Bioprosthetic valves may perforate or tear, resulting in valvular insufficiency. In general, mechanical valves are less susceptible to structural deterioration than are biologic valves.

Thrombi may develop on any type of prosthetic valve but are especially troublesome with mechanical valves. Such thrombi may cause local obstruction of blood flow or serve as a source of systemic emboli. Although anticoagulants are routinely administered to patients with prosthetic valves, they carry with them the additional risk of hemorrhagic complications.

Infective endocarditis, as noted earlier, occurs with increased frequency in prosthetic valves of all types. In mechanical valves the infection typically involves the valve suture line and adjacent perivalvular tissue and may cause the valve to detach. In bioprosthetic valves the valve leaflets as well as the perivalvular tissues may become infected, causing perforation of the leaflets and valvular regurgitation.

Paravalvular leaks may also develop in either type of prosthetic valve. This may occur in the immediate perioperative period or later in the patient's course. Valvular infection is an important cause of paravalvular leaks.

Significant *hemolysis* occurs in a minority of patients with prosthetic valves, particularly in those with mechanical aortic valves, because of the shearing effect of the mechanical valve on erythrocytes. In rare cases the hemolysis is sufficiently severe to require implantation of a different prosthetic valve.

PRIMARY MYOCARDIAL DISEASES

It should be clear from the previous sections that myocardial dysfunction occurs commonly in a number of different conditions, such as coronary artery disease, chronic hypertension, and valvular heart disease. Far less frequent are diseases that are intrinsic to myocardial fibers. Such primary myocardial diseases are a diverse group that includes inflammatory disorders *(myocarditis)*, immunologic diseases, systemic metabolic disorders, muscular dystrophies, and an additional category of idiopathic diseases termed *cardiomyopathies*. Only myocarditis and cardiomyopathies are of sufficient importance to warrant further consideration here.

Myocarditis

Under this category are grouped inflammatory processes of the myocardium that result in injury to the cardiac myocytes. However, the presence of inflammation alone is not diagnostic of myocarditis, because inflammatory infiltrates may also be seen as a secondary phenomenon in conditions such as ischemic injury. In myocarditis, by contrast, the inflammatory process plays a primary role in the development of myocardial injury. Some of the causes of myocarditis are listed in Table 11–5.

Infections are a particularly important cause of myocarditis. In the United States, *viruses* are the most common cause of myocarditis. *Coxsackieviruses A and B* and other enteroviruses probably account for most of these cases. Other less common etiologic agents include cytomegalovirus (CMV), human immunodeficiency virus (HIV), and a host of other agents listed in Table 11–5. Although it is often difficult to isolate the offending virus from the tissues after the onset of clinical symptoms, serologic studies and, more recently, the identification of viral DNA or RNA sequences in the myocardium may identify the culprit. Whether the viruses are the direct cause of the myocardial injury, or they initiate an immune response that cross-reacts with myocardial cells, is unclear in most cases. As with hepatitis viruses (Chapter 16), T cells may damage virus-infected myofibers by reacting against viral antigens expressed on the cell membrane. *Parasites* are an important cause of myocarditis. In particular, Chagas' disease, caused by infection with *Trypanosoma cruzi,* is the most common cause of myocarditis in South America. Other parasitic diseases associated with myocarditis include toxoplasmosis and trichinosis. Bacterial infections, including Lyme disease and diphtheria, are additional infectious causes of myocarditis. In the case of diphtheritic myocarditis, toxins released by *Corynebacterium diphtheriae* appear to be responsible for the myocardial injury. Other causes of myocarditis include cardiac allograft rejection, collagen vascular diseases, drug hypersensitivity, and sarcoidosis.

MORPHOLOGY. In patients who die early after the onset of myocarditis, the heart may be of normal size, but more commonly it is dilated. The myocardium is flabby and pale and often contains small areas of hemorrhage. The histologic appearance varies considerably, depending on the cause of the myocarditis. In acute **viral myocarditis,** the myocardium is edematous and contains an **inflammatory infiltrate dominated by lymphocytes and other mononuclear cells.** Some degree of **myocyte degeneration and/or necrosis** is almost always present. Viral inclusions may be seen in some cases (e.g., CMV myocarditis) but are not a feature of several common forms of viral myocarditis. In more chronic cases, there is marked ventricular dilation. Histologically, inflammation is less conspicuous, while myocardial fibrosis becomes more prominent as cardiac myocytes are lost. At this late stage, myocarditis may be indistinguishable from idiopathic dilated cardiomyopathy, to be described later. In cases of myocarditis caused by **parasites,** the organism is usually demonstrable histologically, as in the case of Chagas' disease, in which trypanosomes directly infect myocardial fibers. In patients with **bacterial myocarditis,** the myocardium contains a neutrophilic infiltrate, sometimes complicated by abscess formation. **Cardiac transplant rejection** is characterized by the presence of interstitial lymphocytes and myocyte degeneration, which in some cases may be difficult to distinguish from infectious myocarditis. Finally, there is a morphologically distinctive myocarditis of unknown cause called **giant cell myocarditis.** As the name indicates, it is characterized by an inflammatory infiltrate in which multinucleate giant cells are prominent. In addi-

---

Table 11–5. MAJOR CAUSES OF MYOCARDITIS

Infections
  Viruses (e.g., coxsackievirus, ECHO, influenza, HIV, cytomegalovirus)
  Chlamydia (e.g., *C. psittaci*)
  Rickettsia (e.g., *R. typhi* [typhus fever])
  Bacteria (e.g., *Corynebacterium* [diphtheria], *Neisseria* [meningococcus], *Borrelia* [Lyme disease])
  Fungi (e.g., *Candida*)
  Protozoa (e.g., Trypanosoma [Chagas' disease], toxoplasmosis)
  Helminths (e.g., trichinosis)

Immune-Mediated Reactions
  Postviral
  Poststreptococcal (rheumatic fever)
  Systemic lupus erythematosus
  Drug hypersensitivity (e.g., methyldopa, sulfonamides)
  Transplant rejection

Unknown
  Sarcoidosis
  Giant cell myocarditis

ECHO, enteric cytopathogenic human orphan; HIV, human immunodeficiency virus.

tion there are lymphocytes, macrophages, and eosinophils, with scattered foci of necrosis.

Clinical Features. The clinical manifestations of myocarditis range from an asymptomatic state to severe congestive heart failure. Arrhythmias are common and may occur in the absence of heart failure. In most cases myocarditis appears to be self-limited, although some patients progress to chronic congestive heart failure months to years after the initial insult. If seen for the first time at such a late stage, they may be considered to have dilated cardiomyopathy.

Cardiomyopathies

The term *cardiomyopathy* (literally, heart muscle disease) could be applied to almost any heart disease, but by convention cardiomyopathy is used to describe *heart disease resulting from a primary abnormality in the myocardium.* This definition is somewhat arbitrary and often frustrating as one attempts to wade through various classification schemes, because some authors exclude any myocardial disorder of known etiology, while others take a more ecumenical view and include any heart disease manifested by primary myocardial dysfunction. Excluded from this definition in almost all classifications, however, are cases of heart failure resulting from hypertension, valvular disease, congenital heart disease, obvious myocarditis, systemic metabolic disturbances, nutritional disorders (e.g., wet beriberi), and hypersensitivity diseases (e.g., acute rheumatic fever). According to many experts, chronic myocardial dysfunction due to ischemia should also be excluded from the cardiomyopathy rubric. However, the term *ischemic cardiomyopathy*, used to describe chronic congestive heart failure caused by coronary artery disease, has gained some popularity. We can leave these complexities to "cardiomyopaths" and resort to the traditional subdivision of cardiomyopathies into three major clinicopathologic groups: *dilated, hypertrophic,* and *restrictive* cardiomyopathy. In many cases these conditions are idiopathic, but in some instances well-defined myocardial diseases may, in the end, resemble those without known causes, both functionally and structurally.

DILATED CARDIOMYOPATHY

This diagnosis is applied to a form of cardiomyopathy characterized by *progressive cardiac hypertrophy, dilation,* and *contractile (systolic) dysfunction.* It is sometimes called congestive cardiomyopathy. This clinicopathologic picture can result from a number of different myocardial insults. *Viral nucleic acids* from coxsackievirus B and other enteroviruses have been detected in the myocardium of some patients, suggesting that, in at least some cases, dilated cardiomyopathy represents a late stage of myocarditis. *Alcohol abuse* is also strongly associated with the development of dilated cardiomyopathy, raising the possibility that ethanol toxicity (Chapter 8), or a secondary nutritional disturbance, may be the cause of the myocardial injury. In yet other cases, a more clearly defined *toxic insult* is the cause of the myocardial failure. Par-

ticularly important in this last group is myocardial injury caused by cobalt and certain chemotherapeutic agents, including doxorubicin (Adriamycin) and other anthracyclines. A special form of dilated cardiomyopathy, termed *peripartum cardiomyopathy*, occurs late in pregnancy or several weeks to months post partum. The cause of peripartum cardiomyopathy is poorly understood but is probably multifactorial. Together, the various "known" causes account for a small fraction of all cases. In most the cause is unknown, and they are appropriately designated as *idiopathic dilated cardiomyopathy*.

Dilated cardiomyopathy may occur at any age but is most common between the ages of 20 and 60 years. Most cases arise sporadically, although familial cases do occur. Dilated cardiomyopathy occurs more frequently in men than in women, possibly reflecting the association between chronic alcohol abuse and cardiomyopathy.

MORPHOLOGY. The heart is enlarged and flabby, with weights in excess of 900 gm. The enlargement is caused by a **combination of dilation and hypertrophy of all chambers** (Fig. 11–19). The substantial dilation and poor contractile function cause stasis of blood in the cardiac chambers and predispose to the development of fragile **mural thrombi** and subsequent emboli. The microscopic features are nonspecific and include myocyte hypertrophy, interstitial fibrosis, wavy fiber change, and (in some cases) a scanty mononuclear inflammatory infiltrate.

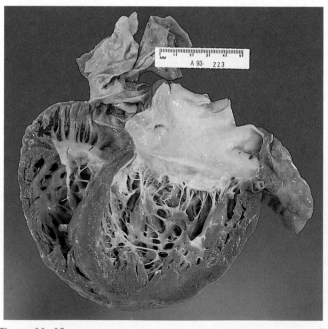

Figure 11–19 ■

Dilated cardiomyopathy with generalized cardiac hypertrophy and dilation. Such changes are usually idiopathic, as in this patient, or the result of a more specific myocardial insult.

Clinical Features. *The fundamental defect in dilated cardiomyopathy is ineffective contraction.* Patients may have an ejection fraction of less than 25% (normal 50% to 65%). Hence, the clinical picture is that of progressive congestive heart failure, which becomes refractory to therapy. An exception to this dismal course occurs in peripartum cardiomyopathy, in which up to half of the patients recover spontaneously. However, the illness may recur with subsequent pregnancies. Idiopathic cases are usually fatal. Death results from severe and intractable heart failure, embolic complications, or ventricular arrhythmias. Cardiac transplantation can be lifesaving in this and other cardiomyopathies.

HYPERTROPHIC CARDIOMYOPATHY

Hypertrophic cardiomyopathy, also referred to as *asymmetric septal hypertrophy* and *idiopathic hypertrophic subaortic stenosis,* is a cardiac disorder characterized by *myocardial hypertrophy, abnormal diastolic filling,* and (in many cases) *intermittent ventricular outflow obstruction.* In contrast to the feebly contracting heart in patients with dilated cardiomyopathy, hypertrophic cardiomyopathy is characterized by powerful, hyperkinetic contractions that rapidly expel blood from the ventricular cavities. In about 50% of cases, the disorder is inherited as an autosomal dominant trait with variable penetrance and expression. In about half of the familial cases, mutations in the gene coding for the heavy chain of β-myosin have been identified on chromosome 14. Additional abnormalities involving chromosomes 1, 11, or 15 have been noted in other cases. Hypertrophic cardiomyopathy may also occur in association with certain other hereditary disorders, including neurofibromatosis, suggesting that this cardiomyopathy, like other forms, is not a single disease entity.

> **MORPHOLOGY.** The essential feature of hypertrophic cardiomyopathy is **myocardial hypertrophy, which is most pronounced in the left ventricle**

and interventricular septum. The degree of hypertrophy varies from patient to patient, even in familial cases, but weights in excess of 800 gm are common. **In most cases the interventricular septum is substantially thicker than the free (lateral) wall of the left ventricle,** a feature best demonstrated in coronal sections through the chamber (Fig. 11–20A). Although disproportionate hypertrophy can involve the entire septum, the hypertrophy is usually most conspicuous in the subaortic region of the septum. Asymmetric hypertrophy is often associated with a significant degree of ventricular outflow obstruction during systole, a feature emphasized in the older designation **idiopathic hypertrophic subaortic stenosis.** In this group of patients, the systolic obstruction is caused by abnormal anterior motion of the mitral valve leaflet(s) during systole. Because of this abnormal systolic anterior motion, there is recurrent, forceful contact between the septum and the anterior leaflet of the mitral valve. This in turn leads to **thickening of the anterior mitral leaflet and adjacent septal endocardium.** Ventricular dilation is uncommon, but the left atrium may be dilated because of impaired diastolic filling of the thickened, rigid left ventricle.

Microscopically, hypertrophic cardiomyopathy is characterized by a **haphazard arrangement of hypertrophied myocytes,** surrounded by loose, basophilic ground substance (Fig. 11–20B). This change is most pronounced in sections taken from the interventricular septum. In later stages of the disease, considerable myocardial fibrosis may develop.

Clinical Features. The basic physiologic abnormality in hypertrophic cardiomyopathy is an *inability to fill a hyper-*

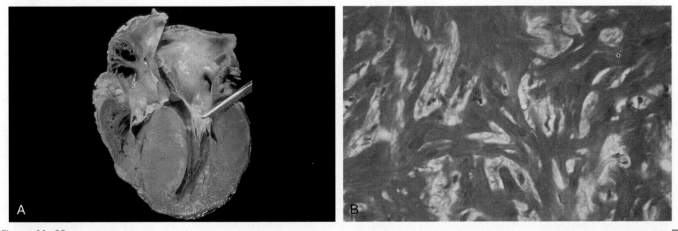

Figure 11–20

Hypertrophic cardiomyopathy. *A,* The ventricular septum is disproportionately thickened and bulges into the lumen of the left ventricle. Contact between the hypertrophic septum and the anterior leaflet of the mitral valve may cause significant left ventricular outflow obstruction. *B,* Microscopic picture shows hypertrophy and extreme disarray of fibers. (Courtesy of Sid Murphree, M.D. Department of Pathology, University of Texas Southwestern Medical School, Dallas, TX.)

trophic left ventricle. Ejection is forceful but ineffective because the amount of blood in the left ventricle is very small. In addition, there may be dynamic obstruction to the left ventricular outflow, as explained above. The limitation of cardiac output and a secondary increase in pulmonary venous pressure cause exertional dyspnea. Auscultation discloses a harsh systolic ejection murmur, caused by anterior motion of the mitral leaflets and by ventricular outflow obstruction. Myocardial ischemia is common, even in the absence of concomitant coronary artery disease, and thus anginal pain is frequent. Hypertrophic cardiomyopathy is associated with an increased incidence of ventricular arrhythmias and sudden death, and is one of the most common causes of sudden unexplained death in young athletes. The risk of infective endocarditis is also increased. In the later stages of the disease, progressive myocardial fibrosis may cause congestive heart failure.

RESTRICTIVE CARDIOMYOPATHY

Restrictive cardiomyopathy is a disorder characterized by a *primary decrease in ventricular compliance, resulting in impaired ventricular filling during diastole.* It is considerably less common than either dilated or hypertrophic cardiomyopathy. Restrictive cardiomyopathy can be caused by any process that reduces myocardial compliance. Worldwide, the most common cause of this form of cardiomyopathy is a disease called *endomyocardial fibrosis,* a disorder of unknown etiology that accounts for up to 10% of cases of childhood heart disease in tropical areas of the world. *Eosinophilic endomyocardial fibrosis,* or Löffler's syndrome, is a rare cause of restrictive cardiomyopathy that may be related to the tropical form of the disease. In the case of Löffler's syndrome, the development of endomyocardial fibrosis has been attributed to proteins released from degranulating eosinophils; whether this process also contributes to the endomyocardial fibrosis in cases seen in the tropics is less clear. Additional important causes of restrictive cardiomyopathy are *cardiac amyloidosis, hemochromatosis,* and *radiation injury* to the heart.

MORPHOLOGY. The appearance of the heart varies with the cause of the restrictive cardiomyopathy. The morphology of cardiac amyloidosis and hemochromatosis is described in detail in Chapters 5 and 16 and will not be repeated here. In patients with **tropical endomyocardial fibrosis** and **Löffler's syndrome,** the atria are typically dilated. The ventricles may be of normal size, although some degree of dilation may occur, particularly in the later stages of the disease. **The endocardium is thickened and opaque,** especially in the left ventricle. The cardiac valves are thickened in some cases, and mural or valvular thrombi may be present. Histologic sections reveal dense endocardial fibrosis, which extends into the underlying myocardium. In cases of endomyocardial fibrosis associated with hypereosinophilia, the endocardium and myocardium may be infiltrated by eosinophils, particularly in the early stages of the disease.

Clinical Features. The physiologic problem in restrictive cardiomyopathy is *a stiff and inelastic ventricle that can be filled only with great effort.* In this aspect it resembles hypertrophic cardiomyopathy. However, unlike the latter, the systole is not forceful. As with other cardiomyopathies, the symptoms in patients with restrictive cardiomyopathy include fatigue, exertional dyspnea, and chest pain. In patients with Löffler's syndrome, systemic emboli may arise from mural or valvular thrombi. The course is often complicated by arrhythmias and atrioventricular blocks, particularly when the myocardial fibrosis or infiltrative process encroaches on the conduction system. Myocardial contractility, although often normal early in the course of the disease, usually declines, causing congestive heart failure in later stages.

CONGENITAL HEART DISEASE

Congenital abnormalities of the heart occur in about 8 per 1000 live births, making them one of the most common types of congenital malformations. With the declining incidence of acute rheumatic fever, congenital heart disease is now the most common cause of heart disease in children in the Western world. Congenital heart diseases encompass a broad spectrum of malformations, ranging from mild lesions that produce only minimal symptoms until adult life, to severe anomalies that cause death in the perinatal period. The cause of most cases of congenital heart disease is unknown. The etiology of congenital malformations in general was discussed in Chapter 7. We will therefore confine our remarks to factors of particular relevance to congenital cardiac malformations.

Genetic factors play an obvious role in some cases, as evidenced by the occurrence of familial forms of congenital heart disease and by well-defined associations between certain chromosomal abnormalities (e.g., trisomies 13, 15, 18, and 21, and the Turner syndrome) and congenital cardiac malformations. *Environmental factors,* such as congenital rubella infection, are responsible for some additional cases. Overall, however, obvious genetic or environmental influences are identifiable in only about 10% of cases of congenital heart disease. In the remaining 90%, the cause is not clearly defined. Multifactorial genetic and environmental factors probably account for the many so-called idiopathic forms.

The major forms of congenital heart disease are listed in Table 11–6. For purposes of discussion, congenital heart diseases can be subdivided into three major groups:

■ Malformations causing a *left-to-right shunt*
■ Malformations causing a *right-to-left shunt* (cyanotic congenital heart diseases)
■ Malformations causing *obstruction*

Within each of these subdivisions, we will consider the pathogenesis, morphology, and clinical manifestations of some of the more common congenital cardiac malformations.

Table 11–6. FREQUENCIES OF CARDIAC MALFORMATIONS IN 1000 CONSECUTIVE CHILDREN*

Malformation	Congenital Heart Disease (%)
Ventricular septal defect	33
Patent ductus arteriosus	10
Pulmonary stenosis	10
Tetralogy of Fallot	9
Aortic stenosis	8
Coarctation of aorta	5
Atrial septal defect	5
Transposition of great arteries	5
Atrioventricular septal defect	4
Truncus arteriosus	1
Tricuspid atresia	1
Total anomalous pulmonary venous connection	1

* Combinations of lesions tabulated with dominant malformation.

Data modified from Moller JH: 1000 consecutive children with a cardiac malformation with 26- to 37-year follow-up. Am J Cardiol 70:661, 1992.

Left-to-Right Shunts

Left-to-right shunts represent the most common type of congenital cardiac malformation. They include *atrial septal defects (ASDs), ventricular septal defects (VSDs),* and *patent (persistent) ductus arteriosus (PDA).* These malformations may be asymptomatic at birth, or they may cause fulminant congestive heart failure. *Cyanosis is not an early feature* of this group of malformations, but it may occur late, after the left-to-right shunt has produced significant pulmonary hypertension to cause a reversal of blood flow through the shunt.

ATRIAL SEPTAL DEFECTS

The atrial septum develops between the fourth and sixth weeks of embryonic life (Fig. 11–21). The initial phase is marked by the growth of a primary septum (*septum primum*) from the dorsal wall of the common atrial chamber toward the developing *endocardial cushions*, as the latter begin to separate the atrial and ventricular cavities. A gap, termed the *ostium primum*, initially separates the developing septum primum from the endocardial cushions. Continued growth and fusion of the septum with endocardial cushions ultimately obliterates the ostium primum; however, at this time a second opening, *ostium secundum,* appears in the central area of the primary septum. This allows continued flow of oxygenated blood from the right atrium to the left, essential for fetal life. As the ostium secundum enlarges, a secondary septum (*septum secundum*) makes its appearance just to the right of the septum primum. The septum secundum proliferates to form a crescent-shaped structure surrounding a space termed the *foramen ovale.* The foramen ovale is guarded on its left side by a flap of tissue derived from the primary septum, which acts as a one-way valve, allowing blood to keep on flowing from right to left during intrauterine life. At the time of birth, as pulmonary vascular resistance falls and systemic arterial pressure increases, pressure in the left atrium rises above that in the right atrium, resulting in functional closure of the foramen ovale. In most individuals the foramen ovale is permanently sealed by fusion of the primary and secondary septa, although a minor degree of patency persists in about 25% of the general population.

Abnormalities in this sequence of events result in the development of various ASDs, which allow free communication between the left and right atria. Three types of ASD are recognized. The most common is the *ostium secundum ASD,* which arises if the septum secundum does not enlarge sufficiently to cover the ostium secundum. *Ostium primum ASDs* occur if the septum primum and endocardial cushions fail to fuse. This defect is often associated with abnormalities in other structures derived from the endocardial cushions, such as the mitral and tricuspid valves. The pathogenesis of the uncommon sinus venous ASD is unclear.

MORPHOLOGY. The ostium secundum ASD appears as a smooth-walled defect in the vicinity of the foramen ovale (Fig. 11–22). This may occur as an isolated lesion, or it may be associated with other cardiac abnormalities. Hemodynamically significant lesions are accompanied by right atrial and ventricular dilation, right ventricular hypertrophy, and dilation of the pulmonary artery, reflecting the effects of a chronically increased volume load on the right side of the heart, and (in some cases) pulmonary hypertension. Ostium primum ASDs occur in the lowermost part of the atrial septum and extend to the mitral and tricuspid valves (Fig. 11–22). An abnormality of the atrioventricular

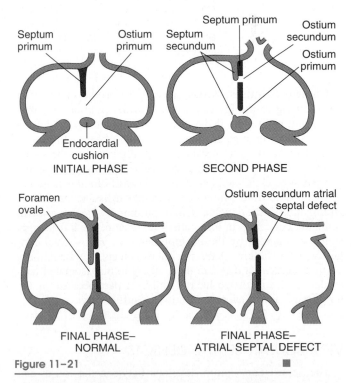

Figure 11–21

Embryogenesis of an atrial septal defect, ostium secundum type.

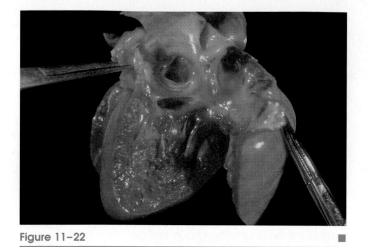

Figure 11-22 ■

Atrial septal defect. This unusual case shows both the ostium secundum and primum defects, and allows comparison of the two. The upper secundum type of atrial septal defect forms an opening in the atrial septal wall in the region of the foramen ovale. The less common ostium primum defect, in contrast, is lower in the atrial septum. (Courtesy of Arthur Weinberg, M.D., Department of Pathology, University of Texas Southwestern Medical School, Dallas, TX.)

valves is usually present, typically in the form of a cleft in the anterior leaflet of the mitral valve or septal leaflet of the tricuspid valve, reflecting the close relationship between development of the septum primum and endocardial cushions. In more severe cases the ostium primum defect is accompanied by a VSD and severe mitral and tricuspid valve deformities, with a resultant **common atrioventricular canal. Sinus venous ASDs** are uncommon. They are located high in the atrial septum and are often accompanied by anomalous drainage of the pulmonary veins into the right atrium or superior vena cava.

Clinical Features. ASDs cause left-to-right shunts after birth, owing to the lower pressures in the pulmonary circulation and right side of the heart. Ostium secundum defects are the most common, accounting for 40% of cases. In general these defects are well tolerated, especially if they are less than 1 cm in diameter, but even larger lesions do not produce any symptoms in childhood because the flow of blood is from left to right. With time, pulmonary vascular resistance increases, culminating in the development of pulmonary hypertension in some patients. This in turn causes reversal of the left-to-right shunt, manifested by the development of cyanosis and congestive heart failure. Ostium primum defects may be initially asymptomatic, but they are more likely to be associated with evidence of congestive heart failure, in part because of the high frequency of associated mitral insufficiency.

VENTRICULAR SEPTAL DEFECTS

The ventricular septum develops between the fourth and eighth weeks of gestation. It is formed by the fusion of an

intraventricular muscular ridge that grows upward from the apex of the heart to a thinner membranous partition that grows downward from the endocardial cushions. The basal (membranous) region is the last part of the septum to develop and is the site where approximately 90% of septal defects are located. *VSDs are the most common congenital heart defects.* Like ASDs, they may occur in isolation (around 30% of cases), but they are encountered most often in association with other cardiac malformations.

MORPHOLOGY. The size and location of VSDs are variable, ranging from minute defects in the muscular or membranous portions of the septum to large defects involving virtually the entire septum (Fig. 11-23). In defects associated with a significant left-to-right shunt, the right ventricle is hypertrophied and often dilated. The diameter of the pulmonary artery is increased owing to the increased volume ejected by the right ventricle. Vascular changes typical of pulmonary hypertension are commonly seen (Chapter 13).

Clinical Features. *Small VSDs may be asymptomatic,* and those in the muscular portion of the septum may close spontaneously during infancy or childhood. *Larger defects, however, cause a severe left-to-right shunt, often complicated by pulmonary hypertension and congestive heart failure.* Progressive pulmonary hypertension, with resultant reversal of the shunt and cyanosis, occurs early and more frequently in patients with VSDs than in those with ASDs; hence, early surgical correction is indicated. A particular risk for those with small or medium-sized defects that produce jet lesions in the right ventricle is superimposed infective endocarditis.

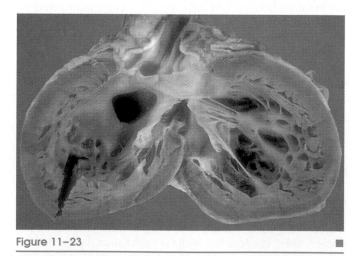

Figure 11-23 ■

Ventricular septal defect, membranous type. Ventricular septal defects may involve any part of the interventricular septum. Most are high in the membranous portion of the septum, as in this case. (Courtesy of Arthur Weinberg, M.D. Department of Pathology, University of Texas Southwestern Medical School, Dallas, TX.)

PATENT DUCTUS ARTERIOSUS

The ductus arteriosus is an arterial channel that courses between the pulmonary artery and aorta. During intrauterine life, the ductus arteriosus permits blood to flow freely from the pulmonary artery to the aorta, thereby bypassing the unoxygenated lungs. Shortly after birth, the ductus begins to constrict in response to increased levels of arterial oxygen, decreasing pulmonary vascular resistance, and declining levels of prostaglandin E_2. In healthy term infants, functional closure is usually complete within 1 to 2 days after birth. Complete, irreversible closure occurs within the first few months of extrauterine life to form the *ligamentum arteriosum*. Ductal closure may be significantly delayed in infants with hypoxia owing to respiratory distress or heart disease. Isolated PDA accounts for about 10% of cases of congenital heart disease. This lesion may also occur in combination with other anomalies, particularly VSDs.

MORPHOLOGY. The usual PDA arises from the left pulmonary artery and joins the aorta just distal to the origin of the left subclavian artery. Its lumen is generally uniform and is lined by smooth endothelium. Oxygenated blood flows from the left ventricle to the lungs and is returned to the left atrium. Because of volume overload, the left atrium and ventricle are dilated and may be hypertrophied. The proximal pulmonary arteries are also dilated. With the development of pulmonary hypertension, atherosclerosis of the main pulmonary arteries and proliferative changes in more distal pulmonary vessels are seen. These are accompanied by right ventricular hypertrophy and dilation, and right atrial dilation.

Clinical Features. PDA causes a high-pressure left-to-right shunt, audible as a harsh waxing and waning murmur sometimes referred to as a "machinery" murmur. As with other left-to-right shunts, the development of pulmonary hypertension is announced by the appearance of cyanosis and congestive heart failure. The high-pressure shunt also predisposes affected individuals to the development of infective endocarditis.

Right-to-Left Shunts

Cardiac malformations associated with right-to-left shunts are distinguished by *cyanosis at or near the time of birth*. This occurs because poorly oxygenated blood from the right side of the heart is introduced directly into the arterial circulation. Two of the most important conditions associated with cyanotic congenital heart disease are *tetralogy of Fallot* and *transposition of the great vessels*.

TETRALOGY OF FALLOT

Accounting for about 10% of all congenital cardiac malformations, tetralogy of Fallot is *the most common cause of cyanotic congenital heart disease*. The four components of the tetralogy are (1) a VSD, (2) a "dextraposed" aortic root that overrides the VSD, (3) right ventricular outflow obstruction, and (4) right ventricular hypertrophy (Fig. 11–24). Abnormal division of the truncus arteriosus into a pulmonary trunk and aortic root has been suggested as the primary event in the development of this malformation, although many details of its pathogenesis remain unsettled.

MORPHOLOGY. The heart is enlarged externally and often "boot" shaped owing to right ventricular hypertrophy. The proximal aorta is often larger than normal and the pulmonary trunk is reduced in diameter. The cardiac chambers on the left side of the heart are of normal size, while the thickness of the right ventricular wall may equal or even exceed that of the left. The VSD lies in the vicinity of the membranous portion of the interventricular septum and may efface all or part of the membranous septum. The aortic valve lies immediately over the VSD. The pulmonary outflow tract is narrowed and, in a few cases, the pulmonic valve itself may be stenotic. Additional abnormalities are present in a significant minority of cases, including PDA or ASD. These are protective because they allow some blood flow to the lungs.

Clinical Features. The hemodynamic consequences of tetralogy of Fallot are a right-to-left shunt, decreased blood flow to the lungs, and increased blood flow through the aorta. *The extent of shunting is determined by the degree of right ventricular outflow obstruction.* If the pulmonic obstruction is

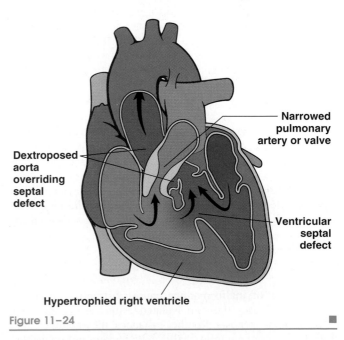

Figure 11–24   ■

Tetralogy of Fallot demonstrating ventricular septal defect, pulmonic stenosis, overriding aorta, and secondary right ventricular hypertrophy. The flow of blood is indicated by *arrows*.

mild, the condition resembles an isolated VSD, because the higher pressure on the left side causes a left-to-right shunt with no cyanosis. Marked stenosis, on the other hand, causes significant cyanosis early in life. As patients with tetralogy of Fallot grow, the pulmonic orifice does not enlarge, despite an overall increase in the size of the heart. Therefore, typically, the degree of stenosis becomes worse with time and is associated with increasing cyanosis. The lungs are protected from excessive hemodynamic load by the pulmonic stenosis, and pulmonary hypertension does not develop. Because of the right-to-left shunt, patients with tetralogy of Fallot are at increased risk for infective endocarditis, systemic emboli, and brain abscesses. Surgical correction of this defect is now possible in almost all instances.

TRANSPOSITION OF THE GREAT ARTERIES

Transposition of the great arteries is the second leading cause of cyanotic congenital heart disease, after tetralogy of Fallot. Because of abnormal truncal septation, *the aorta arises from the right ventricle and the pulmonary artery from the left ventricle.* In its complete form, the pulmonary and systemic circulations are entirely separate, and there is no shunting of blood. However, such a condition is incompatible with extrauterine life; therefore, those who survive after birth must have some type of shunt, such as an ASD, VSD, or PDA, that allows oxygenated blood to reach the aorta.

MORPHOLOGY. Transposition of the great arteries has many variants, and a detailed review of the morphology of this condition is beyond the scope of this chapter. The fundamental lesion, as noted, is abnormal origin of the pulmonary trunk and aortic root. Some degree of right ventricular hypertrophy is usually present because of the increased (systemic) pressure load placed on that chamber. Varying combinations of ASD, VSD, and PDA are seen in patients surviving beyond the neonatal period.

Clinical Features. The predominant manifestation of transposition of the great arteries is cyanosis. The prognosis depends on the degree of intra- or extracardiac shunting and the degree of arterial oxygen saturation. Maneuvers such as atrial balloon septostomy are sometimes used to create shunts that enhance arterial oxygen saturation and allow the patient to survive until definitive surgical correction can be undertaken.

Congenital Obstructive Lesions

A number of malformations cause obstruction of blood flow. In some cases, these are isolated lesions, as in congenital valvular aortic stenosis. In other instances, they are one component of a more complex malformation, as in pulmonic stenosis associated with tetralogy of Fallot. Here we will discuss coarctation of the aorta, a fairly common obstructive anomaly.

COARCTATION OF THE AORTA

Coarctation of the aorta, defined as an abnormal narrowing of the aortic lumen, is one of the most important forms of obstructive congenital heart disease. *In about 50% of cases, this lesion occurs as an isolated cardiac anomaly.* In the remaining cases, coarctation is associated with other malformations, such as PDA, VSD, and ASD. The malformation has also been associated with saccular aneurysms of the central nervous system, and it occurs with increased frequency in patients with Turner syndrome. Coarctation is somewhat more common in males than in females, particularly when it occurs as an isolated lesion. Most cases of coarctation of the aorta can be placed into one of two major categories: preductal and postductal. The postductal type is the more common.

MORPHOLOGY. Preductal coarctation, formerly termed infantile coarctation, is characterized by **narrowing of the so-called aortic isthmus,** the segment of aorta that lies between the left subclavian artery and the point of entry of the ductus arteriosus. In some cases the preductal narrowing takes the form of a fairly distinct ridge; in other cases the entire aortic arch is hypoplastic. The ductus arteriosus is usually patent and is the main source of blood delivered to the distal aorta. Because the right heart is called upon to perfuse the body distal to the site of the coarctation, the right cardiac chambers are often hypertrophic and dilated; the pulmonary trunk is also dilated to accommodate the increased blood flow.

In the more common **postductal,** or **adult-type, coarctation,** the aorta is constricted by a sharply defined ridge of tissue at, or just distal to, the obliterated ductus arteriosus (the ligamentum arteriosum). The constricted segment is made up of smooth muscle and elastic fibers that are continuous with the aortic media and are lined by a thickened layer of intima. The ductus arteriosus is closed. Proximal to the coarctation, the aortic arch and its branch vessels are dilated and, in older patients, often atherosclerotic. The left ventricle is hypertrophic. Collateral flow through the intercostal, phrenic, and epigastric arteries supplies most of the blood to the distal aorta, and these collateral channels are almost always dilated.

Clinical Features. Patients with *preductal coarctation* usually present in infancy, hence the older designation of *infantile* coarctation. Classic features include congestive heart failure and selective cyanosis of the lower extremities, the latter caused by perfusion of the lower part of the body by poorly oxygenated blood delivered via the ductus arteriosus. The femoral pulses are almost invariably weaker than those of the upper extremities, although narrowing of more proximal segments of the aortic root may cause diminished pulses in the upper extremities as well. These patients do not survive the neonatal period without surgical correction.

Postductal coarctation, in contrast, is more likely to present with signs and symptoms in older children and adults. Because the blood reaching the distal aorta in these cases comes from collateral branches connected to the proximal aorta, the oxygen content is normal and selective cyanosis of the lower extremities is not seen. *Hypertension of the upper extremities is seen in most cases, due in part to decreased perfusion of the kidneys and activation of the renin-angiotensin system.* By contrast, blood pressure is low and pulses are weak in the lower extremities. In addition, there are often signs and symptoms of arterial insufficiency in the legs, such as intermittent claudication.

PERICARDIAL DISEASES

Diseases of the pericardium include inflammatory conditions and effusions. These are most frequently seen in conjunction with local myocardial or mediastinal diseases, and in patients with a number of systemic conditions, such as uremia.

Pericarditis

Primary pericarditis is uncommon and usually infectious in origin. *Viruses are responsible for most cases,* although it may also be caused by other organisms, including pyogenic bacteria, mycobacteria, and fungi. An accompanying myocarditis may be present, particularly in the case of viral infections. More often the pericarditis is secondary to acute myocardial infarction, cardiac surgery, or radiation to the mediastinum. *Uremia* is probably the most common systemic disorder associated with pericarditis. Less common secondary causes include rheumatic fever, systemic lupus erythematosus, and metastatic malignancies. The latter are usually associated with a bloody effusion. Pericarditis may (1) cause immediate hemodynamic complications if a significant effusion is present, (2) resolve without significant sequelae, or (3) progress to a chronic fibrosing process.

MORPHOLOGY. The appearance of **acute pericarditis** varies with its cause. In patients with uremia or acute rheumatic fever, the exudate is typically fibrinous and imparts a shaggy, irregular appearance to the pericardial surface ("bread and butter" pericarditis) (Fig. 11–25). A fibrinous exudate may also be seen in cases of viral pericarditis. In acute bacterial pericarditis the pericardial exudate is fibrinopurulent, while in tuberculosis the pericardium contains caseous material. Pericardial metastases are visible grossly as irregular nodular excrescences, often with a shaggy fibrinous exudate and a bloody effusion. In most cases, acute fibrinous or fibrinopurulent pericarditis resolves without any sequelae. However, when there is extensive suppuration or caseation, healing gives rise to chronic pericarditis.

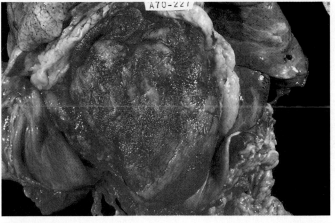

Figure 11–25　■

Acute fibrinous pericarditis. The normally smooth, glistening pericardial surface is covered by shaggy fibrinous exudate. In this case, the pericarditis developed because of uremia and caused a fatal cardiac tamponade.

The appearance of **chronic pericarditis** ranges from delicate adhesions to dense, fibrotic scars that obliterate the pericardial space. In extreme cases the heart is so completely encased by dense scar tissue that it cannot expand normally during diastole, a condition termed **constrictive pericarditis.**

Clinical Features. The manifestations of pericarditis include atypical chest pain, which is often worse on reclining, and a high-pitched friction rub. When associated with significant exudate in the pericardial sac, acute pericarditis may cause signs and symptoms of cardiac tamponade, which include faint distant heart sounds, distended neck veins, declining cardiac output, and shock. Chronic constrictive pericarditis produces a combination of venous distention and low cardiac output, which may be difficult to distinguish from restrictive cardiomyopathy.

Pericardial Effusions

Processes besides inflammation may cause fluid to accumulate in the pericardial space. The nature of the fluid varies with the cause of the effusion. The major types of pericardial effusion and some of their more common causes include

■ *Serous:* congestive heart failure, hypoalbuminemia of any cause
■ *Serosanguineous:* blunt chest trauma, malignancy
■ *Chylous:* mediastinal lymphatic obstruction

Pericardial effusions are often symptomatic. Surprisingly large volumes of fluid can be accommodated if the accumulation occurs slowly. Massive or rapidly developing effusions may cause cardiac tamponade.

Hemopericardium, more properly considered separately from hemorrhagic pericardial effusions, indicates the presence of pure (undiluted) blood in the pericardial sac. Important causes include ruptured aortic aneurysms, ruptured myocardial infarcts, and penetrating traumatic injury to the heart. The escaping blood rapidly fills the pericardial space and leads to cardiac tamponade and death.

CARDIAC TUMORS

The heart, perhaps because of its central role in maintaining life, is largely spared by neoplasms. Those that occur are usually metastatic neoplasms, to be considered first.

Metastatic Neoplasms

Metastatic neoplasms involving the heart are far more common than primary cardiac tumors. Metastases to the heart occur in up to 10% of patients with disseminated cancer. Most often, they involve the pericardium, where they may cause pericarditis and hemorrhagic pericardial effusions. The most common primary neoplasms that metastasize to the heart are carcinomas of the lung and breast, malignant melanomas, and hematopoietic malignancies (lymphomas and leukemias). Metastases may reach the heart via lymphatic, venous, or arterial channels.

Primary Neoplasms

Primary tumors of the heart are rare. The most common types encountered, in descending order of frequency, are myxomas, lipomas, papillary elastofibromas, rhabdomyomas, angiosarcomas, and rhabdomyosarcomas. Only a few merit brief comments.

Myxomas are histologically benign neoplasms that arise most frequently in the left atrium near the fossa ovalis. They appear as sessile or pedunculated lesions, usually covered by an intact endocardium. They occur most often in adults but may arise at any age. Microscopically, they are composed of bland, stellate cells suspended in an edematous, mucopolysaccharide-rich stroma. Immature and mature smooth muscle cells may also be present. Although histologically benign, myxomas may cause significant problems for the patient, either because of the tendency of some lesions to fragment and embolize, or because they may cause a "ball-valve" obstruction of the atrioventricular valves, with resultant syncopal episodes and even sudden death. Surgical resection of such lesions can be lifesaving.

Cardiac rhabdomyomas are the most common primary cardiac tumors of infancy and childhood, often discovered because of obstruction of a valvular orifice. They may occur as apparently isolated lesions, but they are best known for their association with *tuberous sclerosis,* one of the so-called neurocutaneous syndromes. It is likely that these proliferations represent malformations or hamartomas, rather than true neoplasms. Grossly, cardiac rhabdomyomas present as myocardial masses that often project into the ventricular lumen. They

may be solitary or multifocal. Microscopically, they are composed of eosinophilic, polygonal cells, many of which contain large, glycogen-rich cytoplasmic granules. Myofibrils can be demonstrated in such cells under the electron microscope.

Lipomas may occur anywhere in the heart. They most likely represent malformations rather than true neoplasms. Lipoma-like accumulations in the interatrial septum are relatively common and sometimes glorified with the designation *lipomatous hypertrophy*. Although morphologically benign, they have been implicated in some cases of sudden cardiac death.

BIBLIOGRAPHY

Ambrose JA: Plaque disruption and the acute coronary syndromes of unstable angina and myocardial infarction: if the substrate is similar, why is the clinical presentation different? J Am Coll Cardiol 19:1653, 1992.

Buja LM, Willerson JT: The role of coronary artery lesions in ischemic heart disease: insights from recent clinicopathologic, coronary angiographic, and experimental studies. In Virmani R, et al (eds): Cardiovascular Pathology. Philadelphia, WB Saunders, 1991. (A concise, authoritative review of the pathogenesis of coronary artery lesions associated with ischemic heart disease and with the pathophysiology of myocardial ischemia.)

Cannan CR, et al: Natural history of hypertrophic cardiomyopathy. A population-based study, 1976 through 1990. Circulation 92:2488, 1995. (A review of the clinical features and complications, including sudden cardiac death, associated with hypertrophic cardiomyopathy.)

Duncan AK, et al: Cardiovascular disease in elderly patients. Mayo Clin Proc 71:184, 1996. (An overview of the cardiovascular changes associated with aging, and the influence of aging on various forms of cardiac disease.)

Ferencz C, Boughman JA: Congenital heart disease in adolescents and adults. Teratology, genetics, and recurrence rates. Cardiol Clin 11:557, 1993. (A brief review of risk factors and current concepts about the pathogenesis of congenital heart disease.)

Fowler VG, Durack DT: Infective endocarditis. Curr Opin Cardiol 9:389, 1994. (A review of recent literature about the epidemiology and clinical features of infectious endocarditis.)

Fuster V, et al: The pathogenesis of coronary artery disease and the acute coronary syndromes. N Engl J Med 326:242, 310, 1992. (A well-written review of the evolution of coronary atherosclerosis and related lesions associated with myocardial ischemia. Contains an extensive list of useful references.)

Hussain KM, et al: Clinical science review: current aspects of thrombolytic therapy in women with acute myocardial infarction. Angiology 47:23, 1996. (A review of the effectiveness and complications of thrombolytic therapy in myocardial infarction in women compared with men.)

Kaspers EK, et al: The causes of dilated cardiomyopathy: a clinicopathologic review of 673 consecutive patients. J Am Coll Cardiol 23:586, 1994. (A review summarizing an extensive experience with the clinical and morphologic changes associated with dilated cardiomyopathy in a large medical center.)

Keffer JH: Myocardial markers of injury. Evolution and insights. Am J Clin Pathol 105:305, 1996. (An informative review of current trends in laboratory evaluation of acute myocardial infarction and other forms of myocardial injury.)

Keys TF: Early-onset prosthetic valve endocarditis. Cleve Clin J Med 60:455, 1993. (A summary of the risk factors and outcome of infectious endocarditis developing within the first 2 months after valve implantation.)

Payne RM, et al: Toward a molecular understanding of congenital heart disease. Circulation 91:494, 1995. (A review of the incidence and significance of congenital heart disease, and a summary of current ideas about the molecular events underlying its development.)

Van de Werf: Cardiac troponins in acute coronary syndromes. N Engl J Med 335:1388, 1996. (An editorial that summarizes the results of several clinical studies designed to assess the utility of cardiac troponin measurements in diagnosis of ischemic heart disease.)

Virmani R, Roberts WC: Sudden cardiac death. In Virmani R, et al (eds): Cardiovascular Pathology. Philadelphia, WB Saunders, 1991. (A brief but informative review of the various cardiac lesions associated with sudden death.)

Waller BF: The pathology of acute myocardial infarction: definition, location, pathogenesis, effects of reperfusion, complications, and sequelae. Cardiol Clin 6:1, 1988. (A detailed, highly informative presentation of the morphologic features and complications of myocardial infarction.)

Watanakunakorn C, Burkert T: Infective endocarditis at a large community teaching hospital, 1980–1990. A review of 210 episodes. Medicine 72:90, 1993. (A summary of risk factors and pathogens responsible for infectious endocarditis in a large hospital in the midwestern United States.)

Wright JN Jr, Salem D: Sudden cardiac death and the "athlete's heart." Arch Intern Med 155:1473, 1995. (A review of current literature on the cardiovascular response to exercise, and the morphologic lesions associated with sudden cardiac death in younger and older athletes.)

12

The Hematopoietic and Lymphoid Systems

Bleeding Disorders

DISSEMINATED INTRAVASCULAR COAGULATION

Disorders That Affect the Spleen and Thymus

Disorders of the hematopoietic and lymphoid systems encompass a wide range of diseases. They may affect primarily the red cells, the white cells, or the hemostatic mechanisms. *Red cell disorders* are usually reflected in *anemia.* White cell disorders, in contrast, most often involve overgrowth, usually malignant. Hemostatic derangements result in *hemorrhagic diatheses.* Finally, splenomegaly, a feature of several hematopoietic diseases, is discussed at the end of the chapter, as are tumors of the thymus.

Unlike many other organ systems, the lymphohematopoietic system is not confined to a single anatomic site, and hence hematopoietic disorders appear puzzling at first because they involve several anatomically distinct locales. Therefore,

when considering hematopoietic disorders, it is important to remember that the lymphoid and hematopoietic cells are spread throughout the body, and there is constant traffic of cells between various compartments. For example, a patient who is diagnosed, on the basis of a lymph node biopsy, as having a malignant lymphoma may also have neoplastic lymphocytes in the bone marrow and blood and hence be considered to have a leukemia. The malignant lymphoid cells in the marrow may suppress normal production of red cells and platelets, giving rise to anemia and thrombocytopenia; seeding of liver and spleen may cause their enlargement. These apparently diverse manifestations have the same underlying basis.

Red Cell Disorders

Disorders of the red cells usually result in some form of anemia or sometimes in erythrocytosis (i.e., an increase in the number of red cells). *Anemia* is a reduction in the oxygen-

transporting capacity of blood, usually because of a reduction of the total circulating red cell mass to below-normal levels. This is reflected in subnormal hematocrit (HCT) and hemoglobin (Hb) concentrations. In most anemias, erythropoietin production and erythropoiesis are increased, causing erythroid marrow hyperplasia. Increased erythropoiesis can also occur in the spleen and liver of infants (extramedullary hematopoiesis). Classification of anemias is based on the mechanism of production (Table 12–1). Anemias can also be classified on the basis of the appearance of red blood cells (RBCs) in the peripheral blood smear. Factors taken into account in such categorizations are red cell size (normocytic, microcytic, or macrocytic); degree of hemoglobinization, reflected in the color of red cells (normochromic or hypochromic); and several other special features, such as red cell shape. Although these red cell indices are often judged subjectively by the physician, they are also measured objectively and expressed by various terms, as follows:

■

Table 12-2. ADULT REFERENCE RANGES FOR RED BLOOD CELLS*

	Units	Men	Women
Hemoglobin (Hb)	gm/dl	13.6–17.2	12.0–15.0
Hematocrit (HCT)	%	39–49	33–43
Erythrocyte count (RBCs)	×10⁶/mm³	4.3–5.9	3.5–5.0
Reticulocyte count	%	0.5–1.5	
Mean cell volume (MCV)	μm³	76–100	
Mean corpuscular hemoglobin (MCH)	pg	27–33	
Mean corpuscular hemoglobin concentration (MCHC)	gm/dl	33–37	
RBC distribution width (RDW)	—	11.5–14.5	

* Reference ranges vary among laboratories. The reference ranges for the laboratory providing the result should always be used when interpreting a laboratory test. RBC, red blood cell.

■

Table 12-1. CLASSIFICATION OF ANEMIA ACCORDING TO MECHANISM OF PRODUCTION

I. **Blood loss**
  A. Acute: trauma
  B. Chronic: lesions of GI tract, gynecologic disturbances
II. **Increased rate of destruction (hemolytic anemias)**
  A. Intrinsic (intracorpuscular) abnormalities of red cells
    Hereditary:
    1. Disorders of red cell membrane cytoskeleton (e.g., spherocytosis, elliptocytosis)
    2. Red cell enzyme deficiencies
      a. Glycolytic enzymes: pyruvate kinase, hexokinase
      b. Enzymes of hexose monophosphate shunt: G6PD, glutathione synthetase
    3. Disorders of hemoglobin synthesis
      a. Deficient globin synthesis: thalassemia syndromes
      b. Structurally abnormal globin synthesis (hemoglobinopathies): sickle cell anemia, unstable hemoglobins
    Acquired:
    1. Membrane defect: paroxysmal nocturnal hemoglobinuria
  B. Extrinsic (extracorpuscular) abnormalities
    1. Antibody mediated
      a. Isohemagglutinins: transfusion reactions, erythroblastosis fetalis
      b. Autoantibodies: idiopathic (primary), drug-associated, SLE
    2. Mechanical trauma to red cells
      a. Microangiopathic hemolytic anemias: thrombotic thrombocytopenic purpura, DIC
      b. Cardiac traumatic hemolytic anemia
    3. Infections: malaria
III. **Impaired red cell production**
  A. Disturbance of proliferation and differentiation of stem cells: aplastic anemia, pure red cell aplasia, anemia of renal failure, anemia of endocrine disorders
  B. Disturbance of proliferation and maturation of erythroblasts
    1. Defective DNA synthesis: deficiency or impaired utilization of vitamin B₁₂ and folic acid (megaloblastic anemias)
    2. Defective hemoglobin synthesis
      a. Deficient heme synthesis: iron deficiency
      b. Deficient globin synthesis: thalassemias
    3. Unknown or multiple mechanisms: sideroblastic anemia, anemia of chronic infections, myelophthisic anemias due to marrow infiltrations

DIC, disseminated intravascular coagulation; GI, gastrointestinal; G6PD, glucose-6-phosphate dehydrogenase; SLE, systemic lupus erythematosus.

■ *Mean cell volume* (MCV): the average volume of an RBC, expressed in femtoliters (cubic micrometers)
■ *Mean cell hemoglobin* (MCH): the average content (mass) of Hb per RBC, expressed in picograms
■ *Mean cell hemoglobin concentration* (MCHC): the average concentration of Hb in a given volume of packed RBCs, expressed in grams per deciliter
■ *RBC distribution width* (RDW): the coefficient of variation of RBC volume.

RBC indices may be calculated from hematocrit, hemoglobin, and red cell count values, but in most laboratories instruments directly measure or automatically calculate them. Adult reference ranges are shown in Table 12–2. Anemias classified on the basis of morphology and alterations in red cell indices usually correlate with the cause of the red cell deficiency.

HEMORRHAGE: BLOOD LOSS ANEMIA

With acute blood loss, the immediate threat to the patient is hypovolemia (shock) rather than anemia. If the patient survives, hemodilution begins at once and achieves its full effect within 2 to 3 days, unmasking the extent of the red cell loss. If body iron stores are adequate, after several days there is increased erythropoiesis in the marrow, with complete replacement of red cells. *The anemia is normocytic, normochromic.* Marrow compensation is reflected by reticulocytosis in peripheral blood. With chronic blood loss, iron stores are gradually depleted, resulting in anemia of iron deficiency. Because iron deficiency anemia can occur in other clinical settings as well, it is described later in this chapter along with other anemias of diminished erythropoiesis (p 353).

INCREASED RATE OF RED CELL DESTRUCTION: THE HEMOLYTIC ANEMIAS

Shortened survival of red cells may be due either to inherent defects in the erythrocyte (intracorpuscular hemolytic anemia), which are usually inherited, or to external influences (extracorpuscular hemolytic anemia), which are usually acquired. Several examples are listed in Table 12–1.

Before proceeding to discuss the various disorders individually, we will describe certain general features of hemolytic anemias. All are characterized by (1) increased rate of RBC destruction and (2) retention by the body of the products of red cell destruction, including iron. Because the iron is conserved and recycled readily, red cell regeneration can keep pace with the hemolysis. Consequently, these anemias are almost invariably associated with *marked hypercellularity within the marrow* owing to an increase in erythropoiesis. Sometimes there is also extramedullary hematopoiesis in the liver and spleen. Red cell regeneration is demonstrated by an *increase in the reticulocyte count in peripheral blood.*

Destruction of red cells may occur within the vascular compartment (intravascular hemolysis) or within the cells of the mononuclear phagocyte, or reticuloendothelial (RE), system (extravascular hemolysis). *Intravascular hemolysis* is seen in red cells subjected to mechanical trauma or in cells damaged by fixation of complement, as occurs in hemolytic transfusion reactions and in malaria. Whatever the cause, intravascular hemolysis results in hemoglobinemia, hemoglobinuria, and hemosiderinuria. Conversion of the heme pigment to bilirubin may give rise to unconjugated hyperbilirubinemia and jaundice. Massive intravascular hemolysis sometimes leads to acute tubular necrosis (Chapter 14). Levels of *serum haptoglobin,* a protein that binds free Hb, are characteristically low.

Extravascular hemolysis, the more common mode of red cell destruction, takes place largely within the phagocytic cells of the spleen and liver. The mononuclear phagocyte system removes erythrocytes from the circulation whenever red cells are injured or immunologically altered. Because extreme alterations of shape are necessary for red cells to successfully navigate the splenic sinusoids, reduction in deformability makes this passage difficult and leads to splenic sequestration, followed by phagocytosis (Fig. 12–1). This is believed to be an important factor in the pathogenesis of red cell destruction in a variety of hemolytic anemias. Extravascular hemolysis is not associated with hemoglobinemia and hemoglobinuria, but jaundice may result and in long-standing cases may lead to gallstone formation. *Serum haptoglobin* is always decreased, because some Hb invariably escapes into the plasma. In most forms of hemolytic anemia, there is hyperactivity of the mononuclear system, which results in splenomegaly.

Because the pathways for the excretion of excess iron are limited, there is a tendency in hemolytic anemias for abnormal amounts of iron to accumulate, giving rise to systemic he-

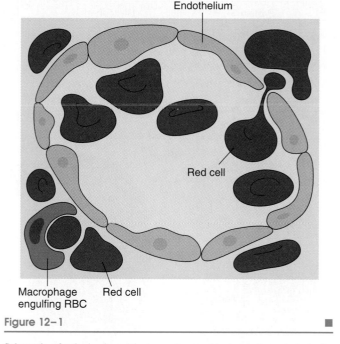

Figure 12–1   ■

Schematic of splenic sinus (electron micrograph). An erythrocyte is in the process of squeezing from the cord into the sinus lumen. Note the degree of deformability required for the red cells to pass through the wall of the sinus.

mosiderosis (Chapter 1) or, in very severe cases, secondary hemochromatosis (Chapter 16).

Hereditary Spherocytosis

This disorder is characterized by an inherited (intrinsic) defect in the red cell membrane that renders the erythrocytes spheroidal, less deformable, and vulnerable to splenic sequestration and destruction. Hereditary spherocytosis (HS) is most commonly transmitted as an autosomal dominant trait; approximately 25% of patients have an autosomal recessive form of the disease that is much more severe than the autosomal dominant form.

Pathogenesis. In HS, the *primary abnormality resides in the proteins that form the skeleton of the red cell membrane.* Several such proteins (Fig. 12–2) form an interlocking but flexible structure on the intracellular face of the cell membrane. They are tethered to the lipid bilayer, serving to stabilize it, and are responsible for the normal shape, strength, and flexibility of the red cell. In most patients, mutations in ankyrin molecule (Fig. 12–2) cause a secondary deficiency of spectrin. These red cells have reduced membrane stability and consequently lose membrane fragments as the cells are exposed to shear stresses in the circulation. Reduction in the membrane substance (and surface area) forces the cells to assume the smallest possible diameter for a given volume— namely, a sphere (Fig. 12–2).

The spleen plays a major role in the destruction of spherocytes. Red cells must undergo extreme degrees of deformation to leave the cords of Billroth and enter the splenic sinusoids. The discoid shape of normal red cells allows

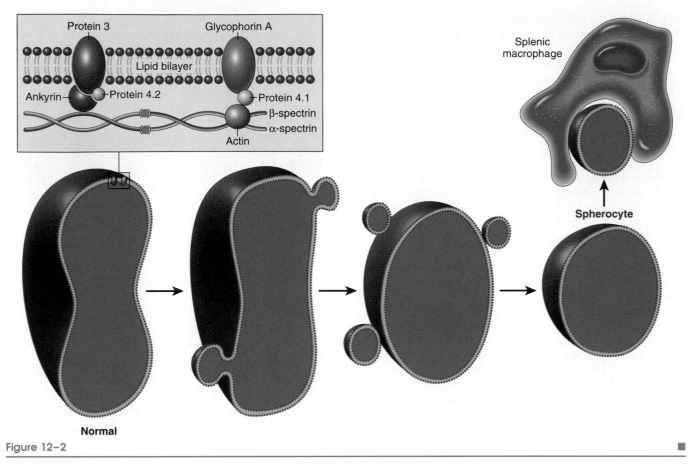

Figure 12–2 ■

Schematic representation of the red cell membrane cytoskeleton, and effects of alterations in the cytoskeletal proteins on the shape of red cells. With mutations that affect the integrity of the membrane cytoskeleton, the normal biconcave erythrocyte loses membrane fragments. To accommodate the loss of surface area, the cell adopts a spherical shape. Such spherocytic cells are less deformable than normal and are therefore trapped in the splenic cords, where they are phagocytosed by macrophages.

considerable latitude for changes in cell shape. In contrast, because of their spheroidal shape and reduced membrane plasticity, spherocytes have great difficulty leaving the splenic cords. The abnormal red cells are sequestered and eventually destroyed by macrophages, which are plentiful in the splenic cords. *The critical role of the spleen in this process is illustrated by the invariably beneficial effect of splenectomy. The red cell defect persists, but the anemia is corrected.*

MORPHOLOGY. On smears, the red cells lack the central zone of pallor because of their spheroidal shape. Spherocytosis, although distinctive, is not diagnostic, because it is seen in any condition that leads to loss of the cell membrane—as, for example, in immune hemolytic anemias, discussed later. To compensate for the excessive red cell destruction, erythropoiesis in the marrow is stimulated. As with other hemolytic anemias, red cell regeneration is demonstrated by reticulocytosis in the peripheral blood. Splenomegaly is greater and more common in HS than in any other form of hemolytic anemia. Splenic weight is usually be-

tween 500 and 1000 gm but may be greater. The enlargement of the spleen results from striking congestion of the cords of Billroth, leaving the splenic sinuses virtually empty. Phagocytosed red cells are frequently seen within hypertrophic macrophages lining the sinusoids and, in particular, within the cords. In long-standing cases there is prominent systemic hemosiderosis.

The other general features of hemolytic anemias described earlier are present with this disorder. In particular, cholelithiasis occurs in 40% to 50% of these patients.

Clinical Course. The characteristic clinical features are *anemia, splenomegaly,* and *jaundice.* The severity of this disorder is highly variable. Asymptomatic cases occur, as do cases characterized by a profound anemia, but in general the anemia is moderate. Because the red cells are spheroidal in shape, there is little margin for expansion of volume when cells are exposed to hypotonic salt solution. As a result, *increased osmotic fragility is a characteristic finding that is helpful in diagnosis.*

The more or less stable clinical course may be punctuated

by an aplastic crisis. These episodes, often triggered by parvovirus infection of developing erythroblasts in the marrow, are associated with cessation of red cell production. There is worsening of anemia and reticulocytopenia. In most cases such episodes are self-limited, but some patients may need blood transfusions.

There is no treatment for HS. In those who are symptomatic, splenectomy is beneficial because the major site of red cell destruction is removed; however, splenectomy must be weighed against the risk of increased susceptibility to infections, particularly in children.

Sickle Cell Anemia

The hemoglobinopathies are a group of hereditary disorders characterized by the presence of a structurally abnormal Hb. More than 300 hemoglobins have been discovered, a third of which are associated with significant clinical manifestations. The prototype and most prevalent hemoglobinopathy results from a mutation in the gene coding for the β-globin chain that causes the formation of the sickle hemoglobin (HbS). The associated disease, sickle cell anemia, is discussed here; other hemoglobinopathies are much less frequent for our consideration.

HbS, like 90% of other abnormal hemoglobins, results from a single amino acid substitution in the globin chain. Hb, as may be recalled, is a tetramer of four globin chains comprising two pairs of similar chains. In the normal adult, Hb is composed of 96% hemoglobin A HbA, ($\alpha_2\beta_2$), 3% HbA$_2$ ($\alpha_2\delta_2$), and 1% fetal hemoglobin (HbF, $\alpha_2\gamma_2$). Substitution of valine for glutamic acid at the sixth position of the β-chain produces HbS. In homozygotes, all HbA is replaced by HbS, whereas in heterozygotes, only about half is replaced.

Incidence. Approximately 8% of American blacks are heterozygous for HbS. In parts of Africa where malaria is endemic, the gene frequency approaches 30%, attributed to the slight protective effect of HbS against *Plasmodium falcipa-*

rum malaria. In the United States, sickle cell anemia affects approximately one of every 600 blacks; worldwide, sickle cell anemia is the most common form of familial hemolytic anemia.

Etiology and Pathogenesis. On deoxygenation, HbS molecules undergo polymerization, a process sometimes called *gelation* or *crystallization.* The change in the physical state of HbS distorts the red cells, which assume an elongated crescentic, or sickle, shape (Fig. 12–3). Sickling of red cells is initially reversible by oxygenation; however, membrane damage occurs with each episode of sickling, and eventually the cells accumulate calcium, lose potassium and water, and become irreversibly sickled, despite adequate oxygenation.

Many factors influence sickling of red cells. The three most important ones are as follows:

■ *The amount of HbS in the cell.* In heterozygotes, approximately 40% of Hb is HbS; the rest is HbA, which interacts only weakly with HbS during the processes of aggregation. Therefore, heterozygotes have little tendency to sickle and are said to have the *sickle cell trait.* In contrast, all of the Hb in homozygotes consists of HbS, and thus homozygotes have full-blown sickle cell anemia.

■ *The presence of hemoglobins other than HbA.* HbC, another mutant β-globin, is fairly common. The carrier rate for HbC in American blacks is about 2.3%, giving the likelihood that one in 1250 newborns will be a double heterozygote for HbS and HbC (i.e., will have the HbS gene from one parent and HbC from the other). HbC has a greater tendency to aggregate with HbS than does HbA, and hence those with HbS and HbC (called *HbSC*) have a more severe disease than do those with the sickle cell trait. Conversely, HbF interacts poorly with HbS, and hence newborns with sickle cell anemia do not manifest the disease until they are 5 to 6 months old, when the HbF falls to adult levels. This, as we will see, can be exploited for the treatment of sickle cell anemia.

■ *The MCHC per cell.* The higher the HbS concentration within the cell, the greater are the chances of contact and

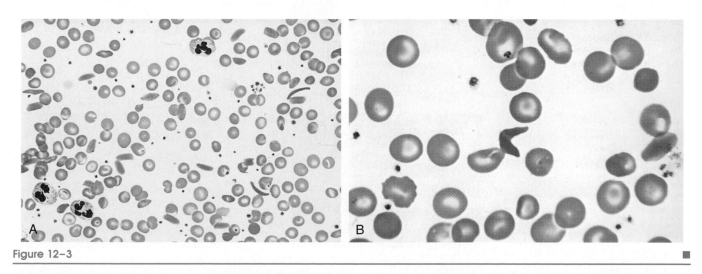

Figure 12–3   ■

Peripheral blood smear from a patient with sickle cell anemia. *A,* Low magnification shows sickle cells, anisocytosis, and poikilocytosis. *B,* Higher magnification shows an irreversibly sickled cell in the center. (Courtesy of Dr. Robert W. McKenna, Department of Pathology, University of Texas Southwestern Medical School, Dallas, TX.)

interaction between HbS molecules. Thus, dehydration, by increasing the MCHC, greatly facilitates sickling and may trigger occlusion of small blood vessels. Conversely, the coexistence of α-thalassemia (described later), characterized by reduced synthesis of globin chains, reduces the MCHC and therefore the severity of sickling.

Two major consequences stem from the sickling of red cells (Fig. 12–4). First, sickled red cells become rigid and therefore susceptible to sequestration and *hemolysis* within the spleen, as already discussed. Their mean life span is reduced from 120 days to approximately 20 days. Second, in addition to hemolytic anemia, sickle cell disease is associated with widespread *microvascular obstructions* and resulting ischemic damage. It is generally assumed that occlusion of small blood vessels results from sickling of cells as they traverse the microvasculature; in addition, recent observations suggest that the presence of HbS is associated with other abnormalities (e.g., increased stickiness of red cells to endothelium owing to up-regulation of adhesion molecules) that play a significant role in the pathogenesis of vascular occlusion.

> **MORPHOLOGY.** The anatomic alterations stem from the following three aspects of the disease: (1) hemolysis, with resultant anemia; (2) increased release of Hb, with bilirubin formation; and (3) capillary stasis, with thrombosis. In peripheral smears, sickled red cells are evident as bizarre, elongated, spindled, or boat-shaped structures (Fig. 12–3). Both the severe anemia and the vascular stasis

lead to fatty changes in the heart, liver, and renal tubules. Erythropoiesis is activated in the bone marrow. Expansion of marrow may lead to resorption of bone with appositional new bone formation on the external aspect of the skull, leading to a "crew-cut" appearance on radiographs. Extramedullary hematopoiesis may appear in the spleen and liver.

In children there is moderate splenomegaly (splenic weight up to 500 gm), caused by congestion of the red pulp with masses of red cells sickled and jammed together. Eventually this splenic erythrostasis leads to enough hypoxic tissue damage, sometimes with frank infarction, to create a shrunken, fibrotic spleen. This process, termed **autosplenectomy,** is seen in all long-standing adult cases. Ultimately, only a small nubbin of fibrous tissue remains of the spleen.

Vascular congestion, thrombosis, and infarction may affect any organ, including bones, liver, kidney, and retina. Approximately 50% of adult patients develop leg ulcers because of hypoxia of the subcutaneous tissues. Cor pulmonale may result from thromboses in the pulmonary vessels. As with the other hemolytic anemias, hemosiderosis and gallstones are common.

Clinical Course. Homozygous sickle cell disease usually becomes apparent after the sixth month of life, as HbF is gradually replaced by HbS. The anemia is severe, with HCT values

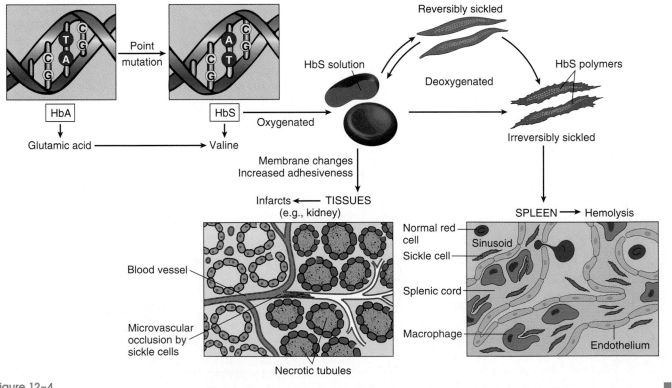

Figure 12–4

Pathophysiology and morphologic consequences of sickle cell anemia.

ranging between 18% and 30% (normal range, 35% to 45%). The chronic hemolysis is associated with marked reticulocytosis and hyperbilirubinemia. From the time of onset, the process runs an unremitting course, punctuated by sudden episodes of so-called crises. The most serious of these are the *vasoocclusive,* or *painful, crises.* The pain in these crises may be localized to the abdomen (sometimes simulating "acute abdomen"), chest, or joints. The painful crises are believed to result from microvascular occlusions and associated hypoxic tissue injury. Such crises may occur without warning or be precipitated by infections, dehydration, and acidosis (all of which favor sickling). Ischemia of the central nervous system may result in stroke. In the course of the disease, virtually any organ may be damaged by such ischemic injury. The other form, *aplastic crisis,* represents a sudden but usually temporary cessation of erythropoiesis. Reticulocytes disappear from the blood, and anemia worsens. As in HS, the aplastic crisis is usually triggered by parvovirus infection of erythroblasts. In addition to these crises, patients with sickle cell disease are very susceptible to infections. The increased susceptibility to infections is probably multifactorial: (1) impaired splenic function—the erythrophagocytosis interferes with bacterial killing; (2) in later stages, total splenic fibrosis removes an important biologic filter of blood-borne microorganisms; and (3) defects in the alternative complement pathway impair opsonization of encapsulated bacteria such as pneumococci. For reasons not entirely clear, patients with sickle cell disease are particularly predisposed to *Salmonella* osteomyelitis.

With full-blown sickle cell disease, at least some sickled erythrocytes can be seen on an ordinary peripheral blood smear. In sickle cell trait, sickling can be induced in vitro by exposing cells to hypoxia. Ultimately, the diagnosis depends on the electrophoretic demonstration of HbS. Prenatal diagnosis of sickle cell anemia can be performed by analyzing the DNA in fetal cells obtained by amniocentesis or biopsy of chorionic villi (Chapter 7).

The clinical course of patients with sickle cell anemia is highly variable. As a result of improvements in supportive care, an increasing number of patients are surviving into adulthood and producing offspring. Approximately 50% survive beyond the fifth decade. Sickle cell trait, in contrast, generally remains entirely asymptomatic unless the patient becomes extremely hypoxic. As mentioned earlier, the presence of HbF in cells retards sickling by inhibiting polymer formation. This observation has been exploited therapeutically. Hydroxyurea, a drug commonly used in cancer chemotherapy, affects erythropoietic stem cells in a manner that results in increased levels of HbF in the newly formed cells. Because HbF retards sickling, treatment with hydroxyurea has been found to be useful in the management of sickle cell disease.

Thalassemia

The thalassemias are a heterogeneous group of genetic disorders of Hb synthesis characterized by a lack of or decreased synthesis of globin chains. In α-thalassemia, α-globin chain synthesis is reduced, whereas in β-thalassemia, β-globin chain synthesis is either absent (designated β^0-thalassemia) or markedly deficient (β^+-thalassemia). Unlike the hemoglobinopathies, which represent qualitative abnormalities, thalassemias result from quantitative abnormalities of globin chain synthesis. The consequences of reduced synthesis of one globin chain derive not only from the low level of intracellular Hb, but also from the relative excess of the other globin chain, as will be discussed later.

Thalassemia is inherited as an autosomal codominant condition. The heterozygous form (*thalassemia minor* or *thalassemia trait*) may be asymptomatic or mildly symptomatic. The homozygous form, *thalassemia major,* is associated with severe hemolytic anemia. The mutant genes are particularly common among Mediterranean, African, and Asian populations.

Molecular Pathogenesis. A complex pattern of molecular defects underlies the thalassemias. Recall that adult Hb, or HbA, contains two α chains and two β chains. The β chains are coded by two β-globin genes, each on one of the two number 11 chromosomes. In contrast, one pair of functional α-globin genes is on each of the two chromosomes 16.

β-Thalassemia. As mentioned earlier, β-thalassemia syndromes can be classified into two categories: (1) β^0-thalassemia, associated with total absence of β-globin chains in the homozygous state, and (2) β^+-thalassemia, characterized by reduced (but detectable) β-globin synthesis in the homozygous state. Sequencing of cloned β-globin genes obtained from thalassemic patients has revealed more than 100 different mutations responsible for β^0- or β^+-thalassemia. Most of these result from single base changes. In contrast to α-thalassemias, described later, *gene deletions rarely underlie β-thalassemias* (Table 12–3).

Details of these mutations and their effects on β-globin synthesis are beyond our scope, but a few illustrative examples will be cited (Fig. 12–5):

■ The promoter region controls the initiation and rate of transcription, and therefore mutations affecting promoter sequences usually lead to reduced globin gene transcription. Because some β-globin is synthesized, patients develop β^+-thalassemia.

■ Mutations in the coding sequences are usually associated with more serious consequences. For example, in some cases a single nucleotide change in one of the exons leads to the formation of a termination, or "stop," codon, which interrupts translation of β-globin messenger RNA (mRNA). Premature termination generates nonfunctional fragments of the β-globin, leading to β^0-thalassemia.

■ *Mutations that lead to aberrant mRNA processing are the most common cause of β-thalassemia.* Most of these affect introns, but some have been located within exons. If the mutation alters the normal splice junctions, splicing does not occur, and all of the mRNA formed is abnormal. Unspliced mRNA is degraded within the nucleus, and β^0-thalassemia results. However, some mutations affect the introns at locations away from the normal intron–exon splice junction. These mutations create new sites that are sensitive to the action of splicing enzymes at abnormal locations—within an intron, for example. Because normal splice sites remain unaffected, both normal and abnormal splicing occur, giving rise to normal as well as abnormal β-globin mRNA. These patients develop β^+-thalassemia.

Two factors contribute to the pathogenesis of anemia in β-thalassemia. Reduced synthesis of β-globin leads to inade-

Table 12–3. CLINICAL AND GENETIC CLASSIFICATION OF THALASSEMIAS

Clinical Nomenclature	Genotype	Disease	Molecular Genetics
β-Thalassemias			
Thalassemia major	Homozygous β^0-thalassemia (β^0/β^0); Homozygous β^+-thalassemia (β^+/β^+)	Severe, requires blood transfusions regularly	Rare gene deletions in β^0/β^0 Defects in transcription, processing, or translation of β-globin mRNA
Thalassemia minor	β^0/β β^+/β	Asymptomatic with mild or no anemia; red cell abnormalities seen	
α-Thalassemia			
Silent carrier	$-\alpha/\alpha\alpha$	Asymptomatic; no red cell abnormality	
α-Thalassemia trait	$--/\alpha\alpha$ (Asian); $-\alpha/-\alpha$ (black African)	Asymptomatic, like thalassemia minor	Gene deletions mainly
HbH disease	$--/-\alpha$	Severe anemia, tetramers of β-globin (HbH) formed in red cells	
Hydrops fetalis	$--/--$	Lethal in utero	

mRNA, messenger RNA.

quate HbA formation, so that the overall Hb concentration (MCHC) per cell is lower, and the cells appear *hypochromic*. Much more important is the *hemolytic component* of β-thalassemia. This is due not to lack of β-globin but to the relative excess of α-globin chains, whose synthesis remains normal. Free α-chains form insoluble aggregates that precipitate within the erythrocytes (Fig. 12–6). These inclusions damage the cell membranes, reduce their plasticity, and render the red cells susceptible to phagocytosis by the mononuclear phagocyte system. Not only are mature red cells susceptible to premature destruction, but also a majority of the erythroblasts within the marrow are destroyed owing to the presence of the inclusions. Such intramedullary destruction of red cells (*ineffective erythropoiesis*) has another untoward effect: it is associated with increased absorption of dietary iron, which contributes to the iron overload in these patients.

α-Thalassemia. The molecular basis of α-thalassemia is quite different from that of β-thalassemia. Most of the α-thal-

assemias are due to deletions of α-globin gene *loci*. Since there are four functional α-globin genes, there are four possible degrees of α-thalassemia, based on loss of one to four α-globin genes from the chromosomes. These cover a wide spectrum of clinical disorders, the severity of which is related to the number of deleted α-globin genes (Table 12–3). Loss of a single α-globin gene is associated with a silent carrier state, whereas deletion of all four α-globin genes is associated with fetal death in utero, because the blood has virtually no oxygen-carrying capacity. The basis of the hemolysis is similar to that in β-thalassemia. With loss of three α-globin genes, there is a relative excess of β-globin or other non–α-globin chains, which form insoluble tetramers within red cells and render the cells vulnerable to phagocytosis and destruction. It should be noted, however, that non-α chains in general form more soluble and less toxic aggregates than do those derived from α chains. Hence the hemolytic anemia and ineffective erythropoiesis tend be less severe in α-thalassemia.

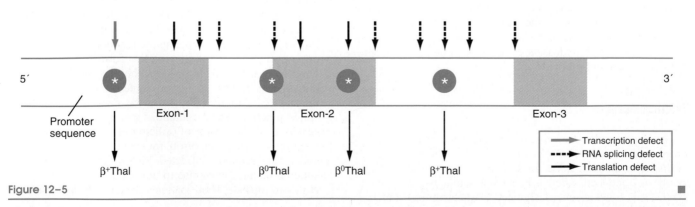

Figure 12–5

Diagrammatic representation of the β-globin gene and some sites where point mutations giving rise to β-thalassemia have been localized. (Modified from Wyngaarden JB, Smith LH, Bennett JC (eds): Cecil Textbook of Medicine, 19th ed. Philadelphia, WB Saunders, 1992.)

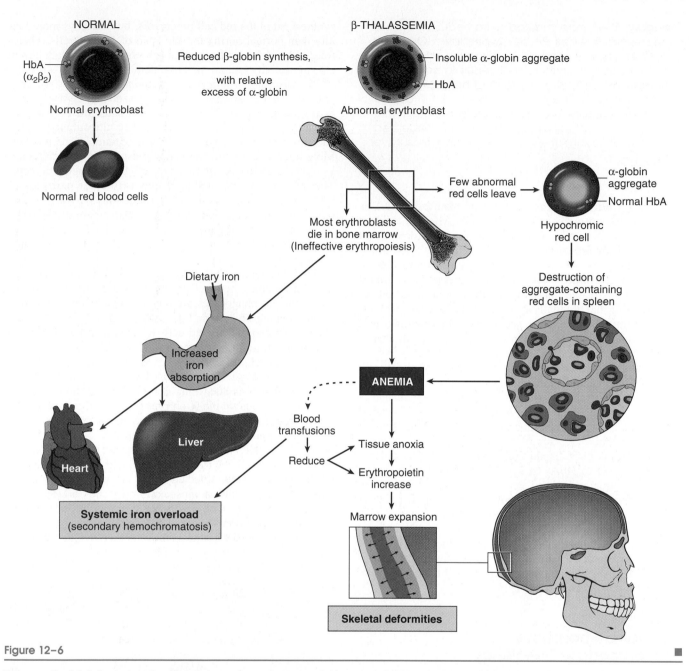

Figure 12–6   ■

Pathogenesis of β-thalassemia major. Note that aggregates of excess α-globin are not visible on routine blood smears. Blood transfusions, on the one hand, correct the anemia and reduce stimulus for erythropoietin secretion and deformities induced by marrow expansion; on the other hand, they add to systemic iron overload.

MORPHOLOGY. Only the morphologic changes in β-thalassemia, which is more common in the United States, will be described. Typically, in thalassemia major the peripheral blood smear shows **microcytic, hypochromic red cells.** Some red cells have an abnormal distribution of Hb, giving them a target-like appearance (target cells). In addition, there is **severe poikilocytosis, anisocytosis, and reticulocytosis.** Normoblasts are present in the peripheral blood.

In β-thalassemia major, the anatomic changes are identical to those of all hemolytic anemias, but especially prominent are hyperactivity of the bone marrow and splenomegaly. The marrow is expanded to the fetal level, so all the fatty marrow may be reactivated. In the red cell series, there is a striking shift toward primitive forms. Massive erythropoiesis within the bone invades the bony cortex, impairs bone growth, and produces **skeletal deformities. Splenomegaly** and **hepato-**

megaly result from marked extramedullary hematopoiesis as well as RE cell hyperplasia. Over the span of years, excessive breakdown of red cells and ineffective erythropoiesis result in **severe hemosiderosis** and, rarely, a form of hemochromatosis (Chapter 16). The iron overload is due in part to excessive dietary iron absorption associated with ineffective erythropoiesis and to the repeated blood transfusions these patients need to survive (Fig. 12–6).

Clinical Course. *Thalassemia major* manifests itself as soon as HbF is normally replaced by HbA. Affected children fail to develop normally, and their growth is retarded almost from birth. They are sustained only by repeated blood transfusions, which not only improve the anemia, but also reduce the skeletal deformities associated with excessive erythropoiesis. With transfusions, survival into the second or third decade is possible, but gradually systemic iron overload develops. Cardiac failure resulting from secondary hemochromatosis is an important cause of death in those who reach adolescence. The average age at death is 17 years.

With *thalassemia minor* there is usually only a mild microcytic hypochromic anemia, and in general these patients have a normal life expectancy. Because *iron deficiency anemia is associated with a similar appearance of red cells,* it should be excluded by appropriate laboratory tests, described later in this chapter. The diagnosis of β-thalassemia minor is made by Hb electrophoresis. In addition to reduced amounts of HbA ($\alpha_2\beta_2$), the level of HbA$_2$ ($\alpha_2\delta_2$) is increased. The diagnosis of β-thalassemia major can generally be made on clinical grounds. The peripheral blood shows a severe microcytic hypochromic anemia, with marked variation in cell shapes (poikilocytosis). The reticulocyte count is increased. Hb electrophoresis shows profound reduction or absence of HbA and increased levels of HbF. The HbA$_2$ level may be normal or increased. Prenatal diagnosis of both forms of thalassemia can be made by DNA probe analysis.

Glucose-6-Phosphate Dehydrogenase Deficiency

The erythrocyte and its membrane are vulnerable to injury by endogenous and exogenous oxidants. Normally, intracellular reduced glutathione (GSH) inactivates such oxidants. Abnormalities of enzymes that participate in the hexose monophosphate shunt or glutathione metabolism reduce the ability of red cells to protect themselves from oxidative injury and lead to hemolytic anemias. The prototype and most prevalent of these anemias is caused by a deficiency of glucose-6-phosphate dehydrogenase (G6PD). The G6PD gene is on the X chromosome, and there is considerable polymorphism at this locus. More than 400 G6PD genetic variants, most of which are not associated with disease, have been identified. In the United States, the G6PD A⁻ variant is associated with hemolytic anemia. It is encountered primarily in blacks. Approximately 10% of black males in the United States are affected. In these individuals, a normal amount of enzyme is synthesized in the red cell precursors, but it decays more rapidly than normal during the life span of the red cells. Therefore, older red cells become progressively more deficient in enzyme activity and are most vulnerable to oxidant stress.

This disorder produces no symptoms unless the red cells are subjected to oxidant injury by exposure to certain drugs, toxins, or infections. The drugs incriminated include antimalarials (e.g., primaquine), sulfonamides, nitrofurantoin, phenacetin, aspirin (in large doses), and vitamin K derivatives. More important are infections that presumably trigger hemolysis owing to release of free radicals from phagocytic cells. The effect of these offending agents is to cause oxidation of GSH to glutathione through the production of hydrogen peroxide. Because regeneration of GSH is impaired in G6PD-deficient cells, hydrogen peroxide accumulates and denatures globin chains by oxidation of sulfhydryl groups. Denatured Hb is precipitated within the red cells in the form of inclusions called *Heinz bodies.* Not only are inclusion-bearing red cells less deformable, their cell membranes are further damaged when splenic phagocytes attempt to "pluck out" the inclusions, creating so-called "bite cells" (Fig. 12–7). All these changes predispose the red cells to becoming trapped in the splenic sinuses and destroyed by the phagocytes.

The drug-induced hemolysis is acute and of variable clinical severity. Typically, patients develop evidence of intravascular hemolysis after a lag period of 2 or 3 days. Because the G6PD gene is on the X chromosome, all the erythrocytes of affected males are deficient in enzyme activity. However, owing to random inactivation of one X chromosome in women (Chapter 7), heterozygous females have two distinct populations of red cells: some normal, and others deficient in G6PD activity. Thus, affected males are more vulnerable to oxidant injury, whereas most carrier females are asymptomatic, except those with a very large proportion of deficient red cells (a condition known as *unfavorable lyonization*). Because the enzyme deficiency is most marked in older red cells,

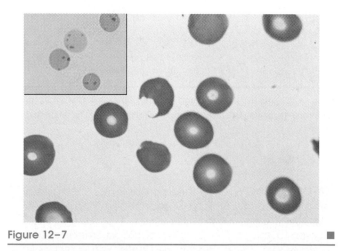

Figure 12–7

Peripheral blood smear from a patient with glucose-6-phosphate dehydrogenase deficiency after exposure to an oxidant drug. *Inset,* Red cells with precipitates of denatured globin (Heinz bodies) revealed by supravital staining. As the splenic macrophages pluck out these inclusions, "bite cells" like the one in this smear are produced. (Courtesy of Dr. Robert W. McKenna, Department of Pathology, University of Texas Southwestern Medical School, Dallas, TX.)

these cells are more susceptible to lysis. As the marrow compensates by producing new (young) red cells, hemolysis tends to abate even if drug exposure continues. In other variants, such as G6PD Mediterranean, found mainly in the Middle East, the enzyme deficiency and the resultant hemolysis are more severe.

Paroxysmal Nocturnal Hemoglobinuria

This rare disorder of unknown etiology is mentioned here because it is the only form of hemolytic anemia that results from an *acquired membrane defect secondary to a mutation that affects myeloid stem cells.* The mutant gene, called *PIG-A,* is required for anchoring several proteins into the cell membrane. These include three proteins that limit the spontaneous activation of complement on the surface of cells. Proliferation of the abnormal clone of myeloid stem cells yields red cells, granulocytes, and platelets that are inordinately sensitive to the lytic activity of complement. These patients have intravascular *hemolysis* and a striking predisposition to *infections* and intravascular *thromboses.* Because paroxysmal nocturnal hemoglobinuria (PNH) is an acquired disorder of stem cells, it sometimes transforms into other stem cell disorders such as acute leukemia and aplastic anemia.

Immunohemolytic Anemias

In these uncommon disorders, the hemolytic anemia is caused by antibodies reactive against normal or altered red cell membranes. Anti–red cell antibodies may arise spontaneously in autoimmune hemolytic anemias, or their formation may be initiated by exogenous agents such as drugs or chemicals. Immunohemolytic anemias are classified on the basis of the nature of the antibody involved and possible associated predisposing conditions, which are presented in simplified form in Table 12–4.

Whatever the cause of antibody formation, the diagnosis of immunohemolytic anemias depends on the demonstration of anti–red cell antibodies. The method most commonly used to detect such antibodies is the *Coombs antiglobulin test,* which is based on the capacity of antihuman antibodies (prepared in animals) to agglutinate red cells. A positive result indicates that the patient's red cells are coated with human antibodies

that can react with the antihuman globulin serum. This is called the *direct Coombs test.* The *indirect Coombs test* is used to detect antibodies in the patient's serum and involves incubating normal red cells with the patient's serum, followed by a direct Coombs test on these incubated red cells.

Warm Antibody Immunohemolytic Anemias. These are characterized by the presence of immunoglobulin G (IgG) (rarely, immunoglobulin A [IgA]) antibodies, which are active at 37°C. Many cases (more than 60%) are idiopathic (primary) and so belong to the category of autoimmune diseases. Approximately one fourth of the cases are so-called secondary because an underlying disease (e.g., systemic lupus erythematosus [SLE]) affects the immune system, or the anemia is induced by drugs. The *pathogenesis of hemolysis in most instances involves opsonization of the red cells by the IgG antibodies and subsequent phagocytosis by splenic macrophages.* Spheroidal cells resembling those found in hereditary spherocytosis are often found in idiopathic immune hemolytic anemia. Presumably, bits of cell membrane are injured and removed during attempted phagocytosis of antibody-coated cells; this reduces surface area and induces *spheroidal conformation.* The spherocytes are then destroyed in the spleen, as described earlier (p 343). The clinical severity of immunohemolytic anemia is quite variable. Most patients have chronic mild anemia with moderate splenomegaly and often require no treatment.

The mechanisms of hemolysis induced by drugs are varied and in some cases poorly understood. Drugs such as α-methyldopa induce an anemia indistinguishable from the primary idiopathic form of hemolytic anemia. Autoantibodies directed against intrinsic red cell antigens, in particular Rh blood group antigens, are formed. Presumably, the drug alters native epitopes and thus allows a bypass of T-cell tolerance to the membrane proteins (see Fig. 5–20). In other cases, drugs such as penicillin act as haptens and induce an antibody response by binding to a red cell membrane protein. Sometimes antibodies are formed against the drug in circulation, and immune complexes damage the red cell membranes as innocent bystanders.

Cold Antibody Immunohemolytic Anemias. These anemias are characterized by the presence of immunoglobulin M (IgM) antibodies, which bind to red cell membranes at temperatures below 30°C, as may be encountered in distal body parts (e.g., hands, toes). Fixation of complement may cause intravascular hemolysis. However, most commonly the antibody- and complement-coated cells are not lysed, because complement is most active at 37°C. When such antibody- and complement-coated cells travel to warmer areas, IgM antibody is released, and the cell is left with a coating of C3b. Because the latter is an opsonin (Chapter 2), the cells are phagocytosed by the mononuclear phagocyte system, especially Kupffer cells, and hence the *hemolysis is extravascular.* Cold agglutinins occur acutely during recovery from mycoplasma pneumonia and infectious mononucleosis. The resulting anemia is mild, transient, and of no clinical import. Chronic cold agglutinin formation and associated hemolytic anemia may also occur in association with lymphoproliferative disorders or as an idiopathic condition. In addition to anemia, Raynaud's phenomenon may occur in these patients owing to agglutination of red cells in the capillaries of exposed parts of the body.

Table 12–4. CLASSIFICATION OF IMMUNOHEMOLYTIC ANEMIAS

Warm Antibody Type
  Primary (idiopathic)
  Secondary: lymphomas and leukemias (CLL and non-Hodgkin's lymphomas), SLE, drugs (e.g., α-methyldopa, penicillin, quinidine)
Cold Antibody Type
  Acute: mycoplasma infection, infectious mononucleosis
  Chronic: idiopathic, associated with lymphomas

Hemolytic Anemias Resulting From Mechanical Trauma to Red Cells

RBCs may be disrupted by physical trauma in a variety of circumstances. *Clinically important are the hemolytic anemias associated with cardiac valve prostheses and with narrowing or obstruction of the vasculature.* Traumatic hemolytic anemia is more severe with artificial, mechanical valves than with bioprosthetic, porcine valves. In patients with prosthetic valves of either type, the red cells are damaged by the shear stresses resulting from the turbulent blood flow and abnormal pressure gradients caused by the valves. Microangiopathic hemolytic anemia, on the other hand, is characterized by mechanical damage to the red cells as they squeeze through abnormally narrowed vessels. Most often the narrowing is caused by widespread deposition of fibrin in the small vessels in association with disseminated intravascular coagulation (DIC) (p 384). Other causes of microangiopathic hemolytic anemia include malignant hypertension, SLE, thrombotic thrombocytopenic purpura, hemolytic-uremic syndrome, and disseminated cancer. Most of these disorders are discussed elsewhere in this book. It suffices to say that common to all of these disorders is the presence of vascular lesions that predispose the circulating red cells to mechanical injury. The morphologic alterations in the injured RBCs may be striking. Thus, "burr cells," "helmet cells," and "triangle cells" may be seen in the peripheral blood film (Fig. 12–8). It should be pointed out that except for thrombotic thrombocytopenic purpura and the related hemolytic uremic syndrome, hemolysis is not a major clinical problem in most instances.

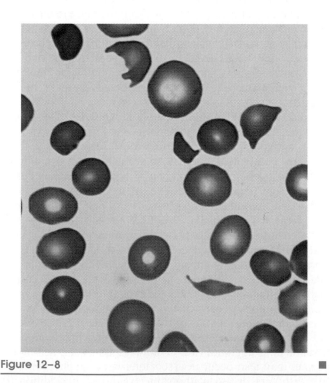

Figure 12–8 ■

Microangiopathic hemolytic anemia. The peripheral blood smear from a patient with hemolytic-uremic syndrome shows several fragmented red cells. (Courtesy of Dr. Robert W. McKenna, Department of Pathology, University of Texas Southwestern Medical School, Dallas, TX.)

Malaria

It has been estimated that 200 million persons suffer from this infectious disease; it is one of the most widespread afflictions of mankind. Malaria is endemic in Asia and Africa, but with widespread jet travel, cases are now reported all over the world. The fact that the eradication of malaria is theoretically feasible makes its prevalence even more unfortunate. Malaria is caused by one of four types of protozoa: *Plasmodium vivax* causes benign tertian malaria; *P. malariae* causes quartan malaria, another benign form; *P. ovale* causes ovale malaria, a relatively uncommon and benign form similar to vivax malaria; and *P. falciparum* causes malignant tertian malaria (falciparum malaria), which has a high fatality rate. All forms are transmitted only by the bite of female *Anopheles* mosquitoes, and humans are the only natural reservoir.

Etiology and Pathogenesis. The life cycle of the plasmodia is a well-understood but complex process. Human liver cells are infected by sporozoites introduced into the blood by mosquito bites. The parasites multiply within liver cells, and after a period of time that varies with the plasmodium species, the infected hepatocytes release merozoites. These in turn enter red cells, where they continue asexual reproduction to produce more merozoites or to give rise to gametocytes that infect the next hungry mosquito. During asexual reproduction in the erythrocytes, the merozoites first develop into trophozoites that are somewhat distinctive for each of the four forms of malaria. Thus, *the specific form of malaria can be recognized in appropriately stained thick smears of peripheral blood.* The asexual phase is completed when the trophozoites give rise to new merozoites, which escape by destroying the red cells.

Clinical Features. The distinctive clinical and anatomic features of malaria are related to the following events:

1. Showers of new merozoites are released from the red cells at intervals of approximately 48 hours for *P. vivax, P. ovale,* and *P. falciparum,* and 72 hours for *P. malariae.* The clinical spikes of shaking, chills, and fever coincide with this release.
2. The parasites destroy large numbers of red cells and thus cause hemolytic anemia.
3. A characteristic brown malarial pigment, probably a derivative of Hb that is identical to hematin, is released from the ruptured red cells along with the merozoites, discoloring principally the spleen, but also the liver, lymph nodes, and bone marrow.
4. Activation of the phagocytic defense mechanisms of the host leads to marked hyperplasia of the mononuclear phagocyte system throughout the body, reflected in massive splenomegaly. Less frequently, the liver may also be enlarged.

Fatal falciparum malaria is characterized by prominent involvement of the brain. Cerebral blood vessels are full of parasitized red cells and are often occluded by microthrombi. The disease may begin suddenly or slowly, but it is rapidly progressive, with the development of high fever, chills, convulsions, shock, and death, usually within days to weeks. In other cases falciparum malaria may pursue a more chronic course but may be punctuated at any time by an uncommon but dramatic complication known as *blackwater fever.* The trigger for this complication is obscure, but it is associated with massive hemolysis, leading to jaundice, hemoglobinemia, and hemoglobinuria. With appropriate chemotherapy, the prognosis for patients with most forms of malaria is good; however, treatment of falciparum malaria is much more difficult because of the emergence of drug-resistant strains. Because of the potentially serious consequences of this disease, early diagnosis and treatment are particularly important but are sometimes delayed in nonendemic settings.

ANEMIAS OF DIMINISHED ERYTHROPOIESIS

Included in this category are anemias that are caused by an inadequate supply to the bone marrow of some substance necessary for hematopoiesis. The most common deficiencies are those of iron, folic acid, or vitamin B_{12}. Infrequently, there is a pyridoxine-responsive anemia or a thiamine-dependent anemia. Another important cause of impaired erythropoiesis is suppression of marrow stem cells, exemplified by aplastic anemia and myelophthisic anemia. In the following sections, some common examples of anemias resulting from nutritional deficiencies and marrow suppression are discussed individually.

Iron Deficiency Anemia

It is estimated that 10% of the population in developed countries and as many as 25% to 50% in developing countries are anemic. Iron deficiency accounts for most of this prevalence. It is without question *the most common form of nutritional deficiency*. The factors responsible for iron deficiency differ somewhat in various populations and can be best considered in the context of normal iron metabolism.

Total body iron content is about 2 gm for women and 6 gm for men. Approximately 80% of functional body iron is found in Hb; the remainder of this pool represents myoglobin and iron-containing enzymes (e.g., catalase and cytochromes). The iron storage pool, represented by hemosiderin and ferritin-bound iron, contains approximately 15% to 20% of total body iron. Stored iron is found in all tissues but particularly in liver, spleen, bone marrow, and skeletal muscle. Because *serum ferritin* is largely derived from the storage pool of iron, its level is a good indicator of the adequacy of body iron stores. *Staining bone marrow* for iron-containing macrophages is another useful and simple method for estimating body iron content. Iron is transported in the plasma by an iron-binding protein called *transferrin*. In normal persons, transferrin is about 33% saturated with iron, yielding serum iron levels that average 120 μg/dl in men and 100 μg/dl in women. Thus, the total iron-binding capacity of serum is in the range of 300 to 350 μg.

Body iron losses are extremely and rigidly limited, ranging from 1 to 2 mg per day lost by shedding of mucosal and skin epithelial cells. *Iron balance, therefore, is maintained largely by regulating the absorption of dietary iron.* The normal daily Western diet contains approximately 10 to 20 mg of iron, most of which is in the form of heme contained in animal products. The remainder is inorganic iron in vegetables. About 20% of heme iron (in contrast to 1% to 2% of nonheme iron) is absorbable, so the average Western diet contains sufficient iron to balance fixed daily losses. The duodenum is the primary site of absorption; there dietary heme iron enters the mucosal cells directly. In contrast, nonheme iron appears to be transported into the cell by a transferrin-independent mechanism involving a luminal mucin that binds the iron and transfers it to cell surface integrins; these in turn deliver the iron to a cytosolic protein called *mobilferrin* (Fig. 12–9). A fraction of the absorbed iron is rapidly delivered to plasma transferrin. The remainder is bound to mucosal ferritin, some to be transferred more slowly to plasma transferrin and some to be lost with exfoliation of mucosal cells. When the body is replete with iron, most of the iron that enters the duodenal epithelium is bound to ferritin and is lost with exfoliation; in iron deficiency, or when there is increased effective or ineffective erythropoiesis, transfer to plasma transferrin is enhanced. How the message is delivered from the body iron stores or bone marrow to the intestinal cells is not clear.

Negative iron balance and consequent anemia may result from low dietary intake, malabsorption, excessive demand, and chronic blood loss:

■ Low dietary intake alone is rarely the cause of iron deficiency in the United States, because the average daily dietary intake of 10 to 20 mg is more than enough for males and about adequate for females. In other parts of the world, however, low intake and poor bioavailability from predominantly vegetarian diets is an important cause of iron deficiency.

■ Malabsorption may occur with sprue and celiac disease or after gastrectomy (Chapter 15).

■ Increased demands not met by normal dietary intake may occur around the world during pregnancy and infancy.

■ Chronic blood loss is the most important cause of iron

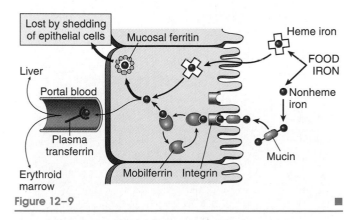

Figure 12–9 ■

Diagrammatic representation of iron absorption. Mucosal uptake of heme and nonheme iron is depicted. When the storage sites of the body are replete with iron and erythropoietic activity is normal, most of the absorbed iron is lost into the gut by shedding of the epithelial cells. Conversely, when body iron needs increase or when erythropoiesis is stimulated, a greater fraction of the absorbed iron is transferred into plasma transferrin, with a concomitant decrease in iron loss through mucosal ferritin.

deficiency anemia in the Western world; this loss may occur from the gastrointestinal tract (e.g., peptic ulcers, colonic cancer, hemorrhoids, hookworm disease) or the female genital tract (e.g., menorrhagia, metrorrhagia, cancers).

Regardless of the cause, the development of the deficiency state occurs insidiously. At first there is depletion of stored iron, which is marked by a *decline in serum ferritin and depletion of stainable iron in the bone marrow.* There follows a decrease in circulating iron, with a low level of serum iron and a rise in the serum transferrin iron-binding capacity. Ultimately, the inadequacy makes its impact on Hb, myoglobin, and other iron compounds. With more significant deficits, impaired work performance and brain function and reduced immunocompetence may develop.

> MORPHOLOGY. Except in unusual circumstances, iron deficiency anemia is relatively mild. The red cells are **microcytic** and **hypochromic,** reflecting the reduced mean corpuscular volume and mean corpuscular Hb concentration (Fig. 12–10). Although there is normoblastic hyperplasia, it is limited by the availability of iron, and hence active marrow is usually only slightly increased in volume. Extramedullary hematopoiesis is uncommon.
>
> In some cases atrophic glossitis is present, giving the tongue a smooth, glazed appearance. When this is accompanied by dysphagia and esopha-geal webs, it constitutes the **Plummer-Vinson syndrome**.

Clinical Course. In most instances iron deficiency anemia is asymptomatic. Nonspecific manifestations, such as weakness, listlessness, and pallor, may be present in severe cases. With long-standing severe anemia, thinning, flattening, and eventually "spooning" of the fingernails sometimes appears.

Diagnostic criteria include low Hb levels; low hematocrit; low mean corpuscular volume; hypochromic, microcytic red cells; low serum ferritin; low serum iron levels; low transferrin saturation; increased total iron-binding capacity; and, ultimately, response to iron therapy. Persons frequently die *with* this form of anemia, but rarely *of* it. It is well to remember that in reasonably adequately nourished persons, microcytic hypochromic anemia is not a disease, but rather a symptom of some underlying disorder.

Anemia of Chronic Disease

This is a common form of anemia that may mimic anemia of iron deficiency. It occurs in a variety of chronic illnesses that include the following:

- Chronic microbial infections such as osteomyelitis, bacterial endocarditis, and lung abscess
- Chronic immune disorders such as rheumatoid arthritis and regional enteritis
- Neoplasms such as Hodgkin's disease and carcinomas of the lung and breast

The common features that characterize anemia in these diverse clinical settings are low serum iron and reduced total iron-binding capacity in association with abundant stored iron in the mononuclear phagocytic cells. This combination suggests that there is some impediment in the transfer of iron from the storage pool to the erythroid precursors. In addition, the compensatory increase in erythropoietin levels is not adequate for the degree of anemia. It appears that the suppression of erythropoiesis and sequestration of iron in the storage compartment result from secretion of interleukin 1 (IL-1), tumor necrosis factor-α, and interferon-γ. Secretion of these cytokines is triggered by the underlying chronic inflammatory or neoplastic disease. The RBCs may be normocytic and normochromic or hypochromic and microcytic, as in anemia of iron deficiency. *The presence of increased storage iron in the marrow macrophages, a high serum ferritin level, and reduced total iron-binding capacity readily rule out iron deficiency as the cause of anemia.* Administration of erythropoietin improves the anemia; treatment of the underlying condition corrects the anemia.

Megaloblastic Anemias

There are two principal types of megaloblastic anemia: one caused by a folate deficiency, and another caused by a lack of vitamin B_{12}. These anemias may be caused by a nutritional deficiency, e.g., of folic acid (folate), or result from impaired absorption, as is the case with vitamin B_{12}. Both of these vi-

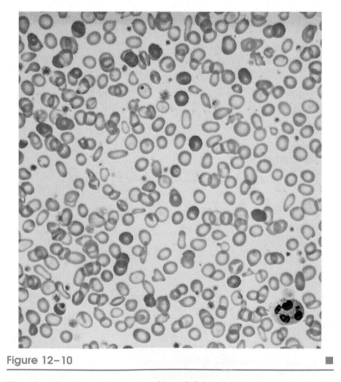

Figure 12–10 ■

Hypochromic microcytic anemia of iron deficiency. Note the small red cells containing a narrow rim of hemoglobin at the periphery. Contrast with the scattered, fully hemoglobinized cells derived from a recent blood transfusion given to the patient. (Courtesy of Dr. Robert W. McKenna, Department of Pathology, University of Texas Southwestern Medical School, Dallas, TX.)

tamins are required for DNA synthesis, and hence the effects of their lack on erythropoiesis are quite similar.

Pathogenesis. The morphologic hallmark of megaloblastic anemias is an enlargement of erythroid precursors that creates *megaloblasts* and correspondingly abnormally large red cells *(macrocytes).* Other proliferating cells, such as granulocyte precursors, are enlarged *(giant metamyelocytes),* yielding enlarged *hypersegmented neutrophils.* Underlying the cellular gigantism, paradoxically, is impairment of DNA synthesis; thus, proliferating cells laboriously synthesize DNA, enlarging their nuclei, but the ultimate mitotic division is delayed. However, synthesis of RNA and cytoplasmic elements proceeds at a normal pace. The nuclei are thus immature, whereas the cytoplasm is fully mature, a situation referred to as *nuclear-cytoplasmic asynchrony.* Because of these maturational derangements, megaloblasts accumulate in the bone marrow, yielding too few erythrocytes, and hence the anemia. Two concomitant processes further aggravate the anemia: (1) ineffective erythropoiesis (a predisposition of megaloblasts to undergo autohemolysis) and (2) increased destruction of the abnormally large red cells by the mononuclear phagocyte system. This increased breakdown of red cells and precursors leads to iron accumulation, mostly in the mononuclear phagocytic cells of the bone marrow. Increased intramedullary destruction may also affect granulocyte and platelet precursors, giving rise to pancytopenia.

MORPHOLOGY. Certain morphologic features are common to all forms of megaloblastic anemias. The **bone marrow** is markedly hypercellular, owing to increased numbers of **megaloblasts.** These cells are larger than normoblasts and have a delicate, finely reticulated nuclear chromatin (suggestive of nuclear immaturity) and an abundant, strikingly basophilic cytoplasm (Fig. 12–11). As the megaloblasts differentiate and begin to acquire Hb, the

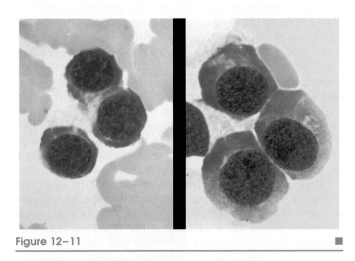

Figure 12–11   ■

Comparison of normoblasts *(left)* and megaloblasts *(right).* The megaloblasts are larger, have relatively immature nuclei with finely reticulated chromatin, and have an abundant basophilic cytoplasm. (Courtesy of Dr. José Hernandez, Department of Pathology, University of Texas Southwestern Medical School, Dallas, TX.)

nucleus retains its finely distributed chromatin and fails to undergo the chromatin clumping typical of an orthochromatic normoblast. Similarly, the granulocytic precursors also demonstrate nuclear-cytoplasmic asynchrony, yielding giant metamyelocytes. Megakaryocytes, too, may be abnormally large, with bizarre multilobed nuclei.

In the **peripheral blood,** the earliest change is usually the appearance of **hypersegmented granulocytes.** These appear even before the onset of anemia. Although the normal number of lobes in a granulocyte nucleus is two or three, with megaloblastic anemias this number may be markedly increased, to five or six. **Erythrocytes are typically large and oval (macroovalocytes), with mean corpuscular volumes over 100 μ^3** (normal 82 to 92 μ^3). Large, misshapen platelets may also be seen. Although macrocytes appear hyperchromic because of their large size, in reality the MCHC is normal. Morphologic changes in other systems, especially the gastrointestinal tract, may also occur, giving rise to some of the clinical features.

FOLATE (FOLIC ACID) DEFICIENCY ANEMIA

Megaloblastic anemia secondary to a lack of folate is not common, but precarious folate levels in the body are surprisingly common among (1) economically deprived persons of all countries who live on marginal diets; (2) pregnant women, whose dietary inadequacies combine with increased metabolic requirements; and (3) alcoholics, the indigent, and the elderly, whose diet is often grossly inadequate.

Ironically, folate is widely prevalent in nearly all raw foods, but it is readily destroyed by 10 to 15 minutes' cooking. Thus, the best sources of folate in the diet are fresh or fresh-frozen vegetables and fruits eaten either uncooked or lightly cooked. Food folates are predominantly in polyglutamate form, and most must be split into monoglutamates for absorption. Acidic foods and conjugase inhibitors found in beans and other legumes hamper absorption by inhibiting intestinal conjugases that catalyze the formation of monoglutamates from polyglutamates. Phenytoin (Dilantin) and a few other drugs also inhibit folate absorption. Others, such as methotrexate, inhibit folate metabolism (see below). The principal site of intestinal absorption is the upper third of the small intestine, so malabsorptive disorders such as celiac disease and tropical sprue, which affect this level of the gut, impair absorption.

The metabolism and physiologic functions of folic acid after absorption are complex. It is sufficient here to note that after absorption, folic acid is transported in the blood mainly as a monoglutamate. Within cells it undergoes conversion to several derivatives, but of principal importance is that it must be reduced to tetrahydrofolate (THF) by a reductase. (This reductase is sensitive to inhibition by folate analogs such as methotrexate, which deprives cells of folate and the capacity to rapidly divide—a property that is the basis for the use of folic acid antagonists as antineoplastic agents.) The primary function of THF is as an acceptor and donor of one-carbon units in a variety of steps involved in DNA synthesis. Several one-carbon transfers are critical to the synthesis of purines, thymidylate, and therefore thymine. Thus, it should be apparent why a deficiency of folate causes the slow DNA synthesis that accounts for megaloblastic anemia.

The onset of the anemia is insidious and is associated with nonspecific symptoms such as weakness and easy fatigability. The clinical picture may be complicated by coexistent deficiency of other vitamins, especially in alcoholics. Since the gastrointestinal tract, like the hematopoietic system, is a site of rapid cell turnover, symptoms referable to the alimentary tract are common and often severe. These include sore tongue and cheilosis. *It should be stressed that in contrast to vitamin B₁₂ deficiency, neurologic abnormalities do not occur.*

The diagnosis of a megaloblastic anemia is readily made from examination of a smear of peripheral blood and bone marrow. The important differentiation between the anemia of folate deficiency and that of vitamin B_{12} deficiency is best accomplished by assays for serum folate and vitamin B_{12} and determination of red cell folate levels.

VITAMIN B_{12} (COBALAMIN) DEFICIENCY ANEMIA: PERNICIOUS ANEMIA

Inadequate levels of vitamin B_{12}, or cobalamin, in the body result in a megaloblastic macrocytic anemia similar hematologically to that of folate deficiency. However, a deficiency of vitamin B_{12} causes at the same time a demyelinating disorder involving the peripheral nerves and, ultimately and most importantly, the spinal cord. There are many causes of vitamin B_{12} deficiency. The term *pernicious anemia (PA),* a relic of the days when the cause and therapy of this condition were unknown, is used to describe vitamin B_{12} deficiency resulting from inadequate gastric production or defective function of intrinsic factor (IF) necessary to absorb B_{12}. IF plays a critical role in the absorption of vitamin B_{12}, as will be evident from the following sequence of events involved in B_{12} absorption:

■ Peptic digestion releases dietary vitamin B_{12}, which is then bound to salivary B_{12}-binding proteins called *cobalophilins,* or *R binders.*
■ R-B_{12} complexes, transported to the duodenum, are split by pancreatic proteases, and the released B_{12} attaches to IF secreted by the parietal cells of the gastric fundic mucosa.
■ The IF-B_{12} complex passes to the distal ileum, where it attaches to the epithelial IF receptors, followed by absorption of vitamin B_{12}.
■ The absorbed B_{12} is bound to transport proteins called *transcobalamins,* which then deliver it to the liver and other cells of the body.

Etiology. Among the many potential causes of cobalamin deficiency, malabsorption is the most common and important. A dietary deficiency of cobalamin is virtually limited to strict vegetarians. This nutrient is abundant in all animal foods, including eggs and dairy products. Indeed, bacterial contamination of water and nonanimal foods may provide adequate amounts of B_{12}; it is stored in the liver and efficiently reabsorbed from the bile, so 20 to 30 years would be required to deplete the normal reserves. Moreover, it is resistant to cooking and boiling. A tiny daily supply, therefore, suffices. Thus, a dietary lack of B_{12} is uncommon; until proved otherwise, *a deficiency of this nutrient (in the Western world) implies PA secondary to inadequate production or function of IF.*

The deranged synthesis of IF appears to be caused by an autoimmune reaction against parietal cells and IF itself, producing gastric mucosal atrophy, described in Chapter 15. Several findings favor the concept of gastric autoimmunity:

1. Autoantibodies are present in the serum and gastric juice of most patients with PA. Three types of antibodies have been found: *parietal canalicular antibodies* bind to the mucosal parietal cells; *blocking antibodies* block the binding of B_{12} to IF; and *binding antibodies* react with IF-B_{12} complex and prevent it from binding to the ileal receptor.
2. The association of PA with other autoimmune diseases such as Hashimoto's thyroiditis, Addison's disease, and type I diabetes mellitus is well documented.
3. There is an increased frequency of serum antibodies to IF in patients who have other autoimmune diseases.

In addition to PA, malabsorption of vitamin B_{12} may result from gastrectomy, which leads to loss of IF-producing cells; resection of ileum, the site of absorption of the IF-B_{12} complex; and disorders that involve the distal ileum, such as regional enteritis, tropical sprue, and Whipple's disease. In individuals over 70 years of age, gastric atrophy and achlorhydria interfere with B_{12} absorption. In the absence of acid-pepsin, the vitamin is not released from its bound form in the diet.

The metabolic defects induced by a cobalamin deficiency seem intertwined with folate metabolism. It seems that *B₁₂ deficiency leads to an "internal folate deficiency"* by reducing the availability of THF, the metabolically active form of folic acid. Although folates are abundant, they are not available in useful form, so DNA synthesis is impaired. This concept is supported by the fact that *the anemia of B_{12} deficiency improves with administration of folates, whereas the anemia of folate deficiency is unaffected by supplementation of vitamin B₁₂.* The biochemical basis of the neuropathy in B_{12} deficiency is unclear. Although both folate and B_{12} deficiency give rise to megaloblastic anemia, neurologic disease does not occur in patients with folate deficiency. It is likely therefore that the function of vitamin B_{12} in the nervous system is independent of its effects on folate metabolism. The neurologic lesions associated with PA comprise, in essence, *demyelination of the posterior and lateral columns of the spinal cord,* sometimes beginning in the peripheral nerves. In time, axonal degeneration may supervene. It is important to note that the severity of neurologic manifestations is not related to the degree of anemia. Indeed, uncommonly, the neurologic disease may occur in the absence of megaloblastic anemia.

Clinical Features. Manifestations of vitamin B_{12} deficiency are nonspecific; as with any other anemia, there is pallor; easy fatigability; and in severe cases, dyspnea and even congestive heart failure. Gastrointestinal symptoms similar to those described under folate deficiency may also be present. Neurologic changes, such as symmetric numbness, tingling, and burning in feet or hands, followed by unsteadiness of gait and loss of position sense, particularly in the toes, may also be present. Although the anemia responds dramatically to parenteral vitamin B_{12}, the neurologic manifestations may often fail to resolve. As discussed in Chapter 15, patients with PA have an increased risk of gastric carcinoma.

The diagnostic features of PA include (1) low serum vitamin B_{12} levels; (2) normal or elevated serum folate levels; (3) histamine-fast gastric achlorhydria (due to loss of gastric parietal cells); (4) inability to absorb an oral dose of cobalamin (the Schilling test); (5) moderate to severe megaloblastic anemia; (6) leukopenia with hypersegmented granulocytes; and (7) most critically, dramatic reticulocytic response (within 2 to 3 days) to parenteral administration of vitamin B_{12}.

Aplastic Anemia

Aplastic anemia is a disorder characterized by the *suppression of multipotent myeloid stem cells, with resultant anemia, thrombocytopenia, and neutropenia (pancytopenia)*. Notwithstanding its name, aplastic anemia should not be confused with selective suppression of erythroid stem cells (pure red cell aplasia), in which anemia is the only manifestation.

Etiology and Pathogenesis. In more than half of cases, aplastic anemia appears without any apparent cause and so is termed *idiopathic*. In other cases, exposure to a known myelotoxic agent can be identified, such as whole body irradiation (as may occur in nuclear plant accidents) or use of myelotoxic drugs. *Drugs and chemicals are the most common causes of secondary aplastic anemia.* With some agents the marrow damage is predictable, dose related, and usually reversible. Included in this category are antineoplastic drugs (alkylating agents, antimetabolites), benzene, and chloramphenicol. In other instances marrow toxicity occurs as an apparent "idiosyncratic" or sensitivity reaction to small doses of known myelotoxic drugs (such as chloramphenicol) or after the use of such agents as phenylbutazone, sulfonamides, or methylphenylethylhydantoin, which are not myelotoxic in other persons.

Aplastic anemia has been reported in patients who have had viral infections. Although several viruses, including the human immunodeficiency virus (HIV), have been implicated, it most often follows viral non-A, non-B hepatitis. Marrow aplasia develops insidiously several months after recovery from non-A, non-B hepatitis and follows a relentless course.

The pathogenetic events leading to marrow failure are obscure, even when a cause can be identified. Two possible mechanisms have been suggested: an intrinsic defect in stem cells, or suppression of normal stem cells by suppressor T cells. Recent studies favor the possibility that some forms of marrow insult cause genetic damage that results in the generation of mutant stem cells with poor proliferative and differentiative capacity. If the altered stem cells dominate, the resultant picture is that of aplastic anemia. The occasional transformation of aplastic anemia into acute leukemia lends credence to this hypothesis. According to this scenario, the presence of suppressor T cells noted in some cases results from an immune response against the genetically damaged stem cells. With such a response, the ability of the mutant stem cell to produce differentiated progeny is further compromised.

> **MORPHOLOGY.** The bone marrow typically is hypocellular, with an increase in the amount of fat. These changes are better appreciated in a bone marrow biopsy than in marrow aspirates. The latter often yield a "dry tap" because of hypocellularity. In marrow biopsy, small foci of lymphocytes and plasma cells may be seen in the fibrous stroma. A number of secondary changes may accompany marrow failure. Hepatic fatty change may result from anemia, and thrombocytopenia and granulocytopenia may give rise to hemorrhages and bacterial infections, respectively. Multiple transfusions may cause hemosiderosis.

Clinical Course. Aplastic anemia usually occurs insidiously; it affects persons of all ages and both sexes. *Anemia* may cause progressive onset of weakness, pallor, and dyspnea. Petechiae and ecchymoses may herald *thrombocytopenia*. *Granulocytopenia* may manifest itself only by frequent and persistent minor infections or by the sudden onset of chills, fever, and prostration. It is important to distinguish aplastic anemia from other causes of pancytopenia, such as "aleukemic leukemia" and myelodysplastic syndromes (p 376). Because pancytopenia is common to these conditions, their clinical manifestations are often indistinguishable; however, with aplastic anemia the marrow is hypocellular owing to stem cell failure, whereas in leukemias and myelodysplasia the marrow is populated by abnormal and immature myeloid cells. *Splenomegaly is characteristically absent* in aplastic anemia; if it is present, the diagnosis of aplastic anemia should be seriously questioned. Typically, the red cells are normocytic and normochromic, although slight macrocytosis is occasionally present; *reticulocytosis is absent*.

The prognosis of marrow aplasia is quite unpredictable. As mentioned earlier, withdrawal of toxic drugs may lead to recovery in some cases. The idiopathic form has a poor prognosis. Bone marrow transplantation is an extremely effective form of therapy, especially in patients younger than 40 years. Older patients benefit from immunosuppressive therapy (e.g., antithymocyte globulin).

Myelophthisic Anemia

This form of marrow failure is caused by extensive replacement of the marrow by tumors or other lesions. This is most commonly associated with metastatic cancer arising from a primary lesion in the breast, lung, prostate, or thyroid. Multiple myeloma, lymphomas, leukemias, advanced tuberculosis, lipid storage disorders, and osteosclerosis are less commonly implicated. Myelophthisic anemia is also seen with progressive fibrosis of the bone marrow (myelofibrosis), discussed later (p 379). The manifestations of marrow infiltration include anemia and thrombocytopenia. The white cell series is less affected. Characteristically, misshapen and immature red cells are seen in the peripheral blood, along with a slightly elevated white cell count (leukoerythroblastosis). Treatment obviously involves the management of the underlying condition.

LABORATORY DIAGNOSIS OF ANEMIAS

The diagnosis of anemia is established by low Hb, reduced HCT, and reduced numbers of RBCs. Examination of peripheral smears allows the categorization of anemias into major morphologic subgroups: normocytic normochromic, microcytic hypochromic, and macrocytic. In addition, abnormalities in red cell shape and size, such as the presence of spherocytes, sickled cells, and fragmented cells, provide additional clues to the etiology of anemia. In suspected hemoglobinopathies, electrophoresis allows detection of abnormal hemoglobins such as HbS by their pattern of migration. Immunologically mediated hemolysis of RBCs is confirmed by Coombs' test. Reticulocyte counts are extremely useful in the work-up of anemias. This simple measurement indicates whether the anemia is caused by impaired red cell production, in which case the reticulocyte count is low, or by increased red cell destruction. The latter is accompanied by reticulocytosis as the marrow undergoes erythroid hyperplasia. Biochemical tests, such as serum iron, serum iron binding capacity, per cent transferrin saturation, and serum ferritin levels, are required to distinguish between hypochromic microcytic anemias caused by iron deficiency, anemia of chronic disease, and thalassemia minor. The distinction between the two major causes of megaloblastic anemias is achieved by measurement of serum and red cell folate and B_{12} levels. Unconjugated hyperbilirubinemia supports the diagnosis of hemolytic anemia but is not useful in distinguishing among various forms. Much more sensitive than serum bilirubin is serum haptoglobin, because its level is markedly reduced in all forms of hemolytic anemia. With the exception of aplastic anemia, the examination of the bone marrow is usually not required for diagnosis of most forms of anemia.

POLYCYTHEMIA

Polycythemia, or *erythrocytosis,* as it is sometimes referred to, denotes an increased concentration of red cells, usually with a corresponding increase in Hb level. Such an increase may be *relative,* when there is hemoconcentration owing to decreased plasma volume, or *absolute,* when there is an increase in total red cell mass. Relative polycythemia results from any cause of dehydration, such as deprivation of water, prolonged vomiting, diarrhea, or excessive use of diuretics. Absolute polycythemia is said to be *primary* when the increase in red cell mass results from an autonomous proliferation of the myeloid stem cells and *secondary* when the red cell progenitors are normal but proliferate in response to increased levels of erythropoietin. Primary polycythemia (polycythemia vera) is one of several expressions of clonal, neoplastic proliferation of myeloid stem cells and is therefore considered later in this chapter with other myeloproliferative disorders. Secondary polycythemias may be caused by an increase in erythropoietin secretion that is physiologically appropriate or by an inappropriate (pathologic) secretion of erythropoietin (Table 12–5).

■

Table 12–5. PATHOPHYSIOLOGIC CLASSIFICATION OF POLYCYTHEMIA

Relative
    Reduced plasma volume (hemoconcentration)
Absolute
    Primary: Abnormal proliferation of myeloid stem cells, normal or low erythropoietin levels (polycythemia vera)
    Secondary: Increased erythropoietin levels
        Appropriate: lung disease, high-altitude living, cyanotic heart disease
        Inappropriate: erythropoietin-secreting tumors (e.g., renal cell carcinoma, hepatoma, cerebellar hemangioblastoma)

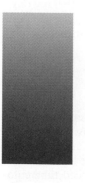

White Cell Disorders

Disorders of white cells may be associated with a deficiency of leukocytes (leukopenias) or with proliferations that may be reactive or neoplastic. Reactive proliferation in response to an underlying primary, often microbial, disease is fairly common. Neoplastic disorders, although less common, are more ominous; they cause approximately 9% of all cancer deaths in adults and a staggering 40% in children younger than 15 years. In the following discussion we first describe some nonneoplastic conditions and then consider in some detail malignant proliferations of white cells.

NON-NEOPLASTIC DISORDERS OF WHITE CELLS

Under this heading are included leukopenias as well as non-specific and specific reactive proliferations.

Leukopenia

A decrease in the peripheral white cell count may occur because of decreased numbers of any of the specific types of leukocytes, but most often it involves the neutrophils (neutropenia). Lymphopenias are much less common; they are associated with congenital immunodeficiency diseases or are acquired in association with specific clinical states, such as treatment with corticosteroids. Only the more common leukopenias that affect granulocytes are discussed here.

NEUTROPENIA/AGRANULOCYTOSIS

A reduction in the number of granulocytes in blood is known as *neutropenia* or sometimes, when severe, as *agranulocytosis*. Characteristically the total white cell count is reduced to 1000 cells per microliter of blood and in some instances to as few as 200 to 300 cells. Affected persons are extremely susceptible to infections, which may be severe enough to cause death.

Etiology and Pathogenesis. The mechanisms that cause neutropenia can be broadly divided into two categories:

■ *Inadequate or ineffective granulopoiesis.* Reduced granulopoiesis may be a manifestation of generalized marrow failure, such as occurs in aplastic anemia and a variety of leukemias. Alternatively, only the committed granulocytic precursors may be affected, most commonly by certain drugs. Like aplastic anemia, granulocytopenia is predictably produced by cancer chemotherapeutic agents; it may also be an idiosyncratic and unpredictable reaction to drugs such as chloramphenicol, sulfonamides, or chlorpromazine. In some cases there is proliferation of CD3+, CD8+ large granular lymphocytes, which seem to suppress myelopoiesis.

■ *Accelerated removal or destruction of neutrophils.* This may be encountered with immune-mediated injury to neutrophils, triggered in some cases by drugs such as aminopyrine, or it may be idiopathic. Increased peripheral utilization may occur in overwhelming bacterial, fungal, or rickettsial infections. An enlarged spleen may also lead to accelerated removal of neutrophils by sequestration.

> **MORPHOLOGY.** Anatomic alterations in bone marrow depend on the underlying basis of the neutropenia. **Marrow hypercellularity** owing to increased numbers of immature granulocytic precursors is seen when the neutropenia is caused by excessive destruction of the mature neutrophils, or in ineffective granulopoiesis such as occurs in mega-loblastic anemia. In contrast, **marrow hypocellularity** is noted when agranulocytosis is caused by agents that affect the committed granulocytic precursors. Erythropoiesis and megakaryopoiesis usually remain at normal levels, but with certain myelotoxic drugs, all marrow elements may be affected.

Clinical Course. The initial symptoms are often malaise, chills, and fever, followed by marked weakness and fatigability. Infections constitute the major problem; they commonly present as ulcerating, necrotizing lesions of the gingiva, floor of the mouth, buccal mucosa, pharynx, or other sites within the oral cavity (agranulocytic angina). All of these lesions often show massive growth of microorganisms, with a relatively poor leukocyte response. In addition to removal of the offending drug and control of infections, current treatment efforts also include administration of recombinant hematopoietic growth factors such as granulocyte colony-stimulating factor (G-CSF). These factors stimulate neutrophil production by the bone marrow.

Reactive Leukocytosis

An increase in the number of white blood cells is a common reaction in a variety of inflammatory states caused by microbial and nonmicrobial stimuli. Leukocytoses are relatively nonspecific and can be classified on the basis of the particular white cell series affected (Table 12–6). As will be discussed later, in some cases reactive leukocytosis may mimic leukemia. Such *leukemoid* reactions must be distinguished from true malignancies of the white cells. Infectious mononucleosis, a form of lymphocytosis caused by Epstein-Barr virus

■

Table 12–6.   CAUSES OF LEUKOCYTOSIS

Polymorphonuclear Leukocytosis	Acute bacterial infections, especially caused by pyogenic bacteria; sterile inflammations caused by, for example, tissue necrosis (myocardial infarction, burns)
Eosinophilic Leukocytosis (Eosinophilia)	Allergic disorders such as asthma, hay fever, allergic skin disease (e.g., pemphigus); parasitic infestations; drug reactions
Monocytosis	Chronic infections (e.g., tuberculosis), bacterial endocarditis, rickettsiosis and malaria; collagen vascular diseases (e.g., systemic lupus erythematosus)
Lymphocytosis	Accompanies monocytosis in many disorders associated with chronic immunologic stimulation; viral infections (e.g., hepatitis, CMV infection, infectious mononucleosis)

CMV, cytomegalovirus.

(EBV) infection, merits separate consideration because it gives rise to a distinctive syndrome.

INFECTIOUS MONONUCLEOSIS

In the Western world, infectious mononucleosis (IM) is an acute, self-limited disease of adolescents and young adults (it delights in college students) that is caused by B lymphocytotropic EBV, a member of the herpesvirus family. The infection is characterized mainly by (1) fever, sore throat, and generalized lymphadenitis; (2) an increase of lymphocytes in blood, many of which have an atypical morphology; and (3) a humoral antibody response to EBV. In passing it should be noted that cytomegalovirus may induce a similar syndrome that can be differentiated only by serologic methods.

Epidemiology and Immunology. EBV is ubiquitous in all human populations. Where economic deprivation results in inadequate living standards, EBV infection early in life is nearly universal. At this age symptomatic disease is uncommon, and despite the fact that infected hosts develop an immune response (described below), more than half of the population continues to be virus shedders, explaining the dissemination of infection. In contrast, in developed countries that enjoy better standards of hygiene, infection is usually delayed until adolescence or young adulthood. Perhaps better standards of health and less underlying intercurrent chronic disease permit a more effective immune response to the EBV, so only about 20% of healthy seropositive persons shed the virus. Concomitantly, only about 50% of those exposed acquire the infection. Transmission to a seronegative "kissing cousin" usually involves direct intimate oral contact. The virus initially penetrates nasopharyngeal, oropharyngeal, and salivary epithelial cells, which are known to possess receptors for EBV, and persists as a subclinical productive infection in the oropharyngeal region. Thus, *the agent is shed in the saliva.* Simultaneously, it spreads to underlying oropharyngeal lymphoid tissue and, more specifically, to B lymphocytes, all of which have receptors for EBV. Infection of B cells may take one of two forms: in a minority of B cells there is productive infection with lysis of infected cells and release of virions; in most cells, however, the virus associates with the host cell genome, giving rise to a latent infection. *B cells that harbor the EBV genome undergo polyclonal activation and proliferation.* They disseminate in the circulation and secrete antibodies with several specificities, including the well-known heterophil anti-sheep RBC antibodies used for the diagnosis of IM.

A normal immune response is extremely important in controlling the proliferation of EBV-infected B cells and cell-free virus. Early in the course of the infection, IgM, and later IgG, antibodies are formed against viral capsid antigens. The latter persist for life. More important in the control of polyclonal B-cell proliferation are cytotoxic CD8+ T cells and natural killer (NK) cells. *Virus-specific cytotoxic T cells appear as atypical lymphocytes in the circulation,* which is characteristic of this disease. It is important to note that in otherwise healthy persons, the fully developed humoral and cellular responses to EBV act as brakes on viral shedding, limiting the number of infected B cells rather than eliminating them. Latent EBV remains in a few B cells as well as in oropharyngeal epithelial cells. As will be seen, impaired immunity in the host can have disastrous consequences.

MORPHOLOGY. The major alterations involve the blood, lymph nodes, spleen, liver, central nervous system, and occasionally other organs. The **peripheral blood** shows absolute lymphocytosis with a total white cell count between 12,000 and 18,000 per microliter, more than 60% of which are lymphocytes. Many of these are large, **atypical lymphocytes,** 12 to 16 μm in diameter, characterized by an abundant cytoplasm containing multiple clear vacuolations and an oval, indented, or folded nucleus (Fig. 12–12). These atypical lymphocytes bear T-cell markers, and are usually sufficiently distinctive to suggest the diagnosis from examination of a peripheral blood smear.

The **lymph nodes** are typically discrete and enlarged throughout the body, principally in the posterior cervical, axillary, and groin regions. Histologically, the lymphoid tissue is flooded by atypical lymphocytes, which occupy the paracortical (T-cell) areas. There is in addition some B-cell reaction, with enlargement of follicles. Occasionally cells resembling Reed-Sternberg cells (p 370) may also be found in the nodes. These are difficult to distinguish from those found in Hodgkin's disease (p 369).

The **spleen** is enlarged in most cases, weighing between 300 and 500 gm. The histologic changes are analogous to those of the lymph nodes, showing a heavy infiltration of atypical lymphocytes. These spleens are especially vulnerable to rupture, possibly resulting in part from infiltration of the trabeculae and capsule by the lymphocytes.

Liver function is almost always transiently impaired to some degree. Histologically, atypical lymphocytes are seen in the portal areas and sinusoids, and

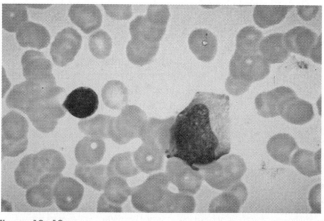

Figure 12–12 ■

Atypical lymphocytes in infectious mononucleosis. The cell on the left is a typical small lymphocyte with a compact nucleus filling the entire cytoplasm. In contrast, an atypical lymphocyte on the right has abundant cytoplasm and a large nucleus with fine chromatin.

scattered, isolated cells or foci of parenchymal necrosis filled with lymphocytes may be present. This histologic picture may be difficult to distinguish from that of viral hepatitis.

Clinical Course. Although classically *IM presents with fever, sore throat, lymphadenitis,* and the other features mentioned earlier, quite often it is more aberrant in behavior. It may present (1) with little or no fever and only malaise, fatigue, and lymphadenopathy, raising the spectre of leukemia-lymphoma; (2) as a fever of unknown origin without significant lymphadenopathy or other localized findings; (3) as hepatitis that is difficult to differentiate from one of the hepatotropic viral syndromes; or (4) as a febrile rash resembling rubella. Ultimately, the diagnosis depends on the following findings, in increasing order of specificity: (1) lymphocytosis with the characteristic atypical lymphocytes in the peripheral blood, (2) a positive heterophil reaction (monospot test), and (3) specific antibodies for EBV antigens (viral capsid antigens, early antigens, or Epstein-Barr nuclear antigen). In most patients, IM resolves within 4 to 6 weeks, but sometimes the fatigue lasts longer. Occasionally one or more complications supervene. These may involve virtually any organ or system in the body. Perhaps most common is marked hepatic dysfunction, with jaundice; elevated hepatic enzyme levels; disturbed appetite; and, rarely, even liver failure. Other complications involve the nervous system, kidneys, bone marrow, lungs, eyes, heart, and spleen (splenic rupture has been fatal). A more serious complication in those suffering from some form of immunodeficiency, such as acquired immunodeficiency syndrome (AIDS), or receiving immunosuppressive therapy (perhaps after transplantation) is that the polyclonal B-cell proliferation may run amok, leading to death. True monoclonal B-cell lymphomas have also appeared, sometimes preceded by polyclonal lymphoproliferation.

X-linked lymphoproliferative syndrome is a rare inherited immunodeficiency characterized by inability to mount an immune response against EBV. Affected boys develop an overwhelming EBV infection that can be fatal.

Reactive Lymphadenitis

Infections and nonmicrobial inflammatory stimuli not only cause leukocytosis, but also involve the lymph nodes, which act as defensive barriers. Here an immune response against foreign antigens develops, a process often associated with lymph node enlargement (lymphadenopathy). The infections that cause lymphadenitis are numerous and varied. In most instances the histologic picture in the nodes is entirely nonspecific, designated acute or chronic nonspecific adenitis. A somewhat distinctive form of lymphadenitis that occurs with cat scratch disease will be described separately.

ACUTE NONSPECIFIC LYMPHADENITIS

This form of lymphadenitis may be confined to a local group of nodes draining a focal infection, or it may be generalized when there is systemic bacterial or viral infection.

Macroscopically, acutely inflamed nodes are swollen, gray-red, and engorged. Histologically, there are large germinal centers containing numerous mitotic figures. When the condition is caused by pyogenic organisms, a neutrophilic infiltrate is seen about the follicles and within the lymphoid sinuses. With severe infections the centers of follicles may undergo necrosis, resulting in the formation of an abscess.

Affected nodes are tender and, when abscess formation is extensive, become fluctuant. The overlying skin is frequently red, and penetration of the infection to the skin may produce draining sinuses. With control of the infection, the lymph nodes may revert to their normal appearance, or scarring may follow more destructive disease.

CHRONIC NONSPECIFIC LYMPHADENITIS

This condition may assume one of three patterns, depending on the causative agent: follicular hyperplasia, paracortical lymphoid hyperplasia, or sinus histiocytosis.

FOLLICULAR HYPERPLASIA. This pattern is often associated with chronic infections caused by organisms that represent B-cell antigens. Large germinal centers develop that contain lymphocytes in varying stages of "blast" transformation. Some causes of follicular hyperplasia are rheumatoid arthritis, toxoplasmosis, and early stages of HIV infection. This form of lymphadenitis may be confused morphologically with follicular (nodular) lymphomas (p 366). Findings that favor a diagnosis of follicular hyperplasia are (1) preservation of the lymph node architecture, with normal lymphoid tissue between germinal centers; (2) marked variation in the shape and size of the lymphoid nodules; (3) a mixed population of lymphocytes in different stages of differentiation; and (4) prominent phagocytic activity in germinal centers.

PARACORTICAL LYMPHOID HYPERPLASIA. This pattern is characterized by reactive changes within the T-cell regions of the lymph node. Parafollicular T cells undergo proliferation and transformation to immunoblasts that may efface the germinal follicles. Paracortical lymphoid hyperplasia is encountered, particularly, in viral infections or after smallpox vaccination, and in immune reactions induced by certain drugs (especially phenytoin (Dilantin)).

SINUS HISTIOCYTOSIS. This reactive pattern is characterized by distention and prominence of the lymphatic sinusoids owing to marked hypertrophy of lining endothelial cells and infiltration with histiocytes. Sinus histiocytosis is often encountered in lymph nodes draining cancers and may represent an immune response to the tumor or its products.

CAT SCRATCH DISEASE

Cat scratch disease is a self-limited lymphadenitis caused by *Bartonella henselae* (formerly *Rochalimaea henselae*). This microbe is related to rickettsiae but, unlike rickettsiae, it can be grown in artificial culture. It is primarily a disease of childhood, with 90% of patients being younger than 18 years. It takes the form of regional lymphadenopathy, most frequently in the axilla and neck. The nodal enlargement appears approximately 2 weeks after a feline scratch or, uncommonly, after a splinter or thorn injury. A raised, inflammatory nodule, vesicle, or eschar may or may not be visible at the site of skin injury. In most patients the lymph node enlargement regresses over the next 2 to 4 months. Rarely, patients develop encephalitis, osteomyelitis, or thrombocytopenia.

The anatomic changes in the lymph node are quite characteristic; initially, **sarcoid-like granulomas are formed that develop central necrosis with accumulation of neutrophils.** These irregular stellate abscesses are similar in appearance to those seen in lymphogranuloma venereum. The microbe is extracellular and can be visualized only with silver stains or electron microscopy. Diagnosis is based on a history of exposure to cats, clinical findings, positive skin test to the microbial antigen, and the distinctive morphologic changes in the lymph nodes.

NEOPLASTIC PROLIFERATIONS OF WHITE CELLS

These represent the most important of the white cell disorders. They can be divided into four somewhat overlapping categories: malignant lymphomas, leukemias, plasma cell dyscrasias and related disorders, and histiocytoses. These can be briefly defined as follows:

■ *Malignant lymphomas* take the form of cohesive tumorous lesions, composed usually of neoplastic lymphocytes and rarely of histiocytes, that typically arise in lymphoid tissue.
■ *Leukemias* are neoplasms of the hematopoietic stem cells that arise in the bone marrow and secondarily flood the circulating blood or other organs.
■ *Plasma cell dyscrasias* and related disorders, usually arising in the bones, take the form of localized or disseminated proliferations of antibody-forming cells (plasma cells).
■ *Histiocytoses* are proliferative lesions of histiocytes and include the rare histiocytic neoplasms that present as malignant lymphomas, mentioned above. A special category of histiocytes, referred to as *Langerhans' cells*, gives rise to a spectrum of clonal neoplastic disorders, some of which behave as disseminated malignant tumors, while others be-

have as localized benign proliferations. This special group is called *Langerhans' cell histiocytoses.*

Malignant Lymphomas

Lymphomas are malignant neoplasms of cells native to lymphoid tissue (i.e., lymphocytes and histiocytes and their precursors and derivatives). The term *lymphoma* is something of a misnomer, because all of these disorders are malignant and, unless controlled by therapy, ultimately lethal.

Two broad groups of lymphomas are recognized: Hodgkin's disease (Hodgkin's lymphoma) and non-Hodgkin's lymphomas (NHLs). Although both arise in the lymphoid tissue, Hodgkin's disease is set apart by the presence in the lesions of the distinctive Reed-Sternberg giant cells (p 370) and by the fact that in the involved nodes, non-neoplastic inflammatory cells frequently outnumber the neoplastic element represented by the RS cell.

NON-HODGKIN'S LYMPHOMAS

Approximately 53,000 cases of NHL will be diagnosed in the United States in 1996, and nearly 23,000 such patients will die, making NHL the sixth leading cause of cancer incidence and death in this country. Even more alarming is the fact that the incidence of NHL is on the increase; some of the increase can be accounted for by the increased incidence of these tumors in patients with AIDS, but there is no satisfactory explanation for the increase in the general population.

NHLs arise in lymphoid tissue, usually in the lymph nodes (65% of cases) or, less frequently, in the lymphoid tissue of parenchymal organs (35%). All variants have the potential for spread to other lymph nodes and into various tissues throughout the body, especially the liver, spleen, and bone marrow. In some cases bone marrow involvement is followed by a spillover of the proliferating cells into the peripheral blood, creating a leukemia-like picture. Conversely, leukemias of lymphoid cells, originating in the bone marrow, may infiltrate lymph nodes as well, creating the histologic picture of lymphoma. Thus, *the distinction between lymphoid leukemias and NHLs may be blurred in certain cases.*

Few areas of pathology have evoked as much controversy and confusion as the classification of NHL. Before we dive into this quagmire, certain important principles relevant to the subgrouping of NHL must be emphasized:

■ As tumors of the immune system, NHLs may originate in T cells, B cells, or histiocytes; the cell of origin can usually be determined on the basis of the phenotypic and molecular characteristics of the tumor cells. Most NHLs (80% to 85%) are of B-cell origin; the remainder are in large part T-cell tumors. Tumors of histiocytes or macrophages are quite uncommon. Tumors of T and B cells represent cells that may have been arrested at any stage along their differentiation pathways (Fig. 12–13). This figure also illustrates the genotypic and phenotypic characteristics that differentiate T and B cells and are useful in subdividing this group of tumors. It will be noted that CD2, CD3, CD4, CD7, and CD8 are useful for identification of T cells and their tumors, and CD10, CD19, CD20, and surface Ig are

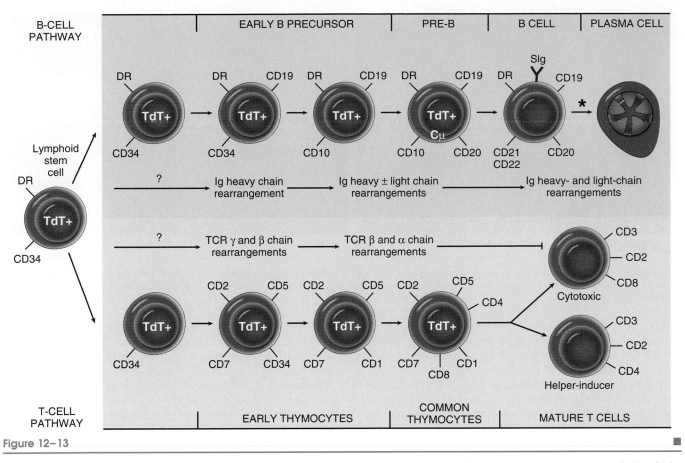

Figure 12-13

Schematic illustration of the phenotypic and genotypic changes associated with the differentiation of B cells and T cells. Not shown are some CD4+, CD8+ cells (common thymocytes) that also express CD3. Stages between resting B cells and plasma are not depicted. CD, cluster designation; TdT, terminal deoxynucleotidyl transferase; Ig, immunoglobulin; TCR, T-cell receptor; DR, HLA-class II antigens.

B-cell markers. In addition to these, CD16 and CD56 are markers for NK cells, whereas CD13, CD14, CD15, and CD64 are myeloid cell antigens. CD34 is expressed on pluripotent stem cells and is retained on the earliest lymphoid and myeloid progenitor cells (Fig. 12-13).

■ Many tumors of B cells recapitulate the follicular pattern of the growth characteristic of normal B cells. Thus, in certain B-cell tumors, the neoplastic cells are clustered into identifiable nodules; these tumors are called *nodular (follicular) lymphomas* (Fig. 12-14A). Other B-cell tumors do not produce nodules, nor do any of the tumors of T cells or histiocytes; instead, they spread diffusely in the lymph nodes. This architecture is referred to as *diffuse lymphoma* (Fig. 12-14B). With either pattern, the normal architecture of the lymph nodes is effaced. As will be discussed later, this simple distinction based on patterns of cell growth is extremely useful. Nodular lymphomas are indolent tumors that are compatible with long survival without treatment; however, they are not curable. In contrast, diffuse lymphomas, regardless of their origin from T or B cells, are aggressive tumors that are rapidly fatal unless treated, but with appropriate therapy, many can be cured.

■ During antigen-induced activation and differentiation, lymphocytes undergo a series of morphologic

changes. Within the B-cell series, for example, the resting B cells have the appearance of a typical small lymphocyte, with a dark, large nucleus; after antigenic challenge, the follicular B cells enlarge, their nucleus develops clefts and folds, and nucleoli become prominent. Many B-cell lymphomas recapitulate these morphologic changes. On the basis of these morphologic characteristics, tumor cells are often described as being small or large with a cleaved nucleus, or blastlike with nucleoli. It should be remembered that these morphologic changes do not imply origin from different cell types; they merely reflect the stage of differentiation or activation at which the tumor cells are "frozen." Most, as stated at the outset, are B-cell tumors.

With this background, we can return to the vexing issue of classification of NHLs. The first to be considered is the Working Formulation for Clinical Use. Proposed in 1982, this classification has been used widely in the United States. It is a clinical classification that divides NHLs into three prognostic groups, designated as low-, intermediate-, and high-grade, based on survival statistics (Table 12-7). Within each prognostic group are several morphologic categories based on the architecture (follicular or diffuse) and the cytologic appearance of cells. No attempt is made to classify malignancies by

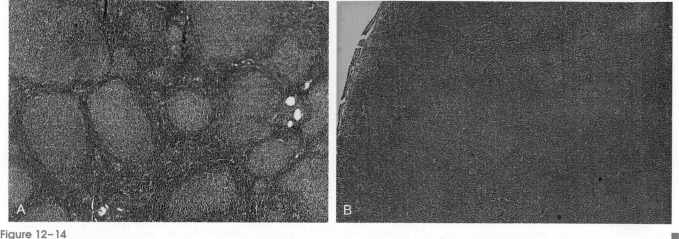

Figure 12–14 ■

Non-Hodgkin's lymphoma. *A,* Nodular pattern; the lymph node is replaced by nodular aggregates of lymphoma cells. *B,* Diffuse pattern; the lymph node is replaced by a diffuse sea of neoplastic lymphoid cells. (Courtesy of Dr. Robert W. McKenna, Department of Pathology, University of Texas Southwestern Medical School, Dallas, TX.)

their cell of origin. The Working Formulation also contains a miscellaneous group to encompass the rare histiocytic tumors and two unusual forms of T-cell neoplasia.

In the past decade it has become apparent that, although simple, the Working Formulation is inadequate in many respects. For example, the subgroup "intermediate lymphoma" includes tumors with distinctly different prognoses. The three diffuse variants within this group are aggressive tumors that, for practical purposes, are treated like high-grade tumors. Furthermore, apparently homogeneous entities such as diffuse small cleaved cell lymphoma include tumors that are quite different in their behavior and prognosis, as will be pointed out later. Finally, several distinct clinicopathologic forms of lymphomas, such as lymphomas of mucosal lymphoid tissue, have no category in the Working Formulation classification. In an attempt to resolve these problems, in 1994 an International Lymphoma Study Group proposed the *R*evised *E*uropean, *A*merican Classification of *L*ymphoid Neoplasms, commonly abbreviated as REAL. This classification includes all

lymphoid neoplasms, including leukemias and multiple myelomas, and segregates them on their basis of origin into three major categories: (1) tumors of B cells, (2) tumors of T cells and NK cells, and (3) Hodgkin's disease. A simplified version of the REAL Classification of B-cell lymphomas, along with equivalent groups of the Working Formulation, is presented in Table 12–8. It is immediately apparent that some entities, such as mantle cell lymphoma, are not formally recognized in the Working Formulation, and conversely, the diffuse large B-cell category of the REAL Classification combines two separate groups of the Working Formulation because of similar origin and prognosis. Thus, there are some *real* advantages to the REAL classification, and studies to establish its clinical value are ongoing. Until they are completed, both classifications are likely to be used. Here we will use an abbreviated version of the Working Formulation but will also include some NHLs that were not recognized in that classification.

As noted in Table 12–7, there are 10 histologic categories in this scheme of classification. However, on the basis of clinicopathologic features, 85% of NHLs seen in the United States can be grouped into one of the following five categories:

- Small lymphocytic lymphomas
- Follicular lymphomas (includes all three follicular subtypes of the Working Formulation)
- Diffuse large cell lymphomas (includes the diffuse mixed large and small cell, diffuse large cell, and diffuse immunoblastic subtypes of Working Formulation)
- Lymphoblastic lymphomas
- Small noncleaved (Burkitt's) lymphoma

In addition, mantle cell lymphoma, not recognized in the Working Formulation, will be described because of its distinctive clinicopathologic features.

Small Lymphocytic Lymphoma

Small lymphocytic lymphoma (SLL) makes up approximately 4% of all NHLs and is the only low-grade lymphoma that does not have a follicular architecture.

Table 12–7. A WORKING FORMULATION OF NON-HODGKIN'S LYMPHOMAS FOR CLINICAL USAGE

Low-Grade
  Small lymphocytic
  Follicular, predominantly small cleaved cell
  Follicular, mixed small cleaved and large cell
Intermediate-Grade
  Follicular, predominantly large cell
  Diffuse, small cleaved cell
  Diffuse, mixed small and large cell
  Diffuse, large cell
High-Grade
  Large cell immunoblastic
  Lymphoblastic
  Small noncleaved cell
Miscellaneous

Table 12–8. REAL CLASSIFICATION OF B-CELL NON-HODGKIN'S LYMPHOMAS AND THE WORKING FORMULATION EQUIVALENTS

REAL Classification of B-Cell Tumors	Working Formulation Equivalent
I. Precursor B-Cell Neoplasms: Precursor B Lymphoblastic Leukemia/Lymphoma	Not included
II. Peripheral B-Cell Neoplasms	
1. B-cell small lymphocytic leukemia/small lymphocytic lymphoma	Low grade—small lymphocytic
2. Lymphoplasmacytic lymphoma/immunocytoma	Low grade—small lymphocytic plasmacytoid
3. Mantle cell lymphoma	No formal equivalent, but included in diffuse small cleaved cell group
4. Follicular center cell lymphoma:	
a. Cytologic grade I	Low grade—follicular, predominantly small cleaved
b. Cytologic grade II	Low grade—follicular, mixed small cleaved and large cell
c. Cytologic grade III	Intermediate grade—follicular large cell
5. Marginal zone B-cell lymphoma	No equivalent
6. Splenic marginal zone lymphoma	No equivalent
7. Hairy cell leukemia	Not included
8. Plasmacytoma/plasma cell myeloma	Not included
9. Diffuse large B-cell lymphoma	Intermediate grade—diffuse large cell and high-grade large cell immunoblastic
10. Burkitt's lymphoma	High-grade—small noncleaved cell

MORPHOLOGY. Cells are compact, small, apparently unstimulated lymphocytes with dark-staining round nuclei, scanty cytoplasm, and little variation in size (Fig. 12–15A). Mitotic figures are rare, and there is little or no cytologic atypia. Bone marrow is involved in almost all cases, and in about 40% of patients the neoplastic cells spill over into blood, evoking a chronic lymphocytic leukemia–like picture. SLL overlaps with chronic lymphocytic leukemia both clinically and morphologically and, in some cases, with Waldenström's macroglobulinemia.

Immunophenotype. Approximately 90% of SLL are tumors of mature B cells, so they display surface IgM (with or without surface immunoglobulin D [IgD]) and the pan–B-cell antigen CD19. However, they also express CD5, an antigen found on all T cells and only rarely on normal B cells. Approximately 10% of patients with SLL have a tumor of T cells.

Clinical Features. SLL (and the related chronic lymphocytic leukemia) occur primarily in older age groups. Patients have generalized lymphadenopathy with mild to moderate enlargement of the liver and spleen; the associated symptoms are mild, and prolonged survival is usual. These patients often have hypogammaglobulinemia, making them prone to infections; curiously, some patients also have autoimmune hemolytic anemia or thrombocytopenia.

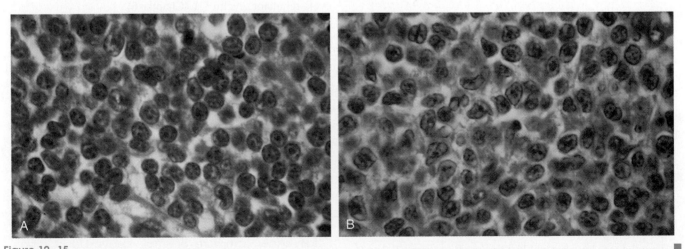

Figure 12–15

Non-Hodgkin's lymphoma. *A,* Small lymphocytic lymphoma. The tumor cells resemble mature, unstimulated lymphocytes, with dark staining round nuclei, scanty cytoplasm, and little variation in size. *B,* Follicular small cleaved cell lymphoma. The neoplastic lymphocytes are only slightly larger than normal lymphocytes. Note, however, that the nuclear contour is angular and indented. (Courtesy of Dr. Robert W. McKenna, Department of Pathology, University of Texas Southwestern Medical School, Dallas, TX.)

Follicular Lymphomas

These tumors, characterized by a nodular or follicular architecture, are extremely common, constituting 40% of adult NHLs in the United States. They include three histologic subtypes of the Working Formulation, described below.

MORPHOLOGY. These are B-cell tumors in which the cells resemble normal antigen-activated B cells in the lymphoid follicles. They are made up of cells that resemble normal follicular center cells, but in varying proportions. **Follicular small cleaved cell lymphoma** is the most common form of follicular NHL. In this variant, the neoplastic B cells are slightly larger than normal lymphocytes, with an angular "cleaved" nuclear contour characterized by prominent indentations and linear infoldings (Fig. 12–15B). Nuclear chromatin is coarse and condensed, and nucleoli are indistinct. Mitoses are infrequent. When the small cleaved cells are admixed with approximately equal numbers of larger cells, the tumors are referred to as **follicular, mixed small cleaved and large cell.** The larger cells are three to four times the size of small lymphocytes and have a vesicular nucleus with nucleoli (an appearance similar to antigen-activated B cells). The nuclear membrane may or may not have infoldings. Least common is the third variant, **follicular, predominantly large cell lymphoma,** in which large cells with cleaved and noncleaved nuclei predominate.

Immunophenotype. As neoplasms of follicular center cells, these tumors express pan–B-cell markers such as CD19 and CD20, and many tumors express the more restricted B-cell marker CD10. Like SLLs, they also express surface immunoglobulins, but unlike SLLs, they do not express CD5.

Clinical Features. The follicular lymphomas have the following distinctive clinical characteristics:

■ They occur predominantly in older persons (rarely before age 20 years).
■ They affect males and females equally.
■ They present with painless lymphadenopathy, which is frequently generalized. Involvement of extranodal (e.g., visceral) sites is uncommon, but bone marrow is frequently involved (75% of cases) at the time of diagnosis.
■ Peripheral blood involvement in the form of frank leukemia is less common than in SLL, but small clonal B-cell populations can be detected in most cases by flow cytometry or molecular techniques.
■ In almost all patients, tumor cells reveal a characteristic translocation t(14;18). The break point on chromosome 18 involves 18q21, where the anti-apoptosis gene *bcl*-2 has been mapped. This translocation causes overexpression of *bcl*-2 (Chapter 6).
■ They have a long natural history (median survival, 7 to 9 years) that appears to be largely unaffected by treatment. Hence, despite their indolent course, *they are not easily curable.* Their lack of response to chemotherapy may be due in part to the anti-apoptosis effect of *bcl*-2, which

prevents tumor cells from being killed by chemotherapeutic agents.
■ In some patients the follicular lymphomas progress to a diffuse high-grade histologic type, with or without treatment. Such a transition reflects the emergence of an aggressive subclone of neoplastic B cells. Progression is usually associated with mutations in the p53 gene. Such transformed tumors lack the curability of de novo diffuse large cell lymphomas, described later.

Mantle Cell Lymphomas

As noted in Table 12–8, these tumors were not recognized in the Working Formulation. Mantle cell lymphomas are B-cell tumors that are believed to arise from the mantle zone of lymphoid follicles rather than from cells in the center of follicles. They comprise approximately 4% of all NHLs.

MORPHOLOGY. Mantle cell lymphomas show a diffuse pattern of lymph node involvement. The tumor cells are slightly larger than normal lymphocytes and have an irregular cleaved or round nucleus. The nucleoli are inconspicuous. Thus, histologically they closely resemble diffuse, small cleaved cell lymphomas of the Working Formulation.

Immunophenotype. The tumor cells express surface IgM and pan–B-cell antigens such as CD19, CD20, and CD22. They differ from follicular center cells by the absence of CD10 and the presence of CD5.

Clinical Features. These tumors occur predominantly in older males and present with disseminated disease. In addition to lymph nodes, spleen, Waldeyer's ring, and bone marrow, extranodal sites such as the gastrointestinal tract are also involved. These tumors are aggressive and incurable, with a median survival of 3 to 5 years. They carry a characteristic t(11;14) translocation that activates the gene encoding the cell cycle regulator, cyclin D1 (Chapter 6).

Diffuse Large Cell Lymphomas

This clinicopathologic grouping includes three histologic subtypes of the Working Formulation: diffuse mixed small and large cell, diffuse large cell, and diffuse immunoblastic lymphomas. Although phenotypically and histologically heterogeneous, they share several clinical features and an aggressive natural history. They account for approximately 50% of all NHLs.

MORPHOLOGY. Two tumors in this group (diffuse mixed and diffuse large cell) may be considered diffuse counterparts of follicular mixed and follicular large cell lymphomas. Accordingly, they contain either a mixture of small cleaved and large (cleaved or noncleaved) cells or predominantly large cells. The small cleaved cell component of the mixed tumors is similar to that described in follicular small cleaved lymphomas. The nuclei of large cleaved cells are irregular in contour, indented, and larger compared with nuclei of normal histiocytes. The nuclear chromatin is dispersed, and nucleoli are inconspicuous. Cytoplasm is scant and pale. Large noncleaved cells are up to four times the size of normal lymphocytes, with a round or oval nucleus and one or two prominent nucleoli (Fig. 12–16). The nuclear chromatin is vesicular, and mitoses are prominent. The amount of cytoplasm is greater than in large cleaved cells.

The cells of the large cell immunoblastic variant are distinct from follicular center cells. They are four to five times larger than a small lymphocyte and have a round or multilobulated large vesicular nucleus with one or two centrally placed prominent nucleoli. The cytoplasm is either deeply staining and pyroninophilic or clear.

Immunophenotype. Immunologically, these lymphomas are heterogeneous. Most are of B-cell origin. Approximately 15% have T-cell surface markers or contain rearranged T-cell-receptor genes indicative of T-cell origin. Rare tumors have markers of macrophages.

Clinical Features. These tumors share the following clinical features that differentiate them from follicular lymphomas:

■ Although they occur mainly in older persons (median age about 60 years), unlike follicular lymphomas, the age range is much wider, and diffuse large cell NHLs constitute about 20% of childhood lymphomas. Most EBV-driven lymphomas that arise in patients with AIDS and other states of immunosuppression are of the diffuse large cell variety.

■ In contrast to patients with follicular lymphomas, patients with these tumors typically present with a rapidly enlarging, often symptomatic mass at a single nodal or extranodal site. Localized disease and extranodal manifestations are more common than in follicular lymphomas. Indeed, involvement of the gastrointestinal tract, skin, bone, or brain may be the presenting feature. Waldeyer's ring of oropharyngeal lymphoid tissue is involved in about 50% of these cases. Involvement of liver and spleen is not common at the time of diagnosis.

■ Bone marrow involvement is relatively uncommon in these patients, especially at the time of diagnosis. With progressive disease, however, the marrow may be involved, and rarely, a leukemic picture may emerge.

■ Approximately 30% of patients have a t(14;18) translocation, with rearrangement of the *bcl*-2 gene. These tumors are believed to have arisen by progression of follicular lymphomas. About one third of diffuse large cell lymphomas show rearrangement of the *bcl*-6 gene, located on 3q27, and in many more there is a mutation in this gene without any cytogenetic alterations. Tumors in which 3q27 is translocated are characterized by involvement of extranodal tissues and seem to have a more favorable prognosis.

■ These diffuse large cell lymphomas are aggressive tumors that are rapidly fatal if untreated. With intensive combination chemotherapy, however, complete remission can be achieved in 60% to 80% of the patients, and of these, approximately 50% remain free of disease for several years and may be considered cured. In contrast, recall that although follicular lymphomas follow an indolent course, they are very difficult to cure. Those that transform into diffuse lymphomas have an extremely poor prognosis, because unlike de novo diffuse lymphomas, their response to aggressive chemotherapy is poor.

Lymphoblastic Lymphoma

This high-grade tumor represents 4% of all NHLs in adults, but 40% of childhood lymphomas. It is closely related to T-cell acute lymphoblastic leukemia (T-ALL).

MORPHOLOGY. Tumor cells are fairly uniform in size, with scanty cytoplasm and nuclei somewhat larger than those of small lymphocytes. The nuclear chromatin is delicate and finely stippled, and nucleoli are either absent or inconspicuous. The nuclear membrane shows deep subdivision, imparting a convoluted (lobulated) appearance in some, but not all, cases. A high mitotic rate with a "starry sky" pattern, produced by the interspersed benign macrophages is typically seen.

Immunophenotype. Tumor cells resemble intrathymic T cells. Most cases are CD7+, CD3+. Terminal deoxynucleotidyl transferase (TdT), an enzyme associated with primitive lymphoid cells, is expressed in all cases.

Clinical Features. Lymphoblastic lymphoma predominantly affects males under the age of 20 years. The presence of a prominent mediastinal mass in 50% to 70% of patients is very characteristic and suggests a thymic origin for this tumor. The disease is rapidly progressive; early dissemination to the bone marrow and thence to blood and meninges leads

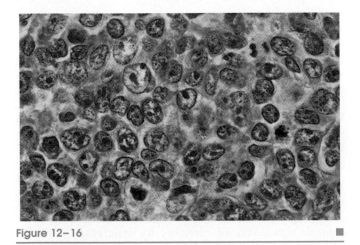

Figure 12–16   ■

Non-Hodgkin's lymphoma, diffuse large cell type. This photomicrograph, taken at the same magnification as Figure 12–15, shows that the tumor cells are larger, with large nuclei and prominent nucleoli. (Courtesy of Dr. Robert W. McKenna, Department of Pathology, University of Texas Southwestern Medical School, Dallas, TX.)

to the evolution of a picture resembling T-ALL. The prognosis is generally poor, but recent attempts to treat this tumor aggressively by utilizing protocols effective in ALL have produced encouraging results.

Small Noncleaved (Burkitt's) Lymphoma

Burkitt's lymphoma is endemic in some parts of Africa and sporadic in other areas, including the United States. Histologically, the African and nonendemic diseases are identical, although there are clinical and virologic differences. The relationship of these disorders to EBV is discussed in Chapter 6.

> **MORPHOLOGY.** Tumor cells are monotonous, intermediate in size between small lymphocytes and large noncleaved cells, and have round or oval nuclei containing two to five prominent nucleoli (Fig. 12–17). The nuclear size approximates that of benign macrophages within the tumor. There is a moderate amount of faintly basophilic or amphophilic cytoplasm, which is intensely pyroninophilic and often contains small, lipid-filled vacuoles. A high mitotic rate is very characteristic of this tumor, as is cell death, accounting for the presence of numerous tissue macrophages with ingested nuclear debris. Because these benign macrophages are often surrounded by a clear space, they create a "starry sky" pattern.

Immunophenotype. These are tumors of B cells that express surface IgM and pan–B-cell markers such as CD19, as well as the CD10 antigen.

Clinical Features. Both the endemic and non-African cases mainly affect children or young adults, accounting for approximately 30% of childhood NHLs in the United States. In

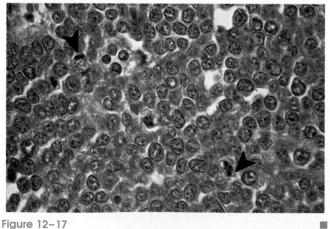

Figure 12–17

Non-Hodgkin's lymphoma, Burkitt's type. The tumor cells and their nuclei are fairly uniform, giving a monotonous appearance. Note the high mitotic activity *(arrowheads)* and prominent nucleoli. The "starry sky" pattern produced by interspersed, lightly staining, normal macrophages is better appreciated at a lower magnification. (Courtesy of Dr. Robert W. McKenna, Department of Pathology, University of Texas Southwestern Medical School, Dallas, TX.)

both forms the disease rarely arises in lymph nodes. In African patients, involvement of the maxilla or mandible is the common mode of presentation, whereas abdominal tumors (bowel, retroperitoneum, ovaries) are more common in North America. Leukemic transformation is uncommon, especially in African cases. Burkitt's lymphoma is a high-grade tumor that may be the fastest growing human neoplasm; however, with aggressive modern chemotherapy, a long-term survival rate of 50% can be expected.

Miscellaneous Non-Hodgkin's Lymphomas

This group includes several uncommon tumors, but only a few are described here, because each is associated with a distinctive clinical presentation.

MALT Lymphoma. This is a special category of extranodal low-grade B-cell tumors that arise most commonly in **m**ucosal-**a**ssociated **l**ymphoid **t**issue (MALT), such as salivary glands, small and large bowel, and lungs, and some nonmucosal sites such as orbit and breast. Most lymphomas that develop in the setting of Sjögren's syndrome, Hashimoto's thyroiditis or *Helicobacter pylori* infection in the stomach belong to this category. Localized MALT tumors can usually be cured by resection.

Mycosis Fungoides and Sézary's Syndrome. These tumors of peripheral CD4+ T cells are characterized by involvement of the skin and therefore belong to the group of *cutaneous T-cell lymphomas.*

Mycosis fungoides presents with an inflammatory premycotic phase and progresses through a plaque phase to a tumor phase. Histologically, there is infiltration of the epidermis and upper dermis by neoplastic T cells, which often have a cerebriform nucleus characterized by marked infolding of the nuclear membrane. With progressive disease, nodal and visceral dissemination appear. Sézary's syndrome is a related condition in which skin involvement is manifested clinically as a generalized exfoliative erythroderma along with an associated leukemia of Sézary cells, which also have a cerebriform nucleus. Circulating Sézary cells can also be identified in as many as 25% of cases of mycosis fungoides in the plaque, or tumor, phase. These are indolent tumors with a median survival time of 8 or 9 years.

Adult T-Cell Leukemia/Lymphoma. This T-cell neoplasm, caused by infection with a retrovirus, human T-cell leukemia virus type 1 (HTLV-1), is endemic in southern Japan and the Caribbean basin, but similar cases have been found sporadically elsewhere, including the southeastern United States. The pathogenesis of this tumor was discussed in Chapter 6. It should be noted that in addition to causing lymphoid malignancies, HTLV-1 infection can also give rise to a progressive demyelinating disease that affects the central nervous system and the spinal cord.

Adult T-cell leukemia/lymphoma is characterized by skin lesions, generalized lymphadenopathy, hepatosplenomegaly, hypercalcemia, and an elevated leukocyte count with multilobed CD4+ lymphocytes. The leukemic cells constitutively express high levels of receptors for interleukin 2 (IL-2). Therefore, targeting of the IL-2 receptor with antibody-toxin conjugates is being tested as a therapeutic approach to this malignancy. In most cases this is an extremely aggressive disease, with a median survival time of about 8 months. Approximately 15% to 20% of patients follow a chronic course;

their disease is clinically indistinguishable from cutaneous T-cell lymphomas.

A summary of the salient clinicopathologic features of the major categories of NHL is presented in Table 12–9.

HODGKIN'S DISEASE

Hodgkin's disease, like NHL, is a disorder involving primarily the lymphoid tissues. It arises almost invariably in a single node or chain of nodes and spreads characteristically to the anatomically contiguous nodes. Nevertheless, it is separated from NHL for several reasons. First, it is *characterized morphologically by the presence of distinctive neoplastic giant cells called Reed-Sternberg (RS) cells* admixed with a variable inflammatory infiltrate. Second, it is often associated with somewhat distinctive clinical features, including systemic manifestations such as fever. Finally, the target cell of neoplastic transformation has yet to be identified with certainty.

Classification. It should be some relief to the student to know that, unlike NHL, there is nearly universal acceptance of a single classification of Hodgkin's disease — the Rye classification. Basically, there are four subtypes: (1) lymphocyte predominance, (2) mixed cellularity, (3) lymphocyte depletion, and (4) nodular sclerosis. Before delineating them, however, we should describe the common denominator among all — the RS cell — and the method used to characterize the extent of the disease in a patient — namely, the staging system.

■

Table 12–9. SUMMARY OF NON-HODGKIN'S LYMPHOMAS

Lymphoma Type or Group	% (In Adults)	Salient Morphology	Immunophenotype	Comments
Small Lymphocytic Lymphoma (SLL)	3–4	Small, unstimulated lymphocytes in a diffuse pattern	>95% B cells	Occurs in old age; generalized lymphadenopathy with marrow involvement and a blood picture resembling CLL; indolent course with prolonged survival
*Follicular Lymphomas**	40	Germinal center cells arranged in a follicular pattern	B cells	Follicular small cleaved cell type most common; occur in older patients; generalized lymphadenopathy; associated with t(14;18); leukemia less common than in SLL; indolent course but difficult to cure
Mantle Cell Lymphoma	3–4	Diffuse pattern with small cleaved cells	B cells	Occurs predominantly in older males; disseminated disease in nodes, spleen, marrow, and GI tract common; t(11;14) is characteristic; aggressive and difficult to cure
Diffuse Large Cell Lymphomas†	40–50	Various cell types; predominantly large germinal center cells; some mixed with smaller cells; others with immunoblastic morphology	~80% B cells ~20% post-thymic T cells	Occur in older patients as well as pediatric age group; greater frequency of extranodal, visceral disease; marrow involvement and leukemia very uncommon at diagnosis and poor prognostic sign; aggressive tumors, but up to 50% are curable
Lymphoblastic Lymphoma	4	Cells somewhat larger than lymphocytes; in many cases nuclei markedly lobulated; high mitotic rate	>95% immature intrathymic T cells	Occurs predominantly in children (40% of all childhood lymphomas); prominent mediastinal mass; early involvement of bone marrow and progression to T-cell ALL; very aggressive
Small Noncleaved (Burkitt's) Lymphoma	<1	Cells intermediate in size between small lymphocytes and immunoblasts; prominent nucleoli; high mitotic rate	B cells	Endemic in Africa; sporadic elsewhere; predominantly affects children; extranodal visceral involvements presenting features; rapidly progressive but responsive to therapy; t(8;14) always present

* Includes all three follicular subtypes of Working Formulation.
† Includes diffuse large cell, diffuse mixed, and large cell immunoblastic lymphomas of the Working Formulation. Other NHLs with diffuse pattern that form distinct clinicopathologic categories (e.g., lymphoblastic lymphomas) not included.

The sine qua non for the histologic diagnosis of Hodgkin's disease is the **RS cell** (Fig. 12–18). However, although necessary, it is not specific for Hodgkin's disease, because it is sometimes found in infectious mononucleosis, mycosis fungoides, and occasionally in NHLs, as well as in other settings. The RS cell has abundant, usually slightly eosinophilic, cytoplasm and ranges in diameter from 15 to 45 μm. It is distinguished principally either by having a multilobate nucleus or by being multinucleate with large, round, prominent nucleoli. **Particularly characteristic are two mirror-image nuclei, each containing a large (inclusion-like) acidophilic nucleolus surrounded by a distinctive clear zone; together they impart an owl-eyed appearance. The nuclear membrane is distinct.**

The staging of Hodgkin's disease (Table 12–10) is of great clinical importance, because the course, choice of therapy, and prognosis are all intimately related to the distribution of the disease. It will become apparent from the ensuing discussion that the more aggressive the variant of the disease, the more likely it is to be in a more advanced stage at the time of diagnosis.

With this background, we can turn to the morphologic classification of Hodgkin's disease into its subgroups and point out some of the salient clinical features of each. Later the manifestations common to all will be presented. The essential morphologic feature that serves to differentiate three subgroups (lymphocyte predominance, mixed cellularity, and lymphocyte depletion) is the frequency of the neoplastic elements (RS cells) relative to the reactive elements, represented by small lymphocytes. The extent of spread and the natural history of untreated Hodgkin's disease appear to be directly related to the ratio of RS cells

to lymphocytes. The fourth subgroup, nodular sclerosis, appears to represent a special expression of the disease that has distinctive clinicopathologic features. The relative frequency of the four histologic subtypes may be gleaned from Table 12–11.

Lymphocyte-Predominance Hodgkin's Disease. This subgroup, comprising about 5% of Hodgkin's disease, is characterized by a large number of mature-looking lymphocytes admixed with a variable number of benign histiocytes (Fig. 12–19). The cells may diffusely flood the lymph nodes and obliterate the normal architecture or may occur within poorly defined nodular areas. Typical RS cells are extremely difficult to find. More common are variant cells that have a delicate multilobed, puffy nucleus that has been likened in appearance to popcorn (**"popcorn cell"**). Other cells, such as eo-

Table 12–10. CLINICAL STAGES OF HODGKIN'S AND NON-HODGKIN'S LYMPHOMAS (ANN ARBOR CLASSIFICATION)* †

Stage	Distribution of Disease
I	Involvement of a single lymph node region (I) or involvement of a single extralymphatic organ or site (I_E)
II	Involvement of two or more lymph node regions on the same side of the diaphragm alone (II) or with involvement of limited contiguous extralymphatic organ or tissue (II_E)
III	Involvement of lymph node regions on both sides of the diaphragm (III), which may include the spleen (III_S), limited contiguous extralymphatic organ or site (III_E), or both (III_{ES})
IV	Multiple or disseminated foci of involvement of one or more extralymphatic organs or tissues with or without lymphatic involvement

* All stages are further divided on the basis of the absence (A) or presence (B) of the following systemic symptoms: significant fever, night sweats, unexplained loss of more than 10% of normal body weight.

† From Carbone PT, et al: Symposium (Ann Arbor): staging in Hodgkin's disease. Cancer Res 31:1707, 1971.

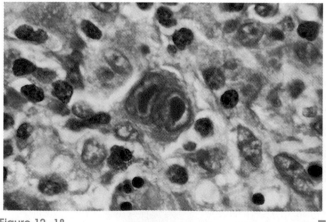

Figure 12–18

Hodgkin's disease. A binucleate Reed-Sternberg cell with large, inclusion-like nucleoli and abundant cytoplasm. It is surrounded by lymphocytes, and an eosinophil can be seen below. (Courtesy of Dr. Robert W. McKenna, Department of Pathology, University of Texas Southwestern Medical School, Dallas, TX.)

Table 12–11. PERCENTAGE OF PATIENTS IN EACH PATHOLOGIC STAGE ACCORDING TO HISTOLOGIC SUBTYPE*

Histologic Subtype	Number of Patients	Pathologic Stage (%)		
		I and II	III	IV
Lymphocyte predominance	55	76	22	2
Mixed cellularity	215	44	47	9
Lymphocyte depletion	21	19	62	19
Nodular sclerosis	628	60	35	5

* From Desforges JF, et al: Hodgkin's disease. N Engl J Med 301:1212, 1979. Reprinted by permission of the New England Journal of Medicine.

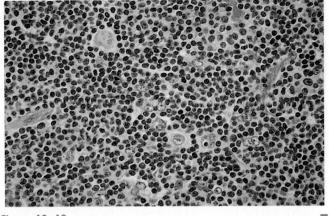

Figure 12–19   ■

Hodgkin's disease, lymphocyte-predominance type. Numerous mature-looking lymphocytes have diffusely infiltrated the node. The large, pale-staining cells, interspersed between the lymphocytes, are the so-called "popcorn" cells. (Courtesy of Dr. Robert W. McKenna, Department of Pathology, University of Texas Southwestern Medical School, Dallas, TX.)

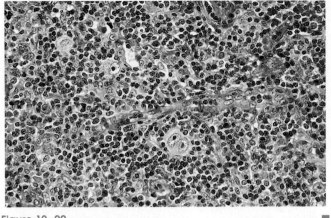

Figure 12–20   ■

Hodgkin's disease, mixed cellularity type. A prominent binucleate Reed-Sternberg cell is surrounded by multiple cell types, including eosinophils (bright red cytoplasm), lymphocytes, and histiocytes. (Courtesy of Dr. Robert W. McKenna, Department of Pathology, University of Texas Southwestern Medical School, Dallas, TX.)

sinophils, neutrophils, and plasma cells, are scanty or absent. The nodular form of lymphocyte-predominance Hodgkin's disease has a more than superficial resemblance to nodular NHLs; indeed, phenotypic studies have revealed that most of the cells .in lymphocyte-predominant Hodgkin's disease are B cells. Hence, this form of Hodgkin's disease is more closely related to follicular lymphomas than to other variants of Hodgkin's disease. Regardless of the precise nosology, the prognosis for patients with this variant is excellent.

Mixed-Cellularity Hodgkin's Disease. This is the most common form of Hodgkin's disease in patients over the age of 50 and is second only to the nodular sclerosis type in overall frequency. It occupies an intermediate clinical position between the lymphocyte-predominance and the lymphocyte-depletion patterns. Typical RS cells are plentiful, but there are fewer lymphocytes than in lymphocyte-predominance disease. This pattern of Hodgkin's disease is rendered distinctive by its heterogeneous cellular infiltrate, which includes eosinophils, plasma cells, and benign histiocytes (Fig. 12–20). The mixed-cellularity form of Hodgkin's disease is more common in males than in females. Compared with the lymphocyte-predominance pattern, more patients with mixed cellularity present with disseminated disease, and these patients more often have systemic manifestations (Table 12–11).

Lymphocyte-Depletion Hodgkin's Disease. This is the least common form of Hodgkin's disease, accounting for less than 5% of cases. It is characterized by a paucity of lymphocytes and a relative abundance of RS cells or their pleomorphic variants. It presents in two morphologic forms, the so-called **diffuse fibrosis** and the **reticular variants**. In

the former, the node is hypocellular and is replaced largely by fibrillar connective tissue. Pleomorphic histiocytes, a few typical and atypical RS cells, and some lymphocytes are scattered within the fibrillar material. The reticular variant is much more cellular and is composed of highly anaplastic, large, pleomorphic cells that resemble RS cells (Fig. 12–21). Only a few typical RS cells can be recognized. Most patients with the lymphocyte-depletion pattern are older, have disseminated involvement (Table 12–11), present with systemic manifestations, and have an aggressive form of the disease. It is currently believed that many cases previously diagnosed as the lymphocyte-de-

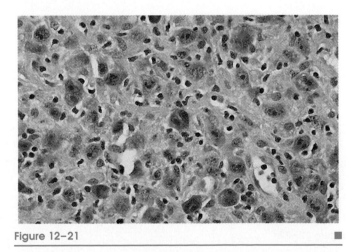

Figure 12–21   ■

Hodgkins' disease, lymphocyte-depletion type. The tumor is composed of highly anaplastic, large, pleomorphic cells that seem to resemble Reed-Sternberg cells. The lymphocytes are sparse. (Courtesy of Dr. Robert W. McKenna, Department of Pathology, University of Texas Southwestern Medical School, Dallas, TX.)

pletion type of Hodgkin's disease are actually aggressive non-Hodgkin's large cell lymphomas.

Nodular Sclerosis Hodgkin's Disease. This is by far the most common histologic form of Hodgkin's disease. It is distinct from the other three forms both clinically and histologically and is characterized morphologically by two features:

■ The presence of a particular variant of the RS cell, the **lacunar cell** (Fig. 12–22). This cell is large and has a single hyperlobate nucleus with multiple small nucleoli and an abundant, pale-staining cytoplasm. In formalin-fixed tissue, the cytoplasm often retracts, giving rise to the appearance of cells lying in clear spaces, or lacunae.

■ The presence in most cases of collagen bands that divide the lymphoid tissue into circumscribed nodules (Fig. 12–23). The fibrosis may be scant or abundant, and the cellular infiltrate may show varying proportions of lymphocytes and lacunar cells. Classic RS cells are infrequent.

Clinically, nodular sclerosis Hodgkin's disease has several distinctive features: it is the only form more common in women, and it has a striking propensity to involve the lower cervical, supraclavicular, and mediastinal lymph nodes. Most of the patients are adolescents or young adults, and they have an excellent prognosis, especially when their disease is in clinical stages I and II.

It is apparent that Hodgkin's disease spans a wide range of histologic patterns and that certain forms, with their characteristic fibrosis, eosinophils, neutrophils, and plasma cells, come deceptively close to simulating an inflammatory reactive process. **The histologic diagnosis, then, of Hodgkin's disease rests on the unmistakable identification of RS cells in most variants and of lacunar cells in the nodular sclerosis pattern. The presence of these cells in the appropri-**

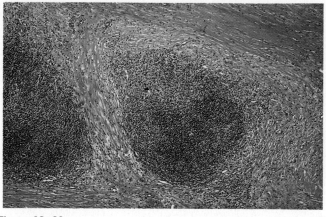

Figure 12–23 ■

Hodgkins' disease, nodular sclerosis type. A low-power view shows well-defined bands of pink, acellular collagen that have subdivided the tumor cells into nodules. (Courtesy of Dr. Robert W. McKenna, Department of Pathology, University of Texas Southwestern Medical School, Dallas, TX.)

ate clinical setting allows the diagnosis of Hodgkin's disease.

In all forms, involvement of the spleen, liver, bone marrow, and other organs and tissues may appear in due course and take the form of irregular, tumor-like nodules of tissue resembling that present in the nodes. At times the spleen is much enlarged and the liver moderately enlarged by these nodular masses. At other times, the involvement is more subtle and becomes evident only on microscopic examination.

Etiology and Pathogenesis. The origins of Hodgkin's disease are unknown. It is now widely accepted that it is a neoplastic disorder and that the RS cells are the transformed cells. However, with the exception of the nodular lymphocyte-predominant variant, which seems to be a tumor of B cells, the origin of the other forms remains an enigma. By both immunohistochemical and molecular analysis, RS cells appear to be monoclonal but of diverse origins. In some cases they seem to arise from B cells and in others, from T cells. No specific markers can be detected in many instances; however, there is consensus that RS cells are not of monocyte-macrophage lineage. Indeed, Hodgkin's disease may be a group of histogenetically distinct disorders that share a common clinicopathologic expression. In all variants there is defective cell-mediated immunity. This is considered to be secondary to dysregulation of the immune system rather than to transformation of a particular cell type.

Given that RS cells represent the malignant component of Hodgkin's disease, what causes the neoplastic transformation? For years, EBV has been suspected as an etiologic agent on the basis of epidemiologic and serologic studies. This notion has been recently bolstered by molecular studies. The EBV genome can be identified in RS cells in 40% to 50% of cases. More importantly, the EBV genome is present in a clonal pattern, making it very unlikely that EBV is a passenger virus that infects RS cells after clonal expansion. The presence of reactive inflammatory cells such as eosinophils is most likely

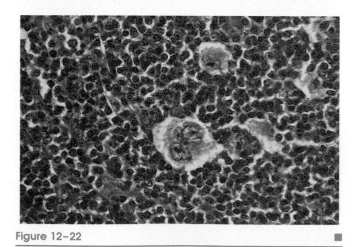

Figure 12–22 ■

Hodgkin's disease, nodular sclerosis type. A distinctive "lacunar cell" with multilobed nucleus containing many small nucleoli is seen lying within a clear space created by retraction of its cytoplasm. It is surrounded by lymphocytes. (Courtesy of Dr. Robert W. McKenna, Department of Pathology, University of Texas Southwestern Medical School, Dallas, TX.)

related to secretion of cytokines such as interleukin 5 (IL-5), by the transformed RS cells. While these studies support the notion that Hodgkin's disease is a monoclonal neoplastic disorder that is strongly associated with EBV, they do not prove that EBV is the causal agent. As in Burkitt's lymphoma and B-cell lymphomas in immunodeficient patients, EBV infection may be one of many steps in the pathogenesis of Hodgkin's disease.

Clinical Course. Hodgkin's disease, like NHLs, usually presents with a painless enlargement of the lymph nodes. Although a definitive distinction between Hodgkin's and NHLs can be made only by examination of a lymph node biopsy specimen, several clinical features favor the diagnosis of Hodgkin's disease (Table 12–12). Younger patients with the more favorable histologic types tend to present in clinical stage I or II (see Table 12–11) and are usually free of systemic manifestations. Patients with disseminated disease (stages III and IV) are more likely to present with systemic complaints such as fever, unexplained weight loss, pruritus, and anemia. As mentioned earlier, these patients generally have the histologically less favorable variants. The outlook after aggressive radiotherapy and chemotherapy for patients with this disease, including those with disseminated disease, has changed considerably. *With current modalities of therapy, the histologic picture has very little impact on the prognosis; instead, clinical stage appears to be the important prognostic indicator.* The 5-year survival rate of patients with stage I-A or II-A disease is close to 100%. Even with advanced disease (stage IV-A or IV-B), a 50% 5-year disease-free survival rate can be achieved. However, the recent therapeutic advances have also brought new problems. Long-term survivors of combined chemotherapy-radiotherapy protocols are at much higher risk of developing acute leukemia, lung cancer, melanomas, and some forms of NHLs.

Leukemias and Myeloproliferative Diseases

The leukemias are malignant neoplasms of the hematopoietic stem cells characterized by diffuse replacement of the bone marrow by neoplastic cells. In most cases the leukemic cells spill over into the blood, where they may be seen in large numbers. These cells may also infiltrate the liver, spleen, lymph nodes, and other tissues throughout the body, causing enlargement of these organs. Although the presence of excessive numbers of abnormal cells in the peripheral blood is the most dramatic manifestation of leukemia, it should be remembered that the leukemias are primary disorders of the bone marrow. Indeed, some patients with a diffusely infiltrated bone marrow may present with leukopenia rather than leukocytosis.

Classification. Leukemias are classified on the basis of the cell type involved and the state of maturity of the leukemic cells. Thus, *acute leukemias* are characterized by replacement of the marrow with very immature cells (called *blasts*) and by a rapidly fatal course in untreated patients. On the other hand, *chronic leukemias* are associated, at least initially, with well-differentiated (mature) leukocytes and with a relatively indolent course. Two major variants of acute and chronic leukemias are recognized: lymphocytic and myelocytic (myelogenous). Thus, a simple classification would have four patterns of leukemia: acute lymphocytic (lymphoblastic) leukemia (ALL), chronic lymphocytic leukemia (CLL), acute myelocytic (myeloblastic) leukemia (AML), and chronic myelocytic leukemia (CML).

Although this classification is widely used and clinically useful, it separates leukemias from closely related neoplastic disorders of hematopoietic stem cells. For example, *it is widely accepted that CML, polycythemia vera, essential thrombocythemia, and myeloid metaplasia represent clonal neoplastic proliferations of the myeloid or, possibly, pluripotent stem cells.* If the erythrocyte precursors dominate, the resulting clinical disorder is classified as *polycythemia vera;* on the other hand, dominance of the granulocytic series is manifested as CML. It seems that the term *chronic myeloproliferative disorders* best describes this constellation of neoplasms originating from the myeloid stem cell. Although the individual chronic myeloproliferative disorders have distinctive clinical features, interconversions and overlaps among some members of this group are well known and further attest to their relatedness.

Analogous to chronic myeloproliferative disorders, it is possible to segregate *chronic lymphoproliferative disorders.* This group includes chronic lymphocytic leukemia and hairy cell leukemia, both neoplastic proliferations of lymphoid cells, most often of B-cell lineage. It will be apparent that as proliferative disorders of lymphoid cells, they are related to the NHLs already discussed. Indeed, there is very little clinical or anatomic difference between CLL and small lymphocytic lymphomas.

In the ensuing discussion, we will follow the traditional, but admittedly imperfect, practice of segregating the acute and chronic leukemias from the chronic myeloproliferative disorders such as polycythemia vera and myeloid metaplasia.

■

Table 12–12.	CLINICAL DIFFERENCES BETWEEN HODGKIN'S AND NON-HODGKIN'S LYMPHOMAS	
Hodgkin's Disease	**Non-Hodgkin's Lymphoma**
More often localized to a single axial group of nodes (cervical, mediastinal, para-aortic)	More frequent involvement of multiple peripheral nodes
Orderly spread by contiguity	Noncontiguous spread
Mesenteric nodes and Waldeyer's ring rarely involved	Waldeyer's ring and mesenteric nodes commonly involved
Extranodal involvement uncommon	Extranodal involvement common

ACUTE LEUKEMIAS

As with all leukemias, the acute ones have their origin in the transformation of hematopoietic stem cells. Acute leukemias are characterized by a paucity of mature cells and an accumulation of leukocyte precursors (leukemic blasts).

Pathophysiology. Morphologic and cell kinetic studies have indicated that in acute leukemias there is a block in differentiation of leukemic stem cells and that the leukemic blasts have a prolonged rather than shortened generation time. Thus, the accumulation of leukemic blasts in acute leukemia results from clonal expansion of the transformed stem cells, as well as a failure of maturation of the progeny into functional end cells. As the leukemic blasts accumulate in the marrow, they suppress normal hematopoietic stem cells. This has two important clinical implications: (1) the major manifestations of acute leukemia result from the paucity of normal red cells, white cells, and platelets; and (2) therapeutically, the aim is to reduce the population of the leukemic clone enough to allow recovery o˘ the few remaining normal stem cells.

Classificati n. Leukemic transformation may affect any stage during ᵗ ᵤe differentiation of pluripotent hematopoietic stem cells. Involvement of the lymphoid series gives rise to ALL, whereas neoplastic transformation of myeloid progenitor cells gives rise to various forms of AML. Each of these two major subtypes is considered separately after discussion of clinical and laboratory features common to all acute leukemias.

Clinical Features. The acute leukemias have the following characteristics:

■ *Abrupt stormy onset.* Most patients present within 3 months of the onset of symptoms.
■ *Symptoms related to depression of normal marrow function.* These include fatigue, owing mainly to anemia; fever, reflecting an infection resulting from an absence of mature leukocytes; and bleeding (petechiae, ecchymoses, epistaxis, gum bleeding) secondary to thrombocytopenia.
■ *Bone pain and tenderness.* These result from marrow expansion with infiltration of the subperiosteum.
■ *Generalized lymphadenopathy, splenomegaly,* and *hepatomegaly.* These reflect dissemination of the leukemic cells; this occurs in all acute leukemias, but more commonly in ALL.
■ *Central nervous system manifestations.* These include headache, vomiting, and nerve palsies resulting from meningeal spread; these features are more common in children than in adults and are more common in ALL than in AML.

Laboratory Findings. Anemia is almost always present. The white blood cell count is variably elevated, sometimes to more than 100,000 cells per microliter, but in about 50% of the patients, it is less than 10,000 cells per microliter. Much more important is the identification of immature white cells, including blast forms, in the circulating blood and the bone marrow, where they make up 60% to 100% of all the cells. The platelet count is usually depressed to less than 100,000 per microliter. Uncommonly there is pancytopenia with few blast cells in the blood (aleukemic leukemia), but the bone marrow is nonetheless flooded with blasts, ruling out aplastic anemia. With this review, we can turn to specific forms of acute leukemia.

Acute Lymphoblastic Leukemia

ALL is primarily a disease of children and young adults. It accounts for 80% of childhood acute leukemias, and the peak incidence is at approximately 4 years of age.

MORPHOLOGY. The nuclei of leukemic blasts in Wright-Giemsa–stained preparations have somewhat coarse and clumped chromatin and one or two nucleoli (Fig. 12–24*B*). In contrast to the blasts of AML, the cytoplasm of ALL blasts contains not azurophilic granules, but large aggregates of periodic acid–Schiff (PAS)–positive material. TdT, a DNA polymerase, is a useful marker because it is present in 95% of cases of ALL and only 5% of cases of AML.

Immunologic Subtypes. Five subtypes, based on the origin of the leukemic lymphoblasts and stage of differentiation, are recognized. Because immunophenotyping has prognostic implications, it is detailed in Table 12–13. Note that most ALLs are of B-cell origin, mainly of the early B precursor type. All B-cell ALLs, regardless of their level of maturity, express the pan–B-cell marker CD19 (Fig. 12–25*C* and *D*). T-cell ALLs are akin to lymphoblastic lymphoma and are associated with prominent mediastinal masses.

Karyotypic Changes. Approximately 90% of patients with ALL have nonrandom karyotypic abnormalities. Most common is hyperdiploidy (>50 chromosomes/cell) in early precursor B-cell ALL. The Philadelphia chromosome (p 377) is present in 2% to 5% of children with ALL and in 25% to 30% of adults with ALL; it carries a very poor prognosis, as does a t(8;14) translocation, characteristic of ALL with a mature B-cell phenotype.

Prognosis. Dramatic advances have been made in the treatment of ALL. The treatment and prognosis depend on the phenotype and karyotype. Children 2 to 10 years of age with early pre-B phenotype and hyperdiploidy have the best prognosis, and most can be cured. Adults (with any phenotype) and children with mature B-cell or immature T-cell disease fare much less well. The presence of translocations worsens the prognosis in all groups.

Acute Myeloblastic Leukemia

AML primarily affects adults. Its incidence increases steadily with age, with the median age being 50 years. It is an extremely heterogeneous disorder, as will be discussed below.

MORPHOLOGY. In most cases myeloblasts can be readily distinguished from lymphoblasts with the usual Wright-Giemsa stain. Such staining reveals delicate nuclear chromatin; three to five nucleoli; and fine, azurophilic, **myeloperoxidase-positive** granules in the cytoplasm (see Fig. 12–24*A*). Distinctive red-staining rodlike structures **(Auer rods)** are present in some cases, more often in the promyelocytic variant. Monocytic differentiation is associated with staining for lysosomal nonspecific esterases. TdT is present in less than 5% of cases.

Classification. AMLs (also called *acute nonlymphocytic leukemias*) are of diverse origin. Some arise from transformation of multipotent stem cells, even though myeloblasts

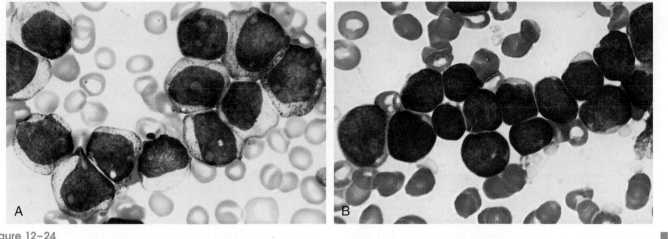

Figure 12-24   ■

Acute leukemia. *A,* Acute myeloblastic leukemia (M1). Myeloblasts have delicate nuclear chromatin, prominent nucleoli, and fine azurophilic granules in the cytoplasm. *B,* Acute lymphoblastic leukemia. Lymphoblasts have fewer nucleoli than do myeloblasts, and the nuclear chromatin is more condensed. Cytoplasmic granules are absent. (Courtesy of Dr. Robert W. McKenna, Department of Pathology, University of Texas Southwestern Medical School, Dallas, TX.)

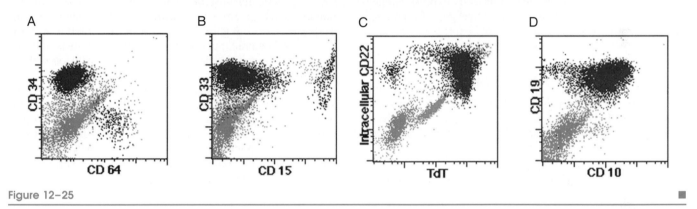

Figure 12-25   ■

Immunophenotype of acute myeloblastic leukemia (AML) and acute lymphoblastic leukemia (ALL) by flow cytometry. *A* and *B* represent the phenotype of AML, M1 type (shown in Fig. 12–24*A*). Note that the myeloblasts represented by red dots express CD34, a marker of multipotential stem cells, but do not express CD64, a marker of mature myeloid cells *(A).* In *B,* the same cells are seen to express CD33, a marker expressed on early myeloid lineage cells, and some cells also express CD15, a marker of more mature myeloid cells. Thus, these blasts are minimally differentiated myeloid cells. *C* and *D* represent the phenotype of ALL (shown in Fig. 12–24*B*). Note that the lymphoblasts represented by red dots express TdT, as well as CD22 *(C).* In *D,* the same cells are seen to express two additional B-cell markers, CD10 and CD19. Thus, these cells represent B lymphoblasts. (Courtesy of Dr. Louis Picker, Department of Pathology, University of Texas Southwestern Medical School, Dallas, TX.)

dominate the picture. In others, the common monocyte-granulocyte precursor is involved, giving rise to myelomonocytic leukemia. Based on the line of differentiation and the maturity of cells, AMLs are divided into eight groups in the widely used French-American-British (FAB) classification. These are listed in Table 12–14, along with their relative frequency and special features. Several cytogenetic changes have been noted in AML; some that are correlated with particular FAB groups and influence prognosis are also indicated in Table 12–14. Of particular interest is the t(15;17) translocation in M3, or acute promyelocytic leukemia. This translocation results in fusion of retinoic acid receptor α (RAR-α) gene on chromosome 7 with a transcriptional unit called *PML* on chromosome 15. This molecular alteration somehow blocks myeloid differentiation that can be overcome by high doses of all-*trans*-retinoic acid (Chapter 8), a vitamin A analog. It is possible, therefore, to induce remission in patients with acute promyelocytic leukemia, by administration of all-*trans*-retinoic acid. Most

patients, however, relapse and require subsequent chemotherapy.

Immunophenotype. The expression of immunologic markers is heterogeneous in AML. Most express some combination of myeloid-associated antigens, such as CD13, CD14, CD15, or CD64. CD33 is expressed on pluripotent stem cells but is retained on myeloid progenitor cells. Hence it is expressed on the most immature of myeloblasts in M0 and M1 (Fig. 12–25*A* and *B*). The diagnostic value of phenotypic markers lies in differentiation from ALL, especially in M0. In addition, monoclonal antibodies reactive with platelet-associated antigens are very helpful in the diagnosis of M7.

Prognosis. AML is a devastating disease. Although the majority of patients achieve remission with intensive chemotherapy, most suffer relapse, and only 15% to 30% enjoy long-term disease-free survival. An increasing number of patients with AML are being treated with allogeneic bone marrow transplantation. Although there are several problems with

Table 12–13. IMMUNOLOGIC CLASSIFICATION OF ACUTE LYMPHOBLASTIC LEUKEMIA

Category	Lymphoid Marker	B-Lineage Markers				T-Lineage Markers			Approximate Frequency (%)
	Tdt	CD19	CD10	Cμ	SIg	CD7	CyCD3	CD2	
B-Lineage									
Early B-precursor	+	+	−	−	−	−	−	−	5–10
	+	+	+	−	−	−	−	−	50–60
Pre-B	+	+	+	+	−	−	−	−	20
Mature B	−	+	±	−	+	−	−	−	1–2
T-Lineage	+	−	−	−	−	+	+	+	15

Tdt = Terminal deoxynucleotidyl transferase; Cμ = cytoplasmic μ; SIg = surface immunoglobulin; CyCD3 = cytoplasmic CD3

bone marrow transplantation, this is the only curative treatment at present.

Biphenotypic Leukemias

Recent phenotypic studies have revealed that in a significant minority of cases, the leukemia cells express antigens typical of both lymphoid and myeloid lineages. The prognostic significance of such "biphenotypic" expression is not yet clear.

MYELODYSPLASTIC SYNDROMES

This term refers to a group of clonal stem cell disorders characterized by maturation defects resulting in ineffective hematopoiesis and an increased risk of transformation to acute myeloblastic leukemias.

In patients with this syndrome, bone marrow is partly or wholly replaced by the clonal progeny of a mutant pluripotent stem cell that retains the capacity to differentiate into red cells, granulocytes, and platelets but in a manner that is both ineffective and disordered. As a result, the bone marrow is usually hypercellular or normocellular, but the peripheral blood shows pancytopenia. The abnormal stem cell clone in the bone marrow is genetically unstable, with a tendency to accumulate mutations and give rise to an acute leukemia. Hence, myelodysplasia may be regarded as a preleukemic condition. Most cases are idiopathic, but some patients develop the syndrome after chemotherapy with alkylating agents, with or without radiation therapy.

Cytogenetic studies reveal that up to 70% of patients have a chromosomally abnormal clone of cells in the marrow. Some common karyotypic abnormalities include a loss of chromosomes 5 or 7 or deletions of their long arms. Morphologically, the marrow is populated by aberrant cells such as megaloblastoid erythroid precursors, bizarre-looking blasts, and micromegakaryocytes, among others.

Table 12–14. FAB CLASSIFICATION OF ACUTE MYELOBLASTIC (MYELOCYTIC) LEUKEMIAS

Class	Morphology	Comments
M0 Minimally differentiated AML	Blasts lack definitive cytologic and cytochemical markers of myeloblasts but express myeloid lineage antigens	2% to 3% of AML
M1 AML without differentiation	Very immature myeloblasts predominate; few granules or Auer rods	20% of AML; Ph¹ chromosome, present in 10% to 15% of cases, worsens prognosis
M2 AML with differentiation	Myeloblasts and promyelocytes predominate; Auer rods present in most cases	30% of AML; presence of t(8;21) translocation associated with good prognosis
M3 Acute promyelocytic leukemia	Hypergranular promyelocytes, often with many Auer rods per cell; may have reniform or bilobed nuclei	5% to 10% of AML; disseminated intravascular coagulation common; presence of t(15;17) translocation is characteristic; responds to retinoic acid therapy
M4 Acute myelomonocytic leukemia	Myelocytic and monocytic differentiation evident; myeloid elements resemble M2; peripheral monocytosis	20% to 30% of AML; presence of inv16 or del 16q associated with better prognosis
M5 Acute monocytic leukemia	Monoblasts (peroxidase-negative, esterase-positive) and promonocytes predominate	10% of AML; usually in children and young adults; gum infiltration common; associated with abnormalities of chromosome 11
M6 Acute erythroleukemia	Bizarre, multinucleated, megaloblastoid erythroblasts predominate; myeloblasts also present	5% of AML; high blood counts and organ infiltration are rare; affected persons are of advanced age
M7 Acute megakaryocytic leukemia	Blasts of megakaryocytic lineage predominate; react with antiplatelet antibodies; myelofibrosis or increased bone marrow reticulin	

Most patients are older males between 50 and 70 years of age. Ten per cent to 40% of these patients develop AML; the remainder are constantly threatened by infections, anemia, and hemorrhages owing to a lack of differentiated myeloid cells. The prognosis is variable; median survival time varies from 9 to 29 months.

CHRONIC MYELOID LEUKEMIA

CML principally affects adults between 25 and 60 years of age and accounts for 15% to 20% of all cases of leukemia. The peak incidence is in the fourth and fifth decades of life.

Pathophysiology. As mentioned earlier, CML is one of the four chronic myeloproliferative disorders. Unlike other myeloproliferative disorders, however, CML is associated with the presence of a *unique chromosomal abnormality,* the Ph[1] (Philadelphia) chromosome. In approximately 90% of patients with CML, the Ph[1] chromosome, usually representing a reciprocal translocation from the long arm of chromosome 22 to another chromosome (usually the long arm of chromosome 9), can be identified in granulocytic, erythroid, and megakaryocytic precursors, as well as B cells and, in some cases, T cells. This finding is *firm evidence for the clonal origin of CML from pluripotent stem cells.* Recall that the translocation responsible for the appearance of Ph[1] chromosome gives rise to a *bcr-c-abl* fusion gene, believed to be critical for neoplastic transformation (Chapter 6). Indeed, most patients who appear to be Ph[1] negative by cytogenetic studies reveal rearrangement of the *bcr* gene at the molecular level. This can be detected by Southern blot analysis or polymerase chain reaction (PCR) technique. While the Ph[1] chromosome is highly characteristic of CML, it should be remembered that by itself it is not diagnostic of this disorder. As stated earlier, the Ph[1] chromosome is found in some cases of AML, as well as in ALL.

Although CML originates in the pluripotent stem cells, granulocyte precursors constitute the dominant cell line. *In contrast to acute leukemias, there is no block in the maturation of leukemic stem cells,* as evidenced by the vast number of granulocytes in the peripheral blood. The basis of the increased myeloid stem cell mass in CML seems to lie in a failure of stem cells to respond to physiologic signals that regulate their proliferation.

Clinical Features. The onset of CML is usually slow, and the initial symptoms may be nonspecific (e.g., easy fatigability, weakness, and weight loss). Sometimes the first symptom is a dragging sensation in the abdomen, caused by the *extreme splenomegaly* that is characteristic of this condition. The laboratory findings are critical in making the diagnosis. Usually there is marked elevation of the leukocyte count, commonly exceeding 100,000 cells per microliter. *The circulating cells are predominantly neutrophils and myelocytes* (Fig. 12–26), *but basophils and eosinophils are also prominent.* A small proportion of myeloblasts, usually less than 5%, can be detected in the peripheral blood. Since CML originates from stem cells, it is not surprising that as many as 50% of patients have *thrombocytosis.* The bone marrow is hypercellular, with hyperplasia of granulocytic and megakaryocytic lineages. The frequency of myeloblasts is increased only slightly. It is sometimes necessary to distinguish CML from a leukemoid reaction, which is also associated with a striking elevation of the granulocyte count in response to infection, stress, chronic in-

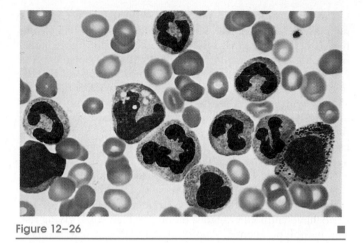

Figure 12–26   ■

Chronic myeloid leukemia. Peripheral blood smear shows many mature neutrophils, some metamyelocytes, and a myelocyte. (Courtesy of Dr. Robert W. McKenna, Department of Pathology, University of Texas Southwestern Medical School, Dallas, TX.)

flammation, and certain neoplasms. *Most important for differentiating leukemoid reactions from CML is the presence of the Ph[1] chromosome* and increased numbers of basophils in the peripheral blood, both of which are quite typical of CML. In addition, the granulocytes in CML are almost completely devoid of alkaline phosphatase.

The course of CML is one of slow progression. Even without treatment, median survival is 3 years. After a variable (and unpredictable) period, approximately 50% of patients enter an accelerated phase, during which there is gradual failure of response to treatment; increasing anemia and thrombocytopenia; acquisition of additional cytogenetic abnormalities; and finally, *transformation into a picture resembling AML* (i.e., blast crisis). In the remaining 50%, blast crises occur abruptly, without an intermediate accelerated phase. It is of interest to note that in 30% of patients, the blasts contain TdT, a marker of primitive lymphoid cells, and express B cell–lineage antigens such as CD10 and CD19. They also reveal clonal rearrangement of immunoglobulin genes. The emergence of B-cell blasts further attests to the origin of CML from a pluripotent stem cell. In the remaining 70% of patients, the blasts exhibit features of myeloblasts. Treatment of CML is unsatisfactory. Although it is possible to induce remission with chemotherapy or interferon-α treatment, the median survival time remains unchanged. *The only curative treatment for CML is allogeneic bone marrow transplantation.* Young patients who undergo transplantation within a year of diagnosis have the best prognosis. It is believed that the therapeutic efficacy of allogeneic bone marrow transplants depends in part on the antileukemic effects of donor T cells, a phenomenon called graft-versus-leukemia effect.

CHRONIC LYMPHOCYTIC LEUKEMIA

CLL, the most indolent of all leukemias, accounts for 30% of leukemias in Western countries. It is quite uncommon in Asia. CLL typically affects persons older than 50 years and shows considerable overlap with SLL.

Pathophysiology. In more than 95% of cases, CLL is a neoplasm of B cells. The leukemic cells bear markers of mature B cells (e.g., IgM, IgD), and either λ or κ light chains, indicating monoclonality. Like all B cells, they also express CD19 and CD20 antigens, but unlike most peripheral B cells, they express the T-cell–associated antigen CD5 (a feature shared with small lymphocytic lymphoma). Only 5% of chronic lymphoid leukemias are truly tumors of T cells, and they express, in addition to CD5, other T-cell markers such as CD2 and CD3. These rare T-cell leukemias are much more aggressive than the B-cell CLLs.

The leukemic B cells fail to respond to antigenic stimulation; hence, many of the patients with CLL have hypogammaglobulinemia. Paradoxically, approximately 15% of patients have antibodies against autologous red cells, giving rise to a hemolytic anemia. Approximately 50% of patients have karyotypic abnormalities, the most common of which is trisomy 12. The presence of chromosomal abnormalities carries a poor prognosis. *To summarize, CLL is characterized by the accumulation of long-lived, nonfunctional B lymphocytes that infiltrate the bone marrow, blood, lymph nodes, and other tissues.*

Clinical Features. CLL is often asymptomatic. When symptoms are present, they are nonspecific and include easy fatigability, weight loss, and anorexia. Because of *hypogammaglobulinemia,* there is increased susceptibility to bacterial infections. *Autoimmune hemolytic anemia* may be present. Generalized *lymphadenopathy* and hepatosplenomegaly are present in 50% to 60% of cases. Total leukocyte count may be increased only slightly or may reach 200,000 per microliter. In all cases, there is *absolute lymphocytosis* of small, mature-looking lymphocytes. Only a small fraction of lymphocytes are large ones with indented nuclei and nucleoli. The course and prognosis of CLL are extremely variable. Many patients live more than 10 years after diagnosis and die of unrelated causes; the median survival is 4 to 6 years. Unlike CML, transformation to acute leukemia with blast crisis is rare.

HAIRY CELL LEUKEMIA

This uncommon form of chronic B-cell leukemia is distinguished by the presence of leukemic cells that have fine, hair-like cytoplasmic projections, best recognized under the phase contrast microscope but also visible in routine blood smears. A cytochemical feature that is quite characteristic of hairy cells is the presence of tartrate-resistant acid phosphatase in neoplastic B cells. The hairy cells express surface Ig with a single light chain, confirming clonality. In addition, B-cell antigens, including CD19 and CD20, are expressed.

Hairy cell leukemia occurs mainly in older males, and its *manifestations result largely from infiltration of bone marrow and spleen.* Splenomegaly, which is often massive, is the most common and sometimes the only abnormal physical finding. *Pancytopenia,* resulting from marrow failure and splenic sequestration, is seen in more than half the cases. Hepatomegaly is less common and not as marked, and lymphadenopathy is distinctly rare. *Leukocytosis is not a common feature,* being present in only 15% to 20% of patients. Hairy cells can be identified in the peripheral blood smear in most cases. The course of this disease is chronic, and the median survival time

is 4 years. Because of pancytopenia, infections are a major problem. Splenectomy raises the peripheral blood count and so provides at least a temporary relief from symptoms. However, additional chemotherapy is always needed. Several agents are effective, including α-interferons and purine nucleosides; these cause durable and complete responses in most cases.

ETIOLOGY AND PATHOGENESIS OF LEUKEMIAS AND LYMPHOMAS

As with many other forms of cancer, several environmental agents have been implicated in the causation of leukemias and lymphomas. Well-established influences include ionizing radiations and chemicals. Exposure to radiation—occupational, therapeutic, or accidental—increases the incidence of several leukemias (with the curious exception of CLL). The increased risk of leukemias and NHLs after treatment with alkylating agents is also well established. The risk is even greater if both irradiation and chemotherapy have been used, as, for example, in the treatment of Hodgkin's disease.

Two viruses, HTLV-1 and EBV, have been associated with acute T-cell leukemia/lymphoma and Burkitt's lymphoma, respectively. The possible mechanisms of transformation by these viral agents were discussed earlier in Chapter 6. As with all neoplasms, mutations in oncogenes, tumor suppressor genes, and genes that regulate apoptosis are important in the causation of leukemias and lymphomas. Of particular relevance to this group of disorders are mutations in cyclin D1, *bcl*-2, c-*myc,* c-*abl,* and RAR-α, discussed previously.

MYELOPROLIFERATIVE DISORDERS

The concept that myeloproliferative disorders result from clonal neoplastic proliferations of the multipotent myeloid stem cells has already been discussed (p 373). It was mentioned in our earlier presentation that four disorders—CML, polycythemia vera, myeloid metaplasia with myelofibrosis, and essential thrombocythemia—are included in this group. CML was discussed along with other leukemias. Of the remaining three, only polycythemia vera and myeloid metaplasia with myelofibrosis are presented here. Essential thrombocythemia occurs too infrequently to merit further discussion.

Polycythemia Vera

As with all myeloproliferative disorders, polycythemia vera is associated with excessive proliferation of erythroid, granulocytic, and megakaryocytic elements, all derived from a single neoplastic stem cell. However, in polycythemia vera, the erythroid precursors dominate, so there is an *absolute increase in red cell mass.* This should be contrasted with *relative polycythemia,* which results from hemoconcentration. Furthermore, unlike other forms of absolute polycythemia that result from increased secretion of erythropoietin, polycythemia vera is associated with low but detectable levels of erythropoietin in the serum. It seems that the growth of neoplastic erythroid stem cells is autonomous and erythropoietin independent. In patients with polycythemia vera, such stem cells coexist with normal, erythropoietin-dependent, progenitor cells.

MORPHOLOGY. The major anatomic changes stem from the increase in blood volume and viscosity brought about by the erythrocytosis. Plethoric congestion of all tissues and organs is characteristic of polycythemia vera. The liver is enlarged and frequently contains foci of myeloid metaplasia. The spleen is slightly enlarged in about 75% of patients, up to 250 to 300 gm, and is quite firm. The splenic sinuses are packed with red cells, as are all the vessels within the spleen.

Consequent to the increased viscosity and vascular stasis, thromboses and infarctions are common; they affect most often the heart, spleen, and kidneys. Hemorrhages occur in about a third of these patients, probably owing to excessive distention of blood vessels and abnormal platelet function. They usually affect the gastrointestinal tract, oropharynx, or brain. Although these hemorrhages are said on occasion to be spontaneous, more often they follow some minor trauma or surgical procedure. Peptic ulceration has been described in about a fifth of these patients.

The bone marrow is hypercellular, with hyperplasia of erythroid, myeloid, and megakaryocytic cells. In addition, some degree of marrow fibrosis is present in 10% of patients at the time of diagnosis. This may increase if the disease progresses to myelofibrosis. If the disease changes its course, the marrow reflects the alterations and may become leukemic or fibrotic, as discussed below.

Clinical Course. Polycythemia vera appears insidiously, usually in late middle age (40 to 60 years). Patients with this disorder classically are plethoric and often somewhat cyanotic. There may be an intense pruritus, resulting perhaps from histamine released as a result of an increase in basophils. The excess histamine may also account for the peptic ulceration seen in these patients. Other complaints are referable to the thrombotic and hemorrhagic tendencies and to hypertension. *Headache, dizziness, gastrointestinal symptoms, hematemesis, and melena are common.* Owing to the high rate of cell turnover, symptomatic gout is seen in 5% to 10% of cases, although many more patients have hyperuricemia.

The diagnosis is usually made in the laboratory. Red cell counts range from 6 to 10 million per microliter, and the hematocrit may approach 60%. Since there is hyperproliferation of granulocytic precursors as well as megakaryocytes in the bone marrow, the white cell count may be as high as 50,000/mm^3, and the platelet count is often greater than 400,000/mm^3. Basophil counts are frequently elevated. The platelets are morphologically and functionally abnormal in most cases. Giant forms and megakaryocytic fragments are seen in the blood. About 30% of patients develop thrombotic complications, usually affecting the brain or heart. Hepatic vein thrombosis, giving rise to the Budd-Chiari syndrome (Chapter 16), is not uncommon. Minor hemorrhages (e.g., epistaxis and bleeding from gums) are common; life-threatening hemorrhages occur in 5% to 10% of patients. In patients who receive no treatment, death resulting from these vascular episodes occurs within

months after diagnosis; however, if the red cell mass can be maintained near normal by phlebotomies, median survival of 10 years can be achieved.

Prolonged survival with treatment has revealed that the *natural history of polycythemia vera involves a gradual transition to a "spent phase," during which the clinical and anatomic features of myeloid metaplasia with myelofibrosis develop.* Approximately 15% to 20% of patients undergo such a transformation after an average interval of 10 years. This transition is brought about by creeping fibrosis in the bone marrow (myelofibrosis) and a shift of hematopoiesis to the spleen, which enlarges markedly. This is perhaps the most striking example of conversion of one myeloproliferative disorder to another. As in CML, another myeloproliferative disease, certain patients with polycythemia vera develop a terminal acute myeloblastic leukemia. However, the incidence of this transition is much lower than in CML and is estimated to be about 2% in patients who are treated with phlebotomy alone and about 15% in those who receive myelosuppressive treatment with chlorambucil or marrow irradiation with radioactive phosphorus. Presumably, the increase is related to the mutagenic effects of these therapeutic agents.

Myeloid Metaplasia With Myelofibrosis

In this chronic myeloproliferative disorder, the proliferation of the neoplastic myeloid stem cells occurs principally in the spleen (myeloid metaplasia), and in the fully developed syndrome, the bone marrow is hypocellular and fibrotic (myelofibrosis). Sometimes polycythemia vera and, less often, CML "burn out," as it were, and terminate in a myelofibrotic pattern. In many patients, however, extramedullary hematopoiesis in the spleen and marrow fibrosis arise insidiously without an identifiable preceding syndrome or toxic cause for marrow destruction and fibrosis; the term *agnogenic (idiopathic) myeloid metaplasia* is sometimes used to describe this condition.

Although marrow fibrosis is characteristic of this condition, the fibroblasts are not clonal descendants of the transformed stem cells. Instead, marrow fibrosis is secondary to derangements in hematopoietic cells, particularly megakaryocytes. It is believed that *marrow fibroblasts are stimulated to proliferate by platelet-derived growth factor and transforming growth factor β released from neoplastic megakaryocytes.* These two growth factors are known to be mitogenic for fibroblasts. It is postulated that the proliferation of neoplastic stem cells begins within the marrow and that there is subsequent seeding of the spleen and other organs such as the liver. As the disease progresses, marrow fibrosis occurs secondary to the elaboration of fibroblast growth factors mentioned above. By the time the patient comes to clinical attention, fibroblasts have already taken over the marrow, and the spleen remains the major site of myeloproliferation. This scheme is supported by the finding of hypercellular bone marrow with prominent megakaryocytes early in the course of this disease.

MORPHOLOGY. The principal site of the extramedullary hematopoiesis is the **spleen,** which is usually markedly enlarged, sometimes up to 4000 gm. As with most causes of massive splenomegaly, multiple subcapsular infarcts may be present. Histologically **there is trilineage proliferation affecting normoblasts, granulocyte precursors, and megakaryocytes; however, megakaryocytes are usually prominent owing to their large size and nuclear morphology.** Sometimes disproportional activity of any one of the three major cell lines is seen.

The **liver** may be moderately enlarged, with foci of extramedullary hematopoiesis. The **lymph nodes** are only rarely the site of blood cell formation and usually are not enlarged.

The **bone marrow** in a typical case is **hypocellular and shows diffuse fibrosis.** However, the marrow is hypercellular in early cases, with equal representation of the three major cell lines. Megakaryocytes are often prominent and may show dysplastic changes.

Clinical Course. Myeloid metaplasia may begin with a blood picture suggestive of polycythemia vera or myelogenous leukemia, or it may arise as an apparently primary disease. Most patients have moderate to severe anemia. The white cell count may be normal, reduced, or markedly elevated. Early in the course of the disease, the platelet count is normal or elevated, but eventually patients develop thrombocytopenia. The *peripheral blood smear appears markedly abnormal* (Fig. 12–27). Red cell abnormalities include the

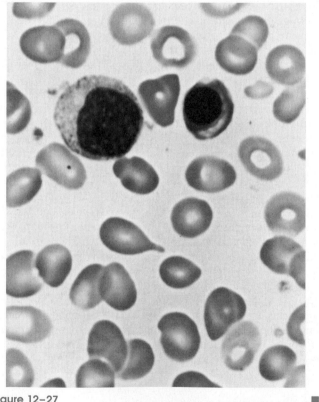

Figure 12–27 ■

Myeloid metaplasia with myelofibrosis. A peripheral blood smear shows a teardrop red cell in the center field. An immature myeloid *(left)* and a nucleated red cell *(right)* are seen. (Courtesy of Dr. José Hernandez, Department of Pathology, University of Texas Southwestern Medical School, Dallas, TX.)

presence of immature forms and bizarre shapes (poikilocytes, teardrop cells). Immature white cells (myelocytes and metamyelocytes) are also seen in the peripheral blood. Basophils are usually increased. Platelets are often abnormal in size and shape and defective in function. In some cases the clinical and blood picture may resemble CML, but the *Ph¹ chromosome is absent.* In addition, patients with myelophthisic anemia, in which marrow fibrosis results from an identifiable cause of marrow injury, may also present with similar findings in the peripheral blood; hence a careful history must be taken to exclude such causes. Owing to a high rate of cell turnover, hyperuricemia and gout may complicate the picture. The outcome of myeloid metaplasia is variable. There is constant threat of infections, as well as thrombotic and hemorrhagic episodes owing to platelet abnormalities. Splenic infarctions are therefore common. As many as 5% to 15% of patients eventually suffer a blast crisis resembling AML. The median survival time overall is 4 to 5 years.

Plasma Cell Dyscrasias and Related Disorders

The plasma cell dyscrasias are a group of disorders that have in common the *expansion of a single clone of immunoglobulin-secreting cells and a resultant increase in serum levels of a single homogeneous immunoglobulin or its fragments.* The homogeneous immunoglobulin identified in the blood is often referred to as an *M component.* Because a common feature of the various plasma cell dyscrasias is the presence in the serum of excessive amounts of immunoglobulins, these disorders have also been called *monoclonal gammopathies.* In many cases these dyscrasias behave as malignant diseases, although it should be remembered that M components are also seen in otherwise normal elders, a condition called monoclonal gammopathy of undetermined significance. Collectively, these disorders account for about 15% of deaths from malignant white cell disease; they are most common in middle-aged and elderly persons.

The plasma cell dyscrasias can be divided into six major variants: (1) multiple myeloma, (2) localized plasmacytoma (solitary myeloma), (3) Waldenström's macroglobulinemia, (4) heavy-chain disease, (5) primary or immunocyte-associated amyloidosis, and (6) monoclonal gammopathy of undetermined significance. Each of these disorders will be briefly characterized before the morphologic features of the more common forms are presented.

Multiple Myeloma. Multiple myeloma, by far the most common of the malignant plasma cell dyscrasias, is a *clonal proliferation of neoplastic plasma cells in the bone marrow that is usually associated with multifocal lytic lesions throughout the skeletal system.* The proliferation of neoplastic plasma cells, also called *myeloma cells,* is triggered in large part by the cytokine interleukin 6 (IL-6), produced by fibroblasts and macrophages in the bone marrow stroma. This finding is of importance because high serum levels of IL-6 are associated with poor prognosis; as a corollary, antibodies against IL-6 may prove useful in the treatment of multiple myeloma.

In approximately 60% of patients, the M component is IgG; in 20% to 25%, IgA; rarely, it is IgM, IgD, or IgE. In the remaining 15% to 20% of cases, the plasma cells produce *only* κ or λ light chains, which, because of their low molecular weight, are readily excreted in urine, where they are termed *Bence Jones proteins.* In these patients, Bence Jones proteinuria without serum M component is present *(light-chain disease).* However, in up to 80% of patients, the malignant plasma cells synthesize complete immunoglobulin molecules as well as excess light chains, and therefore both Bence Jones proteins and serum M components are present.

Localized Plasmacytoma. This designation refers to the presence of a single lesion in the skeleton or in the soft tissues. Solitary skeletal myeloma tends to occur in the same locations as multiple myeloma, whereas the extraosseous lesions usually form tumorous masses in the upper respiratory tract (sinuses, nasopharynx, larynx). Modest elevations in the levels of M protein are demonstrable in some of these patients. Those with solitary skeletal myelomas usually have occult lesions elsewhere. The patients may remain stable for several years, but after a lapse of 10 to 20 years, most develop disseminated disease. Extraosseous (soft tissue) plasmacytomas rarely disseminate. They represent limited disease that can be readily cured by local resection.

Waldenström's Macroglobulinemia. This disease is best regarded as a hybrid of small lymphocytic lymphoma (SLL) and multiple myeloma. In multiple myeloma the neoplastic B cells are fully differentiated into immunoglobulin-secreting plasma cells, whereas in SLL the malignant B cells are arrested prior to acquisition of secretory capacity. Between the two is Waldenström's macroglobulinemia, which involves B cells that are sufficiently differentiated to secrete immunoglobulins but not enough to look like plasma cells. Interestingly, the morphologic and clinical features of Waldenström's macroglobulinemia overlap those of both SLL and myeloma. Like myeloma, there is an M component, which in most cases is due to the production of monoclonal IgM. However, unlike myeloma (but resembling lymphoma), the neoplastic B lymphocytes diffusely infiltrate the lymphoid organs, including bone marrow, lymph nodes, and spleen.

Heavy-Chain Disease. This is an extremely rare plasma cell dyscrasia in which only heavy chains are produced. These may be of the IgG, IgA, or IgM class. Except for the presence of an M component, the disease often mimics a lymphoma-leukemia, and in this respect it resembles Waldenström's macroglobulinemia. However, the precise characteristics depend to some extent on which heavy chain is involved. With IgG heavy-chain disease, there is diffuse lymphadenopathy and hepatosplenomegaly. IgA heavy-chain disease shows a predilection for the lymphoid tissues that are normally the site of IgA synthesis, such as the small intestine and respiratory tract.

Primary or Immunocyte-Associated Amyloidosis. It may be recalled that monoclonal proliferation of plasma cells, with excessive production of light chains, underlies this form of amyloidosis (Chapter 5). The amyloid deposits (AL type) consist of partially degraded light chains.

Monoclonal Gammopathy of Undetermined Significance. M proteins can be detected in the serum of 1% to 3% of asymptomatic, healthy persons over age 50 years. The term *monoclonal gammopathy of undetermined significance (MGUS)* is applied to this dysproteinosis without any associated disease. This is the most common monoclonal gammopathy. Approximately 20% of patients with MGUS develop a well-defined plasma cell dyscrasia (myeloma, Waldenström's macroglobulinemia, or amyloidosis) over a period of 10 to 15 years. The diagnosis of MGUS should be made with caution and after careful exclusion of all other specific forms of monoclonal gammopathies. In general, patients with MGUS have less than 3 gm/dl of monoclonal protein in the serum and no Bence Jones proteinuria.

MORPHOLOGY. Multiple myeloma presents most often as multifocal destructive bone lesions throughout the skeletal system. Although any bone may be affected, the following distribution was found in a large series of cases: vertebral column, 66%; ribs, 44%; skull, 41%; pelvis, 28%; femur, 24%; clavicle, 10%; and scapula, 10%. These focal lesions generally begin in the medullary cavity, erode the cancellous bone, and progressively destroy the cortical bone. The bone resorption results from the secretion of osteoclast-activating factors (e.g., IL-1, TNF-α, lymphotoxin) by myeloma cells. Pathologic fractures are often produced by plasma cell lesions; they are most common in the vertebral column but may affect any of the numerous bones suffering erosion and destruction of their cortical substances. Most commonly, the lesions appear radiographically as punched-out defects, usually 1 to 4 cm in diameter (Fig. 12–28), but in some cases only diffuse demineralization is evident. Microscopic examination of the marrow reveals an increased number of plasma cells, constituting 10% to 90% of all cells in the marrow. The neoplastic plasma cells may resemble normal ma-

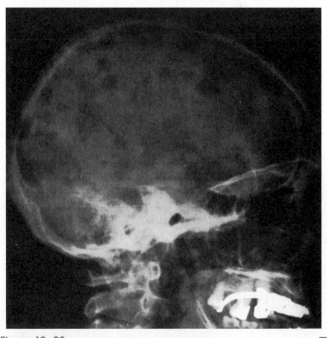

Figure 12–28   ■

Multiple myeloma of the skull (radiograph, lateral view). The sharply punched-out bone defects are most obvious in the calvarium.

ture plasma cells, but sometimes more immature forms are found that may even resemble lymphocytes. With progressive disease, plasma cell infiltrations of soft tissues may be encountered in the spleen, liver, kidneys, lungs, and lymph nodes, or more widely.

Renal involvement, generally called **myeloma nephrosis,** is one of the more distinctive features of multiple myeloma. Microscopically, interstitial infiltrates of abnormal plasma cells may be encountered. Proteinaceous casts are prominent in the distal convoluted tubules and collecting ducts. Most of these casts are made up of Bence Jones proteins, but they may also contain complete immunoglobulins, Tamm-Horsfall protein, and albumin. Some casts have tinctorial properties of amyloid. This is not surprising, in view of the fact that AL amyloid is derived from Bence Jones proteins (Chapter 5). The casts are usually surrounded by multinucleate giant cells derived from fusion of infiltrating macrophages. Very often the cells that line tubules containing casts become necrotic or atrophic because of the toxic actions of free light chains (Bence Jones proteins). Metastatic calcification may be encountered within the kidney because of the **hypercalcemia** that frequently accompanies multiple myeloma. When complicated by amyloidosis, typical glomerular lesions associated with renal amyloidosis are present. Pyelonephritis may occur owing to the increased susceptibility of these patients to infections.

In contrast to multiple myeloma, Waldenström's **macroglobulinemia and heavy-chain disease are not associated with lytic skeletal lesions.** Instead, the neoplastic cells diffusely infiltrate the bone marrow, lymph nodes, spleen, and sometimes the liver. Infiltrations of other organs have also been reported. The cellular infiltrate consists of lymphocytes, plasma cells, lymphocytoid plasma cells, and several other hybrid forms. The remaining forms of plasma cell dyscrasias have either already been described (e.g., primary amyloidosis (Chapter 5)) or are too rare for further description.

Clinical Course. The clinical manifestations of the plasma cell dyscrasias are varied. They result from the destructive or otherwise damaging effect of the infiltrating neoplastic cells in various tissues and from the effects of the abnormal immunoglobulins secreted by the tumors. In multiple myeloma, the pathologic effects of tumorous masses of plasma cells predominate, whereas in Waldenström's macroglobulinemia, most of the signs and symptoms result from the IgM macroglobulins in the serum.

The peak age of incidence of multiple myeloma is between 50 and 60 years. The major clinical features of this disease are as follows:

■ Bone pain, resulting from infiltration by neoplastic plasma cells, is extremely common. Pathologic fractures and hypercalcemia occur, with focal bone destruction and diffuse

resorption. Hypercalcemia may cause neurologic manifestations such as confusion and lethargy; it also contributes to renal disease. Anemia results from marrow replacement as well as from inhibition of hematopoiesis by tumor cells.

■ Recurrent infections with bacteria such as *Staphylococcus aureus,* *Streptococcus pneumoniae,* and *Escherichia coli* are serious clinical problems. They result from severe suppression of normal immunoglobulin secretion.

■ Excessive production and aggregation of myeloma proteins may lead to the hyperviscosity syndrome (described below).

■ As many as 50% of patients suffer renal insufficiency. It results from multiple factors, such as recurrent bacterial infections and hypercalcemia, but most importantly from the toxic effects of Bence Jones proteins on cells lining the tubules.

■ Amyloidosis develops in 5% to 10% of patients.

The diagnosis of multiple myeloma can be readily made by the characteristic focal, punched-out radiologic defects in the bone, especially when these are present in the vertebrae or calvarium. Electrophoresis of the serum and urine is an important diagnostic tool in suspected cases. In 99% of cases a monoclonal spike of complete immunoglobulin or immunoglobulin light chain can be detected in the serum, in the urine, or in both. In the remaining 1% of cases, monoclonal immunoglobulins can be found within the plasma cell masses but not in the serum or urine. Such cases are sometimes called *nonsecretory myelomas.*

Waldenström's macroglobulinemia affects somewhat older persons, with the peak incidence being between the sixth and seventh decades. Most clinical symptoms of this disease can be traced to the presence of IgM globulins. Because of their size and increased concentration, the macroglobulins form large aggregates that greatly increase the viscosity of blood, giving rise to the *hyperviscosity syndrome.* This is characterized by the following features:

■ Visual impairment, related to the striking tortuosity and distention of retinal veins; retinal hemorrhages and exudates may also contribute to the visual problems.

■ Neurologic problems such as headaches, dizziness, deafness, and stupor, stemming from sluggish blood flow and sludging.

■ Bleeding, related to the formation of complexes between macroglobulins and clotting factors as well as interference with platelet functions.

■ Cryoglobulinemia, related to precipitation of macroglobulins at low temperatures and producing symptoms such as Raynaud's phenomenon and cold urticaria.

Multiple myeloma and Waldenström's macroglobulinemia are progressive diseases, with median survival in the range of 2 to 4 years.

Histiocytoses

LANGERHANS' CELL HISTIOCYTOSIS

The term *histiocytosis* is an "umbrella" designation for a variety of proliferative disorders of histiocytes or macrophages. Some, such as the rare histiocytic lymphomas mentioned earlier, are clearly malignant. Others, such as the reactive histiocytic proliferations in lymph nodes, are clearly benign. Between these two extremes is a small cluster of conditions characterized by proliferation of a special type of cell called *Langerhans' cells* (Chapter 5). Langerhans' histiocytoses are clonal proliferations of dendritic antigen-presenting cells readily seen in the skin, but also present in other organs. It is to these disorders that our attention is now directed, albeit briefly because of their relative rarity.

In the past these disorders were referred to as *histiocytosis X* and subdivided into three categories: Letterer-Siwe syndrome, Hand-Schüller-Christian disease, and eosinophilic granuloma. These three conditions are now believed to represent different expressions of the same basic disorder. The proliferating cell in all forms is the Langerhans' cell of marrow origin that is normally found in the epidermis. These specialized antigen-presenting cells are human leukocyte antigen DR (HLA-DR) positive and express the CD1 antigen. *Characteristic is the presence of HX bodies (Birbeck granules) in the cytoplasm.* Under the electron microscope, these are seen to have a pentalaminar, rodlike, tubular structure, with characteristic periodicity and sometimes a dilated terminal end (tennis-racket appearance). Under the light microscope, the proliferating Langerhans' cells in these disorders do not resemble their normal dendritic counterparts. Instead, they have abundant, often vacuolated, cytoplasm, with vesicular nuclei. This appearance is more akin to that of tissue histiocytes (macrophages) and hence the term *Langerhans' histiocytosis.*

As mentioned previously, Langerhans' cell histiocytosis presents as one of three clinicopathologic entities: Acute disseminated Langerhans' cell histiocytosis, unifocal eosinophilic granuloma, or multifocal eosinophilic granuloma.

Acute disseminated Langerhans' cell histiocytosis (Letterer-Siwe disease) usually occurs before 2 years of age but occasionally may involve adults. The dominant clinical feature is the development of cutaneous lesions that resemble seborrheic skin eruptions, secondary to infiltrations of Langerhans' histiocytes. Most of those affected have concurrent hepatosplenomegaly, lymphadenopathy, pulmonary lesions, and eventually, destructive osteolytic bone lesions. Extensive infiltration of the marrow often leads to anemia, thrombocytopenia, and predisposition to recurrent infections such as otitis media and mastoiditis. Hence, the clinical picture may resemble that of an acute leukemia. The course of untreated disease is rapidly fatal. With intensive chemotherapy, 50% of patients survive 5 years.

Both unifocal and multifocal Langerhans' cell histiocytosis (unifocal and multifocal eosinophilic granuloma) are characterized by expanding, erosive accumulations of Langerhans' cells, usually within the medullary cavities of bones. Histiocytes are variably admixed with eosinophils, lymphocytes, plasma cells, and neutrophils. The eosinophilic component ranges from scattered mature cells to sheetlike masses of cells. Virtually any bone in the skeletal system may be involved, most commonly the calvarium, ribs, and femur. Similar lesions may be found in the skin, lungs, or stomach, either as unifocal lesions or as components of the multifocal disease.

Unifocal lesions usually affect the skeletal system. They may be asymptomatic or may cause pain and tenderness and, in some instances, pathologic fractures. This is an indolent disorder that may heal spontaneously or may be cured by local excision or irradiation.

Multifocal Langerhans' cell histiocytosis usually affects children, who present with fever; diffuse eruptions, particularly on the scalp and in the ear canals; and frequent bouts of otitis media, mastoiditis, and upper respiratory tract infections. An infiltrate of Langerhans' cells may lead to mild lymphadenopathy, hepatomegaly, and splenomegaly. In about 50% of patients, involvement of the posterior pituitary stalk of the hypothalamus leads to diabetes insipidus. The combination of calvarial bone defects, diabetes insipidus, and exophthalmos is referred to as the *Hand-Schüller-Christian triad.* Many patients experience spontaneous regression; others can be treated with chemotherapy.

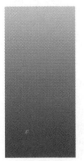

Bleeding Disorders

These disorders are characterized by spontaneous bleeding or excessive bleeding after trauma. Such abnormal hemorrhage may have as its cause (1) increased fragility of the vessels, (2) inadequacy of hemostatic responses in the form of either platelet deficiency or dysfunction, or (3) derangement in the clotting mechanism. Before embarking on a discussion of these three forms of bleeding disorders, it would be profitable to review normal hemostasis and the common laboratory tests used in the evaluation of a bleeding diathesis.

It should be recalled from the discussion in Chapter 4 that the normal hemostatic response involves the blood vessel wall, the platelets, and the clotting cascade. The various tests used in the initial evaluation of patients with bleeding disorders are as follows:

■ *Bleeding time.* This represents the time taken for a standardized skin puncture to stop bleeding. Measured in minutes, this procedure provides an in vivo assessment of platelet response to limited vascular injury. The reference range depends on the actual method employed and varies from 2 to 9 minutes. It is abnormal when there is a defect in platelet numbers or function.

■ *Platelet counts.* These are obtained on anticoagulated blood by using an electronic particle counter. The reference range is 150 to 450 × 10³/mm³. Counts outside this range must be confirmed by a visual inspection of a peripheral blood smear.

■ *Prothrombin time (PT).* Measured in seconds, this procedure tests the adequacy of the extrinsic and common coagulation pathways. It represents the time needed for plasma to clot in the presence of an exogenously added source of tissue thromboplastin (e.g., brain extract) and Ca⁺⁺ ions. A prolonged PT may result from a deficiency of factors V, VII, or X; prothrombin; or fibrinogen.

■ *Partial thromboplastin time (PTT).* This test is designed to assess the integrity of the intrinsic and common clotting pathways. In this test, the time (in seconds) needed for the plasma to clot in the presence of kaolin, cephalin, and calcium is measured. Kaolin serves to activate the contact-dependent factor XII, and cephalin substitutes for platelet phospholipids. Prolongation of PTT may occur owing to a deficiency of factors V, VIII, IX, X, XI, or XII; prothrombin; or fibrinogen.

In addition to these, more specialized tests include measurement of the levels of specific clotting factors, fibrinogen, and fibrin split products; determination of the presence of circulating anticoagulants; and platelet function tests. With this overview, we can return to the three important categories of bleeding disorders.

Increased fragility of the vessels is associated with severe vitamin C deficiency (scurvy) (Chapter 8), as well as with a large number of infectious and hypersensitivity vasculitides. These include meningococcemia, infective endocarditis, the rickettsial diseases, typhoid, and Henoch-Schönlein purpura. Some of these conditions are discussed in other chapters; others are beyond the scope of this book. A hemorrhagic diathesis that is purely the result of vascular fragility is characterized by (1) the apparently spontaneous appearance of petechiae and ecchymoses in the skin and mucous membranes (probably owing to minor trauma), (2) a normal platelet count and tests of coagulation (PT, PTT), and (3) a bleeding time that is usually normal.

Deficiencies of platelets (thrombocytopenia) are important causes of hemorrhagic disorders. They may occur in a variety of clinical settings that are discussed later. Here we would like to point out that there are disorders in which platelet function is impaired, despite a normal platelet count. Such qualitative defects are seen in uremia, after aspirin ingestion, in von Willebrand disease, and in a variety of rare inherited disorders. Thrombocytopenia and platelet dysfunction are similar to increased vascular fragility in that petechiae and ecchymoses are present, as well as easy bruising, nosebleeds, excessive bleeding from minor trauma, and menorrhagia. Similarly, PT and PTT are normal, although in contrast to the vascular disorders, the bleeding time is always prolonged.

A bleeding diathesis based purely on a *derangement in the intricate clotting mechanism* differs in several respects from that resulting from defects in the vessel walls or in platelets. PT, PTT, or both, are prolonged, whereas the bleeding time is normal. Petechiae and other evidence of bleeding from very minor surface trauma are usually absent. However, massive hemorrhage may follow operative or dental procedures or severe trauma. Moreover, hemorrhages into areas of the body subject to trauma, such as the joints of the lower extremities, are characteristic. In this category is a group of congenital coagulation disorders.

One of the most complex of the bleeding diatheses, disseminated intravascular coagulation (DIC), discussed below, involves consumption of both platelets and the clotting factors, so it presents laboratory and clinical features of both thrombocytopenia and a coagulation disorder. von Willebrand disease also involves derangements in both modalities.

In this section the following hemorrhagic disorders are discussed: DIC (consumption of fibrinogen and platelets), thrombocytopenia (deficiency of platelets), and coagulation disorders (deficiency in clotting factors).

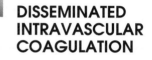

DISSEMINATED INTRAVASCULAR COAGULATION

DIC is an acute, subacute, or chronic thrombohemorrhagic disorder that occurs as a secondary complication in a variety of diseases. *It is characterized by activation of the coagulation sequence, leading to formation of thrombi throughout the microcirculation. As a consequence of the widespread thromboses, there is consumption of platelets and coagulation factors and, secondarily, activation of fibrinolysis.* Thus, DIC may give rise either to tissue hypoxia and microinfarcts caused by myriad microthrombi or to a bleeding disorder related to pathologic activation of fibrinolysis and depletion of the elements required for hemostasis (hence the term *consumption coagulopathy*), or to both derangements. This entity is probably a more important cause of bleeding than all of the congenital coagulation disorders, which will be discussed later.

Etiology and Pathogenesis. Before presenting the specific disorders associated with DIC, we will discuss in a general way the pathogenetic mechanisms by which intravascular clotting can occur. Reference to earlier comments on normal blood coagulation (Chapter 4) may be helpful at this point. It suffices here to recall that clotting may be initiated by either of two pathways: the extrinsic pathway, which is triggered by the release of tissue factor (tissue thromboplastin), or the intrinsic pathway, which involves the activation within the blood of factor XII by surface contact, collagen, or other negatively charged substances. Both pathways lead to the generation of thrombin. Clot-inhibiting influences include the rapid clearance of activated clotting factors by the mononuclear phagocytic system or by the liver, activation of endogenous anticoagulants (e.g., protein C), and activation of fibrinolysis.

Two major mechanisms may trigger DIC: (1) release of tissue factor or thromboplastic substances into the circulation and (2) widespread injury to endothelial cells (Fig. 12–29).

The tissue thromboplastic substances released into the circulation may be derived from a variety of sources—for example from the placenta in obstetric complications, from the cytoplasmic granules in the leukemic cells of acute promyelocytic leukemia, or from neoplastic cells in mucin-secreting adenocarcinomas. Carcinomas may also release other thromboplastic substances, such as proteolytic enzymes, mucin, and other undefined tumor products. In gram-negative sepsis (an important cause of DIC), endotoxins cause increased synthesis, membrane exposure, and release of tissue factor from monocytes. Furthermore, activated monocytes release IL-1 and TNF-α, both of which increase the expression of tissue factor on endothelial cell membranes and simultaneously decrease the expression of thrombomodulin. The latter, you may recall, activates protein C, an anticoagulant (Chapter 4). The result is both activation of the extrinsic clotting system and inhibition of coagulation control.

Endothelial cell injury can initiate DIC by causing release of tissue factor and by promoting platelet aggregation and activation of the intrinsic coagulation cascade as a result of the exposure of subendothelial collagen. Even subtle damage to the endothelium can unleash procoagulant activity by enhancing membrane expression of tissue factor. Widespread endothelial injury may be produced by deposition of antigen-antibody complexes (e.g., in SLE), temperature extremes (e.g., in heat stroke or burns), or by microorganisms (e.g., meningococci and rickettsiae). As discussed in Chapter 4, endothelial injury is an important consequence of endotoxemia, and not surprisingly, DIC is a frequent complication of gram-negative sepsis.

Several additional disorders associated with DIC are listed

Table 12–15.   MAJOR DISORDERS ASSOCIATED WITH DIC

Obstetric Complications
Abruptio placentae
Retained dead fetus
Septic abortion
Amniotic fluid embolism
Toxemia
Infections
Gram-negative sepsis
Meningococcemia
Rocky Mountain spotted fever
Histoplasmosis
Aspergillosis
Malaria
Neoplasms
Carcinomas of pancreas, prostate, lung, and stomach
Acute promyelocytic leukemia
Massive Tissue Injury
Traumatic
Burns
Extensive surgery
Miscellaneous
Acute intravascular hemolysis, snakebite, giant hemangioma, shock, heat stroke, vasculitis, aortic aneurysm, liver disease

DIC, disseminated intravascular coagulation.

in Table 12–15. Of these, *DIC is most likely to follow sepsis, obstetric complications, malignancy, and major trauma.* The initiating factors in these conditions are multiple and often interrelated. For example, in obstetric conditions, tissue factor derived from the placenta, retained dead fetus, or amniotic fluid may enter the circulation; however, shock, hypoxia, and

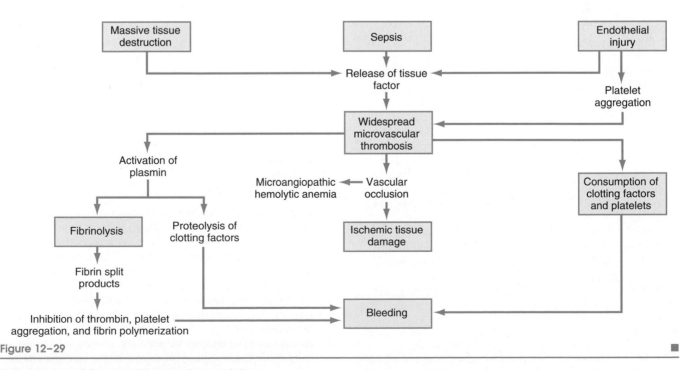

Figure 12–29

Pathophysiology of disseminated intravascular coagulation.

acidosis often coexist and may cause widespread endothelial injury. Supervening infections may complicate the problem further.

Whatever the pathogenetic mechanism, DIC has two consequences. First, *there is widespread fibrin deposition within the microcirculation.* This leads to ischemia in the more severely affected or more vulnerable organs and to hemolysis as the RBCs are traumatized while passing through the fibrin strands *(microangiopathic hemolytic anemia).* Second, a *bleeding diathesis* ensues as the platelets and clotting factors are consumed and there is secondary release of plasminogen activators. Plasmin not only can cleave fibrin (fibrinolysis), it can also digest factors V and VIII, thereby reducing their concentration further. In addition, fibrinolysis leads to the formation of fibrin degradation products, which have an inhibitory effect on platelet aggregation, have antithrombin activity, and impair fibrin polymerization, all of which contribute to the hemostatic failure (Fig. 12–29).

MORPHOLOGY. The anatomic changes of DIC are related, on the one hand, to widespread fibrin deposition and, on the other, to hemorrhage.

The **microthrombi** are found principally in the arterioles and capillaries of the kidneys, adrenals, brain, and heart, but no organ is spared, and the lungs, liver, and gastrointestinal mucosa may also be prominently involved. The glomeruli contain small fibrin thrombi, which may evoke only a reactive swelling of the endothelial cells or may be surrounded by a florid focal glomerulitis. The resultant ischemia leads to microinfarcts in the renal cortex. In severe cases the ischemia may even extend to destroy the entire cortex and cause bilateral renal cortical necrosis. Involvement of the adrenal glands reproduces the picture of the **Waterhouse-Friderichsen syndrome** (Chapter 20). Microinfarcts are also commonly encountered in the brain, surrounded by microscopic or gross foci of hemorrhage. These may give rise to bizarre neurologic signs. Similar changes are seen in the heart and often in the anterior pituitary. It has been suggested that DIC may contribute to **Sheehan's postpartum pituitary necrosis** (Chapter 20).

When the underlying disorder is toxemia of pregnancy, the placenta is the site of capillary thromboses and, occasionally, florid degeneration of the vessel walls. Such changes are in all likelihood responsible for the premature loss of cytotrophoblasts and syncytiotrophoblasts that characterizes this condition.

The bleeding tendency associated with DIC is manifested not only by larger than expected hemorrhages near foci of infarction, but also by diffuse petechiae and ecchymoses, which may be found on the skin, serosal linings of the body cavities, epicardium, endocardium, lungs, and mucosal lining of the urinary tract.

Clinical Course. The clinical picture is an apparent paradox, with a bleeding tendency in the face of evidence of widespread coagulation. It is almost impossible to detail all the potential clinical manifestations. In general, *acute DIC (e.g., that associated with obstetric complications) is dominated by a bleeding diathesis, whereas chronic DIC (such as may occur in a patient with cancer) tends to present with thrombotic complications.* Typically, the abnormal clotting occurs only in the microcirculation, although large vessels are involved occasionally. The manifestations may be minimal, or there may be shock, with acute renal failure, dyspnea, cyanosis, convulsions, and coma. Hypotension is characteristic. Most often, attention is called to the presence of a bleeding diathesis by prolonged and copious postpartum bleeding or by the presence of petechiae and ecchymoses on the skin. These may be the only manifestations, or there may be severe hemorrhage into the gut or urinary tract. Laboratory evaluation reveals *thrombocytopenia and prolongation of PT and PTT* (owing to consumption of platelets, clotting factors, and fibrinogen). *Fibrin split products* are increased in the plasma.

The prognosis for patients with DIC is highly variable and depends on the underlying disorder as well as on the degree of intravascular clotting, the activity of the mononuclear phagocyte system, and the amount of fibrinolysis. In some cases it can be life threatening; in others it can be treated with anticoagulants such as heparin or coagulants contained in fresh-frozen plasma. The underlying disorder must be treated simultaneously to prevent the progressive derangement of hemostasis.

THROMBOCYTOPENIA

Thrombocytopenia is characterized by spontaneous bleeding, a prolonged bleeding time, and normal PT and PTT. A platelet count of 100,000 per microliter or less is generally considered to constitute thrombocytopenia, although spontaneous bleeding does not become evident until the count falls below 20,000 per microliter. Platelet counts in the range of 20,000 to 50,000 may lead to post-traumatic bleeding. Thrombocytopenia is associated with bleeding from small blood vessels. Petechiae or sometimes large ecchymoses are commonly found in the skin and mucous membranes of the gastrointestinal and urinary tracts, but no site is immune. Bleeding into the central nervous system constitutes a major hazard in patients whose platelet count is markedly depressed. The etiologic groups of thrombocytopenia are listed in Table 12–16. Of these, reduced production and increased destruction are the most important categories.

■ A decrease in the production of platelets is associated with various forms of marrow failure or injury; these include idiopathic aplastic anemias, drug-induced marrow failure, and marrow infiltration by tumors. Thrombocytopenia is also an important hazard after bone marrow transplantation. Platelet recovery occurs much more slowly than recovery of other lineages. In all of these settings, the cytopenia is associated with a decrease in marrow megakaryocytes.

■ Accelerated destruction of platelets is often immunologically mediated, resulting from formation of antiplatelet antibodies or adsorption of immune complexes formed in the

Table 12-16.   CAUSES OF THROMBOCYTOPENIA

I. Decreased production of platelets
 Generalized disease of bone marrow
  Aplastic anemia: congenital and acquired
  Marrow infiltration: leukemia, disseminated cancer
 Selective impairment of platelet production
  Drug-induced: alcohol, thiazides, cytotoxic drugs
  Infections: measles, HIV
 Ineffective megakaryopoiesis
  Megaloblastic anemia
  Paroxysmal nocturnal hemoglobinuria

II. Decreased Platelet Survival
 Immunologic destruction
  Autoimmune: idiopathic thrombocytopenic purpura, SLE
  Isoimmune: post-transfusion and neonatal
  Drug-associated: quinidine, heparin, sulfa compounds
  Infections: infectious mononucleosis, HIV infection, CMV
 Nonimmunologic destruction
  Disseminated intravascular coagulation
  Thrombotic thrombocytopenic purpura
  Giant hemangiomas
  Microangiopathic hemolytic anemias

III. Sequestration
 Hypersplenism
IV. Dilutional

SLE, systemic lupus erythematosus; HIV, human immunodeficiency virus; CMV, cytomegalovirus.

circulation. Antibody-mediated destruction of platelets may be associated with well-known autoimmune diseases such as SLE, or it may appear as an apparently isolated derangement (idiopathic thrombocytopenic purpura). Some of the drug-induced thrombocytopenias are also suspected to be immunologically mediated.

■ Excessive destruction of platelets is mediated in some cases by nonimmunologic means. As mentioned earlier, excessive utilization of platelets occurs in DIC. Other nonimmunologic causes include prosthetic heart valves and the rare disorder called thrombotic thrombocytopenic purpura, described later. Whatever the cause of accelerated destruction, the bone marrow reveals a normal or a compensatory increase in megakaryocytes. Hence, bone marrow examination allows a ready distinction between the two major categories of thrombocytopenia.

Thrombocytopenia is one of the most common hematologic manifestations of AIDS. It may occur early in the course of HIV infection and is believed to result from immune complex–mediated injury of platelets and HIV-mediated suppression of megakaryocytes.

Idiopathic Thrombocytopenic Purpura

A disorder of autoimmune origin, idiopathic thrombocytopenic purpura (ITP) most often occurs as an apparently isolated derangement but sometimes as a first manifestation of SLE. Although an acute, self-limited form that follows viral infections has been described in children, most patients are adult females between the ages of 20 and 40 years.

Antiplatelet immunoglobulins directed against platelet membrane glycoproteins IIb/IIIa complex or Ib have been identified in most patients with ITP. In some patients such autoantibodies may bind to megakaryocytes and impair platelet production as well. In most cases megakaryocyte injury is not significant enough to deplete their numbers. The spleen plays an important role in the pathogenesis of this disorder. It is the major site of production of the antiplatelet antibodies and destruction of the IgG-coated platelets. *In more than two thirds of patients, splenectomy is followed by the return of normal platelet counts and complete remission of the disease.* The spleen usually appears remarkably normal, with only minimal, if any, enlargement. The presence of splenomegaly or lymphadenopathy should lead one to consider other possible diagnoses. Histologically, the marrow may appear normal but usually reveals increased numbers of megakaryocytes, some of which have only a single nucleus and are thought to be young. A similar marrow picture is noted in most forms of thrombocytopenia that result from accelerated platelet destruction. The importance of marrow examination is to rule out thrombocytopenia resulting from marrow failure.

The onset of ITP is usually insidious. The patients manifest petechiae, easy bruisability, epistaxis, gum bleeding, and hemorrhages after minor trauma. More serious intracerebral or subarachnoid hemorrhages are much less common, especially in patients treated with steroids. The diagnosis is based on clinical features, the presence of thrombocytopenia, marrow examination, and exclusion of secondary causes of thrombocytopenia. Tests for specific antiplatelet antibodies are not widely available.

Thrombotic Microangiopathies: Thrombotic Thrombocytopenic Purpura and Hemolytic-Uremic Syndrome

The term *thrombotic microangiopathies* encompasses a spectrum of clinical syndromes that includes thrombotic thrombocytopenic purpura (TTP) and hemolytic uremic syndrome (HUS). Traditionally, *TTP has been characterized by its occurrence in adult females and the pentad of fever, thrombocytopenia, microangiopathic hemolytic anemia, transient neurologic deficits, and renal failure.* HUS, like TTP, is also associated with microangiopathic hemolytic anemia and thrombocytopenia but is distinguished from it by the absence of neurologic symptoms, the dominance of acute renal failure, and onset in childhood (Chapter 14). Recent studies have blurred these distinctions, because many adults with TTP lack one or more of the five criteria, and some patients with HUS have fever and neurologic dysfunction. *Fundamental to both of these conditions is widespread formation of hyaline thrombi in the microcirculation that are composed primarily of dense aggregates of platelets that are surrounded by fibrin.* The development of myriads of platelet aggregates causes thrombocytopenia, and the narrowing of blood vessels by the thrombi results in microangiopathic hemolytic anemia.

Although these disorders may have diverse causes, endothelial injury and activation of intravascular thrombosis seem to be the initiating mechanisms. The trigger for endothelial injury in HUS is a toxin released by certain strains of *E. coli.* Thus, HUS most commonly follows gastroenteritis caused by *E. coli* 0157:H7. The affected children present with bloody diarrhea, and a few days later HUS makes its appearance. TTP shares several clinical features with HUS, but unlike the latter, there is no evidence of previous bacterial infection, and hence the cause of endothelial injury remains obscure. It should be noted that while DIC and the thrombotic microangiopathies share features such as microvascular occlusions and microangiopathic hemolytic anemias, they are pathogenetically distinct. In TTP and HUS, unlike in DIC, activation of the coagulation cascade is not of primary importance, and hence results of laboratory tests of coagulation, such as PT and PTT, are usually normal.

COAGULATION DISORDERS

These disorders result from either congenital or acquired deficiencies of clotting factors. The latter, which are much more common and relatively straightforward, are considered first.

Acquired coagulation disorders are usually associated with deficiencies of multiple clotting factors. As discussed in Chapter 8, *vitamin K deficiency* may be associated with a severe coagulation defect, because this nutrient is essential for the synthesis of prothrombin and clotting factors VII, IX, and X. The liver is the site of synthesis of several coagulation factors; thus, *parenchymal diseases of the liver* are among the most common causes of hemorrhagic diatheses. In addition, several liver diseases are associated with complex derangements of platelet function and fibrinogen metabolism, all of which contribute to the coagulopathy in liver disease.

Hereditary deficiencies have been identified for each of the coagulation factors. These deficiencies characteristically occur singly. Hemophilia A, resulting from deficiency of factor VIII, and hemophilia B (Christmas disease), resulting from deficiency of factor IX, are transmitted as X-linked recessive disorders, whereas most others are autosomal disorders. Most of these conditions are rare; only von Willebrand disease, hemophilia A, and hemophilia B are sufficiently common to warrant further consideration.

Deficiencies of Factor VIII–von Willebrand Factor Complex

Hemophilia A and von Willebrand disease, two of the most common inherited disorders of bleeding, are caused by qualitative or quantitative defects involving factor VIII–von Willebrand factor (vWF) complex. Before we can discuss these disorders, it is essential to review the structure and function of these proteins.

Plasma factor VIII–vWF is a complex made up of two separate proteins that can be distinguished by functional, biochemical, and immunologic criteria. One component, which is required for the activation of factor X in the intrinsic co-

agulation pathway, is called *factor VIII procoagulant protein,* or *factor VIII* (Fig. 12–30). Deficiency of factor VIII gives rise to hemophilia. Through noncovalent bonds, factor VIII is linked to a much larger protein, von Willebrand factor. The latter, which forms approximately 99% of the factor VIII–vWF complex, is not a discrete protein but exists in the form of a series of high-molecular-weight multimers. vWF can bind to collagen as well as to platelet membrane glycoproteins Ib and IIb/IIIa and therefore can "glue" these structures together (Fig. 12–30). Indeed, *the most important function of vWF in vivo is to facilitate the adhesion of platelets to subendothelial collagen.* Thus, vWF is crucial to the normal process of hemostasis, and its absence in von Willebrand disease leads to a bleeding diathesis. In addition to its function in platelet adhesion, vWF also serves as a carrier for factor VIII. When factor VIII is activated by thrombin, it dissociates from vWF

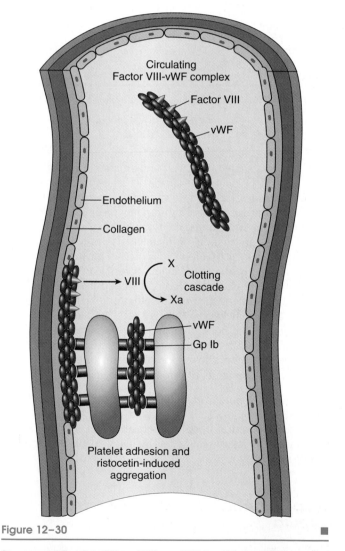

Figure 12–30 ■

Structure and function of factor VIII–von Willebrand factor (vWF) complex. Factor VIII is synthesized by the liver and vWF in the endothelial cells. The two circulate as a complex in the circulation. Factor VIII takes part in the coagulation cascade by activating factor X. vWF causes adhesion of platelets to subendothelial collagen, primarily via Gp Ib platelet receptor. Ristocetin activates Gp Ib receptors in vitro and causes platelet aggregation if vWF is present.

and serves its coagulant function. vWF can be assayed by immunologic techniques or by the so-called ristocetin aggregation test. Ristocetin (once used as an antibiotic) binds to platelets in vitro and activates vWF receptors on their surface. This leads to platelet aggregation if vWF is available to "bridge" the platelets (Fig. 12–30). Thus, ristocetin-induced platelet aggregation can be used as a bioassay for vWF.

The two components of the factor VIII–vWF complex are coded by separate genes and are synthesized by different cells. Although vWF is produced by both endothelial cells and megakaryocytes, the former cells are the major source of plasma vWF. Factor VIII can be synthesized by several tissues, but liver is the major source of this protein. *To summarize, the two components of factor VIII–vWF complex, synthesized separately, come together and circulate in the plasma as a unit that serves to promote clotting as well as the platelet–vessel wall interactions necessary to ensure hemostasis.* With this background we can turn to the discussion of diseases resulting from deficiencies of factor VIII–vWF complex.

VON WILLEBRAND DISEASE

Von Willebrand disease is characterized clinically by spontaneous bleeding from mucous membranes, excessive bleeding from wounds, menorrhagia, and a prolonged bleeding time in the presence of a normal platelet count. In most cases it is transmitted as an autosomal dominant disorder, but several rare autosomal recessive variants have been identified. Its precise incidence is difficult to estimate, because in many instances the clinical manifestations are mild and the diagnosis requires sophisticated tests; it may well be the most common inherited bleeding disorder.

Without delving into great complexities, we can state that the classic and most common variant (type I) of von Willebrand disease is characterized by a reduced quantity of circulating vWF. Because vWF stabilizes factor VIII by binding to it, a deficiency of vWF is associated with a secondary decrease in the levels of factor VIII. The less common form of von Willebrand disease, type II, is characterized by a selective loss of intermediate- and high-molecular-weight multimers of vWF. Because these multimers are the most active form of vWF, there is a functional deficiency. To summarize, patients with von Willebrand disease have a compound defect involving platelet function and the coagulation pathway. However, except in those most severely affected (e.g., homozygous patients), the effects of factor VIII deficiency that characterize hemophilia, such as bleeding into the joints, are uncommon.

FACTOR VIII DEFICIENCY (HEMOPHILIA A, CLASSIC HEMOPHILIA)

Hemophilia A is the most common hereditary disease associated with serious bleeding. It is caused by a reduced amount or reduced activity of factor VIII. As an X-linked recessive trait, it occurs in males or in homozygous females. However, excessive bleeding has been described in heterozygous females, presumably owing to extremely unfavorable lyonization (inactivation of the normal X chromosome in most of the cells). *Approximately 30% of cases are due to new mutations and hence do not have a family history.* Overt clinical symptoms develop only in the presence of severe deficiency (less than 1% factor VIII activity). Mild (1% to 5% activity) or moderate (5% to 75% activity) degrees of deficiency are usually asymptomatic, although post-traumatic bleeding may be somewhat excessive. The variable degrees of deficiency in the level of factor VIII procoagulant are related to the type of mutation in the factor VIII gene. As with thalassemia, several genetic lesions (e.g., deletions, splice junction mutations, nonsense mutations) have been identified. To add to the complexities, in about 10% of patients levels of factor VIII appear normal by immunoassay, but the coagulant activity detected by bioassay is low. In these patients a mutation causes the synthesis of an antigenically normal but functionally abnormal protein. Approximately 15% of the most severely affected patients have antibodies against factor VIII.

In all symptomatic cases there is a tendency toward easy bruising and massive hemorrhage after trauma or operative procedures. In addition, "spontaneous" hemorrhages are frequently encountered in regions of the body normally subject to trauma, particularly the joints, where they are known as *hemarthroses*. Recurrent bleeding into the joints leads to progressive deformities that may be crippling. *Petechiae are characteristically absent.* Typically, patients with hemophilia A have a normal bleeding time, normal platelet counts, and a normal prothrombin time, with a prolonged PTT that is corrected by mixing with normal plasma. If antibody against factor VIII is present in the patient's plasma, then mixing fails to correct the PTT. Factor VIII assays are required for diagnosis.

Treatment of hemophilia A involves infusion of factor VIII derived from human plasma. Replacement therapy, however, is not an unalloyed blessing. It carries with it the risk of transmission of viral diseases. As discussed in Chapter 5, before 1985 thousands of hemophiliacs received factor VIII preparations contaminated with HIV. Subsequently many became seropositive and developed AIDS. However, with current blood banking practices, the risk of HIV transmission has been virtually eliminated, but the threat of other undetected infections remains. Ultimately, the only safe factor VIII will be one derived from a cloned human gene. Clinical trials with recombinant factor VIII are in progress.

Factor IX Deficiency (Hemophilia B, Christmas Disease)

Severe factor IX deficiency is a disorder that is clinically indistinguishable from hemophilia A. Moreover, it is also inherited as an X-linked recessive trait and may occur asymptomatically or with associated hemorrhage. It is much less common than hemophilia A. The PTT is prolonged; bleeding time is normal. Identification of Christmas disease (named after the first patient with this condition, not the holy day) is possible only by assay of the factor levels.

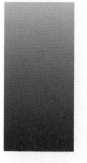

Disorders That Affect the Spleen and Thymus

Splenomegaly

The spleen is frequently involved in a wide variety of systemic diseases. In virtually all cases the splenic changes are secondary to disease that is primary elsewhere, and in almost all instances the presentation of the splenic lesion is enlargement. Excessive destruction by the spleen of red cells, leukocytes, and platelets may ensue. Evaluation of splenomegaly is a common clinical problem that is aided considerably by knowledge of the usual limits of splenic enlargement caused by the disorders being considered. Obviously, it would be erroneous to attribute enlargement of the spleen into the pelvis to vitamin B_{12} deficiency and equally erroneous to accept as classic a case of chronic myeloid leukemia unless there is significant splenomegaly. As an aid to diagnosis, then, we present the following list of disorders, classified according to the degree of splenomegaly characteristically produced:

A. Massive splenomegaly (weight more than 1000 gm)
　1. Chronic myeloproliferative disorders (chronic myeloid leukemia, myeloid metaplasia with myelofibrosis)
　2. Chronic lymphocytic leukemia (less massive)
　3. Hairy cell leukemia
　4. Lymphomas
　5. Malaria
　6. Gaucher disease
　7. Primary tumors of the spleen (rare)
B. Moderate splenomegaly (weight 500 to 1000 gm)
　1. Chronic congestive splenomegaly (portal hypertension or splenic vein obstruction)
　2. Acute leukemias (inconstant)
　3. Hereditary spherocytosis
　4. Thalassemia major
　5. Autoimmune hemolytic anemia
　6. Amyloidosis
　7. Niemann-Pick disease
　8. Langerhans' histiocytosis
　9. Chronic splenitis (especially with infective endocarditis)
　10. Tuberculosis, sarcoidosis, typhoid
　11. Metastatic carcinoma or sarcoma
C. Mild splenomegaly (weight less than 500 gm)
　1. Acute splenitis
　2. Acute splenic congestion

3. Infectious mononucleosis
4. Miscellaneous acute febrile disorders, including septicemia, systemic lupus erythematosus, and intra-abdominal infections

The microscopic changes associated with most of the previously mentioned diseases need not be described here, because they have been discussed in the relevant sections of this and other chapters.

An enlarged spleen may remove excessive amounts of one or more of the formed elements of blood, resulting in anemia, leukopenia, or thrombocytopenia. This is referred to as *hypersplenism* and may be associated with many of the diseases of the spleen listed previously. In some cases, however, hypersplenism is associated with an apparently normal spleen, without any known cause for splenic hyperfunction. These cases are labeled *primary hypersplenism.*

Disorders of the Thymus

As is well known, the thymus is a central lymphoid organ that plays a critical role in T-cell differentiation. It is not surprising, therefore, that the thymus can be involved in lymphomas, particularly those of T-cell lineage. These were discussed earlier in this chapter. Here we will focus on the two most frequent (albeit uncommon) disorders of the thymus: thymic hyperplasias and thymomas.

HYPERPLASIA

The normal thymus is devoid of lymphoid follicles. *Hyperplasia of the thymus is characterized by the appearance of lymphoid follicles within the medulla.* Immunochemical staining techniques reveal that the follicles are rich in immunoglobulins. Thymic hyperplasia is present in most patients with myasthenia gravis and is also present in various other autoimmune diseases such as SLE and rheumatoid arthritis. The relationship between the thymus and myasthenia gravis is discussed in Chapter 21; for now, it suffices that T cells generated in the thymus and sensitized to its myoid cells cooperate with B cells in the lymphoid follicles to produce the autoantibodies that underlie the autoimmune reaction to acetylcholine receptors at the neuromuscular junction, a characteristic of this grave neuromuscular disorder. Significantly, removal of a hyperplastic thymus is beneficial early in the disease.

THYMOMA

Although the normal thymus is a lymphoepithelial organ, the term *thymoma* is restricted to tumors in which epithelial cells constitute the neoplastic element. Scant or abundant thymic lymphocytes may also be present in these tumors, but they are normal, non-neoplastic thymocytes. Lymphomas arising in the lymphoid elements of the thymus gland are therefore not classified as thymomas. Numerous subtypes of thymoma have been established, based on cytologic and biologic criteria. A commonly used classification is as follows:

- Benign thymoma: cytologically and biologically benign
- Malignant thymoma
  - Type I: cytologically benign but biologically aggressive and capable of local invasion and, rarely, distant spread
  - Type II, also called *thymic carcinoma*: cytologically malignant with all of the features of cancer and comparable behavior

MORPHOLOGY. Macroscopically, thymomas are lobulated, firm, gray-white masses up to 15 to 20 cm in longest dimension. Most appear encapsulated, but in about 20% to 25% there is apparent penetration of the capsule and infiltration of perithymic tissues and structures.

Microscopically, virtually all thymomas are made up of a mixture of epithelial cells and a variable infiltrate of non-neoplastic lymphocytes. The relative proportions of the epithelial and lymphocytic components are of little significance. In **benign thymomas,** the epithelial cells tend to resemble those of the medulla and are often elongated or spindle shaped, producing what is called a **medullary thymoma.** Frequently there is an admixture of the plumper, rounder, cortical-type epithelial cells, and some are composed largely of such cells. This pattern of thymoma often has few lymphocytes. Some experts would call this pattern a **mixed thymoma.** The medullary and mixed patterns account for 60% to 70% of all thymomas.

The designation **malignant thymoma type I** implies a cytologically benign tumor that is locally invasive and sometimes has the capacity for widespread metastasis. These tumors account for about 20% to 25% of all thymomas. They are composed of varying proportions of epithelial cells and lymphocytes; the epithelial cells, however, tend to be of the cortical variety, with abundant cytoplasm and rounded vesicular nuclei. Palisading of these cells about blood vessels is sometimes seen. Some spindled epithelial cells may be present as well. **The critical distinguishing feature of these neoplasms is penetration of the capsule with invasion into surrounding structures.**

Malignant thymoma type II is better designated **thymic carcinoma.** These represent about 5% of thymomas. In contrast to the type I malignant thymomas, these are cytologically malignant. Macroscopically, they are usually fleshy, obviously invasive masses sometimes accompanied by metastases to such sites as the lungs. Most are **squamous cell carcinomas, either well or poorly differentiated.** The next most common malignant pattern is the so-called **lymphoepithelioma,** composed of cytologically anaplastic cortical-type epithelial cells scattered against a dense background of benign-appearing lymphocytes. Some of these tumors contain the EBV genome and hence resemble nasopharyngeal carcinomas.

Clinical Features. All thymomas are rarities, the malignant more so than the benign. They may arise at any age but typically occur in middle adult life. In a large series, about 30% were asymptomatic; 30% to 40% produced local manifestations such as a computed tomography–demonstrable mass in the anterosuperior mediastinum associated with cough, dyspnea, and superior vena caval syndrome; and the remainder were associated with some systemic disease, principally myasthenia gravis. Some 15% to 20% of patients with this disorder have a thymoma. Removal of the tumor often leads to improvement in the neuromuscular disorder. Additional associations with thymomas include hypogammaglobulinemia, SLE, pure red cell aplasia, and nonthymic cancers.

BIBLIOGRAPHY

Aisenberg AC: Coherent view of non-Hodgkin's lymphoma. J Clin Oncol 13:2656, 1995. (The title accurately reflects this excellent review, which provides a practical yet scientific view of the pathology of non-Hodgkin's lymphomas.)

Boyce TG, et al: *Escherichia coli* 0157:H7 and the hemolytic-uremic syndrome. N Engl J Med 333:364, 1995. (A very good article on the etiology and pathogenesis of the hemolytic-uremic syndrome.)

Conrad ME, Umbreit JN: A concise review: iron absorption—the mucin-mobilferrin-integrin pathway. A competitive pathway for metal absorption. Am J Hematol 42(1):67, 1993. (A good discussion of the proteins involved in the absorption of iron from the gut.)

Delabie J, et al: Hodgkin's disease: a monoclonal lymphoproliferative disorder? Histopathology 27:93, 1995. (An excellent short review of the etiology and pathogenesis of Hodgkin's disease.)

Devine SM, Larson RA: Acute leukemia in adults: recent developments in diagnosis and treatment. CA Cancer J Clin 44:326, 1994. (A well-written review of acute ALL and AML in adults.)

Dimopoulos MA, Alexanian R: Waldenström's macroglobulinemia. Blood 83:1452, 1994. (Excellent review of the clinical features of Waldenström's macroglobulinemia.)

Foon KA: Chronic lymphoid leukemias: recent advances in biology and therapy. Stem Cells 13:1, 1995. (A concise review of chronic lymphoproliferative disorders, including CLL, hairy cell leukemia, and T-cell leukemia.)

Haluska FG, et al: The cellular biology of the Reed-Sternberg cell. Blood 84:1005, 1994. (A scholarly and detailed discussion of the pathogenesis of Hodgkin's disease.)

Hoyer LW: Hemophilia A. N Engl J Med 330:38, 1994. (A very good basic and clinical review of hemophilia A.)

Klein B, et al: Interleukin-6 in human multiple myeloma. Blood 85:863, 1995. (An article summarizing the recent developments in the pathogenesis of multiple myeloma.)

Krantz SB: Pathogenesis and treatment of the anemia of chronic disease. Am J Med Sci 307:353, 1994. (A discussion of the multiple factors that underlie anemia of chronic disease.)

Lyons SE, Ginsburg D: Molecular and cellular biology of von Willebrand factor. Trends Cardiovasc Med 4:34, 1994. (A short article describing the structure, synthesis, and function of vWF, as well as the diseases resulting from its lack.)

Pui Ching-Hon: Childhood leukemias. N Engl J Med 332:1618, 1995. (An up-to-date account of the clinical, phenotypic, and karyotypic features of acute leukemias in children.)

Segal GH, et al: CD5-expressing B-cell non-Hodgkin's lymphomas with bcl-1 gene rearrangement have a relatively homogeneous immunophenotype and are associated with an overall poor prognosis. Blood 85:1570, 1995. (A paper describing the utility of phenotypic and molecular markers in the clinical management of one form of NHL.)

Schechter AN, Rodgers GP: Sickle cell anemia—basic research reaches the clinic. N Engl J Med 332:1372, 1995. (An editorial summarizing recent advances in the treatment of sickle cell anemia by hydroxyurea.)

Schwartz RS: *PIG-A*—the target gene in paroxysmal nocturnal hemoglobinuria. N Engl J Med 330:283, 1994. (An editorial explaining the molecular basis of hemolysis and other abnormalities in paroxysmal nocturnal hemoglobinuria and the implications for other more common disorders of stem cells, such as aplastic anemia and acute leukemias.)

Willman CL, et al: Langerhans'-cell histiocytosis (histiocytosis X)—a clonal proliferative disease. N Engl J Med 331:154, 1994. (A paper documenting the clonal nature of Langerhans' histiocytosis, thus settling the nature of these disorders.)

Young NS: Agranulocytosis. JAMA 271:935, 1994. (A practical approach to the etiology and management of agranulocytosis.)

Young NS, Barrett AJ: The treatment of severe acquired aplastic anemia. Blood 85:3367, 1995. (A balanced perspective on the causes and management of aplastic anemias.)

13

Lungs and the Upper Respiratory Tract

Thanks are due to Dr. Mary F. Lipscomb for the use of material from her chapter "The Respiratory System" in the fifth edition of this book.

The major function of the lung is to excrete carbon dioxide from blood and replenish oxygen. The chest wall and diaphragm act as bellows to move air in and out of the lungs, allowing gas exchange across the alveolocapillary membrane. Obviously, opportunities for disease in this important organ system are legion. A common approach in the study of lung pathology, and one that provides the framework for this chapter, is to organize lung diseases into those affecting (1) the airways, (2) the interstitium, and (3) the pulmonary vascular system. This division into discrete compartments is, of course, deceptively neat. In reality, disease in one compartment is generally accompanied by alterations of morphology and function in another.

The respiratory system includes, in addition to the lungs, (1) the diaphragm and muscles of the chest wall, (2) the regulatory neural circuits, (3) the pleural spaces, and (4) the upper respiratory tract (the nasopharynx and trachea, including the larynx). Diseases affecting the first two will not be discussed, but those affecting the pleura and upper respiratory tract will be considered after a discussion of the diseases of lung. We begin our discussion with atelectasis, because it can complicate many primary lung disorders.

ATELECTASIS (COLLAPSE)

Atelectasis, also known as collapse, is loss of lung volume due to inadequate *expansion of airspaces*. It is associated with shunting of inadequately oxygenated blood from pulmonary arteries into veins, thus giving rise to a ventilation-perfusion imbalance and hypoxia. On the basis of the underlying mechanism or the distribution of alveolar collapse, atelectasis is divided into the following categories (Fig. 13–1).

Resorption Atelectasis. Resorption atelectasis occurs when an obstruction prevents air from reaching distal airways. The air already present gradually becomes absorbed, and alveolar collapse follows. Depending on the level of airway obstruction, an entire lung, a complete lobe, or one or more segments may be involved. The most frequent cause of resorption collapse is obstruction of a bronchus by a mucous or mucopurulent plug. This frequently occurs postoperatively but may also complicate bronchial asthma, bronchiectasis, or chronic bronchitis. Sometimes obstruction is caused by the aspiration of foreign bodies, particularly in children, or blood clots during oral surgery or anesthesia. Airways may also be obstructed by tumors (especially bronchogenic carcinoma), by enlarged lymph nodes (as from tuberculosis), and (rarely) by vascular aneurysms.

Compression Atelectasis. Compression atelectasis (sometimes called *passive* or *relaxation atelectasis*) is usually associated with accumulations of fluid, blood, or air within the pleural cavity, which mechanically collapse the adjacent lung. This is a frequent occurrence with pleural effusions, caused most commonly by congestive heart failure. Leakage of air into the pleural cavity (pneumothorax) also leads to compression atelectasis. Basal atelectasis resulting from the elevated position of the diaphragm commonly occurs in bedridden patients, in patients with ascites, and in surgical patients during and after the operation.

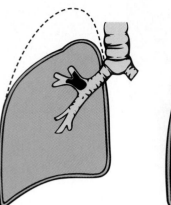
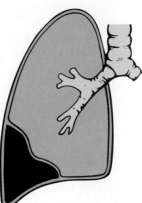

Resorption   Compression

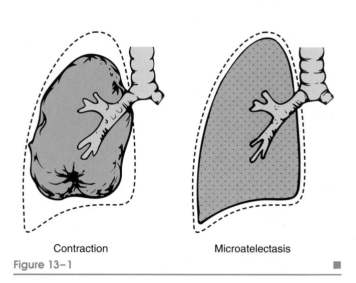

Contraction   Microatelectasis

Figure 13–1 ■

Various forms of atelectasis in adults.

Microatelectasis. Microatelectasis (or nonobstructive atelectasis) is a generalized loss of lung expansion due to a complex set of events, the most important of which is loss of surfactant. Microatelectasis is present in both adult and neonatal respiratory distress syndromes and in several lung diseases associated with interstitial inflammation. It is also believed to contribute to postsurgical atelectasis.

Contraction Atelectasis. Contraction (or cicatrization) atelectasis occurs when either local or generalized fibrotic changes in the lung or pleura hamper expansion and increase elastic recoil during expiration.

Atelectasis (except that caused by contraction) is potentially reversible and should be treated promptly to prevent hypoxemia and superimposed infection of the collapsed lung.

OBSTRUCTIVE AND RESTRICTIVE LUNG DISEASES

Diffuse pulmonary diseases can be classified in two categories: (1) obstructive disease (airway disease), characterized by limitation of airflow usually resulting from an increase in resistance due to partial or complete obstruction at any level; and (2) restrictive disease, characterized by reduced expansion of lung parenchyma accompanied by decreased total lung capacity.

The *major obstructive disorders* (excluding tumors or inhalation of a foreign body) are *asthma, emphysema, chronic bronchitis, bronchiectasis, cystic fibrosis,* and *bronchiolitis.* In patients with these diseases, total lung capacity and forced vital capacity (FVC) are either normal or increased, but the hallmark is a decreased expiratory flow rate, usually measured by forced expiratory volume at 1 second (FEV_1). Thus, *the ratio of FEV_1 and FVC is characteristically decreased.* Expiratory obstruction may result either from anatomic airway narrowing, classically observed in asthma, or from loss of elastic recoil, characteristic of emphysema.

In contrast, in *restrictive diseases,* FVC is reduced and the expiratory flow rate is normal or reduced proportionately. Hence, *the ratio of FEV_1 and FVC is near normal.* The restrictive defect occurs in two general conditions: (1) *extrapulmonary disorders* that affect the ability of the chest wall to act as a bellows (e.g., severe obesity, kyphoscoliosis, and neuromuscular disorders, such as the Guillain-Barré syndrome [Chapter 23], that affect the respiratory muscles) and (2) *acute* or *chronic interstitial lung diseases.* The classic acute restrictive disease is adult respiratory distress syndrome (ARDS). *Chronic* restrictive diseases include the pneumoconioses (Chapter 8), sarcoidosis, and idiopathic pulmonary fibrosis (IPF).

OBSTRUCTIVE LUNG DISEASES

Asthma

Asthma is characterized by episodic, reversible bronchospasm resulting from an exaggerated bronchoconstrictor response to various stimuli. The basis of bronchial hyperreactivity is not entirely clear, but it is widely believed to result from persistent bronchial inflammation. Hence, bronchial asthma is best considered a chronic inflammatory disorder of the airways. Clinically, asthma is manifested by episodic dyspnea, cough, and wheezing (a soft whistling sound during expiration). This common disease affects about 5% of adults and 7% to 10% of children.

Because asthma is a heterogeneous disease triggered by a variety of inciting agents, there is no universally accepted simple classification. Nevertheless, it is customary to classify asthma into two major categories based on the presence or absence of an underlying immune disorder:

1. *Extrinsic asthma,* in which the asthmatic episode is typically initiated by a type I hypersensitivity reaction induced by exposure to an extrinsic antigen (Chapter 5). Three types of extrinsic asthma are recognized: *atopic asthma, occupational asthma* (many forms), and *allergic bronchopulmonary aspergillosis* (bronchial colonization with *Aspergillus* organisms followed by development of immunoglobulin E [IgE] antibodies). Atopic asthma is the most common type of asthma; its onset is usually in the first two decades of life, and it is commonly associated with other allergic manifestations in the patient as well as in other family members. Serum IgE levels are usually elevated, as is the blood eosinophil count.

2. *Intrinsic asthma,* in which the triggering mechanisms are nonimmune. In this form, a number of stimuli that have little or no effect in normal subjects can trigger bronchospasm. Such factors include aspirin; pulmonary infections, especially those caused by viruses; cold; psychological stress; exercise; and inhaled irritants such as sulfur dioxide. These patients are said to have an asthmatic diathesis. It must be emphasized, however, that, because of inherent tracheobronchial hyperreactivity, a person who has extrinsic asthma is also susceptible to developing an asthmatic attack when exposed to one of the mentioned agents. Thus, in many cases a neat distinction between intrinsic and extrinsic asthma is not possible.

Pathogenesis. As emphasized at the outset, the common denominator underlying all forms of asthma is an exaggerated bronchoconstrictor response (also called *increased airway reactivity*) to a variety of stimuli. Bronchial hyperresponsiveness can be readily demonstrated in the form of increased sensitivity to bronchoconstrictive agents such as histamine or methacholine (a cholinergic agonist).

Although the importance of increased airway reactivity is established, the basis of the abnormal bronchial response is not fully understood. Most current evidence suggests that *bronchial inflammation is the substrate for hyperresponsiveness.* Persistent inflammation of bronchi, manifested by the presence of inflammatory cells (particularly eosinophils, lymphocytes, and mast cells) and by damage to the bronchial epithelium, is a constant feature of bronchial asthma.

What causes the bronchial inflammation? In allergic or atopic asthma, it is readily explained by type I hypersensitivity reactions, but the cause is much less clear in patients with so-called intrinsic asthma. Because the basis of bronchial inflammation is better understood in allergic (atopic) asthma, this will be considered first.

Atopic Asthma. The details of type I hypersensitivity were discussed in an earlier chapter (Chapter 5), so only mechanisms of particular importance in the pathogenesis of asthma are reviewed here (Fig. 13–2). Like all type I hypersensitivity reactions, allergic asthma is driven by sensitization of CD4+ cells of the T_H2 type. It may be recalled that T_H2 cells release cytokines, such as interleukin 4 and 5 (IL-4 and IL-5), that favor the synthesis of IgE, growth of mast cells (IL-4), and growth and activation of eosinophils (IL-5). *IgE, mast cells, and eosinophils are key players in allergic asthma.* Attacks of atopic asthma often demonstrate two phases: an early phase, beginning 30 to 60 minutes after inhalation of antigen and then remitting, followed 4 to 8 hours later by a more protracted late phase. As might be expected, the initial triggering of mast cells occurs on the mucosal surface; the resultant mediator release opens mucosal intercellular junctions, allowing penetration of the antigen to more numerous mucosal mast cells. In addition, direct stimulation of subepithelial vagal (parasympathetic) receptors provokes reflex bronchoconstriction. As detailed in Chapter 5, mast cell activation leads to the release of a variety of primary and secondary mediators.

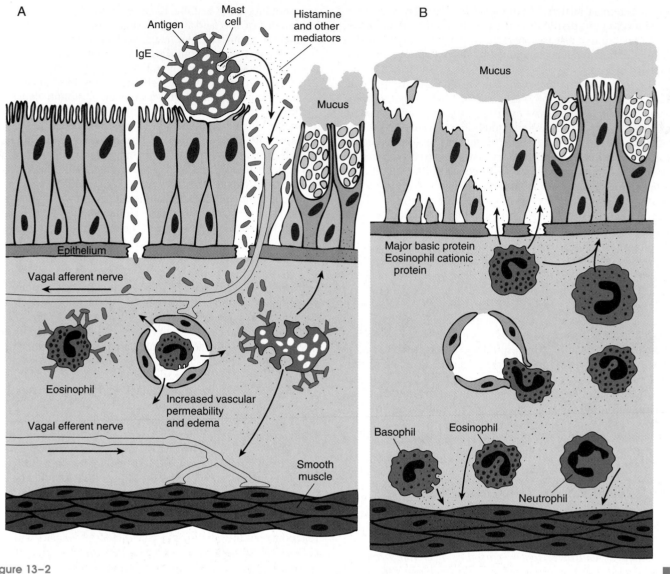

Figure 13-2

A model for immediate and late stages of allergic asthma. *A,* The immediate reaction is triggered by Ag-induced cross-linking of IgE bound to IgE receptors (FcRϵ) on mast cells (and possibly FcRϵ-expressing eosinophils and macrophages) in the airways. These cells release preformed mediators that open tight junctions between epithelial cells. Antigen can then enter the mucosa to activate mucosal mast cells and eosinophils, which in turn release additional mediators. Collectively the mediators, either directly or via neuronal reflexes, induce bronchospasm, increased vascular permeability, and mucus production and also recruit additional mediator-releasing cells from the blood. *B,* The arrival of recruited cells signals the initiation of the late stage of asthma, in which residual antigen binding to IgE *(not shown)* may trigger a fresh round of mediator release. Factors, particularly from eosinophils, may also stimulate release of mediators from other inflammatory cells and cause damage to the epithelium. (Reproduced with permission. Modified from Lichtenstein L: The nasal late phase response— an in vivo model. HOSPITAL PRACTICE 23(1):119, 1988. ©1988, The McGraw-Hill Companies. Illustration by Ilil Arbel.)

Those considered important in the pathogenesis of asthma include

■ Leukotrienes C_4, D_4, and E_4; these are extremely potent mediators that cause prolonged bronchoconstriction, increase vascular permeability, and increase mucin secretion.

■ Prostaglandin D_2 (PGD_2), which elicits bronchoconstriction and vasodilatation.

■ Eosinophilic and neutrophilic chemotactic factors, and leukotriene B_4, which recruit and activate eosinophils and neutrophils.

■ Platelet-activating factor (PAF), which causes aggregation

of platelets and release of histamine from their granules; in the presence of IL-5, it is also strongly chemotactic for eosinophils.

Together these mediators induce bronchoconstriction, edema, and mucus secretion; these initial reactions are followed by the late phase, which is dominated by additional recruitment of leukocytes: basophils, neutrophils, and eosinophils. Such recruitment is favored by release of cytokines, such as tumor necrosis factor-α from mast cells, that up-regulate adhesion molecules on vascular endothelium and also on inflammatory cells. Not only do these cells release additional waves of mediators and thus intensify the initial response, they also cause epithelial cell damage. Epithelial cells themselves are sources of mediators, such as endothelin and nitric oxide (NO), that can cause smooth muscle contraction and relaxation, respectively. Loss of epithelial integrity, by reducing available NO, may thus contribute to airway hyperresponsiveness. *Eosinophils* are particularly important in the late phase. As mentioned earlier their accumulation at sites of allergic inflammation is favored by mast cell–derived chemotactic factors, IL-5, and PAF. Recent studies have implicated several chemokines in eosinophil chemotaxis. The most potent of these appears to be *eotaxin,* produced in part by activated bronchial epithelial cells. The accumulated eosinophils exert a variety of effects. Their armamentarium of mediators is as extensive as that of mast cells and in addition they produce major basic protein (MBP) and eosinophil cationic protein (ECP), which are toxic to the epithelial cells. Activated eosinophils also produce leukotriene C_4 and PAF and directly activate mast cells to release mediators. Thus, eosinophils can amplify and sustain the inflammatory response without additional exposure to the triggering antigen.

Intrinsic Asthma. The mechanism of bronchial inflammation and hyperresponsiveness is much less clear in patients with intrinsic (nonatopic) asthma. Incriminated in such cases are *viral infections of the respiratory tract and inhaled air pollutants such as sulfur dioxide, ozone, and nitrogen dioxide.* These agents increase airway hyperreactivity in both normal and asthmatic subjects. In the latter, however, the bronchial response, manifested as spasm, is much more severe and sustained. In some of these patients, bronchial hyperresponsiveness is superimposed on clinically manifest chronic bronchitis, referred to as *chronic asthmatic bronchitis* (discussed later). In such patients the distinction between chronic bronchitis and asthma is hazy and clinically irrelevant.

In closing, it should be mentioned that bronchial hyperresponsiveness has also been ascribed to some fundamental defect in autonomic regulation, but the possible existence and importance of an underlying abnormality in the autonomic control of bronchial constriction is still unproved.

MORPHOLOGY. The morphologic changes in asthma have been described in patients who die of prolonged severe attacks (status asthmaticus) and in mucosal biopsies of patients challenged with allergens. In fatal cases, grossly, the lungs are overdistended because of overinflation, and there may be small areas of atelectasis. **The most striking macroscopic finding is occlusion of bronchi and bronchioles by thick, tenacious mucous plugs.** Histologically, the mucous plugs contain whorls of shed epithelium (Curschmann's spirals). Numerous eosinophils and Charcot-Leyden crystals (collections of crystalloids made up of eosinophil proteins) are also present. In addition, characteristic histologic findings in both nonfatal and fatal cases include

■ Edema, hyperemia, and an inflammatory infiltrate in the bronchial walls, with prominent eosinophils, which may constitute 5% to 50% of the cellular infiltrate. Also present are mast cells and

basophils, macrophages, lymphocytes, plasma cells, and some neutrophils; many of the lymphocytes are CD4+ cells of the T_H2 type that secrete IL-4 and IL-5.
■ Patchy necrosis and shedding of epithelial cells.
■ An increase in collagen immediately beneath the basement membrane, giving the appearance of a thickened basement membrane. This change is believed to result from cytokine-mediated activation of myofibroblasts that secrete collagen.
■ An increase in size of the submucosal mucous glands (or increased numbers of goblet cells in bronchiolar epithelium).
■ Hypertrophy and hyperplasia of the smooth muscle in the bronchial wall (Fig. 13–3).

Clinical Course. An attack of asthma is characterized by severe dyspnea with wheezing; the chief difficulty lies in expiration. The victim labors to get air into the lungs and then cannot get it out, so that there is progressive hyperinflation of the lungs with air trapped distal to the bronchi, which are constricted and filled with mucus and debris. In the usual case, attacks last from 1 to several hours and subside either spontaneously or with therapy, usually bronchodilators and corticosteroids. Intervals between attacks are characteristically free from respiratory difficulty, but persistent, subtle respiratory deficits can be detected by spirometric methods. Occasionally,

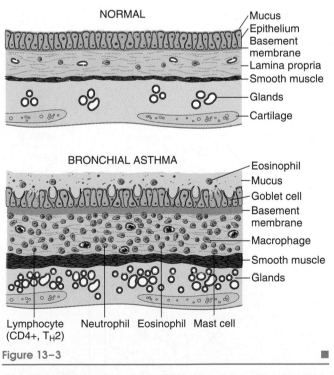

Figure 13–3   ■

Comparison of a normal bronchiole with that in a patient with asthma. Note the accumulation of mucus in the bronchial lumen resulting from an increase in the number of mucus-secreting goblet cells in the mucosa and hypertrophy of submucosal mucous glands. In addition, there is intense chronic inflammation due to recruitment of eosinophils, macrophages, and other inflammatory cells. Basement membrane underlying the mucosal epithelium is thickened and there is hypertrophy and hyperplasia of smooth muscle cells.

a severe paroxysm occurs that does not respond to therapy and persists for days and even weeks *(status asthmaticus)*. The associated hypercapnia, acidosis, and severe hypoxia may be fatal, although in most cases the disease is more disabling than lethal. In recent years, however, there has been an alarming increase in deaths from severe asthma. The basis of this trend is not clear.

Chronic Obstructive Pulmonary Diseases

Despite the wide use of the designation chronic pulmonary obstructive disease (COPD), there is no general agreement on its precise definition. According to some, it is defined strictly on the basis of pulmonary function tests and is said to exist when there is objective evidence of persisting (and irreversible) airflow obstruction. Others use the term more broadly to include two common conditions: chronic bronchitis and emphysema, recognizing that in some cases either of these conditions can exist without significant airflow obstruction. Despite these uncertainties, one thing is clear: *by the time patients with chronic bronchitis or emphysema develop sufficient dyspnea (breathlessness) to seek medical attention, airway obstruction can be readily demonstrated.* Furthermore, as will be emphasized again, these two conditions often coexist, so on practical clinical grounds the grouping of chronic bronchitis and emphysema under the rubric of COPD is justified.

EMPHYSEMA

Emphysema is characterized by *permanent enlargement* of the airspaces distal to the terminal bronchioles accompanied by *destruction of their walls.* There are several conditions in which enlargement of airspaces is not accompanied by destruction; this is more correctly called *overinflation.* For example, the distention of airspaces in the opposite lung after unilateral pneumonectomy is compensatory overinflation rather than emphysema.

The relationship between chronic bronchitis and emphysema is complicated, but the use of precise definitions has helped bring some order to what was once chaos. At the outset, it should be emphasized that the definition of emphysema is a morphologic one, whereas chronic bronchitis (see later) is defined on the basis of clinical features such as the presence of chronic and recurrent cough with excess mucus secretion. Although chronic bronchitis may exist without demonstrable emphysema and almost pure emphysema may occur (particularly in patients with inherited α_1-antitrypsin deficiency), the two diseases usually coexist because the major pathogenic mechanism, cigarette smoking, is common to both. Predictably, when the two entities coexist, the clinical and physiologic features overlap.

Types of Emphysema. Emphysema is defined not only in terms of the anatomic nature of the lesion but also according to its distribution in the lobule and acinus. Recall that an acinus is the part of the lung distal to the terminal bronchiole, and a cluster of three to five acini is referred to as a lobule.

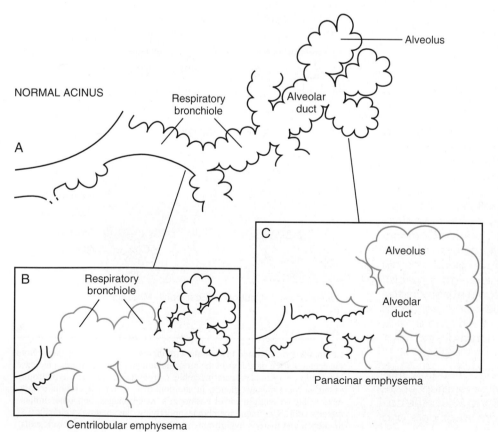

NORMAL ACINUS

A

B
Centrilobular emphysema

C
Panacinar emphysema

Figure 13–4 ■

A, Diagram of normal structures within the acinus, the fundamental unit of the lung. A terminal bronchiole *(not shown)* is immediately proximal to the respiratory bronchiole. *B,* Centrilobular emphysema with dilation that initially affects the respiratory bronchioles. *C,* Panacinar emphysema with initial distention of the peripheral structures (i.e., the alveolus and alveolar duct); the disease later extends to affect the respiratory bronchioles.

There are three types of emphysema: (1) centriacinar, (2) panacinar, and (3) distal acinar. The first two are more important, but their differentiation is often difficult in advanced disease, and so they are diagrammed in Figure 13–4 and briefly described below.

Centriacinar (Centrilobular) Emphysema. The distinctive feature of this type of emphysema is the pattern of involvement of the lobules: the central or proximal parts of the acini, formed by respiratory bronchioles, are affected, while distal alveoli are spared. Thus, both emphysematous and normal airspaces exist within the same acinus and lobule (Fig. 13–5A). The lesions are more common and severe in the upper lobes, particularly in the apical segments. In severe centriacinar emphysema the distal acinus also becomes involved, and so, as noted, the differentiation from panacinar emphysema becomes difficult.

Panacinar (Panlobular) Emphysema. In this type of emphysema the acini are uniformly enlarged from the level of the respiratory bronchiole to the terminal blind alveoli (Fig. 13–5B). In contrast to centriacinar emphysema, panacinar emphysema tends to occur more commonly in the lower lung zones and is the type of emphysema that occurs in α_1-antitrypsin deficiency.

Distal Acinar (Paraseptal) Emphysema. In this form the proximal portion of the acinus is normal but the distal part is dominantly involved. The emphysema is more striking adjacent to the pleura, along the lobular connective tissue septa, and at the margins of the lobules. It occurs adjacent to areas

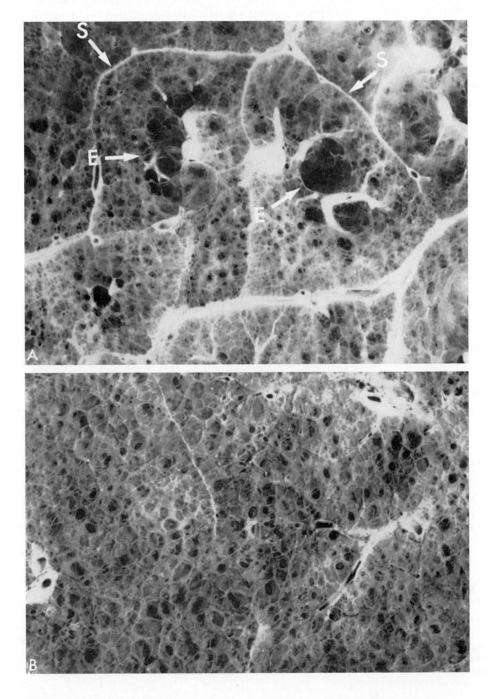

Figure 13–5   ■

A, Centrilobular emphysema (magnification ×5). The pulmonary arteries contain injected barium. The emphysematous foci (E) abut the arteries, but normal alveolar spaces are adjacent to the septa (S). *B,* Panacinar emphysema (×5) demonstrates a more generalized distribution of the permanently enlarged emphysematous foci. Compare with *A.* (From Bates DV, et al: Respiratory Function in Disease, 2nd ed. Philadelphia, WB Saunders, 1971.)

of fibrosis, scarring, or atelectasis and is usually more severe in the upper half of the lungs. The characteristic findings are the presence of multiple, contiguous, enlarged airspaces that range in diameter from less than 0.5 mm to more than 2.0 cm, sometimes forming cystlike structures that with progressive enlargement are referred to as bullae. This type of emphysema probably underlies many of the cases of spontaneous pneumothorax in young adults.

Incidence. Emphysema is a common disease, but its precise incidence is difficult to estimate because a definite diagnosis, which is based on morphology, can be made only by examination of the lungs at autopsy. It is generally agreed that emphysema is present in approximately 50% of adults who come to autopsy. Most of those found to have emphysema at autopsy are asymptomatic. Emphysema, especially centriacinar, is much more common and more severe in men than in women. *There is a clear association between heavy cigarette smoking and emphysema,* and the most severe type occurs in those who smoke heavily. Although emphysema does not become disabling until the fifth to eighth decades of life, ventilatory deficits may become clinically evident decades earlier.

Pathogenesis. The genesis of the two common forms of emphysema, centriacinar and panacinar, is not completely understood. The most plausible hypothesis to explain alveolar wall destruction and airspace enlargement invokes *excess protease or elastase activity unopposed by appropriate antiprotease regulation* (Fig. 13–6).

This hypothesis is based on the observation that patients with a genetic deficiency of the antiprotease α_1-antitrypsin have a markedly enhanced tendency to develop pulmonary emphysema, which is compounded by smoking. About 2% of all patients with emphysema have this defect. α_1-Antitrypsin, normally present in serum, tissue fluids, and macrophages, is a major inhibitor of proteases (particularly elastase) secreted by neutrophils during inflammation. This enzyme is encoded by codominantly expressed genes on the proteinase inhibitor (Pi) locus on chromosome 14. The Pi locus is extremely polymorphic, with many different alleles. Most common is the normal (M) allele and the corresponding PiMM phenotype. Approximately 0.012% of the U.S. population is homozygous for the Z allele (PiZZ), associated with markedly decreased serum levels of α_1-antitrypsin. Many of these persons develop symptomatic emphysema.

The following sequence is postulated:

1. Neutrophils (the principal source of cellular elastase) are normally sequestered in peripheral capillaries, including those in the lung, and a few gain access to the alveolar spaces.
2. Any stimulus that increases either the number of leukocytes (neutrophils and macrophages) in the lung or the release of their elastase-containing granules increases elastolytic activity.
3. With low levels of serum α_1-antitrypsin, elastic tissue destruction is unchecked and emphysema results.

Thus, emphysema is seen to result from the destructive effect of high protease activity in subjects with low antiprotease activity. This hypothesis is strongly supported by studies in experimental animals in which intratracheal instillation of the proteolytic enzymes papain and, more important, human neutrophil elastase results in the degradation of elastin accompanied by the development of emphysema.

The protease-antiprotease hypothesis also helps explain the effect of cigarette smoking in the production of emphysema, particularly the centriacinar form in subjects with normal α_1-antitrypsin levels:

■ Smokers have accumulation of neutrophils and macrophages in their alveoli.
■ Smoking stimulates release of elastase from neutrophils.
■ Smoking enhances elastase activity in macrophages; macrophage elastase is not inhibited by α_1-antitrypsin, and indeed can proteolytically digest this antiprotease.
■ Oxidants in cigarette smoke and oxygen free radicals secreted by neutrophils inhibit α_1-antitrypsin and thus decrease net antielastase activity in smokers.

In summary, it is likely that the impaction of smoke particles, predominantly at the bifurcation of respiratory bronchioles, results in the influx of neutrophils and macrophages, both of which secrete elastase. An increase in the elastase activity localized in the centriacinar region, together with the smoke-induced decrease of α_1-antitrypsin activity, causes the centriacinar pattern of emphysema seen in smokers. This schema also explains the additive influence of smoking and α_1-antitrypsin deficiency in inducing serious obstructive airway disease.

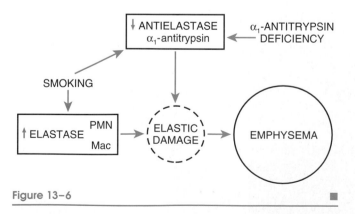

Figure 13–6

Protease-antiprotease mechanism of emphysema. Smoking inhibits antielastase and favors the recruitment of leukocytes and release of elastase. PMN, polymorphonuclear leukocytes; Mac, alveolar macrophages.

MORPHOLOGY. The diagnosis and classification of emphysema depend largely on the macroscopic appearance of the lung. Panacinar emphysema, when well developed, produces pale, voluminous lungs that often obscure the heart when the anterior chest wall is removed at autopsy. The macroscopic features of centriacinar emphysema are less impressive. The lungs are a deeper pink and less voluminous, unless the disease is well advanced. Generally, in centriacinar emphysema the upper two thirds of the lungs is more severely affected than the lower lungs, and in extreme cases emphysematous bullae may be grossly visible (Fig. 13–7).

Histologically, there is thinning and destruction of

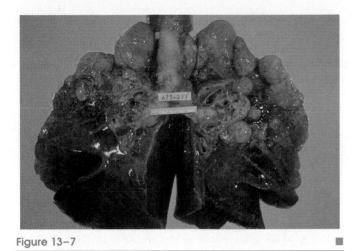

Figure 13–7   ■

Bullous emphysema with large apical and subpleural bullae. (From the teaching collection of the Department of Pathology, University of Texas Southwestern Medical School, Dallas, TX.)

alveolar walls. With advanced disease, adjacent alveoli become confluent, creating large airspaces (Fig. 13–8). Terminal and respiratory bronchioles may be deformed because of the loss of septa that help tether these structures in the parenchyma. With the loss of elastic tissue in the surrounding alveolar septa, there is reduced radial traction on the small airways. As a result, they tend to collapse during expiration—an important cause of chronic airflow obstruction in severe emphysema. In addition to alveolar loss, the number of alveolar capillaries is diminished. There is fibrosis of respiratory bronchioles and there may also be evidence of accompanying bronchitis and bronchiolitis.

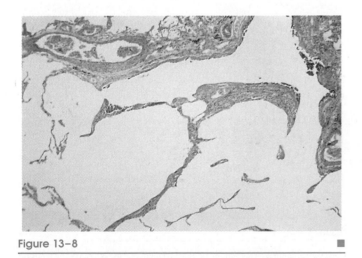

Figure 13–8   ■

Pulmonary emphysema. There is marked enlargement of airspaces, with thinning and destruction of alveolar septa. (From the teaching collection of the Department of Pathology, University of Texas Southwestern Medical School, Dallas, TX.)

Clinical Course. Dyspnea is usually the first symptom; it begins insidiously but is steadily progressive. In patients with underlying chronic bronchitis or chronic asthmatic bronchitis, cough and wheezing are initial complaints. Weight loss is common and may be so severe as to suggest a hidden malignant tumor. Pulmonary function tests reveal reduced FEV_1 with normal or near-normal FVC. Hence, the ratio of FEV_1 to FVC is reduced.

The classic presentation in individuals who have no "bronchitic" component is one in which the patient is barrel-chested and dyspneic, with obviously prolonged expiration, sitting forward in a hunched-over position, attempting to squeeze the air out of the lungs with each expiratory effort. In these patients, air space enlargement is severe and diffusing capacity is low. Dyspnea and hyperventilation are prominent, so that until very late in the disease gas exchange is adequate and blood gas values are relatively normal. Because of prominent dyspnea and adequate oxygenation of hemoglobin, these patients are sometimes called "pink puffers."

On the other extreme are patients with emphysema who also have pronounced chronic bronchitis and a history of recurrent infections with purulent sputum. They usually have less prominent dyspnea and respiratory drive, so they retain carbon dioxide, become hypoxic, and are often cyanotic. For reasons not entirely clear, they tend to be obese. Often they seek medical help after the onset of congestive heart failure (cor pulmonale, Chapter 11) and associated edema. Patients with this clinical picture are sometimes unflatteringly called "blue bloaters."

Most patients with emphysema and COPD fall somewhere between these two classic extremes. In all patients chronic hypoxemia can lead to pulmonary vascular spasm, pulmonary hypertension, and cor pulmonale. Death from emphysema is related to (1) pulmonary failure with respiratory acidosis, hypoxia, and coma; or (2) right-sided heart failure.

CONDITIONS RELATED TO EMPHYSEMA. Several conditions resemble emphysema or are inappropriately referred to as such.

Compensatory emphysema is a term used to designate the compensatory dilation of alveoli in response to loss of lung substance elsewhere, such as occurs in residual lung parenchyma after surgical removal of a diseased lung or lobe.

Senile emphysema refers to the overdistended lungs of elders, which result from age-related alterations of the internal geometry of the lung (e.g., larger alveolar ducts and smaller alveoli). There is no significant tissue destruction, and a better designation for such aging lungs would be **senile hyperinflation.**

Obstructive overinflation refers to the condition in which the lung expands because air is trapped within it. A common cause is subtotal obstruction by a tumor or foreign object. Obstructive overinflation can be a life-threatening emergency if the affected portion extends sufficiently to compress the remaining normal lung.

Mediastinal (interstitial) emphysema designates

the entrance of air into the connective tissue stroma of the lung, mediastinum, and subcutaneous tissue. This may occur spontaneously with a sudden increase in intraalveolar pressure (as with vomiting or violent coughing) that causes a tear, with dissection of air into the interstitium. Sometimes it occurs in children with whooping cough. It is particularly apt to occur in patients on respirators who have partial bronchiolar obstruction or in persons who suffer a perforating injury (e.g., a fractured rib). When the interstitial air enters the subcutaneous tissue, the patient may literally blow up like a balloon, with marked swelling of the head and neck and crackling crepitation all over the chest. In most instances the air is resorbed spontaneously when the site of entry is sealed.

CHRONIC BRONCHITIS

Chronic bronchitis is common among cigarette smokers and urban dwellers in smog-ridden cities; some studies of men in the 40- to 65-year age group indicate that 20% to 25% have the disease. The diagnosis of chronic bronchitis is made on clinical grounds: it is defined as *a persistent productive cough for at least 3 consecutive months in at least 2 consecutive years.* It can occur in several forms:

■ Most patients have *simple chronic bronchitis:* the productive cough raises mucoid sputum, but airflow is not obstructed.

■ If the sputum contains pus, presumably because of secondary infections, the patient is said to have *chronic mucopurulent bronchitis.*

■ Some patients with chronic bronchitis may demonstrate hyperresponsive airways and intermittent episodes of asthma. This condition, termed *chronic asthmatic bronchitis,* is often difficult to distinguish from atopic asthma.

■ A small subpopulation of bronchitic patients develop chronic outflow obstruction as measured by pulmonary function tests. They are said to have *chronic obstructive bronchitis.*

The morphologic basis of airflow obstruction in chronic bronchitis is twofold: (1) inflammation, fibrosis, and resultant narrowing of bronchioles ("small airway disease"); and (2) coexistent emphysema. It is generally believed that while small airway disease (chronic bronchiolitis) does contribute to airflow obstruction, chronic bronchitis with significant airflow obstruction is almost always complicated by emphysema. Between 5% and 15% of smokers develop physiologic evidence of COPD, and many of these present initially with chronic bronchitis. At present, it is not possible to determine which cigarette smokers, including those with chronic bronchitis, will develop clinically significant COPD, with its potentially dire consequences.

Pathogenesis. The distinctive feature of chronic bronchitis is hypersecretion of mucus that starts in the large airways. Although the single most important causative factor is cigarette smoking, other air pollutants, such as sulfur dioxide and nitrogen dioxide, may contribute. These irritants, directly or through neurohumoral pathways, *induce hypersecretion of the bronchial mucous glands, cause hypertrophy of mucous glands,* and *lead to metaplastic formation of mucin-secreting goblet cells in the surface epithelium of bronchi.* Microbial infection is often present but plays a secondary role, chiefly by maintaining the inflammation and exacerbating symptoms.

MORPHOLOGY. Grossly, the mucosal lining of the larger airways is usually hyperemic and swollen by edema fluid. It is often covered by a layer of mucinous or mucopurulent secretions. The smaller bronchi and bronchioles may also be filled with similar secretions. Histologically, the diagnostic feature of chronic bronchitis in the trachea and larger bronchi is **enlargement of the mucus-secreting glands** (Fig. 13–9). The magnitude of the increase in size is assessed by the ratio of the thickness of the submucosal gland layer to that of the bronchial wall (Reid index). Often, an increased number of goblet cells is seen in the lining epithelium, with concomitant loss of ciliated epithelial cells. Squamous metaplasia frequently develops (Fig. 13–9), followed by dysplastic changes in the lining epithelial cells, a sequence of events that may lead to the evolution of bronchogenic carcinoma. A variable density of inflammatory cells, largely mononuclear but sometimes admixed with neutrophils, is frequently present in the bronchial mucosa. **Chronic bronchiolitis** (small airway disease), characterized by goblet cell metaplasia (normally the number of goblet cells is small in peripheral airways), inflammation, fibrosis in the walls, and smooth muscle hyperplasia, is also present.

Clinical Course. In patients with chronic bronchitis, a prominent cough and the production of sputum may persist

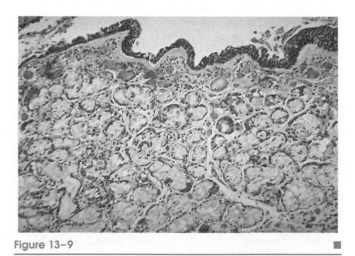

Figure 13–9 ■

Chronic bronchitis. The lumen of the bronchus is above. Note the marked thickening of the mucous gland layer (approximately twice normal) and squamous metaplasia of lung epithelium. (From the teaching collection of the Department of Pathology, University of Texas Southwestern Medical School, Dallas, TX.)

indefinitely without ventilatory dysfunction. However, as alluded to earlier, some patients develop significant COPD with outflow obstruction. This is accompanied by hypercapnia, hypoxemia, and (in severe cases) cyanosis. Differentiation of this form of COPD from that caused by emphysema can be made in the classic case, but, as mentioned, many patients have both conditions. With progression, chronic bronchitis is complicated by cardiac failure (Chapter 11). Recurrent infections and respiratory failure are constant threats.

Bronchiectasis

Bronchiectasis is the permanent dilation of bronchi and bronchioles due to destruction of the muscle and elastic supporting tissue, resulting from or associated with chronic necrotizing infections. It is not a primary disease but rather is secondary to persisting infection or obstruction caused by a variety of conditions. Once developed, it gives rise to a characteristic symptom complex dominated by cough and expectoration of copious amounts of purulent sputum. Diagnosis depends on an appropriate history along with radiographic demonstration of bronchial dilation. The conditions that most commonly predispose to bronchiectasis include

1. *Bronchial obstruction.* Common causes are tumors, foreign bodies, and occasionally mucous impaction. Under these conditions, the bronchiectasis is localized to the obstructed lung segment. Bronchiectasis can also complicate atopic asthma and chronic bronchitis.
2. *Congenital or hereditary conditions.* Only a few are cited:

■ In cystic fibrosis, widespread severe bronchiectasis results from obstruction and infection due to the secretion of abnormally viscid mucus. This is an important and serious complication (Chapter 7).
■ In immunodeficiency states, particularly immunoglobulin deficiencies, bronchiectasis is prone to develop because of an increased susceptibility to repeated bacterial infections; localized or diffuse bronchiectasis can occur.
■ Kartagener's syndrome, an autosomal recessive disorder, is frequently associated with bronchiectasis and sterility in males. Structural abnormalities of the cilia impair mucociliary clearance in the airways, leading to persistent infections, and reduce the mobility of spermatozoa.

3. *Necrotizing,* or *suppurative, pneumonia* may predispose to bronchiectasis. In the past, it was sometimes a sequela to childhood pneumonias complicating measles, whooping cough, and influenza. Although this form of postinfective bronchiectasis is no longer common in the United States, it continues to be an important problem in underdeveloped countries.

Pathogenesis. Two processes are critical and intertwined in the pathogenesis of bronchiectasis: (1) obstruction and (2) chronic persistent infection. Either of these two processes may come first. Normal clearance mechanisms are hampered by obstruction, so secondary infection soon follows; conversely, chronic infection in time causes damage to bronchial walls, leading to weakening and dilation. For example, obstruction due to a bronchogenic carcinoma or a foreign body impairs clearance of secretions, providing a fertile soil for superimposed infection. The resultant inflammatory damage to the bronchial wall and the accumulating exudate further distend the airways, leading to irreversible dilation. Conversely, a persistent necrotizing inflammation in the bronchi or bronchioles may cause obstructive secretions, inflammation throughout the wall (with peribronchial fibrosis and scarring traction on the walls), and eventually the train of events already described.

In the usual case a mixed flora can be cultured from the involved bronchi, including staphylococci, streptococci, pneumococci, enteric organisms, anaerobic and microaerophilic bacteria, and (particularly in children) *Haemophilus influenzae* and *Pseudomonas aeruginosa.*

> **MORPHOLOGY.** Bronchiectatic involvement of the lungs usually affects the lower lobes bilaterally, particularly those air passages that are most vertical. When tumors or aspiration of foreign bodies lead to bronchiectasis, involvement may be sharply localized to a single segment of the lungs. Usually, the most severe involvement is found in the more distal bronchi and bronchioles. The airways may be dilated to as much as four times their usual diameter, and on gross examination of the lung can be followed almost to the pleural surfaces (Fig. 13–10). (By contrast, in normal lungs

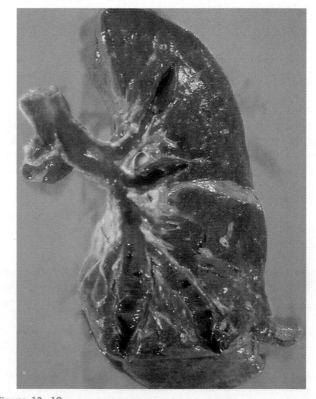

Figure 13–10   ■

Bronchiectasis. Dilated bronchi extend almost to the pleura in the left lower lung lobe. (From the teaching collection of the Department of Pathology, University of Texas Southwestern Medical School, Dallas, TX.)

the bronchioles cannot be followed by ordinary gross examination beyond a point 2 to 3 cm from the pleural surfaces.)

The histologic findings vary with the activity and chronicity of the disease. In the full-blown, active case an intense acute and chronic inflammatory exudate within the walls of the bronchi and bronchioles, and desquamation of lining epithelium, cause extensive areas of ulceration. Fibrosis of the bronchial and bronchiolar walls and peribronchiolar fibrosis develop in more chronic cases. When healing occurs, the lining epithelium may regenerate completely; however, usually so much injury has occurred that abnormal dilation and scarring persist. In some instances **the necrosis destroys the bronchial or bronchiolar walls and forms a lung abscess.**

Clinical Course. The clinical manifestations consist of severe, persistent cough with expectoration of mucopurulent, sometimes fetid, sputum. The sputum may contain flecks of blood; frank hemoptysis can occur. Symptoms are often episodic and are precipitated by upper respiratory tract infections or the introduction of new pathogenic agents. Clubbing of the fingers may develop. In cases of severe, widespread bronchiectasis, significant obstructive ventilatory defects develop, with hypoxemia, hypercapnia, pulmonary hypertension, and (rarely) cor pulmonale. Metastatic brain abscesses and reactive amyloidosis are other, less frequent complications of bronchiectasis.

 ## RESTRICTIVE LUNG DISEASES

Restrictive lung diseases are characterized by reduced compliance (i.e., more pressure is required to expand the lungs because they are stiff). Although chest wall abnormalities, some of which were mentioned earlier, can also cause restrictive disease, this discussion will concentrate on parenchymal causes.

Before we discuss the individual disorders, it is useful to consider two general features of restrictive pulmonary diseases, beginning with a brief review of the microanatomy of the septal wall.

■ As noted in Figure 13–11, only a thin basement membrane, scant pericapillary interstitial tissue, and the cytoplasm of two very flat cells, endothelium and alveolar epithelium, are interposed between air and blood. The initiating injury in these diseases usually affects either of these two cell types, although with chronicity changes in the interstitium tend to dominate the picture. Because of prominent changes in the interstitium, these disorders are often referred to as *interstitial lung disease*. It should be evident from Figure 13–11, however, that because of their intimate relationship, changes in the interstitium can affect both alveoli and capillaries.

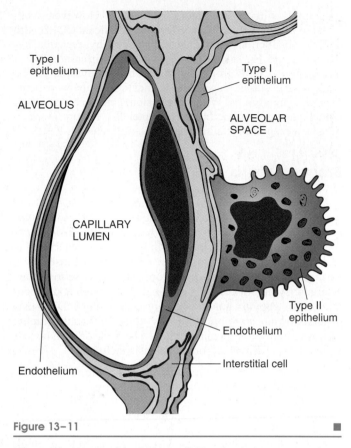

Figure 13–11 ■

Microscopic structure of the alveolar wall. Note that the basement membrane *(yellow)* is thin on one side and widened where it is continuous with the interstitial space. Portions of interstitial cells are shown.

■ The important signs and symptoms of restrictive lung disease can be inferred from the morphologic changes. Interstitial fluid or fibrosis produces a "stiff lung," which in turn reduces lung compliance and necessitates increased effort of breathing (dyspnea). Furthermore, damage to the alveolar epithelium and interstitial vasculature produces abnormalities in the ventilation-perfusion ratio, leading to hypoxia. For example, damaged or underventilated air units (alveoli) may still be perfused, and, conversely, with damage to the capillaries, underperfusion of ventilated airspaces occurs. With progression, patients develop severe hypoxia and respiratory failure, often in association with pulmonary hypertension and cor pulmonale (Chapter 11).

Restrictive lung disease can be either (1) acute, associated with an abrupt decrement in respiratory function and demonstrable pulmonary edema, often with accompanying inflammation; or (2) chronic, associated with insidious development of respiratory dysfunction. Chronic restrictive lung disorders demonstrate variable amounts of chronic inflammation and fibrosis; in addition, some reveal unique features described later. In the discussion that follows, we first consider adult respiratory distress syndrome, the prototypic and most important acute restrictive lung disease, and then several examples of chronic interstitial disorders.

Acute Restrictive Lung Diseases

ADULT RESPIRATORY DISTRESS SYNDROME: DIFFUSE ALVEOLAR DAMAGE

Adult respiratory distress syndrome (ARDS) is a clinical syndrome characterized by the acute onset of respiratory distress accompanied by (1) decreased arterial oxygen pressure, (2) decreased lung compliance, and (3) the development of diffuse pulmonary infiltrates on radiographs, without evidence of primary left-sided heart failure. *Diffuse alveolar damage is the morphologic counterpart of ARDS.* It is associated with diffuse alveolar endothelial and epithelial injury and, usually, pulmonary edema. Diffuse alveolar damage occurs in a multitude of clinical settings (Table 13–1), all characterized by a cascade of events that lead to a common pattern of acute injury of the alveolocapillary membrane.

Pathogenesis. Some conditions that lead to ARDS primarily damage the alveolar epithelium, but in most the endothelium is the primary target; ultimately both are involved. In some clinical settings the toxins responsible for the damage can be identified. For example, ARDS following exposure to high oxygen concentrations results from injurious oxygen-derived free radicals; however, in many instances, including some common conditions (Table 13–1), the specific toxic agent has not been identified. Nevertheless, *there is compelling evidence that neutrophils—and most likely macrophages—are involved in mediating the injury in most cases.* The postulated sequence of events in gram-negative sepsis, an important cause of ARDS, is illustrated in Figure 13–12. Endotoxin triggers the release of TNF-α (Chapter 4) from monocytes and alveolar macrophages, and activates the alternate pathway of complement to generate C5a. This complement component up-regulates the expression of adhesion molecules on neutrophils (Chapter 2), whereas TNF-α activates endothelial cells to up-regulate adhesion molecules and to produce

cytokines. The up-regulation of adhesion molecules on neutrophils and endothelial cells causes "sticking" of neutrophils to the endothelium and thus leads to sequestration of neutrophils in lung capillaries. The activated neutrophils, and possibly macrophages, release powerful mediators, including oxygen free radicals, proteases, leukotrienes, and prostaglandins, which damage the endothelium, increase vascular permeability, and trigger coagulation. *Collectively, the consequences of all these mediators and reactions are interstitial edema and necrosis of endothelial and epithelial cells.* Early in the course of ARDS there is little evidence of generalized thrombosis, but within 72 hours disseminated intravascular coagulation (DIC) may become evident and complicate the clinical picture.

MORPHOLOGY. The anatomic changes in diffuse alveolar damage are remarkably consistent, whatever the precipitating condition. On gross examination early in the disease, the lungs resemble the liver; they are dark red, firm, airless, and heavy. Very late in the course, with deposition of collagen, they become diffusely gray as a result of fibrosis. Microscopically, the process may be divided into exudative, proliferative (or repair), and fibrotic phases. In the exudative phase there is capillary congestion, interstitial and intraalveolar edema and hemorrhage, necrosis of alveolar epithelial cells, and (particularly with sepsis) collections of neutrophils in capillaries. The alveolar ducts are dilated, and alveoli tend to collapse, in all likelihood owing to a secondary impairment of surfactant synthesis (microatelectasis, p 394). Fibrin thrombi may be present in capillaries and large vessels. **The most characteristic finding, however, is hyaline membranes, particularly lining the distended alveolar ducts** (Fig. 13–13). Such membranes consist of protein-rich edema fluid admixed with remnants of necrotic epithelial cells. Overall, the picture is remarkably similar to that seen in respiratory distress syndrome in the newborn (Chapter 7). The proliferative phase, readily appreciated by day 10, is marked by proliferation of type II pneumocytes and interstitial fibroblasts. The latter also invade the exudates that have accumulated in the airspaces. Finally, the progressive fibrosis involving the interstitium and alveolar space may result in marked distortion of lung parenchyma, leading sometimes to diffuse interstitial fibrosis interspersed with dilated and distorted airspaces (honeycomb lung).

Table 13–1. CONDITIONS ASSOCIATED WITH DEVELOPMENT OF *ARDS*

Infection	Inhaled Irritants
*Sepsis	Oxygen toxicity
*Diffuse pulmonary infections: Viral, mycoplasma, and *Pneumocystis* pneumonia; miliary tuberculosis	Smoke
	Irritant gases and chemicals
	Chemical Injury
	Heroin or methadone overdose
*Gastric aspiration	Acetylsalicylic acid
Physical Injury	Barbiturate overdose
*Mechanical trauma, including head injuries	Paraquat
Pulmonary contusions	**Hematologic Conditions**
Near drowning	Multiple transfusions
Fractures with fat embolism	DIC
Burns	**Pancreatitis**
Ionizing radiation	**Uremia**
	Cardiopulmonary Bypass

* More than 50% of cases of ARDS are associated with these four conditions.
ARDS, adult respiratory distress syndrome; DIC, disseminated intravascular coagulation.

Clinical Course. The prognosis of ARDS is grim, and in the past mortality rates approached 100%. With improved methods of management, mortality is still around 50%; the toll exacted by sepsis is higher. The more severe the initial permeability leak in alveolocapillary membranes, the poorer is the prognosis. Patients who develop associated hypoxic multisystem failure (especially cardiac, renal, or hepatic) gen-

ENDOTOXIN EXPOSURE

PMN SEQUESTRATION AND DIFFUSE ALVEOLAR DAMAGE

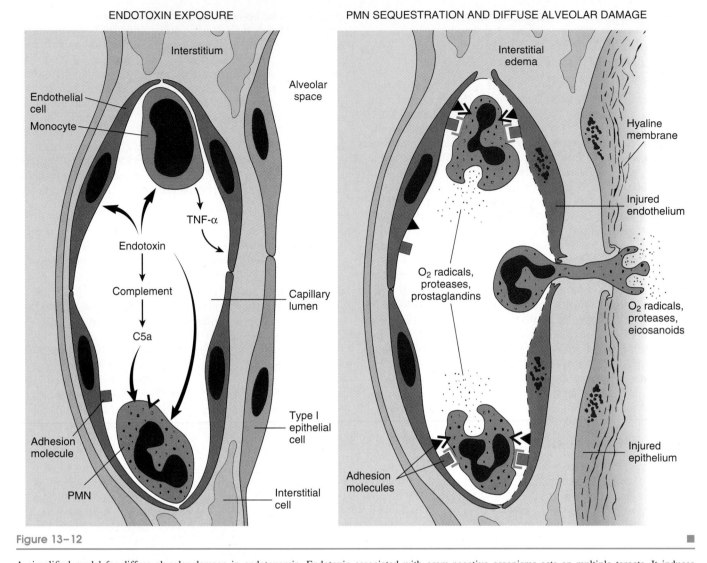

Figure 13–12

A simplified model for diffuse alveolar damage in endotoxemia. Endotoxin associated with gram-negative organisms acts on multiple targets. It induces monocytes and lung macrophages to release mediators, including tumor necrosis factor α (TNF-α) and chemotactic peptides (e.g., leukotriene B$_4$, interleukin 8). Endotoxin-induced activation of complement via the alternate pathway releases C5a, which together with bacterial lipopolysaccharide and TNF-α activates polymorphonuclear neutrophil leukocytes (PMNs) and up-regulates expression of adhesion molecules. Endotoxin also activates endothelial cells to up-regulate adhesion molecules that facilitate binding of neutrophils. Activation of PMNs results in the release of oxidants, proteases, and prostaglandins. The net result is the sequestration of PMNs in pulmonary capillaries, damage to endothelial and epithelial cells, and the development of interstitial edema and alveolar hyaline membranes.

erally have an especially poor outcome. A confounding clinical problem is that the high levels of oxygen sometimes used to treat hypoxemia may lead to additional alveolar damage owing to oxygen toxicity.

The alveolar exudates also provide a rich culture medium for microorganisms, and secondary infections are common. Should the patient survive the acute stage, diffuse interstitial fibrosis may occur and continue to compromise respiratory function. However, in most patients who survive the acute insult and are spared the chronic sequelae, normal respiratory function returns within 4 to 6 months.

Chronic Restrictive Lung Diseases

The chronic restrictive (interstitial) diseases of the lung parenchyma are a heterogeneous group with little uniformity regarding terminology and classification. Many entities are of unknown cause and pathogenesis; some have an intra-alveolar as well as an interstitial component, and there is frequent overlap in histologic features among the different conditions. Nevertheless, the presence of similar clinical signs, symptoms, radiographic alterations, and pathophysiologic changes justifies their consideration as a group. As stated earlier, *these patients have reduced FVC with proportionate reduction of FEV₁, and hence (unlike the situation in obstructive lung diseases) the FEV₁ to FVC ratio is not reduced.*

Chronic restrictive lung disorders account for about 15% of noninfectious diseases seen by pulmonary physicians. They can be divided into two broad categories (Table 13–2), those with known causes and those of unknown cause, and further divided on the basis of the presence or absence of granulomas. This distinction is of some utility when diagnosis is made

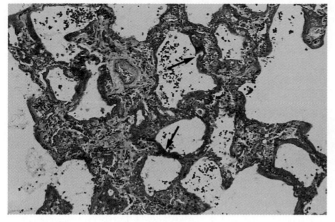

Figure 13–13

Diffuse alveolar damage (adult respiratory distress syndrome). Some alveoli are collapsed; others are distended. Many are lined by bright pink hyaline membranes *(arrows).*

from biopsy tissue. The most common conditions are those caused by specific environmental agents, sarcoidosis, IPF, and the collagen vascular diseases. The remainder have more than 150 different causes and associations in addition to those listed here.

The chronic interstitial diseases probably evolve over time from low-grade inflammation that may resemble a more limited form of ARDS. Indeed, some agents (e.g., radiation and bleomycin) in large doses can cause ARDS, and in smaller doses and after repeated exposure can lead to interstitial fibrosis and restrictive lung disease. Some of the more common and prototypic forms of chronic restrictive disease are described next.

Table 13–2. MAJOR CATEGORIES OF CHRONIC INTERSTITIAL LUNG DISEASE WITH SELECTED EXAMPLES

Known Etiology	Unknown Etiology
A. Lung Response: Alveolitis, Interstitial Inflammation, and Diffuse Fibrosis	
†Environmental agents: Asbestos, fumes, gases	†Collagen vascular diseases: Scleroderma, rheumatoid arthritis, systemic lupus erythematosus, dermatomyositis, mixed connective tissue disease
Ionizing radiation	
Following ARDS	
Drugs: Busulfan, bleomycin	
	†Idiopathic pulmonary fibrosis
	Goodpasture's syndrome
	Idiopathic pulmonary hemosiderosis
B. Lung Response: As in A But With Granulomas	
Beryllium	†Sarcoidosis
Hypersensitivity pneumonitis	Eosinophilic granuloma
	Wegener's granulomatosis

Adapted from Reynolds HY: Interstitial lung diseases. In Isselbacher KJ, et al (eds): Harrison's Principles of Internal Medicine, 13th ed. New York, McGraw-Hill, 1994, p 1206.
† Most common causes.

IDIOPATHIC PULMONARY FIBROSIS

Idiopathic pulmonary fibrosis (IPF) refers to a poorly understood pulmonary disorder of unknown cause characterized histologically by diffuse interstitial fibrosis, which in advanced cases results in severe hypoxemia and cyanosis. There are at least 20 synonyms for this entity (e.g., chronic interstitial pneumonitis, Hamman-Rich syndrome, diffuse or cryptogenic fibrosing alveolitis). Males are affected more often than females, and most patients are between 30 and 50 years old when the condition is diagnosed. It should be stressed that similar clinical and pathologic findings may be noted with well-defined entities such as asbestosis, the connective tissue diseases, and a number of other conditions (Table 13–2). Therefore, known causes must be ruled out before the appellation "idiopathic" is used.

The proposed sequence of events in IPF begins with some form of alveolar wall injury, which results in interstitial edema and accumulation of inflammatory cells (alveolitis). If the injury is mild and self-limited, resolution with restoration of normal architecture follows. However, with persistence of the injurious agent, a cascade of cellular interactions involving lymphocytes, macrophages, neutrophils, and alveolar epithelial cells leads to proliferation of fibroblasts and progressive fibrosis of both the alveolar septa and the alveolar exudate. It is suspected that immune mechanisms trigger this sequence of events (Fig. 13–14). In some patients, circulating immune complexes may bind to the Fc receptors of alveolar macrophages and stimulate them. In other instances, macrophages are activated by cytokines derived from T cells responding to unknown antigens. Regardless of whether the macrophages are driven by T cells or immune complexes, they secrete factors, such as IL-8 and leukotrienes, that recruit and activate neutrophils. The soluble mediators released from macrophages and recruited neutrophils injure alveolar epithelial cells and degrade connective tissue. Alveolar macrophages from patients with IPF secrete a host of other factors, including fibroblast growth factor, TGF-β, and platelet-derived growth factor (PDGF), which can attract fibroblasts as well as stimulate their proliferation, thus setting in motion a repair response. It is now believed that alveolar epithelial cells are not merely passive targets in this process. Destruction of type I pneumocytes is often accompanied by proliferation of type II pneumocytes. These cells secrete chemotactic factors (e.g., macrophage chemotactic protein 1) that attract macrophages and T cells. In addition, they can contribute to fibrosis by secreting PDGF and other fibrogenic cytokines, such as TGF-β.

To summarize, IPF is initiated by unknown injurious agents that cause alveolitis and also induce an immune response. Intra-alveolar inflammation causes epithelial cell injury and triggers a fibrogenic response in which lymphocytes, macrophages, and type II pneumocytes all participate (Fig. 13–14.)

MORPHOLOGY. The morphologic changes vary according to the stage of the disease. In early cases the lungs are firm; microscopically, they show pulmonary edema, intraalveolar exudate, hyaline membranes, and infiltration of the alveolar septa with mononuclear cells. Type I pneumocytes

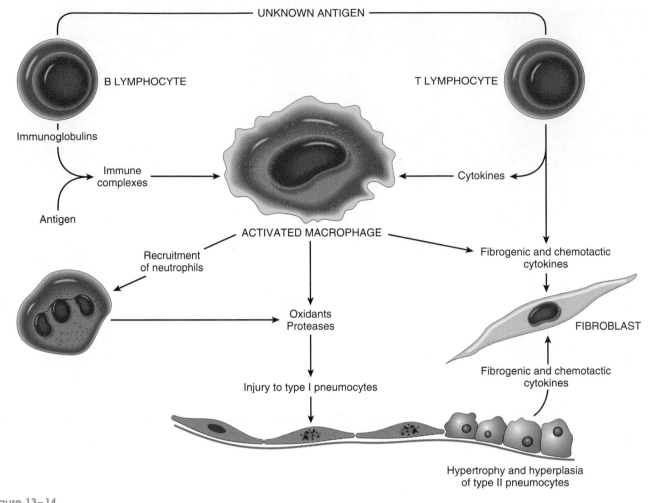

Figure 13–14 ■

A possible schema of the pathogenesis of idiopathic pulmonary fibrosis.

are particularly susceptible to injury. Subsequently, there is hyperplasia of type II pneumocytes, which appear as cuboidal or even columnar cells lining the alveolar spaces. With advancing disease, there is organization of the intraalveolar exudate by fibrous tissue, as well as thickening of the alveolar septa owing to fibrosis and variable amounts of inflammation. At this stage the lungs demonstrate alternating areas of fibrosis and normal tissue. In the end the lung consists of spaces lined by cuboidal or columnar epithelium separated by inflammatory fibrous tissue, an appearance referred to as honeycomb lung (Fig. 13–15). There is also intimal thickening of the pulmonary arteries and lymphoid infiltration in the fibrotic interstitium.

Clinically, patients exhibit respiratory difficulty and, in advanced cases, hypoxemia and cyanosis. The septal fibrosis constitutes a significant alveolocapillary block. Cor pulmonale and cardiac failure may result. The progression in individ-

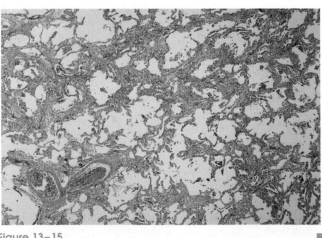

Figure 13–15 ■

Idiopathic pulmonary fibrosis. The alveolar walls are thickened by fibrosis. In addition, there is an interstitial infiltrate of mononuclear cells. Not seen at this magnification is hyperplasia of type II pneumocytes lining the airspaces. Note also irregularly dilated airspaces. Alternating areas of fibrosis and dilation give rise to the honeycomb appearance noted on gross examination.

ual cases is unpredictable. In some patients the disease remits spontaneously; in a few it progresses very rapidly, leading to fibrosis in a matter of weeks, whereas in others it develops over many years. The median survival is about 5 years.

SARCOIDOSIS

Although considered here as an example of a restrictive lung disease with granulomatous tissue response, it should be remembered that sarcoidosis is a *multisystem disease of unknown cause characterized by noncaseating granulomas in many tissues and organs.* Other diseases, including mycobacterial or fungal infections and berylliosis, sometimes also produce noncaseating granulomas; therefore, the histologic *diagnosis of sarcoidosis is one of exclusion.* Although the multisystem involvement of sarcoidosis can present in many clinical guises, bilateral hilar lymphadenopathy or lung involvement (or both), visible on chest radiographs, is the major presenting manifestation in most cases. Eye and skin involvement each occur in about 25% of cases and may occasionally be the presenting feature of the disease.

Sarcoidosis occurs worldwide, but the frequency varies in different populations. In the United States it occurs in 1 to 4 per 10,000 and is 10 times more prevalent in blacks.

Etiology and Pathogenesis. The distinctive granulomatous tissue response seen in sarcoidosis suggests that the disease represents a cell-mediated immune response to an unidentified antigen. Many causal agents have been proposed as the immunogen (atypical mycobacteria, pine pollen, and so forth), but none has been proved to be the cause. Several features support a role for a deranged immune response to one or more still unidentified agents in the pathogenesis of sarcoidosis:

■ Most patients manifest cutaneous anergy to common skin test antigens (e.g., *Candida,* mumps, purified protein derivative [PPD]) to which normal persons have been exposed and sensitized.
■ The number of peripheral blood T lymphocytes is often decreased, resulting in an absolute lymphopenia, and the CD4 to CD8 ratio may be reduced to less than 0.8 (normal 0.9 to 2.5).
■ Bronchoalveolar lavage fluids from patients with active sarcoid lung lesions demonstrate an increased number of T lymphocytes, with a CD4 to CD8 T-cell ratio of up to 10:1. CD4+ T cells demonstrate cell surface activation markers, including the IL-2 receptor (IL-2R), and lavage fluids contain detectable levels of secreted IL-2 and IL-2R.
■ Circulating B cells are normal in number, but the serum contains excess polyclonal immunoglobulins, secreted by B cells in lymphoid tissues.

All of these findings are consistent with a cell-mediated immune response (type IV hypersensitivity reaction) to an unidentified antigen. The depletion of CD4+ T cells in the peripheral blood and cutaneous anergy is most likely due to the recruitment of the CD4+ T cells into the lesions. Still unexplained is the distribution of lesions.

MORPHOLOGY. Virtually any organ may be affected; the most common morphologic changes will be described.

Lymph nodes are involved in almost all cases, commonly the hilar and paratracheal ones, but any node in the body may be involved, particularly those in the head and neck. The tonsils are affected in about one quarter to one third of cases. The nodes are characteristically enlarged and discrete, and sometimes lobulated (when viewed on chest radiographs, the bilateral hilar lymphadenopathy is referred to as "potato nodes"). Histologically, all involved nodes show classic noncaseating granulomas (Fig. 13–16). These are made up of aggregates of tightly clustered epithelioid cells, often with Langhans' or foreign body–type giant cells. The granulomas are surrounded by a rim of lymphocytes, mostly CD4+ helper T cells. Very rarely, central necrosis is present. In chronic disease the granulomas may become enclosed within fibrous rims or eventually be replaced by hyaline fibrous scars. Two other microscopic features are often present in the granulomas: (1) Schaumann bodies, laminated concretions composed of calcium and proteins; and (2) asteroid bodies, stellate inclusions enclosed within giant cells. Their presence is not required for diagnosis of sarcoidosis; they may also occur in granulomas of other origins.

The lungs are a common site of involvement. In approximately one third of all patients, pulmonary infiltrates and hilar adenopathy can be seen in chest radiographs. Microscopic lesions are distributed throughout the parenchyma, usually bilaterally, with some tendency to localize in the walls of peribronchiolar and perivenular lymphatics. The granulomas may be cellular, with collections of macrophages surrounded by lymphocytic infiltrates, or they may exhibit variable amounts of fibrosis. In a minority of patients the granulomas are eventually replaced by diffuse interstitial fibro-

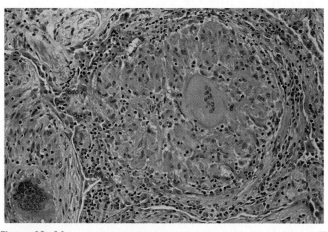

Figure 13–16 ■

Characteristic sarcoid noncaseating granulomas in lung with many giant cells. (Courtesy of Dr. Ramon Bianco, Department of Pathology, Brigham and Women's Hospital, Boston.)

sis accompanied by pulmonary artery sclerosis and cor pulmonale.

Skin lesions are encountered in one third to one half of the cases. Sarcoidosis of the skin assumes a variety of macroscopic appearances (e.g., discrete subcutaneous nodules; focal, slightly elevated, erythematous plaques; violaceous indurated lesions involving ear, lips, or nose). Lesions may also appear on the mucous membranes of the oral cavity and upper respiratory tract. In all instances, these lesions reveal noncaseating granulomas.

Involvement of the eye, lacrimal glands, and salivary glands occurs in about one fifth to one half of the cases. The ocular involvement takes the form of iritis or iridocyclitis and may be unilateral or bilateral. As a consequence, corneal opacities, glaucoma, and (less commonly) total loss of vision may develop. The posterior uveal tract is also affected, with resultant choroiditis, retinitis, and optic nerve involvement. These ocular lesions are frequently accompanied by inflammation in the lacrimal glands, with suppression of lacrimation. When bilateral sarcoidosis of the parotid, submaxillary, and sublingual glands occurs, the combined uveoparotid involvement is designated **Mikulicz's syndrome.**

The spleen may appear unaffected grossly, but in about three quarters of cases it contains granulomas. In approximately 20% it becomes enlarged.

The liver demonstrates microscopic granulomatous lesions, usually in portal triads, about as often as the spleen, but only about one third of the patients demonstrate hepatomegaly or abnormal liver function.

Less frequently affected organs include kidneys, bones, joints, muscles, and endocrine glands. Bone lesions, usually involving the short bones of the hands and feet, can be identified in 3% to 5% of patients. Sometimes there is hypercalcemia and hypercalciuria. This is not related to bone destruction but rather is due to increased calcium absorption secondary to production of active vitamin D by the mononuclear phagocytes in the granulomas.

Clinical Course. In many patients the disease is entirely asymptomatic, discovered on routine chest films as bilateral hilar adenopathy or as an incidental finding at autopsy. In others, peripheral lymphadenopathy, cutaneous lesions, eye involvement, splenomegaly, or hepatomegaly may be presenting manifestations. In about two thirds of symptomatic cases, there is a gradual appearance of respiratory symptoms (shortness of breath, cough, or vague substernal discomfort) or constitutional signs and symptoms (fever, fatigue, weight loss, anorexia, night sweats). Occasionally, the presentation takes the form of a systemic hypersensitivity reaction with fever, erythema nodosum, and polyarthritis associated with bilateral hilar adenopathy or, alternatively, eye and salivary gland involvement (Mikulicz's syndrome). Because of the

variable and nondiagnostic clinical features, resort is frequently made to lung or lymph node biopsy. *The presence of noncaseating granulomas is suggestive of sarcoidosis, but other identifiable causes of granulomatous inflammation must be excluded.*

Sarcoidosis follows an unpredictable course characterized by either progressive chronicity or periods of activity interspersed with remissions. The remissions may be spontaneous or initiated by steroid therapy and are often permanent. Overall, 65% to 70% of affected patients recover with minimal or no residual manifestations. Twenty per cent develop permanent lung dysfunction or visual impairment. Of the remaining 10% to 15%, most succumb to progressive pulmonary fibrosis and cor pulmonale.

HYPERSENSITIVITY PNEUMONITIS

Hypersensitivity pneumonitis is an immunologically mediated inflammatory lung disease that primarily affects the alveoli and is therefore often called *allergic alveolitis*. Most often it is an occupational disease that results from heightened sensitivity to inhaled antigens in the form of organic dusts such as moldy hay (Table 13–3). Unlike bronchial asthma, in *which bronchi are the focus of immunologically mediated injury, the damage in hypersensitivity pneumonitis occurs at the level of alveoli.* Hence, it presents as a predominantly restrictive lung disease with decreased diffusing capacity, lung compliance, and total lung volume. The occupational exposures are diverse, but each syndrome shares common clinical and pathologic findings, and probably very similar pathophysiology.

Hypersensitivity pneumonitis may present either as an *acute reaction* with fever, cough, dyspnea, and constitutional complaints 4 to 8 hours after exposure or as a *chronic disease*

■

Table 13–3. SELECTED CAUSES OF HYPERSENSITIVITY PNEUMONITIS

Syndrome	Exposure	Antigens
Microbes Contaminating Vegetable Matter or Water		
Farmer's lung	Moldy hay	Various actinomycetes, *Aspergillus* spp.
Bagassosis	Moldy pressed sugar cane (bagasse)	Thermophilic actinomycetes
Maple bark disease	Maple bark	*Cryptostroma corticale*
Humidifier lung	Cool-mist humidifier	Thermophilic actinomycetes, *Aureobasidium pullulans,* protozoal proteins
Animal Products		
Pigeon breeder's lung	Pigeons	Pigeon serum proteins in droppings
Chemicals		
Trimellitic anhydride pneumonia	Chemical industry	Haptenated protein

with insidious onset of cough, dyspnea, malaise, and weight loss. In all probability, acute syndromes result from the combination of (1) a direct irritant effect, (2) activation of the alternate complement pathway (perhaps because the inhaled material is contaminated by endotoxin), and (3) immune complex- and T cell-mediated injury. The chronic form of the disease is mediated almost entirely by delayed hypersensitivity reactions.

> **MORPHOLOGY.** The histopathology of both acute and chronic forms of hypersensitivity pneumonitis demonstrates mononuclear cell infiltrates in the alveoli and alveolar walls and around terminal bronchioles. Lymphocytes predominate, but plasma cells and large foamy macrophages are also present. In acute forms of the disease, variable numbers of neutrophils may also be seen. Interstitial noncaseating granulomas reflecting type IV hypersensitivity reaction are present in more than two thirds of cases. In advanced chronic cases, diffuse interstitial fibrosis occurs.

The clinical course is variable. If antigenic exposure is terminated after acute attacks of the disease, fever and cough usually last a few days, and constitutional complaints clear in several weeks. The chronic form of the disease resolves more slowly, and most patients continue to experience mild to moderate symptoms. In a small number of cases (about 5%), respiratory failure and death may occur.

DIFFUSE PULMONARY HEMORRHAGE SYNDROMES

Hemorrhage in the lung is a dramatic complication of some interstitial and vascular lung disorders. These so-called pulmonary hemorrhage syndromes include (1) Goodpasture's syndrome, (2) idiopathic pulmonary hemosiderosis, and (3) vasculitis-associated hemorrhage.

Goodpasture's syndrome is an uncommon but intriguing condition characterized by a crescentic, usually rapidly progressive, glomerulonephritis (Chapter 14) and hemorrhagic interstitial pneumonitis. Both the renal and pulmonary lesions are caused by antibodies to antigens common to glomerular and pulmonary basement membranes. These antibodies can be detected in the serum of over 90% of patients. The immunopathogenesis of Goodpasture's syndrome and the changes in the glomeruli are discussed in Chapter 14. It suffices to say that most cases begin clinically with respiratory symptoms, principally hemoptysis, and with radiographic evidence of bilateral fluffy infiltrates.

> Microscopic examination of the lungs demonstrates focal necrosis of alveolar walls associated with intra-alveolar hemorrhages, fibrous thickening of the septa, and hypertrophy of septal lining cells. The once dismal prognosis for this disease has been markedly improved by plasma-
> pheresis and immunosuppressive therapy. Plasma exchange removes offending antibodies, and immunosuppressive drugs inhibit antibody production. With severe renal disease, renal transplantation is eventually required.

Idiopathic pulmonary hemosiderosis is an uncommon pulmonary disease of uncertain cause that usually presents with insidious onset of productive cough, hemoptysis, anemia, and weight loss, and with pulmonary infiltrates on x-ray examination. Microscopically, the lung reveals intra-alveolar hemorrhage with hemosiderin-filled macrophages. There is mild to moderate interstitial fibrosis. The pulmonary manifestations are similar to those of Goodpasture's syndrome, but there is no associated renal disease or circulating anti-basement membrane antibody. Clinically, the course is usually mild to moderate, with periods of activity followed by prolonged remissions, and often spontaneous remission.

Vasculitis-associated hemorrhage is infrequent but can occur in some conditions, most commonly in systemic lupus erythematosus, Wegener's granulomatosis, and microscopic polyangitis (microscopic polyarteritis) (Chapter 10). In this group there is necrotizing inflammation of the pulmonary capillaries. Although pulmonary manifestations in lupus are common, pulmonary hemorrhage occurs in only 2%. In Wegener's granulomatosis, mild intra-alveolar hemorrhage is present in up to 50% of cases, but massive hemorrhage is much less frequent. Alveolar hemorrhage occurs in about one third of patients with microscopic polyangitis.

■ VASCULAR LUNG DISEASES

Pulmonary Thromboembolism, Hemorrhage, and Infarction

The embolization of venous and right-sided cardiac thrombi to the lungs is an extremely important clinical problem. Indeed, pulmonary thromboembolism is the most common preventable cause of death in hospitalized patients. In total, thromboembolism causes approximately 50,000 deaths per year in the United States. Even when not directly fatal, it can complicate the course of other diseases. The true incidence of nonfatal pulmonary embolism is not known. Some emboli undoubtedly occur outside the hospital in ambulatory patients and are small and clinically silent. Even among hospitalized patients, not more than one third are diagnosed before death. Moreover, when the diagnosis of a fatal pulmonary embolism is made clinically, postmortem examination fails to document the presence of emboli in approximately 50% of cases. Unfortunately, autopsy data on the incidence of pulmonary emboli vary widely, ranging from less than 1% to the extreme of 64%. If only fatal pulmonary emboli are considered, they are detected at postmortem examination in about 0.3% of hospitalized patients who have medical diseases, 1% of patients who have undergone surgery, and 5% to 8% of patients with hip fractures.

More than 95% of all pulmonary emboli arise from thrombi

within the large deep veins of the lower legs, typically originating in the popliteal vein and larger veins above it. Thromboemboli do not commonly arise from superficial or smaller leg veins. Even when a patient has a well-documented pulmonary embolus, deep vein thrombosis can be identified clinically in only 20% to 70% of instances; this variation reflects whether or not invasive procedures such as venography were used.

The influences that predispose to venous thrombosis in the legs were discussed in Chapter 4, but the following risk factors should be emphasized: (1) prolonged bed rest (particularly with immobilization of the legs), (2) surgery on the legs (as following knee surgery), (3) severe trauma (including burns or multiple fractures), (4) congestive heart failure, (5) women in the period around parturition or who take birth control pills with high estrogen content (those who are carriers of a mutation in the coagulant factor V are particularly vulnerable) (Chapters 4 and 8), and (6) disseminated cancer.

The pathophysiologic consequences of thromboembolism in the lung depend largely on the size of the embolus, which in turn dictates the size of the occluded pulmonary artery, and on the cardiopulmonary status of the patient. There are two important consequences of embolic pulmonary arterial occlusion: (1) an increase in pulmonary artery pressure due to blockage of flow and, possibly, vasospasm caused by neurogenic mechanisms and/or release of mediators (e.g., thromboxane A_2 and serotonin); and (2) ischemia of the downstream pulmonary parenchyma. Thus, occlusion of a *major vessel* results in a sudden increase in pulmonary artery pressure, diminished cardiac output, right-sided heart failure (acute cor pulmonale), or even death. Usually hypoxemia develops, as a result of multiple mechanisms:

■ *Perfusion of lung zones that have become atelectatic.* The alveolar collapse occurs in the ischemic areas because of a reduction in surfactant production, and because pain associated with embolism leads to reduced movement of the chest wall; in addition, some of the pulmonary blood flow is redirected through areas of the lung that are normally hypoventilated.
■ The decrease in cardiac output causes a *widening of the difference in arterial-venous oxygen saturation.*
■ *Right-to-left shunting* of blood may occur in some patients through a patent foramen ovale, present in 30% of normal persons.

If *smaller vessels* are occluded, the result is less catastrophic and the event may even be clinically silent.

Recall that lung is oxygenated not only by the pulmonary arteries but also by bronchial arteries and directly from air in the alveoli. If the bronchial circulation is normal and adequate ventilation is maintained, the resultant decrease in blood flow does not cause tissue necrosis. Indeed, ischemic necrosis (infarction) resulting from pulmonary thromboembolism is the exception rather than the rule, occurring in as few as 10% of cases. It occurs only if there is compromise in cardiac function or bronchial circulation, or if the region of the lung at risk is underventilated owing to underlying pulmonary disease.

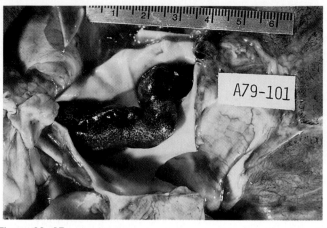

Figure 13–17 ■

Large saddle embolus from the femoral vein lying astride the main left and right pulmonary arteries. (From the teaching collection of the Department of Pathology, University of Texas Southwestern Medical School, Dallas, TX.)

MORPHOLOGY. The morphologic consequences of pulmonary embolism, as noted, depend on the size of the embolic mass and the general state of the circulation. Large emboli impact in the main pulmonary artery or its major branches or lodge astride the bifurcation as a saddle embolus (Fig. 13–17). Death usually follows so suddenly from hypoxia or acute failure of the right side of the heart (acute cor pulmonale) that there is no time for morphologic alterations in the lung.

Smaller emboli become impacted in medium-sized and small pulmonary arteries. With adequate circulation and bronchial arterial flow, the vitality of the lung parenchyma is maintained, but the alveolar spaces may fill with blood to produce pulmonary hemorrhage as a result of ischemic damage to the endothelial cells.

With compromised cardiovascular status, as may occur with congestive heart failure, **infarction** results. The more peripheral the embolic occlusion, the more likely is infarction. About three fourths of all infarcts affect the lower lobes, and more than half are multiple. They vary in size from lesions barely visible to involvement of large parts of a lobe. Characteristically, they are wedge shaped, with their base at the pleural surface and the apex pointing toward the hilus of the lung. Pulmonary infarcts are typically hemorrhagic and appear as raised, red-blue areas in the early stages (Fig. 13–18). The adjacent pleural surface is often covered by a fibrinous exudate. If the occluded vessel can be identified, it is usually found near the apex of the infarcted area. The red cells begin to lyse within 48 hours, and the infarct pales, eventually becoming red-brown as hemosiderin is produced. In time, fibrous replacement begins at the margins as a gray-white peripheral zone and

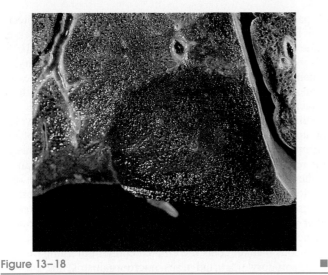

Figure 13–18   ■

A recent small, roughly wedge-shaped hemorrhagic pulmonary infarct.

eventually converts the infarct into a scar that is contracted below the level of the lung substance. Histologically, the hallmark of fresh infarcts is coagulative necrosis of the lung parenchyma in the area of hemorrhage.

Clinical Course. The clinical consequences of pulmonary thromboembolism are summarized here:

■ Most pulmonary emboli (60% to 80%) are clinically silent because they are small; the embolic mass is rapidly removed by fibrinolytic activity, and the bronchial circulation sustains the viability of the affected lung parenchyma until this is accomplished.

■ In 5% of cases, sudden death, acute right-sided heart failure (acute cor pulmonale), or cardiovascular collapse (shock) may occur when more than 60% of the total pulmonary vasculature is obstructed by a large embolus or multiple, simultaneous, small emboli. Massive pulmonary embolism is one of the few causes of literally instantaneous death, even before the patient experiences chest pain or dyspnea.

■ Obstruction of relatively small to medium pulmonary branches (10% to 15% of cases) that behave as end-arteries causes pulmonary infarction when some element of circulatory insufficiency is present. Typically, patients who sustain an infarct manifest dyspnea, the basis of which is not fully understood.

■ In a small but significant subset of patients (less than 3%), recurrent multiple emboli lead to pulmonary hypertension, chronic right-sided heart strain (chronic cor pulmonale), and, in time, pulmonary vascular sclerosis with progressively worsening dyspnea.

Emboli usually resolve after the initial acute insult. They contract, and endogenous fibrinolytic activity may cause total lysis of the thrombus. However, in the presence of an underlying predisposing factor, a small innocuous embolus may presage a larger one, and *patients who have experienced one*

pulmonary embolus have a 30% chance of developing a second. Thus, recognition and appropriate preventive treatment are essential. Prophylactic therapy includes early ambulation for postoperative and postpartum patients, elastic stockings, and isometric leg exercises for bedridden patients. Anticoagulation is warranted for persons at high risk. Patients with pulmonary embolism are given thrombolytic and anticoagulation therapy.

Pulmonary Hypertension and Vascular Sclerosis

Pulmonary hypertension is most often caused by a decrease in the cross-sectional area of the pulmonary vascular bed, but it may also result from increased pulmonary vascular blood flow. It is most frequently *secondary* to (1) chronic obstructive or interstitial lung disease, (2) recurrent pulmonary emboli, or (3) heart disease in which there is a left-to-right shunt. Rarely (less than 5% of cases), pulmonary hypertension exists even though all known causes of increased pulmonary pressure can be excluded; this is referred to as primary, or *idiopathic, pulmonary hypertension*. Distinction of primary hypertension from that caused by recurrent thromboembolism may be particularly difficult, but angiography and radioisotope scanning may be helpful. Table 13–4 provides an overview of causes of pulmonary hypertension.

Because many of the diseases that give rise to secondary pulmonary vascular hypertension have already been discussed, only primary pulmonary hypertension is considered here. It should be stated at the outset that the mechanism of primary pulmonary hypertension is not known. According to current thinking, chronic vasoconstriction resulting from vascular hyperreactivity gives rise to pulmonary hypertension and, in time, its morphologic counterpart, intimal and medial vascular hypertrophy. The importance of vascular hyperreactivity is supported by the fact that about 10% of patients with primary pulmonary hypertension suffer from vasospastic disorders such as Raynaud's phenomenon (Chapter 10). In

■

Table 13–4.   CAUSES OF PULMONARY HYPERTENSION AND VASCULAR SCLEROSIS

Secondary Pulmonary Hypertension
Cardiac disease: Left-to-right shunts: septal defects; mechanical obstructions; atrial myxoma, mitral stenosis
Inflammatory vascular disease: Scleroderma and other connective tissue diseases; other forms of vasculitis
Lung disease: Chronic hypoxia: high-altitude hypoxia, extraparenchymal restrictive lung diseases (obesity); chronic hypoxia with destruction of vascular bed: COPD, chronic interstitial fibrosing diseases, pneumoconiosis
Recurrent thromboembolism*
Primary Pulmonary Hypertension
Plexiform pulmonary arteriopathy (30%–70% of cases)
Thrombotic pulmonary arteriopathy (20%–50% of cases)*
Pulmonary venoocclusive disease (~10% of cases)

* These two diseases are difficult to distinguish clinically or morphologically.
COPD, chronic obstructive pulmonary disease.

addition, pulmonary vascular resistance can sometimes be rapidly decreased with vasodilators. The hyperreactivity is believed to be secondary to endothelial dysfunction and injury, idiopathic in most cases but sometimes associated with autoimmune diseases such as scleroderma and systemic lupus erythematosus. Endothelial dysfunction manifests as reduced production of prostacyclin and NO and increased generation of endothelin, all of which promote vasoconstriction. Endothelial cells may also elaborate growth factors that induce migration and proliferation of smooth muscle cells, responsible for vascular thickening.

MORPHOLOGY. Vascular alterations in all forms of pulmonary sclerosis (primary and secondary) involve the entire arterial tree and include (1) in the main elastic arteries, atheromas similar to those in systemic atherosclerosis; (2) in medium-sized muscular arteries, proliferation of myointimal cells and smooth muscle cells, causing thickening of the intima and media with narrowing of the lumina; and (3) in smaller arteries and arterioles, thickening, medial hypertrophy, and reduplication of the internal and external elastic membranes. In these vessels the wall thickness may exceed the diameter of the lumen, which is sometimes narrowed to the point of near obliteration. In patients with severe, long-standing primary pulmonary hypertension, additional changes take the form of plexiform lesions and necrotizing arteritis with fibrinoid necrosis and thrombosis. The plexiform lesions consist of a multichanneled outpouching of the pulmonary arterial wall. These may represent aneurysmal dilation of the vessel wall or reparative lesions in areas of previous fibrinoid necrosis.

Clinical Course. *Secondary pulmonary vascular sclerosis* may develop at any age. The clinical features reflect the underlying disease, usually pulmonary or cardiac, with accentuation of respiratory insufficiency and right-sided heart strain. *Primary pulmonary vascular sclerosis,* on the other hand, is almost always encountered in young persons, more commonly women, and is marked by fatigue, syncope (particularly on exercise), dyspnea on exertion, and sometimes chest pain. These patients eventually develop severe respiratory insufficiency and sometimes cyanosis. In patients with primary pulmonary hypertension, death usually results from right-sided heart failure within a few years of the diagnosis. Some amelioration of the respiratory distress can be achieved by vasodilators, but without lung transplantation the prognosis is grim.

PULMONARY INFECTIONS

Pulmonary infections in the form of pneumonia are responsible for one sixth of all deaths in the United States. This is not surprising because (1) the epithelial surfaces of the lung are constantly exposed to liters of variously contaminated air;

(2) nasopharyngeal flora are regularly aspirated during sleep, even by healthy persons; and (3) other common lung diseases render the lung parenchyma vulnerable to virulent organisms. It is therefore a small miracle that the normal lung parenchyma remains sterile. This attests to the efficiency of a series of pulmonary defense mechanisms. We will briefly review these to facilitate an understanding of lung infections.

Pulmonary defenses can be divided into those that involve the upper airways (from the nasopharynx to the level of the terminal bronchioles) and those that involve the lower airways (the respiratory bronchioles and distal airspaces). They can be further categorized into those that are immune and those that are not. Nonimmunologic defense mechanisms are important not only in protecting against microbes but also in removing other particulates. Microorganisms in the air drawn through the nose may be filtered out by vibrissae lining the mucosa. A mucous blanket coats the ciliated epithelium lining the upper respiratory tract and traps microorganisms; the coordinated beating of the cilia propels the debris-laden mucous layer to the pharynx, where it can be swallowed or expectorated. Coughing enhances the function of this mucociliary elevator.

In the air-exchanging spaces of the lung comprising the lower respiratory tract, mucous and ciliated cells are absent, so resident alveolar macrophages serve as the primary defense mechanism. If this vigilant cell is overwhelmed, it secretes mediators that increase vascular permeability and local levels of complement and recruit neutrophils. A primary immune response is initiated in the regional lymph nodes. A humoral response gives rise to IgA, which finds its way to the surface of the trachea, bronchi, and bronchioles. This immunoglobulin effectively blocks the epithelial attachment of a number of pathogenic microorganisms, including mycoplasmas and viruses. Serum immunoglobulins of all classes enter the alveolar lining fluid, particularly in the presence of local inflammation. Induction of cell-mediated immunity generates sensitized T cells, which accumulate in the interstitium and alveolar spaces. If the host is immune to the microorganism because of previous exposure, immune defenses amplify the nonspecific mechanisms. These mechanisms are summarized in Figure 13–19. From this review it can be predicted that abnormalities affecting either nonimmune or immune defense mechanisms predispose to lung infections.

Defects in nonimmune defenses (including neutrophil and complement defects) and humoral immunodeficiency typically lead to an increased incidence of infections with pyogenic bacteria. On the other hand, cell-mediated immune defects lead to increased infections with intracellular microbes such as mycobacteria and herpesviruses as well as with microorganisms of very low virulence such as *Pneumocystis carinii.* Several of these infectious agents will be discussed after a general review of pneumonias.

Pneumonia can be very broadly defined as any infection in the lung (Table 13–5). It may present as acute, fulminant clinical disease or as chronic disease with a more protracted course. A given pathogen usually causes only one of these forms of pneumonia (Table 13–5). *Acute pneumonias* may be caused by pyogenic bacteria that induce primarily neutrophilic exudates in alveoli, bronchioles, and bronchi or by a miscellaneous group of microorganisms that induce predominantly peribronchiolar and interstitial mononuclear inflammation. As

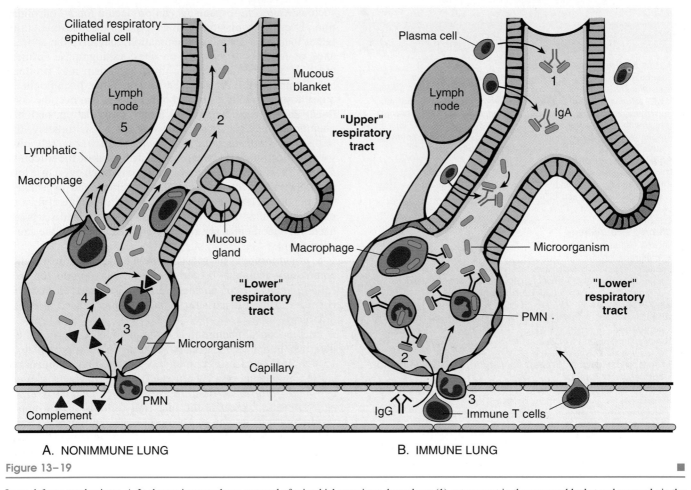

Figure 13–19   ■

Lung defense mechanisms. *A,* In the nonimmune lung, removal of microbial organisms depends on (1) entrapment in the mucous blanket and removal via the mucociliary elevator, (2) phagocytosis by alveolar macrophages that can kill and degrade organisms and remove them from the airspaces by migrating onto the mucociliary elevator, or (3) phagocytosis and killing by neutrophils recruited by macrophage factors. 4, Serum complement may enter the alveoli and be activated by the alternate pathway to provide the opsonin C3b that enhances phagocytosis. 5, Organisms, including those ingested by phagocytes, may reach the draining lymph nodes to initiate immune responses. *B,* Additional mechanisms operate in the immune lung. 1, Secreted IgA can block attachment of the microorganism to epithelium in the upper respiratory tract. 2, In the lower respiratory tract, serum antibodies (IgM, IgG) are present in the alveolar lining fluid. They activate complement more efficiently by the classic pathway, yielding C3b *(not shown).* In addition, IgG is opsonic. 3, The accumulation of immune T cells is important for controlling infections by viruses and other intracellular microorganisms.

commonly used, the term *pneumonia* usually refers to the acute bacterial pneumonias, whereas the term *pneumonitis* is reserved for inflammatory conditions that primarily affect the interstitium and present clinically as "atypical" pneumonias. In contrast to these two forms of acute pneumonias, *chronic pneumonias* are usually caused by fungi, parasites, and intracellular bacteria as well as by the filamentous bacteria, *Nocardia* and *Actinomyces* species. With this background we can discuss pulmonary infections by individual bacterial, viral, and fungal agents. This presentation follows the general sequence outlined in Table 13–5.

Acute Bacterial Pneumonias

Bacterial pneumonias are typically associated with intraalveolar exudation resulting in *consolidation* (solidification) of lung parenchyma. They tend to conform to one of two anatomic and radiographic patterns, referred to as *lobar pneumonia* and *bronchopneumonia*. In lobar pneumonia the contiguous airspaces of part or all of a lobe are homogeneously filled with an exudate that can be visualized on radiographs as a lobar or segmental consolidation, and is thus sometimes referred to as *airspace pneumonia* (Fig. 13–20A). In contrast, bronchopneumonia implies a patchy distribution of inflammation that generally involves more than one lobe (Fig. 13–20B). This pattern results from an initial infection of the bronchi and bronchioles with extension into the adjacent alveoli. Certain organisms tend to cause bronchopneumonia, whereas others such as *Streptococcus pneumoniae* tend to produce a lobar pattern. More than 90% of lobar pneumonias are caused by *S. pneumoniae,* sometimes referred to as *pneumococcus,* so this pattern is usually predictive of this specific pathogen. It should be noted, however, that the causal associations are not clear-cut. For example, less commonly, other bacteria

Table 13-5. LUNG INFECTIONS

Acute Bacterial Pneumonias

Community-acquired, often following influenza: *Streptococcus pneumoniae* (single most common cause), *Haemophilus influenzae*, *Staphylococcus aureus*, *Klebsiella pneumoniae* and other gram-negative rods, *Legionella pneumophilia*, aspiration pneumoniae with mixed aerobes and anaerobes, *Moraxella catarrhalis*

Hospital-acquired (nosocomial): *Pseudomonas* spp., other gram-negative bacilli, *S. aureus*, commonly penicillin resistant

Atypical Pneumonias

Mycoplasma pneumoniae

Viruses: Children: respiratory syncytial virus, parainfluenza virus; adults: influenza A and B, adenovirus (in military recruits)

Chlamydia (C. psittaci, C. trachomatis, and *C. pneumoniae)*

Rickettsiae *(Coxiella burnetii, Rickettsia rickettsii)*

Chronic Pneumonias

Nocardia spp.

Actinomyces spp.

Granulomatous: *Mycobacterium tuberculosis* and atypical mycobacteria, *Histoplasma capsulatum, Coccidioides immitis, Blastomyces dermatitidis, Paracoccidioides brasiliensis*

Lung Abscesses

Mixed anaerobes, with or without accompanying aerobes (particularly *Streptococcus* spp.)

Aerobes, uncommonly isolated alone: *S. aureus, Streptococcus* spp., *K. pneumoniae, Nocardia* spp.

Pneumonias Largely Limited to Neutropenic or Immunosuppressed Persons*

Cytomegalovirus

Pneumocystis carinii (particularly in AIDS)

Mycobacterium avium-intracellulare

Invasive aspergillosis

Invasive candidiasis

* These patients are also at increased risk for the development of pneumonias caused by most of the other agents in this listing, particularly gram-negative bacilli.

■

such as *Klebsiella* organisms can produce a lobar consolidation. Even mycoplasmas, which typically cause interstitial rather than intra-alveolar inflammation, may give the appearance of lobar consolidation on chest radiographs. Furthermore, as will be discussed, a given organism may produce bronchopneumonia in one setting and lobar pneumonia in other hosts. Sometimes bronchopneumonia can become confluent and induce almost total lobar consolidation, or lobar pneumonia may not involve an entire lobe. Ultimately, the terms *bronchopneumonia* and *lobar pneumonia* merely give some indication of the anatomic distribution of the infection and the likely causative agent, but there is much overlap. More significant is the total amount of involvement and, especially, the identity of the specific invader and its vulnerability to particular antibiotics. Therefore, in the ensuing discussion, bacterial pneumonias are categorized on the basis of the causative agent.

S. pneumoniae is the most common bacterial cause of acute community-acquired bacterial pneumonia, producing socalled *pneumococcal pneumonia.* This is described first and is followed by a discussion of pneumonias caused by other organisms.

Pneumococcal pneumonia occurs in all age groups, but elders and infants are particularly vulnerable. Approximately 15% to 25% of cases of community-acquired pneumonias are caused by pneumococci. *Individuals with underlying congestive heart failure, COPD, diabetes, or alcoholism are especially prone.* Typically, the infection follows a viral upper respiratory tract infection. The onset is abrupt, with high fever and an episode of a severe shaking chill accompanied by pleuritic chest pain and a cough productive of rusty-colored purulent sputum.

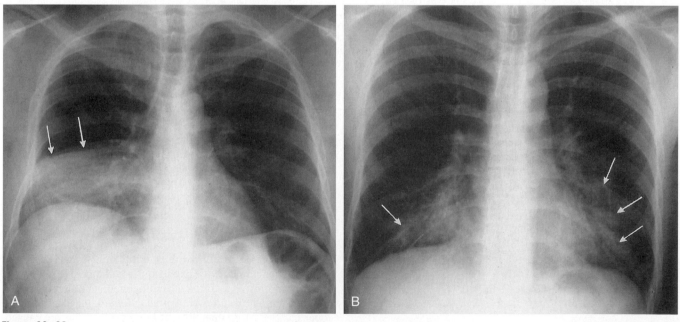

Figure 13-20

■

A, Chest radiograph of lobar pneumonia involving the right lower lobes. Arrows demonstrate the interlobar fissure. *B,* Radiograph of bronchopneumonia illustrating the patchy distribution of the infiltrates. The arrows demonstrate patches in the right and left lower lobes. (Courtesy of Dr. Michael Landay, Department of Radiology, University of Texas Southwestern Medical School, Dallas, TX.)

MORPHOLOGY. With pneumococcal lung infection, either pattern of pneumonia, lobar or bronchopneumonia, may occur; the latter is much more prevalent at the extremes of age. Regardless of the distribution of the pneumonia, because pneumococcal lung infections usually originate by aspiration of pharyngeal flora (20% of adults harbor *S. pneumoniae* in their throats), the lower lobes or the right middle lobe are most frequently involved.

In the preantibiotic era, pneumococcal pneumonia involved whole or almost whole lobes and evolved through four stages: congestion, red hepatization, gray hepatization, and resolution. Early antibiotic therapy alters or halts this typical progression, so if the patient dies the anatomic changes seen at autopsy may not conform to the classic stages.

During the first stage, that of congestion, the affected lobe(s) is (are) heavy, red, and boggy; histologically, vascular congestion can be seen, with proteinaceous fluid, scattered neutrophils (Fig. 13–21), and many bacteria in the alveoli. Within a few days the stage of red hepatization ensues, in which the lung lobe is liver-like in consistency; the alveolar spaces are packed with neutrophils, red cells, and fibrin; and the pleura usually demonstrates a fibrinous or fibrinopurulent exudate. In the next stage, gray hepatization, the lung is dry, gray, and firm, and the fibrinous exudate persists within the alveoli but is relatively depleted of red cells (Fig. 13–22). Resolution follows in uncomplicated cases, as exudates within the alveoli are enzymatically digested and either resorbed or expectorated, leaving the basic architecture intact. The pleural reaction may similarly resolve or undergo organization, leaving fibrous thickening or permanent adhesions.

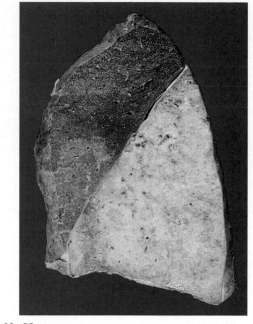

Figure 13–22   ■

Gross view of lobar pneumonia with gray hepatization. The lower lobe is uniformly consolidated.

In the bronchopneumonic pattern, foci of inflammatory consolidation are distributed in patches throughout one or several lobes, most frequently bilateral and basal. Well-developed lesions up to 3 or 4 cm in diameter are slightly elevated and are gray-red to yellow; confluence of these foci may occur in severe cases, producing the appearance of a lobar consolidation. The lung substance immediately surrounding areas of consolidation is usually hyperemic and edematous, but the large intervening areas are generally normal. Pleural involvement is less common than in lobar pneumonia. Histologically, the reaction consists of focal suppurative exudate that fills the bronchi, bronchioles, and adjacent alveolar spaces (Fig. 13–23).

With appropriate therapy, complete restitution of the lung is the rule for both forms of pneumococcal pneumonia, but in occasional cases complications may occur: (1) tissue destruction and necrosis may lead to **abscess** formation; (2) suppurative material may accumulate in the pleural cavity, producing an **empyema**; (3) organization of the intraalveolar exudate may convert areas of the lung into solid fibrous tissue; and (4) bacteremic dissemination may lead to **meningitis, arthritis,** or **infective endocarditis.** Complications are much more likely with serotype 3 pneumococci.

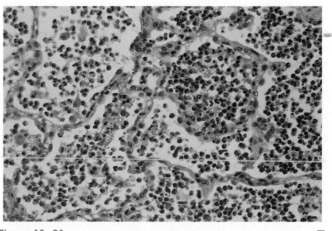

Figure 13–21   ■

Acute pneumonia at the stage of early red hepatization with congested septal capillaries and extensive white cell exudation into alveoli. Fibrin nets have not yet formed.

Examination of Gram-stained sputum is an important step in the diagnosis of acute pneumonia. The presence of numerous neutrophils containing the typical gram-positive, lancet-shaped diplococci is good evidence of pneumococcal pneu-

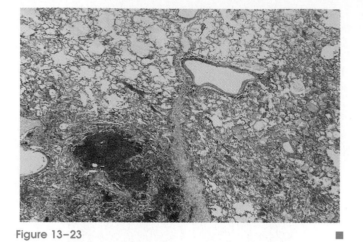

Figure 13–23 ■

Bronchopneumonia. Lower lung fields show a pink area of consolidation in which the alveoli are filled with an exudate. A large purple aggregate within the area of consolidation represents bronchiole filled with neutrophils. In the upper field, relatively normal alveoli can be seen.

monia, but it must be remembered that *S. pneumoniae* is a part of the endogenous flora, and therefore false-positive results may be obtained by this method. Isolation of pneumococci from blood cultures is more specific. During early phases of illness, blood cultures may be positive in 20% to 30% of patients.

Pneumococcal pneumonias respond readily to penicillin treatment, but there is an increasing awareness of penicillin-resistant strains of pneumococci, so whenever possible antibiotic sensitivity should be determined.

Haemophilus influenzae, a small, gram-negative coccobacillus long known to be a common cause of meningitis in children, is increasingly recognized as an important lung pathogen. Encapsulated *H. influenzae* type b is also an important cause of epiglottitis in children. Both unencapsulated and encapsulated forms are important causes of bronchopneumonias after viral infections and in patients with chronic pulmonary diseases such as cystic fibrosis, chronic bronchitis, and bronchiectasis. The morphologic changes are indistinguishable from those of other bacterial bronchopneumonias. *H. influenzae* pneumonia is typically milder than other forms of pneumonia, has a more insidious onset, and in adults rarely results in abscess formation or empyema. Children are more likely to develop empyema and extrapulmonary complications such as otitis media, epiglottitis, arthritis, pericarditis, or meningitis.

Staphylococcus aureus is also an important cause of secondary bacterial pneumonia in children and healthy adults after viral respiratory illnesses: measles in children and influenza in both children and adults. *S. aureus* may also cause a primary pneumonia in persons with chronic pulmonary disease, a particularly serious problem in hospitalized patients who are intubated or suffer aspiration. Hospital-acquired infections are of particular concern because the causative strains are frequently penicillin resistant and a significant minority (5%) are unresponsive to most antibiotics. Staphylococcal pneumonia occurring in association with right-sided staphylococcal endocarditis is a serious complication of intravenous

drug abuse. Most often *S. aureus* causes bronchopneumonia with formation of multiple abscesses, but occasionally it can produce a lobar pattern of consolidation.

Klebsiella pneumoniae is the most common cause of gram-negative bacillary pneumonia, most frequently among debilitated and malnourished persons, particularly chronic alcoholics. The onset is abrupt and prostrating, similar to that of pneumococcal pneumonia, and it may be even more severe. Thick and gelatinous sputum is characteristic because the organism produces an abundant viscid capsular polysaccharide and the patient may have difficulty coughing it up. *The pattern of pneumonia is frequently lobar* and there is a propensity for distention of the lobes, seen as bulging of the interlobar fissures on radiographs. Even with treatment, this type of pneumonia carries a considerably greater mortality rate than does pneumococcal pneumonia. If the patient survives, complete resolution is less frequent, and abscesses, fibrosis, and bronchiectasis may remain.

Legionella pneumophila, the agent of legionnaires' disease, received its colorful name by being recognized first after an epidemic of frequently fatal pneumonia among delegates to the 1976 American Legion convention in Philadelphia. The spread of infection was traced to a contaminated water-cooled air-conditioning system in the convention hotel. It soon became evident, however, that legionnaires' disease occurs endemically and sporadically and is *a common cause of severe pneumonia requiring hospitalization. L. pneumophila* is also frequently involved in hospital-acquired respiratory infections.

Legionella species are gram-negative rods that are ubiquitous in water, particularly standing tepid or warm water. Inhalation of airborne contaminated droplets is the likely mode of spread. *Legionella* pneumonia is unusual in children and is more common in elders and persons with some predisposing condition such as cardiac, renal, immunologic, or hematologic disease. Organ transplant recipients are particularly susceptible. The clinical presentation is indistinguishable from that of pneumonias caused by other bacteria. However, *Legionella* pneumonia is a severe form of lung infection with a fatality rate of about 15%. Mortality is even higher in those who are immunosuppressed. Diagnosis is made by culture of organisms and by direct identification of the bacteria by fluorescent antibody techniques in samples obtained by transtracheal aspiration or bronchoalveolar lavage. *Legionella* antigens are excreted in urine, and thus their detection in urine is helpful, especially in patients who have been partially treated. The diagnosis can also be made retrospectively by demonstrating a rise in antibody titer in acute- and convalescent-phase serum.

Pseudomonas aeruginosa, a common cause of nosocomial (hospital-acquired) pneumonia, occurs almost exclusively in persons who have some defect in natural defenses. It is particularly prone to occur in patients rendered neutropenic, usually by chemotherapy for hematopoietic malignancies; in patients with extensive burns or cystic fibrosis; and in patients requiring mechanical ventilation. *Pseudomonas* pneumonia occurs with or without bacteremia. Nonbacteremic *Pseudomonas* pneumonia presents as a diffuse bronchopneumonia with abscess formation and a high incidence of empyema reminiscent of staphylococcal pneumonia. Bacteremic *Pseudomonas* pneumonia is a progressive, necrotizing pneumonia with prominent blood vessel invasion and consequent extrapulmonary manifestations. Both forms of pneumonia are associated with a high mortality rate.

Aspiration bronchopneumonia occurs in markedly debilitated patients or those who aspirate gastric contents either while unconscious (e.g., after a stroke) or during repeated vomiting. The resultant pneumonia is partly chemical, owing to the extremely irritating effects of the gastric acid, and partly bacterial. The bacterial component is a mixture of anaerobic and microaerophilic organisms normally present in the oral cavity. This type of pneumonia is often necrotizing, pursues a fulminant clinical course, and is a frequent cause of death in patients predisposed to aspiration. In those who survive, abscess formation is a common complication.

Moraxella catarrhalis (formerly *Branhamella catarrhalis*) was once considered a harmless commensal in the nasopharynx. It is now implicated in invasive infectious diseases, including pneumonia, in adults who have underlying COPD. The pneumonia resembles that caused by *H. influenzae*.

Primary Atypical Pneumonias

The concept of primary atypical pneumonia was set forth in 1938 with the description of eight cases in which pharyngitis and systemic flulike symptoms evolved into laryngitis and finally tracheobronchitis and pneumonia. Unlike "typical" acute pneumonias, sputum production was modest, there were no physical findings of consolidation, the white cell count was only moderately elevated, and bacteria and influenza A viruses could not be isolated. In retrospect, these cases were probably caused by *Mycoplasma pneumoniae*. This agent is the most common cause of atypical pneumonias, particularly at times when influenza A epidemics are not present in the community. A similar syndrome may occur with a number of other agents, including viruses, chlamydiae, and rickettsiae. Among these, *Chlamydia pneumoniae* is being increasingly recognized as an important cause of community-acquired atypical pneumonias. Nearly all of these agents can also cause a primarily upper respiratory tract infection with coryza (inflammation with diffuse discharge from the nasal mucosa), pharyngitis, laryngitis, and tracheobronchitis. The common pathogenetic mechanism is attachment of the organisms to the respiratory epithelium followed by necrosis of the cells and an inflammatory response. When the process extends to alveoli there is usually *interstitial* inflammation, but there may also be some outpouring of fluid into alveolar spaces so that on chest films the changes may mimic bacterial pneumonia. Damage to and denudation of the respiratory epithelium inhibits mucociliary clearance and predisposes to secondary bacterial infections. Viral infections of the respiratory tract are well known for this complication.

Mycoplasma infections are particularly common among children and young adults. They occur sporadically or as local epidemics in closed communities (schools, military camps, prisons). Viral lower respiratory tract infections may occur at any age, and in adults they are most often caused by influenza viruses A and B (Table 13–5). Less common offenders are parainfluenza and respiratory syncytial viruses, the latter especially in infants and children. Adenovirus pneumonias are particularly common in young army recruits. A number of other viruses are sometimes implicated, including those that cause measles and chickenpox. Much depends on the resistance of the host, so atypical pneumonias range from mild to severe. More serious lower respiratory tract infection is favored by infancy, old age, malnourishment, alcoholism, and immunosuppression. Not surprisingly, viruses and mycoplasmas are frequently involved in outbreaks of infection in hospitals.

MORPHOLOGY. Regardless of cause, the morphologic patterns in atypical pneumonias are similar. The process may be patchy, or it may involve whole lobes bilaterally or unilaterally. Macroscopically, the affected areas are red-blue, congested, and subcrepitant. Histologically, the inflammatory reaction is largely confined within the walls of the alveoli (Fig. 13–24). The septa are widened and edematous; they usually contain a mononuclear inflammatory infiltrate of lymphocytes, histiocytes, and occasionally plasma cells. In contrast to bacterial pneumonias, alveolar spaces are remarkably free of cellular exudate. In severe cases, however, full-blown **diffuse alveolar damage with hyaline membranes may develop.** In less severe, uncomplicated cases, subsidence of the disease is followed by reconstitution of the native architecture. Superimposed bacterial infection, as expected, results in a mixed histologic picture.

Clinical Course. The clinical course of primary atypical pneumonia is extremely varied, even among cases caused by a single pathogen. It may masquerade as a severe upper respiratory infection or "chest cold" that goes undiagnosed, or it may present as a fulminant, life-threatening infection in immunocompromised patients. More typically, the onset is that of an acute, nonspecific febrile illness characterized by fever, headache, and malaise, and later on cough with minimal sputum. Chest radiographs usually reveal transient, ill-defined patches, mainly in the lower lobes. Physical findings are char-

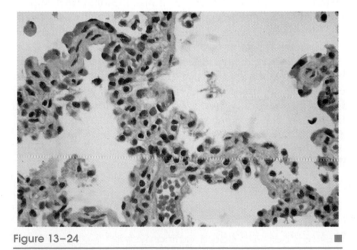

Figure 13–24 ■

Viral pneumonia. The thickened alveolar walls are heavily infiltrated with mononuclear leukocytes.

acteristically minimal, indistinguishable from bronchopneumonia, although, particularly with *Mycoplasma*, lobar consolidations may occur. Because the edema and exudation are both in a strategic position to cause an alveolocapillary block, there may be respiratory distress seemingly out of proportion to the physical and radiographic findings.

Identifying the causative agent is difficult. Indeed, in most cases the pathogen remains undetermined. Culture of the organism is possible but is often difficult. Rising titers of specific antibodies point to the diagnosis, but these results are usually obtained after the patient has begun to recover. Elevations in the titers of cold agglutinins occur in mycoplasmal infection, but this is present in only 50% of cases. Because this test is not specific, it is of only historic interest. Tests for *Mycoplasma* antigens and polymerase chain reaction (PCR) testing for *Mycoplasma* DNA are under development. As a practical matter, patients with community-acquired pneumonia, for which a bacterial agent seems unlikely, are treated with an antibiotic (erythromycin) effective against *Mycoplasma* and *Chlamydia pneumoniae* because these are the most common treatable pathogens.

The prognosis for uncomplicated cases is good; generally, complete recovery is the rule. The most serious infections, caused by influenza viruses in infirm and elderly persons, are often complicated by bacterial superinfection.

Actinomycosis and Nocardiosis

The agents that most commonly cause actinomycosis (*Actinomyces israelii*) and nocardiosis (*Nocardia asteroides*) are bacteria belonging to the order Actinomycetales. These organisms produce chronic infections that are more indolent than those caused by pyogenic bacteria.

A. israelii is a normal anaerobic inhabitant of the oral cavity. There are three classic patterns of actinomycosis: (1) *cervicofacial* (involving the jaw extending into the neck), (2) *thoracic,* and (3) *abdominal and pelvic. A. israelii,* an anaerobe, becomes pathogenic whenever there is devitalization of tissues and reduced oxygen tension. Thus, actinomycosis may develop in the jaw and neck after an intraoral infection or dental surgery, or in the lung or gastrointestinal tract, superimposed on an antecedent disorder (e.g., lung abscess, ulceroinflammatory disease of the gut) that provides a favorable environment for its growth.

Nocardia organisms are aerobic and are not usually normal inhabitants of the oral cavity. They are weakly acid fast (as compared with the mycobacteria), which distinguishes them from other actinomycetes. *Nocardia* infections usually take the form of acute bronchopneumonia with abscess formation, although they may occasionally simulate tuberculosis. Sometimes there is associated empyema. *Nocardia* has a propensity to disseminate and in one third of cases may infect the brain, where it typically causes abscesses.

MORPHOLOGY. The gross appearance of the lesions caused by both actinomycetes is essentially intense suppuration with abscess formation. Within the suppurative exudate, **A. israelii grows in col**ony formation with a tangled mass of filaments surrounded by radiating, sometimes terminally clubbed, organisms. These colonies are grossly visible as yellow to gray "sulfur granules." The branching filaments of *Nocardia* organisms rarely form colonies. Typical of both organisms is great chronicity, burrowing spread of the infection, and (sometimes) the development of penetrating sinus tracts. Thus, lesions in the lung produced by both *A. israelii* and *Nocardia* resemble bronchopneumonia with abscess formation. In time, the abscesses are enclosed by a fibroblastic reaction, but sometimes fistulous sinus tracts penetrate to the pleural cavities or even through the chest wall. The fibroblastic response is much more pronounced in actinomycosis. A similar sequence occurs wherever the organisms become implanted.

The diagnosis must be suspected whenever there is persistent suppurative chronic infection with abscess formation. It can be confirmed by identification of sulfur granules within the inflammatory exudate (actinomycosis) or the characteristic acid-fast forms in smears of exudate (nocardiosis) or culture of the causative agents.

Tuberculosis

Tuberculosis is a communicable chronic granulomatous disease caused by *Mycobacterium tuberculosis.* It usually involves the lungs but may affect any organ or tissue in the body. Typically, the centers of tubercular granulomas undergo caseous necrosis.

Epidemiology. Among medically and economically deprived persons throughout the world, tuberculosis remains a leading cause of death. It is estimated that 1.7 billion individuals are infected worldwide, with 8 to 10 million new cases and 3 million deaths per year. The World Health Organization estimates that tuberculosis causes 6% of all deaths worldwide. In the Western world, deaths due to tuberculosis peaked in 1800 and steadily declined throughout the 1800s and 1900s. However, in 1984 the decline in new cases stopped abruptly, a change that resulted from the increased incidence of tuberculosis in human immunodeficiency virus (HIV)–infected persons. Currently, it is estimated that about 25,000 new cases with active tuberculosis arise in the United States annually, and there is an alarming increase in the proportion of patients infected by multidrug-resistant tubercle bacilli.

It is important that *infection* be differentiated from *disease.* Infection implies seeding of some focus with organisms, which may or may not cause clinically significant tissue damage (i.e., disease). Although other routes may be involved, most infections are acquired by direct person-to-person transmission of airborne droplets of organisms from an active case to a susceptible host. In most persons an asymptomatic focus of pulmonary infection appears that is self-limited, although, uncommonly, primary tuberculosis may result in the development of fever and pleural effusion. Generally, the only evidence of infection, if any remains, is a tiny, telltale fibrocalcific nodule at the site of the infection. Viable organisms may remain dormant in such loci for decades, and possibly for the life of the host. Such persons are infected but do not have active disease and so cannot transmit organisms to others. Yet when their defenses are lowered, the infection may reactivate to produce communicable and potentially life-threatening disease.

Infection with *M. tuberculosis* typically leads to the development of delayed hypersensitivity, which can be detected by the tuberculin (Mantoux) test. About 2 to 4 weeks after the infection has begun, intracutaneous injection of 0.1 ml of purified protein derivative (PPD) induces a visible and palpable induration (at least 5 mm in diameter) that peaks in 48 to 72 hours. Sometimes, more PPD is required to elicit the reaction, and unfortunately, in some responders, the standard dose may produce a large, necrotizing lesion. *A positive tuberculin test result signifies cell-mediated hypersensitivity to tubercular antigens.* It does not differentiate between infection and disease. The possibility has been raised, but not proved, that a positive reaction requires that viable organisms persist in the latent focus of infection. It is well recognized that *false-negative reactions (or skin test anergy) may be produced by certain viral infections, sarcoidosis, malnutrition, Hodgkin's disease, immunosuppression, and (notably) overwhelming active tuberculous disease.* False-positive reactions may also result from infection by atypical mycobacteria.

About 80% of the population in certain Asian and African countries are tuberculin positive. By contrast, in 1980, 5% to 10% of the U.S. population reacted positively to tuberculin, indicating the marked difference in rates of exposure to the tubercle bacillus. Of the approximately 15 million persons exposed to tubercle bacilli in the United States, only 23,000 developed active disease in 1986. Thus, *only a small fraction of those who contract an infection develop active disease.*

Tuberculosis flourishes wherever there is poverty, crowding, and chronic debilitating illness. Similarly, elders, with their weakened defenses, are vulnerable. In the United States, tuberculosis is a disease of the elderly, the urban poor, patients with acquired immunodeficiency syndrome (AIDS), and those belonging to minority communities. American blacks, Native Americans, the Inuit (from Alaska), Hispanics, and immigrants from Southeast Asia have higher attack rates than other segments of the population. Whether this disparity can be ascribed entirely to socioeconomic factors or is in part genetic in origin is not known. Certain diseases also increase the risk: diabetes mellitus, Hodgkin's disease, chronic lung disease (particularly silicosis), malnutrition, alcoholism, and immunosuppression. *In areas of the world where HIV infection is prevalent, this infection has become the single most important risk factor for the development of tuberculosis.* Most, perhaps all, of these predisposing conditions are related to a decrease in the capacity to develop and maintain T cell–mediated immunity against the infectious agent.

Etiology. Mycobacteria are slender rods that are acid fast (i.e., they have a high content of complex lipids that readily bind the Ziehl-Neelsen [carbol fuchsin] stain and subsequently stubbornly resist decolorization). *M. tuberculosis hominis* is responsible for most cases of tuberculosis; the reservoir of infection is usually found in humans with active pulmonary disease. Transmission is usually direct, by inhalation of airborne organisms in aerosols generated by expectoration or by exposure to contaminated patient secretions.

Oropharyngeal and intestinal tuberculosis contracted by drinking milk contaminated with *M. bovis* is now rare in developed nations but still seen in countries that have tuberculous dairy cows and unpasteurized milk. Both *M. hominis* and *M. bovis* species are obligate aerobes whose slow growth is retarded by a pH lower than 6.5 and by long-chain fatty acids, hence the difficulty of finding tubercle bacilli in the centers of large caseating lesions where anaerobiosis, low pH, and increased levels of fatty acids are present. Other mycobacteria, particularly *M. avium-intracellulare*, are much less virulent than *M. tuberculosis* and rarely cause disease in immunocompetent individuals. However, in patients with AIDS, these strains are frequently found, affecting 10% to 30% of patients.

Pathogenesis. There are three important considerations in understanding the pathogenesis of tuberculosis: (1) the basis of virulence of the organism, (2) the relationship of hypersensitivity (as expressed by a positive skin test result) to immunity against the infection, and (3) the pathogenesis of the caseation necrosis.

The virulence of the tubercle bacillus is not related to any known endotoxin. Although mycosides (complex lipids and linked carbohydrates) such as the "cord factor" have been shown to be toxic in animals, there is no clear evidence of their role in human disease. Virulent strains possess certain sulfated glycolipids that prevent fusion of phagosomes containing bacilli to lysosomes, and may thus insulate the ingested bacteria from the battery of lysosomal enzymes. However, to date, no virulence gene has been identified, and it is generally believed that the tissue destruction in tuberculosis is mediated largely by the host immune response.

The development of cell-mediated, or type IV, hypersensitivity to the tubercle bacillus probably explains the organism's destructiveness in tissues and also the emergence of resistance to the organisms. On initial exposure to the organism, the inflammatory response is nonspecific, resembling the reaction to any form of bacterial invasion. Within 2 or 3 weeks, coincident with the appearance of a positive skin reaction, the reaction becomes granulomatous, and the centers of granulomas become caseous, forming typical "soft tubercles." The sequence of events following an initial lung infection (discussed in Chapter 5) is outlined in Figure 13–25 and summarized here:

■ Antigen from the tubercle bacillus reaches draining lymph nodes and is presented to T cells. CD4+ cells of the T_H1 type are sensitized and recirculate to the site of infection. Critical in this initial generation of sensitized T_H1 cells is elaboration of IL-12 by the macrophages.

■ Sensitized CD4+ cells release cytokines when exposed to antigen at the site of infection.

■ Monocytes are recruited and activated (particularly by γ-interferon from the CD4+ cells) to kill or inhibit the growth of the organism.

■ In response to cytokines and possibly the constituents of the cell wall of the bacillus, some of the activated macrophages form granulomas, which may subsequently entrap the residual microorganisms.

■ CD4+ helper T cells also facilitate the development of CD8+ cytotoxic T cells, which can not only kill tuberculosis-infected macrophages but also produce IFN-γ.

Thus, it is apparent that *the development of hypersensitivity*

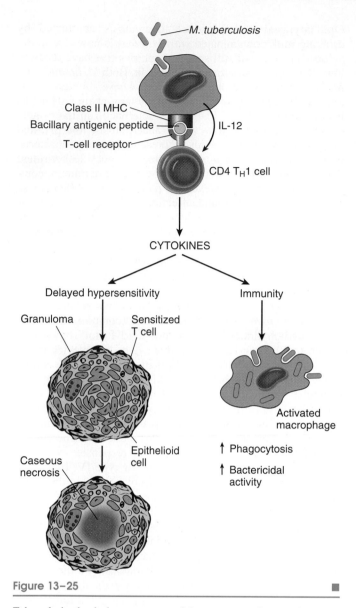

Figure 13–25

Tuberculosis: the dual consequences of the emergence of macrophage activation and sensitization. MHC, major histocompatibility complex.

is a requisite for granuloma formation and for enhanced resistance to the organisms. Whether hypersensitivity and resistance are separate but concurrent functions or are interdependent is uncertain. In addition to the role of CD4+ T_H1 cells, recent evidence indicates that T cells with the $\gamma\delta$ T-cell receptor (Chapter 5) that are normally found at many mucosal sites may also be involved in resistance against tubercle bacilli. However, the central role of CD4+ cells in host resistance against tuberculosis is affirmed by the increased incidence of this scourge in HIV-infected individuals.

As mentioned, typical granulomas in tuberculosis have central caseation (soft tubercles), although sometimes there is no caseation (hard tubercles). What induces the caseation remains a mystery. Most likely the products derived from sensitized T cells or activated macrophages are responsible for the necrosis.

In summary, the appearance of hypersensitivity signals the acquisition of immunity and resistance to the organism. At the same time, however, hypersensitivity is accompanied by the caseating destructive response to the tubercle bacillus. Thus, the sensitized host more rapidly mobilizes a defensive reaction but suffers enhanced necrosis of tissue. Whether the protective or destructive response predominates determines whether the primary focus of infection remains localized and disseminated organisms are destroyed, or whether disabling disease appears.

PRIMARY TUBERCULOSIS

Primary tuberculosis is the form of disease that develops in a previously unexposed, and therefore unsensitized, person. Elders and profoundly immunosuppressed persons may lose their sensitivity to the tubercle bacillus and so may develop primary tuberculosis more than once. With primary tuberculosis, the source of the organism is exogenous. About 5% of those newly infected develop significant disease.

MORPHOLOGY. In countries where bovine tuberculosis and infected milk have largely disappeared, primary tuberculosis almost always begins in the lungs. Typically, the inhaled bacilli implant in the distal airspaces of the lower part of the upper lobe or the upper part of the lower lobe, usually close to the pleura. As sensitization develops, a 1- to 1.5-cm area of gray-white inflammatory consolidation emerges, **the Ghon focus.** In most cases the center of this focus undergoes caseation necrosis. Tubercle bacilli, either free or within phagocytes, drain to the regional nodes, which also often caseate. **This combination of parenchymal lesion and nodal involvement is referred to as the Ghon complex** (Fig. 13–26). During the first few weeks, there is also lymphatic and hematogenous dissemination to other parts of the body. In approximately 95% of cases, development of cell-mediated immunity controls the infections. Hence, the Ghon complex undergoes progressive fibrosis, often followed by calcification, and despite seeding of other organs, no lesions develop.

Histologically, **sites of active involvement are marked by a characteristic granulomatous inflammatory reaction that forms both caseating and noncaseating tubercles** (Fig. 13–27). Individual tubercles are microscopic; it is only when multiple granulomas coalesce that they become macroscopically visible. The granulomas are usually enclosed within a fibroblastic rim punctuated by lymphocytes. Multinucleate giant cells are present in the granulomas.

The chief implications of primary tuberculosis are that (1) it induces hypersensitivity and increased resistance; (2) the foci of scarring may harbor viable bacilli for years, perhaps for life, and thus be the nidus for reactivation at a later time

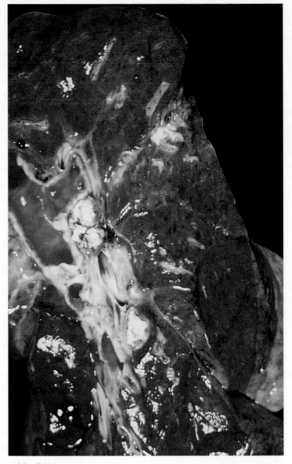

Figure 13–26   ■

Primary pulmonary tuberculosis, Ghon complex. The gray-white parenchymal focus is under the pleura in the lower part of the upper lobe. Hilar lymph nodes with caseation are seen on the left.

when host defenses are compromised; and (3) uncommonly, the disease may develop without interruption into so-called progressive primary tuberculosis or disseminated disease. This occurs in individuals who are immunocompromised because of a well-defined illness such as AIDS or because of nonspecific impairment of host defenses, as may occur in malnourished children or in the elderly. Certain racial groups, such as Eskimos, are also more prone to develop progressive primary tuberculosis. With DNA fingerprinting of *M. tuberculosis* isolates, it is now possible to determine the source of infection and hence the likelihood that clinical disease is a manifestation of a recent primary infection. When such studies were performed in two groups of patients with AIDS, it was found that 35% to 40% of patients were infected by genetically identical mycobacteria, clearly indicating that they were all recently infected from a single source, presumably someone to whom all were exposed. It seems from such studies that the incidence of progressive primary infection is probably quite high in HIV-infected patients.

In progressive primary tuberculosis, the primary focus enlarges, caseates, and cavitates, sometimes spreading through the airways or lymphatics to multiple sites within the lung. Blood-borne dissemination may give rise to miliary tuberculosis. These consequences also occur in secondary tuberculosis and so are described later.

SECONDARY TUBERCULOSIS (REACTIVATION TUBERCULOSIS)

Secondary (or postprimary) tuberculosis is the pattern of disease that arises in a previously sensitized host. It may follow shortly after primary tuberculosis, but more commonly it arises from reactivation of dormant primary lesions many decades after initial infection, particularly when host resistance is weakened. It may also result from exogenous reinfection

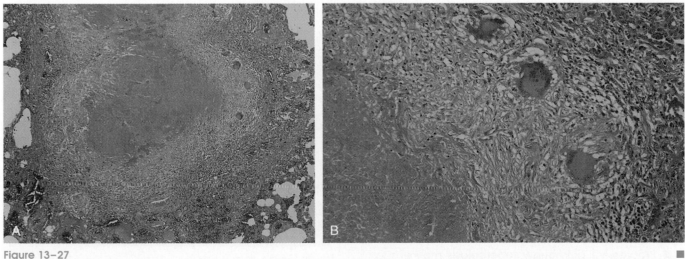

Figure 13–27   ■

A characteristic tubercle at low magnification *(A)* and in detail *(B),* to illustrate central granular caseation surrounded by epithelioid and multinucleated giant cells.

because of waning of the protection afforded by the primary disease or because of a large inoculum of virulent bacilli. Whatever the source of the organism, only a few patients (less than 5%) with primary disease subsequently develop secondary tuberculosis.

Secondary pulmonary tuberculosis is classically localized to the apex of one or both upper lobes. The reason is obscure but may relate to high oxygen tension in the apices. Because of the preexistence of hypersensitivity, the bacilli excite a prompt and marked tissue response that tends to wall off the focus. As a result of this localization, the regional lymph nodes are less prominently involved early in the developing disease than they are in primary tuberculosis. On the other hand, cavitation occurs readily in the secondary form, resulting in dissemination along the airways. Indeed, cavitation is almost inevitable in neglected secondary tuberculosis, and erosion into an airway becomes an important source of infectivity because the patient now raises sputum containing bacilli. *It is noteworthy that in patients with HIV infection who are known to have been previously exposed to tuberculosis, reactivation disease does not usually present with apical lesions; cavitation is distinctly uncommon and mediastinal lymphadenopathy usually occurs.* Thus, in these markedly immunodeficient persons, the pattern of reactivation tuberculosis is more like that of primary tuberculosis. Because of impaired T-cell immunity in AIDS, dissemination of tuberculosis occurs in about 50% of cases. It is also noteworthy that, in patients with AIDS, primary or reactivation tuberculosis occurs early in the course of the disease, before a significant decline in CD4+ cells occurs. Evidently, the defects in the function of memory T cells that predate reduction in CD4+ cells are sufficient to tilt the balance in favor of *M. tuberculosis* (Chapter 5). This is in contrast to infections with atypical mycobacteria, which raise their ugly heads only in patients with marked reduction (<100 cells/mm³) of CD4+ cells.

MORPHOLOGY. The initial lesion is usually a small focus of consolidation, less than 2 cm in diameter, within 1 to 2 cm of the apical pleura. Such foci are sharply circumscribed, firm, gray-white to yellow areas that have a variable amount of central caseation and peripheral fibrosis. In favorable cases the initial parenchymal focus undergoes progressive fibrous encapsulation, leaving only fibrocalcific scars. Histologically, the active lesions show characteristic coalescent tubercles with central caseation. Although tubercle bacilli can be demonstrated by appropriate methods in early exudative and caseous phases of granuloma formation, it is usually impossible to find them in the late, fibrocalcific stages. Localized, apical, secondary pulmonary tuberculosis may heal with fibrosis either spontaneously or after therapy, or the disease may progress and extend along several different pathways:

■ **Progressive pulmonary tuberculosis** may ensue. The apical lesion enlarges with expansion of the area of caseation. Erosion into a bronchus evacuates the caseous center, creating a ragged, ir-

regular cavity lined by caseous material that is poorly walled off by fibrous tissue (Fig. 13–28). Erosion of blood vessels may result in hemoptysis. With adequate treatment, the process may be arrested, and healing by fibrosis may distort the pulmonary architecture. Irregular cavities, now free of caseation necrosis, may remain or collapse in the surrounding fibrosis. If the treatment is inadequate, or if host defenses are impaired, the infection may spread by direct expansion, via dissemination through airways, lymphatic channels, or the vascular system. **Miliary pulmonary disease** occurs when organisms drain through lymphatics into the lymphatic ducts, which empty into the venous return to the right side of the heart and thence into the pulmonary arteries. Individual lesions are either microscopic or small, visible (2-mm) foci of yellow-white consolidation scattered through the lung parenchyma. Miliary lesions may expand and coalesce to yield almost total consolidation of large regions or even whole lobes of the lung. With progressive pulmonary tuberculosis, the pleural cavity is invariably involved, and serous **pleural effusions**, **tuberculous empyema**, or **obliterative fibrous pleuritis** may develop.

■ **Endobronchial, endotracheal, and laryngeal tuberculosis** may develop when infective material is spread either through lymphatic channels or from expectorated infectious material. The mucosal lining may be studded with minute granulomatous lesions, sometimes apparent only on microscopic examination.

■ **Systemic miliary tuberculosis** ensues when infective foci in the lungs seed the pulmonary venous return to the heart; the organisms subsequently disseminate through the systemic arterial system. Almost every organ in the body may be seeded. Lesions resemble those in the lung. Miliary tuberculosis is most prominent in the liver, bone mar-

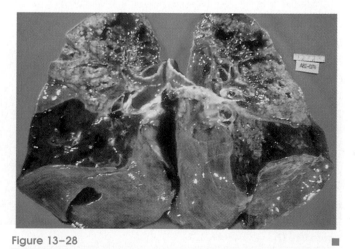

Figure 13–28 ■

Secondary pulmonary tuberculosis. The upper parts of both lungs are riddled with gray-white areas of caseation and multiple areas of softening and cavitation.

row, spleen, adrenals, meninges, kidneys, fallopian tubes, and epididymis (Fig. 13–29).

■ **Isolated-organ tuberculosis** may appear in any one of the organs or tissues seeded hematogenously and may be the presenting manifestation of tuberculosis. Organs typically involved include the meninges (tuberculous meningitis), kidneys (renal tuberculosis), adrenals (formerly an important cause of Addison's disease), bones (osteomyelitis), and fallopian tubes (salpingitis). When the vertebrae are affected, the disease is referred to as Pott's disease.

■ In years past, **intestinal tuberculosis** contracted by the drinking of contaminated milk was fairly common as a primary focus of tuberculosis. It was often preceded by tuberculous involvement of the oropharyngeal lymphoid tissue with spread to the lymph nodes in the neck (scrofula). In developed countries today, intestinal tuberculosis is more often a complication of protracted advanced secondary tuberculosis, secondary to the swallowing of coughed-up infective material. Typically, the organisms are trapped in mucosal lymphoid aggregations of the small and large bowel, which then undergo inflammatory enlargement with ulceration of the overlying mucosa, particularly in the ileum.

The many patterns of tuberculosis are depicted in Figure 13–30.

Clinical Course. Localized secondary tuberculosis may be asymptomatic. When manifestations appear, they are usually *insidious* in onset; there is gradual development of both systemic and localizing symptoms. Systemic symptoms are probably related to cytokines released by activated macrophages (e.g., TNF-α and IL-1). They often appear early in the course and include malaise, anorexia, weight loss, and fever. Commonly the *fever is low grade* and remittent (appearing late each afternoon and then subsiding), and night sweats occur. With progressive pulmonary involvement, increasing amounts

of sputum, at first mucoid and later purulent, appear. When cavitation is present, the sputum contains tubercle bacilli. Some degree of *hemoptysis* is present in about half of all cases of pulmonary tuberculosis. *Pleuritic pain* may result from extension of the infection to the pleural surfaces. The diagnosis is based in part on the history and on physical and radiographic findings of consolidation or cavitation in the apices of the lungs. Ultimately, however, *tubercle bacilli must be identified.* Acid-fast smears and cultures of the sputum of patients suspected of having tuberculosis should be performed. Because conventional cultures may take up to 10 weeks to become positive, there is much interest in the new DNA-based diagnostic techniques. PCR amplification of *M. tuberculosis* DNA allows rapid diagnosis, and such a test has been approved for use in the United States. However, culture remains the gold standard because it also allows testing of drug susceptibility. As stated earlier, multidrug resistance is now seen more commonly, and hence currently all newly diagnosed U.S. cases are treated with multiple agents. Extrapulmonary tuberculosis, which in the past was noted in approximately 15% of newly diagnosed cases, is seen in 60% to 80% of patients with AIDS. Miliary tuberculosis is difficult to diagnose, often presenting, particularly in elders and AIDS patients, as a fever of unknown origin in the absence of apparent active pulmonary disease. The diagnosis may depend on identifying granulomas containing acid-fast bacilli in bone marrow or liver biopsy.

The prognosis is generally good if infections are localized to the lungs, except when they are caused by drug-resistant strains or occur in aged, debilitated, or immunosuppressed persons, who are at high risk for developing miliary tuberculosis. Amyloidosis may appear in persistent cases.

Fungal Infections

Many pathogenic fungi (e.g., the dermatophytes) limit their activities to the skin, producing superficial mycoses. Those that cause systemic infections (deep mycoses) are, of course, of greater medical concern. The dimorphic fungi—*Histoplasma capsulatum, Coccidioides immitis,* and *Blastomyces dermatitidis*—all cause pulmonary disease in ostensibly normal hosts after inhalation of the infective forms of the organism. As would be expected, the infections are likely to be more severe in immunosuppressed persons. The nonseptate hyphal fungi belonging to the order Mucorales and the mold-like fungus *Aspergillus* are strictly opportunistic infectious agents. They are particularly aggressive in patients with decreased numbers or functions of phagocytes. The yeastlike fungi—*Candida* species and *Cryptococcus neoformans*—can cause disease in otherwise healthy hosts, but they are best considered opportunistic infectious agents because they clearly cause more serious infection in immunocompromised patients. All systemic fungi can infect the lung, although extrapulmonary disease may be more frequent and clinically more important with some fungi.

HISTOPLASMOSIS

Histoplasmosis, one of the most common systemic fungal infections in the United States, is endemic in the Ohio and

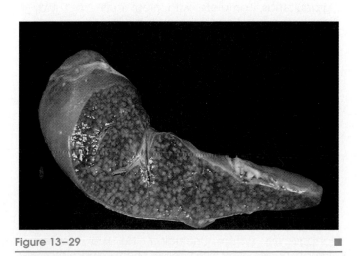

Figure 13–29 ■

Miliary tuberculosis of the spleen. The cut surface shows numerous gray-white granulomas.

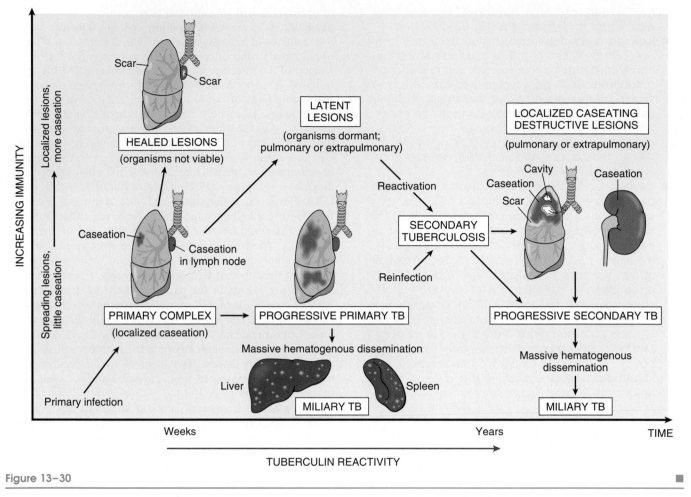

Figure 13–30 ■

The natural history and spectrum of tuberculosis. (Adapted from a sketch provided by Dr. R. K. Kumar, The University of New South Wales, School of Pathology, Sydney, Australia.)

central Mississippi River Valleys and along the Appalachian Mountains in the southeastern United States. Warm, moist soil, enriched by droppings from bats and birds, provides the ideal medium for the growth of the mycelial form, which produces infectious spores. When airborne and inhaled, the spores germinate into the parasitic yeast form in the lungs. *The infection mimics tuberculosis both clinically and histologically.* In most normal adults the infection is asymptomatic and takes the form of a peripheral pulmonary lesion associated with hilar lymphadenopathy, recapitulating the Ghon complex of tuberculosis. Exposed persons develop a positive histoplasmin skin reaction (analogous to the tuberculin test). The primary infection may undergo fibrosis and calcification and be discovered only by radiography in a person with a positive histoplasmin skin test result who is tuberculin negative. In children or adults with lowered resistance or defective immune responses, disseminated extrapulmonary disease develops.

MORPHOLOGY. The round to oval histoplasma yeast forms, 2 to 5 μm in diameter, infect and multiply within mononuclear phagocytes. The pri-

mary pulmonary nodules, composed of aggregates of macrophages stuffed with organisms, are associated with similar lesions in the regional lymph nodes. These lesions develop into small granulomas complete with giant cells, and may develop central necrosis and later fibrosis and calcification. The similarity to tuberculosis is striking, and differentiation requires identification of the yeast forms (best seen with periodic acid–Schiff (PAS) or silver stains). In the vulnerable host chronic cavitary disease develops in the upper lobe, resembling the secondary form of tuberculosis. In infants or immunocompromised adults, particularly those with HIV infection, histoplasmosis develops into disseminated disease (analogous to miliary tuberculosis). Under these circumstances, when T cell–mediated immunity is markedly impaired, there is no granuloma formation. Instead, focal collections of phagocytes stuffed with yeast forms are seen within cells of the mononuclear phagocyte system, including the liver, spleen, lymph nodes, lymphoid tissue of the gastrointestinal tract, and bone marrow. The adrenals and meninges may also be involved, and in about 25% of cases ulcers form in the nose and mouth, on the tongue, or in the larynx.

Clinical Course. The clinical manifestations of histoplasmosis are almost indistinguishable from those of tuberculosis. The infection may be asymptomatic, or it may cause fever, malaise, and myalgias and be readily mistaken for "flu." With more extensive pulmonary involvement, cough, hemoptysis, and even dyspnea and chest pain may appear. Disseminated disease is a hectic, febrile illness with hepatosplenomegaly, anemia, leukopenia, and thrombocytopenia. Although the histoplasmin skin test and elevated serum antibody titers are helpful, the diagnosis of active infection is best made by direct visualization of the organism in the lesion and by culture of sputum, bone marrow, or liver biopsy. *Detection of a capsular antigen in body fluids or urine is a specific and sensitive test for disseminated disease.*

COCCIDIOIDOMYCOSIS

Coccidioidomycosis, or "cocci," as some call it, is caused by *C. immitis.* It results from inhalation of infective arthrospores and is endemic in the southwest and far west of the United States, particularly in the San Joaquin Valley, where it is known as valley fever. There, almost 80% of the population are coccidioidin skin test positive (analogous to the tuberculin test). Coccidioidomycosis, like histoplasmosis and tuberculosis, takes the form of (1) *an asymptomatic pulmonary infection (about 60% of exposed persons),* (2) *progressive pulmonary disease,* or (3) *miliary disease.*

MORPHOLOGY. The primary pulmonary form consists of a small focus of consolidation. Spread to the hilar lymph nodes simulates the Ghon complex of tuberculosis. The sites of infection are usually marked by granulomas, which often have central caseation and giant cells. **Fungi appearing as thick-walled, nonbudding spherules, 20 to 60 μm in diameter (often filled with small endospores),** can be visualized around the necrotic debris, or sometimes within macrophages or giant cells. A pyogenic reaction is imposed when the spherules rupture and release endospores. In most instances the lesions heal by progressive fibrosis and calcification and the infection is asymptomatic. In about 40% of patients the disease produces symptoms such as fever, chills, cough, and pleuritic chest pain, mimicking a pneumonia caused by a mycoplasmal infection or virus. Often such persons have hypersensitivity reactions such as erythema nodosum or multiforme, polyarthritis, pleuritis, and pericarditis. Progressive disease is marked by more disseminated involvement of the lungs and coalescent areas of consolidation. In less than 1%, miliary (hematogenous) dissemination follows with spread to the skin, bones, adrenals, lymph nodes, spleen, liver, and meninges. Systemic spread is

more likely to occur in blacks, Asians, or Filipinos than in Caucasians, unless they have underlying AIDS.

The clinical diagnosis can be suspected with a positive coccidioidin skin test, which develops within 10 days to 3 weeks of infection, and is further supported by the presence of specific antibodies within the first month of infection. Diagnosis is confirmed by culture of the organism.

CANDIDIASIS

Candida albicans is the most frequent disease-causing fungus. It is a normal inhabitant of the oral cavity, gastrointestinal tract, and vagina in many individuals. The spectrum of candidiasis is broad. *C. albicans* most frequently causes superficial, bothersome infections of the mouth, nails, and genital tract (vaginitis in females), and in the perianal area of infants (diaper rash), but in immunosuppressed persons it can cause widespread mucocutaneous involvement or become systemic, producing abscesses in many organs. In fungemic states the source of infection is often contaminated indwelling intravenous lines, surgical drains, or urinary tract catheters. In many cases in which *Candida* is consistently isolated from the blood, the patient improves when the infecting source is simply removed, particularly if he or she is not severely immunosuppressed.

The most common pattern of candidiasis takes the form of a superficial infection on mucosal surfaces of the oral cavity (thrush) or vagina. Florid proliferation of the fungi creates gray-white, dirty-looking superficial membranes composed of matted organisms and inflammatory debris. Deep to the surface there is mucosal hyperemia and inflammation. This form of candidiasis is seen in newborns, diabetics, debilitated patients, and persons receiving broad-spectrum antibiotics that destroy competing normal bacterial flora. However, vaginal candidiasis may develop in otherwise healthy women; it is particularly common in pregnant women and in those who take oral contraceptives. A more erosive chronic mucocutaneous candidiasis occurs, particularly in the esophagus, in the gravely ill or in association with any hematologic or T-cell derangement that markedly impairs the inflammatory-immune response. *Oral thrush, often accompanied by esophageal candidiasis, is extremely common in patients with AIDS.*

Invasive candidiasis implies blood-borne dissemination of organisms to various tissues or organs. Common patterns include (1) renal abscesses, (2) myocardial abscesses and endocarditis, (3) brain involvement (most commonly meningitis, but parenchymal microabscesses occur), (4) endophthalmitis (virtually any eye structure can be involved), (5) hepatic abscesses, and (6) pulmonary lesions (manifest as irregular or "cannonball" abscesses of varying sizes, which are sometimes hemorrhagic owing to vascular invasion).

Blood-borne dissemination and miliary abscess formation is likely to occur when there is extensive tissue trauma or neutrophil defects. Patients receiving chemotherapy for acute lymphoblastic leukemia are particularly susceptible because of neutropenia associated with bone marrow suppression. In patients who have valvular heart disease or a prosthetic heart valve, or who are heroin addicts, candidemia is particularly prone to cause *Candida* endocarditis, which then serves as a continuing source of seeding via the bloodstream.

OTHER FUNGAL INFECTIONS

Blastomycosis, caused by *B. dermatitidis,* is most easily remembered as being similar to histoplasmosis and coccidioidomycosis. It may take the form of an asymptomatic primary pulmonary infection, progressive pulmonary disease, or (rarely) disseminated miliary disease.

Similarly, the histologic changes are most often granulomatous but may be suppurative in particularly vulnerable hosts. "Blasto," however, has the following differences from "cocci":

■ The pathogen is smaller (5 to 25 μm in diameter), round to oval, and thick walled and reproduces by budding rather than endosporulation.

■ The endemic area is confined in the United States to areas overlapping with those where histoplasmosis is found.

■ There is no reliable skin test, and serologic tests are relatively insensitive. Diagnosis requires culture from clinical specimens.

■ Dissemination frequently involves the skin in the form of indolent papules or enlarging fungating ulcers.

■ Cutaneous infections frequently induce striking pseudoepitheliomatous hyperplasia, which is easily mistaken for squamous cell carcinoma.

Cryptococcosis, caused by *C. neoformans,* rarely occurs in otherwise healthy persons. It almost always represents an opportunistic infection in immunocompromised hosts, particularly those with AIDS, leukemia, lymphoma, or Hodgkin's disease. The fungus, a 5- to 10-μm yeast, has a thick, gelatinous capsule and reproduces by budding. Like the previously described systemic fungi, the infective form is most likely present in the soil and is acquired by inhalation. *The fungus initially localizes in the lungs and then disseminates to other sites, particularly the meninges.* Sites of involvement are marked by a variable tissue response, which ranges from florid proliferation of gelatinous organisms with a minimal or absent inflammatory cell infiltrate (in immunodeficient hosts) to a granulomatous reaction (in the more reactive host). In immunosuppressed patients, masses of fungi grow in gelatinous masses within the meninges or small, cystlike spaces in the gray matter (Fig. 13–31), the so-called soap-bubble lesions. Diagnosis can be made in about 70% of cases by adding India ink to a drop of centrifuged spinal fluid to demonstrate the yeast cell body surrounded by the halo of the polysaccharide capsule. However, the most sensitive test is based on detection of cryptococcal antigen by utilizing antibodies to cryptococcal polysaccharide attached to latex particles. Results of the latex agglutination test are positive in more than 95% of cases and should be confirmed by culture.

Mucormycosis and *invasive aspergillosis* are uncommon infections limited to immunocompromised hosts, particularly those with diabetes or leukemia-associated neutrophil defects and those receiving steroid treatment. Both diseases are caused by fungi that assume mycelial forms in lesions. In mucormycosis the hyphae are nonseptate and branch at right angles; in aspergillosis the hyphae are septate and branch at more acute angles. In mucormycosis the organisms prefer-

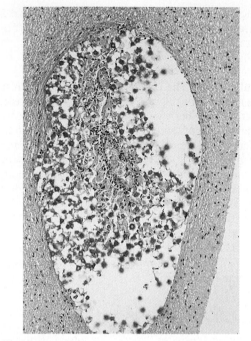

Figure 13–31 ■

Mucicarmine stain of cryptococci (staining red) in a Virchow-Robin perivascular space of the brain (soap-bubble lesion).

entially localize in the nose (from which they may rapidly spread to the sinuses and brain), lungs, and gastrointestinal tract. *Aspergillus* species favor the lungs, from whence they may disseminate. Both agents cause a nondistinctive, suppurative, sometimes granulomatous reaction with a *predilection for invading blood vessel walls, causing vascular necrosis and infarction.*

In addition to the invasive aspergillosis seen in severely compromised patients, two other forms of pulmonary aspergillosis may occur. The first consists of colonization of pulmonary cavities (e.g., ectatic bronchi or lung cysts), to create fungus balls; these may act as ball valves, occluding the cavity and thus predisposing to infection and hemoptysis. The second takes the form of allergic bronchopulmonary aspergillosis; in this form patients with asthma develop an exacerbation of symptoms due to development of type I hypersensitivity against the fungus growing in the bronchi.

Lung Abscess

Lung abscess refers to a localized area of suppurative necrosis within the pulmonary parenchyma. The causative organism may be introduced into the lung by any of the following mechanisms:

■ *Aspiration of infective material* from carious teeth or infected sinuses or tonsils, particularly likely during oral surgery, anesthesia, coma, or alcoholic intoxication and in debilitated patients with depressed cough reflexes.

■ *Aspiration of gastric contents,* usually accompanied by infectious organisms from the oropharynx.

■ As a *complication of acute bacterial pneumonias,* particularly those caused by *S. aureus, K. pneumoniae, Pseudomonas* species, and occasionally type 3 pneumococci. Mycotic infections and bronchiectasis may also lead to lung abscesses.

■ *Bronchial obstruction,* particularly with bronchogenic carcinoma obstructing a bronchus or bronchiole. Impaired drainage, distal atelectasis, and aspiration of blood and tumor fragments all contribute to the development of abscesses. An abscess may also form within an excavated necrotic portion of a tumor.

■ *Septic embolism,* from septic thrombophlebitis or from infective endocarditis of the right side of the heart.

In addition, lung abscesses may result from hematogenous spread of bacteria in disseminated pyogenic infection. When all the above pathogenetic pathways are excluded, there are still many cases of mysterious origin, referred to as *primary cryptogenic lung abscesses.*

Anaerobic bacteria are present in almost all lung abscesses, sometimes in vast numbers, and they are the exclusive isolates in one third to two thirds of cases. The most frequently encountered anaerobes are commensals normally found in the oral cavity, principally species of *Bacteroides, Fusobacterium, Peptococcus,* and microaerophilic streptococci. Often there is a mixed anaerobic-aerobic infection; the most commonly isolated aerobic organisms are *S. aureus,* β-hemolytic streptococci, *Nocardia,* and many different gram-negative organisms.

MORPHOLOGY. Abscesses vary in diameter from a few millimeters to large cavities of 5 to 6 cm. The localization and number of abscesses depend on their mode of development. Pulmonary abscesses resulting from aspiration of infective material are much more common on the right side (more vertical airways) than on the left, and most are single. On the right side they tend to occur in the subapical and axillary portions of the upper lobe and in the apical portion of the lower lobe, because these locations reflect the likely course of aspirated material when the patient is recumbent. Abscesses that develop in the course of pneumonia or bronchiectasis are commonly multiple, basal, and diffusely scattered. Septic emboli and abscesses arising from hematogenous seeding are commonly multiple and may affect any region of the lungs.

As the focus of suppuration enlarges, it almost inevitably ruptures into airways. Thus, the contained exudate may be partially drained, producing an air fluid level on radiographic examination. Occasionally, abscesses rupture into the pleural cavity and produce bronchopleural fistulas, the consequence of which is pneumothorax or empyema. Other complications arise from embolization of septic material to the brain, giving rise to meningitis or brain abscess. Histologically, as expected with any abscess, there is suppuration surrounded by variable amounts of fibrous scarring and mononuclear infiltration (lymphocytes, plasma cells, macrophages), depending on the chronicity of the lesion.

Clinical Course. The manifestations of a lung abscess are much like those of bronchiectasis and include a prominent cough that usually yields copious amounts of foul-smelling, purulent, or sanguineous sputum; occasionally hemoptysis occurs. Spiking fever and malaise are common. Clubbing of the fingers, weight loss, and anemia may all occur. Infective abscesses occur in 10% to 15% of patients with bronchogenic carcinoma; thus, when a lung abscess is suspected in an older patient, underlying carcinoma must be considered. Secondary amyloidosis may develop in chronic cases. Treatment includes antibiotic therapy and, if needed, surgical drainage. Overall, the mortality rate is in the range of 10%.

Cytomegalovirus Infections

Cytomegalovirus (CMV), a member of the herpesvirus family, may produce a variety of disease manifestations, depending partly on the age of the infected host but even more on the host's immune status. Cells infected by the virus exhibit gigantism of both the entire cell and its nucleus. Within the nucleus is an enlarged inclusion, which gives the name to the classic form of symptomatic disease that occurs in neonates, cytomegalic inclusion disease (CID). Although classic CID is a multisystem disease, CMV infections are discussed here because in immunosuppressed adults, particularly AIDS patients, and recipients of allogeneic bone marrow transplants, CMV pneumonitis is a serious problem. Transmission of CMV occurs by several mechanisms:

■ Transplacentally from a newly acquired or chronic asymptomatic infection in the mother.

■ During the first year of life, by transmission of the virus through cervical or vaginal secretions at birth, or later, through breast milk from a mother who has active infection.

■ During preschool years, especially in day care centers, through saliva. Toddlers so infected readily transmit the virus to their parents.

■ After 15 years of age, the venereal route is the dominant mode of transmission, but spread may also occur via respiratory secretions and the fecal-oral route

■ Iatrogenic transmission occurs through organ transplants or by blood transfusions.

In healthy young children and adults the disease is nearly always asymptomatic. In surveys around the world, 50% to 100% of adults demonstrate anti-CMV antibodies in the serum, indicating exposure. Typically, in such seropositive but asymptomatic individuals, the virus remains latent within leukocytes, which are the major reservoirs. Occasionally, some immunocompetent adults develop an infectious mononucleosis–like illness, with fever, atypical lymphocytosis, lymphadenopathy, and hepatomegaly accompanied by abnormal liver function test results, suggesting mild hepatitis.

Congenital Infections. Infection acquired in utero may take many forms. In approximately 90% of cases it is asymptomatic, but in some, mainly those who acquire the virus from a mother with primary infection (who does not have protective immunoglobulins), classic CID develops. Affected infants may suffer intrauterine growth retardation (Chapter 7), be profoundly ill, and manifest jaundice, hepatosplenomegaly, anemia, bleeding due to thrombocytopenia, and encephalitis.

> In fatal cases the brain is often smaller than normal (microcephaly) and may show foci of calcification. Histologically, the characteristic enlargement of cells can be appreciated. In the glandular organs, the parenchymal epithelial cells are affected; in the brain, the neurons; in the lungs, the alveolar macrophages and epithelial and endothelial cells; and in the kidneys, the tubular epithelial and glomerular endothelial cells. Affected cells are strikingly enlarged, often to a diameter of 40 μm, and they show cellular and nuclear polymorphism. Prominent intranuclear basophilic inclusions spanning half the nuclear diameter are usually set off from the nuclear membrane by a clear halo (Fig. 13–32). Within the cytoplasm of these cells, smaller basophilic inclusions may also be seen.

Those infants who survive usually bear permanent residual effects, including mental retardation and various neurologic impairments. The congenital infection is not always devastating, however, and may take the form of interstitial pneumonitis, hepatitis, encephalitis, or a hematologic disorder. Most infants with this milder form of CID recover, although a few may develop mental retardation later. Uncommonly, a totally asymptomatic infection may be followed months to years later by neurologic sequelae, including delayed-onset mental retardation, hearing deficits, and cerebral calcifications.

CMV in Immunosuppressed Individuals. This occurs most commonly in three groups of patients:

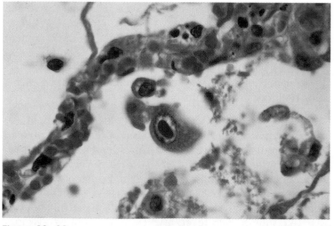

Figure 13–32 ■

Cytomegalovirus infection of the lung. A typical distinct nuclear and ill-defined cytoplasmic inclusion is seen. (Courtesy of Dr. Arlene Sharpe, Brigham & Women's Hospital, Boston, MA.)

■ *Recipients of organ transplants* (heart, liver, kidney) from seropositive donors. These patients typically receive immunosuppressive therapy, and the CMV is usually derived from the donor organ, but reactivation of latent CMV infection in the host may also occur.

■ *Recipients of allogeneic bone marrow transplants.* These patients are immunosuppressed not only because of drug therapy but also because of graft-versus-host disease. In this setting, there is usually reactivation of latent CMV in the recipient.

■ *Patients with AIDS.* These immunosuppressed individuals have reactivation of latent infection and are also infected by their sexual partners.

In all these settings, serious, life-threatening disseminated CMV infections primarily affect the lungs, gastrointestinal tract, and retina; the central nervous system is usually spared.

In the pulmonary infection, an interstitial mononuclear infiltrate with foci of necrosis develops, accompanied by the typical enlarged cells with inclusions. The pneumonitis can progress to full-blown adult respiratory distress syndrome. Intestinal necrosis and ulceration can develop and be extensive, leading to debilitating diarrhea. CMV chorioretinitis can occur either alone or in combination with involvement of the lungs and intestinal tract. Diagnosis of CMV infections is made by demonstration of characteristic morphologic alterations, isolation of the virus, rising antiviral antibody titer, and PCR-based detection of the viral genome. An overview of the many outcomes of infection is offered in Figure 13–33.

Pneumocystis Pneumonia

P. carinii, an opportunistic infectious agent long considered to be a protozoan, is now believed to be more closely related to fungi. Serologic evidence indicates that virtually all persons are exposed to *Pneumocystis* during the first few years of life, but in most the infection remains latent. Reactivation and clinical disease occurs almost exclusively in those who are immunocompromised. Indeed, *P. carinii* is an extremely common cause of infection in patients with AIDS and may also infect severely malnourished infants and immunosuppressed persons. *Pneumocystis* infections are largely confined to the lung, where they produce interstitial pneumonitis.

> Microscopically, involved areas of the lung demonstrate intra-alveolar foamy, pink-staining exudate (with hematoxylin and eosin), and the septa are thickened by edema and a minimal mononuclear infiltrate (Fig. 13–34). Special stains are required to visualize the organism in either the trophozoite or encysted form. Silver stains of tissue sections reveal cup-shaped cyst walls in the alveolar exudates. If sputum production can be successfully induced in the patient, Giemsa or methylene blue stains can demonstrate the trophozoite forms of the organism (about 6 μm in diameter with long filopodia) in about 50% of patients. The

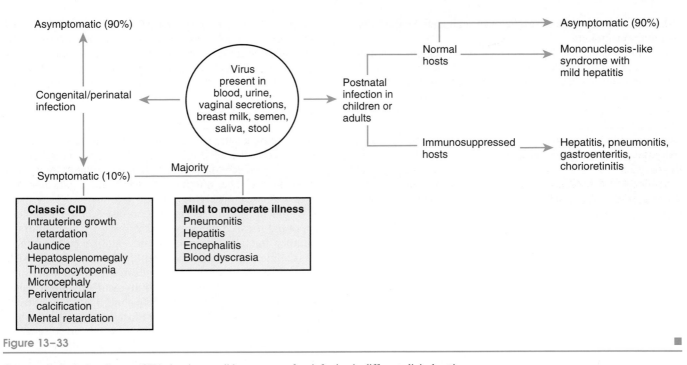

Figure 13–33   ■

Cytomegalic inclusion disease (CID) showing possible outcomes of an infection in different clinical settings.

most sensitive and effective method of diagnosis is to identify the organism in bronchoalveolar lavage fluids or in a transbronchial biopsy.

Fever, dry cough, and dyspnea occur in 90% to 95% of patients, who typically demonstrate bilateral perihilar and basilar infiltrates. Hypoxia is frequent; pulmonary function studies show a restrictive lung defect. If treatment is initiated before widespread involvement, the outlook for recovery is good; however, because residual organisms are likely to remain, particularly in AIDS patients, relapses are common unless the underlying immunosuppression is reversed.

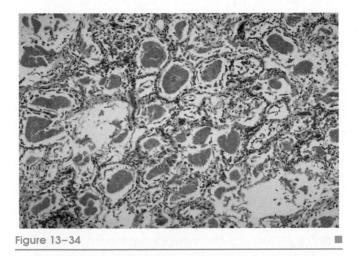

Figure 13–34   ■

Pneumocystis pneumonia. The alveoli are filled with a characteristic foamy exudate. There is a sparse mononuclear cell infiltrate in the alveolar septa.

LUNG TUMORS

Although lungs are frequently the site of metastases from cancers in extrathoracic organs, primary lung cancer is also a common disease. Ninety-five per cent of primary lung tumors arise from the bronchial epithelium (bronchogenic carcinomas); the remaining 5% are a miscellaneous group that includes bronchial carcinoids, mesotheliomas, bronchial gland neoplasms, mesenchymal malignancies (e.g., fibrosarcomas, leiomyomas), lymphomas, and a few benign lesions. The most common benign lesions are spherical, small (3- to 4-cm), discrete hamartomas that often show up as "coin" lesions on chest radiographs. They consist mainly of mature cartilage but are often admixed with fat, fibrous tissue, and blood vessels in varying proportions.

Bronchogenic Carcinoma

Bronchogenic carcinoma (bronchial carcinoma) is without doubt the number one cause of cancer-related deaths in industrialized countries. It has long held this position among males in the United States, accounting for about one third of cancer deaths in men, and it has become the leading cause of cancer deaths in women. In 1996, lung cancer was expected to cause 158,700 deaths in the United States alone. The rate of increase among males is slowing down, but it continues to accelerate among females (Chapter 6). These statistics are undoubtedly related to the causal relationship of cigarette smoking and bronchogenic carcinoma. The peak incidence of lung cancer occurs between ages 40 and 70 years; currently, the male to female ratio is about 2:1. Male cigarette smokers are about 10 times more likely to die of bronchogenic carcinoma than are nonsmokers.

The four major histologic types of bronchogenic carcinomas are squamous cell carcinoma, adenocarcinoma, large cell undifferentiated carcinoma, and small cell carcinoma. It has become apparent that for most therapeutic decisions the first three can be lumped into a category termed non–small cell lung carcinoma (NSCLC) to distinguish them from small cell lung cancer (SCLC). In some cases there is a combination of histologic patterns. This classification is summarized in Table 13–6.

Etiology and Pathogenesis. Like all cancers, lung cancers result from genetic changes that affect oncogenes and tumor suppressor genes. SCLCs are characterized by changes in several oncogenes, including amplification of the *myc* family. L-*myc* amplification is associated with particularly aggressive behavior. Mutational inactivation of the tumor suppressor genes p53 and *Rb* are also common in SCLC. In addition, all SCLCs have a deletion of the short arm of chromosome 3 (3p14-25), where at least three distinct tumor suppressor genes are suspected to reside. The genetic alterations in NSCLC are somewhat different. Alterations in *myc*, p53, and *Rb* are present, but less frequently than in SCLC. On the other hand, mutations of K-*ras*, not seen in SCLC, are found in about 30% of adenocarcinomas, and the activation of these oncogenes is associated with poor prognosis.

As with colorectal cancers, there seems to be a temporal sequence in the accumulation of specific mutations. For example, inactivation of the putative cancer suppressor genes located on 3p seems to be a very early event, whereas activation of the *ras* oncogene occurs relatively late. More important, it appears that loss of heterozygosity at 3p occurs not only in preinvasive lesions such as carcinomas in situ, but also in areas of hyperplasia, suggesting that large areas of the respiratory mucosa are mutagenized after exposure to carcinogens ("field effect"). On this fertile soil, those cells that accumulate additional mutations ultimately develop into cancer.

With regard to carcinogenic influences, there is strong evidence that smoking and, to a much lesser extent, other environmental insults are the main culprits responsible for the genetic changes that give rise to lung cancers. First, the evidence relating to cigarette smoking will be given, followed by a few brief comments on the less important factors.

An impressive body of evidence—statistical, clinical, and experimental—incriminates cigarette smoking. Statistically, there is a nearly linear correlation between the frequency of lung cancer and pack-years of cigarette smoking. The increased risk becomes 20 times greater among habitual heavy smokers (40 or more cigarettes a day for a span of years) compared with nonsmokers. About 80% of lung cancers occur in active smokers or those who stopped recently. Cessation of cigarette smoking for at least 15 years brings the risk down almost to control levels. Passive smoking (proximity to cigarette smokers) increases the risk to approximately twice that of nonsmokers. The smoking of pipes and cigars also increases the risk, but only modestly.

The *clinical evidence* is largely composed of the documentation of progressive alterations in the lining epithelium of the respiratory tract in habitual cigarette smokers. In essence, there is a linear correlation between the intensity of exposure to cigarette smoke and the appearance of ever more worrisome epithelial changes, beginning with atypical squamous metaplasia, then dysplasia, and ultimately abnormalities approaching carcinoma in situ, followed in most instances by the bad news.

The *experimental evidence,* although it mounts with each passing year, lacks one important link: it has not so far been possible to produce lung cancer in an experimental animal by exposing it to cigarette smoke. Nonetheless, cigarette smoke condensate is a witches' brew of tumorigenic delicacies such as polycyclic hydrocarbons and other potent mutagens and carcinogens. Despite the lack of an experimental model, the chain of evidence linking cigarette smoking to lung cancer grows ever stronger.

Other influences may act in concert with smoking or may by themselves be responsible for some lung cancers; witness the increased incidence of this form of neoplasia in miners of radioactive ores; asbestos workers; and workers exposed to dusts containing arsenic, chromium, uranium, nickel, vinyl chloride, and mustard gas. *Heavy smokers exposed to asbestos have an approximately 55 times greater risk of lung cancer than do nonsmokers not exposed to asbestos.*

Despite the fact that smoking and other environmental factors are paramount in the causation of lung cancer, it is well known that all persons exposed to tobacco smoke do not develop cancer. It is very likely that the mutagenic effect of carcinogens is conditioned by hereditary (genetic) factors. Recall that many chemicals (procarcinogens) require metabolic activation via the P-450 monooxygenase enzyme system for conversion into ultimate carcinogens (Chapter 6). There is evidence that the function of this enzyme system is under genetic control, and conceivably persons who efficiently metabolize the procarcinogens incur the greatest exposure and risk of developing lung cancer.

■

Table 13–6. HISTOLOGIC CLASSIFICATION OF BRONCHOGENIC CARCINOMA AND APPROXIMATE INCIDENCE

I. Non-Small Cell Lung Carcinoma (NSCLC) (70%–75%)
1. Squamous cell (epidermoid) carcinoma (25%–30%)
2. Adenocarcinoma, including bronchioloalveolar carcinoma (30%–35%)
3. Large cell carcinoma (10%–15%)

II. Small Cell Lung Carcinoma (SCLC) (20%–25%)

III. Combined Patterns (5%–10%)
Most frequently
  Mixed squamous cell carcinoma and adenocarcinoma
  Mixed squamous cell carcinoma and SCLC

MORPHOLOGY. Bronchogenic carcinomas in the various histologic categories share several features:

■ The majority arise in the lining epithelium of major bronchi, usually close to the hilus of the lung.
■ All patterns are associated with cigarette smok-

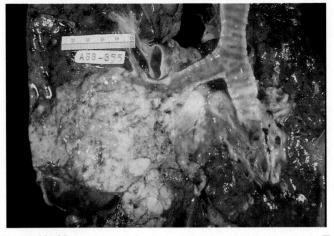

Figure 13–35   ■

Bronchogenic carcinoma. The gray-white tumor tissue is seen infiltrating the lung substance. Histologically, this large tumor mass was identified as a squamous cell carcinoma.

the lumen of a major bronchus, often producing distal atelectasis and infection. Simultaneously, the lesion invades surrounding pulmonary substance (Fig. 13–35).

Histologically, these tumors range from well-differentiated squamous cell neoplasms showing keratin pearls (Fig. 13–36) and intercellular bridges to poorly differentiated neoplasms having only minimal residual squamous cell features.

Adenocarcinomas are most common in patients under the age of 40, women, and nonsmokers. They may occur as central lesions like the squamous cell variant but are usually more peripherally located, many arising in relation to peripheral lung scars. The basis of this association with lung scars is not clear. In general, these tumors grow slowly and form smaller masses than do the other subtypes, but they tend to metastasize widely at an early stage. Histologically, they assume a variety of forms, including typical adenocarcinomas with mucus secretion (relatively uncommon) and papillary or bronchioloalveolar patterns (more common). The latter two are believed to have a common origin from bronchiolar epithelium, but they have different patterns of growth structure.

Bronchioloalveolar carcinomas involve peripheral parts of the lung, either as a single nodule or, more often, as multiple diffuse nodules that may coalesce to produce pneumonia-like consolidation. They derive their name from their growth pattern as seen under the microscope. The tumor cells grow along preexisting structures such as bronchioles and alveoli. Sometimes there are papillary folds and invasion into interstitial spaces. Tumor cells are tall and columnar, sometimes with intracellular mucus. Most are well differentiated, with little anaplasia.

Large cell carcinomas constitute a group of neoplasms that lack cytologic differentiation and probably represent squamous cell or glandular neoplasms that are too undifferentiated to permit

ing; the strongest association is with squamous cell and small cell carcinomas.

- All are aggressive, locally invasive, widely metastasizing neoplasms (particularly SCLC) with a propensity for spread to the liver, adrenals, brain, and bones, although almost every organ in the body can be affected.
- All varieties, especially SCLC, have the capacity to synthesize bioactive products, producing paraneoplastic syndromes.

These tumors begin as small mucosal lesions, usually firm and gray-white, that may form intraluminal masses, invade the bronchial mucosa, or form large bulky masses pushing into adjacent lung parenchyma. Some large masses undergo cavitation due to central necrosis or develop focal areas of hemorrhage. Finally, these tumors may extend to the pleura, invade the pleural cavity and chest wall, and spread to adjacent intrathoracic structures. More distant spread can occur via the lymphatics or the hematogenous route.

Squamous cell carcinomas are more common in men than in women; they tend to arise centrally in major bronchi and eventually spread to local hilar nodes, but they disseminate outside the thorax later than other histologic types. Large lesions may undergo central necrosis, giving rise to cavitation. Squamous cell carcinomas are often preceded for years by atypical metaplasia or dysplasia in the bronchial epithelium, which then transforms to carcinoma in situ, a phase that may last for several years. By this time, atypical cells may be identified in cytologic smears of sputum or in bronchial lavage fluids or brushings, although the lesion is asymptomatic and undetectable on radiographs. Eventually the small neoplasm reaches a symptomatic stage, when a well-defined tumor mass begins to obstruct

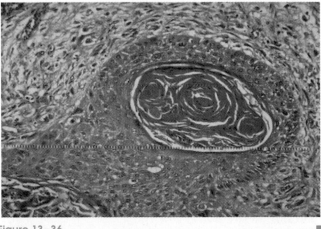

Figure 13–36   ■

Bronchogenic carcinoma, squamous cell type. An area of keratin formation is seen in this well-differentiated tumor.

categorization. The cells are large, are usually anaplastic, and have large vesicular nuclei. They have a poor prognosis because of their tendency to spread to distant sites early in their course.

Small cell lung carcinomas are more common in men than in women and are strongly associated with cigarette smoking. They generally appear as pale gray, centrally located masses with extension into the lung parenchyma and early involvement of the hilar and mediastinal nodes. These cancers are composed of small, dark, round-to-oval, lymphocyte-like cells (albeit larger than lymphocytes) that have scant cytoplasm and hyperchromatic nuclei, among which mitoses are numerous (Fig. 13–37). This is the classic "oat" cell. In some cases the tumor cells are spindle shaped or fusiform. Penetration of submucosal vessels is often seen.

SCLCs are rapidly growing lesions that tend to infiltrate widely and metastasize early in their course and so are rarely resectable. These tumors are derived from neuroendocrine cells of the lung, which are characterized by expression of neuron-specific enolase, neurosecretory granules (detected by electron microscopy), neurofilaments, and the ability to secrete a host of polypeptide hormones including adrenocorticotropic hormone (ACTH), calcitonin, gastrin-releasing peptide, and chromogranin A. Hence, these tumors are associated with a variety of paraneoplastic syndromes.

Combined patterns require no further comment, but it should be noted that a significant minority of bronchogenic carcinomas reveal more than one line of differentiation, sometimes several (Table 13–6), suggesting that all are derived from a multipotential progenitor cell.

For all of these neoplasms, one can trace involvement of successive chains of nodes about the carina, in the mediastinum, and in the neck (scalene nodes) and clavicular regions, and, sooner or later, distant metastases. Involvement of the supraclavicular node (Virchow's node) is particularly characteristic and sometimes calls attention to an occult primary tumor. These cancers, when advanced, often extend into the pericardial or pleural spaces, leading to inflammation and effusions. They may compress or infiltrate the superior vena cava to cause either venous congestion or the full-blown vena caval syndrome. Apical neoplasms may invade the brachial or cervical sympathetic plexus to cause severe pain in the distribution of the ulnar nerve or to produce Horner's syndrome (ipsilateral enophthalmos, ptosis, meiosis, and anhidrosis). Such apical neoplasms are sometimes called Pancoast's tumors, and the combination of clinical findings Pancoast's syndrome. Pancoast's tumor is often accompanied by destruction of the first and second ribs and sometimes thoracic vertebrae. As with other cancers, tumor-node-metastases (TNM) categories have been established to indicate the size and spread of the primary neoplasm.

Clinical Course. Bronchogenic carcinomas are silent, insidious lesions that more often than not have spread so as to be unresectable before they produce symptoms. In some instances, chronic cough and expectoration call attention to still localized, resectable disease. When hoarseness, chest pain, superior vena caval syndrome, pericardial or pleural effusion, or persistent segmental atelectasis or pneumonitis makes its appearance, the prognosis is grim. Too often the tumor presents with symptoms emanating from metastatic spread to the brain (mental or neurologic changes), liver (hepatomegaly), or bones (pain). Although the adrenals may be nearly obliterated by metastatic disease, adrenal insufficiency (Addison's disease) is uncommon because islands of cortical cells sufficient to maintain adrenal function usually persist.

Overall, NSCLCs have a better prognosis than SCLCs. When NSCLCs (squamous cell carcinomas or adenocarcinomas) are detected prior to metastases or local spread, cure is possible by lobectomy or pneumonectomy. SCLCs, on the other hand, have invariably spread by the time they are first detected, even if the primary tumor appears small and localized. Thus, surgical resection is not a viable treatment. They are very sensitive to chemotherapy but invariably recur. Median survival even after treatment is 1 year.

It is variously estimated that about 3% to 10% of all lung cancer patients develop clinically overt paraneoplastic syndromes. These include (1) hypercalcemia due to secretion of a parathyroid hormone–related peptide (osteolytic lesions may also cause hypercalcemia, but this would not be a paraneoplastic syndrome [Chapter 6]); (2) Cushing's syndrome (from increased production of ACTH); (3) syndrome of inappropriate secretion of antidiuretic hormone (SIADH); (4) neuromuscular syndromes, including a myasthenic syndrome, peripheral neuropathy, and polymyositis; (5) clubbing of the fingers and hypertrophic pulmonary osteoarthropathy; and (6) hematologic manifestations, including migratory thrombophlebitis, nonbacterial endocarditis, and DIC. Secretion of calcitonin and other ectopic hormones has also been documented by assays, but these products usually do not provoke distinc-

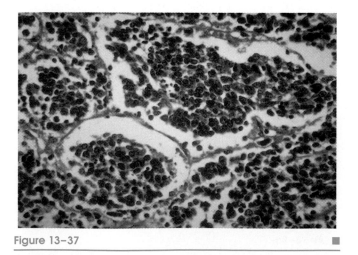

Figure 13–37 ■

Small cell lung carcinoma. There are nests of small round, oval cells with deep, basophilic nuclei.

tive syndromes. *Hypercalcemia is most often encountered with squamous cell neoplasms, the hematologic syndromes with adenocarcinomas. The remaining syndromes are much more common with small cell neoplasms, but exceptions abound.*

Bronchial Carcinoid

Bronchial carcinoids show the neuroendocrine differentiation of Kulchitsky cells in the bronchial mucosa and resemble intestinal carcinoids (Chapter 15). The cells contain dense core neurosecretory granules in their cytoplasm and rarely may secrete hormonally active polypeptides. They occasionally occur as part of multiple endocrine neoplasia (Chapter 20). Bronchial carcinoids appear at an early age (mean 40 years) and represent about 5% of all pulmonary neoplasms. In happy contrast to bronchogenic carcinomas, they are often resectable and curable.

> Most bronchial carcinoids originate in mainstem bronchi and grow in one of two patterns: (1) an obstructing polypoid, spherical, intraluminal mass; or (2) a mucosal plaque penetrating the bronchial wall to fan out in the peribronchial tissue—the so-called collar-button lesion. Even these penetrating lesions push into the lung substance along a broad front and are therefore reasonably well demarcated. About 30% of these tumors metastasize to hilar nodes, and a few to more distant sites such as liver. Histologically, these neoplasms, like their counterparts in the intestinal tract, are composed of uniform cuboidal cells that have regular round nuclei with few mitoses and little or no anaplasia. Occasional tumors are less well differentiated and may resemble small cell carcinomas. In these cases, it can be difficult to differentiate the highly malignant small cell cancer from the much more indolent carcinoid.

Most bronchial carcinoids present with findings related to their intraluminal growth (i.e., they cause cough, hemoptysis, and recurrent bronchial and pulmonary infections). Some are asymptomatic and discovered by chance on chest radiographs. Only rarely do they induce the carcinoid syndrome. In any case, because they are slow-growing lesions that rarely spread beyond the local hilar nodes, these tumors are amenable to conservative resection. The reported 5- to 10-year survival rate ranges from 50% to 95%, but late recurrences sometimes develop.

 PLEURAL LESIONS

Lesions of the pleura may be inflammatory or neoplastic. Although inflammatory processes are far more common, we will begin our discussion with the more ominous, but fortunately rare, malignant tumor of the pleura.

Malignant Mesothelioma

Malignant mesothelioma is a rare cancer of mesothelial cells, usually arising in the parietal or visceral pleura but less commonly in the peritoneum, and (rarely) elsewhere. It has assumed great importance because it is related to occupational exposure to asbestos in the air (Chapter 8). Approximately 50% of the patients have a history of exposure to asbestos. Those who work directly with asbestos (shipyard workers, miners, insulators) are at greatest risk, but malignant mesotheliomas have appeared in persons whose only exposure was living in proximity to an asbestos factory or being a relative of an asbestos worker. The latent period for developing mesotheliomas is long, often 25 to 40 years. As stated earlier, *the combination of cigarette smoking and asbestos exposure greatly increases the risk of bronchogenic carcinoma, but it does not increase the risk of developing mesotheliomas.*

The basis for the carcinogenicity of asbestos is still a mystery. Clearly, the physical form of the asbestos is critical; very nearly all cases are related to exposure to amphibole asbestos, which has long, straight fibers, and not to serpentine chrysotile (Chapter 8). Asbestos is not removed or metabolized, and hence the fibers remain in the body for life. Thus, there is a lifetime risk after exposure that does not diminish with time (unlike smoking, in which the risk decreases after cessation). Asbestosis of the lungs occurs concurrently in only 20% of cases.

> **MORPHOLOGY.** Mesotheliomas are often preceded by extensive pleural fibrosis and plaque formation, readily seen in computed tomographic scans. Mesothelial cell proliferation causes pleural effusion. Malignant mesotheliomas begin in a localized area and in the course of time spread widely, either by contiguous growth or by seeding of the effusion and opposing pleural surfaces. At autopsy, the affected lung is typically ensheathed by a yellow-white, firm, sometimes gelatinous layer of tumor that obliterates the pleural space (Fig. 13–38). Distant metastases are rare. The neoplasm

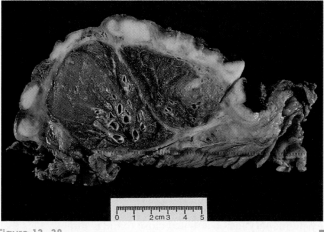

Figure 13–38

Malignant mesothelioma. Note the thick, firm, white, pleural tumor that ensheathes this bisected lung.

may directly invade the thoracic wall or the subpleural lung tissue. Normal mesothelial cells are biphasic, giving rise to pleural lining cells as well as the underlying fibrous tissue. Therefore, histologically, mesotheliomas conform to one of three patterns: (1) sarcomatoid, in which spindled and sometimes fibroblastic-appearing cells grow in nondistinctive sheets; (2) epithelial, in which cuboidal cells line tubular and microcystic spaces, into which small papillary buds project (resembling an adenocarcinoma); and (3) biphasic, the most common pattern, having both sarcomatoid and epithelioid areas.

Pleural Effusion and Pleuritis

Pleural effusion, the presence of fluid in the pleural space, can be either a transudate or an exudate. A pleural effusion that is a transudate is termed *hydrothorax.* Hydrothorax from congestive heart failure is probably the most common cause of fluid in the pleural cavity. An exudate, characterized by a specific gravity greater than 1.020 and, often, inflammatory cells, suggests pleuritis. The four principal causes of pleural exudate are (1) microbial invasion via either direct extension of a pulmonary infection or blood-borne seeding; (2) cancer: bronchogenic carcinoma, metastatic neoplasms to the lung or pleural surface, mesothelioma; (3) pulmonary infarction; and (4) viral pleuritis. Other, less common causes of exudative pleural effusions are seen in patients with systemic lupus erythematosus, rheumatoid arthritis, or uremia and in those who have undergone thoracic surgery. Cancer should be suspected as the underlying cause of an exudative effusion in any patient over the age of 40, particularly when there is no febrile illness, no pain, and a negative tuberculin test result. These effusions characteristically are large and frequently are serosanguineous. Cytologic examination may reveal malignant and inflammatory cells.

Whatever the cause, transudates and serous exudates are usually resorbed without residual effects if the inciting cause is controlled or remits. In contrast, fibrinous, hemorrhagic, and suppurative exudates may lead to fibrous organization, yielding adhesions or fibrous pleural thickening, and sometimes minimal to massive calcifications.

Pneumothorax, Hemothorax, and Chylothorax

Pneumothorax refers to air or other gas in the pleural sac. It may occur in young, apparently healthy adults, usually men without any known pulmonary disease (simple or spontaneous pneumothorax), or as a result of some thoracic or lung disorder (secondary pneumothorax), such as emphysema or a fractured rib. Secondary pneumothorax occurs with rupture of any pulmonary lesion situated close to the pleural surface that allows inspired air to gain access to the pleural cavity. Such pulmonary lesions include emphysema, lung abscess, tuberculosis, carcinoma, and many other, less common processes.

Mechanical ventilatory support with high pressure may also trigger secondary pneumothorax.

There are several possible complications of pneumothorax. A ball-valve leak may create a tension pneumothorax that shifts the mediastinum. Compromise of the pulmonary circulation may follow and may even be fatal. If the leak seals and the lung is not re-expanded within a few weeks (either spontaneously or through medical or surgical intervention), so much scarring may occur that it can never be fully re-expanded. In these cases, serous fluid collects in the pleural cavity and creates hydropneumothorax. With prolonged collapse, the lung becomes vulnerable to infection, as does the pleural cavity when communication between it and the lung persists. Empyema is thus an important complication of pneumothorax (pyopneumothorax). Secondary pneumothorax tends to be recurrent if the predisposing condition remains. What is less readily understood is that simple pneumothorax is also recurrent.

Hemothorax refers to the collection of whole blood (in contrast to bloody effusion) in the pleural cavity, and is almost always a fatal complication of a ruptured intrathoracic aortic aneurysm. With hemothorax, in contrast to bloody pleural effusions, the blood clots within the pleural cavity.

Chylothorax is a pleural collection of a milky lymphatic fluid containing microglobules of lipid. The total volume of fluid may not be large, but chylothorax is always significant because it implies obstruction of the major lymph ducts, usually by an intrathoracic cancer (e.g., a primary or secondary mediastinal neoplasm, such as a lymphoma).

LESIONS OF THE UPPER RESPIRATORY TRACT

Acute Infections

Acute infections of the upper respiratory tract are among the most common afflictions of man, most frequently presenting as the common cold. The clinical features are well known to all: nasal congestion accompanied by watery discharge; sneezing; scratchy, dry sore throat; and a slight increase in temperature that is more pronounced in young children. The most common pathogens are rhinoviruses, but coronaviruses, respiratory syncytial viruses, parainfluenza and influenza viruses, adenoviruses, enteroviruses, and even group A β-hemolytic streptococci have also been implicated. In a significant number of cases (around 40%) the cause cannot be determined; perhaps new viruses will be discovered. Most of these infections occur in the fall and winter and are self-limiting (usually lasting for a week or less). In a minority of cases, colds may be complicated by the development of bacterial otitis media or sinusitis.

In addition to the common cold, infections of the upper respiratory tract may present with signs and symptoms localized to the pharynx, epiglottis, or larynx. *Acute pharyngitis,* manifesting as a sore throat, may be caused by a host of agents. Mild pharyngitis with minimal physical findings frequently accompanies a cold and is the most common form of pharyngitis. More severe forms with tonsillitis, associated with marked hyperemia and exudates, occur with β-hemolytic streptococci and adenovirus infections. In the latter infection, the conjunctiva may also be inflamed. Herpes simplex and coxsackievirus A may produce pharyngeal vesicles and ulcers. Pharyngitis is also an important component of infectious mononucleosis caused by Epstein-Barr virus (EBV).

Acute *bacterial epiglottitis* is a syndrome predominantly of young children who have an infection of the epiglottis by *H. influenzae,* in which pain and airway obstruction are the major findings. The onset is abrupt. Failure to appreciate the need to maintain an open airway for a child with this condition can be fatal.

Acute laryngitis can result from inhalation of irritants or may be due to allergic reactions. It may also be caused by the agents that produce the common cold and usually involve the pharynx and nasal passages as well as the larynx. Brief mention should be made of two uncommon but important forms of laryngitis: *tuberculous* and *diphtheritic*. The former is almost always a consequence of protracted active tuberculosis, during which infective sputum is coughed up. Diphtheritic membranous laryngitis has fortunately become uncommon because of the widespread immunization of young children against diphtheria toxin. After it is inhaled, *Corynebacterium diphtheriae* implants on the mucosa of the upper airways and elaborates a powerful exotoxin that causes necrosis of the mucosal epithelium accompanied by a dense fibrinopurulent exudate that creates the classic superficial, dirty gray membrane of diphtheria. The major hazards of this infection are sloughing and aspiration of the membrane (causing obstruction of major airways) and absorption of bacterial exotoxins (producing myocarditis, peripheral neuropathy, or other tissue injury).

In children, influenza A and B viruses and respiratory syncytial virus are important causes of laryngotracheobronchitis, more commonly known as *croup*. Although self-limited, croup may cause disturbing inspiratory stridor and harsh persistent cough. In occasional cases the laryngeal inflammatory reaction may narrow the airway sufficiently to cause respiratory failure. Viral infections in the upper respiratory tract predispose the patient to secondary bacterial infection, particularly by staphylococci, streptococci, and *H. influenzae.*

Nasopharyngeal Carcinoma

This rare neoplasm merits comment because of (1) the strong epidemiologic links to EBV and (2) the high frequency of this form of cancer in Chinese people, which raises the possibility of viral oncogenesis on a background of genetic susceptibility. EBV infects the host by first replicating in the nasopharyngeal epithelium (and then infecting nearby tonsillar B lymphocytes). In some persons this leads to transformation of the epithelial cells. Unlike the case with Burkitt's lymphoma (Chapter 12), another EBV-associated tumor, the EBV genome is found in virtually all nasopharyngeal carcinomas, including those that occur outside the endemic areas in Asia.

The three histologic variants are squamous cell carcinoma, nonkeratinizing carcinoma, and undifferentiated carcinoma; the last-mentioned is the most common and the one most closely linked with EBV. The undifferentiated neoplasm is characterized by large epithelial cells having indistinct cell borders and prominent nuclei. It should be recalled that in infectious mononucleosis, EBV directly infects B lymphocytes, after which a marked proliferation of reactive T lymphocytes causes atypical lymphocytosis, seen in the peripheral blood, and enlarged lymph nodes (Chapter 12). Similarly, in nasopharyngeal carcinomas a striking influx of mature lymphocytes can often be seen. These neoplasms are therefore referred to as "lymphoepitheliomas," a true misnomer because the lymphocytes are not part of the neoplastic process, nor is the tumor benign. Nasopharyngeal carcinomas invade locally, spread to cervical lymph nodes, and then metastasize to distant sites. They tend to be radiosensitive, and 5-year survival rates of 50% are reported for even advanced cancers.

Laryngeal Tumors

A variety of non-neoplastic, benign, and malignant neoplasms of squamous epithelial and mesenchymal origin may arise in the larynx, but only vocal cord nodules, papillomas, and squamous cell carcinomas are sufficiently common to merit comment. In all these conditions, the most common presenting feature is hoarseness.

NONMALIGNANT LESIONS

Vocal cord nodules ("polyps") are smooth, hemispheric protrusions (usually less than 0.5 cm in diameter) located, most often, on the true vocal cords. They are composed of fibrous tissue and covered by stratified squamous mucosa that is usually intact but can be ulcerated by contact trauma with the other vocal cord. These lesions occur chiefly in heavy smokers or singers (singer's nodes), suggesting that they are the result of chronic irritation or abuse.

Laryngeal papilloma is a benign neoplasm, usually on the true vocal cords, that forms a soft, raspberry-like excrescence rarely more than 1 cm in diameter. Histologically, it consists of multiple, slender, finger-like projections supported by central fibrovascular cores and covered by an orderly, typical, stratified squamous epithelium. When the papilloma is on the free edge of the vocal cord, trauma may lead to ulceration that can be accompanied by hemoptysis.

Papillomas are usually single in adults but are often multiple in children, in whom they are referred to as *juvenile laryngeal papillomatosis*. These lesions are caused by human papillomavirus types 6 and 11, do not become malignant, and often spontaneously regress at puberty. In children, the papillomas tend to recur after excision. Cancerous transformation is rare.

CARCINOMA OF THE LARYNX

Carcinoma of the larynx represents only 2% of all cancers. It most commonly occurs after age 40 years and is more common in men (7:1) than in women. Environmental influences are very important in its causation; nearly all cases occur in smokers, and alcohol and asbestos exposure may also play roles.

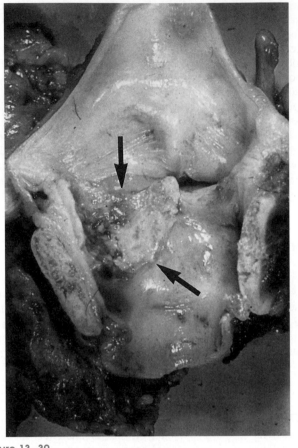

Figure 13–39 ■

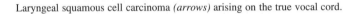

Laryngeal squamous cell carcinoma *(arrows)* arising on the true vocal cord.

About 95% of laryngeal carcinomas are typical squamous cell lesions. Rarely, adenocarcinomas are seen, presumably arising from mucous glands. The tumor usually develops directly on the vocal cords, but it may arise above or below the cords, on the epiglottis or aryepiglottic folds, or in the piriform sinuses. Those confined within the larynx proper are termed *intrinsic,* whereas those that arise or extend outside the larynx are called *extrinsic.* Squamous cell carcinomas of the larynx follow the growth pattern of all squamous cell carcinomas. They begin as in situ lesions that later appear as pearly gray, wrinkled plaques on the mucosal surface, ultimately ulcerating and fungating (Fig. 13–39). The degree of anaplasia of these laryngeal tumors is highly variable. Sometimes massive tumor giant cells and multiple bizarre mitotic figures are seen. As expected with lesions arising from recurrent exposure to environmental carcino-

gens, adjacent mucosa may demonstrate squamous cell hyperplasia with foci of dysplasia, or even carcinoma in situ.

Carcinoma of the larynx manifests itself clinically by persistent hoarseness. At presentation about 60% of these cancers are confined to the larynx; as a result the prognosis is better than for those that have spread into adjacent structures. Later, laryngeal tumors may produce pain, dysphagia, and hemoptysis. Patients with this condition are extremely vulnerable to secondary infection of the ulcerating lesion. With surgery, radiation, or combined therapeutic treatments many patients can be cured, but about one third die of the disease. The usual cause of death is infection of the distal respiratory passages or widespread metastases and cachexia.

BIBLIOGRAPHY

Barnes PJ: Is asthma a nervous disease? Chest 107:S119, 1995. (An examination of the role of autonomic nerves in the pathogenesis of asthma.)

Drobniewski FA, et al: Tuberculosis and AIDS. J Med Microbiol 43:85, 1995. (A discussion of tuberculosis in patients with AIDS.)

Fulkerson WJ, et al: Pathogenesis and treatment of the adult respiratory distress syndrome. Arch Intern Med 156:29, 1996. (A clinically oriented review with an excellent discussion of the pathogenesis and mediators of lung injury.)

Gazdar AF: The molecular and cellular basis of human lung cancer. Anticancer Res 14:261, 1994. (A very good review of the genetic alterations in lung cancer.)

Hanshaw JB: Cytomegalovirus infections. Pediatr Rev 16:43, 1995. (A concise discussion of the entire spectrum of diseases resulting from cytomegalovirus infection.)

Hopewell PC: A clinical view of tuberculosis. Radiol Clin North Am 33:641, 1995. (A review of the clinical spectrum of tuberculosis.)

Howarth PH: The airway inflammatory response in allergic asthma and its relationship to clinical disease. Allergy 50 (Suppl 22):13, 1995. (An excellent review of the role of bronchial inflammation in the pathogenesis of airway hyperresponsiveness.)

Hutchinson DC: Pulmonary emphysema. BMJ 309:1244, 1994. (A succinct editorial on the pathogenesis of emphysema.)

Kita H, Gleich GJ: Commentary. Chemokines active on eosinophils: potential roles in allergic inflammation. J Exp Med 183:2421, 1996. (A summary of the chemotactic factors that recruit eosinophils to the sites of allergic inflammation, including bronchial asthma.)

Kumar RK, Lykke AWJ: Messages and handshakes: cellular interactions in pulmonary fibrosis. Pathology 27:18, 1995. (An excellent discussion of the pathogenesis of pulmonary fibrosis.)

Skerrett SJ: Host defenses against respiratory infection. Med Clin North Am 78:941, 1994. (A scholarly discussion of the defense mechanisms that protect the normal lung from infection.)

Smith AL, et al: Extensive areas of aneuploidy are present in the respiratory epithelium of lung cancer patients. Br J Cancer 73:203, 1996. (A very provocative analysis of changes in the normal respiratory epithelium in patients with lung cancer, providing evidence for "field effects" caused by carcinogen exposure.)

Thurlbeck WM: Chronic airflow obstruction. In Thurlbeck WM, Churg J (eds): Pathology of Lung, 2nd ed. New York, Thieme Medical, 1995, p 739. (A detailed discussion by a leader in the field of the entire spectrum of diseases characterized by chronic airflow obstruction.)

Weissler JC: Sarcoidosis: immunology and clinical management. Am J Med Sci 307:233, 1994. (An excellent review of the pathogenesis and clinical features of sarcoidosis.)

14

The Kidney and Its Collecting System

The kidney is a structurally complex organ that has evolved to subserve a number of important functions: excretion of the waste products of metabolism, regulation of body water and salt, maintenance of appropriate acid balance, and secretion of a variety of hormones and autocoids. Diseases of the kidney are as complex as its structure, but their study is facilitated by dividing them into those that affect the four basic morphologic components: glomeruli, tubules, interstitium, and blood vessels. This traditional approach is useful because the early manifestations of diseases that affect each of these components tend to be distinctive. Further, some components appear to be more vulnerable to specific forms of renal injury; for example, glomerular diseases are often immunologically mediated, whereas tubular and interstitial disorders are more likely to be caused by toxic or infectious agents. Nevertheless, some disorders affect more than one structure. In addition, the anatomic interdependence of structures in the kidney implies that damage to one almost always secondarily affects the others. Thus, severe glomerular damage impairs the flow through the peritubular vascular system; conversely, tubular destruction, by increasing intraglomerular pressure, may induce glomerular atrophy. Thus, whatever the origin, there is a tendency for all forms of chronic renal disease ultimately to destroy all four components of the kidney, culminating in chronic renal failure and what has been called *end-stage contracted kidneys*. The functional reserve of the kidney is large, and much damage may occur before functional impairment is evident. For these reasons, the early signs and symptoms are particularly important to the clinician, and these are referred to in the discussion of individual diseases.

CLINICAL MANIFESTATIONS OF RENAL DISEASES

The clinical manifestations of renal disease can be grouped into reasonably well defined syndromes. Some are peculiar to glomerular diseases; others are present in diseases that affect any one of the components. Before we list the syndromes, a few terms must be clarified.

Azotemia is a biochemical abnormality that refers to an elevation of blood urea nitrogen (BUN) and creatinine levels and is largely related to a decreased glomerular filtration rate (GFR). Azotemia is produced by many renal disorders, but it also arises from extrarenal disorders. *Prerenal azotemia* is encountered when there is hypoperfusion of the kidneys, which impairs renal function *in the absence of parenchymal damage*. Similarly, *postrenal azotemia* is seen whenever urine flow is obstructed below the level of the kidney. Relief of the obstruction is followed by prompt correction of the azotemia.

When azotemia becomes associated with a constellation of clinical signs and symptoms and biochemical abnormalities, it is termed *uremia*. Uremia is characterized not only by failure of renal excretory function but also by a host of metabolic and endocrine alterations incident to renal damage. There is, in addition, secondary gastrointestinal (e.g., uremic gastroenteritis), neuromuscular (e.g., peripheral neuropathy), and cardiovascular (e.g., uremic fibrinous pericarditis) involvement.

We can now turn to a brief description of the major renal syndromes:

1. *Acute nephritic syndrome* is a glomerular syndrome dominated by the acute onset of usually grossly visible hematuria (red blood cells in urine), mild to moderate proteinuria, and hypertension; it is the classic presentation of acute poststreptococcal glomerulonephritis (GN).
2. The *nephrotic syndrome* is characterized by heavy proteinuria (more than 3.5 gm per day), hypoalbuminemia, severe edema, hyperlipidemia, and lipiduria (lipid in the urine).
3. *Asymptomatic hematuria* or *proteinuria*, or a combination of these two, is usually a manifestation of subtle or mild glomerular abnormalities.
4. *Acute renal failure* (ARF) is dominated by oliguria or anuria (no urine flow), with recent onset of azotemia. It can result from glomerular injury (such as crescentic GN), interstitial injury, or acute tubular necrosis.
5. *Chronic renal failure*, characterized by prolonged symptoms and signs of uremia, is the end result of all chronic renal diseases.
6. *Urinary tract infection* (UTI) is characterized by bacteriuria and pyuria (bacteria and leukocytes in the urine). The infection may be symptomatic or asymptomatic, and it may affect the kidney (*pyelonephritis*) or the bladder (*cystitis*) only.
7. *Nephrolithiasis* (renal stones) is manifested by renal colic, hematuria, and recurrent stone formation (p 464).

In addition to these renal syndromes, *urinary tract obstruction* and *renal tumors,* discussed later, represent specific anatomic lesions that often have varied manifestations.

GLOMERULAR DISEASES

Glomerular diseases constitute some of the major problems encountered in nephrology; indeed, chronic GN is one of the most common causes of chronic renal failure in humans. Recall that the glomerulus consists of an anastomosing network of capillaries invested by two layers of epithelium. The visceral epithelium is incorporated into and becomes an intrinsic part of the capillary wall, whereas the parietal epithelium lines Bowman's space (urinary space), the cavity in which plasma filtrate first collects. The glomerular capillary wall is the filtering membrane and consists of the following structures (Figs. 14–1 and 14–2):

1. A thin layer of fenestrated *endothelial cells*, each fenestrum being about 70 to 100 nm in diameter.
2. A *glomerular basement membrane* (GBM) with a thick, electron-dense central layer, the *lamina densa*, and thinner, electron-lucent peripheral layers, the *lamina rara interna* and *lamina rara externa*. The GBM consists of collagen (mostly type IV), laminin, polyanionic proteoglycans, fibronectin, and several other glycoproteins.
3. The *visceral epithelial cells* (podocytes), structurally complex cells that possess interdigitating processes embedded in and adherent to the lamina rara externa of the basement membrane. Adjacent *foot processes* (pedicels) are sepa-

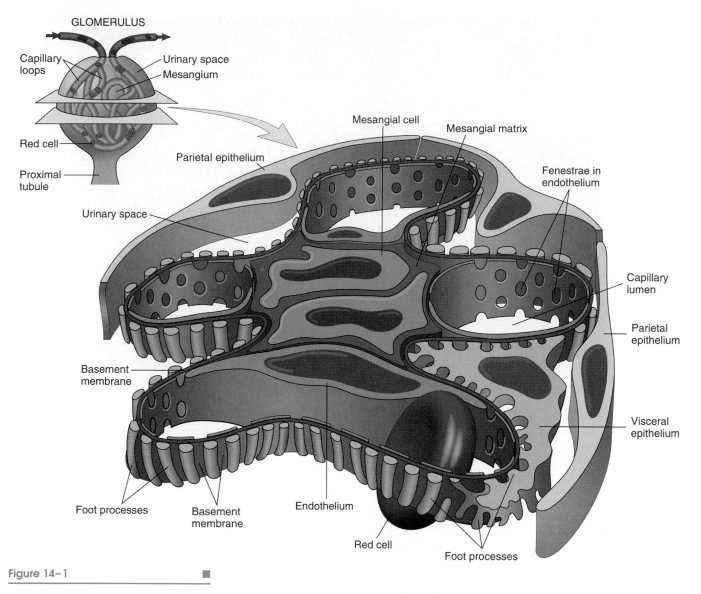

GLOMERULUS

Capillary loops

Urinary space

Mesangium

Red cell

Proximal tubule

Parietal epithelium

Urinary space

Mesangial cell

Mesangial matrix

Fenestrae in endothelium

Capillary lumen

Parietal epithelium

Basement membrane

Visceral epithelium

Foot processes

Basement membrane

Endothelium

Red cell

Foot processes

Figure 14–1   ■

Schematic representation of a glomerular lobe.

rated by 20- to 30-nm wide *filtration slits*, which are bridged by a thin diaphragm.

4. The entire glomerular tuft is supported by *mesangial cells* lying between the capillaries. Basement membrane–like mesangial matrix forms a meshwork through which the mesangial cells are scattered. These cells, of mesenchymal origin, are contractile and phagocytic, and capable of proliferation, of laying down both matrix and collagen, and of secreting a number of biologically active mediators, as we shall see.

The major characteristics of glomerular filtration are an extraordinary high permeability to water and small solutes and an almost complete impermeability to molecules of the size of albumin (± 3.6 nm radius; 70,000 kD). The latter characteristic, called glomerular barrier function, discriminates among protein molecules depending on their size (the larger, the less permeable) and charge (the more cationic, the more

permeable). This size- and charge-dependent barrier function is accounted for by the complex structure of the capillary wall, the integrity of the GBM, and the many anionic moieties present within the wall, including the acidic proteoglycans of the GBM and the sialoglycoproteins of epithelial and endothelial cell coats. The *visceral epithelial cell* is critical to the maintenance of glomerular barrier function: its filtration slit diaphragm presents a distal diffusion barrier to the filtration of proteins, and it is the cell type that is largely responsible for synthesis of GBM components.

Glomeruli may be injured by a variety of factors and in the course of a number of systemic diseases. Immune diseases such as systemic lupus erythematosus (SLE), vascular disorders such as hypertension and polyarteritis nodosa, metabolic diseases such as diabetes mellitus, and some purely hereditary conditions such as Fabry's disease often affect the glomerulus. These are termed *secondary glomerular diseases* to differentiate them from those in which the kidney is the only or pre-

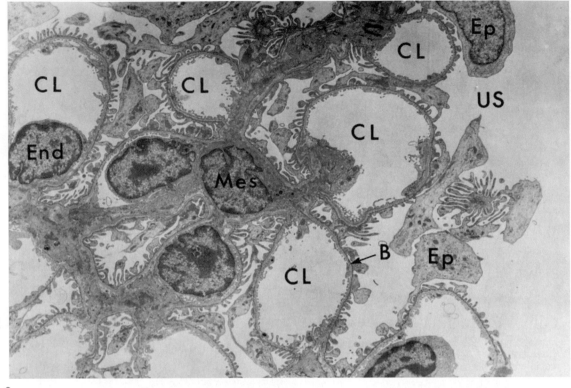

Figure 14–2

Low-power electron micrograph of rat glomerulus. CL, capillary lumen; End, endothelium; Mes, mesangium; B, basement membrane; Ep, visceral epithelial cells with foot processes; US, urinary space.

dominant organ involved. The latter constitute the various types of *primary GN* or *glomerulopathy*. Here we shall discuss the various types of primary GN. The glomerular alterations in systemic diseases are covered in other parts of this book.

Table 14–1 lists the most common forms of GN that have reasonably well defined morphologic and clinical manifestations.

Pathogenesis of Glomerular Diseases

Although we know little of etiologic agents or triggering events, it is clear that immune mechanisms underlie most cases of primary GN and many of the secondary glomerular involvements. Experimentally, GN can be readily induced by antigen-antibody reactions, and glomerular deposits of immunoglobulins, often with various components of complement, are found in more than 70% of patients with GN. Cell-mediated immune mechanisms also play a role in certain glomerular diseases.

Two forms of antibody-associated injury have been established: (1) injury resulting from *deposition of soluble circulating antigen-antibody complexes* in the glomerulus and (2) injury by *antibodies reacting in situ within the glomerulus,* either with insoluble fixed (intrinsic) glomerular antigens or with molecules planted within the kidney (Fig. 14–3). In

addition cytotoxic antibodies directed against glomerular cell components may cause glomerular injury. These pathways are not mutually exclusive, and in humans all may contribute to injury.

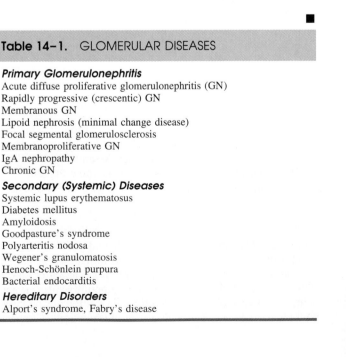

Table 14–1. GLOMERULAR DISEASES

Primary Glomerulonephritis
Acute diffuse proliferative glomerulonephritis (GN)
Rapidly progressive (crescentic) GN
Membranous GN
Lipoid nephrosis (minimal change disease)
Focal segmental glomerulosclerosis
Membranoproliferative GN
IgA nephropathy
Chronic GN

Secondary (Systemic) Diseases
Systemic lupus erythematosus
Diabetes mellitus
Amyloidosis
Goodpasture's syndrome
Polyarteritis nodosa
Wegener's granulomatosis
Henoch-Schönlein purpura
Bacterial endocarditis

Hereditary Disorders
Alport's syndrome, Fabry's disease

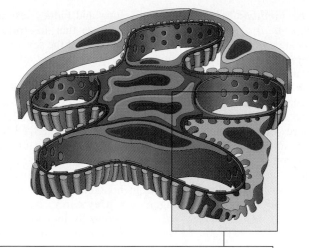

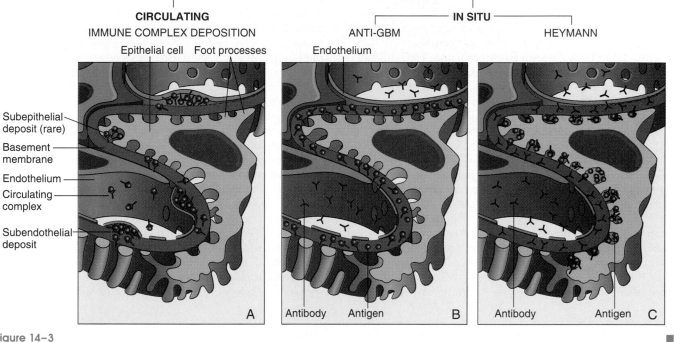

CIRCULATING

IMMUNE COMPLEX DEPOSITION

Epithelial cell   Foot processes

Subepithelial deposit (rare)

Basement membrane

Endothelium

Circulating complex

Subendothelial deposit

A

IN SITU

ANTI-GBM

Endothelium

Antibody   Antigen   B

HEYMANN

Antibody   Antigen   C

Figure 14–3   ■

Antibody-mediated glomerular injury can result either from the deposition of circulating immune complexes *(A)* or from formation in situ of complexes *(B* and *C)*. Anti–glomerular basement membrane (GBM) disease *(B)* is characterized by linear immunofluorescence patterns, whereas circulating and other lesions induced in situ develop granular patterns.

CIRCULATING IMMUNE COMPLEX NEPHRITIS

The pathogenesis of immune complex diseases (type III hypersensitivity reactions) was discussed in detail in Chapter 5. Here we shall briefly review the salient features that relate to glomerular injury. With circulating immune complex disease, the glomerulus may be considered an "innocent by-stander" because it does not incite the reaction. The antigen is not of glomerular origin. It may be endogenous, as in the glomerulopathy associated with SLE, or it may be exogenous, as is likely in the GN that follows certain bacterial (strepto-coccal), viral (hepatitis B), parasitic *(Plasmodium falciparum* malaria), and spirochetal *(Treponema pallidum)* infections. Sometimes the inciting antigen is unknown.

Whatever the antigen may be, antigen-antibody complexes are formed in the circulation and are then trapped in the glo-meruli, where they produce injury, in large part through the binding of complement, although complement-independent injury may also occur (see later). The glomerular lesions usu-ally consist of leukocytic infiltration in glomeruli and prolif-eration of endothelial, mesangial, and parietal epithelial cells. Electron microscopy reveals the complexes as electron-dense deposits or clumps that lie either in the mesangium, between the endothelial cells and the GBM (subendothelial deposits), or between the outer surface of the GBM and the podocytes (subepithelial deposits). Deposits may be located at more than one site in a given case. The presence of immunoglobulins and complement in these deposits can be demonstrated by immunofluorescence microscopy. *When fluorescinated anti-*

immunoglobulin or anticomplement antibodies are used, the immune complexes are seen as granular deposits in the glomerulus (Fig. 14–4A). Once deposited in the kidney, immune complexes may eventually be degraded, mostly by infiltrating monocytes and phagocytic mesangial cells, and the inflammatory changes may then subside. Such a course occurs when the exposure to the inciting antigen is short-lived and limited, as in most cases of poststreptococcal GN. However, if a continuous shower of antigens is provided, repeated cycles of immune complex formation, deposition, and injury may occur, leading to chronic GN. In some cases the source of chronic antigenic exposure is clear, such as in SLE, in which autoimmune injury to the tissues constantly releases nuclear and cytoplasmic antigens. In other cases, however, the antigen is unknown.

IMMUNE COMPLEX NEPHRITIS IN SITU

As noted, antibodies in this form of injury react directly with fixed or planted antigens in the glomerulus.

Anti–Glomerular Basement Membrane. The best-established model is so-called classic anti-GBM nephritis (see Fig. 14–3B). In this type of injury, antibodies are directed against fixed antigens in the GBM. It has its experimental counterpart in the nephritis of rabbits called *Masugi's nephritis* or *nephrotoxic serum nephritis*. This is produced by injecting rats with anti-GBM antibodies produced by immunization of rabbits with rat kidney. Although in the experimental model anti-GBM antibodies are produced by injecting "foreign" kidney antigens into an animal, *spontaneous anti-GBM nephritis in humans results from the formation of autoantibodies directed against GBM*. The antibodies directly bind along the GBM to create a *"linear pattern,"* as seen with immunofluorescent techniques, in contrast to the granular pattern described for other forms of antibody-mediated nephritis (Fig. 14–4B). Sometimes the anti-GBM antibodies cross-react with basement membranes of lung alveoli, resulting in simultaneous lung and kidney lesions *(Goodpasture's syndrome)*. It must be clear that this form of GN is an autoimmune disease, so any one of the several mechanisms discussed earlier (Chapter 5) in relation to autoimmunity may be involved in triggering the disease.

Anti-GBM nephritis accounts for less than 5% of human GN. It is established as the cause of injury in Goodpasture's syndrome (Chapter 13). Many instances of anti-GBM nephritis are characterized by very severe glomerular damage and the development of rapidly progressive crescentic GN. The basement membrane antigen responsible for classic anti-GBM nephritis of Goodpasture's syndrome is a component of the noncollagenous domain of the α-3 chain of collagen type IV.

Heymann's Nephritis. The Heymann model of rat GN was originally induced by immunizing animals with preparations of proximal tubular brush border. The rats develop antibodies to brush border antigens and a membranous type of GN that closely resembles human membranous GN (p 447). This is characterized on immunofluorescence by diffuse deposition of immunoglobulins and complement in a *granular* (rather than linear) pattern along the GBM. It is now clear that the GN results from the reaction of antibodies to an antigen-complex located in the coated pits of visceral epithelial cells of the glomerulus in a discontinuous distribution, and cross-reactive with a brush border antigen. The antigen consists of a large protein, $\pm$ 330 kD, called *megalin*, having homology to the LDL receptor, complexed to a smaller 44-kD protein, called *receptor-associated protein*. Heymann's nephritis most closely resembles human membranous GN, in which the epithelial cell antigen also appears to be a homologue of the megalin complex.

Antibodies may also react in situ with previously "planted" nonglomerular antigens, which may localize in the kidney by interacting with various intrinsic components of the glomerulus. Planted antigens include cationic molecules that bind to glomerular capillary anionic sites; DNA, which has an affinity for GBM components; bacterial products, such as endostrep-

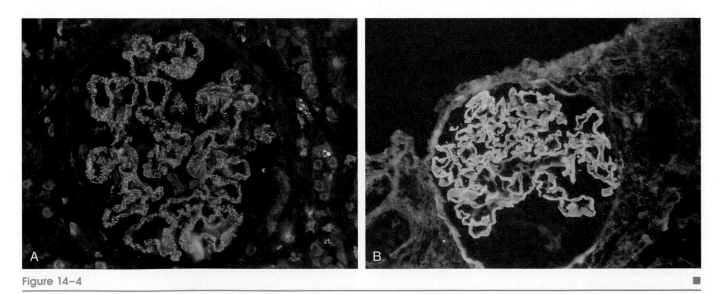

Figure 14–4

Two patterns of deposition of immune complexes as seen by immunofluorescence microscopy: *A,* Granular, characteristic of circulating and in situ immune complex nephritis; *B,* linear, characteristic of classic anti-GBM disease.

tosin, a protein of group A streptococci; large aggregated proteins (e.g., aggregated IgG), which deposit in the mesangium because of their size; and immune complexes themselves, since they continue to have reactive sites for further interactions with free antibody, free antigen, or complement. Most of these planted antigens induce a granular pattern of immunoglobulin deposition by fluorescence microscopy.

Several factors affect glomerular localization of antigen, antibody, or complexes. The molecular charge and size of these reactants are clearly important. The pattern of localization is also affected by changes in glomerular hemodynamics, mesangial function, and the integrity of the charge-selective barrier in the glomerulus. These influences may well explain the variable pattern of immune reactant deposition and histologic change in GN. Studies in experimental models have shown that complexes deposited in the proximal zones of the GBM (endothelium or subendothelium) elicit an inflammatory reaction in the glomerulus with infiltration of leukocytes. In contrast, antibodies directed to distal zones of the GBM (epithelium and subepithelium) are largely noninflammatory and elicit lesions similar to those of Heymann's or membranous GN.

To conclude the discussion of antibody-mediated injury, it must be stated that antigen-antibody deposition in the glomerulus is a major pathway of glomerular injury, and that immune reactions in situ, trapping of circulating complexes, interactions between these two events, and local hemodynamic and structural determinants in the glomerulus all contribute to the morphologic and functional alterations in GN.

CELL-MEDIATED IMMUNE GLOMERULONEPHRITIS

There is increasing evidence that sensitized T cells, formed during the course of a cell-mediated immune reaction, can cause glomerular injury. The idea is an attractive one, as it may account for the instances of GN in which either there are no immune deposits or the deposits do not correlate with the severity of damage.

MEDIATORS OF IMMUNE INJURY

Once immune reactants are localized in the glomerulus, how does glomerular damage ensue? *Glomerular damage is reflected physiologically by loss of glomerular barrier function manifested by proteinuria, and in some instances by reductions in glomerular filtration rate.* One well-established pathway is the *complement-leukocyte–mediated mechanism* (Fig. 14–5A). Activation of complement initiates the generation of chemotactic agents (mainly C5a) and the recruitment of neutrophils and monocytes. Neutrophils release proteases, which cause GBM degradation; oxygen-derived free radicals, which cause cell damage; and arachidonic acid metabolites, which contribute to the reductions in GFR. However, this mechanism applies only to some types of GN, since many types show few neutrophils in the damaged glomeruli. Some models suggest complement- but not neutrophil-dependent injury, owing to an effect of the *C5–C9 lytic component* (membrane attack complex) of complement, which causes epithelial

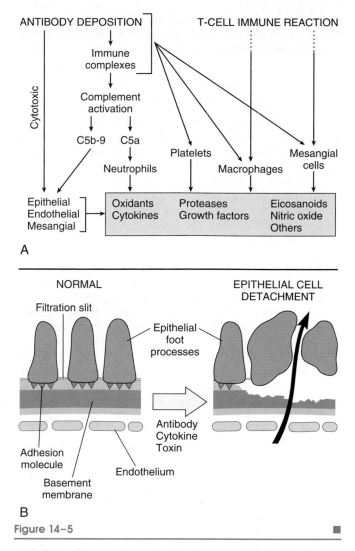

A, Mediators of immune glomerular injury (see text). B, Epithelial cell injury. The postulated sequence is a consequence of antibodies to epithelial cell antigens, or toxins, or cytokines or other factors causing injury and detachment of epithelial cells, and protein leakage through defective GBM and filtration slits. (Adapted from Couser WG: Mediation of immune glomerular injury. Am Soc Nephrol 1:13, 1990.)

cell detachment and stimulates mesangial and epithelial cells to secrete damaging chemical mediators.

In addition to producing immune complexes, antibodies directed to glomerular cell antigens may cause direct cytotoxicity. Such cytotoxic antibodies may mediate damage in those disorders in which immune complexes are not found. Other mediators of glomerular damage include (1) *monocytes and macrophages*, which infiltrate the glomerulus in antibody- and cell-mediated reactions, and, when activated release a vast number of biologically active molecules; (2) *platelets*, which aggregate in the glomerulus during immune-mediated injury and release prostaglandins and growth factors; (3) *resident glomerular cells* (epithelial, mesangial, and endothelial), which can be stimulated to secrete mediators such as cytokines (interleukin 1), arachidonic acid metabolites, growth factors, nitric oxide, and endothelin; and (4) *fibrin-related products*, which cause leukocyte infiltration and glomerular cell proliferation. In essence, virtually all the mediators described in our discussion of inflammation in Chapter 2 may contribute to glomerular injury.

OTHER MECHANISMS OF GLOMERULAR INJURY

Other mechanisms may contribute to glomerular damage in certain primary renal disorders. Two that deserve special mention are epithelial cell injury and renal ablation glomerulopathy.

Epithelial Cell Injury. This can be induced by antibodies to visceral epithelial cell antigens; by toxins, as in an experimental model of proteinuria induced by puromycin aminonucleoside; conceivably by certain cytokines; or by still poorly characterized factors, as is the case in focal glomerulosclerosis (p 449). Such injury is reflected by morphologic changes in the visceral epithelial cells, which include loss of foot processes, vacuolization, retraction and detachment of cells from the GBM; and functionally by proteinuria. It is hypothesized that the detachment of visceral epithelial cells is caused by loss of its adhesive interactions with the basement membrane, and that this detachment leads to protein leakage (Fig. 14–5B).

Renal Ablation Glomerulopathy. Once any renal disease, glomerular or otherwise, destroys sufficient functioning nephrons to reduce the GFR to about 30% to 50% of normal, progression to end-stage renal failure often proceeds inexorably, although the rate varies. Such patients develop proteinuria, and their kidneys show widespread *glomerulosclerosis*. Such progressive sclerosis may be initiated, at least in part, by the adaptive changes that occur in the relatively unaffected glomeruli of diseased kidneys. The remaining glomeruli undergo hypertrophy to maintain renal function. This is associated with hemodynamic changes, including increases in single-nephron glomerular filtration rate, blood flow, and transcapillary pressure (capillary hypertension). The additional load on the intact glomeruli leads ultimately to endothelial and epithelial cell injury, increased glomerular permeability to proteins, accumulation of proteins and lipids in the mesangial matrix, and fibrin deposition. This is followed by proliferation of mesangial cells, increased deposition of mesangial matrix, and sclerosis of glomeruli. The latter results in further reductions in nephron mass and a vicious cycle of continuing glomerulosclerosis.

We now turn to a consideration of specific types of GN and the glomerular syndromes they produce.

Glomerular Syndromes and Disorders

THE NEPHROTIC SYNDROME

The nephrotic syndrome refers to a clinical complex made up of the following: (1) *massive proteinuria,* with the daily loss in the urine of 3.5 gm or more of protein; (2) *generalized edema,* the most obvious clinical manifestation; (3) *hypoalbuminemia,* with plasma albumin levels less than 3 gm per deciliter; and (4) *hyperlipidemia and lipiduria.* At the onset there is little or no azotemia, hematuria, or hypertension.

The components of the nephrotic syndrome bear a logical relationship to one another. The initial event is a derangement in the capillary walls of the glomeruli, resulting in increased permeability to the plasma proteins. It will be remembered from the previous discussion of the normal kidney that the glomerular capillary wall, with its endothelium, GBM, and visceral epithelial cells, acts as a barrier through which the glomerular filtrate must pass. Any increased permeability resulting from either structural or physicochemical alterations allows protein to escape from the plasma into the glomerular filtrate. Massive proteinuria may result. With long-standing or extremely heavy proteinuria, the serum albumin tends to become depleted, resulting in hypoalbuminemia and a reversed albumin-globulin ratio. The generalized edema of the nephrotic syndrome is in turn largely a consequence of the drop in osmotic pressure produced by hypoalbuminemia. As fluid escapes from the vascular tree into the tissues, there is a concomitant drop in plasma volume, with diminished glomerular filtration. Compensatory secretion of aldosterone, along with the reduced glomerular filtration rate, and reduction of secretion of natriuretic peptides promotes retention of salt and water by the kidneys, thus further aggravating the edema. By repetition of this chain of events, massive amounts of edema (termed *anasarca*) may accumulate. The genesis of the hyperlipidemia is more obscure. Presumably hypoalbuminemia triggers increased synthesis of lipoproteins in the liver. There is also abnormal transport of circulating lipid particles and impairment of peripheral breakdown of lipoproteins. The lipiduria in turn reflects the increased GBM permeability to lipoproteins.

The relative frequencies of the several causes of the nephrotic syndrome vary according to age. *In children under 15 years of age, for example, the nephrotic syndrome is almost always caused by a lesion primary to the kidney, whereas among adults it may often be associated with a systemic disease.* Table 14–2 represents a composite derived from several

■

Table 14–2. CAUSES OF NEPHROTIC SYNDROME

	Prevalence* (%)	
	Children	Adults
Primary Glomerular Disease		
Membranous glomerulonephritis (GN)	5	40
Lipoid nephrosis	65	15
Focal segmental glomerulosclerosis	10	15
Membranoproliferative GN	10	7
Other proliferative GN (focal, "pure mesangial," IgA nephropathy)	10	23
Systemic Diseases		
Diabetes mellitus		
Amyloidosis		Most common systemic causes
Systemic lupus erythematosus		
Drugs (gold, penicillamine, "street heroin")		
Infections (malaria, syphilis hepatitis, B, AIDS)		
Malignancy (carcinoma, melanoma)		
Miscellaneous (bee-sting allergy, hereditary nephritis)		

*Approximate prevalence of primary disease is 95% in children, 60% in adults. Approximate prevalence of systemic disease is 5% in children, 40% in adults.

studies of the causes of the nephrotic syndrome, and is therefore only approximate. As the table indicates, the most frequent *systemic* causes of the nephrotic syndrome are SLE, diabetes, and amyloidosis. The renal lesions produced by these disorders are described elsewhere in this text. The most important of the *primary* glomerular lesions that characteristically lead to the nephrotic syndrome are *lipoid nephrosis (minimal change disease)* and *membranous GN*. The former is most important in children; the latter in adults. Two other primary lesions, *focal glomerulosclerosis* and *membranoproliferative GN*, also produce the nephrotic syndrome. These four lesions are discussed individually below. The fifth possible primary cause of this syndrome, *proliferative GN*, is not considered in this section because this lesion frequently presents with the nephritic syndrome.

MINIMAL CHANGE DISEASE (LIPOID NEPHROSIS)

This relatively benign disorder is the most frequent cause of the nephrotic syndrome in children. *It is characterized by glomeruli that have a normal appearance under the light microscope but disclose diffuse loss of visceral epithelial foot processes when viewed with the electron microscope.* Although it may develop at any age, this condition is most common between ages 2 and 3 years.

Pathogenesis. The pathogenesis of lipoid nephrosis is shrouded in mystery. There is no evidence for either an immune complex or an anti-GBM mechanism, but the ultrastructural changes in glomerular epithelial cells clearly point to primary epithelial cell injury. In addition, certain clinical features such as the association with atopy, viral infections, and the dramatic response to corticosteroids suggest a disorder of T-cell function. The current hypothesis is that such an immune defect results in the elaboration of a circulating factor, perhaps a cytokine, secreted by lymphocytes or macrophages, which causes epithelial injury, loss of glomerular polyanionic molecules, and proteinuria. Indeed such factors are currently under investigation (Fig. 14–5B).

MORPHOLOGY. With the light microscope the glomeruli appear nearly normal (Fig. 14–6A). The cells of the proximal convoluted tubules are often heavily laden with lipids, but this is secondary to tubular reabsorption of the lipoproteins passing through the diseased glomeruli. This appearance of the proximal convoluted tubules is the basis for the older term for this disorder, **lipoid nephrosis.** Even with the electron microscope, the GBM appears normal. The only obvious glomerular abnormality is the uniform and diffuse loss of the foot processes of the podocytes (Fig. 14–6C). The cytoplasm of the podocytes thus appears smeared over the external aspect of the GBM, obliterating the network of arcades between the podocytes and the GBM. There are also epithelial cell vacuolization, microvillus formation, and occasional focal detachments. The changes in the podocytes are completely reversible after remission of the proteinuria.

Clinical Course. The disease manifests itself by the insidious development of the nephrotic syndrome in an otherwise healthy child. There is no hypertension, and renal function is preserved in most patients. The protein loss is usually confined to the smaller serum proteins, chiefly albumin (selective proteinuria). The prognosis in children with this disorder is good. More than 90% of cases respond to a short course of corticosteroid therapy; however, proteinuria recurs in more than two thirds of the initial responders, some of whom become steroid dependent. Less than 5% develop chronic renal failure after 25 years. Because of its responsiveness to therapy in children, lipoid nephrosis must be differentiated from the other causes of the nephrotic syndrome in nonresponders. Adults also respond to steroid therapy, but relapses are more common.

MEMBRANOUS GLOMERULONEPHRITIS (MEMBRANOUS NEPHROPATHY)

This slowly progressive disease, most common between ages 30 and 50 years, *is characterized morphologically by the presence of subepithelial immunoglobulin-containing deposits along the GBM.* Early in the disease, the glomeruli may appear normal by light microscopy, but well-developed cases show *diffuse thickening of the capillary wall.*

Membranous GN (MGN) may occur in association with known disorders or agents (secondary MGN): (1) infections (chronic hepatitis B, syphilis, schistosomiasis, malaria); (2) malignant epithelial tumors, particularly carcinoma of the lung and colon and melanoma; (3) SLE; (4) exposure to inorganic salts (gold, mercury); (5) drugs (penicillamine, captopril); and (6) metabolic disorders (diabetes mellitus, thyroiditis). In about 85% of cases the condition is truly idiopathic (primary).

Pathogenesis. Membranous GN is a form of chronic immune complex nephritis. Although circulating complexes of known exogenous (e.g., hepatitis B) or endogenous (DNA in SLE) antigen can cause MGN, it is now thought that most idiopathic forms are induced by antibodies reacting in situ to endogenous or planted glomerular antigens.

The lesions bear a striking resemblance to those of experimental Heymann's nephritis, which, as you may recall, is induced by antibodies to a megalin antigenic complex, and a similar antigen is present in humans (p 444). Susceptibility to Heymann's nephritis in rats and MGN in humans is linked to the HLA locus, which influences the ability to elaborate antibodies to the *nephritogenic* antigen. Thus idiopathic MGN, like Heymann's nephritis, is considered an autoimmune disease linked to susceptibility genes and caused by antibodies to a renal autoantigen.

Begging the question of the nature of the immune deposits, how does the glomerular capillary wall become leaky? In the absence of neutrophils, monocytes, or platelets and the virtually uniform presence of complement, current work points to a direct action of C5b–9, the membrane attack complex of complement (p 443).

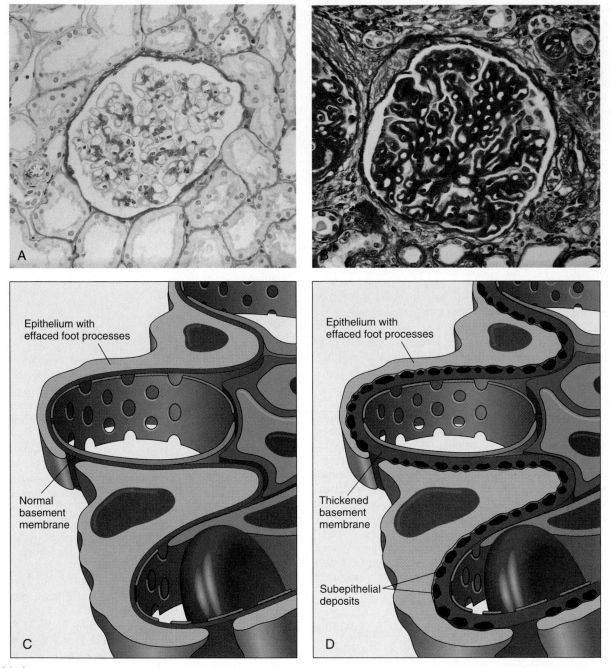

Figure 14-6

Lipoid nephrosis *(A and C)* and membranous glomerulonephritis (GN) *(B and D)*. Note that under the light microscope the periodic acid–Schiff (PAS)–stained glomerulus appears normal, with a thin basement membrane, in lipoid nephrosis *(A)*. Compare this with the diffuse thickening of the basement membrane in membranous GN *(B)*. Lipoid nephrosis exhibits diffuse loss of foot processes of visceral epithelial cells *(C)*, whereas membranous GN *(D)* is characterized by electron-dense subepithelial deposits.

MORPHOLOGY. Seen by light microscopy, the basic change appears to be diffuse thickening of the GBM (Fig. 14–6B). By electron microscopy, the apparent thickening is caused in part by subepithelial deposits that nestle against the GBM and are separated from each other by small, spikelike protrusions of GBM matrix ("spike and dome" pattern, (Fig. 14–6D). As the disease progresses, these spikes close over the deposits, incorporating them into the GBM. In addition, the podocytes lose their foot processes. The consequent close apposition of the podocytes to the GBM contributes to the appearance of GBM thickening on light microscopy. Later in the disease, the incorporated deposits are catabolized and eventually disappear, leaving for a time cavities within the GBM. These are later filled in by deposition of GBM-like material. With further progression, the glomeruli become sclerosed and finally become completely hyalinized. Fluorescence microscopy shows typical granular deposition of immunoglobulins and complement along the GBM (see Fig. 14–4A).

Clinical Course. The onset is characterized by the insidious development of the nephrotic syndrome, usually without antecedent illness; however, proteinuria may be present without the full-blown nephrotic syndrome. In contrast to minimal change disease, the proteinuria is nonselective and does not usually respond to corticosteroid therapy. Globulins are lost in the urine, as are the smaller albumin molecules. MGN follows a notoriously variable and often indolent course. Overall, although proteinuria persists in over 60% of patients, only about 40% of patients suffer progressive disease terminating in renal failure after 2 to 20 years. An additional 10% to 30% have a more benign course with partial or complete remission of proteinuria.

FOCAL SEGMENTAL GLOMERULOSCLEROSIS

Focal segmental glomerulosclerosis (FSG) is characterized histologically by sclerosis affecting some but not all glomeruli and involving only segments of each glomerulus. This histological picture is often associated with the nephrotic syndrome and can occur in 4 settings: (1) in association with other known conditions, such as human immunodeficiency virus (HIV) infection and heroin addiction (HIV nephropathy, heroin addiction nephropathy); (2) as a secondary event in other forms of GN (e.g., IgA nephropathy); (3) as a component of glomerular ablation nephropathy (described earlier); or (4) as a primary disease.

Primary (or idiopathic) FSG accounts for approximately 10% of all cases of the nephrotic syndrome. *In children it is important to distinguish this cause of the nephrotic syndrome from lipoid nephrosis (minimal change disease),* because the clinical course is markedly different. Unlike the case with lipoid nephrosis, patients with this lesion have a higher incidence of hematuria and hypertension, their proteinuria is nonselective, and in general their response to corticosteroid therapy is poor. At least 50% of patients develop end-stage failure within 10 years of diagnosis. Adults in general fare even less well than children.

Pathogenesis. The pathogenesis of primary focal glomerulosclerosis is unknown. Some investigators have suggested that focal glomerulosclerosis is a variant, albeit an aggressive one, of minimal change disease. Others believe it to be a distinct clinicopathologic entity. In any case, *the characteristic disruption of visceral epithelial cells is thought to represent the hallmark of FSG.* The hyalinosis and sclerosis described below represent entrapment of plasma proteins and lipids in hyperpermeable foci, and mesangial cell reaction to such proteins and to fibrin deposits. The recurrence of proteinuria in patients with focal sclerosis who receive renal allografts, sometimes within 24 hours of transplantation, suggests a circulating mediator as the cause of the epithelial damage, and

indeed such a permeability-increasing mediator has recently been isolated from these patients.

MORPHOLOGY. The disease first affects only some of the glomeruli (hence the term focal) and initially only the juxtamedullary glomeruli. With progression, eventually all levels of the cortex are affected. Histologically, focal glomerulosclerosis is characterized by lesions occurring in some tufts within a glomerulus and sparing of the others (hence the term segmental). Thus, the involvement is both focal and segmental (Fig. 14–7). The lesions exhibit increased mesangial matrix, collapsed basement membranes, deposition of hyaline masses (hyalinosis), and of lipid droplets. Occasionally, glomeruli are completely sclerosed (global sclerosis). In affected glomeruli, immunofluorescent microscopy reveals deposits of immunoglobulins, usually IgM, and complement in the mesangium. On electron microscopy, the visceral epithelial cells exhibit loss of foot processes, as in lipoid nephrosis, but also a **greater degree of epithelial cell detachment** with denudation of underlying GBM.

In time, progression of the disease leads to total sclerosis of the glomeruli with pronounced tubular atrophy and interstitial fibrosis. This advanced picture is difficult to differentiate from other forms of chronic GN, described later.

There is little tendency for spontaneous remission of idiopathic FSG, and responses to corticosteroid therapy are poor. Progression to renal failure occurs at varying rates, and about 50% of patients suffer renal failure after 10 years.

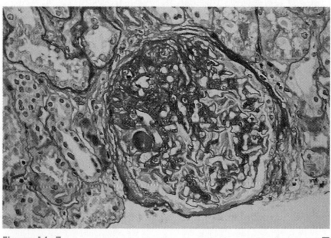

Figure 14–7   ■

High-power view of focal segmental glomerulosclerosis (PAS stain), seen as a hyaline mass that has replaced a portion of the glomerulus. (Courtesy of Dr. H. Rennke, Department of Pathology, Brigham and Women's Hospital, Boston.)

MEMBRANOPROLIFERATIVE GLOMERULONEPHRITIS

Membranoproliferative GN (MPGN) is manifested histologically by alterations in the basement membrane and mesangium and by proliferation of glomerular cells. It accounts for 5% to 10% of cases of idiopathic nephrotic syndrome in children and adults. Some patients present only with hematuria or proteinuria in the non-nephrotic range; others have a combined nephrotic-nephritic picture. Two major types of MPGN (I and II) are recognized on the basis of distinct ultrastructural, immunofluorescent, and probably pathogenic findings.

MORPHOLOGY. By light microscopy, both types are similar. The glomeruli are large and show proliferation of mesangial cells as well as infiltrating leukocytes (Fig. 14–8A). They have a lobular appearance. The GBM is thickened, and the glomerular capillary wall often shows a double-contour or "tramtrack" appearance, especially evident in silver or periodic acid–Schiff (PAS) stains. This is caused by "splitting" of the basement membrane because of the inclusion within it of processes of mesangial cells extending into the peripheral capillary loops, so-called *mesangial interposition* (Fig. 14–8B).

Types I and II have different ultrastructural and immunofluorescent features (Fig. 14–8B). **Type I MPGN** (two thirds of cases) is characterized by subendothelial electron-dense deposits. By immunofluorescence, C3 is deposited in a granular pattern, and IgG and early complement components (C1q and C4) are often also present, suggesting an immune complex pathogenesis.

In **type II lesions,** the lamina densa of the GBM is transformed into an irregular, ribbon-like, extremely electron-dense structure, owing to the deposition of dense material of unknown composition in the GBM proper, giving rise to the term **dense-deposit disease.** C3 is present in irregular granular-linear foci in the basement membranes and mesangium in characteristic circular aggregates (mesangial rings). IgG is usually absent, as are the early-acting complement components (C1q and C4).

Pathogenesis. Although there is considerable overlap, different pathogenic mechanisms are involved in the evolution of type I and type II disease. Most cases of type I MPGN

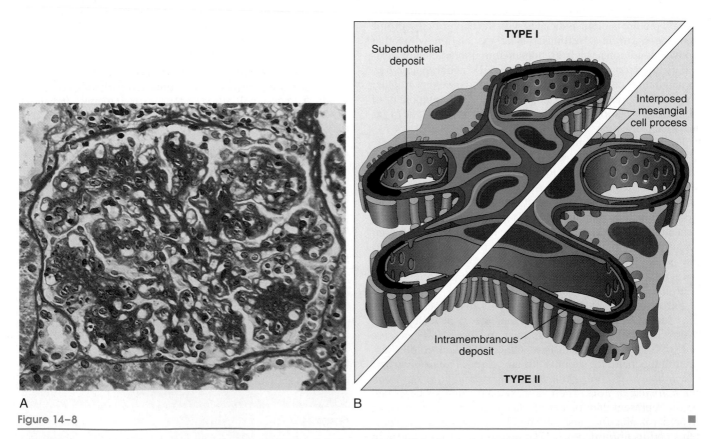

A   B

Figure 14–8

A, Membranoproliferative GN, showing mesangial cell proliferation, basement membrane thickening, leukocyte infiltration, and accentuation of lobular architecture. *B,* Schematic representation of patterns in the two types of membranoproliferative GN. In type I there are subendothelial deposits; type II is characterized by intramembranous dense deposits (dense deposit disease). In both, mesangial interposition gives the appearance of split basement membranes when viewed in the light microscope.

appear to be caused by a chronic immune complex reaction, but the inciting antigen is not known. Type I MPGN also occurs in association with hepatitis B and C antigenemia, SLE, infected atrioventricular shunts, and secondary infections. The pathogenesis of type II MPGN is less clear. The serum of patients with type II MPGN has a factor called *C3 nephritic factor* (C3NeF), which can activate the alternative complement pathway. This factor is an immunoglobulin that reacts with C3 convertase of the alternative complement pathway and serves to stabilize it, thus activating the pathway and resulting in the elaboration of biologically active complement fragments. C3NeF is thus an autoantibody and, as in other autoimmune diseases, there is a genetic predisposition to the development of MPGN. The hypocomplementemia, more marked in type II, is contributed in part by excessive consumption of C3 and in part by reduced synthesis of C3 by the liver. It is still not clear how the complement abnormality induces the glomerular changes.

Clinical Course. The principal mode of presentation is the nephrotic syndrome, although MPGN may begin as acute nephritis or more insidiously as mild proteinuria. The prognosis of MPGN is uniformly poor. In one study, none of 60 patients followed for 1 to 20 years showed complete remission. Forty per cent progressed to end-stage renal failure, 30% had variable degrees of renal insufficiency, and the remaining 30% had persistent nephrotic syndrome without renal failure. Type II disease has a worse prognosis, and it tends to recur in transplant recipients. Like many other glomerulonephritides, MPGN, usually of type I, may occur in association with other known disorders *(secondary MPGN),* such as SLE, hepatitis B and C infection, chronic liver disease, and certain malignancies.

THE NEPHRITIC SYNDROME

The nephritic syndrome is a clinical complex, usually of acute onset, characterized by (1) *hematuria* with red cell and hemoglobin casts in the urine, (2) some degree of *oliguria* and azotemia, and (3) *hypertension.* Although there may also be some proteinuria and even edema, these are usually not sufficiently marked to cause the nephrotic syndrome. The lesions that cause this syndrome have in common proliferation of the cells within the glomeruli, often accompanied by a leukocytic infiltrate. This inflammatory reaction injures the capillary walls, permitting escape of red cells into the urine, and induces hemodynamic changes that lead to a reduction in the glomerular filtration rate. The reduced glomerular filtration rate is manifested clinically by oliguria, reciprocal fluid retention, and azotemia. Hypertension is probably a result of both the fluid retention and some augmented renin release from the ischemic kidneys.

The acute nephritic syndrome may be produced by systemic disorders such as SLE or may be the result of primary glomerular disease. The latter, which is more common, is exemplified by acute diffuse proliferative GN, discussed below.

Acute Proliferative (Poststreptococcal, Postinfectious) Glomerulonephritis

Diffuse proliferative GN (PGN), one of the more frequent of the glomerular disorders, is typically caused by immune complexes. The inciting antigen may be exogenous or endog-

enous. The prototype exogenous pattern is postinfectious GN, whereas that produced by an endogenous antigen is lupus nephritis, seen in SLE (Chapter 5). Infections by organisms other than the streptococci may also be associated with diffuse PGN. These include certain pneumococcal and staphylococcal infections as well as a number of common viral diseases such as mumps, measles, chickenpox, and hepatitis B.

The classic case of poststreptococcal GN develops in a child 1 to 4 weeks after the patient recovers from a group A streptococcal infection. Only certain "nephritogenic" strains of the β-hemolytic streptococci are capable of evoking glomerular disease. In most cases the initial infection is pharyngitis or a skin infection.

Pathogenesis. It is generally agreed that acute poststreptococcal GN is mediated by deposition of immune complexes. *Typical features of immune complex disease, such as hypocomplementemia and granular deposits of IgG and complement on the GBM, are seen.* Nevertheless, the nature of the pathogenic antigen remains mysterious, and it is not clear whether circulating or complexes formed in situ are the predominant forms. Streptococcal antigens, altered GBM, and altered forms of IgG have been implicated at one time or another.

> **MORPHOLOGY.** Under the light microscope, the most characteristic change is a fairly uniformly increased cellularity of the glomerular tufts affecting nearly all glomeruli, hence the term *diffuse* (Fig. 14-9A). The increased cellularity is caused both by proliferation and swelling of endothelial and mesangial cells and by a neutrophilic and monocytic infiltrate. Sometimes there are thrombi within the capillary lumina and necrosis of the capillary walls. In a few cases there may also be "crescents" (p 452) inside Bowman's capsule. In general, these are an ominous finding. When they involve most of the glomeruli, the pattern merges with that of rapidly progressive GN, to be discussed. In the early stages of the disease, the electron microscope shows the immune complexes arrayed as subendothelial, intramembranous, or most often subepithelial "humps" nestled against the GBM (Fig. 14-9B). Immunofluorescence studies reveal IgG and complement within the deposits. These deposits are usually cleared over a period of about 2 months.

Clinical Course. The onset of the kidney disease tends to be abrupt, heralded by malaise, a slight fever, nausea, and the nephritic syndrome. In the usual case, oliguria, azotemia, and hypertension are only mild to moderate. Characteristically, there is gross hematuria, the urine appearing smoky brown rather than bright red. Some proteinuria is a constant feature of the disease and, as mentioned earlier, it may occasionally be severe enough to produce the nephrotic syndrome. Serum complement levels are low and serum antistreptolysin O titers elevated in poststreptococcal cases.

Complete recovery occurs in most children in epidemic cases. A very few children (less than 1%) develop rapidly

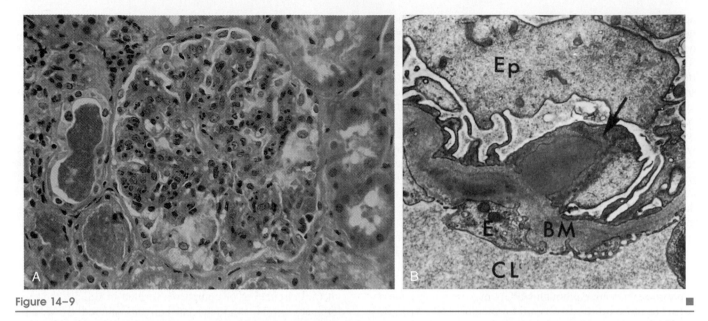

Figure 14-9

Poststreptococcal GN. *A*, Glomerular hypercellularity is due to intracapillary leukocytes and proliferation of intrinsic glomerular cells. Note the red cell casts in the tubules. *B*, Typical electron-dense subepithelial "hump" and intramembranous deposits.

progressive GN or chronic renal disease. The prognosis in sporadic cases is less clear. In adults, 15% to 50% of cases become chronic, depending on the clinical and histologic severity. In contrast, the prevalence of chronicity after sporadic cases of acute GN in children is much lower.

Rapidly Progressive (Crescentic) Glomerulonephritis

Rapidly progressive glomerulonephritis (RPGN) is a clinicopathologic syndrome and not a specific etiologic form of GN. Clinically it is characterized by rapid and progressive loss of renal function associated with severe oliguria and (if untreated) death from renal failure within weeks to months. *Regardless of the cause, the histologic picture is characterized by the presence of crescents in most of the glomeruli* (crescentic GN). These are produced in part by proliferation of the parietal epithelial cells of Bowman's capsule and in part by infiltration of monocytes and macrophages.

Pathogenesis. RPGN may be caused by a number of different diseases, some restricted to the kidney and others systemic. Although no single mechanism can explain all cases, there is little doubt that in most cases the glomerular injury is immunologically mediated. Thus, a practical classification divides RPGN into three groups on the basis of immunologic findings (Table 14–3). In each group the disease may be associated with a known disorder, or it may be idiopathic.

Type I RPGN is best remembered as *anti-GBM disease* and hence is characterized by linear deposits of IgG and, in many cases, C3 on the GBM, as previously described. In some of these patients the anti-GBM antibodies cross-react with pulmonary alveolar basement membranes to produce the clinical picture of pulmonary hemorrhages associated with renal failure. These patients are said to have *Goodpasture's syndrome,* to distinguish their condition from the idiopathic cases in which renal involvement occurs in the absence of pulmonary disease. It is important to recognize type I RPGN, because

these patients are benefited by plasmapheresis, which serves to remove pathogenic antibodies from the circulation.

Type II RPGN is an *immune complex–mediated disease.* It can be a complication of any of the immune complex nephritides, including poststreptococcal GN, SLE, IgA nephropathy, and Henoch-Schönlein purpura. In some cases immune complexes can be demonstrated, but the underlying cause is undetermined. In all of these cases, immunofluorescence studies reveal the characteristic ("lumpy bumpy") granular pattern of staining. These patients cannot usually be helped by plasmapheresis, and they require treatment for the underlying disease.

Type III RPGN, also called *pauci-immune type,* is defined by the lack of anti-GBM antibodies or immune complexes by immunofluorescence and electron microscopy. Most of these patients have antineutrophil cytoplasmic antibody (ANCA) in the serum, which, as we have seen (Chapter 10), plays a role in some vasculitides. Hence, in some cases type III RPGN is

Table 14–3. RAPIDLY PROGRESSIVE GLOMERULONEPHRITIS (RPGN)

Type I RPGN (Anti-GBM)
  Idiopathic
  Goodpasture's syndrome
Type II RPGN (Immune Complex)
  Idiopathic
  Systemic lupus erythematosus
  Post infectious
  Henoch-Schönlein purpura
Type III RPGN (Pauci-immune)
  Idiopathic
  Wegener's granulomatosis
  Polyarteritis

a component of a systemic vasculitis such as polyarteritis no-dosa or Wegener's granulomatosis. In many cases, however, pauci-immune crescentic GN is isolated and hence idiopathic.

It should be obvious from this discussion that, although all three types of RPGN may be associated with a well-defined renal or extrarenal disease, in many cases (approximately 50%) it is idiopathic. Of these cases, about one fourth have anti-GBM disease (RPGN type I) without lung involvement; another one fourth have type II RPGN; and the remainder are pauci-immune or type III RPGN. *The common denominator in all types of RPGN is severe glomerular injury.*

MORPHOLOGY. The kidneys are enlarged and pale, often with petechial hemorrhages on the cortical surfaces. Depending on the underlying cause, the glomeruli may show focal necrosis and thrombosis, diffuse or focal endothelial prolifera-tion, and mesangial proliferation. However, the his-tologic picture is dominated by the formation of distinctive crescents (Fig. 14–10). Crescents are formed by proliferation of parietal cells and by migration of monocytes into Bowman's space. The crescents eventually obliterate Bowman's space and compress the glomeruli. Fibrin strands are prominent between the cellular layers in the cres-cents, and there is evidence that the escape of fibrin into Bowman's space incites crescent forma-tion. Electron microscopy may disclose subepithe-lial deposits in some cases, as expected, but in all cases it shows distinct ruptures in the GBM. In time, most crescents undergo sclerosis.

Clinical Course. The onset of RPGN is much like that of the nephritic syndrome except that the oliguria and azotemia are more pronounced. Ninety per cent of these patients be-

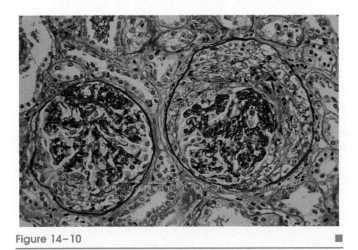

Figure 14–10   ■

Crescentic GN (PAS stain). Note the collapsed glomerular tufts and the cres-cent-shaped mass of proliferating cells and leukocytes internal to Bowman's capsule. (Courtesy of Dr. M. A. Venkatachalam, Department of Pathology, University of Texas Health Sciences Center, San Antonio, TX.)

come anephric and require long-term dialysis or transplanta-tion. The prognosis can be roughly related to the number of crescents: patients with crescents in less than 80% of the glomeruli have a slightly better prognosis than those with higher percentages of crescents. Plasma exchange benefits some patients, particularly those with Goodpasture's syn-drome.

IgA Nephropathy (Berger's Disease)

This condition usually affects children and young adults, and begins as an episode of gross hematuria occurring within a day or two of a nonspecific upper respiratory tract infection. Typically, the hematuria lasts several days and then subsides, only to recur every few months. It is often associated with loin pain. *IgA nephropathy is one of the most common causes of recurrent microscopic or gross hematuria and the most common glomerular disease worldwide.*

The pathogenic hallmark is the deposition of IgA in the mesangium. Some have considered Berger's disease to be a variant of *Henoch-Schönlein purpura,* often characterized by IgA deposition in the mesangium. In contrast to Berger's dis-ease, which is purely a renal disorder, Henoch-Schönlein pur-pura is a systemic syndrome involving the skin (purpuric rash), gastrointestinal tract (abdominal pain), joints (arthritis), and kidneys.

Pathogenesis. The pathogenesis is unknown, but there are certain clues. IgA, the main immunoglobulin in mucosal se-cretions, is at low levels in normal serum but increased in patients with IgA nephropathy. In addition, circulating IgA-containing immune complexes are present in some patients. A genetic influence is suggested by the occurrence of this condition in families and in HLA-identical siblings, and by the increased frequency of certain HLA and complement phe-notypes in some populations. The prominent mesangial dep-osition of IgA suggests entrapment of IgA immune complexes in the mesangium, and the absence of Clq and C4 in glomeruli points to activation of the alternative complement pathway. Taken together, these clues suggest a genetic or acquired ab-normality of immune regulation, leading to increased mucosal IgA synthesis in response to respiratory or gastrointestinal ex-posure to environmental agents (e.g., viruses, bacteria, food proteins). IgA and IgA complexes are then entrapped in the mesangium, where they activate the alternative complement pathway and initiate glomerular injury. In support of this sce-nario, IgA nephropathy occurs with increased frequency in patients with celiac disease in whom intestinal mucosal de-fects are seen, and in liver disease where there is defective hepatobiliary clearance of IgA complexes (*secondary IgA nephropathy*).

MORPHOLOGY. Histologically, the lesions vary con-siderably. The glomeruli may be normal or may show mesangial widening and segmental prolifer-ation confined to some glomeruli (focal GN); dif-fuse mesangial proliferation (mesangioprolif-erative); or (rarely) overt crescentic GN. The characteristic immunofluorescent picture is of **mesangial deposition of IgA,** often with C3 and properdin and smaller amounts of IgG or IgM (Fig. 14–11). Early complement components are usually absent. Electron microscopy confirms the presence of electron-dense deposits in the mesangium.

Clinically, IgA nephropathy is a heterogeneous disease. Although most children have a benign course, the disease appears to be slowly progressive in adults. It is estimated that chronic renal failure develops in more than 50% of cases over a period of 20 years.

Hereditary Nephritis

Hereditary nephritis refers to a group of hereditary familial renal diseases associated primarily with glomerular injury. The best-studied entity is *Alport's syndrome,* in which nephritis is accompanied by nerve deafness and various eye disorders, including lens dislocation, posterior cataracts, and corneal dystrophy. Males tend to be affected more frequently and more severely than females and are more likely to progress to renal failure. Patients present at age 5 to 20 years with gross or microscopic hematuria and proteinuria, and overt renal failure occurs between 20 and 50 years of age. The inheritance is heterogeneous, being either X-linked or autosomal dominant in most pedigrees.

Histologically, there is segmental glomerular proliferation or sclerosis, or both, and an increase in mesangial matrix. In some kidneys, glomerular or tubular epithelial cells take on a foamy appearance owing to accumulation of neutral fats and mucopolysaccharides **(foam cells).** With progression, there is increasing glomerulosclerosis, vascular narrowing, tubular atrophy, and interstitial fibrosis. With the electron microscope, the basement

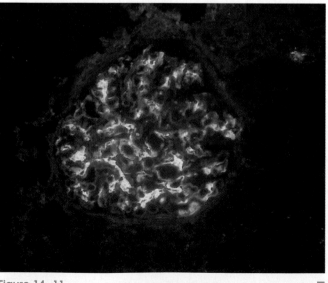

Figure 14–11 ■

IgA nephropathy showing characteristic immunofluorescence deposition of IgA, principally in mesangial regions.

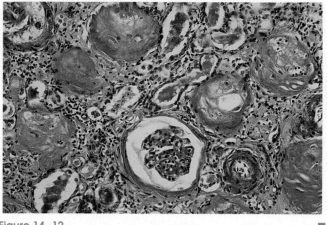

Figure 14–12 ■

Chronic GN. A Masson trichrome preparation shows complete replacement of virtually all glomeruli by blue-staining collagen. (Courtesy of Dr. M. A. Venkatachalam, Department of Pathology, University of Texas Health Sciences Center, San Antonio, TX.)

membrane of glomeruli and tubules shows irregular foci of thickening or attenuation, with pronounced splitting and lamination of the lamina densa.

The basement membrane defect has been traced in patients with X-linked disease to mutations in the gene encoding the α-5 chain of collagen type IV, interfering with the structure and permeability of the GBM. Additional mutations in a newly discovered α-6 chain occur in some patients.

CHRONIC GLOMERULONEPHRITIS

Having discussed various forms of glomerular disease, we should now turn to one of their unfortunate outcomes, chronic GN. It is an important cause of end-stage renal disease presenting as chronic renal failure. Thirty to 50% of all patients who require chronic hemodialysis or renal transplantation have the diagnosis of chronic GN.

By the time chronic GN is discovered, the glomerular changes are so far advanced that it is difficult to discern the nature of the original lesion. It probably represents the end stage of a variety of entities, prominent among which are focal glomerulosclerosis, membranous GN, and membranoproliferative GN. It has been estimated that perhaps 20% of cases arise with no history of symptomatic renal disease. Although chronic GN may develop at any age, it is usually first noted in young and middle-aged adults.

MORPHOLOGY. Classically, the kidneys are symmetrically contracted and their surfaces are red-brown and diffusely granular.

Microscopically, the feature common to all cases is advanced scarring of the glomeruli and Bowman's spaces, sometimes to the point of complete replacement or hyalinization of the glomeruli (Fig. 14–12). This obliteration of the glomeruli is the end point of all cases, and it is impossible to ascertain from such kidneys the nature of the earlier lesion.

The obstruction to blood flow between afferent and efferent arterioles secondary to glomerular damage must of necessity have an impact on the other elements of the kidney. There is, then, marked interstitial fibrosis, associated with atrophy and replacement of many of the tubules in the cortex. The small and medium-sized arteries are frequently thick walled, with narrowed lumina, secondary to hypertension. Lymphocytic (and, rarely, plasma cell) infiltrates are present in the interstitial tissue. As damage to all structures progresses, it may become difficult to ascertain whether the primary lesion was glomerular, vascular, or interstitial. Such markedly damaged kidneys are thus designated "end-stage kidneys."

Clinical Course. Most often, chronic GN develops insidiously and is discovered only late in its course, after the onset of renal insufficiency. Very frequently, renal disease is first suspected with the discovery of proteinuria, hypertension, or azotemia on routine medical examination. In some patients the course is punctuated by transient episodes of either the nephritic or the nephrotic syndrome. Some of these patients may seek medical attention for the edema. As the glomeruli become obliterated, the avenue for protein loss is progressively closed, and the nephrotic syndrome thus becomes less common with more advanced disease. Some proteinuria, however, is constant in all cases. Hypertension is very common and its effects may dominate the clinical picture. Although microscopic hematuria is usually present, grossly bloody urine is infrequent.

Without treatment, the prognosis is poor; relentless progression to uremia and death is the rule. The rate of progression is extremely variable, however, and 10 years or more may elapse between onset of the first symptoms and death. Renal dialysis and renal transplants, of course, alter this course and allow long-term survival.

DISEASES AFFECTING TUBULES AND INTERSTITIUM

Most forms of tubular injury also involve the interstitium, so the two are discussed together. Under this heading we present diseases characterized by (1) inflammatory involvement of the tubules and interstitium (interstitial nephritis) and (2) ischemic or toxic tubular injury, leading to *acute tubular necrosis* and *acute renal failure*.

Tubulointerstitial Nephritis

Tubulointerstitial nephritis (TIN) refers to a group of inflammatory diseases of the kidneys that primarily involve the interstitium and tubules. The glomeruli may be spared altogether or affected only late in the course. In most cases of TIN caused by bacterial infection the renal pelvis is promi-

nently involved, hence the more descriptive term *pyelonephritis* (from *pyelo,* pelvis). The term *interstitial nephritis* is generally reserved for cases that are noninfectious in origin. These include tubular injury resulting from drugs, metabolic disorders such as hypokalemia, physical injury such as irradiation, and immune reactions. On the basis of clinical features and the character of the inflammatory exudate, TIN, regardless of the etiologic agent, can be divided into acute and chronic categories. In the following section we present PN first, followed by other noninfectious forms of interstitial nephritis.

ACUTE PYELONEPHRITIS

Acute pyelonephritis, a common suppurative inflammation of the kidney and the renal pelvis, is caused by bacterial infection. It is an important manifestation of urinary tract infection (UTI), which implies involvement of the lower (cystitis, prostatitis, urethritis) or upper (pyelonephritis) urinary tract, or both. As we shall see, pyelonephritis is almost always associated with infection of the lower urinary tract. The latter, however, may remain localized without extending to involve the kidney. UTIs are extremely common clinical problems.

Pathogenesis. The principal causative organisms are the enteric gram-negative rods. *Escherichia coli* is by far the most common one. Other important organisms are species of *Proteus, Klebsiella, Enterobacter,* and *Pseudomonas;* these are usually associated with recurrent infections, especially in patients who undergo urinary tract manipulations. Staphylococci and *Streptococcus faecalis* may also cause pyelonephritis, but this is uncommon.

There are two routes by which bacteria can reach the kidneys: through the bloodstream (hematogenous) and from the lower urinary tract (ascending infection). Although *hematogenous spread* is the far less common of the two, acute pyelonephritis may result from seeding of the kidneys by bacteria in the course of septicemia or infective endocarditis (Fig. 14–13). *Ascending infection* from the lower urinary tract is the most important route by which the bacteria reach the kidney. The first step in the pathogenesis of ascending infection appears to be colonization of the distal urethra (and the introitus in females) by gram-negative coliform bacteria. From here the organisms must gain access to the bladder, moving against the flow of urine. This may occur during urethral instrumentation, including catheterization and cystoscopy, which are important predisposing factors in the pathogenesis of UTIs. In the absence of instrumentation, UTI most commonly affects females, in whom the short urethra, and trauma to the urethra during sexual intercourse, facilitate the entry of bacteria into the urinary bladder. Ordinarily, bladder urine is sterile and remains so owing to antimicrobial properties of the bladder mucosa and owing to the flushing action associated with periodic voiding of urine. With outflow obstruction or bladder dysfunction, however, the natural defense mechanisms of the bladder are overwhelmed, setting the stage for UTI. Obstruction at the level of the urinary bladder results in incomplete emptying and increased residual volume of urine. In the presence of stasis, bacteria introduced into the bladder (as by catheterization) can multiply undisturbed, without being unceremoniously flushed out or destroyed by the bladder wall. From the contaminated bladder urine, the bacteria ascend along the

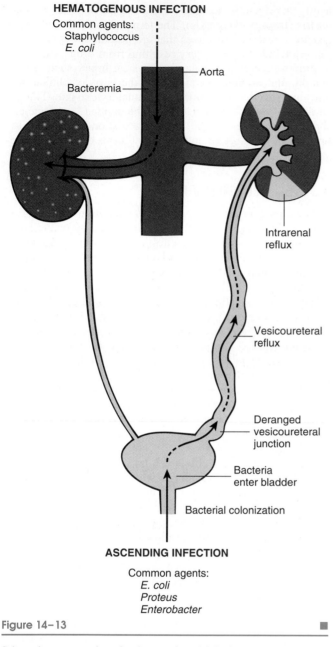

HEMATOGENOUS INFECTION

Common agents:
    Staphylococcus
    E. coli

Bacteremia — Aorta

Intrarenal reflux

Vesicoureteral reflux

Deranged vesicoureteral junction

Bacteria enter bladder

Bacterial colonization

ASCENDING INFECTION

Common agents:
    E. coli
    Proteus
    Enterobacter

Figure 14–13 ■

Schematic representation of pathways of renal infection. Hematogenous infection results from bacteremic spread. More common is ascending infection, which results from a combination of urinary bladder infection, vesicoureteral reflux, and intrarenal reflux.

ureters to infect the renal pelvis and parenchyma. Accordingly, UTI is particularly frequent among patients with urinary tract obstruction, as may occur with benign prostatic hypertrophy and uterine prolapse.

Although obstruction is an important predisposing factor in the pathogenesis of ascending infection, it is *incompetence of the vesicoureteral orifice* that allows bacteria to ascend the ureter into the pelvis. The normal ureteral insertion into the bladder is a competent one-way valve that prevents retrograde flow of urine, especially during micturition, when the intravesical pressure rises. An incompetent vesicoureteral orifice allows the reflux of bladder urine into the ureters (*vesicoure-*

teral reflux [VUR]). The effect of VUR is similar to that of an obstruction in that after voiding there is residual urine in the urinary tract, which favors bacterial growth. Furthermore, VUR affords a ready mechanism by which the infected bladder urine can be propelled up to the renal pelves and farther into the renal parenchyma through open ducts at the tips of the papillae (*intrarenal reflux*).

Besides the various predisposing factors already discussed (obstruction, VUR, pregnancy, and instrumentation of the urinary tract), diabetes tends to increase the risk of serious complications of pyelonephritis, including septicemia, necrotizing papillitis, and recurrence of infection.

> **MORPHOLOGY.** One or both kidneys may be involved. The affected kidney may be normal in size or enlarged. **Characteristically, discrete, yellowish, raised abscesses are grossly apparent on the renal surface** (Fig. 14–14). They may be widely scattered or limited to one region of the kidney, or they may coalesce to form a single large area of suppuration.

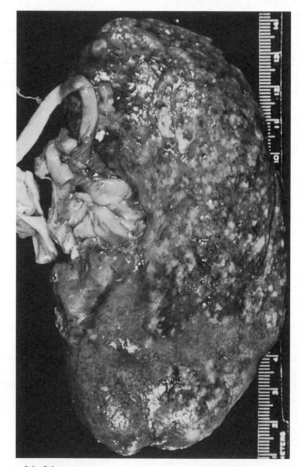

Figure 14–14 ■

Acute pyelonephritis. The cortical surface is studded with focal pale abscesses, more numerous in the upper pole and midregion of the kidney; the lower pole is relatively unaffected. Between the abscesses there is dark congestion of the renal surface.

The characteristic histologic feature of acute pyelonephritis is suppurative necrosis or abscess formation within the renal substance. In the early stages the suppurative infiltrate is limited to the interstitial tissue, but later abscesses rupture into tubules. Large masses of neutrophils frequently extend within involved nephrons into the collecting ducts, giving rise to the characteristic white cell casts found in the urine. Typically, the glomeruli appear to be resistant to the infection.

When the element of obstruction is prominent, the suppurative exudate may be unable to drain and thus fills the renal pelvis, calyces, and ureter, producing **pyonephrosis.**

A second (and fortunately infrequent) form of pyelonephritis is necrosis of the renal papillae, known as **necrotizing papillitis** or **papillary necrosis.** This is particularly common among diabetics who develop acute pyelonephritis and may also complicate acute pyelonephritis when there is significant urinary tract obstruction. It is also seen with the chronic interstitial nephritis associated with analgesic abuse (p 458). This lesion consists of a combination of ischemic and suppurative necrosis of the tips of the renal pyramids (renal papillae). **The pathognomonic gross feature of necrotizing papillitis is sharply defined gray-white to yellow necrosis of the apical two thirds of the pyramids.** One, several, or all papillae may be affected. Microscopically, the papillary tips show characteristic coagulative necrosis, with surrounding neutrophilic infiltrate.

When the bladder is involved in a UTI, as is often the case, **acute** or **chronic cystitis** results. In long-standing cases associated with obstruction, the bladder may be grossly hypertrophic, with trabeculation of its walls, or it may be thinned and markedly distended from retention of urine.

Clinical Course. When uncomplicated acute pyelonephritis is clinically apparent, the onset is usually sudden, with pain at the costovertebral angle and systemic evidence of infection, such as chills, fever, and malaise. *Urinary findings include pyuria and bacteriuria.* In addition, there are usually indications of bladder and urethral irritation (dysuria, frequency, urgency). Even without antibiotic treatment, the disease tends to be benign and self-limited. The symptomatic phase of the disease usually lasts no longer than a week, although bacteriuria may persist much longer. In cases involving predisposing influences, the disease may become recurrent or chronic, particularly when it is bilateral. The development of necrotizing papillitis is associated with a much poorer prognosis. These patients have evidence of overwhelming sepsis, and often renal failure.

CHRONIC PYELONEPHRITIS AND REFLUX NEPHROPATHY

Chronic pyelonephritis is defined here as *a morphologic entity in which predominantly interstitial inflammation and scarring of the renal parenchyma is associated with grossly visible scarring and deformity of the pelvicalyceal system.* Chronic pyelonephritis is an important cause of chronic renal failure. It can be divided into two forms: chronic obstructive and chronic reflux associated.

Chronic Obstructive Pyelonephritis. We have seen that obstruction predisposes the kidney to infection. Recurrent infections superimposed on diffuse or localized obstructive lesions lead to recurrent bouts of renal inflammation and scarring, which eventually cause chronic pyelonephritis. The disease can be bilateral, as with congenital anomalies of the urethra (posterior urethral valves), resulting in fatal renal insufficiency unless the anomaly is corrected; or unilateral, such as occurs with calculi and unilateral obstructive anomalies of the ureter.

Reflux Nephropathy (Chronic Reflux–Associated Pyelonephritis). This is the more common form of chronic pyelonephritic scarring and results from superimposition of a UTI on congenital vesicouretral reflux and intrarenal reflux. Reflux may be unilateral or bilateral; thus, the resultant renal damage either may cause scarring and atrophy of one kidney or may involve both and lead to chronic renal insufficiency. Whether vesicouretral reflux causes renal damage in the absence of infection (sterile reflux) is uncertain, because it is difficult clinically to rule out remote infection in a patient first seen with pyelonephritic scarring.

MORPHOLOGY. One or both kidneys may be involved, either diffusely or patchily. **Even when involvement is bilateral, the kidneys are not equally damaged and therefore are not equally contracted. This uneven scarring is useful in differentiating chronic pyelonephritis from the more symmetrically contracted kidneys caused by benign nephrosclerosis and chronic GN. The hallmark of chronic pyelonephritis is scarring involving the pelvis or calyces, or both, leading to papillary blunting and marked calyceal deformities** (Fig. 14–15).

The microscopic changes are largely nonspecific, and similar alterations may be seen with other tubulointerstitial disorders such as analgesic nephropathy. The parenchyma shows the following features:

- Uneven interstitial fibrosis and an inflammatory infiltrate of lymphocytes, plasma cells, and occasionally neutrophils.
- Dilation or contraction of tubules, with atrophy of the lining epithelium. Many of the dilated tubules contain pink to blue, glassy-appearing casts known as *colloid casts* that suggest the appearance of thyroid tissue, hence the descriptive term *"thyroidization."* Often, neutrophils are seen within tubules.
- Chronic inflammatory infiltration and fibrosis involving the calyceal mucosa and wall.
- Vascular changes similar to those of hyaline or proliferative arteriolosclerosis caused by the frequent association with hypertension.

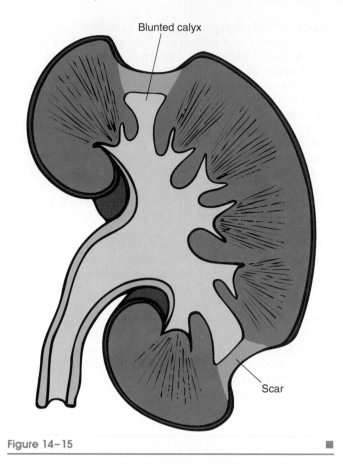

Blunted calyx

Scar

Figure 14–15 ■

Typical coarse scars of chronic pyelonephritis associated with vesicoureteral reflux. The scars are usually polar and are associated with underlying blunted calyces.

■ Although glomeruli are usually normal, in some cases, glomerular lesions, which are similar morphologically to those present in idiopathic focal glomerulosclerosis, are seen. Such cases are often associated with proteinuria.

Clinical Course. Many patients with chronic pyelonephritis come to medical attention relatively late in the course of the disease because of the gradual onset of renal insufficiency or because signs of kidney disease are noticed on routine laboratory tests. Often the renal disease is heralded by the development of hypertension. Pyelograms are characteristic: they show the affected kidney to be asymmetrically contracted, with some degree of blunting and deformity of the calyceal system (caliectasis). Renal cortical scanning with radioactive technetium (Tc) can also detect early scarring. The presence or absence of significant bacteriuria is not particularly helpful diagnostically; its absence certainly should not rule out chronic pyelonephritis. If the disease is bilateral and progressive, tubular dysfunction occurs with loss of concentrating ability, manifested by polyuria and nocturia.

As noted earlier, some patients with chronic pyelonephritis or reflux nephropathy ultimately develop glomerular lesions of focal segmental glomerulosclerosis. These are associated with proteinuria and eventually lead to progressive chronic

renal failure. Such glomerular lesions may be caused by adaptive responses that occur in glomeruli as a result of reductions of renal mass (p 446).

DRUG-INDUCED INTERSTITIAL NEPHRITIS

In this era of antibiotics and analgesics, drugs have emerged as important causes of renal injury. Two forms of tubulointerstitial nephritis caused by drugs are recognized.

Acute Drug-Induced Interstitial Nephritis. This is an adverse reaction to a constantly increasing number of drugs. Acute tubulointerstitial nephritis most frequently occurs with synthetic penicillins (methicillin, ampicillin), other synthetic antibiotics (rifampin), diuretics (thiazides), nonsteroidal anti-inflammatory agents (phenylbutazone), and miscellaneous drugs (phenindione, cimetidine). The disease begins about 15 days (range, 2 to 40 days) after exposure to the drug and is characterized by *fever, eosinophilia* (which may be transient), *a skin rash* in about 25% of patients, and *renal abnormalities.* Renal findings include hematuria, mild proteinuria, and leukocyturia (including eosinophils). A *rising serum creatinine level or acute renal failure with oliguria develops in about 50% of cases,* particularly in older patients. It is important to recognize drug-induced renal failure, because withdrawal of the offending drug is followed by recovery, although it may take several months for renal function to return to normal.

MORPHOLOGY. The abnormalities are in the interstitium, which shows pronounced edema and infiltration by mononuclear cells, principally lymphocytes and macrophages (Fig. 14–16). Eosinophils and neutrophils may be present, often in large numbers. With some drugs (e.g., methicillin, thiazides), interstitial granulomas with giant cells may be seen. The glomeruli are normal except in some cases caused by nonsteroidal anti-inflammatory agents when minimal change disease and the nephrotic syndrome develop concurrently.

Pathogenesis. Many features of the disease suggest an immune mechanism. Clinical evidence of hypersensitivity includes the latent period, the eosinophilia and skin rash, the fact that the onset of nephropathy is not dose related, and the recurrence of hypersensitivity after re-exposure to the same or a cross-reactive drug. IgE serum levels are increased in some patients, suggesting type I hypersensitivity. The mononuclear or granulomatous infiltrate, together with positive skin tests to drug haptens, suggests a type IV hypersensitivity reaction.

The most likely sequence of pathogenetic events is that the drugs act as haptens, which, during secretion by tubules, covalently bind to some cytoplasmic or extracellular component of tubular cells and become immunogenic. The resultant injury is then due to IgE- and cell-mediated immune reactions to tubular cells or their basement membranes.

Analgesic Nephropathy. Patients who consume large quantities of analgesics may develop chronic interstitial nephritis, *often associated with renal papillary necrosis.* Al-

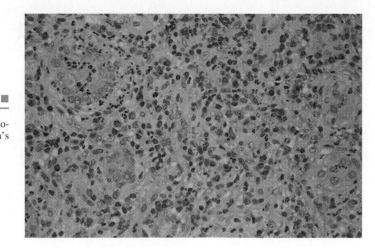

Figure 14–16 ■

Drug-induced interstitial nephritis, with prominent eosinophilic and mononuclear infiltrate. (Courtesy of Dr. Helmut Rennke, Brigham and Women's Hospital, Boston.)

though at times ingestion of single types of analgesics has been incriminated, most patients who develop this nephropathy consume mixtures containing some combination of phenacetin, aspirin, acetaminophen, caffeine, or codeine for long periods. Analgesic nephropathy is most common in Western Europe and some parts of Australia; in the United States the incidence is relatively low, being highest in the southeast.

Pathogenesis. The pathogenesis of the renal lesions is not entirely clear. Papillary necrosis is the initial event, and the interstitial nephritis in the overlying renal parenchyma is a secondary phenomenon. Acetaminophen, a phenacetin metabolite, injures cells by both *covalent binding* and *oxidative damage*. The ability of aspirin to inhibit prostaglandin synthesis suggests that this drug may induce its potentiating effect by inhibiting the vasodilatory effects of prostaglandin and predisposing the papilla to ischemia. Thus, the papillary damage may be due to a combination of direct toxic effects of phenacetin metabolites as well as ischemic injury to both tubular cells and vessels.

MORPHOLOGY. The necrotic papillae appear yellowish-brown owing to the accumulation of breakdown products of phenacetin and other lipofuscin-like pigments. Later on, the papillae may shrivel, be sloughed off, and drop into the pelvis. Microscopically the papillae show coagulative necrosis associated with loss of cellular detail but preservation of tubular outlines. Foci of dystrophic calcification may occur in the necrotic areas. The cortex drained by the necrotic papillae shows tubular atrophy, interstitial scarring, and inflammation. The small vessels in the papillae and urinary tract submucosa exhibit characteristic PAS-positive basement membrane thickening (analgesic microangiopathy).

Common clinical features of analgesic nephropathy include chronic renal failure, hypertension, and anemia. The anemia results in part from damage to red cells by phenacetin metabolites. Cessation of analgesic intake may stabilize or even improve renal function. A complication of analgesic abuse is the increased incidence of *transitional cell carcinoma* of the renal pelvis in patients who survive the renal failure.

Acute Tubular Necrosis

Acute tubular necrosis (ATN) is a clinicopathologic entity characterized morphologically by destruction of tubular epithelial cells and clinically by acute suppression of renal function. It is the most common cause of acute renal failure (ARF). ARF signifies an acute suppression of renal function and urine flow, falling, within 24 hours, to less than 400 ml (oliguria). Other causes of ARF include: (1) severe glomerular diseases such as RPGN, (2) diffuse renal vessel diseases such as polyarteritis nodosa and malignant hypertension, (3) acute papillary necrosis associated with acute pyelonephritis, (4) acute drug-induced interstitial nephritis, and (5) diffuse cortical necrosis. Here we discuss ATN; the other causes of ARF are discussed elsewhere in this chapter.

ATN is a reversible renal lesion that arises in a variety of clinical settings. Most of these, ranging from severe trauma to acute pancreatitis to septicemia, have in common a period of inadequate blood flow to the peripheral organs, usually accompanied by marked hypotension and shock. The pattern of ATN associated with shock is called *ischemic ATN*. Mismatched blood transfusions and other hemolytic crises, as well as myoglobinuria, also produce a picture resembling ischemic ATN. The second pattern, called *nephrotoxic ATN*, is caused by a variety of poisons, including heavy metals (e.g., mercury); organic solvents (e.g., carbon tetrachloride); and a multitude of drugs such as gentamicin, other antibiotics, and radiographic contrast agents. Because of the many precipitating factors, ATN occurs quite frequently. Moreover, its reversibility adds to its clinical importance because proper management means the difference between full recovery and death.

Pathogenesis. The critical events in both ischemic and nephrotoxic ATN are believed to be (1) tubular injury and (2) persistent and severe disturbances in blood flow as depicted in Figure 14–17.

■ Tubular epithelial cells are particularly sensitive to anoxia and are also vulnerable to toxins. Several factors predispose the tubules to toxic injury, including a vast electri-

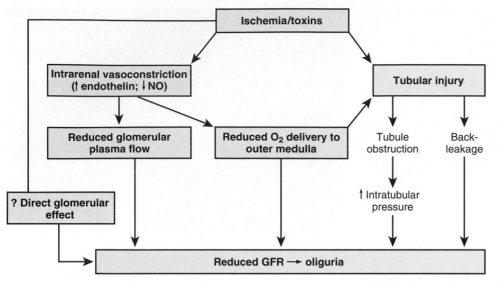

Figure 14–17 ■

Postulated sequence in acute renal failure (see text). NO, nitric oxide; GFR, glomerular filtration rate. (Modified from Brady HR, et al: Acute renal failure. In Brenner BM (ed): Brenner and Rector's The Kidney, Vol II, 5th ed. Philadelphia, WB Saunders, 1996, p 1210.)

cally charged surface for tubular reabsorption, active transport systems for ions and organic acids, and the capability for effective concentration. Ischemia causes numerous structural alterations in epithelial cells; loss of cell polarity appears to be a functionally important early event. Damage to the tubules and the resultant tubular debris could block urine outflow and eventually increase intratubular pressure, thereby decreasing the glomerular filtration rate. Additionally, fluid from the damaged tubules could leak into the interstitium, resulting in increased interstitial pressure and collapse of the tubule.

■ Ischemic renal injury is also characterized by severe hemodynamic alterations that cause reduced glomerular filtration rate. The major one is intrarenal *vasoconstriction,* which results in both reduced glomerular plasma flow and reduced oxygen delivery to the functionally important tubules in the outer medulla (thick ascending limb and straight segment of the proximal tubule) (Fig. 14–17). Although a number of vasoconstrictor pathways have been implicated in this phenomenon (e.g., renin-angiotensin, norepinephrine), the current opinion is that vasoconstriction is mediated by *sublethal endothelial injury,* leading to increased release of the endothelial vasoconstrictor *endothelin* and decreased production of the vasodilator *nitric oxide.* Finally, there is also some evidence of a direct effect of ischemia or toxins on the glomerulus, causing a reduced glomerular ultrafiltration coefficient, possibly due to mesangial contraction.

MORPHOLOGY. Ischemic ATN is characterized by necrosis of short segments of the tubules. Most of the lesions are seen in the straight portions of the proximal tubule and the ascending thick limbs, but no segment of the proximal or distal tubules is spared. Tubular necrosis is often subtle, requiring careful histologic examination; it is usually associated with the difficult-to-discern rupture of the basement membrane **(tubulorrhexis).** A striking

additional finding is the presence of proteinaceous casts in the distal tubules and collecting ducts. They consist of Tamm-Horsfall protein (secreted normally by tubular epithelium) along with hemoglobin and other plasma proteins. When crush injuries have produced ATN, the casts are composed of myoglobin. The interstitium usually discloses generalized edema along with an inflammatory infiltrate consisting of polymorphonuclear leukocytes, lymphocytes, and plasma cells. The histologic picture in **toxic ATN** is basically similar, with some differences. Necrosis is most prominent in the proximal tubule, and the tubular basement membranes are generally spared.

If the patient survives for a week, epithelial regeneration becomes apparent in the form of mitotic activity in the persisting tubular epithelial cells. Except where the basement membrane is destroyed, regeneration is total and complete.

Clinical Course. The clinical course of ATN may be divided into initiating, maintenance, and recovery stages. The *initiating* phase, lasting for about 36 hours, is usually dominated by the inciting medical, surgical, or obstetric event in the ischemic form of ATN. The only indication of renal involvement is a slight decline in urine output with a rise in blood urea nitrogen. At this point, oliguria could be explained on the basis of a transient decrease in blood flow to the kidneys.

The *maintenance* phase begins anywhere from the second to the sixth day. Urine output falls dramatically, usually to between 50 and 400 ml per day. Sometimes it declines to only a few milliliters per day, but complete anuria is rare. Oliguria may last only a few days or may persist as long as 3 weeks. The clinical picture is dominated by the signs and symptoms of uremia and fluid overload. In the absence of careful supportive treatment or dialysis, patients may die during this phase. With good care, however, survival is the rule.

The *recovery* is ushered in by a steady increase in urine

volume, reaching up to about 3 liters per day over the course of a few days. Because tubular function is still deranged, serious electrolyte imbalances may occur during this phase. There also appears to be increased vulnerability to infection. For these reasons, about 25% of deaths from ATN occur during this phase.

During the final phase, there is a progressive return of the patient's well-being. Urine volume returns to normal; however, subtle functional impairment of the kidneys, particularly of the tubules, may persist for months. With modern methods of care, patients who do not succumb to the underlying precipitating problem have a 90% to 95% chance of recovering from ATN.

DISEASES INVOLVING BLOOD VESSELS

Nearly all diseases of the kidney involve the renal blood vessels secondarily. Systemic vascular disease, such as various forms of arteritis, also involves renal blood vessels, and often the effects on the kidney are clinically important. These were considered in Chapter 10. The kidney is intimately involved in the pathogenesis of both essential and secondary hypertension, as discussed in detail in Chapter 10. Here we shall cover the two renal lesions associated with benign and malignant hypertension.

BENIGN NEPHROSCLEROSIS

Benign nephrosclerosis, the term used for the renal changes in benign hypertension, is always associated with hyaline arteriolosclerosis. Some degree of benign nephrosclerosis, albeit mild, is present at autopsy in many persons over 60 years of age. The frequency and severity of the lesions are increased in young age groups in association with hypertension and diabetes mellitus.

The kidneys are symmetrically atrophic, each weighing 110 to 130 gm, with a surface of diffuse, fine granularity that resembles grain leather.

MORPHOLOGY. Microscopically, the basic anatomic change is hyaline thickening of the walls of the small arteries and arterioles, known as **hyaline arteriolosclerosis.** This appears as a homogeneous, pink hyaline thickening, at the expense of the vessel lumina, with loss of underlying cellular detail (Fig. 14–18). The narrowing of the lumina results in markedly decreased blood flow through the affected vessels and thus produces ischemia in the organ served. All structures of the kidney show ischemic atrophy. In far-advanced cases of benign nephrosclerosis the glomerular tufts may become obliterated by homogeneous hyalinization. Diffuse tubular atrophy and interstitial fibrosis are present. Often there is a scant interstitial lymphocytic infiltrate. The larger blood vessels (interlobar and arcuate arteries) show reduplication of internal elas-

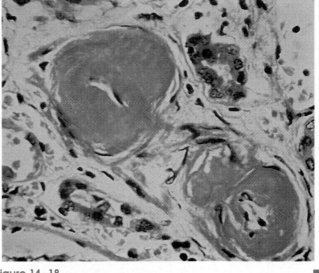

Figure 14–18   ■

Benign nephrosclerosis. High-power view of two arterioles with hyaline deposition, marked thickening of the walls, and a narrowed lumen. (Courtesy of Dr. M. A. Venkatachalam, Department of Pathology, University of Texas Health Sciences Center, San Antonio, TX.)

tic lamina along with fibrous thickening of the media (fibroelastic hyperplasia).

It should be remembered that many renal diseases cause hypertension, which in turn may lead to benign nephrosclerosis. Thus, this renal lesion is often seen superimposed on other primary kidney diseases.

Because this renal lesion alone rarely causes severe damage to the kidney, it very infrequently leads to uremia and death. Nonetheless, there is usually some functional impairment, such as loss of concentrating ability or a variably diminished glomerular filtration rate. A mild degree of proteinuria is a constant finding. Usually these patients die from hypertensive heart disease or cerebrovascular accidents rather than from renal disease.

MALIGNANT HYPERTENSION AND MALIGNANT NEPHROSCLEROSIS

Malignant hypertension is far less common than benign hypertension, occurring in only about 5% of patients with elevated blood pressure. It may arise de novo (i.e., without pre-existing hypertension) or may appear suddenly in a person who had mild hypertension.

Pathogenesis. The basis for this turn for the worse in hypertensive subjects is unclear, but the following sequence of events is suggested. The initial event appears to be some form of vascular damage to the kidneys. This most commonly results from long-standing benign hypertension, with eventual injury to the arteriolar walls, or it may spring from arteritis. In either case, the result is increased permeability of the small vessels to fibrinogen and other plasma proteins, endothelial injury, and platelet deposition. This leads to the appearance of *fibrinoid necrosis* of arterioles and small arteries, and intravascular thrombosis. Mitogenic factors from platelets (e.g., platelet-derived growth factor) and plasma cause intimal smooth hyperplasia of vessels, resulting in the hyperplastic arteriolosclerosis typical of malignant hypertension and further narrowing of the lumina. The kidneys become markedly ischemic. With severe involvement of the renal afferent arterioles, the renin-angiotensin system receives a powerful stimulus, and indeed *patients with malignant hypertension have markedly elevated levels of plasma renin.* This then sets up a self-perpetuating cycle in which angiotensin II causes intrarenal vasoconstriction, and the attendant renal ischemia perpetuates renin secretion. Aldosterone levels are also elevated, and salt retention undoubtedly contributes to the elevation of blood pressure. The consequences of the markedly elevated blood pressure on the blood vessels throughout the body are known as *malignant arteriolosclerosis,* and the renal disorder as malignant nephrosclerosis.

MORPHOLOGY. The kidney may be essentially normal in size or slightly shrunken, depending on the duration and severity of the hypertensive disease. Small, pinpoint petechial hemorrhages may appear on the cortical surface from rupture of arterioles or glomerular capillaries, giving the kidney a peculiar flea-bitten appearance.

The microscopic changes reflect the pathogenetic events described earlier. Damage to the small vessels is manifested as **fibrinoid necrosis** of the arterioles (Fig. 14–19*A*). The vessel walls appear to take on a homogeneous, granular eosinophilic appearance masking underlying detail. Also, there is often a sprinkling of inflammatory cells, giving rise to the term **necrotizing arteriolitis.** The inflammation is presumably secondary to vascular damage. A different response is seen in the interlobular arteries and larger arterioles, where the proliferation of intimal cells produces an onion-skin appearance (Fig. 14–19*B*). This name is derived

from the concentric arrangement of cells whose origin is believed to be intimal smooth muscle, although this issue is not finally settled. This lesion, called **hyperplastic arteriolosclerosis,** causes marked narrowing of arterioles and small arteries, to the point of total obliteration. Necrotizing arteriolitis may extend to involve the glomeruli **(necrotizing glomerulitis).** Microthrombi may be seen within the glomeruli as well as necrotic arterioles.

Clinical Course. The full-blown syndrome of *malignant hypertension is characterized by diastolic pressures greater than 120 mm Hg, papilledema, encephalopathy, cardiovascular abnormalities, and renal failure.* Most often, the early symptoms are related to increased intracranial pressure and include headaches, nausea, vomiting, and visual impairments, particularly the development of scotomas, or spots before the eyes. At the onset of rapidly mounting blood pressure there is marked proteinuria and microscopic, or sometimes macroscopic, hematuria but no significant alteration in renal function. Soon, however, renal failure makes its appearance. The syndrome is a true medical emergency that requires prompt institution of aggressive antihypertensive therapy before the irreversible renal lesions develop. About 50% of patients survive at least 5 years, and further progress is still being made. Ninety per cent of deaths are caused by uremia and others by cerebral hemorrhage or cardiac failure.

THROMBOTIC MICROANGIOPATHIES

As described in Chapter 12, these represent clinical syndromes characterized morphologically by widespread thrombosis in the microcirculation, and clinically by *microangiopathic hemolytic anemia, thrombocytopenia,* and, in certain instances, *renal failure.* The diseases include (1) childhood hemolytic-uremic syndrome (HUS), (2) various forms of adult HUS, and (3) thrombotic thrombocytopenic purpura. Central to the pathogenesis of these disorders is *endothelial injury and activation*, with resultant intravascular thrombosis.

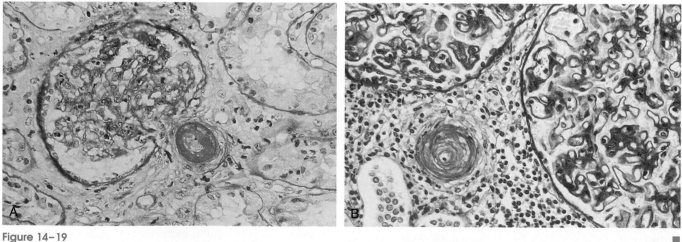

Figure 14–19

Malignant hypertension. *A,* Fibrinoid necrosis of afferent arteriole (Periodic acid–Schiff stain). *B,* Hyperplastic arteriolitis (onion-skin lesion). (Courtesy of Dr. Helmut Rennke, Brigham and Women's Hospital, Boston.)

Childhood HUS is the best characterized of the renal syndromes. As many of 75% of cases follow intestinal infection with verocytotoxin-producing *E. coli* such as in epidemics caused by ingestion of infected ground meat (hamburgers). (Verocytotoxins are so called because they cause damage to vero cells in culture.) *The disease is one of the main causes of acute renal failure in children.* It is characterized by the sudden onset, usually after a gastrointestinal or flu-like prodromal episode, of bleeding manifestations (especially hematemesis and melena), severe oliguria, hematuria, microangiopathic hemolytic anemia, and (in some patients) prominent neurologic changes.

The pathogenesis of this syndrome is related to the effects of verocytotoxin on endothelium, causing increased adhesion of leukocytes, increased endothelin production and loss of endothelial nitric oxide (both favoring vasoconstriction), and (in the presence of cytokines, such as tumor necrosis factor), endothelial lysis. The resultant endothelial effects enhance thrombosis, most prominent in interlobular and afferent arterioles and glomerular capillaries, as well as vasoconstriction, resulting in the characteristic microangiopathy.

If the renal failure is managed properly with dialysis, most patients recover in a matter of weeks. The long-term (15- to 25-year) prognosis, however, is not uniformly favorable, as about 25% of children eventually develop renal insufficiency.

CYSTIC DISEASES OF THE KIDNEY

Cystic diseases of the kidney are a heterogeneous group comprising hereditary, developmental but nonhereditary, and acquired disorders. As a group, they are important for several reasons: (1) they are reasonably common and often present diagnostic problems for clinicians, radiologists, and pathologists; (2) some forms, such as adult polycystic disease, are major causes of chronic renal failure; and (3) they can occasionally be confused with malignant tumors. Here we shall briefly mention simple cysts, the most common form, and discuss in some detail polycystic kidney disease.

Simple Cysts

These generally innocuous lesions occur as multiple or single cystic spaces that vary in diameter within a wide range. Commonly, they are 1 to 5 cm; translucent; lined by a gray, glistening, smooth membrane; and filled with clear fluid. Microscopically, these membranes are composed of a single layer of cuboidal or flattened cuboidal epithelium, which in many instances may be completely atrophic. The cysts are usually confined to the cortex. Rarely, large massive cysts up to 10 cm in diameter are encountered.

Simple cysts are a common postmortem finding that has no clinical significance. The main importance of cysts lies in their differentiation from kidney tumors, when they are discovered either incidentally or because of hemorrhage and pain during life. Radiographic studies show that, in contrast to renal tumors, renal cysts have smooth contours, are almost always

avascular, and give fluid rather than solid signals on ultrasonography.

Dialysis-associated acquired cysts occur in the kidneys of patients with end-stage renal disease who have undergone prolonged dialysis. They are present in both cortex and medulla and may bleed, causing hematuria. Occasionally, renal adenomas or even adenocarcinomas arise in the walls of these cysts.

Autosomal Dominant (Adult) Polycystic Kidney Disease

Adult polycystic kidney disease (APKD) is *characterized by multiple expanding cysts of both kidneys that ultimately destroy the intervening parenchyma.* It is seen in approximately one in 1000 persons and accounts for 10% of cases of chronic renal failure. This disease is genetically heterogeneous. It can be caused by inheritance of at least two autosomal dominant genes of very high penetrance. In 90% of families (APKD-1) the defective gene is on the short arm of chromosome 16. This gene encodes a large ($\pm$ 460 kD) and complex cell-membrane associated protein, called *polycystin*, that is mainly extracellular. The polycystin molecule has regions of homology to proteins known to be involved in cell-cell or cell-matrix adhesion (e.g., lectin-like domains, fibronectin-like domains). How mutations in this protein cause cyst formation is at present unclear, but it is thought that the resultant defects in cell-matrix interactions may lead to alterations in growth, differentiation, and matrix production by tubular epithelial cells, and cyst formation. The APKD-2 gene, implicated in 10% of all cases, resides on chromosome 4 but has not yet been definitively identified.

MORPHOLOGY. The kidneys may achieve enormous size, and weights of up to 4 kg for each kidney have been recorded. These very large kidneys are readily palpable abdominally as masses extending into the pelvis. On gross examination the kidney seems to be composed solely of a mass of cysts of varying sizes up to 3 or 4 cm in diameter with no intervening parenchyma. The cysts are filled with fluid, which may be clear, turbid, or hemorrhagic (Fig. 14–20).

Microscopic examination reveals some normal parenchyma dispersed among the cysts, which may arise at any level of the nephron, from tubules to collecting ducts, and therefore have a variable, often atrophic lining. Occasionally, Bowman's capsules are involved in the cyst formation, and in these cases glomerular tufts may be seen within the cystic space. The pressure of the expanding cysts leads to ischemic atrophy of the intervening renal substance. Evidence of superimposed hypertension or infection is common.

Clinical Course. Polycystic kidney disease in adults usually *does not produce symptoms until the fourth decade,* by

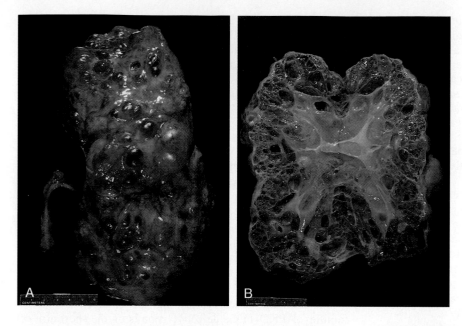

Figure 14–20 ■

Autosomal dominant adult polycystic kidney, viewed from the external surface *(A)* and bisected *(B)*. The kidney is markedly enlarged (note the centimeter rule) with numerous dilated cysts.

which time the kidneys are quite large. The most common complaint of the patient is *flank pain* or at least a heavy, dragging sensation. Acute distention of a cyst, either by intracystic hemorrhage or by obstruction, may cause excruciating pain. Sometimes attention is first drawn to the lesion by palpation of an abdominal mass. *Intermittent gross hematuria* commonly occurs. The most important complications, because of their deleterious effect on already marginal renal function, are *hypertension and urinary infection.* Hypertension of varying severity develops in about 75% of patients. Saccular (berry) aneurysms of the circle of Willis are present in 10% to 30% of patients, and these individuals show a high incidence of subarachnoid hemorrhage. Asymptomatic liver cysts occur in one third of patients.

Although the disease is ultimately fatal, the outlook is generally better than with most chronic renal diseases. The condition tends to be relatively stable and progresses very slowly. End-stage renal failure occurs at about age 50, but there is wide variation in the course of this disorder, and nearly normal life spans are reported. Those who develop renal failure are treated by renal transplantation. Death usually results from uremia or hypertensive complications.

Autosomal Recessive (Childhood) Polycystic Kidney Disease

This rare developmental anomaly is genetically distinct from adult polycystic kidney disease, having autosomal recessive inheritance. Perinatal, neonatal, infantile, and juvenile subcategories have been defined, depending on time of presentation and the presence of associated hepatic lesions. The first two are most common; serious manifestations are usually present at birth, and young infants may succumb rapidly to renal failure. Kidneys exhibit numerous small cysts in the cortex and medulla that give the kidney a spongelike appearance. Dilated, elongated channels at right angles to the cortical surface completely replace the medulla and cortex. The cysts

have a uniform lining of cuboidal cells, reflecting their origin from the collecting tubules. The disease is invariably bilateral. *In almost all cases, there are multiple epithelium-lined cysts in the liver as well as proliferation of portal bile ducts.* Patients who survive infancy develop liver cirrhosis (congenital hepatic fibrosis).

■ URINARY OUTFLOW OBSTRUCTION

Renal Stones

Urolithiasis is calculus formation at any level in the urinary collecting system, but most often calculi arise in the kidney. It is a frequent disorder, as evidenced by the finding of stones in about 1% of all autopsies. Symptomatic urolithiasis is most common in males. A familial tendency toward stone formation has long been recognized.

Pathogenesis. About 75% of renal stones are composed of either calcium oxalate or calcium oxalate mixed with calcium phosphate. Another 15% are composed of magnesium ammonium phosphate, and 10% are either uric acid or cystine stones. In all cases, there is an organic matrix of mucoprotein that makes up about 2.5% of the stone by weight (Table 14–4).

The cause of stone formation is often obscure, particularly in the case of calcium-containing stones. Probably involved is a confluence of predisposing conditions. *The most important cause is increased urine concentration of the stone's constituents, so that it exceeds their solubility in urine (supersaturation).* As shown in Table 14–4, 50% of the patients who develop *calcium stones* have hypercalciuria that is not associated with hypercalcemia. Most in this group absorb calcium from the gut in excessive amounts and promptly excrete it in the urine, and some have a primary renal defect of calcium reabsorption. In 5% to 10% of patients there is hypercalcemia

Table 14–4. PREVALENCE OF VARIOUS TYPES OF RENAL STONES

Stone	Percentage of All Stones
Calcium oxalate (phosphate)	75
Idiopathic hypercalciuria (50%)	
Hypercalcemia and hypercalciuria (10%)	
Hyperoxaluria (5%)	
Enteric (4.5%)	
Primary (0.5%)	
Hyperuricosuria (20%)	
No known metabolic abnormality (15%–20%)	
Struvite (Mg, NH_3, Ca, PO_4)	10–15
Renal infection	
Uric acid	6
Associated with hyperuricemia	
Associated with hyperuricosuria	
Idiopathic (50% of uric acid stones)	
Cystine	1–2
Others or unknown	±10

(due to hyperparathyroidism, vitamin D intoxication, sarcoidosis) and consequent hypercalciuria. In 20% of this subgroup there is excessive excretion of uric acid in the urine, which favors calcium stone formation; presumably the urates provide a nidus for calcium deposition. In 5% there is hyperoxaluria or hypercitraturia, and in the remainder there is no known metabolic abnormality.

The causes of the other types of renal stones are better understood. *Magnesium ammonium phosphate (struvite) stones* almost always occur in patients with a persistently alkaline urine, owing to urinary tract infections. In particular, the ureasplitting bacteria, such as *Proteus vulgaris* and the staphylococci, predispose the patient toward urolithiasis. Moreover, bacteria may serve as particulate nidi for the formation of any kind of stone. In avitaminosis A, desquamated squames from the metaplastic epithelium of the collecting system act as nidi.

Gout and diseases involving rapid cell turnover, such as the leukemias, lead to high uric acid levels in the urine and the possibility of *uric acid stones*. About half of the patients with uric acid stones, however, have neither hyperuricemia nor increased urine urate but an unexplained tendency to excrete a persistently acid urine (under pH 5.5) favoring stone formation. *Cystine stones* are almost invariably associated with a genetically determined defect in the renal transport of certain amino acids, including cystine. In contrast to magnesium ammonium phosphate stones, both uric acid and cystine stones are more likely to form when the urine is relatively acidic.

Urolithiasis may also conceivably result from the lack of influences that normally inhibit mineral precipitation. Inhibitors of crystal formation in urine include pyrophosphate, mucopolysaccharides, diphosphonates, and a glycoprotein called *nephrocalcin*, but no deficiency of any of these substances has been consistently demonstrated in patients with urolithiasis.

MORPHOLOGY. Stones are unilateral in about 80% of patients. Common sites of formation are renal pelves, calyces, and the bladder. Often, many stones are found in one kidney. They tend to be small (average diameter 2 to 3 mm) and may be smooth or jagged. Occasionally, progressive accretion of salts leads to the development of branching structures known as **staghorn calculi,** which create a cast of the renal pelvis and calyceal system. These massive stones are usually composed of magnesium ammonium phosphate.

Clinical Course. Stones may be present without producing either symptoms or significant renal damage. This is particularly true with large stones lodged in the renal pelvis. Smaller stones may pass into the ureter, producing a typical intense pain known as *renal or ureteral colic,* characterized by paroxysms of flank pain radiating toward the groin. Often at this time there is *gross hematuria*. The clinical significance of stones lies in their capacity to obstruct urine flow or to produce sufficient trauma to cause ulceration and bleeding. In either case, they *predispose the patient to bacterial infection.* Fortunately, in most cases the diagnosis is readily made radiologically.

Hydronephrosis

Hydronephrosis refers to dilation of the renal pelvis and calyces, with accompanying atrophy of the parenchyma, caused by obstruction to the outflow of urine. The obstruction may be sudden or insidious, and it may occur at any level of the urinary tract, from the urethra to the renal pelvis. The most common causes are as follows:

A. *Congenital:* Atresia of the urethra, valve formations in either ureter or urethra, aberrant renal artery compressing the ureter, renal ptosis with torsion, or kinking of the ureter.
B. *Acquired:*
  1. Foreign bodies: Calculi, necrotic papillae.
  2. Tumors: Benign prostatic hypertrophy, carcinoma of the prostate, bladder tumors (papilloma and carcinoma), contiguous malignant disease (retroperitoneal lymphoma, carcinoma of the cervix or uterus).
  3. Inflammation: Prostatitis, ureteritis, urethritis, retroperitoneal fibrosis.
  4. Neurogenic: Spinal cord damage with paralysis of the bladder.
  5. Normal pregnancy: Mild and reversible.

Bilateral hydronephrosis occurs only when the obstruction is below the level of the ureters. If blockage is at the ureters or above, the lesion is unilateral. Sometimes obstruction is complete, allowing no urine to pass; usually it is only partial.

Even with complete obstruction, glomerular filtration persists for some time, and the filtrate subsequently diffuses back into the renal interstitium and perirenal spaces, whence it ultimately returns to the lymphatic and venous systems. Because of the continued filtration, the *affected calyces and pelvis become dilated,* often markedly so. The unusually high pressure thus generated in the renal pelvis, as well as that transmitted back through the collecting ducts, causes compression of the renal vasculature. Both arterial insufficiency and venous stasis result, although the latter is probably more important. The most severe effects are seen in the papillae, because they are subjected to the greatest increases in pressure. Accordingly, *the initial functional disturbances are largely tubular, manifested primarily by impaired concentrating ability.* Only later does glomerular filtration begin to diminish. Experimental studies indicate that serious irreversible damage occurs in about 3 weeks with complete obstruction, and in 3 months with incomplete obstruction.

MORPHOLOGY. **Bilateral** hydronephrosis (as well as unilateral hydronephrosis when the other kidney is already damaged or absent) leads to renal failure, and the onset of uremia tends to abort the natural course of the lesion. In contrast, **unilateral** involvements display the full range of morphologic changes, which vary with the degree and speed of obstruction. With subtotal or intermittent obstruction, the kidney may be massively enlarged (lengths in the range of 20 cm) and the organ may consist almost entirely of the greatly distended pelvicalyceal system. The renal parenchyma itself is compressed and atrophied, with obliteration of the papillae and flattening of the pyramids (Fig. 14–21). On the other hand, when **obstruction is sudden and complete, glomerular filtration is compromised relatively early, and as a consequence, renal function may cease while dilation is still comparatively slight.** Depending on the level of the obstruction, one or both ureters may also be dilated **(hydroureter).**

Microscopically, the early lesions show tubular dilation, followed by atrophy and fibrous replacement of the tubular epithelium with relative spar-ing of the glomeruli. Eventually, in severe cases the glomeruli also become atrophic and disappear, converting the entire kidney into a thin shell of fibrous tissue. With sudden and complete obstruction, there may be coagulative necrosis of the renal papillae, similar to the changes of necrotizing papillitis. In uncomplicated cases, the accompanying inflammatory reaction is minimal. Complicating pyelonephritis, however, is common.

Clinical Course. *Bilateral* complete obstruction produces anuria, which is soon brought to medical attention. When the obstruction is below the bladder, the dominant symptoms are those of bladder distention. Paradoxically, incomplete bilateral obstruction causes polyuria rather than oliguria, as a result of defects in tubular concentrating mechanisms, and this may obscure the true nature of the disturbance. Unfortunately, *unilateral* hydronephrosis may remain completely silent for long periods unless the other kidney is for some reason not functioning. Often the enlarged kidney is discovered on routine physical examination. Sometimes the basic cause of the hydronephrosis, such as renal calculi or an obstructing tumor, produces symptoms that indirectly draw attention to the hydronephrosis. Removal of obstruction within a few weeks usually permits full return of function; however, with time the changes become irreversible.

TUMORS

Many types of benign and malignant tumors occur in the urinary tract. In general, benign tumors such as small (rarely over 2.5 cm in diameter) *cortical adenomas* or *medullary fibromas* (interstitial cell tumors) have no clinical significance. The most common malignant tumor of the kidney is renal cell carcinoma, followed in frequency by Wilms' tumors and by primary tumors of the calyces and pelves. Other types of renal cancer are extremely rare and need not be discussed here. Tumors of the lower urinary tract are about twice as common as renal cell carcinomas; they are described at the end of this section.

Renal Cell Carcinoma

Renal cell carcinoma is the type of neoplasm usually meant by the term *cancer of the kidney*. It is an adenocarcinoma arising from tubular epithelial cells, and represents 80% to 90% of all malignant tumors of the kidney and 2% of all cancers in adults. The lesions are most common from the sixth to seventh decades, and men are affected twice as often as women. Although no neoplasm has an absolutely predictable course, renal cell carcinoma distinguishes itself by being especially variable in its behavior. There is a *greater frequency in cigarette smokers, and familial forms have been reported.* About two thirds of patients with von Hippel-Lindau syndrome (VHL), characterized by hemangioblastomas of the central nervous system and retina, develop bilateral, often

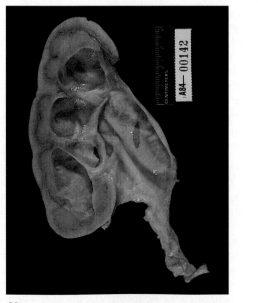

Figure 14–21 ■

Hydronephrosis of the kidney, with marked dilation of the pelvis and calyces and thinning of renal parenchyma.

multiple renal cell carcinomas. The VHL gene is a tumor suppressor gene on chromosome 3p25, and t(3;8) and t(3;11) translocations are also often found in familial cases of non-papillary renal cell carcinoma; mutations and deletions of the VHL gene have also been reported in sporadic cases. *Thus, the VHL gene, or a gene related to VHL on chromosome 3, may be involved in renal carcinogenesis.*

MORPHOLOGY. These cancers are usually large by the time they are discovered and appear as spherical masses 3 to 15 cm in diameter. They may arise anywhere in the kidney. The cut surface is yellow-gray-white, with prominent areas of cystic softening or of hemorrhage, either fresh or old (Fig. 14–22). The margins of the tumor are well defined; however, at times small processes project into the surrounding parenchyma and small satellite nodules are found in the surrounding substance, providing clear evidence of the aggressiveness of these lesions. As the tumor enlarges, it may fungate through the walls of the collecting system, extending through the calyces and pelvis as far as the ureter. Even more frequently, the tumor invades the renal vein and grows as a solid column within this vessel, sometimes extending in serpentine fashion as far as the inferior vena cava and even into the right side of the heart. Occasionally there is direct invasion into the perinephric fat and adrenal gland.

Depending on the amount of lipid and glycogen present, the tumor cells may appear almost

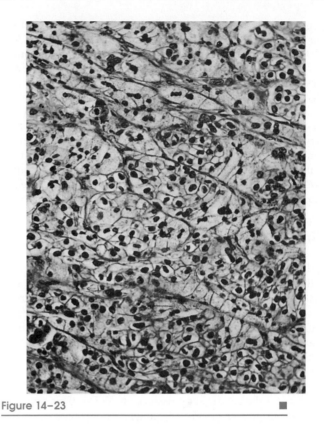

Figure 14–23

High-power detail of the clear cell pattern of renal cell carcinoma.

totally vacuolated or may be solid. The classic vacuolated (lipid-laden) or **clear cells** are demarcated only by their cell membranes; the nuclei are usually pushed basally and are small (Fig. 14–23). At the other extreme are the **granular cells,** resembling the tubular epithelium, which have round, small, regular nuclei enclosed within granular pink cytoplasm. These cells may show great regularity of cytologic detail. Some tumors exhibit marked degrees of anaplasia, with numerous mitotic figures, and giant cells. Between the extremes of clear cells and solid cells, all intergradations may be found. The cellular arrangement, too, varies widely; the cells may form abortive tubules or papillary patterns, or they may cluster in cords or disorganized masses. The stroma is usually scant but highly vascularized.

Clinical Course. Renal cell carcinomas have several peculiar clinical characteristics that create especially difficult but challenging diagnostic problems. The symptoms vary, but the *most frequent presenting manifestation is hematuria, occurring in more than 50% of cases.* Macroscopic hematuria tends to be intermittent and fleeting, superimposed on a steady microscopic hematuria. In other patients the tumor may declare itself simply by virtue of its size, when it has grown large enough to produce flank pain and a palpable mass. Extrarenal effects are fever and polycythemia, both of which may be associated with a renal cell carcinoma but which, because they

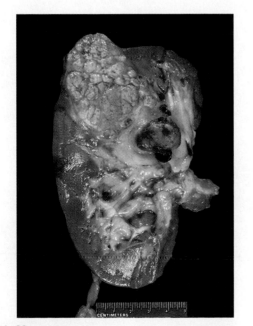

Figure 14–22

Renal cell carcinoma: typical cross-section of yellowish, spherical neoplasm in one pole of the kidney. Note the tumor in the dilated, thrombosed renal vein.

are nonspecific, may be misinterpreted for some time before their true significance is appreciated. Polycythemia affects 5% to 10% of patients with this disease. It results from elaboration of erythropoietin by the renal tumor. Uncommonly, these tumors produce a variety of hormone-like substances, resulting in hypercalcemia, hypertension, Cushing's syndrome, or feminization or masculinization. In many patients the primary tumor remains silent and is discovered only after its metastases have produced symptoms. The prevalent locations for metastases are the lungs and the bones. It must be apparent that renal cell carcinoma presents in many fashions, some quite devious, *but the triad of painless hematuria, long-standing fever, and dull flank pain is characteristic.*

Wilms' Tumor

Although Wilms' tumor occurs infrequently in adults, it is the third most common organ cancer in children under the age of 10 years. It is therefore one of the major cancers of children. These tumors contain a variety of cell and tissue components, all derived from the mesoderm. Wilms' tumor, like retinoblastoma, may arise sporadically or be familial, with the susceptibility to tumorigenesis inherited as an autosomal dominant trait. Many tumors are associated with deletions in the short arm of chromosome 11 (11p13) and resultant loss or mutations of the cancer suppressor gene WT-1. This tumor is discussed in greater detail in Chapter 7 along with other tumors of children.

Tumors of the Urinary Bladder and Collecting System (Renal Calyces, Pelvis, Ureter, and Urethra)

The entire urinary collecting system from renal pelvis to urethra is lined with transitional epithelium, so its epithelial tumors assume similar morphologic patterns. Tumors in the collecting system above the bladder are relatively uncommon; those in the bladder, however, are an even more frequent cause of death than are kidney tumors. Nevertheless, in the individual case, a small lesion in the ureter, for example, may cause urinary outflow obstruction and have greater clinical significance than a much larger mass in the capacious bladder. We shall consider first the range of histologic patterns *as they occur in the urinary bladder,* and then their clinical implications.

MORPHOLOGY. Tumors arising in the urinary bladder range from small benign papillomas to large invasive cancers (Fig. 14–24). The very rare benign **papillomas** are small (0.2- to 1.0-cm), frondlike structures, having a delicate fibrovascular core covered by multilayered, well-differentiated transitional epithelium. In some of these lesions the covering epithelium appears as normal as the mucosal surface whence these tumors arise; such lesions are usually solitary, almost invariably noninvasive, and benign and rarely recur once removed.

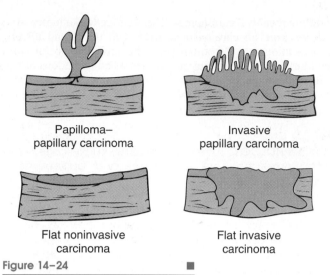

Papilloma–
papillary carcinoma

Invasive
papillary carcinoma

Flat noninvasive
carcinoma

Flat invasive
carcinoma

Figure 14–24 ■

Four morphologic patterns of bladder tumor.

Transitional cell carcinomas range from papillary to flat, noninvasive to invasive, and extremely well differentiated (grade I, Fig. 14–25) to highly anaplastic aggressive cancers (grade III). Grade I carcinomas are always papillary, rarely invasive but may recur after removal. Whether the regrowth is a true recurrence or a second primary growth is uncertain. Increasing degrees of cellular atypia and anaplasia are encountered in papillary exo-

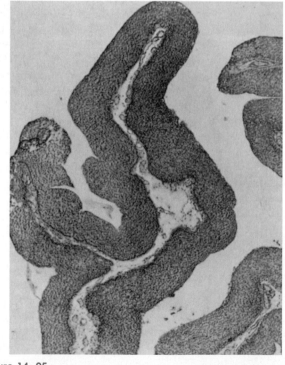

Figure 14–25 ■

Grade I papillary transitional cell carcinoma of the bladder. The delicate papilla is covered by orderly transitional epithelium.

phytic growths, accompanied by increase in size of the lesion and evidence of invasion of the submucosal or muscular layers. These tumors are unequivocally transitional cell carcinomas, grade II or grade III. Grade III cancers can be papillary or occasionally flat, may cover larger areas of the mucosal surface, invade deeper, and have a shaggier necrotic surface. Occasionally these cancers show foci of squamous cell differentiation, but only 5% of bladder cancers are true **squamous cell carcinomas.** Carcinomas of grades II and III infiltrate surrounding structures, spread to regional nodes, and on occasion metastasize widely.

In addition to overt carcinoma, an **in situ stage of bladder carcinoma** can be recognized, often in patients with previous or simultaneous papillary or invasive tumors. Indeed, wide areas of atypical hyperplasia and dysplasia may be present. It is now thought that these epithelial changes and cancers in situ are caused by the generalized influence of a putative carcinogen on urothelium and that they may be the precursors of invasive carcinomas in some patients. However, despite the presence of wide areas of epithelial lesions, the bladder tumors, even when multiple, are monoclonal in origin. Apparently, clonal descendants of a single transformed cell can seed multiple areas of the mucosa.

Clinical Course. *Painless hematuria is the dominant clinical presentation* of all these tumors. Because most arise in the bladder, we shall consider these first. They affect men about three times as frequently as women and usually develop between the ages of 50 and 70 years. Although most occur in persons with no known history of exposure to industrial solvents, bladder tumors are 50 times more common in those exposed to β-naphthylamine. Cigarette smoking, chronic cystitis, schistosomiasis of the bladder, and certain drugs (cyclophosphamide) are also believed to induce higher attack rates.

The clinical significance of bladder tumors depends on several factors: obviously on their histologic grade and differentiation, and (most important) on the depth of invasion of the lesion. Except for the clearly benign papillomas, all tend stubbornly to recur after removal and tend to kill by infiltrative obstruction of ureters rather than by metastasis. Lesions that invade the ureteral or urethral orifices cause urinary tract obstruction. In general, with low-grade shallow lesions, the prognosis after removal is good, but when deep penetration of the bladder wall has occurred, the 5-year survival rate is less than 20%. Overall 5-year survival is 57%.

Although papillary and cancerous neoplasms of the lining epithelium of the collecting system occur much less frequently in the renal pelvis than in the bladder, they nonetheless make up 5% to 10% of primary renal tumors. Painless hematuria is the most characteristic feature of these lesions, but in their critical location they produce pain in the costovertebral angle as hydronephrosis develops. Infiltration of the walls of the pelvis, calyces, and renal vein worsens the prognosis. Despite removal of the tumor by nephrectomy, less than 50% of patients survive for 5 years. Cancer of the ureter is fortunately the rarest of the tumors of the collecting system. The 5-year survival rate is less than 10%.

BIBLIOGRAPHY

Bonventre JV: Mechanisms of ischemic acute renal failure. Kidney Int 47:1160, 1995.

Brenner BM (ed): Brenner and Rector's The Kidney, 5th ed. Philadelphia, WB Saunders, 1996. (A comprehensive book of renal medicine.)

Cotran RS: Tubulointerstitial Nephropathies. New York, Churchill Livingstone, 1986. (A review of tubulointerstitial diseases, including reflux nephropathy, obstructive uropathy, and drug-induced interstitial diseases.)

Galla JH: IgA nephropathy. Kidney Int 47:377, 1995. (A review of the subject, emphasizing pathogenesis.)

Harris PC, et al: Polycystic kidney disease 1: Identification and analysis of the primary defect. J Am Soc Nephrol 6:1125, 1995. (An account of the APKD-1 gene.)

Heptinstall RH: Pathology of the Kidney, 4th ed. Boston, Little, Brown, 1992. (A classic illustrated written text of renal pathology.)

Hill G (ed): Uropathology. New York, Churchill Livingstone, 1989. (A multiauthor book dealing with pathology of the lower urinary tract; new edition in press).

Lamm DL, Torti FM: Bladder Cancer 1996. CA 46:93, 1996. (An easy-to-read article that presents an overview of the etiology, clinical features, and treatment of bladder cancer.)

Linas SL (ed): Ischemic nephropathy. Semin Nephrol. 16:1, 1996. (A compendium of short updates on the consequences of ischemia on renal function.)

Motzer RJ, et al: Medical progress: renal cell carcinoma. N Engl J Med 335:865, 1996.

Murphy WM (ed): Urological Pathology, 2nd ed. Philadelphia, WB Saunders, 1997. (A comprehensive review of lesions of the lower urinary tract.)

Murphy WM, et al: Tumors of the Kidney, Bladder and Related Urinary Structures. AFIP Atlas of Tumor Pathology. Washington, DC, American Registry of Pathology, 1994.

Tisher C, Brenner BM: Renal Pathology, with Clinical and Pathological Correlations. Philadelphia, JB Lippincott, 1994. (A multiauthor renal pathology reference work.)

15

The Oral Cavity and Gastrointestinal Tract

James M. Crawford, MD, PhD

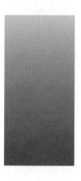

Oral Cavity

Diseases of the oral cavity can be broadly divided into two groups: those affecting the soft tissues (including the salivary glands) and those that involve the teeth. Only the more common conditions affecting the soft tissues are considered in this chapter. Excluded are extraoral diseases that sometimes involve the mouth and pharynx, such as diphtheria, lichen planus, and leukemia, as well as dental disorders.

ULCERATIVE AND INFLAMMATORY LESIONS

Although several ulcerative and inflammatory conditions are discussed here, it is well to remember that mechanical trauma and cancer may produce ulcerations in the oral cavity and must be considered in the differential diagnosis.

Aphthous Ulcers (Canker Sores). These lesions are extremely common, small (usually less than 5 mm in diameter), painful, shallow ulcers. Characteristically, they take the form of rounded, superficial erosions, often covered with a gray-white exudate and having an erythematous rim. They appear singly or in groups on the nonkeratinized oral mucosa, particularly the soft palate, buccolabial mucosa, floor of the mouth, and lateral borders of the tongue. They are more common in the first two decades of life and are often apparently triggered by stress, fever, ingestion of certain foods, and activation of inflammatory bowel disease. Although the cause remains unknown, an autoimmune basis is suspected. Self-limited, they usually resolve within a few weeks, but they may recur in the same or a different location.

Herpesvirus Infection. Herpetic stomatitis is an extremely common infection caused by herpes simplex virus type 1 (HSV-1). The pathogen is transmitted from person to person, most often by kissing; by middle life over three fourths of the population have been infected. In most adults, the primary infection is asymptomatic, but the virus persists in a dormant state within ganglia about the mouth (e.g., trigeminal). With reactivation (fever, sun or cold exposure, respiratory tract infection, trauma), solitary or multiple small (less than 5 mm in diameter) vesicles containing clear fluid appear. They are most often on the lips or about the nasal orifices and are well known as "cold sores" or "fever blisters." They soon rupture, leaving shallow, painful ulcers that heal within a few weeks, but recurrences are common. Histologically, the vesicles begin as an intraepithelial focus of intercellular and intracellular edema. The infected cells become ballooned and develop intranuclear acidophilic viral inclusions. Sometimes adjacent cells fuse to form giant cells or polykaryons. Necrosis of the infected cells and the focal collections of edema fluid account for the intraepithelial vesicles seen clinically (Fig. 15–1). Identification of the inclusion-bearing cells or polykaryons in smears of blister fluid constitutes the diagnostic *Tzanck test* for HSV infection; antiviral agents may accelerate healing.

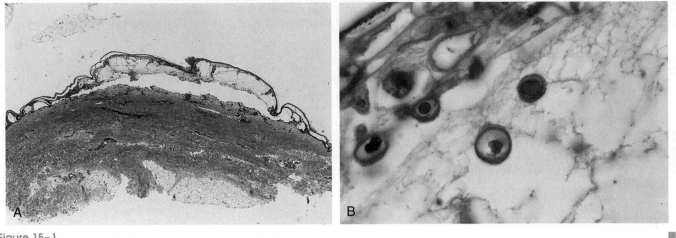

Figure 15-1 ■

Herpesvirus pharyngitis. *A,* Herpesvirus blister in mucosa. *B,* High-power view of cells from blister in *A,* showing glassy intranuclear herpes simplex inclusion bodies.

When primary HSV-1 infection occurs in a prepubescent child or immunocompromised adult, a more virulent disseminated eruption is likely, marked by multiple vesicles throughout the oral cavity, including the pharynx (herpetic gingivostomatitis). In the worst case, viremia may seed the brain (encephalitis) or produce disseminated visceral lesions. In passing, it should be noted that HSV-1 may localize in many other sites, including the conjunctivae (keratoconjunctivitis) and the esophagus, when a nasogastric tube is introduced through an infected oral cavity. HSV-2 (the agent of herpes genitalis), on the other hand, is transmitted sexually and produces vesicles on the genital mucous membranes and external genitalia that have the same histologic characteristics as those that occur about the mouth.

Fungal Infection. *Candida albicans* is a normal inhabitant of the oral cavity found in 30% to 40% of the population; it causes disease only when there is some impairment of the usual protective mechanisms. Oral candidiasis (thrush, moniliasis) is a common fungal infection among persons rendered vulnerable by diabetes mellitus, anemia, antibiotic or glucocorticoid therapy, some form of immunodeficiency, or debilitating illnesses such as disseminated cancer. Typically, *oral candidiasis takes the form of an adherent white, curdlike, circumscribed plaque anywhere within the oral cavity.* The pseudomembrane can be scraped off to reveal an underlying granular erythematous inflammatory base. Histologically, the pseudomembrane is composed of a myriad of fungal organisms superficially attached to the underlying mucosa. In milder infections there is minimal ulceration, but in severe cases the entire mucosa may be denuded. The fungi can be identified within these pseudomembranes as boxcar-like chains of tubular cells producing pseudohyphae from which bud ovoid yeast forms, typically 2 to 4 μm in greater diameter.

In the particularly vulnerable host, candidiasis may spread into the esophagus, especially when a nasogastric tube has been introduced, or it may produce widespread visceral lesions when the fungus gains entry into the bloodstream. Disseminated candidiasis is a life-threatening infection that must be treated aggressively. For poorly understood reasons, local candidal lesions may appear in the vagina, not only in predisposed persons but also in apparently healthy young women, particularly ones who are pregnant or using oral contraceptives.

Acquired Immunodeficiency Syndrome (AIDS). AIDS and less advanced forms of human immunodeficiency virus (HIV) infection are often associated with lesions in the oral cavity. They may take the form of candidiasis, herpetic vesicles, or some other microbial infection (producing gingivitis or glossitis). Of particular interest are the intraoral lesions of Kaposi's sarcoma and hairy leukoplakia. Kaposi's sarcoma, as described in Chapter 10, is a multifocal, systemic disease that eventually evolves into highly vascular tumor nodules. Although Kaposi's sarcoma may occur in the absence of HIV infection, it affects about 20% of AIDS patients, particularly homosexual or bisexual males. More than 50% of those afflicted develop intraoral purpuric discolorations or violaceous, raised, nodular masses; sometimes this involvement constitutes the presenting manifestation.

Hairy leukoplakia is an uncommon lesion seen virtually only in persons infected with HIV. It constitutes white confluent patches, anywhere on the oral mucosa, that have a "hairy" or corrugated surface resulting from marked epithelial thickening. It is caused by Epstein-Barr virus infections of epithelial cells. Occasionally, the development of hairy leukoplakia calls attention to the existence of the underlying HIV infection.

LEUKOPLAKIA

As generally used, the term *leukoplakia refers to a whitish, well-defined, mucosal patch or plaque caused by epidermal thickening or hyperkeratosis.* The term is not applied to other white lesions, such as those caused by candidiasis or lichen planus among many others.

The plaques are more frequent among older men and are most often on the vermilion border of the lower lip, buccal

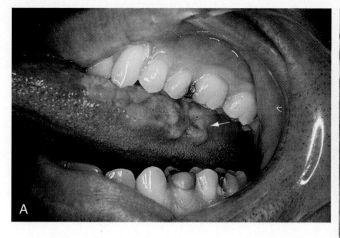

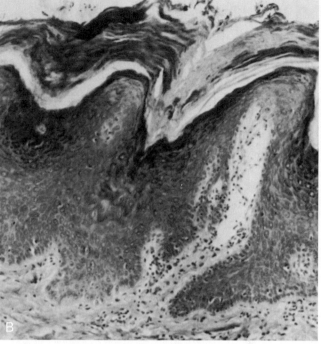

Figure 15–2 ■

A, Leukoplakia of the tongue in a smoker. Microscopically, this lesion showed severe dysplasia with transformation to squamous cell carcinoma in the posterior elevated portion *(arrow). B,* Microscopic appearance of leukoplakia (from another case) reveals marked surface hyperkeratosis and thickening of the mucosa but no dysplasia.

mucosa, and the hard and soft palates and less frequently on the floor of the mouth and other intraoral sites. They appear as localized, sometimes multifocal or even diffuse, smooth or roughened, leathery, white, discrete areas of mucosal thickening. On microscopic evaluation they vary from banal hyperkeratosis without underlying epithelial dysplasia to mild to severe dysplasia bordering on carcinoma in situ (Fig. 15–2). Only histologic evaluation distinguishes among these changes. The lesions are of unknown cause except that there is a *strong association with the use of tobacco,* particularly pipe smoking and smokeless tobacco (pouches, snuff, chewing). Less strongly implicated are *chronic friction* as from ill-fitting dentures or jagged teeth, *alcohol abuse,* and irritant foods. More recently, human papillomavirus antigen has been identified in some tobacco-related lesions, raising the possibility that the virus and tobacco act in concert in the induction of these lesions.

Oral leukoplakia is an important finding because 5% to 15% (depending somewhat on location) undergo transformation to squamous cell carcinoma. It is impossible to distinguish the innocent lesion from the ominous one on visual inspection. The transformation rate is greatest with lip and tongue lesions and lowest with those on the floor of the mouth. Those lesions that display significant dysplasia on microscopic examination have a greater probability of cancerous transformation.

Two somewhat related lesions must be differentiated from oral leukoplakia. Hairy leukoplakia, described earlier and seen virtually only in patients with AIDS, has a corrugated or "hairy" surface rather than the white, opaque thickening of oral leukoplakia and has not been related to the development of oral cancer. *Erythroplasia* refers to red, velvety, often granular, circumscribed areas that may or may not be elevated, having poorly defined, irregular boundaries. Histologically, erythroplasia almost invariably reveals marked epithelial dysplasia (the malignant transformation rate is more than 50%),

so recognition of this lesion becomes even more important than identification of oral leukoplakia.

CANCERS OF THE ORAL CAVITY AND TONGUE

The overwhelming preponderance of oral cavity cancers are squamous cell carcinomas. Although they represent only about 3% of all cancers in the United States, they are disproportionately important. Almost all are readily accessible to biopsy and early identification, but about half kill within 5 years and indeed may have already metastasized by the time the primary lesion is discovered. These cancers tend to occur later in life and are rare before age 40. The various influences thought to be important in development of these cancers are summarized in Table 15–1.

■

Table 15–1. RISK FACTORS FOR ORAL CANCER

Factor	Comments
Leukoplakia, erythroplasia	See text discussion
Tobacco use	Best-established influence, particularly pipe smoking and smokeless tobacco
Alcohol abuse	Less strong influence than tobacco
Human papillomavirus types 16, 18, and 11	Identified by molecular probes in some cases
Protracted irritation	Weakly associated
Plummer-Vinson syndrome	Association questionable

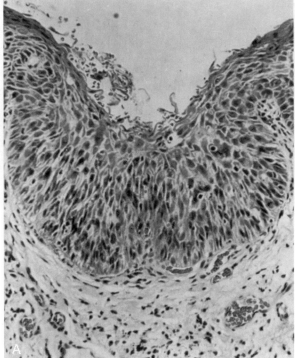

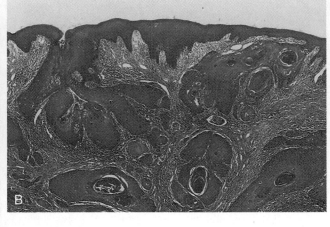

Figure 15–3 ■

A, Oral carcinoma in situ shows nuclear pleomorphism in all strata of the epithelium. B, Oral squamous cell carcinoma. Invasive tumor islands show formation of keratin pearls. (A, Courtesy of Dr. L.R. Eversole, Professor and Chairman, Department of Oral Diagnostic Sciences, College of Dentistry, University of Florida, Gainesville, FL.)

The three predominant sites of origin of oral cavity carcinomas are (in order of frequency) the (1) vermilion border of the lateral margins of the lower lip, (2) floor of the mouth, and (3) lateral borders of the mobile tongue. Early lesions appear as pearly white to gray, circumscribed thickenings of the mucosa closely resembling leukoplakic patches (Fig. 15–2A). They then may grow in an exophytic fashion to produce readily visible and palpable nodular and eventually fungating lesions, or they may assume an endophytic, invasive pattern with central necrosis to create a cancerous ulcer. The squamous cell carcinomas are usually moderately to well differentiated keratinizing tumors (Fig. 15–3). Before the lesions become advanced it may be possible to identify epithelial atypia, dysplasia, or carcinoma in situ in the margins, suggesting origin from leukoplakia or erythroplasia. Spread to regional nodes is present at the time of initial diagnosis only rarely with lip cancer, in about 50% of cases of tongue cancer, and in more than 60% of those with cancer of the floor of the mouth. More remote spread to tissues or organs in the thorax or abdomen is less common than extensive regional spread.

Clinical Features. These lesions may cause local pain or difficulty in chewing, but many are relatively asymptomatic and so the lesion (very familiar to the exploring tongue) is ignored. It is tragic that so many are not discovered until beyond cure. The 5-year survival rates, despite surgery and radiation, vary from 91% for lip cancer to about 30% for cancers of the base of the tongue, pharynx, and floor of the mouth.

SALIVARY GLAND DISEASES

Although diseases primary to the major salivary glands are in general uncommon, the parotids bear the brunt of these involvements. Among the many possible disorders, attention is restricted here to sialadenitis and salivary gland tumors.

Sialadenitis

Inflammation of the major salivary glands may be of viral, bacterial, or autoimmune origin. Dominant among these causations is the infectious viral disease *mumps,* which may produce enlargement of all the major salivary glands but predominantly the parotids. This paramyxovirus usually produces a diffuse, interstitial inflammation marked by edema and a mononuclear cell infiltration and, sometimes, by focal necrosis. Although childhood mumps is self-limited and rarely leaves residua, mumps in adults may be accompanied by pancreatitis or orchitis; the latter sometimes causes permanent sterility.

Presumed *autoimmune sialadenitis,* which is almost invariably bilateral, is seen in Sjögren's syndrome, which is discussed in Chapter 5. All of the salivary glands (major and minor), as well as the lacrimal glands, may be affected in this disorder, which induces dry mouth (*xerostomia*) and dry eyes (*keratoconjunctivitis sicca*). The combination of salivary and lacrimal gland inflammatory enlargement, which is usually painless, and xerostomia, whatever the cause, is sometimes referred to by the eponymic term *Mikulicz' syndrome,* embracing sarcoidosis, leukemia, lymphoma, and idiopathic lymphoepithelial hyperplasia.

Bacterial sialadenitis most often occurs secondary to ductal obstruction resulting from stone formation *(sialolithiasis).* The sialadenitis may be largely interstitial or cause focal areas of suppurative necrosis or even abscess formation.

Salivary Gland Tumors

The salivary glands give rise to a surprising diversity of tumors, about 80% of which occur within the parotid glands and most of the others in the submandibular glands. Males and females are affected about equally, usually in the sixth or seventh decade of life. In the parotids 70% to 80% of these tumors are benign, whereas in the submaxillary glands only half are benign. Thus, it is evident that *a neoplasm in the submaxillary glands is more ominous than one in the parotids.* The dominant tumor arising in the parotids is the benign pleomorphic adenoma, which is sometimes called a mixed tumor of salivary gland origin. Much less frequent is the papillary cystadenoma lymphomatosum (Warthin's tumor). Collectively, these two types account for three fourths of parotid tumors. Whatever the type, they present clinically as a mass causing a swelling at the angle of the jaw. Among the diverse cancers of parotid glands, the two dominant types are (1) malignant mixed tumors arising either de novo or in preexisting, benign, pleomorphic adenomas and (2) mucoepidermoid carcinoma. Only the benign pleomorphic adenoma and Warthin's tumor are sufficiently common to merit description.

Pleomorphic Adenoma (Mixed Tumor of Salivary Glands). This benign tumor, the most common tumor of salivary glands, is a slow-growing, well-demarcated, apparently encapsulated lesion rarely exceeding 6 cm in greatest dimension. Most often arising in the superficial parotid, it usually causes painless swelling at the angle of the jaw and can be readily palpated as a discrete mass. It is nonetheless often present for years before being brought to medical attention. Despite its encapsulation, histologic examination often reveals multiple projections of tumor cells penetrating the capsule. Adequate margins of resection are thus necessary to prevent recurrences. This may require sacrifice of the facial nerve, which courses through the parotid gland. On average, about 10% of excisions are followed by recurrence.

The characteristic histologic feature is heterogeneity. Epithelial elements form ducts, acini, tubules, strands, or sheets of cells, which are intermingled with a loose, often myxoid connective tissue stroma sometimes containing islands of apparent chondroid or, rarely, bone (Fig. 15–4). The epithelial cells are small and dark and range from cuboidal to spindle forms. Immunohistochemical evidence suggests that all of the diverse cell types within these tumors, including those within the stroma, are of myoepithelial derivation. When primary or recurrent benign tumors are present for many years (10 to 20 years), malignant transformation may occur, referred to then as a **malignant mixed salivary gland tumor.** Malignancy is less common in the parotid gland (15%) than in the submandibular glands (40%).

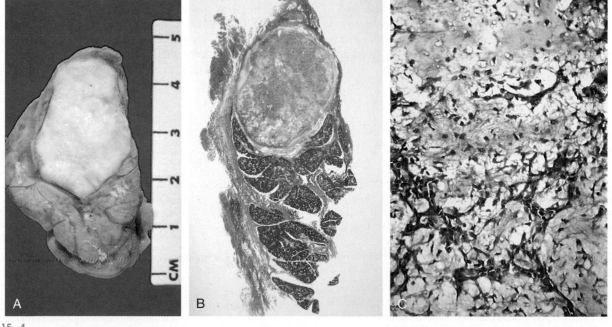

Figure 15–4   ■

Pleomorphic adenoma. *A,* A well-demarcated tumor in the parotid gland. *B,* Low-power view showing a well-demarcated tumor with normal parotid acini below. *C,* High-power view showing amorphous myxoid stroma resembling cartilage, with interspersed islands and strands of myoepithelial cells. (Courtesy of E. Lee, MD, Department of Pathology, University of Texas Southwestern Medical Center, Dallas, TX.)

Warthin's Tumor (Papillary Cystadenoma Lymphomatosum, Cystadenolymphoma). This infrequent benign tumor occurs virtually only in the parotid gland. It is generally a small, well-encapsulated, round to ovoid mass that on transection often reveals mucin-containing cleftlike or cystic spaces within a soft gray background. Microscopically, it exhibits two characteristic features: (1) a two-tiered epithelial layer lining the branching, cystic, or cleftlike spaces; and (2) an immediately subjacent, well-developed lymphoid tissue sometimes forming germinal centers. A recurrence rate of about 10% is attributed to incomplete excision, multicentricity, or a second primary tumor. Malignant transformation is rare and controversial.

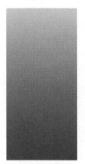

Esophagus

Lesions of the esophagus run the gamut from highly lethal cancers to bland esophagitis yet evoke a remarkably limited range of symptoms. All produce *dysphagia* (difficulty in swallowing), which is attributed either to deranged esophageal motor function or to narrowing or obstruction of the lumen. *Heartburn* (retrosternal burning pain) usually reflects regurgitation of gastric contents into the lower esophagus. Less commonly, *hematemesis* (vomiting of blood) and *melena* (blood in the stools) are evidence of severe inflammation, ulceration, or laceration of the esophageal mucosa. Massive hematemesis may reflect life-threatening rupture of esophageal varices.

stitutes 95% of cases; protrusion of the stomach above the diaphragm creates a bell-shaped dilation, bounded below by the diaphragmatic narrowing. In *paraesophageal hernias,* a separate portion of the stomach, usually along the greater curvature, enters the thorax through the widened foramen. The cause of this deranged anatomy is obscure.

On the basis of radiographic studies, hiatal hernias are reported in 1% to 20% of adult subjects, increasing in incidence with age. Only about 9% of these adults, however, suffer from heartburn or regurgitation of gastric juices into the mouth. These symptoms more likely result from incompetence of the lower esophageal sphincter than from the hiatal hernia per se

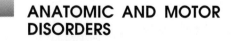

ANATOMIC AND MOTOR DISORDERS

Both esophageal anatomy and motor function may be affected secondarily by many esophageal disorders. Anatomic disorders encountered infrequently are summarized in Table 15–2. The more common conditions are described below.

Hiatal Hernia

In this disorder, separation of the diaphragmatic crura and widening of the space between the muscular crura and the esophageal wall permits a dilated segment of the stomach to protrude above the diaphragm. Two anatomic patterns are recognized (Fig. 15–5): the axial, or sliding, hernia, and the nonaxial, or paraesophageal, hiatal hernia. The *sliding hernia* con-

Table 15–2. SELECTED ANATOMIC DISORDERS OF ESOPHAGUS

Disorder	Clinical Presentation and Anatomy
Stenosis	Adult with progressive dysphagia to solids and eventually to all foods; a lower esophageal narrowing, which is usually the result of chronic inflammatory disease, including gastroesophageal reflux
Atresia, fistula	Newborn with aspiration, paroxysmal suffocation, pneumonia; esophageal atresia (absence of a lumen) and tracheoesophageal fistulas may occur together
Mucosal webs	Episodic dysphagia to solid foods; a (presumably) acquired mucosal membrane partially occluding the esophagus
Diverticula	Episodic food regurgitation, especially nocturnal, sometimes pain is present; an acquired outpouching of the esophageal wall

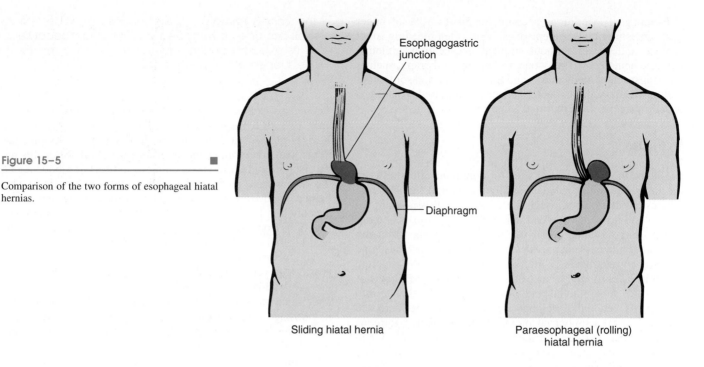

Figure 15–5

Comparison of the two forms of esophageal hiatal hernias.

Sliding hiatal hernia

Paraesophageal (rolling) hiatal hernia

and are accentuated by positions favoring reflux (bending forward, lying supine) and obesity. Although most patients with sliding hiatal hernias do not have reflux esophagitis (discussed later), those with severe reflux esophagitis are likely to have a sliding hiatal hernia. Other complications affecting both types of hiatal hernias include mucosal ulceration, bleeding, and even perforation. Paraesophageal hernias rarely induce reflux, but they can become strangulated or obstructed.

Achalasia

The term *achalasia* means "failure to relax" and in the present context denotes incomplete relaxation of the lower esophageal sphincter in response to swallowing. This produces functional obstruction of the esophagus, with consequent dilation of the more proximal esophagus. Manometric studies show three major abnormalities in achalasia: (1) aperistalsis, (2) partial or incomplete relaxation of the lower esophageal sphincter with swallowing, and (3) increased resting tone of the lower esophageal sphincter. There is near consensus that the muscles of the esophagus are inherently normal and that there is some derangement in the innervation of the lower esophageal sphincter. Secondary achalasia may arise from pathologic processes that impair esophageal function. The classic example is Chagas' disease, caused by *Trypanosoma cruzi*, which causes destruction of the myenteric plexus of the esophagus, duodenum, colon, and ureter. In most instances, however, achalasia occurs as a primary disorder of uncertain etiology.

In primary achalasia there is progressive dilation of the esophagus above the level of the lower esophageal sphincter. The wall of the esophagus may be of normal thickness, thicker than normal owing to hypertrophy of the muscularis, or markedly thinned out by dilation. The myenteric ganglia are usually absent from the body of the esophagus but may or may not be reduced in number in the region of the lower esophageal sphincter. Although this is not a mucosal disease, stasis of food may produce inflammation, ulceration, or fibrotic thickening proximal to the lower esophageal sphincter.

Achalasia is characterized clinically by progressive dysphagia and inability to completely convey food to the stomach. Nocturnal regurgitation and aspiration of undigested food may occur. It usually becomes manifest in young adulthood, but it may appear in infancy or childhood. The most serious aspect of this condition is the hazard of developing esophageal squamous cell carcinoma, reported to occur in about 5% of patients, typically at an earlier age than those without this disease.

Lacerations (Mallory-Weiss Syndrome)

Longitudinal tears in the esophagus at the esophagogastric junction are termed *Mallory-Weiss tears* and are encountered most frequently in chronic alcoholics after a bout of severe retching or vomiting. The presumed pathogenesis is inadequate relaxation of the musculature of the lower esophageal sphincter during vomiting, with stretching and tearing of the esophagogastric junction during propulsive expulsion of gastric contents. The tears may involve only the mucosa or may penetrate the wall. Infection of the defect may lead to an inflammatory ulcer or to mediastinitis.

Esophageal lacerations account for 5% to 10% of upper gastrointestinal bleeding episodes. Most often bleeding is not profuse and ceases without surgical intervention, although massive hematemesis may occur. Supportive therapy, such as vasoconstrictive medications and transfusions, and sometimes balloon tamponade, is usually all that is required. Healing is usually prompt, with minimal to no residua.

Varices

One of the few potential sites for communication between the intra-abdominal splanchnic circulation and the systemic venous circulation is through the esophagus. When portal venous blood flow into the liver is impeded by cirrhosis or other causes, the resultant portal hypertension induces the formation of collateral bypass channels wherever the portal and systemic systems communicate. Portal blood flow is thereby diverted through the coronary veins of the stomach into the plexus of esophageal subepithelial and submucosal veins, thence into the azygos veins and the superior vena cava. The increased pressure in the esophageal plexus produces dilated tortuous vessels called varices. *Varices occur in approximately two thirds of all cirrhotic patients and are most often associated with alcoholic cirrhosis.*

Varices appear primarily as tortuous dilated veins lying primarily within the submucosa of the distal esophagus and proximal stomach. The net effect is irregular protrusion of the overlying mucosa into the lumen, although varices are collapsed in surgical or postmortem specimens (Fig. 15–6). When the varix is unruptured, the mucosa may be normal, but often it is eroded and inflamed because of its exposed position, further weakening the tissue support of the dilated veins.

Variceal rupture produces massive hemorrhage into the lumen, as well as suffusion of blood into the esophageal wall. Varices produce no symptoms until they rupture. Among patients with advanced cirrhosis of the liver, half the deaths result from rupture of a varix, either as a direct consequence of the hemorrhage or from the hepatic coma triggered by the hemorrhage. However, even when varices are present, they account for less than half of all episodes of hematemesis. Bleeding from concomitant gastritis, peptic ulcer, or esophageal laceration accounts for most of the remainder.

The factors leading to rupture of a varix are unclear: silent erosion of overlying thinned mucosa, increased tension in progressively dilated veins, and vomiting with increased intra-abdominal pressure are likely to be involved. Once begun, the hemorrhage rarely subsides spontaneously, and endoscopic injection of thrombotic agents (sclerotherapy) or balloon tamponade is usually required. When varices bleed, 40% of patients die in the first episode. Among those who survive, rebleeding occurs in over half within 1 year, with a similar rate of mortality for each episode.

ESOPHAGITIS

Injury to the esophageal mucosa with subsequent inflammation is a common condition worldwide. In northern Iran, the prevalence of esophagitis is over 80%; it is also extremely high in regions of China. The basis of this prevalence is unknown. In the United States and other Western countries, esophagitis is present in 10% to 20% of the adult population. The inflammation may have many origins: prolonged gastric intubation, uremia, ingestion of corrosive or irritant substances, and radiation or chemotherapy, among others. However, *the overwhelming preponderance of cases in Western countries are attributable to reflux of gastric contents (reflux esophagitis).* There are many presumed contributory factors:

■ Decreased efficacy of esophageal antireflux mechanisms
■ Inadequate or slowed esophageal clearance of refluxed material
■ The presence of a sliding hiatal hernia
■ Increased gastric volume, contributing to the volume of refluxed material
■ Impaired reparative capacity of the esophageal mucosa by prolonged exposure to gastric juices

Any one of these influences may assume primacy in an individual case, but more than one is likely to be involved in most instances.

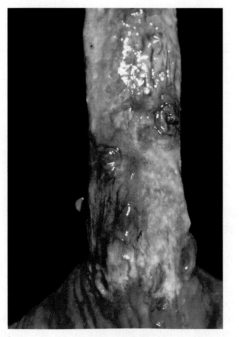

Figure 15–6 ■

Esophageal varices: a view of the everted esophagus and gastroesophageal junction, showing dilated submucosal veins (varices). The blue-colored varices have collapsed in this postmortem specimen.

The anatomic changes depend on the causative agent and on the duration and severity of the

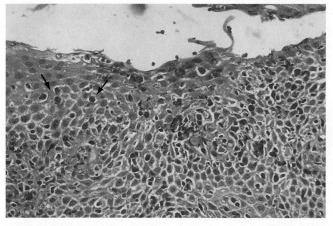

Figure 15–7 ■

Reflux esophagitis showing the superficial portion of the mucosa. Numerous eosinophils *(arrows)* are present within the mucosa, and the stratified squamous epithelium has not undergone complete maturation owing to ongoing inflammatory damage.

exposure. Mild esophagitis may appear macroscopically as simple hyperemia. The mucosa in severe esophagitis exhibits confluent epithelial erosions or total ulceration. Three histologic features are characteristic of uncomplicated **reflux esophagitis** (Fig. 15–7), although only one or two may be present: (1) eosinophils, with or without neutrophils, in the epithelial layer; (2) basal zone hyperplasia; and (3) elongation of lamina propria papillae. Intraepithelial neutrophils are markers of more severe injury.

Clinical Features. The dominant manifestation of reflux disease is heartburn, sometimes accompanied by regurgitation of a sour brash. Rarely, chronic symptoms are punctuated by attacks of severe chest pain mimicking a heart attack. *The severity of symptoms is not related closely to the presence and degree of anatomic esophagitis.* Although largely limited to adults older than age 40, reflux esophagitis is occasionally seen in infants and children. The potential consequences of severe reflux esophagitis are bleeding, development of stricture, and Barrett's esophagus, with its predisposition to malignancy.

BARRETT'S ESOPHAGUS

Barrett's esophagus is a complication of long-standing gastroesophageal reflux, occurring in up to 11% of patients with symptomatic reflux disease, as well as in some patients with asymptomatic reflux. *Barrett's esophagus is defined as replacement of the normal distal stratified squamous mucosa by abnormal metaplastic columnar epithelium containing goblet cells.* Prolonged and recurrent gastroesophageal reflux is

thought to produce inflammation and eventually ulceration of the squamous epithelial lining. Healing then apparently occurs by ingrowth of stem cells and re-epithelialization. In the microenvironment of an abnormally low pH in the distal esophagus, the cells differentiate into an abnormal columnar epithelium that is thought to be more resistant to injury from refluxing gastric contents. In addition to the symptomatology of reflux esophagitis, the chief clinical significance of Barrett's esophagus relates to a 30- to 40-fold increase in the risk of developing adenocarcinoma. Secondary complications also include local ulceration with bleeding and stricture.

Barrett's esophagus is apparent as a red, velvety mucosa between the smooth, pale pink esophageal squamous mucosa and the more lush light brown gastric mucosa. It may exist as tongues extending up from the gastroesophageal junction, as an irregular circumferential band displacing the squamocolumnar junction cephalad, or as isolated patches (islands) in the distal esophagus (Fig. 15–8). **Microscopically, the esophageal squamous epithelium is replaced by metaplastic columnar epithelium,** as depicted in Figure 15–9. **Barrett's mucosa may be quite focal and variable from one site to the next, often necessitating repeated endoscopy and biopsy for definitive diagnosis.** Critical to the pathologic evaluation of patients with Barrett's mucosa is the recognition of dysplastic changes in the mucosa that may be precursors of cancer.

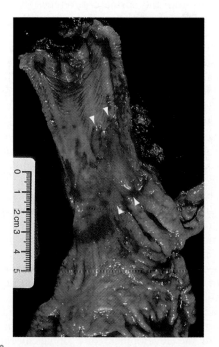

Figure 15–8 ■

Barrett's esophagus: gross view of distal esophagus *(top)* and proximal stomach *(bottom),* showing granular zone of Barrett's esophagus *(arrowheads).*

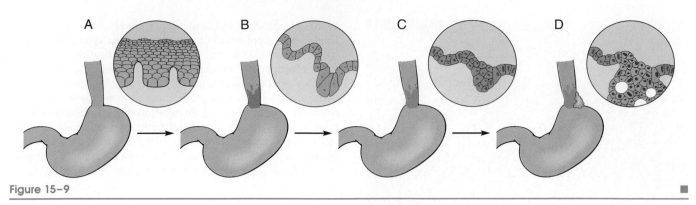

Figure 15–9

Schematic of Barrett's esophagus. *A,* The normal esophagus is lined by stratified squamous epithelium. *B,* Prolonged gastroesophageal reflux leads to metaplastic replacement of the squamous epithelium in the distal esophagus by a columnar type of epithelium, which is gastric, intestinal, or mixed in composition. *C,* In patients with long-standing Barrett's esophagus, the columnar epithelium may become dysplastic, leading eventually to the development of invasive adenocarcinoma *(D).*

ESOPHAGEAL CARCINOMA

Benign tumors may arise in the esophagus from both the squamous mucosa and underlying mesenchyme. However, these are overshadowed by cancer of the esophagus, of which most are squamous cell carcinomas and the remainder are adenocarcinomas. In the United States, most cases occur in adults over the age of 50 with a male-to-female ratio of 3 : 1. There are striking and puzzling differences in the incidence of esophageal carcinoma worldwide. In the United States, there are about 6 new cases per 100,000 population per year, accounting for 1% to 2% of all cancer deaths. In regions of Asia extending from the northern provinces of China to the Caspian littoral in Iran, the prevalence is well over 100 per 100,000, and 20% of cancer deaths are due to esophageal carcinoma, females being affected more often than males. In the United States there is a three- to fourfold higher incidence of esophageal cancer among blacks than among whites. These epidemiologic contrasts must contain causative clues that remain to be deciphered.

Etiology and Pathogenesis. The environmental and dietary factors associated with *squamous cell carcinoma* are presented in Table 15–3. An important contributing factor is retarded passage of food through the esophagus, prolonging mucosal exposure to potential carcinogens such as those contained in tobacco and alcoholic beverages. There is a well-defined predisposing role for chronic esophagitis, itself associated with alcohol and tobacco. However, different influences must underlie the very high incidence of this tumor among the orthodox Moslems of Iran, who neither drink nor smoke. Other environmental factors are invoked, particularly diet, without much direct causal evidence. The role of genetic predisposition is extremely ill defined, but the rare genetic syndrome of tylosis, characterized by excess keratin formation in the skin of the palm and soles, carries an almost certain probability of the development of esophageal cancer. *Barrett's esophagus is the only recognized precursor of esophageal adenocarcinoma.*

Links have been drawn between the previously mentioned risk factors and molecular changes. For example, the tumor suppressor gene *p53* is abnormal in up to 50% of squamous cell carcinomas and is correlated with the use of tobacco and alcohol. The frequency of *p53* mutations in Barrett's esophagus increases with increasing degrees of mucosal dysplasia. In fact, alterations or loss of *p53* and other tumor suppressor genes can be identified in most esophageal cancers.

Squamous cell carcinomas are usually preceded by a long prodrome of mucosal epithelial dysplasia followed by carcinoma in situ and, ultimately, by the emergence of invasive cancer. Early overt lesions appear as small, gray-white, plaquelike thickenings or elevations of the mucosa. In months to years, these lesions become tumorous, taking one of three forms: (1) polypoid fungating masses that protrude into the lumen; (2) necrotizing can-

Table 15–3. RISK FACTORS FOR SQUAMOUS CELL CARCINOMA OF THE ESOPHAGUS

Esophageal Disorders
Long-standing esophagitis
Achalasia
Plummer-Vinson syndrome (esophageal webs, microcytic hypochromic anemia, atrophic glossitis)
Life Style
Alcohol consumption
Tobacco abuse
Dietary
Deficiency of vitamins
   (A, C, riboflavin, thiamine, pyridoxine)
Deficiency of trace metals (zinc, molybdenum)
Fungal contamination of foodstuffs
High content of nitrites/nitrosamines
Genetic Predisposition
Tylosis (hyperkeratosis of palms and soles)

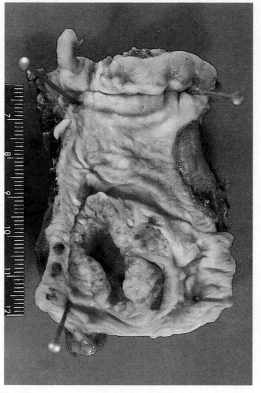

Figure 15–10   ■

Large ulcerated squamous cell carcinoma of the esophagus.

cerous ulcerations that extend deeply and sometimes erode into the respiratory tree, aorta, or elsewhere (Fig. 15–10); and (3) diffuse infiltrative neoplasms that impart thickening and rigidity to the wall and narrowing of the lumen. Whichever the pattern, about 20% arise in the cervical and upper thoracic esophagus, 50% in the middle third, and 30% in the lower third.

Adenocarcinomas appear to arise from dysplastic mucosa in the setting of Barrett's esophagus. They are usually in the distal esophagus and may invade the subjacent gastric cardia. They represent one fourth of all esophageal carcinomas in the United States and more than one half of those in the distal third of the esophagus. Initially appearing as flat or raised patches on an otherwise intact mucosa, they may develop into large nodular masses or exhibit deeply ulcerative or diffusely infiltrative features. Microscopically, most tumors are mucin-producing glandular tumors exhibiting intestinal-type features, in keeping with the morphology of the preexisting metaplastic mucosa. The occasional development of tumors of other alimentary cell types supports the concept that Barrett's epithelium arises from multipotential cells.

Clinical Features. Esophageal carcinoma is insidious in onset and produces dysphagia and obstruction gradually and late. Weight loss, anorexia, fatigue, and weakness appear, followed by pain, usually related to swallowing. Diagnosis is usually made by imaging techniques and endoscopic biopsy. Because these cancers extensively invade the rich esophageal lymphatic network and adjacent structures, surgical excision rarely is curative. Thus, there is emphasis on routine screening procedures, particularly for those with manifestations of chronic esophagitis or known Barrett's esophagus. In the fortunate patient, early esophageal cancer is detected that is confined to the mucosa or submucosa and is therefore amenable to surgical treatment.

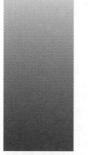

Stomach

Gastric disorders frequently cause clinical disease, ranging from bland chronic gastritis to the anything but bland gastric carcinoma. Gastric infection with *Helicobacter pylori* represents perhaps the most common gastrointestinal infection. Occasionally, congenital anomalies are encountered, which are summarized in Table 15–4.

In keeping with the limited sensory apparatus of the alimentary tract, gastric disorders give rise to symptoms similar to esophageal disorders, primarily *heartburn* and *vague epigastric pain*. With breach of the gastric mucosa and bleeding, *hematemesis* or *melena* may ensue. Unlike esophageal bleeding, however, blood quickly congeals and turns brown in the acid environment of the stomach lumen. Vomited blood hence has the appearance of coffee grounds.

Table 15–4. CONGENITAL GASTRIC ANOMALIES

Condition	Comment
Pyloric stenosis	1 in 300 to 900 live births
	Male to female ratio 3 : 1
	Pathology: muscular hypertrophy of pyloric smooth muscle wall
	Symptoms: persistent, nonbilious projectile vomiting in young infant
Diaphragmatic hernia	Rare
	Pathology: herniation of stomach and other abdominal contents into thorax through a diaphragmatic defect
	Symptoms: acute respiratory embarassment in newborn
Gastric heterotopia	Uncommon
	Pathology: a nidus of gastric mucosa in the esophagus or small intestine ("ectopic rest")
	Symptoms: asymptomatic, or an anomalous peptic ulcer in adult

GASTRITIS

This diagnosis is both overused and often missed—overused when it is applied loosely to any transient upper abdominal complaint in the absence of validating evidence and missed because most patients with chronic gastritis are asymptomatic. *Gastritis is simply defined as inflammation of the gastric mucosa.* By far the majority of cases are *chronic gastritis,* but occasionally distinct forms of *acute gastritis* are encountered. Because there is continued dispute about the classification of gastritis, we will adhere to this simple distinction between types.

Chronic Gastritis

Chronic gastritis is defined as the presence of chronic mucosal inflammatory changes leading eventually to mucosal atrophy and epithelial metaplasia. It is notable for distinct causal subgroups and for patterns of histologic alterations that vary in different parts of the world. In the Western world, the prevalence of histologic changes indicative of chronic gastritis exceeds 50% in the later decades of adult life.

Pathogenesis. By far the most important etiologic association is chronic infection by the bacillus *Helicobacter pylori* (Fig. 15–11). This organism is a worldwide pathogen that has the highest infection rates in developing countries. Prevalence of infection among adults in Puerto Rico exceeds 80%; American adults older than age 50 exhibit prevalence rates approaching 50%. In areas where the infection is endemic, it seems to be acquired in childhood and persists for decades. Most individuals with the infection also have the associated gastritis but are asymptomatic.

H. pylori is a noninvasive, non–spore-forming, S-shaped gram-negative rod measuring approximately 3.5 × 0.5 μm.

The mechanisms by which gastritis develops remain unclear but may relate to the combined influence of bacterial enzymes and toxins and release of noxious chemicals by the recruited neutrophils. Patients with chronic gastritis and *H. pylori* usually improve when treated with antimicrobial agents, and relapses are associated with reappearance of this organism.

Other forms of chronic gastritis are much less common in the United States. A chronic gastritis of unknown cause that produces extensive multifocal atrophy is endemic in some parts of the world such as Japan. *Autoimmune gastritis* results from autoantibodies to the gastric gland parietal cells, in particular to the acid-producing enzyme H^+,K^+-ATPase. The autoimmune injury leads to gland destruction and mucosal atrophy, with concomitant loss of acid and intrinsic factor production. The resultant deficiency of intrinsic factor leads to pernicious anemia, as further discussed in Chapter 12. This form of gastritis is seen most often in Scandinavia, in association with other autoimmune disorders such as Hashimoto's thyroiditis and Addison's disease.

Regardless of the histologic distribution of chronic gastritis, the inflammatory changes consist of a lymphocytic and plasma cell infiltrate in the lamina propria, occasionally accompanied by neutrophilic inflammation of the neck region of the mucosal pits. The inflammation may be accompanied by variable gland loss and mucosal atrophy. When present, *H. pylori* organisms are found nestled within the mucous layer overlying the superficial mucosal epithelium (Fig. 15–12). In the autoimmune variant, loss of parietal cells is particularly prominent. Two additional features are of note. **Intestinal metaplasia** refers to the replacement of gastric epithelium with columnar and goblet cells of intestinal variety. This is significant, because gastric intestinal type carcinomas (see later) appear to arise from **dysplasia** of this metaplastic epithelium. Second, *H. pylori*–induced proliferation of **lymphoid tissue** within the gastric mucosa has been implicated as a precursor of gastric lymphoma.

Clinical Features. Chronic gastritis usually causes few or no symptoms; upper abdominal discomfort and nausea and vomiting can occur. When severe parietal cell loss occurs in the setting of autoimmune gastritis, hypochlorhydria or achlorhydria (referring to levels of gastric luminal hydrochloric acid) and hypergastrinemia are characteristically present. Individuals with chronic gastritis from other causes may be hypochlorhydric, but because parietal cells are never completely destroyed, these patients do not develop achlorhydria or pernicious anemia. Serum gastrin levels are usually within the normal range or only modestly elevated. Most important is the relationship of chronic gastritis to the development of peptic ulcer and gastric carcinoma. Most patients with a peptic ulcer, whether duodenal or gastric, have *H. pylori* infection. The long-term risk of gastric carcinoma for persons with autoimmune gastritis is in the range of 2% to 4%, which is considerably above that of the normal population.

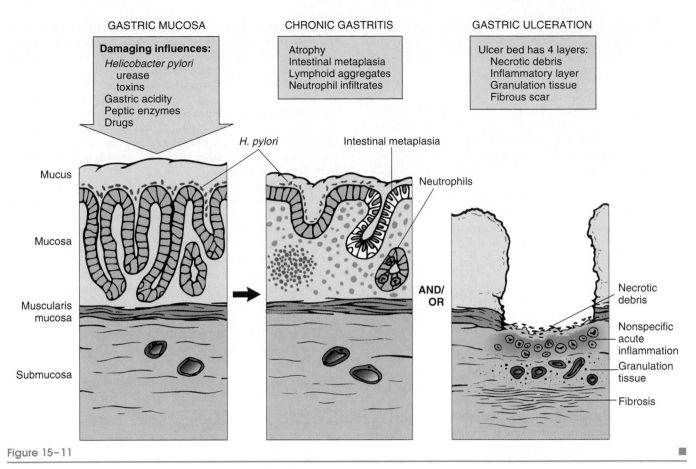

Figure 15–11

Schematic presentation of the presumed action of *Helicobacter pylori* in the development of chronic gastritis and peptic ulcerations. The histologic features of the two disease conditions are depicted.

Acute Gastritis

Acute gastritis is an acute mucosal inflammatory process, usually of a transient nature. The inflammation may be accompanied by hemorrhage into the mucosa and, in more se-

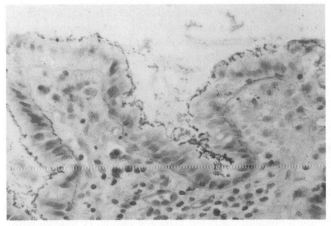

Figure 15–12

Helicobacter pylori gastritis. A Steiner silver stain demonstrates the numerous darkly stained *Helicobacter* organisms along the luminal surface of the gastric epithelial cells. Note that there is no tissue invasion by bacteria.

vere circumstances, by sloughing of the superficial mucosal epithelium *(erosion).* This severe erosive form of the disease is an important cause of acute gastrointestinal bleeding.

Pathogenesis. The pathogenesis is poorly understood, in part because normal mechanisms for gastric mucosal protection are not totally clear. Acute gastritis is frequently associated with the following:

- Heavy use of nonsteroidal anti-inflammatory drugs (NSAIDs), particularly aspirin
- Excessive alcohol consumption
- Heavy smoking
- Treatment with cancer chemotherapeutic drugs
- Uremia
- Systemic infections (e.g., salmonellosis)
- Severe stress (e.g., trauma, burns, surgery)
- Ischemia and shock
- Suicide attempts with acids and alkali
- Mechanical trauma (e.g., nasogastric intubation)
- After distal gastrectomy with reflux of bilious material

One or more of the following influences are thought to be operative in these varied settings: disruption of the adherent mucous layer, stimulation of acid secretion with hydrogen ion back-diffusion into the superficial epithelium, decreased production of bicarbonate buffer by superficial epithelial cells, reduced mucosal blood flow, and direct damage to the epithelium. Not surprisingly, mucosal insults can act synergistically. Finally, acute infection with *H. pylori* induces neutrophilic inflammation of the gastric mucosa, but this event usually escapes the notice of the patient.

> There is a spectrum of severity ranging from localized (as occurs in nonsteroidal anti-inflammatory agent–induced injury) to diffuse, and from superficial inflammation to involvement of the entire mucosal thickness with hemorrhage and focal erosions. Concurrent erosion and hemorrhage is readily visible by endoscopy and is termed **acute erosive gastritis**. All variants are marked by mucosal edema and an inflammatory infiltrate of neutrophils and possibly by chronic inflammatory cells. Regenerative replication of epithelial cells in the gastric pits is usually prominent. Provided that the noxious event is short lived, acute gastritis may disappear within days with complete restitution of the normal mucosa.

Clinical Features. Depending on the severity of the anatomic changes, acute gastritis may be entirely asymptomatic, may cause variable epigastric pain with nausea and vomiting, or may present as overt hematemesis, melena, and potentially fatal blood loss. Overall, *it is one of the major causes of hematemesis, particularly in alcoholics.* Even in certain other settings, the condition is quite common; as many as 25% of persons who take daily aspirin for rheumatoid arthritis develop acute gastritis at some time in their course, many with occult or overt bleeding.

GASTRIC ULCERATION

Ulcers are defined as a breach in the mucosa of the alimentary tract that extends through the muscularis mucosa into the submucosa or deeper. This is to be contrasted to *erosions,* in which there is loss of the superficial epithelium of the mucosa. Erosions may heal within days, whereas healing of ulcers takes much longer. Although ulcers may occur anywhere in the alimentary tract, none are as prevalent as the peptic ulcers that occur in the duodenum and stomach.

Peptic Ulcers

Peptic ulcers are chronic, most often solitary, lesions that occur in any portion of the gastrointestinal tract exposed to the aggressive action of acid-peptic juices. At least 98% of peptic ulcers are either in the first portion of the duodenum or in the stomach, in a ratio of about 4 : 1.

Epidemiology. Peptic ulcers are remitting, relapsing lesions that are most often diagnosed in middle-aged to older adults, but they may first become evident in young adult life. They often appear without obvious precipitating influences and may then, after a period of weeks to months of active disease, heal. *Even with healing, however, the propensity to develop peptic ulcers remains.* Thus, it is difficult to obtain accurate data on the prevalence of active disease. Best estimates suggest that in the American population, about 2% of males and 1.5% of females have peptic ulcers.

Genetic or racial influences appear to play little or no role in the causation of peptic ulcers. Duodenal ulcers are more frequent in patients with alcoholic cirrhosis, chronic obstructive pulmonary disease, chronic renal failure, and hyperparathyroidism. With respect to the last two conditions, hypercalcemia, whatever its cause, stimulates gastrin production and, therefore, acid secretion.

Pathogenesis. There are two key facts. First, *the fundamental requisite for peptic ulceration is mucosal exposure to gastric acid and pepsin.* Second, *there is a very strong causal association with H. pylori infection.* Despite the clarity of these two statements, the actual pathogenesis of mucosal ulceration remains murky. It is best perhaps to consider that peptic ulcers are induced by imbalance between the gastroduodenal mucosal defenses and the countervailing aggressive forces that overcome such defenses, as depicted in Figure 15–13. Both sides of the imbalance are considered.

The array of *host mechanisms* that prevent the gastric mucosa from being digested like a piece of meat include the following:

■ Secretion of mucus by surface epithelial cells
■ Secretion of bicarbonate into the surface mucus, to create a buffered surface microenvironment
■ Secretion of acid- and pepsin-containing fluid from the gastric pits as "jets" through the surface mucous layer, entering the lumen directly without contacting surface epithelial cells
■ Rapid gastric epithelial regeneration
■ Robust mucosal blood flow, to sweep away hydrogen ions that have back-diffused into the mucosa from the lumen and to sustain the high cellular metabolic and regenerative activity
■ Mucosal elaboration of prostaglandins, which help maintain mucosal blood flow

H. pylori infection is present in virtually all patients with duodenal ulcers and about 70% of those with gastric ulcers. Furthermore, antibiotic treatment of *H. pylori* infection promotes healing of ulcers and tends to prevent their recurrence. Hence much interest is focused on the possible mechanisms by which this tiny noninvasive spiral organism tips the balance of mucosal defenses. Some likely possibilities include

■ Secretion by *H. pylori* of a *urease* that generates free ammonia and a *protease* that breaks down glycoproteins in the gastric mucus. The organisms also elaborate phospholipases, which damage surface epithelial cells and may release bioactive leukotrienes and eicosanoids.
■ Neutrophils attracted by *H. pylori* release myeloperoxidase, which produces hypochlorous acid, yielding, in turn, monochloramine in the presence of ammonia. Both hypochlorous acid and monochloramine can destroy mammalian cells.
■ Both mucosal epithelial cells and lamina propria endothelial cells are prime targets for the destructive actions of *H. pylori* colonization. Thrombotic occlusion of surface capillaries is also promoted by a bacterial platelet-activating factor.

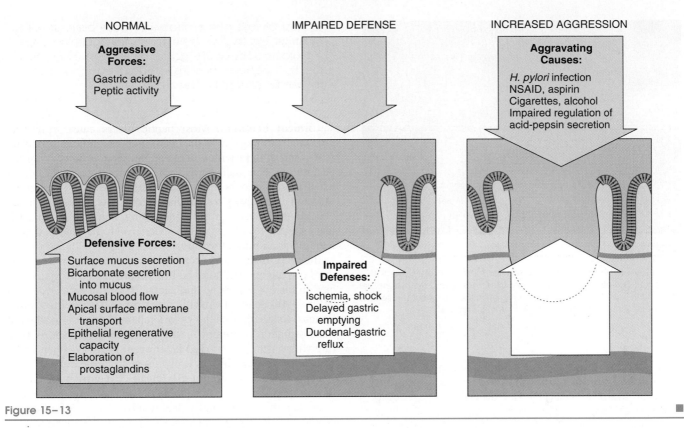

Figure 15-13   ■

Diagram of aggravating causes of, and defense mechanisms against, peptic ulceration.

■ In addition to elaboration of enzymes, *H. pylori* may release other factors (including lipopolysaccharide) that recruit inflammatory cells to the mucosa. The chronically inflamed mucosa is more susceptible to acid injury.

■ Finally, damage to the mucosa is thought to permit leakage of tissue nutrients into the surface microenvironment, thereby sustaining the bacillus.

Only 10% to 20% of individuals worldwide infected with *H. pylori* actually develop peptic ulcer. Hence, a key enigma is why most are spared and some are susceptible. Perhaps there are unknown interactions with *H. pylori* and the mucosa that occur only in some individuals. Another perplexing observation is that in patients with duodenal ulcer *H. pylori* is more readily isolated from the gastric antrum than from the duodenum. It has been suggested that antral infection releases inflammatory mediators that drain downstream and injure the duodenal mucosa. *Suffice it to say that while the link between* H. pylori *infection and gastric and duodenal ulcers is established, the interactions leading to ulceration remain to be deciphered.*

Other events may act alone or in concert with *H. pylori* to promote peptic ulceration. The *Zollinger-Ellison syndrome* (Chapter 20) is associated with multiple peptic ulcerations in the stomach, duodenum, and even jejunum, owing to excess gastrin secretion by a tumor and, hence, excess gastric acid production. Chronic use of nonsteroidal anti-inflammatory agents and aspirin suppresses mucosal prostaglandin synthesis; aspirin also is a direct irritant. Cigarette smoking impairs mucosal blood flow and healing. Alcohol has not been proved

to directly cause peptic ulceration, but alcoholic cirrhosis is associated with an increased incidence of peptic ulcers. *Corticosteroids* in high dose and with repeated use promote ulcer formation. Finally, there are compelling arguments that personality and psychological stress are important contributing factors, even though data on cause and effect are lacking.

All peptic ulcers, whether gastric or duodenal, have an identical gross and microscopic appearance. **By definition, they are defects in the mucosa that penetrate at least into the submucosa, and usually into the muscularis propria or deeper. Most are round, sharply punched-out craters 2 to 4 cm in diameter** (Fig. 15-14); those in the duodenum tend to be smaller, and occasional gastric lesions are significantly larger. Favored sites are the anterior and posterior walls of the first portion of the duodenum and the lesser curvature of the stomach. The location within the stomach is dictated by the extent of the associated gastritis: antral gastritis is most common, and the ulcer is often along the lesser curvature at the margin of the inflamed area and the upstream acid-secreting mucosa of the corpus. Occasional gastric ulcers occur on the greater curvature or anterior or posterior walls of the stomach, the very same locations of most ulcerative cancers.

Classically, **the margins of the crater are perpen-**

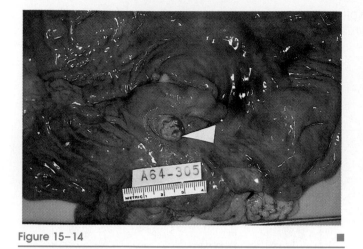

Figure 15–14 ■

Peptic ulcer of the duodenum. Note that the ulcer is small (2 cm) with a sharply punched-out appearance. Unlike cancerous ulcers, the margins are not elevated. The ulcer base shows a small amount of blood but is otherwise clean. Compare with the ulcerated carcinoma in Figure 15–17.

dicular and there is some mild edema of the immediately adjacent mucosa, but unlike cancerous ulcers, there is no significant elevation or beading of the edges. The surrounding mucosal folds may radiate like wheel spokes. The base of the crater appears remarkably clean, owing to peptic digestion of the inflammatory exudate and necrotic tissue. Infrequently, an eroded artery is visible in the ulcer (usually associated with a history of significant bleeding). If the ulcer crater penetrates through the duodenal or gastric wall, a localized or generalized peritonitis may develop. Alternatively, the perforation is sealed by an adjacent structure such as adherent omentum, liver, or pancreas.

The histologic appearance varies with the activity, chronicity, and degree of healing. In a chronic, open ulcer, four zones can be distinguished (Fig. 15–15): (1) the base and margins have a thin layer of necrotic fibrinoid debris underlain by (2) a zone of active nonspecific inflammatory infiltration with neutrophils predominating, underlain by (3) granulation tissue, deep to which is (4) fibrous, collagenous scar that fans out widely from the margins of the ulcer. Vessels trapped within the scarred area are characteristically thickened and occasionally thrombosed, but in some instances they are widely patent. With healing, the crater fills with granulation tissue, followed by reepithelialization from the margins and more or less restoration of the normal architecture (hence the prolonged healing times). Extensive fibrous scarring remains.

Chronic gastritis is virtually universal among patients with peptic ulcer disease, occurring in 85% to 100% of patients with duodenal ulcers and 65% of patients with gastric ulcers. *H. pylori* infection is almost always demonstrable in these patients with gastritis. This feature is helpful in distinguishing peptic ulcers from acute gastric ulceration (discussed next), because gastritis in adjacent mucosa is generally absent in the latter condition.

Clinical Features. Most peptic ulcers cause epigastric gnawing, burning, or boring pain, but a significant minority first come to light with complications such as hemorrhage or perforation. The pain tends to be worse at night and occurs usually 1 to 3 hours after meals during the day. Classically, the pain is relieved by alkalis or food, but there are many exceptions. Nausea, vomiting, bloating, belching, and significant weight loss (raising the specter of some hidden malignancy) are additional manifestations.

Bleeding is the chief complication, occurring in up to one third of patients, and may be life threatening. Perforation occurs in far fewer patients but accounts for the greater portion of the 3000 deaths from this disease per year in the United States. Obstruction of the pyloric channel is rare. Malignant transformation is unknown with duodenal ulcers and is very rare with gastric ulcers. The latter event is always open to the possibility that carcinoma was present from the outset.

Peptic ulcers are notoriously chronic, recurrent lesions — they more often impair the quality of life than shorten it. When untreated, the average individual requires 15 years for healing of a peptic ulcer. Nevertheless, with present-day therapies (including antibiotics active against *H. pylori*), most ulcer victims can be helped if not cured, and they usually escape the surgeon's knife.

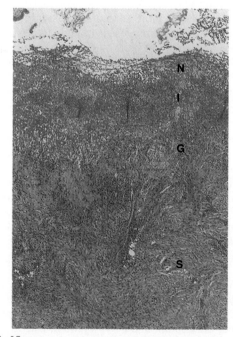

Figure 15–15 ■

Medium-power detail of the base of a nonperforated peptic ulcer, demonstrating the layers of necrosis (N), inflammation (I), granulation tissue (G), and scar (S) moving from the luminal surface at the top to the muscle wall at the bottom.

Acute Gastric Ulceration

Focal, acutely developing gastric mucosal defects may appear after severe stress and are designated *stress ulcers*. Generally, there are multiple lesions located mainly in the stomach and occasionally in the duodenum. Stress ulcers are most commonly encountered in the following conditions:

- Severe trauma, including major surgical procedures, sepsis, or grave illness of any type
- Extensive burns (the ulcers are then referred to as Curling's ulcers)
- Traumatic or surgical injury to the central nervous system or an intracerebral hemorrhage (the ulcers are then called Cushing's ulcers)
- Chronic exposure to gastric irritant drugs, particularly nonsteroidal anti-inflammatory agents and corticosteroids

The pathogenesis of these lesions is uncertain and may vary with the setting. The systemic acidosis that can accompany severe trauma and burns, for example, may contribute to mucosal compromise presumably by lowering the intracellular pH of mucosal cells already rendered hypoxic by impaired mucosal blood flow. With cranial lesions, direct stimulation of vagal nuclei by increased intracranial pressure is proposed, because gastric acid hypersecretion has been documented in these patients.

Acute stress ulcers are usually circular and small (less than 1 cm in diameter). The ulcer base is frequently stained a dark brown by the acid digestion of extruded blood. Unlike chronic peptic ulcers, acute stress ulcers are found anywhere in the stomach. They may occur singly, but more often they are multiple, throughout the stomach and duodenum (Fig. 15–16). Microscopically, acute stress ulcers are abrupt lesions, with essentially unremarkable adjacent mucosa. They range in depth from very superficial lesions (erosion) to deeper lesions that involve the entire mucosal thickness (true ulceration). The shallow erosions are, in essence, an extension of acute erosive gastritis. The deeper lesions comprise well-defined ulcerations but are not precursors of chronic peptic ulcers. Even the deeper lesions do not penetrate the muscularis propria.

Clinical Features. A high percentage of patients admitted to hospital intensive care units with sepsis, severe burns, or trauma acutely develop superficial gastric erosions or ulcers. These may be of limited clinical consequence or life threatening. Although prophylactic antacid regimens and blood transfusions may blunt the impact of stress ulceration, the single most important determinant of clinical outcome is the ability to correct the underlying condition. The gastric mucosa can recover completely if the patient does not succumb to the primary disease.

TUMORS

As with the remainder of the gastrointestinal tract, tumors arising from the mucosa predominate over mesenchymal tumors. These are broadly classified into polyps and carcinoma.

Gastric Polyps

The term polyp is applied to any nodule or mass that projects above the level of the surrounding mucosa. Occasionally, a lipoma or leiomyoma arising in the wall of the stomach may protrude from under the mucosa to produce an apparent polypoid lesion. However, *the use of this term in the gastrointestinal tract is generally restricted to mass lesions arising in the mucosa.* Gastric polyps are uncommon and are found in about 0.4% of adult autopsies, as compared with colonic polyps, which are seen in 25% to 50% of older persons. In the stomach, these lesions are most frequently (1) hyperplastic polyps (80% to 85%), (2) fundic gland polyps (about 10%), and (3) adenomatous polyps (about 5%). All three types arise in the setting of chronic gastritis and so are seen in the same patient populations. Hyperplastic and fundic gland polyps are essentially innocuous. In contrast, there is a definite risk of an adenomatous polyp harboring adenocarcinoma, which increases with polyp size.

Hyperplastic polyps arise from an exuberant reparative response to chronic mucosal damage and hence are composed of a hyperplastic mucosal epithelium and an inflamed edematous stroma. They are not true neoplasms. Fundic gland polyps are small collections of dilated corpus-type glands

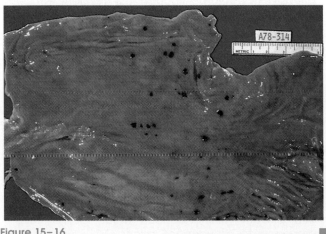

Figure 15–16 ■

Multiple stress ulcers of the stomach, highlighted by the dark digested blood in their bases.

thought to be small hamartomas. On the other hand, the less common adenomas contain dysplastic epithelium. As with colonic adenomas, to be described later, adenomas are true neoplasms.

Gastric Carcinoma

Among the malignant tumors that occur in the stomach, carcinoma is overwhelmingly the most important and the most common (90% to 95%). Next in order of frequency are lymphomas and carcinoids (4% and 3%, respectively, discussed later in this chapter) and mesenchymal spindle cell tumors (2%).

Epidemiology and Classification. Gastric carcinoma is a worldwide disease with a widely varying incidence. Japan, Colombia, Costa Rica, and Hungary have a particularly high incidence. Nevertheless, in most countries there has been a steady decline in both the incidence and the mortality of gastric cancer. Yet it remains among the leading killer cancers, representing 3% of all cancer deaths in the United States. This is attributable to its dismal 5-year survival rate, which remains at less than 10%.

Gastric cancers exhibit two morphologic types, denoted intestinal and diffuse. The *intestinal variant* is thought to arise from gastric mucous cells that have undergone intestinal metaplasia in the setting of chronic gastritis. This pattern of cancer tends to be better differentiated and is the more common type in high-risk populations. *Intestinal-type carcinoma is the pattern that is progressively diminishing in frequency in the United States.* In contrast, the *diffuse variant* is thought to arise de novo from native gastric mucus cells, is not associated with chronic gastritis, and tends to be poorly differentiated. Most importantly, *diffuse gastric carcinoma has not significantly changed in frequency in the past 60 years and now constitutes approximately half of gastric carcinomas in the United States.* Whereas the intestinal-type carcinoma occurs primarily after age 50 years with a 2:1 male predominance, the diffuse carcinoma occurs at an earlier age with no male predominance. It would almost appear that there are two quite distinct forms of gastric carcinoma.

Pathogenesis. The major factors thought to affect the genesis of this form of cancer are environmental, as summarized in Table 15–5. Several points are worthy of emphasis. Risk factors for the increasingly more common diffuse carcinoma are largely unknown. The predisposing influences for the intestinal-type adenocarcinoma are many, but their relative importance is changing. For example, dietary factors have changed drastically in recent years with the increased use of refrigeration worldwide, markedly decreasing the need for food preservation by the use of nitrates, smoking, and salt. Refrigeration also makes possible the increased availability of vegetables and fruit, a potential source of protective antioxidants. Chronic gastritis associated with *H. pylori* infection remains a major risk factor for gastric carcinoma. As with peptic ulcer disease, genetic makeup has not emerged as a major factor.

Changes in multiple oncogenes and tumor-suppressor genes

Table 15–5. RISK FACTORS FOR GASTRIC CARCINOMA

Intestinal-Type Adenocarcinoma
Diet
  Nitrites derived from nitrates (found in food and drinking water, and used as preservatives in prepared meats) may undergo nitrosation to form nitrosamines and nitrosamides
  Smoked foods and pickled vegetables
  Excessive salt intake
  Decreased intake of fresh vegetables and fruits: antioxidants present in these foods may be protective by inhibition of nitrosation
Infection with *Helicobacter pylori*
  Chronic gastritis with intestinal metaplasia
Pernicious anemia
  Chronic gastritis with intestinal metaplasia
Altered anatomy
  After subtotal distal gastrectomy
Diffuse Carcinoma
Risk factors undefined
Infection with *Helicobacter pylori* and chronic gastritis often absent
Slightly increased association with blood group A

have been documented in gastric cancer, as has genomic instability. The mutations and allelic losses in *p53* and in other genes are similar to those encountered in colon carcinogenesis, which is discussed in detail later. In addition, growth factor receptors are also expressed, for example that for transforming growth factor α. However, unifying concepts for the initiation and progression of gastric cancer have not yet emerged.

The location of gastric carcinomas within the stomach is as follows: pylorus and antrum, 50% to 60%; cardia, 25%; and the remainder in the body and fundus. The lesser curvature is involved in about 40% and the greater curvature in 12%. **Thus, a favored location is the lesser curvature of the antropyloric region.** Although less frequent, an ulcerative lesion on the greater curvature is more likely to be malignant.

Gastric carcinoma is classified on the basis of depth of invasion, macroscopic growth pattern, and histologic subtype. The morphologic feature having the greatest impact on clinical outcome is the **depth of invasion. Early gastric carcinoma is defined as a lesion confined to the mucosa and submucosa, regardless of the presence or absence of perigastric lymph node metastases. Advanced gastric carcinoma is a neoplasm that has extended below the submucosa into the muscular wall** and has perhaps spread more widely. Gastric mucosal **dysplasia** is the presumed precursor lesion of early gastric cancer, which then in turn progresses to "advanced" lesions.

The three macroscopic growth patterns of gas-

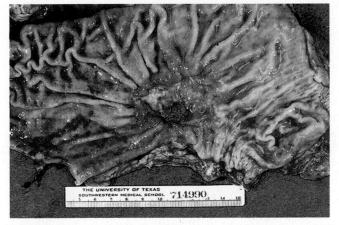

Figure 15-17 ■

Ulcerative gastric carcinoma. The ulcer is large with irregular, heaped-up margins. There is extensive excavation of the gastric mucosa with a necrotic gray area in the deepest portion. Compare with the benign peptic ulcer in Figure 15-14.

tric carcinoma, which may be evident at both the early and advanced stages, are (1) **exophytic,** with protrusion of a tumor mass into the lumen; (2) **flat or depressed,** in which there is no obvious tumor mass within the mucosa; and (3) **excavated,** whereby a shallow or deeply erosive crater is present in the wall of the stomach. Exophytic tumors may contain portions of an adenoma. Flat or depressed malignancy presents only as regional effacement of the normal surface mucosal pattern. Excavated cancers may mimic, in size and appearance, chronic peptic ulcers, although more advanced cases exhibit heaped-up margins (Fig. 15-17). Uncommonly, a broad region of the

gastric wall, or the entire stomach, is extensively infiltrated by malignancy. The rigid and thickened stomach is termed a *leather bottle stomach,* or **linitis plastica;** metastatic carcinoma from the breast and lung may generate a similar picture.

The histologic subtypes of gastric cancer have been variously subclassified, but **the two most important types are the intestinal type and diffuse type** (Fig. 15-18). **The intestinal variant is composed of malignant cells forming neoplastic intestinal glands resembling those of colonic adenocarcinoma. The diffuse variant is composed of gastric-type mucus cells that generally do not form glands but rather permeate the mucosa and wall as scattered individual "signet-ring" cells or small clusters in an "infiltrative" growth pattern.**

Whatever the histologic variant, all gastric carcinomas eventually penetrate the wall to involve the serosa, spread to regional and more distant lymph nodes, and metastasize widely. For obscure reasons, the earliest lymph node metastasis may sometimes involve a supraclavicular lymph node (Virchow's node). Another somewhat unusual mode of intraperitoneal spread in females is to both the ovaries, giving rise to the so-called **Krukenberg tumor.**

Clinical Features. Early gastric carcinoma is generally asymptomatic and can be discovered only by repeated endoscopic examinations in persons at high risk, as is the practice in Japan. Advanced carcinoma also may be asymptomatic, but it often first comes to light because of abdominal discomfort or weight loss. Uncommonly, these neoplasms cause dysphagia when they are located in the cardia, or obstructive symptoms when they arise in the pyloric canal. The only hope for cure is early detection and surgical removal.

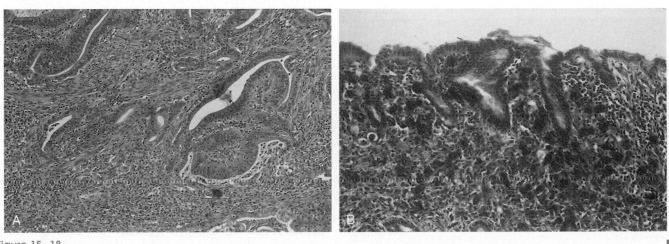

Figure 15-18 ■

Gastric cancer. *A,* Intestinal type demonstrating gland formation by malignant cells, which are invading the muscular wall of the stomach. (H & E.) *B,* Diffuse type demonstrating individual red, mucin-containing malignant cells in the lamina propria of an intact mucosa. (Mucicarmine stain.)

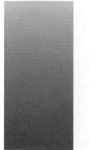

Small and Large Intestines

Many conditions, such as infections, inflammatory diseases, and tumors, affect both the small and large intestines. These two organs are therefore considered together. Collectively, disorders of the intestines account for a large portion of human disease.

DEVELOPMENTAL ANOMALIES

These deviations from the norm are uncommon, but sometimes dramatic, sources of clinical disease. In the small intestine the major anomalies are as follows:

■ *Atresia or stenosis*, the former being complete failure of development of the intestinal lumen and the latter representing only narrowing. Both defects usually involve only a segment of bowel.
■ *Duplication* usually takes the form of well-formed saccular to tubular cystic structures, which may or may not communicate with the lumen of the small intestine.
■ *Meckel's diverticulum* is the most common and innocuous of the anomalies. It results from failure of involution of the omphalomesenteric duct, leaving a persistent blind-ended tubular protrusion up to 5 to 6 cm long (Fig. 15–19). The diameter is variable, sometimes approximating

that of the small intestine itself. Such diverticula are usually in the ileum within about 2 feet (85 cm) of the cecum and are composed of all layers of the normal small intestine. They generally are asymptomatic, save when they permit bacterial overgrowth that depletes vitamin B_{12}, producing a syndrome similar to pernicious anemia. Rarely, pancreatic rests are found in a Meckel's diverticulum, and in about half of the cases there are heterotopic islands of functioning gastric mucosa. Peptic ulceration in the adjacent intestinal mucosa sometimes is responsible for mysterious intestinal bleeding or symptoms resembling acute appendicitis.
■ In *omphalocele*, a congenital defect of the periumbilical abdominal wall leaves behind a membranous sac, into which the intestines herniate.

In the *large intestine*, the major anomalies are

■ *Malrotation* of the developing bowel, preventing the intestines from assuming their normal intra-abdominal positions. The cecum, for example, may be found anywhere in the abdomen, including the left upper quadrant, rather than in its normal position in the right lower quadrant. The large intestine is predisposed to volvulus (discussed later). Confusing clinical syndromes may arise when appendicitis presents as left upper quadrant pain.
■ *Hirschsprung disease*, leading to congenital megacolon.

Hirschsprung Disease: Congenital Megacolon

Distention of the colon to greater than 6 or 7 cm in diameter (megacolon) occurs as a congenital and as an acquired disorder. Hirschsprung disease (congenital megacolon) results when, during development, the caudad migration of neural crest–derived cells along the alimentary tract arrests at some point before reaching the anus. Hence, an aganglionic segment is left that lacks both Meissner's submucosal and Auerbach's myenteric plexuses. This causes functional obstruction and progressive distention of the colon proximal to the affected segment. In most instances, only the rectum and sigmoid are aganglionic, but in about a fifth of cases a longer segment, and rarely the entire colon, is affected.

Genetically, Hirschsprung disease is heterogeneous, and several different defects that lead to the same outcome have been identified. This anomaly occurs in approximately 1 in

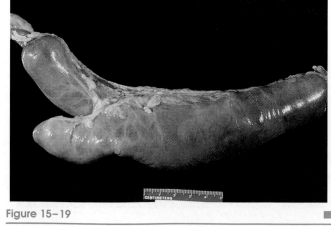

Figure 15–19 ■

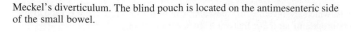

Meckel's diverticulum. The blind pouch is located on the antimesenteric side of the small bowel.

5000 to 8000 live births; males predominate 4 : 1. It is much more frequent in those with other congenital anomalies such as hydrocephalus, ventricular septal defect, and Meckel's diverticulum.

> The critical lesion is the lack of ganglion cells, and of ganglia, in the muscle wall and submucosa of the affected segment. The affected segment is not distended—it is the upstream, properly innervated segment that undergoes dilation. Thus, when only the distal colon is affected, the remainder of the colon becomes massively distended, sometimes achieving a diameter of 15 to 20 cm. The wall may be thinned by distention or in some cases is thickened by compensatory muscle hypertrophy. The mucosal lining of the distended portion may be intact or have shallow, so-called **stercoral ulcers** produced by impacted, inspissated feces.

Clinical Features. In most cases a delay occurs in the initial passage of meconium, which is followed by vomiting in 48 to 72 hours. When a very short distal segment of the rectum alone is involved, the obstruction may not be complete and may not produce manifestations until later in infancy, in the form of alternating periods of obstruction and passage of diarrheal stools. The principal threat to life is superimposed enterocolitis with fluid and electrolyte disturbances. More rarely, the distended colon perforates, usually in the thin-walled cecum. The diagnosis is established by documenting the absence of ganglion cells in the nondistended bowel segment.

Acquired megacolon may result from (1) Chagas' disease, in which the trypanosomes directly invade the bowel wall to destroy the plexuses, (2) organic obstruction of the bowel by a neoplasm or inflammatory stricture, (3) toxic megacolon complicating ulcerative colitis or Crohn's disease (discussed later), or (4) a functional psychosomatic disorder. Except for the trypanosomal Chagas' disease, in which the inflammatory involvement of the ganglia is evident, the remaining forms of megacolon are not associated with any deficiency of mural ganglia.

■ VASCULAR DISORDERS

Ischemic Bowel Disease

Ischemic lesions may be restricted to the small or large intestine or may affect both, depending on the particular vessel or vessels involved. Acute occlusion of one of the three major supply trunks of the intestines—celiac, superior, and inferior mesenteric arteries—may lead to infarction of extensive segments of intestine. However, *insidious loss of one vessel may be without effect,* owing to the rich anastomotic interconnections between the vascular beds. Lesions within the end-arteries that penetrate the gut wall produce small, focal ischemic lesions. As illustrated in Figure 15–20, the severity of injury ranges from *transmural infarction* of the gut, involving all visceral layers, to *mural infarction* of the mucosa and submucosa, sparing the muscular wall, to *mucosal infarction*, if the lesion extends no deeper than the muscularis mucosae.

Almost always, transmural infarction implies acute occlusion of a major mesenteric artery. Mural or mucosal infarction more often results from either physiologic hypoperfusion or more localized anatomic defects and may be acute or chronic. Mesenteric venous thrombosis is a less frequent cause of vascular compromise. The predisposing conditions for all three forms of ischemia are as follows:

- *Arterial thrombosis:* severe atherosclerosis (usually at the origin of the mesenteric vessel), systemic vasculitis, dissecting aneurysm, angiographic procedures, aortic reconstructive surgery, surgical accidents, hypercoagulable states, and oral contraceptives
- *Arterial embolism:* cardiac vegetations (as with endocarditis, or myocardial infarction with mural thrombosis), angiographic procedures, and aortic atheroembolism
- *Venous thrombosis:* hypercoagulable states induced, for example, by oral contraceptives or antithrombin III deficiency, intraperitoneal sepsis, the postoperative state, vascular-invasive neoplasms (particularly hepatocellular carcinoma), cirrhosis, and abdominal trauma

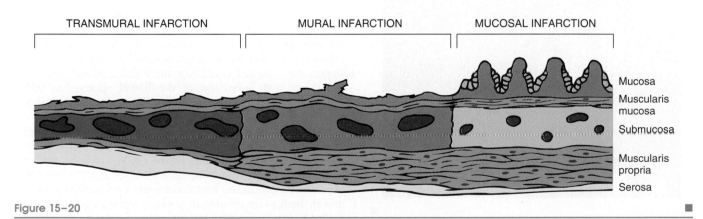

TRANSMURAL INFARCTION   MURAL INFARCTION   MUCOSAL INFARCTION

Mucosa
Muscularis mucosa
Submucosa
Muscularis propria
Serosa

Figure 15–20   ■

Acute ischemic bowel disease. Schematic of the three levels of severity, diagrammed for the small intestine.

■ *Nonocclusive ischemia:* cardiac failure, shock, dehydration, vasoconstrictive drugs (such as digitalis, vasopressin, propranolol)

■ *Miscellaneous:* radiation injury, volvulus, stricture, and internal or external herniation

Transmural intestinal infarction may involve a short or long segment, depending on the particular vessel affected and the patency of the anastomotic supply. Whether the occlusion is arterial or venous, the infarction always has a dark red hemorrhagic appearance because of reflow of blood into the damaged area (Fig. 15–21). The ischemic injury usually begins in the mucosa and extends outward; within 18 to 24 hours there is a thin, fibrinous exudate over the serosa. With arterial occlusion the demarcation from adjacent normal bowel is fairly sharply defined, but with venous occlusion the margins are less distinct. Histologically, the changes are those that would be anticipated, with marked edema, interstitial hemorrhage, necrosis, and sloughing of the mucosa. Within 24 hours intestinal bacteria produce outright gangrene and sometimes perforation of the bowel.

Mural and mucosal infarction characteristically are marked by multifocal lesions interspersed with spared areas. Their location depends in part on the extent of preexisting atherosclerotic narrowing of the arterial supply; lesions can be scattered over large regions of the small or large intestines. Affected foci may or may not be visible from the serosal surface, because by definition the ischemia does not affect the entire thickness of the bowel. When the bowel is opened, hemorrhagic edematous thickening of the mucosa, sometimes with superficial ulcerations, is seen. Histologic features are those of acute injury: edema, hemorrhage, and outright necrosis of the affected tissue

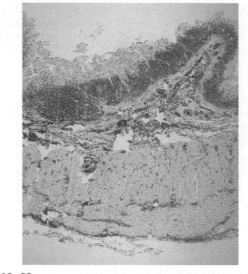

Figure 15–22 ■

Mucosal infarction of the small bowel. The mucosa is hemorrhagic, and there is no epithelial layer. The remaining layers of the bowel are intact.

layers (Fig. 15–22). Inflammation develops at the margins of the lesions, and an inflammatory fibrin-containing exudate **(pseudomembrane),** usually secondary to bacterial superinfection, may coat the affected mucosa. Alternatively, **chronic vascular insufficiency may produce a chronic inflammatory and ulcerative condition, mimicking idiopathic inflammatory bowel disease** (discussed later).

Clinical Features. Ischemic bowel injury is most common in the later years of life. With the transmural lesions, there is the sudden onset of abdominal pain, often out of proportion to the physical signs. Sometimes the pain is accompanied by bloody diarrhea. The onset of pain tends to be more sudden with mesenteric embolism than with arterial or venous thrombosis. Because this condition may progress to shock and vascular collapse within hours, the diagnosis must be made promptly, and making it requires a high index of suspicion in the appropriate setting (e.g., recent major abdominal surgery, recent myocardial infarct, atrial fibrillation, or manifestations suggestive of some form of vegetative endocarditis). The mortality rate with infarction of the bowel approaches 90%, largely because the window of time between onset of symptoms and perforation due to gangrene is so small.

In contrast, mural and mucosal ischemia may appear only as unexplained abdominal distention or gastrointestinal bleeding, sometimes accompanied by the gradual onset of abdominal pain or discomfort. Suspicion is raised if the patient has experienced conditions that favor acute hypoperfusion of the bowel, such as an episode of severe cardiac decompensation or shock. Mucosal and mural infarction are not by themselves fatal, and, indeed, if the cause or causes of hypoperfusion can be corrected, the lesions may heal.

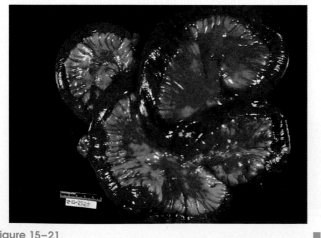

Figure 15–21 ■

Infarcted small bowel, secondary to acute thrombotic occlusion of the superior mesenteric artery.

Angiodysplasia

Tortuous dilations of submucosal and mucosal blood vessels are seen most often in the cecum or right colon, usually only after the sixth decade of life. They are prone to rupture and bleed into the lumen. *Such lesions account for 20% of significant lower intestinal bleeding.* The hemorrhage may be chronic and intermittent and only cause severe anemia, but rarely it is acute and massive.

These lesions sometimes are part of a systemic disorder such as hereditary hemorrhagic telangiectasia (Osler-Weber-Rendu syndrome) or limited scleroderma, sometimes called the CREST syndrome (Chapter 5). Most often, they are isolated lesions thought to develop over decades as the result of mechanical factors operative in the colonic wall. As penetrating veins pass through the muscularis they are subject to intermittent occlusion during peristaltic contractions, but the thicker-walled arteries remain patent, thus producing venous distention and ectasia.

Hemorrhoids

Hemorrhoids are variceal dilations of the anal and perianal submucosal venous plexuses. They are common after age 50 and develop in the setting of persistently elevated venous pressure within the hemorrhoidal plexus. Common predisposing conditions are straining at stool in the setting of chronic constipation and the venous stasis of pregnancy in younger women. More rarely, hemorrhoids may reflect portal hypertension, usually due to cirrhosis of the liver (Chapter 16).

Varicosities in the superior and middle hemorrhoidal veins appear above the anorectal line and are covered by rectal mucosa *(internal hemorrhoids).* Those that appear below the anorectal line represent dilations of the inferior hemorrhoidal plexus and are covered by anal mucosa *(external hemorrhoids).* Both are thin-walled, dilated vessels that commonly bleed, sometimes masking bleeding from far more serious proximal lesions. They may become thrombosed, particularly when subject to trauma from passage of stool. Finally, internal hemorrhoids may prolapse during straining at stool and then become trapped by the compressive anal sphincter, leading to sudden, extremely painful, edematous hemorrhagic enlargement or strangulation.

DIARRHEAL DISEASES

Diarrheal diseases of the bowel make up a veritable Augean stable of entities. Many are caused by microbiologic agents; others arise in the setting of malabsorptive disorders and idiopathic inflammatory bowel disease (discussed in a subsequent section). Consideration should first be given to the conditions known as *diarrhea* and *dysentery.*

Diarrhea and Dysentery

Although a precise definition of diarrhea is elusive, an increase in stool mass, stool frequency, or stool fluidity is per- ceived as diarrhea by most patients. For many individuals, this consists of daily stool production in excess of 250 gm, containing 70% to 95% water. Over 14 liters of fluid may be lost per day in severe cases of diarrhea, equivalent to the circulating blood volume! Diarrhea is often accompanied by pain, urgency, perianal discomfort, and incontinence. *Low-volume, painful, bloody diarrhea is known as dysentery.*

Diarrheal disorders are categorized as follows:

■ *Secretory diarrhea:* net intestinal fluid secretion that is isotonic with plasma and persists during fasting.
■ *Osmotic diarrhea:* excessive osmotic forces exerted by luminal solutes that abate with fasting.
■ *Exudative diseases:* output of purulent, bloody stools that persists on fasting; stools are frequent but may be small or large volume.
■ *Malabsorption:* output of voluminous, bulky stools with increased osmolarity owing to unabsorbed nutrients and excess fat (steatorrhea); it usually abates on fasting.
■ *Deranged motility:* highly variable features regarding stool output, volume, and consistency; other forms of diarrhea must be excluded.

The major causes of diarrhea are presented in Table 15–6; selected entities are discussed here. It is important to bear in mind that multiple mechanisms may be operative in the same patient.

Infectious Enterocolitis

Intestinal diseases of microbial origin are marked principally by diarrhea and sometimes by ulceroinflammatory changes in the small or large intestine. *Infectious enterocolitis is a global problem of staggering proportions, causing more than 12,000 deaths per day among children in developing countries, thereby accounting for one half of all deaths worldwide in children younger than 5 years of age.* Although far less prevalent in industrialized nations, infectious enterocolitis still exhibits attack rates of one to two illnesses per person (child and adult) per year, second only to the common cold in frequency.

Among the most common offenders in developed countries are rotavirus and Norwalk virus and enterotoxigenic *Escherichia coli.* However, many pathogens can cause diarrhea; the major offenders vary with the age, nutrition, and immune status of the host, environment (living conditions, public health measures), and special predispositions such as foreign travel, exposure to more virulent organisms while hospitalized, and wartime dislocation. In 40% to 50% of cases, the specific agent cannot be isolated.

Worldwide, intestinal parasitic disease and protozoal infections are major causes of chronic or recurrent infectious enterocolitis. Collectively, they affect more than one half of the world's population, because they are endemic in less favored nations. Of the various lower alimentary tract infections, only selected examples are described here.

Viral Gastroenteritis. Viral infection of surface epithelium in the small intestine destroys these cells and their absorptive function. (The term *gastroenteritis* is widely used but is somewhat of a misnomer, because the stomach is affected minimally or not at all.) Repopulation of the small intestinal villi

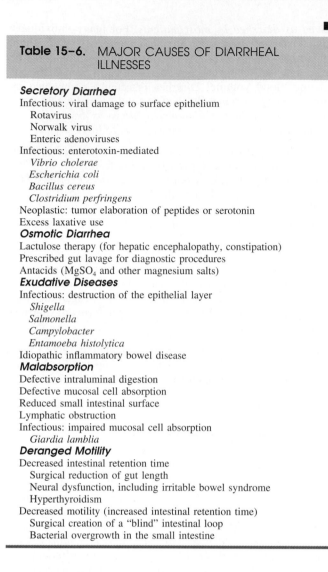

Table 15-6. MAJOR CAUSES OF DIARRHEAL ILLNESSES

Secretory Diarrhea
Infectious: viral damage to surface epithelium
 Rotavirus
 Norwalk virus
 Enteric adenoviruses
Infectious: enterotoxin-mediated
 Vibrio cholerae
 Escherichia coli
 Bacillus cereus
 Clostridium perfringens
Neoplastic: tumor elaboration of peptides or serotonin
Excess laxative use

Osmotic Diarrhea
Lactulose therapy (for hepatic encephalopathy, constipation)
Prescribed gut lavage for diagnostic procedures
Antacids ($MgSO_4$ and other magnesium salts)

Exudative Diseases
Infectious: destruction of the epithelial layer
 Shigella
 Salmonella
 Campylobacter
 Entamoeba histolytica
Idiopathic inflammatory bowel disease

Malabsorption
Defective intraluminal digestion
Defective mucosal cell absorption
Reduced small intestinal surface
Lymphatic obstruction
Infectious: impaired mucosal cell absorption
 Giardia lamblia

Deranged Motility
Decreased intestinal retention time
 Surgical reduction of gut length
 Neural dysfunction, including irritable bowel syndrome
 Hyperthyroidism
Decreased motility (increased intestinal retention time)
 Surgical creation of a "blind" intestinal loop
 Bacterial overgrowth in the small intestine

---

with immature enterocytes and relative preservation of crypt secretory cells leads to net secretion of water and electrolytes, compounded by an osmotic diarrhea from incompletely absorbed nutrients. Symptomatic disease is caused by several distinct groups of viruses:

■ *Rotavirus* accounts for an estimated 140 million cases and 1 million deaths worldwide per year. The affected population is children 6 to 24 months of age; spread is by fecal-oral contamination.
■ Small round structured viruses, of which *Norwalk virus* is the prototype, are responsible for most cases of nonbacterial food-borne epidemic gastroenteritis in older children and adults. Infection in young children is unusual.
■ Additional viruses accounting for infectious diarrhea in children, almost always by person-to-person contact, include several subtypes of *adenovirus* (Ad40 and Ad41), *calicivirus*, and *astrovirus*.

Bacterial Enterocolitis. Several mechanisms underlying bacterial diarrheal illness were discussed briefly in Chapter 9 but are worthy of emphasis at this time:

■ *Ingestion of preformed toxin,* present in contaminated food. Major offenders of food poisoning are *Staphylococcus aureus,* *Vibrio* species, and *Clostridium perfringens.* One may also ingest preformed neurotoxins, exemplified by *Clostridium botulinum.*
■ *Infection by toxigenic organisms,* which proliferate within the gut lumen and elaborate an enterotoxin.
■ *Infection by enteroinvasive organisms,* which proliferate, invade, and destroy mucosal epithelial cells.

The latter two mechanisms involve bona fide bacterial replication in the gut and depend on three key bacterial properties:

1. *The ability to adhere to the mucosal epithelial cells.* To produce disease, ingested organisms must adhere to the mucosa; otherwise they are swept away by the fluid stream. Adherence is often mediated by plasmid-coded *adhesins*—rigid, wiry proteins expressed on the surface of the organism.
2. *The ability to elaborate enterotoxins.* Enterotoxigenic organisms produce polypeptides that cause diarrhea. The polypeptides may be secretagogues, which activate secretion without inducing cell damage; cholera toxin, elaborated by *Vibrio cholerae,* is the prototype toxin of this type. Alternatively, they may be cytotoxins, which cause direct epithelial cell necrosis, as exemplified by Shiga's toxin.
3. *The capacity to invade.* Enteroinvasive organisms such as *Shigella* possess a large virulence plasmid that confers the capacity for epithelial cell invasion. This is followed by intracellular proliferation, cell lysis, and cell-to-cell spread. Other organisms such as *Salmonella typhi* and *Yersinia enterocolitica* pass through mucosal epithelial cells en route to lymphatics and the bloodstream.

The major bacteria giving rise to *bacterial enterocolitis* are presented in Table 15–7.

Given the multitude of bacterial pathogens, the pathologic manifestations of small intestinal and colonic bacterial disease are quite variable. **Most bacterial infections exhibit a general nonspecific pattern of damage to the surface epithelium, with an increased mitotic rate in mucosal crypts and decreased maturation of surface epithelial cells. There follows hyperemia and edema of the lamina propria and variable neutrophilic infiltration into the lamina propria and epithelial layer.** In more severe infections with cytotoxin-producing or enteroinvasive bacteria, progressive destruction of the mucosa leads to erosion, ulceration, and severe submucosal inflammation. Notable features of particular infections include the following:

■ *Escherichia coli* (a particularly versatile organism):
 ■ Enterotoxigenic strains (ETEC) affect the small intestine, with histologic features similar to *Vibrio cholerae* (described later).
 ■ The enterohemorrhagic strain (EHEC) 0157:H7 produces most severe disease in the right colon, with hemorrhage and ulceration.

Table 15-7.   MAJOR CAUSES OF BACTERIAL ENTEROCOLITIS

Organism	Pathogenic Mechanism	Source	Clinical Features
Escherichia coli			Traveler's diarrhea, including:
ETEC	Cholera-like toxin, no invasion	Food, water	Watery diarrhea
EHEC	Shiga-like toxin, no invasion	Undercooked beef products	Hemorrhagic colitis, hemolytic uremic syndrome (Chapter 14)
EPEC	Attachment, enterocyte effacement, no invasion	Weaning foods, water	Watery diarrhea, infants and toddlers
EIEC	Invasion, local spread	Cheese, water, person-to-person	Fever, pain, diarrhea, dysentery
Salmonella	Invasion, translocation, lymphoid inflammation, dissemination	Milk, beef, eggs, poultry	Fever, pain, diarrhea or dysentery, bacteremia, extraintestinal infection, common source outbreaks
Shigella	Invasion, local spread	Person-to-person, low-inoculum	Fever, pain, diarrhea, dysentery, epidemic spread
Campylobacter	?Toxins, invasion	Milk, poultry, animal contact	Fever, pain, diarrhea, dysentery, food sources, animal reservoirs
Yersinia enterocolitica	Invasion, translocation, lymphoid inflammation, dissemination	Milk, pork	Fever, pain, diarrhea, mesenteric lymphadenitis, extraintestinal infection, food sources
Vibrio cholerae, other *Vibrio* species	Enterotoxin, no invasion	Water, shellfish, person-to-person spread	Watery diarrhea, cholera, pandemic spread
Clostridium difficile	Cytotoxin, local invasion	Nosocomial environmental spread	Fever, pain, bloody diarrhea, after antibiotic use, nosocomial acquisition
Clostridium perfringens	Enterotoxin, no invasion	Meat, poultry, fish	Watery diarrhea, food sources, "pigbel"
Mycobacterium tuberculosis	Invasion, mural inflammatory foci with necrosis and scarring	Contaminated milk, swallowing of coughed-up organisms	Chronic abdominal pain, complications of malabsorption, stricture, perforation, fistulae, hemorrhage

ETEC, enterotoxigenic *E. coli;* EHEC, enterohemorrhagic *E. coli;* EPEC, enteropathogenic *E. coli;* EIEC, enteroinvasive *E. coli.*

- Enteropathogenic strains (EPEC) affect the small intestine, producing villus blunting.
- Enteroinvasive strains (EIEC) affect the colon, with histologic features similar to *Shigella*.
- *Salmonella* species are a major cause of common-source outbreaks of enterocolitis, producing localized mucosal disease primarily in the ileum and colon (as with *S. enteritidis, S. typhimurium,* and others). *S. typhimurium* is the archetypal organism that invades Peyer's patches and produces local ulceration over massively enlarged lymphoid tissue. Life-threatening systemic illness is the hallmark of *S. typhi*, whereby small intestinal invasion leads to systemic dissemination **(typhoid fever)**. Typhoid fever is a protracted disease featuring **bacteremia** (first week), widespread reticuloendothelial involvement with **splenomegaly** and **foci of necrosis in the liver** (second week), and **ulceration of Peyer's patches with intestinal bleeding and shock** (third week). **Gallbladder colonization** produces a chronic carrier state; chronic infection also may affect the joints, bones, meninges, and other sites.
- *Shigella* affects primarily the distal colon, producing acute mucosal inflammation and erosion.

- *Campylobacter jejuni* (and other species) affects the small intestine, appendix, and colon, producing multiple superficial ulcers, mucosal inflammation, and exudates.
- *Yersinia enterocolitica* and *Y. pseudotuberculosis* affect the ileum, appendix, and colon. Peyer's patch invasion leads to mesenteric lymph node enlargement with necrotizing granulomas. Systemic spread may lead to peritonitis, pharyngitis, and pericarditis.
- *Vibrio cholerae* (cholera) affects the small intestine, especially more proximally. The mucosa is essentially intact, with only mucus-depleted crypts.
- *Clostridium difficile* is a normal gut organism, but cytotoxin-producing strains may emerge after systemic antibiotic use. A distinctive **pseudomembranous colitis** is produced, which derives its name from the plaquelike adhesion of fibrinopurulent debris and mucus to the damaged superficial mucosa (Fig. 15-23). These are not true "membranes," because the coagulum is not an epithelial layer.
- *Clostridium perfringens* exhibits features similar to *V. cholerae*, but with some epithelial damage.

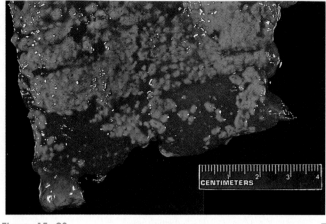

Figure 15-23 ■

Pseudomembranous colitis. Plaques of yellow fibrin and inflammatory debris are adherent to a reddened colonic mucosa.

> Some strains produce a severe necrotizing enterocolitis with perforation (**pigbel**).
> ■ Ingested *Mycobacterium tuberculosus* incites chronic inflammation and granuloma formation in mucosal lymphoid tissue—particularly Peyer's patches in the terminal ileum—and regional lymph nodes (Chapter 13).

Protozoal Infection. *Entamoeba histolytica* is a dysentery-causing protozoan parasite spread by fecal-oral spread. Amebae invade the crypts of colonic glands and burrow down into the submucosa (Fig. 15-24); the organisms then fan out laterally to create a flask-shaped ulcer with a narrow neck and broad base. There may be very little inflammatory infiltrate within the ulcer. In about 40% of patients with amebic dysentery, parasites penetrate portal vessels and embolize to the liver to produce solitary, or less often multiple, discrete hepatic abscesses, some exceeding 10 cm in diameter. Some

patients may present with amebic liver abscesses, without a clinical history of amebic dysentery. As with the intestinal lesions, there is a scant inflammatory reaction at the margin. The liquefied tissue in the fibrin-lined cavity may be dark-chocolate colored because of hemorrhage. Occasional amebic abscesses are encountered in the lung, heart, kidneys, and even brain. Such abscesses remain long after the acute intestinal illness has passed.

Giardia lamblia is an intestinal protozoan spread by fecal contaminated water. *Giardia* attach to the small intestinal mucosa but do not appear to invade (Fig. 15-25). Small intestinal morphology may range from virtually normal to marked blunting of the villi with a mixed inflammatory infiltrate in the lamina propria. A malabsorptive diarrhea appears to result from mucosal cell injury by mechanisms that are not understood.

Clinical Features. The clinical features of viral and protozoal infection have been briefly noted already. At the risk of oversimplification, bacterial enterocolitis takes the following forms:

■ *Ingestion of preformed bacterial toxins.* Symptoms develop within a matter of hours; explosive diarrhea and acute abdominal distress herald an illness that passes within a day or so. Ingested systemic neurotoxins, as from *C. botulinum*, may produce rapid, and fatal, respiratory failure.

■ *Infection with enteric pathogens.* With ingestion of enteric pathogens, an incubation period of several hours to days is followed by *diarrhea and dehydration* if the primary pathogenic mechanism is a secretory enterotoxin or *dysentery* if the primary mechanism is a cytotoxin or an enteroinvasive process. Traveler's diarrhea (e.g., Montezuma's revenge, turista) usually occurs after ingestion of fecally contaminated food or water; it begins abruptly and subsides within 2 to 3 days.

■ *Insidious infection. Yersinia* and *Mycobacterium* may also present as subacute diarrheal illnesses mimicking Crohn's disease. All enteroinvasive organisms can mimic, or even

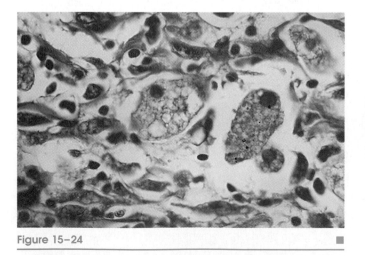

Figure 15-24 ■

Amebiasis of the colon with three *Entamoeba histolytica* trophozoites within the submucosa.

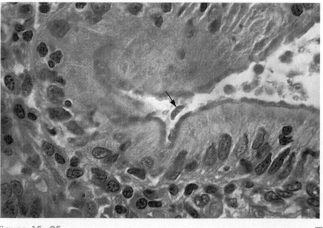

Figure 15-25 ■

Giardia lamblia. Trophozoite *(arrow)* of the organism immediately adjacent to the duodenal surface epithelium; note the double nuclei. The other luminal material is mucus (bluish) and an erythrocyte displaced by the biopsy procedure. (H & E.)

precipitate, acute onset of idiopathic inflammatory bowel disease (discussed later).

In general, bacterial enterocolitis is a more severe illness than viral disease. The complications of bacterial enterocolitis result from massive fluid loss or destruction of the intestinal mucosal barrier, and include dehydration, sepsis, and perforation. In the most severe cases, death ensues rapidly without quick intervention, particularly in the very young.

A distressing gastrointestinal emergency in neonates, particularly those who are premature or of low birth weight, is *necrotizing enterocolitis.* This acute, necrotizing inflammation of the small and large intestines is thought to result from a combination of functional immaturity of the neonatal gut, colonization and invasion by pathogenic organisms, and secondary ischemic injury. A small portion of terminal ileum and ascending colon may be affected, or the entire small and large intestines may be involved. The injury is initially mucosal, but in severe cases the entire bowel wall becomes hemorrhagic and gangrenous, necessitating surgical resection. In a typical case, there is abdominal distention, tenderness, ileus, and diarrhea with occult or frank blood. Onset of gangrene and perforation are immediately life threatening.

Malabsorption Syndromes

Malabsorption is characterized by suboptimal absorption of fats, fat-soluble and other vitamins, proteins, carbohydrates, electrolytes and minerals, and water. At the most basic level, it is the result of disturbance of at least one of these normal digestive functions:

1. *Intraluminal digestion,* in which proteins, carbohydrates, and fats are enzymatically broken down. The process begins in the mouth with saliva, receives a major boost from gastric peptic digestion, and continues in the small intestine, assisted by pancreatic enzyme secretion and the emulsive action of bile.
2. *Terminal digestion,* which involves the hydrolysis of carbohydrates and peptides by disaccharidases and peptidases, respectively, in the brush border of the small intestinal mucosa.
3. *Transepithelial transport,* in which nutrients, fluid, and electrolytes are transported across the epithelium of the small intestine for delivery to the intestinal vasculature. Absorbed fatty acids are converted to triglycerides and are assembled with cholesterol and apoprotein B into chylomicrons for delivery to the intestinal lymphatic system.

A host of disorders interrupt the above sequence either directly or indirectly (Table 15–8). The malabsorptive disorders most commonly encountered in the United States are chronic pancreatitis, celiac sprue, and Crohn's disease. The first two and selected other conditions are highlighted here; Crohn's disease is discussed in a later section.

Pancreatic insufficiency, primarily from chronic pancreatitis or cystic fibrosis, is a major cause of *defective intraluminal digestion.* Excessive growth of normal bacteria within the proximal small intestine *(bacterial overgrowth)* also impairs intraluminal digestion and can damage mucosal epithelial cells. Immunologic deficiencies, inadequate gastric acid-

■

Table 15–8.   THE MAJOR MALABSORPTION SYNDROMES

Defective Intraluminal Digestion
Digestion of fats and proteins
   Pancreatic insufficiency, due to pancreatitis or cystic fibrosis
   Zollinger Ellison syndrome, with inactivation of pancreatic enzymes by excess gastric acid secretion
Solubilization of fat, due to defective bile secretion
   Ileal dysfunction or resection, with decreased bile salt uptake
   Cessation of bile flow from obstruction, hepatic dysfunction
Nutrient preabsorption or modification by bacterial overgrowth
Primary Mucosal Cell Abnormalities
Defective terminal digestion
   Disaccharidase deficiency (lactose intolerance)
   Bacterial overgrowth, with brush border damage
Defective transepithelial transport
   Abetalipoproteinemia
Reduced Small Intestinal Surface
Gluten-sensitive enteropathy (celiac sprue)
Short-gut syndrome, following surgical resections
Crohn's disease
Lymphatic Obstruction
Lymphoma
Tuberculosis and tuberculous lymphadenitis
Infection
Acute infectious enteritis
Parasitic infestation
Tropical sprue
Whipple's disease *(Tropheryma whippelii)*
Iatrogenic
Subtotal or total gastrectomy
Distal ileal resection or bypass

ity, and intestinal stasis, as from surgical alteration of small intestinal anatomy, predispose to bacterial overgrowth. Typical features of defective intraluminal digestion are an *osmotic diarrhea* from undigested nutrients and *steatorrhea,* which is excess output of undigested fat in stool. The intestinal mucosa in bacterial overgrowth either is normal or is minimally damaged.

The classic example of defective mucosal cell absorption is *lactose intolerance.* The inherited deficiency of disaccharidase is rare but is of great consequence because in infants it produces milk intolerance, leading to diarrhea, weight loss, and failure to thrive. The acquired deficiency is common among adults, particularly North American blacks. Aside from the need to avoid milk products, the disorder is of minimal consequence. The intestinal mucosa is morphologically normal. Diagnosis is most readily made by measurement of breath hydrogen level, which reflects bacterial overgrowth in the presence of excess intraluminal carbohydrate.

The rare autosomal recessive deficiency of apolipoprotein B *(abetalipoproteinemia)* renders the mucosal epithelial cell unable to export lipid, because this protein is synthesized by these cells for assembly of dietary lipids into chylomicrons for export to intestinal lymphatics. Hence, mucosal absorptive cells contain vacuolated lipid inclusions, but the mucosa is otherwise normal. This deficiency causes diarrhea and steatorrhea in infancy and significant failure to thrive. There are systemic lipid membrane abnormalities as well, readily observed in circulating erythrocytes as a characteristic burr cell transformation termed *acanthocytosis.*

Gluten-sensitive enteropathy, also known as celiac sprue, is the prototype of a noninfectious cause of malabsorption due to a reduction in small intestinal absorptive surface area. The basic disorder in celiac sprue is sensitivity to gluten, the component of wheat and related grains (oat, barley, and rye) that contains the water-insoluble protein gliadin. This disease exhibits a strong genetic susceptibility, including familial clustering and a strong association with the HLA-DQw2 histocompatibility antigen. The small intestinal mucosa, when exposed to gluten, accumulates large numbers of B cells and plasma cells sensitized to gliaden; accumulation of lymphocytes in gastric and colonic mucosa also may occur. In addition to filling the lamina propria, lymphocytes also cross into the epithelial space, with accompanying damage to surface enterocytes. Total flattening of mucosal villi (and hence loss of surface area) is the outcome.

The prevalence of this disease is 1:2000 to 1:3000 in European white populations, but it is rare in Asians. Because gliadin cross-reacts with a fragment of the E1b protein of type 12 adenovirus, it has been proposed that celiac sprue arises, in part, from environmental exposure to this virus. The age of presentation with symptomatic diarrhea and malnutrition varies from infancy to mid-adulthood; removal of gluten from the diet is met with dramatic improvement. There is, however, a long-term risk of malignant disease on the order of a twofold increase over the usual rate. Intestinal lymphomas, especially T-cell lymphomas, are disproportionately represented; other malignancies include gastrointestinal and breast carcinomas.

Tropical sprue and *Whipple's disease* are two disorders that exemplify malabsorption syndromes arising from intestinal infection. Tropical sprue is so named because this celiac-like disease occurs almost exclusively in persons living in or visiting the tropics. No specific causal agent has been clearly identified, but the appearance of malabsorption within days or a few weeks of an acute diarrheal enteric infection strongly implicates an infectious process, as does prompt response to broad-spectrum antibiotic therapy. Small intestinal changes vary from near normal to a severe diffuse enteritis with villus flattening. In contrast to celiac sprue, injury is seen at all levels of the small intestine.

Whipple's disease is a rare, systemic infection that may involve any organ of the body but principally affects the intestine, central nervous system, and joints. The hallmark of Whipple's disease is a small intestinal mucosa laden with distended macrophages in the lamina propria. The macrophages contain rod-shaped bacilli by electron microscopy, now identified as a gram-positive actinomycete, *Tropheryma whippelii.* Similar macrophages are found in the brain, the synovium of affected joints, and elsewhere. At each of these sites, inflammation is essentially absent. Occurring principally in males in the fourth to fifth decades of life, Whipple's disease is a malabsorptive syndrome occasionally accompanied by lymphadenopathy, hyperpigmentation, polyarthritis, and obscure central nervous system complaints. Response to antibiotic therapy is usually prompt, although some patients have a protracted course.

Clinical Features. Clinically, the malabsorption syndromes resemble each other more than they differ. The passage of abnormally bulky, frothy, greasy, yellow or gray stools is a prominent feature of malabsorption, accompanied by weight loss, anorexia, abdominal distention, borborygmi and flatus, and muscle wasting. The consequences of malabsorption affect many organ systems:

■ *Hematopoietic system:* anemia from iron, pyridoxine, folate or vitamin B_{12} deficiency (vitamin B_{12} is normally absorbed in the ileum), and bleeding from vitamin K deficiency (a fat-soluble vitamin)

■ *Musculoskeletal system:* osteopenia and tetany from defective calcium, magnesium, vitamin D, and protein absorption

■ *Endocrine system:* amenorrhea, impotence, and infertility from generalized malnutrition; and hyperparathyroidism from protracted calcium and vitamin D deficiency

■ *Skin:* purpura and petechiae from vitamin K deficiency; edema from protein deficiency; dermatitis and hyperkeratosis from deficiencies of vitamin A (also fat soluble), zinc, essential fatty acids, and niacin; mucositis from vitamin deficiencies

■ *Nervous system:* peripheral neuropathy from vitamin A and B_{12} deficiencies.

IDIOPATHIC INFLAMMATORY BOWEL DISEASE

Crohn's disease (CD) and ulcerative colitis (UC) are chronic relapsing disorders of unknown origin. These diseases share many common features and are collectively known as idiopathic inflammatory bowel disease (IBD). *CD is a granulomatous disease that may affect any portion of the gastrointestinal tract from esophagus to anus but most often involves the small intestine and colon. UC is a nongranulomatous disease limited to the colon.* Before considering these diseases separately, the pathogenesis of these two forms of IBD will be considered.

Etiology and Pathogenesis. The normal intestine is in a steady state of "physiologic" inflammation, representing a dynamic balance between (1) factors that activate the host immune system, such as luminal microbes, dietary antigens, and endogenous inflammatory stimuli; and (2) host defenses that down-regulate inflammation and maintain the integrity of the mucosa. The search for the cause or causes of loss of this balance in CD and UC has revealed many parallels, not the least of which is that *both diseases remain unexplained,* and are thus best designated as *idiopathic.* Although CD and UC share important pathophysiologic features, there are sufficient differences to justify regarding them as two separate diseases. Attempts to explain their origin have included investigation of the following:

■ *Genetic predisposition.* Familial aggregations in IBD have been observed repeatedly. However, with minor exceptions, attempts to identify associations with HLA haplotypes have been unsuccessful.

■ *Abnormal structure of the intestinal mucosa.* Intrinsic defects in mucosal structure are suggested by increased intestinal permeability to polyethylene glycol in some patients (and relatives) with CD and by alterations in mucin glycoproteins in UC patients and their family members.

■ *Infectious causes.* The history of IBD research is littered with candidate pathogens, including measles virus, chlamydia, atypical bacteria, and mycobacteria. Although causal relationships have not been established, these antigens may provoke an abnormal host response.

■ *Abnormal host immunoreactivity. It is hypothesized that the intestinal immune system is inappropriately activated by luminal or mucosal antigens,* either through abnormal function of mucosal epithelial cells as antigen-presenting cells or abnormal regulation of the cross-talk between immune cells in the intestinal mucosa. The occurrence of IBD in mice lacking selected immunoregulatory cytokines (interleukin-2, interleukin-10) or of the α or β chains of the T-cell receptor supports this concept.

Inflammation is the final common pathway for the pathogenesis of IBD. Both the clinical manifestations of IBD and the morphologic changes are ultimately the result of activation of inflammatory cells—neutrophils initially and mononuclear cells later in the course. The products of these inflammatory cells cause nonspecific tissue injury. *Inflammation causes (1) impaired integrity of the mucosal epithelial barrier, (2) loss of surface epithelial cell absorptive function, and (3) activation of crypt epithelial cell secretion.* The inflammation ultimately causes outright mucosal destruction, which leads to obvious loss of mucosal barrier and absorptive function. Collectively, these events give rise to the intermittent bloody diarrhea that is characteristic of these diseases. Most therapeutic interventions act entirely or partly through nonspecific downregulation of the immune system.

Crohn's Disease

Early descriptions of CD emphasized the sharply segmental transmural fibrosis and thickening of the terminal ileum, giving rise to the designation *terminal ileitis.* Recognition that other sharply delineated small intestinal segments might be affected, with intervening unaffected ("skip") areas, led to the alternative name *regional enteritis.* It now is clear that this disease may affect any level of the alimentary tract; thus the eponymic name *Crohn's disease* is preferred. Moreover, active cases of CD are often accompanied by extraintestinal complications of immune origin, such as iritis and uveitis, sacroiliitis, migratory polyarthritis, erythema nodosum, hepatic pericholangitis and sclerosing cholangitis, and various renal disorders secondary to trapping of the ureters in the inflammatory process, including nephrolithiasis and predisposition to urinary tract infections. Systemic amyloidosis is a rare late consequence. Thus, *CD must be viewed as a systemic disease with predominant gastrointestinal involvement.*

Epidemiology. Worldwide in distribution, CD is much more prevalent in the United States, Great Britain, and Scandinavia than in Central Europe and is rare in Asia and Africa. In the United States, its annual incidence is 1 to 3 per 100,000, which is slightly less frequent than ulcerative colitis. The incidence and prevalence of CD has been steadily rising in the United States and Western Europe. It occurs at any age, from young childhood to advanced age, but the peak incidence is between the second and third decades of life, with a minor peak in the sixth and seventh decades. Females are affected slightly more often than males. Whites appear to develop the disease two to five times more often than do nonwhites. In the United States, CD occurs three to five times more often among Jews than among non-Jews.

In CD, there is gross involvement of the small intestine alone in about 40% of cases, of small intestine and colon in 30%, and of the colon alone in about 30%. CD may involve the duodenum, stomach, esophagus, and even mouth, but these sites are distinctly uncommon. **When fully developed, CD is characterized by (1) sharply delimited and typically transmural involvement of the bowel by an inflammatory process with mucosal damage, (2) the presence of noncaseating granulomas in 40% to 60% of cases, and (3) fissuring with formation of fistulae.** In diseased segments, the serosa becomes granular and dull gray, and often the mesenteric fat wraps around the bowel surface **("creeping fat"). The intestinal wall is rubbery and thick, the result of edema, inflammation, fibrosis, and hypertrophy of the muscularis propria.** As a result, the lumen is almost always narrowed; in the small intestine this is evidenced radiographically as the "string sign," a thin stream of barium passing through the diseased segment. Strictures may occur in the colon but are usually less severe. **A classic feature of CD is the sharp demarcation of diseased bowel segments from adjacent uninvolved bowel. When multiple bowel segments are involved, the intervening bowel is essentially normal ("skip" lesions).**

In the intestinal mucosa, early disease exhibits focal mucosal ulcers resembling canker sores (aphthous ulcers), edema, and loss of the normal mucosal texture. With progressive disease, ulcers coalesce into long, serpentine linear ulcers, which tend to be oriented along the axis of the bowel (Fig. 15–26). Because the intervening mucosa tends to be relatively spared, it acquires a coarsely textured, cobblestone appearance. **Narrow fissures develop between the folds of the mucosa,** often penetrating deeply through the bowel wall all the way to the serosa. This may lead to adhesions with adjacent loops of bowel. Further extension of fissures leads to **fistula or sinus tract formation,** either to an adherent viscus, to the outside skin, or into a blind cavity to form a localized abscess.

By microscopic examination, the mucosa exhibits several characteristic features (Fig. 15–27): (1) **inflammation,** with neutrophilic infiltration into the epithelial layer and accumulation within crypts to form **crypt abscesses;** (2) **ulceration,** which is the usual outcome of active disease; and (3) **chronic mucosal damage** in the form of architectural distortion, atrophy, and metaplasia (including rudimentary gastric metaplasia in the intestine). **Granulomas are an inconstant finding but may be present anywhere in the alimentary tract, even in**

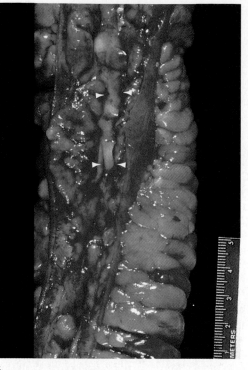

Figure 15–26 ■

Crohn's disease of the ileum showing narrowing of the lumen, bowel wall thickening, serosal extension of mesenteric fat ("creeping fat"), and linear ulceration of the mucosal surface *(arrowheads).*

patients with CD limited to one bowel segment. Conversely, the absence of granulomas does not preclude a diagnosis of CD. In diseased segments, the muscularis mucosa and muscularis propria are usually markedly thickened and fibrosis affects all tissue layers.

Particularly important in patients with long-standing chronic disease are dysplastic changes appearing in the mucosal epithelial cells. These may be focal or widespread, tend to increase with time, and are thought to be related to a fivefold to sixfold increased risk of carcinoma, particularly of the colon.

Clinical Features. The presentation of CD is highly variable and ultimately unpredictable. The dominant manifestations are recurrent episodes of diarrhea, crampy abdominal pain, and fever lasting days to weeks. These manifestations usually begin insidiously, but in some instances, particularly in young persons, the onset of the pain is so abrupt and the diarrhea so mild that abdominal exploration is performed with a diagnosis of appendicitis. Some melena is present in about 50% of cases with colon involvement; it is usually mild but sometimes massive. In most patients, after an initial attack, the manifestations remit either spontaneously or with therapy, but characteristically they are followed by relapses, and intervals between successive attacks grow shorter. In 10% to 20% of patients the symptom-free interval after the initial attack may last for decades, and for a very fortunate few the

first attack is the last. Alternatively, chronic pain may be severe, leading to marked weight loss. Superimposed on this course are the potential development of malabsorption and some of the extraintestinal manifestations mentioned earlier.

The debilitating consequences of CD include (1) *fistula formation* to other loops of bowel, the urinary bladder, vagina, or perianal skin; (2) *abdominal abscesses* or peritonitis; and (3) *intestinal stricture* or obstruction, necessitating surgical intervention. Rare but devastating events are massive intestinal bleeding, toxic dilation of the colon, or carcinoma of the colon or small intestine. Although the increased risk for carcinoma is significant, it is substantially less than that associated with ulcerative colitis.

Ulcerative Colitis

Ulcerative colitis (UC) is an ulceroinflammatory disease affecting the colon but limited to the mucosa and submucosa except in the most severe cases. UC begins in the rectum and extends proximally in a continuous fashion, sometimes involving the entire colon. Like CD, UC is a systemic disorder associated in some patients with migratory polyarthritis, sacroiliitis, ankylosing spondylitis, uveitis, hepatic involvement (pericholangitis and primary sclerosing cholangitis), and skin

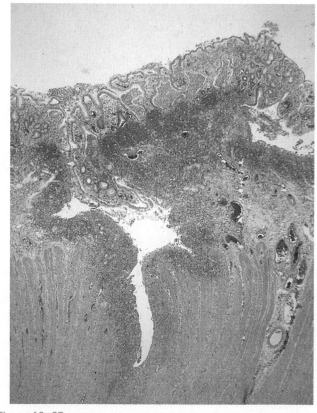

Figure 15–27 ■

Crohn's disease of the colon showing a deep fissure extending into the muscle wall, a second, shallow ulcer (on the upper right) and relative preservation of the intervening mucosa. Abundant lymphocyte aggregates are present, evident as dense blue patches of cells at the interface between mucosa and submucosa.

lesions. There are several important differences between UC and CD:

■ In UC, well-formed granulomas are absent.
■ UC does not exhibit skip lesions.
■ The mucosal ulcers in UC rarely extend below the submucosa, and there is surprisingly little fibrosis.
■ Mural thickening does not occur in UC, and the serosal surface is usually completely normal.
■ Patients with UC are at greater risk for carcinoma.

Some of the distinctive features of CD and UC are depicted in Figure 15–28 and compared in Table 15–9.

Epidemiology. UC is somewhat more common than CD in the United States and Western countries, with an incidence of 4 to 6 per 100,000 population, but it is infrequent in Asia, Africa, and South America. As with CD, the incidence of this condition has risen in recent decades. In the United States it is more common among whites than among nonwhites and exhibits no particular sex predilection. The disease may arise at any age, with a peak incidence between ages 20 and 25 years. Individuals with UC and ankylosing spondylitis have an increased frequency of HLA-B27, but this association is related to the spondylitis and not to UC.

As noted, UC involves the rectum or rectosigmoid in about 80% of cases and extends proximally in a retrograde fashion to involve the entire colon (pancolitis) in the more severe cases (about 10%). When there is active inflammation, the mucosa may exhibit hyperemia, edema, and granularity with friability and easy bleeding. With severe disease, there is extensive and broad-based ulceration of the mucosa in the distal colon or throughout its length (Fig. 15–29). Isolated islands of regenerating mucosa bulge upward to create **pseudopolyps.** Often the undermined edges of adjacent ulcers interconnect to create tunnels covered by tenuous mucosal bridges. As with CD, the ulcers of UC are frequently aligned along the axis of the colon, but rarely do they replicate the linear serpentine ulcers of CD. In rare cases, the muscularis propria is so compromised as to permit perforation and pericolonic abscess formation. Exposure of the muscularis propria and neural plexus to fecal material also may lead to complete shutdown of neuromuscular function. When this occurs, the colon progressively swells and becomes gangrenous **(toxic megacolon).** With indolent chronic disease or with healing of active disease, progressive mucosal atrophy leads to a flattened and attenuated mucosal surface.

The pathologic features of UC are those of mucosal inflammation, ulceration, and chronic mucosal damage (Fig. 15–30). First, **a diffuse, predominantly mononuclear inflammatory infiltrate in the lamina propria is almost universally present,** even at the time of clinical presentation. Neutrophilic infiltration of the epithelial layer may produce collections of neutrophils in crypt lumina **(crypt ab-**

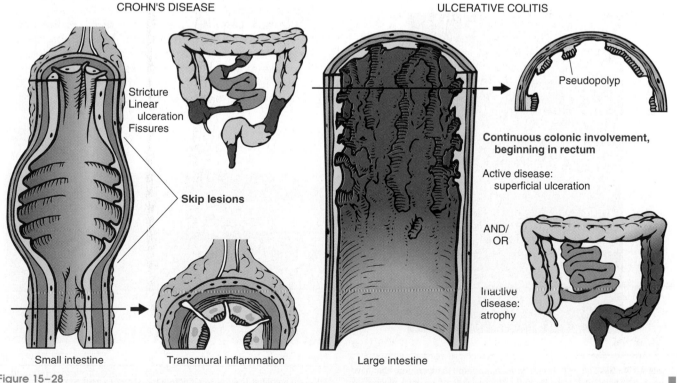

CROHN'S DISEASE

ULCERATIVE COLITIS

Stricture
Linear
ulceration
Fissures

Skip lesions

Pseudopolyp

Continuous colonic involvement, beginning in rectum

Active disease:
superficial ulceration

AND/
OR

Inactive
disease:
atrophy

Small intestine   Transmural inflammation   Large intestine

Figure 15–28   ■

The distribution patterns of Crohn's disease and ulcerative colitis are compared, as well as the different conformations of the ulcers and wall thickenings.

Table 15-9. DISTINCTIVE FEATURES OF CROHN'S DISEASE AND ULCERATIVE COLITIS*

Feature	Crohn's Disease (Small Intestine)	Crohn's Disease (Colon)	Ulcerative Colitis
Macroscopic			
Bowel region	Ileum ± colon†	Colon ± ileum	Colon only
Distribution	Skip lesions	Skip lesions	Diffuse
Stricture	Early	Variable	Late/rare
Wall appearance	Thickened	Variable	Thin
Dilation	No	Yes	Yes
Microscopic			
Pseudopolyps	None to slight	Marked	Marked
Ulcers	Deep, linear	Deep, linear	Superficial
Lymphoid reaction	Marked	Marked	Mild
Fibrosis	Marked	Moderate	Mild
Serositis	Marked	Variable	Mild to none
Granulomas	Yes (40% to 60%)	Yes (40% to 60%)	No
Fistulae/sinuses	Yes	Yes	No
Clinical			
Fat/vitamin malabsorption	Yes	Yes, if ileum	No
Malignant potential	Yes	Yes	Yes
Response to surgery‡	Poor	Fair	Good

* Not all features present in a single case.
† Crohn's disease can occur elsewhere in the small intestine as well.
‡ Based on likelihood of disease recurrence following surgical removal of a diseased segment.

scesses). These are not specific for UC and may be observed in CD or any active inflammatory colitis. Unlike CD, there are no granulomas, although rupture of crypt abscesses may incite a foreign body reaction in the lamina propria. Second, **further destruction of the mucosa leads to** **outright ulceration, extending into the submucosa and sometimes leaving only the raw, exposed muscularis propria.** Third, with remission of active disease, granulation tissue fills in the ulcer craters, followed by regeneration of the mucosal epithelium. **Submucosal fibrosis and mucosal architectural disarray and atrophy remain as residua of healed disease.**

The most serious complication of UC is the development of colon carcinoma. Two factors govern the risk: duration of the disease and its extent. It is believed that with 10 years of disease limited to the left colon the risk is minimal, and at 20 years the risk is on the order of 2%. With pancolitis,

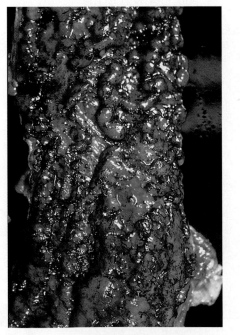

Figure 15-29

Ulcerative colitis. The pale, irregular regions comprise ulcerations that have in many instances coalesced, leaving virtual islands of residual mucosa. A tendency toward pseudopolyp formation is already evident. The darker material is adherent mucus stained by feces.

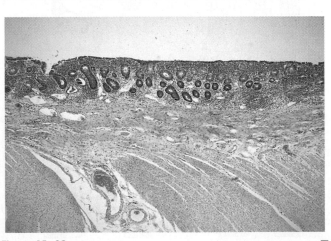

Figure 15-30

Ulcerative colitis. Low-power micrograph showing marked chronic inflammation of the mucosa with atrophy of colonic glands, moderate submucosal fibrosis, and a normal muscle wall.

the risk of carcinoma is 10% at 20 years and 15% to 25% by 30 years.

Clinical Features. Ulcerative colitis is a chronic relapsing and remitting disorder marked by attacks of bloody mucoid diarrhea that may persist for days, weeks, or months and then subside, only to recur after an asymptomatic interval of months to years or even decades. Presentation is usually insidious, with cramps, tenesmus, and colicky lower abdominal pain that is relieved by defecation. Some patients manifest fever and weight loss. Grossly bloody stools are more common with UC than with CD, and the blood loss may be considerable. In the fortunate patient, the first attack is the last. At the other end of the spectrum, the explosive initial attack may lead to such serious bleeding and fluid and electrolyte imbalance as to constitute a medical emergency. Intercurrent infectious illnesses, as with enterotoxin-forming *Clostridium difficile*, may first bring UC to light; they do not precipitate the disease.

Extraintestinal manifestations, particularly migratory polyarthritis, are more common with UC than with CD. Uncommon but *life-threatening complications* include severe diarrhea and electrolyte derangements, massive hemorrhage, severe colonic dilation (toxic megacolon) with potential rupture, and perforation with peritonitis. Inflammatory strictures of the colorectum, while uncommon, must be differentiated from cancer.

Diagnosis can usually be made by endoscopic examination and biopsy. Specific infectious causes must always be ruled out. The most feared long-term complication of UC is cancer. The sequential mucosal changes from dysplasia to invasive carcinoma provide the rationale for surveillance programs of repeated colonoscopies and multiple biopsies aimed at detecting dysplasia for possible prophylactic colectomy.

COLONIC DIVERTICULOSIS

A diverticulum is a blind pouch leading off the alimentary tract, lined by mucosa, that communicates with the lumen of the gut. Congenital diverticula have all three layers of the bowel wall (mucosa, submucosa, and most notably the muscularis propria) and are distinctly uncommon. The prototype is *Meckel's diverticulum,* described earlier.

Virtually all other diverticula are acquired and either lack or have an attenuated muscularis propria. *Acquired diverticula may occur anywhere in the alimentary tract, but by far the most common location is the colon,* giving rise to *diverticular disease* of the colon, also called *diverticulosis.* The colon is unique in that the outer longitudinal muscle coat is not complete but is gathered into three equidistant bands (the taeniae coli). Where nerves and arterial vasa recta penetrate the inner circular muscle coat alongside the taeniae, focal defects in the muscle wall are created. The connective tissue sheaths accompanying these penetrating vessels provide potential sites for herniations.

Colonic diverticulosis is relatively infrequent in native populations of non-Western countries. Although unusual in West-

ern adults younger than 30 years of age, in those over the age of 60 the prevalence approaches 50%. This disparity is attributed to the consumption of a refined, low-fiber diet in Western societies, resulting in reduced stool bulk with increased difficulty in passage of intestinal contents. Exaggerated spastic contractions of the colon isolate segments of the colon (segmentation) in which the intraluminal pressure becomes markedly elevated, with consequent herniation of the bowel wall through the anatomic points of weakness. Thus, *two factors are thought to be important in the genesis of diverticular protrusions: (1) exaggerated peristaltic contractions with abnormal elevation of intraluminal pressure and (2) focal defects peculiar to the normal muscular colonic wall.*

Most colonic diverticula are **small, flasklike or spherical outpouchings, usually 0.5 to 1 cm in diameter** (Fig. 15–31A). They are in the sigmoid colon in approximately 95% of patients. Infrequently, more proximal levels and sometimes the entire colon are affected. Isolated cecal diverticula also occur. The exaggerated peristalsis often induces muscular hypertrophy in affected segments, with unusually prominent taenia coli and circular muscle bundles. Most diverticula penetrate between the bundles of circular muscle fibers adjacent to the mesenteric and lateral taeniae at sites of penetrating blood vessels. They frequently dissect into the appendices epiploicae and therefore may be inapparent on casual external inspection.

In the uninflamed state the walls are usually very thin, made up largely of mucosa and submucosa enclosed within fat or an intact peritoneal covering (Fig. 15–31B). Inflammatory changes may supervene to produce both diverticulitis and peridiverticulitis. Perforation may lead to localized peritonitis or abscess formation. When multiple closely adjacent diverticula become inflamed, the bowel wall may be encased by fibrous tissue, with narrowing of the lumen producing a remarkable resemblance to a cancerous stricture.

Clinical Features. In most persons, diverticular disease is asymptomatic and is discovered only at autopsy or by chance during a laparoscopy or barium enema for some other problem. In only about a fifth of the cases does intermittent cramping or sometimes continuous left-side lower quadrant discomfort appear, with a sensation of never being able to completely empty the rectum. Superimposed diverticulitis accentuates the symptoms and produces left lower quadrant tenderness and fever. Other less common complications include minimal, chronic intermittent bleeding or, rarely, brisk hemorrhage, perforation with pericolic abscess, or fistula formation.

The treatment of this condition merits brief mention because it bears on its pathogenesis. A high-fiber diet is recommended on the theory that the increased stool bulk reduces the exaggerated peristalsis as the source of discomfort. Whether a high-fiber diet prevents disease progression or protects against superimposed diverticulitis is unclear.

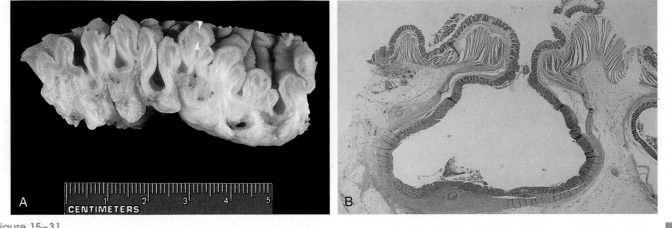

Figure 15–31 ■

Diverticulosis. *A,* Section through the sigmoid colon showing multiple saclike diverticula protruding through the muscle wall into the mesentery. The muscularis in between the diverticular protrusions is markedly thickened *(arrowheads). B,* Low-power micrograph of diverticulum of the colon showing protrusion of mucosa and submucosa through the muscle wall. A dilated blood vessel at the base of the diverticulum was a source of bleeding; some blood clot is present within the diverticular lumen.

BOWEL OBSTRUCTION

The major causes of intestinal obstruction are listed in Table 15–10. Although any part of the gut may be involved, because of its narrow lumen, the small bowel is most commonly affected. Four entities—hernias, intestinal adhesions, intussusception, and volvulus—account for at least 80% of the cases.

A weakness or defect in the wall of the peritoneal cavity may permit protrusion of a pouchlike, serosa-lined sac of peritoneum, called a *hernial sac.* The usual sites of weakness are anteriorly at the inguinal and femoral canals, at the umbilicus, and in surgical scars. Rarely, retroperitoneal hernias may occur, chiefly about the ligament of Trietz. *Hernias are of concern because segments of viscera frequently intrude and become trapped in them (external herniation).* This is particularly true with inguinal hernias, which have narrow orifices and large sacs. The most frequent intruders are small bowel

loops, but portions of omentum or large bowel also may become trapped. Pressure at the neck of the pouch may impair venous drainage of the trapped viscus. The ensuant stasis and edema increase the bulk of the herniated loop, leading to permanent trapping *(incarceration).* Further compromise of their blood supply and drainage leads to infarction of the trapped segment *(strangulation).*

Surgical procedures, infection, and even endometriosis often cause localized or more general peritoneal inflammation (peritonitis). With healing, *adhesions* may develop between bowel segments or the abdominal wall and operative site. These fibrous bridges can create closed loops through which the intestines may slide and become trapped *(internal herniation).* The sequence of events is much the same as with external hernias.

Intussusception denotes telescoping of a proximal segment of bowel into the immediately distal segment. In children, intussusception sometimes occurs without apparent anatomic basis, perhaps related to excessive peristaltic activity. In adults, such telescoping often points to an intraluminal mass (e.g., tumor) that becomes trapped by a peristaltic wave and pulls its point of attachment along with it into the distal segment. Not only does intestinal obstruction ensue, but the vascular supply may be so compromised as to cause infarction of the trapped segment.

Volvulus refers to twisting of a loop of bowel or other structure (e.g., ovary) about its base of attachment, constricting the venous outflow and sometimes the arterial supply as well. Volvulus affects the small bowel most often and rarely the redundant sigmoid. Intestinal obstruction and infarction may follow.

Table 15–10.	MAJOR CAUSES OF INTESTINAL OBSTRUCTION

Mechanical Obstruction
   Hernias, internal or external
   Adhesions
   Intussusception
   Volvulus
   Tumors
   Inflammatory strictures
   Obstructive gallstones, fecaliths, foreign bodies
   Congenital stricture, atresias
   Congenital bands
   Meconium in cystic fibrosis
   Imperforate anus
Pseudo-obstruction
   Paralytic ileus (e.g., postoperative)
   Vascular: bowel infarction
   Myopathies and neuropathies (e.g., Hirschsprung disease)

TUMORS OF THE SMALL AND LARGE INTESTINES

Epithelial tumors of the intestines are a major cause of morbidity and mortality worldwide. The colon, including the rec-

* Benign and malignant counterparts of the most common neoplasms in the intestines.

tum, is host to more primary neoplasms than any other organ in the body. Colorectal cancer ranks second only to bronchogenic carcinoma among the cancer killers. Adenocarcinomas constitute the vast majority of colorectal cancers and represent 70% of all malignancies arising in the gastrointestinal tract. Curiously, the small intestine is an uncommon site for benign or malignant tumors despite its great length and its vast pool of dividing mucosal cells. The classification of intestinal tumors is the same for the small and large bowel and is summarized in Table 15–11.

Before embarking on our discussion, several concepts pertaining to terminology must be emphasized (Fig. 15–32):

■ A *polyp* is a tumorous mass that protrudes into the lumen of the gut; traction on the mass may create a stalked, or *pedunculated,* polyp. Alternatively, the polyp may be *sessile,* without a definable stalk.

■ Polyps may be formed as the result of abnormal mucosal maturation, inflammation, or architecture. These polyps are *non-neoplastic* and do not have malignant potential; an example is the hyperplastic polyp.

■ Those polyps that arise as the result of epithelial proliferation and dysplasia are termed *adenomatous polyps* or *adenomas. They are true neoplastic lesions ("new growth") and are precursors of carcinoma.*

■ Some polypoid lesions may be caused by submucosal or mural tumors. However, as with the stomach, the term *polyp* unless otherwise specified refers to lesions arising from the epithelium of the mucosa.

Non-Neoplastic Polyps

The overwhelming majority of intestinal polyps occur sporadically, particularly in the colon, and increase in frequency with age. Non-neoplastic polyps represent about 90% of all epithelial polyps in the large intestine and are found in more than half of all persons age 60 years or older. Most are *hyperplastic polyps,* which are small (less than 5 mm in diameter), nipple-like, hemispheric, smooth protrusions of the mucosa. They may occur singly but are more often multiple. Although they may be anywhere in the colon, well over half are found in the rectosigmoid region. Histologically, they contain abundant crypts lined by well-differentiated goblet or absorptive epithelial cells, separated by a scant lamina propria. Although large hyperplastic polyps may rarely coexist with foci of adenomatous change, *the usual small, hyperplastic polyp has virtually no malignant potential.*

Juvenile polyps are essentially hamartomatous proliferations, mainly of the lamina propria, enclosing widely spaced, dilated cystic glands. They occur most frequently in children younger than 5 years old but also are found in adults of any age; in the latter group they may be called *retention polyps.* Irrespective of terminology, the lesions are usually large in children (1 to 3 cm in diameter) but smaller in adults; they are rounded, smooth, or slightly lobulated and sometimes have a stalk up to 2 cm long. In general, they occur singly and in the rectum, and being hamartomatous they have no malignant potential. Juvenile polyps may be the source of rectal bleeding and in some cases become twisted on their stalks to undergo painful infarction. *Peutz-Jeghers* polyps are uncommon hamartomatous polyps that occur as part of the rare autosomal dominant Peutz-Jeghers syndrome, characterized in addition by melanotic mucosal and cutaneous pigmentation. This condition, like the familial polyposis syndromes to be described later, is associated with an increased risk of both intestinal and extraintestinal malignancies.

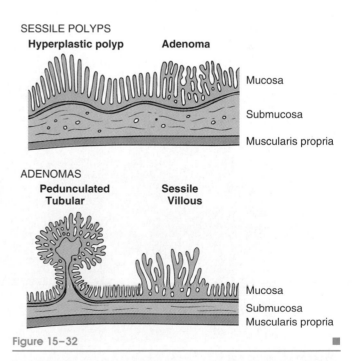

Figure 15–32 ■

Diagrammatic representation of two forms of sessile polyp (hyperplastic polyp and adenoma) and of two types of adenoma (pedunculated and sessile). There is only a loose association between the tubular architecture for pedunculated adenomas and the villous architecture for sessile polyps.

Adenomas

Adenomas are neoplastic polyps that range from small, often pedunculated tumors to large lesions that are usually sessile. Because the incidence of adenomas in the small intestine is very low, this discussion focuses on those adenomas that arise in the colon. The prevalence of colonic adenomas is 20% to 30% before age 40, rising to 40% to 50% after age 60. Males and females are affected equally. There is a well-defined familial predisposition to sporadic adenomas, accounting for about a fourfold greater risk for adenomas among first-degree relatives, and also a fourfold greater risk of colorectal carcinoma in any patient with adenomas.

All adenomatous lesions arise as the result of epithelial proliferation and dysplasia, which may range from mild to so severe as to constitute carcinoma in situ. Furthermore, there is strong evidence that most, and perhaps all, invasive colorectal adenocarcinomas arise in preexisting adenomatous lesions. Adenomatous polyps are segregated into three subtypes on the basis of the epithelial architecture:

■ *Tubular adenomas:* mostly tubular glands
■ *Villous adenomas:* villous projections
■ *Tubulovillous adenoma:* a mixture of the above

Tubular adenomas are by far the most common; 5% to 10% of adenomas are tubulovillous, and only 1% are villous. Most tubular adenomas are small and pedunculated; villous adenomas tend to be large and sessile. Conversely, most pedunculated polyps are tubular, and large sessile polyps usually exhibit villous features.

The malignant risk with an adenomatous polyp is correlated with three interdependent features: polyp size, histologic architecture, and severity of epithelial dysplasia, as follows:

■ Cancer is rare in tubular adenomas smaller than 1 cm in diameter.
■ The likelihood of cancer is high (approaching 40%) in sessile villous adenomas more than 4 cm in diameter.
■ Severe dysplasia, when present, is often found in villous areas.

However, among these variables, *maximum diameter is the chief determinant of the risk of an adenoma's harboring carcinoma;* architecture does not provide substantive independent information.

Tubular adenomas may arise anywhere in the colon, but about half are found in the rectosigmoid, the proportion increasing with age. In about half of the instances they occur singly, but in the remainder two or more lesions are distributed at random. Most adenomas have slender stalks 1 to 2 cm long and raspberry-like heads (Fig. 15–33A) and rarely exceed 2.5 cm in diameter. Histologically, the stalk is covered by normal colonic mucosa but the head is composed of neoplastic epithelium, forming branching glands lined by tall, hyperchromatic, somewhat disorderly cells, which may or may not show mucin secretion (Fig. 15–33B). In some instances there are small foci of villous architecture. In the clearly benign lesion, the branching glands are well separated by lamina propria and the level of dysplasia or cytologic

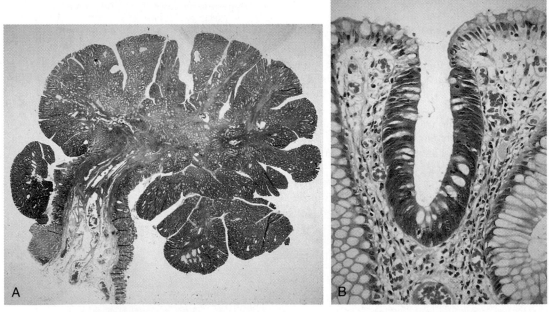

Figure 15–33 ■

A, Pedunculated adenoma showing a fibrovascular stalk lined by normal colonic mucosa, and a head that contains abundant dysplastic epithelial glands, hence the blue color. *B,* A small focus of adenomatous epithelium in an otherwise normal (mucin-secreting, clear) colonic mucosa, showing how the dysplastic columnar epithelium (deeply stained) can populate a colonic crypt ("tubular" architecture).

atypia is slight. However, all degrees of dysplasia may be encountered, ranging up to cancer confined to the mucosa (**intramucosal carcinoma**) or **invasive carcinoma** extending into the submucosa of the stalk. A frequent finding in any adenoma is superficial erosion of the epithelium, the result of mechanical trauma.

Villous adenomas are the larger and more ominous of the epithelial polyps. They tend to occur in older persons, most commonly in the rectum and rectosigmoid, but they may be located elsewhere. They generally are sessile, up to 10 cm in diameter, velvety or cauliflower-like masses projecting 1 to 3 cm above the surrounding normal mucosa. The histology is that of frondlike villiform extensions of the mucosa covered by dysplastic, sometimes very disorderly, sometimes piled-up, columnar epithelium (Fig. 15–34). All degrees of dysplasia may be encountered, and invasive carcinoma is found in up to 40% of these lesions, the frequency being correlated with the size of the polyp.

Tubulovillous adenomas are composed of a broad mix of tubular and villous areas. They are intermediate between the tubular and the villous lesions in their frequency of having a stalk or being sessile, their size, the degree of dysplasia, and the risk of harboring intramucosal or invasive carcinoma.

Clinical Features. The smaller adenomas are usually asymptomatic, until such time that occult bleeding leads to clinically significant anemia. Villous adenomas are much more frequently symptomatic because of overt or occult rectal bleeding. The most distal villous adenomas may secrete sufficient amounts of mucoid material rich in protein and potassium to produce hypoproteinemia or hypokalemia. Adenomas of the small intestine may present with anemia or rarely intussusception or obstruction. Adenomas in the immediate vicinity of the ampulla of Vater may produce biliary obstruction. On discovery, all adenomas, regardless of their location in the alimentary tract, are to be considered potentially malignant; thus, in practical terms, prompt and adequate excision is mandated.

Familial Polyposis Syndromes

Familial polyposis syndromes are uncommon autosomal dominant disorders. Their importance lies in the propensity for malignant transformation and in the insights that such transformation has provided in unraveling the molecular basis of colorectal cancer. In *familial adenomatous polyposis* (FAP), patients typically develop 500 to 2500 colonic adenomas that carpet the mucosal surface (Fig. 15–35); a minimum number of 100 is required for the diagnosis. Multiple adenomas may also be present elsewhere in the alimentary tract. Most polyps are tubular adenomas; occasional polyps have villous features. Polyps usually become evident in adolescence or early adulthood. *The risk of colonic cancer is virtually 100% by mid life, unless a prophylactic colectomy is performed.* The genetic defect underlying FAP has been localized to chromosome 5q21, as discussed later; *Gardner's syndrome* and the much rarer *Turcot's syndrome* appear to share the same genetic defect as FAP. These syndromes differ from each other with respect to the occurrence of extraintestinal tumors in the latter two: osteomas, gliomas, and soft tissue tumors, to name a few.

Hereditary nonpolyposis colorectal cancer (HNPCC) is an autosomal dominant familial syndrome (described by Henry Lynch, hence the alternative name of Lynch's syndrome) characterized by an increased risk of colorectal cancer and extraintestinal cancer, particularly of the endometrium (in

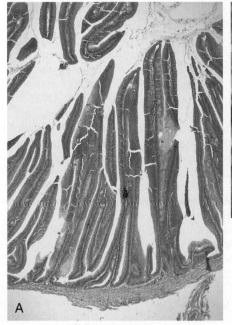

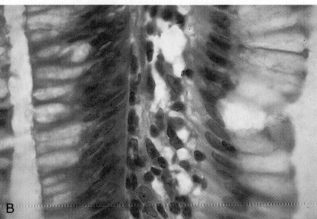

Figure 15–34   ■

A, Sessile adenoma with villous architecture. Each frond is lined by dysplastic epithelium. *B,* Portion of a villous frond with dysplastic columnar epithelium on the left and normal colonic columnar epithelium on the right.

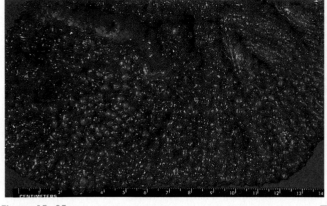

Figure 15–35 ■

Familial adenomatous polyposis in an 18-year-old woman. The mucosal surface is carpeted by innumerable polypoid adenomas.

women). Adenomas do occur in low numbers, but considerably earlier than in the general adult population. The colonic malignancies are typically located proximal to the splenic flexure, are often multiple, and do not arise in preexisting adenomas.

Colorectal Carcinoma

A great majority (98%) of all cancers in the large intestine are adenocarcinomas. They represent one of the prime challenges to the medical profession, because they almost always arise in adenomatous polyps that are generally curable by resection. With an estimated 150,000 new cases per year, and about 58,000 deaths, this disease accounts for nearly 15% of all cancer-related deaths in the United States.

Epidemiology. The peak incidence for colorectal cancer is 60 to 70 years of age; fewer than 20% of cases occur before the age of 50 years. When colorectal cancer is found in a young person, preexisting ulcerative colitis or one of the polyposis syndromes must be suspected. Adenomas are the presumed precursor lesion; the frequency with which colorectal cancer arises de novo from flat colonic mucosa remains undefined but appears to be low. Males are affected about 20% more often than females.

Colorectal carcinoma has a worldwide distribution, with the highest incidence rates in the United States, Canada, Australia, New Zealand, Denmark, Sweden, and other "developed" countries. Its incidence is substantially lower, up to 30-fold, in India, South America, and Africa. The incidence in Japan, which formerly was very low, has now risen to the intermediate levels observed in the United Kingdom. Environmental factors, particularly dietary practices, are implicated in these striking geographic contrasts. The dietary factors receiving the most attention are (1) a low content of unabsorbable vegetable fiber, (2) a corresponding high content of refined carbohydrates, (3) a high fat content (as from meat), and (4) decreased intake of protective micronutrients such as vitamins A, C, and E. It is theorized that reduced fiber content leads to decreased stool bulk, increased fecal retention in the bowel, and an altered bacterial flora of the intestine. Potentially toxic oxidative byproducts of carbohydrate degradation by bacteria are therefore present in higher concentrations in the small stools and are held in contact with the colonic mucosa for longer periods of time. Moreover, high fat intake enhances the synthesis of cholesterol and bile acids by the liver, which in turn may be converted into potential carcinogens by intestinal bacteria. Refined diets also contain less of vitamins A, C, and E, which may act as oxygen radical scavengers. Intriguing as these scenarios are, they remain unproven.

The Adenoma-Carcinoma Sequence. The development of carcinoma from adenomatous lesions is referred to as the adenoma-carcinoma sequence and is documented by these observations:

■ Populations that have a high prevalence of adenomas have a high prevalence of colorectal cancer, and vice versa.
■ The distribution of adenomas within the colorectum is more or less comparable to that of colorectal cancer.
■ The peak incidence of adenomatous polyps antedates by some years the peak for colorectal cancer.
■ When invasive carcinoma is identified at an early stage, surrounding adenomatous tissue is often present.
■ The risk of cancer is directly related to the number of adenomas, and hence the virtual certainty of cancer in patients with familial polyposis syndromes.
■ Programs that assiduously follow patients for the development of adenomas, and remove all that are identified, reduce the incidence of colorectal cancer.

Colorectal Carcinogenesis. Virtually all colorectal carcinomas exhibit genetic alterations, the study of which has provided deep insights into the general mechanisms of carcinogenesis. This topic was covered in detail in Chapter 6; but concepts specifically pertinent to colorectal carcinogenesis are described here (Fig. 15–36).

Adenomatous Polyposis Coli (APC). The inherited defect underlying FAP and Gardner's syndromes has been mapped to chromosome 5q21, where the APC tumor suppressor gene has been identified. The encoded protein is believed to play a role in cell adhesion. Mutation of APC is an early event in the evolution of sporadic colon cancer as well.

Hereditary Nonpolyposis Colon Carcinoma (HNPCC). Inherited mutations in any of four genes that are involved in DNA repair are putatively responsible for the familial syndrome of HNPCC. These human mismatch repair genes, *hMSH2* (chromosome 2p22), *hMLH1* (chromosome 3p21), *hPMS1* (chromosome 2q31-33), and *hPMS2* (chromosome 7p22), are involved in genetic "proofreading" during DNA replication. There are 50,000 to 100,000 dinucleotide repeat sequences in the human genome, and mutations in mismatch repair genes can be detected by the presence of widespread alterations in these repeats; this is referred to as *microsatellite instability.* Patients who inherit one mutant DNA repair gene have normal repair activity owing to the remaining wild type allele. However, cells in some organs (colon, stomach, endometrium) are susceptible to a second, somatic mutation that inactivates the wild type allele. Mutation rates up to 1000 times normal ensue, such that most of the HNPCC tumors show microsatellite instability. Ten to 15% of sporadic colon cancers also have mutations in similar DNA repair genes, implicating somatic (acquired) mutations in these tumors as well.

Methylation Abnormalities. A separate early recognizable

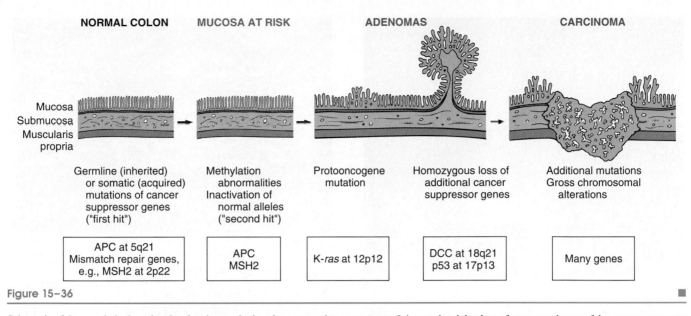

Figure 15-36   ■

Schematic of the morphologic and molecular changes in the adenoma-carcinoma sequence. It is postulated that loss of one normal copy of the cancer suppressor gene APC and loss of DNA repair genes (e.g., MSH2) occur early. Indeed, individuals may be born with one mutant allele, rendering them extremely likely to develop colon cancer. This is the "first hit" according to Knudson's hypothesis. The loss of the normal copy of APC or MSH2 follows ("second hit"). Mutations of the oncogene K-*ras* seem to occur next. Additional mutations inactivate the tumor suppressor genes DCC and p53, leading finally to the emergence of carcinoma, in which additional mutations occur. It is important to note that while there seems to be a temporal sequence of changes, as shown, the accumulation of mutations, rather than their occurrence in a specific order, is more important.

change in colonic neoplasms is loss of methyl groups in DNA (hypomethylation).

K-ras. The K-*ras* gene (Chapter 6) is the most frequently observed activated oncogene in adenomas and colon cancers. K-*ras* (chromosome 12p12) plays a role in intracellular signal transduction and is mutated in fewer than 10% of adenomas less than 1 cm, in 50% of adenomas larger than 1 cm, and in 50% of carcinomas.

DCC. A tumor suppressor gene located on 18q21, termed *DCC* (*D*eleted in *C*olon *C*ancer) is frequently inactivated in colon cancer. The encoded protein, a cell adhesion molecule, normally is widely expressed on the colonic mucosa; its expression is reduced or absent in 70% to 75% of colon cancers.

p53. Losses at chromosome 17p have been found in 70% to 80% of colon cancers, yet similar losses are infrequent in adenomas. These chromosomal deletions affect *p53*, suggesting that mutations in *p53* occur late in colon carcinogenesis. The critical role of *p53* in cell cycle regulation was discussed in Chapter 6.

These considerations have led to the formulation of a multistage, "multi-hit" concept for colon cancer carcinogenesis. APC mutations are usually the earliest and possibly the initiating event in about 80% of sporadic colon cancers. During the progression from adenoma to carcinoma, additional mutations ensue, but not necessarily in order. A single sequence of events does not appear to be operative; rather, cumulative alterations in the genome lead to progressive increases in size, level of dysplasia, and invasive potential of neoplastic lesions.

The distribution of cancers in the colorectum appears to be changing in the United States: there is a well-defined shift toward the right colon, particularly in the elderly. About 25% of carcinomas are in the cecum or ascending colon and a similar proportion in the rectum and distal sigmoid. An additional 25% are in the descending colon and proximal sigmoid; the remainder are scattered elsewhere. No longer are more than half of colorectal cancers readily detectable by digital or proctosigmoidoscopic examination. Most often carcinomas occur singly and have frequently obliterated their adenomatous origins. When multiple carcinomas are present, they are often at widely disparate sites in the colon. Whereas most cases occur sporadically, 1% to 3% of colorectal carcinomas occur in patients with familial adenomatous polyposis or inflammatory bowel disease.

Although all colorectal carcinomas begin as in situ lesions, they evolve into different morphologic patterns. **Tumors in the proximal colon tend to grow as polypoid, fungating masses that extend along one wall of the capacious cecum and ascending colon** (Fig. 15-37). Obstruction is uncommon. **When carcinomas in the distal colon are discovered, they tend to be annular, encircling lesions that produce so-called napkin ring constrictions of the bowel and narrowing of the lumen** (Fig. 15-38); the margins of the napkin ring are classically heaped up. Both forms of neoplasm directly penetrate the bowel wall over the course of time (probably years) and may appear as firm masses on the serosal surface.

Regardless of their gross appearance, all colon carcinomas are microscopically similar. Almost all are adenocarcinomas that range from well-differ-

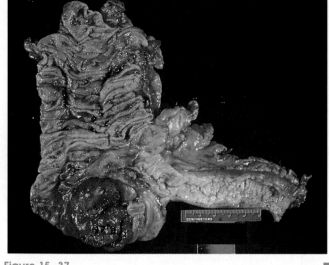

Figure 15–37 ■

Carcinoma of the cecum. The fungating carcinoma projects into the lumen but has not caused obstruction.

entiated (Fig. 15–39) to undifferentiated, frankly anaplastic masses. Many tumors produce mucin, which is secreted into the gland lumina or into the

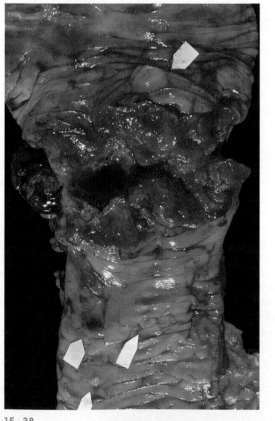

Figure 15–38 ■

Carcinoma of the descending colon. This circumferential tumor has heaped-up edges and an ulcerated central portion. The arrows identify separate mucosal polyps.

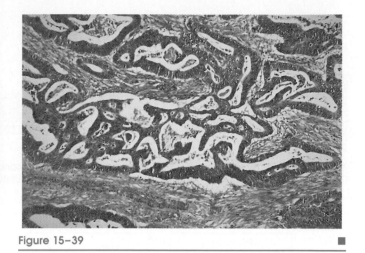

Figure 15–39 ■

Invasive adenocarcinoma of colon showing malignant glands infiltrating the muscle wall.

interstitium of the gut wall. Because these secretions dissect through the gut wall, they facilitate extension of the cancer and worsen the prognosis. Cancers of the anal zone are predominantly squamous cell in origin.

Clinical Features. Colorectal cancers remain asymptomatic for years; symptoms develop insidiously and frequently have been present for months, sometimes years, before diagnosis. Cecal and right colonic cancers most often are called to clinical attention by the appearance of fatigue, weakness, and iron deficiency anemia. Left-sided lesions may produce occult bleeding, changes in bowel habit, or crampy left lower quadrant discomfort. Although anemia in females may arise from gynecologic causes, it is a clinical maxim that *iron deficiency anemia in an older male means gastrointestinal cancer until proved otherwise.*

All colorectal tumors spread by direct extension into adjacent structures, and by metastasis through the lymphatics and blood vessels. In order of preference, the favored sites for metastasis are the regional lymph nodes, liver, lungs, and bones, followed by many other sites including the serosal membrane of the peritoneal cavity. In general, the disease has spread beyond the range of curative surgery in 25% to 30% of patients. Carcinomas of the anal region are locally invasive and metastasize to regional lymph nodes and distant sites.

The detection and diagnosis of colorectal neoplasms relies on a variety of methods, beginning with digital rectal examination and fecal testing for occult blood loss. Barium enema, sigmoidoscopy, and colonoscopy usually require confirmatory biopsy for diagnosis. Computed tomography and other radiographic studies are usually employed to assess metastatic spread. Elevated blood levels of carcinoembryonic antigen are of little diagnostic value, because they reach significant levels only after the tumor has achieved considerable size and has very likely spread. Moreover, "positive" carcinoembryonic antigen levels may be produced by carcinomas of the lung, breast, ovary, urinary bladder, and prostate, as well as such non-neoplastic disorders as alcoholic cirrhosis, pancreatitis, and ulcerative colitis. Instead, this marker has its greatest value in monitoring for possible recurrence of the neoplasm after resection of the primary tumor.

The single most important prognostic indicator of colorectal carcinoma is the extent of the tumor at the time of diagnosis. A widely used staging system is that described by Astler and Coller in 1954 (Table 15–12 and Fig. 15–40), which represents a modification of classifications proposed by Dukes and Kirklin. Staging can be applied only after the neoplasm has been resected and the extent of spread determined by surgical exploration and anatomic examination. Surgery performed for cure slightly improves the 5-year survival rates originally published by Astler and Coller. It is evident that the challenge is to discover these neoplasms when curative resection is possible, preferably in their "infancy" when they are still adenomatous polyps.

Small Intestinal Neoplasms

Whereas the small bowel represents 75% of the length of the alimentary tract, its tumors account for only 3% to 6% of gastrointestinal tumors, with a slight preponderance of benign tumors. The annual death rate in the United States is under 1000, representing only about 1% of gastrointestinal malignancies. The most frequent benign tumors in the small intestine are stromal tumors of predominantly smooth muscle origin, adenomas, and lipomas, followed by various neurogenic, vascular, and hamartomatous epithelial lesions. Small intestinal adenocarcinomas and carcinoids have a roughly equal incidence.

ADENOCARCINOMA OF THE SMALL INTESTINE

These tumors grow in a napkin-ring encircling pattern or as polypoid fungating masses, in a manner similar to colonic

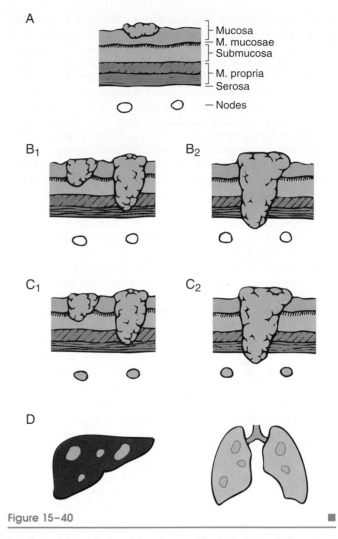

Figure 15–40   ■

Pathologic staging of colorectal cancer according to the Astler-Coller system. Staging is based on the extent of local invasion and the presence of lymph node metastases (*A* to *C*) and distant visceral metastases (*D*).

cancers. Most small bowel carcinomas arise in the duodenum (including the ampulla of Vater). Cramping pain, nausea, vomiting, and weight loss are the common presenting signs and symptoms, but such manifestations generally appear late in the course of these cancers. Most have already penetrated the bowel wall, invaded the mesentery or other segments of the gut, spread to regional nodes, and sometimes metastasized to the liver and more widely by the time of diagnosis. Despite these problems, wide en bloc excision of these cancers yields a 5-year survival rate of about 70%. Duodenal lesions in the periampullary region may lead to obstructive jaundice early in their course.

CARCINOID TUMORS

Cells generating bioactive compounds, particularly peptide and nonpeptide hormones, are normally dispersed along the length of the gastrointestinal tract mucosa and play a major role in coordinated gut function. Although they are derived from epithelial stem cells in the mucosal crypts, they are des-

Table 15–12.   **ASTLER-COLLER CLASSIFICATION OF CARCINOMA OF THE COLON AND RECTUM**

Tumor Stage	Histologic Features of the Neoplasm	Five-Year Survival
A	Limited to the mucosa	100%
B1	Extending into the muscularis propria but not penetrating through it; uninvolved nodes	67%
B2	Penetrating through the muscularis propria; uninvolved nodes	54%
C1	Extending into the muscularis propria but not penetrating through it; involved nodes	43%
C2	Penetrating through the muscularis propria; involved nodes	22%
D	Distant metastatic spread	Very low

From Astler VB, Coller FA: The prognostic significance of direct extension of carcinoma of the colon and rectum. Ann Surg 139:846, 1954. Tumor stage "D" is not routinely included, but was an addition by Turnbull RB Jr, et al: Cancer of the colon: the influence of the no-touch isolation technic on survival rates. Ann Surg 166:420, 1967. Incorrectly assigned eponyms include Dukes', Modifed Dukes', and Dukes'-Kirklin.

ignated *neuroendocrine* because phenotypically they resemble many neuronal (e.g., anterior pituitary) and endocrine (e.g., pancreatic islet) cells. Neuroendocrine cells are abundant in other organs, including the lungs, but the great preponderance of tumors arising from these cells are in the gut. A scattering of tumors arises in the pancreas or peripancreatic tissue, lungs, biliary tree, and even liver. The peak incidence of these neoplasms is in the sixth decade, but they may appear at any age. They comprise less than 2% of colorectal malignancies but almost half of small intestinal malignant tumors.

Although all carcinoids are potentially malignant tumors, the tendency for aggressive behavior correlates with the site of origin, the depth of local penetration, and the size of the tumor. For example, *appendiceal and rectal carcinoids infrequently metastasize,* even though they may show extensive local spread. By contrast, 90% of ileal, gastric, and colonic carcinoids that have penetrated halfway through the muscle wall have spread to lymph nodes and distant sites at the time of diagnosis, especially those greater than 2 cm in diameter.

As with normal neuroendocrine cells, the cells of carcinoid tumors can synthesize and secrete a variety of bioactive products and hormones. Although multiple factors may be synthesized by a single tumor, when a tumor secretes a predominant product to cause a clinical syndrome, it may be called by that name (e.g., gastrinoma, somatostatinoma, and insulinoma).

The appendix is the most common site of gut carcinoid tumors, followed by the small intestine (primarily ileum), rectum, stomach, and colon. However, the rectum may represent up to half of those that come to clinical attention. In the appendix they appear as bulbous swellings of the tip, which frequently obliterate the lumen. Elsewhere in the gut, they appear as intramural or submucosal masses that create small, polypoid, or plateau-like elevations rarely more than 3 cm in diameter (Fig. 15–41A). The overlying mucosa may be intact or ulcerated, and the tumors may permeate the bowel wall to invade the mesentery. Those that arise in the stomach and ileum are frequently multicentric, but the remainder tend to

be solitary lesions. **A characteristic feature is a solid, yellow-tan appearance on transection.** The tumors are exceedingly firm, owing to striking desmoplasia; and when these fibrosing lesions penetrate the mesentery of the small bowel they may cause sufficient angulation or kinking to cause obstruction. When present, visceral metastases are usually small, dispersed nodules and rarely achieve the size seen with the primary lesions. Notably, **rectal and appendiceal carcinoids almost never metastasize.**

Histologically, the neoplastic cells may form discrete islands, trabeculae, strands, glands, or undifferentiated sheets. Whatever their organization the tumor cells are monotonously similar, having a scant, pink granular cytoplasm and a round-to-oval stippled nucleus. In most tumors there is minimal variation in cell and nuclear size, and mitoses are infrequent or absent (Fig. 15–41B). By electron microscopy (Fig. 15–41C) the cells in most tumors contain cytoplasmic, well-formed, membrane-bounded secretory granules with osmophilic centers (dense-core granules). Most carcinoids can be shown to contain chromogranin A, synaptophysin, and neuron-specific enolase. Specific hormonal peptides may occasionally be identified by immunocytochemical techniques.

Clinical Features. Gastrointestinal carcinoids are frequently asymptomatic, including virtually all that arise in the appendix. Only rarely do carcinoids produce local symptoms, owing to angulation or obstruction of the small intestine. However, the secretory products of some carcinoids may produce a variety of syndromes or endocrinopathies. Gastric, peripancreatic, and pancreatic carcinoids can release their products directly into the systemic circulation and can produce the Zollinger-Ellison syndrome by excess elaboration of gastrin, Cushing's syndrome due to ACTH secretion, hyperinsulinism, and others. In some instances, these tumors may be under 1.0 cm in size and extremely difficult to find, even during surgical exploration.

Some neoplasms are associated with a distinctive *carcinoid*

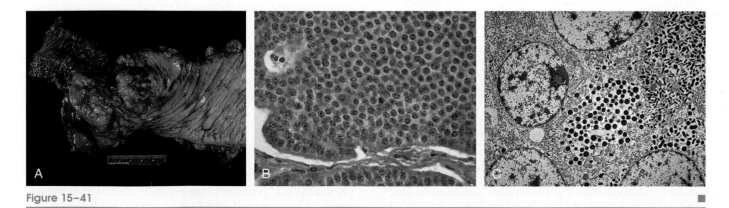

Figure 15–41 ■

Carcinoid tumor. *A,* Multiple protruding tumors are present at the ileocecal junction. *B,* The tumor cells exhibit a monotonous morphology, with a delicate intervening fibrovascular stroma. (H & E.) *C,* Electron micrograph showing dense core bodies in the cytoplasm.

Table 15-13. CLINICAL FEATURES OF THE CARCINOID SYNDROME

Vasomotor disturbances
    Cutaneous flushes and apparent cyanosis (most patients)
Intestinal hypermotility
    Diarrhea, cramps, nausea, vomiting (most patients)
Asthmatic bronchoconstrictive attacks
    Cough, wheezing, dyspnea (about one third of patients)
Hepatomegaly
    Nodular, related to hepatic metastases (some cases)
Systemic fibrosis
    Cardiac involvement
        Pulmonic and tricuspid valve thickening and stenosis
        Endocardial fibrosis, principally in right ventricle
        (Bronchial carcinoids affect the left side)
    Retroperitoneal and pelvic fibrosis
    Collagenous pleural and intimal aortic plaques

syndrome, detailed in Table 15–13. The syndrome occurs in about 1% of all patients with carcinoids and in 20% of those with widespread metastases. The precise basis of the carcinoid syndrome is uncertain, but most manifestations are thought to arise from elaboration of serotonin (5-hydroxytryptamine [5-HT]). Elevated levels of 5-HT and its metabolite, 5-hydroxyindoleacetic acid (5-HIAA) are present in the blood and urine of most patients with the classic syndrome; 5-HT is degraded in the liver to functionally inactive 5-HIAA. Thus, with gastrointestinal carcinoids, hepatic dysfunction resulting from metastases must be present for the development of the syndrome. The possibility that other secretory products such as histamine, bradykinin, and prostaglandins contribute to the manifestations of this syndrome has not been excluded.

The 5-year survival rate for carcinoids (excluding appendiceal) is approximately 90%. Even with small bowel tumors that have spread to the liver, it is better than 50%. However, widespread disease usually causes death.

GASTROINTESTINAL LYMPHOMA

Any segment of the gastrointestinal tract may be involved secondarily by systemic dissemination of non-Hodgkin lymphomas. However, up to 40% of lymphomas arise in sites other than lymph nodes, and the gut is the most common extranodal location; 1% to 4% of all gastrointestinal malignancies are lymphomas. By definition, primary gastrointestinal lymphomas exhibit no evidence of liver, spleen, or bone marrow involvement at the time of diagnosis; regional lymph node involvement may be present. Sporadic lymphomas are the most common form in the Western Hemisphere and appear to arise from the B cells of mucosa-associated lymphoid tissue (MALT). This type of gastrointestinal lymphoma usually affects adults, lacks a sex predilection, and may arise anywhere in the gut: stomach (55% to 60% of cases), small intestine (25% to 30%), proximal colon (10% to 15%), and distal colon (up to 10%). The appendix and esophagus are only rarely involved. For most gastrointestinal lymphomas, no specific associations with predisposing diseases or pathologic lesions have been reported. However, it has been proposed that lymphomas of MALT arise in the setting of mucosal lymphoid activation, as may result from *Helicobacter*-associated chronic gastritis.

The symptoms of gastrointestinal lymphoma are nonspecific. They may be related to the effects of a mass lesion but more often are simply malaise, loss of appetite, and weight loss. Primary gastrointestinal lymphomas generally have a better prognosis than do those arising in other sites, because combined surgery, chemotherapy, or radiation therapy offer reasonable hopes of cure.

Appendix

Diseases of the appendix loom large in surgical practice; appendicitis is the most common acute abdominal condition the surgeon is called on to treat. Despite the preeminence of this diagnostic entity, a differential diagnosis must include virtually every acute process that can occur within the abdominal cavity, as well as some emergent conditions affecting organs of the thorax. On occasion, a tumor arises in the appendix, necessitating abdominal exploration.

Acute Appendicitis

Surveys indicate that approximately 10% of persons in the United States and other Western countries develop appendicitis at some time. No age is immune, but the peak incidence is in the second and third decades, although lately a second smaller peak is appearing among elders. Males are affected more often than females in a ratio of 1.5 : 1.

Pathogenesis. Appendiceal inflammation is associated with obstruction in 50% to 80% of cases, usually in the form of a fecalith and, less commonly, a gallstone, tumor, or ball of worms (*Oxyuriasis vermicularis*). With continued secretion of mucinous fluid, the build-up of intraluminal pressure presumably is sufficient to cause collapse of the draining veins. Obstruction and ischemic injury then favors bacterial proliferation with additional inflammatory edema and exudation, further embarrassing the blood supply. Nevertheless, a significant minority of inflamed appendices have no demonstrable luminal obstruction, and the pathogenesis of the inflammation remains unknown.

At the earliest stages, only a scant neutrophilic exudate may be found throughout the mucosa, submucosa, and muscularis propria. Subserosal vessels are congested, and often there is a modest perivascular neutrophilic infiltrate. The inflammatory reaction transforms the normal glistening serosa into a dull, granular, red membrane; this transformation signifies **early acute appendicitis** for the operating surgeon. At a later stage, a prominent neutrophilic exudate generates a fibrinopurulent reaction over the serosa (Fig. 15–42). As the inflammatory process worsens, there is abscess formation within the wall, along with ulcerations and foci of necrosis in the mucosa. This state constitutes **acute suppurative appendicitis.** Further ap-

pendiceal compromise leads to large areas of hemorrhagic green ulceration of the mucosa, and green-black gangrenous necrosis through the wall extending to the serosa, creating **acute gangrenous appendicitis** that is quickly followed by rupture and suppurative peritonitis.

The histologic criterion for the diagnosis of acute appendicitis is neutrophilic infiltration of the muscularis. Usually, neutrophils and ulcerations are also present within the mucosa.

Clinical Features. Acute appendicitis is the easiest and most difficult of abdominal diagnoses. The classic case is marked by (1) mild periumbilical discomfort, followed by (2) anorexia, nausea, and vomiting, soon associated with (3) right lower quadrant tenderness, which in the course of hours is transformed into (4) a deep constant ache or pain in the right lower quadrant. Fever and leukocytosis appear early in the course. Regrettably, a large number of cases are not classic. The condition can be remarkably silent, particularly in the aged, or can fail to reveal localizing right-sided lower quadrant signs, as when the appendix is retrocecal or when there is malrotation of the colon. Moreover, the following disorders may present many of the clinical features of acute appendicitis: (1) mesenteric lymphadenitis after a viral systemic infection, (2) gastroenteritis with mesenteric adenitis, (3) pelvic inflammatory disease with tubo-ovarian involvement, (4) rupture of an ovarian follicle at the time of ovulation, (5) ectopic pregnancy, (6) Meckel's diverticulitis, and other conditions as well. Thus, despite all efforts, surgeons remove normal appendices 20% to 25% of the time. However, *it is generally conceded that it is better to have a substantial negative diagnostic error than to risk the morbidity and mortality (about 2%) of appendiceal perforation.*

Tumors of the Appendix

Carcinoids (discussed earlier) are the most common form of neoplasia in the appendix. The only other lesions worthy of mention are mucocele of the appendix and mucinous neoplasms.

Mucocele refers to dilation of the lumen of the appendix by mucinous secretion. It is caused by non-neoplastic obstruction of the lumen and is usually associated with a fecalith in the lumen, permitting the slow accumulation of sterile mucinous secretions. Eventually, the distention induces atrophy of the mucin-secreting mucosal cells and the secretions stop. This condition is usually asymptomatic; rarely a mucocele ruptures, spilling otherwise innocuous mucin into the peritoneum.

Mucinous neoplasms range from the benign *mucinous cystadenoma,* to *mucinous cystadenocarcinoma,* which invades the wall, to a form of disseminated intraperitoneal cancer called *pseudomyxoma peritonei.* The cystadenoma is histologically identical to analogous tumors in the ovary (Chapter 19). The malignant mucin-secreting neoplasms (cystadenocarcinomas) invade the wall, allowing tumor cells to implant throughout the peritoneal cavity, which becomes filled with mucin (pseudomyxoma peritonei).

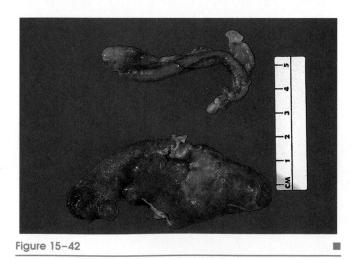

Figure 15–42 ■

Acute appendicitis. The inflamed appendix shown below is red, swollen, and covered with a fibrinous exudate. For comparison, a normal appendix is shown above.

BIBLIOGRAPHY

Oral Cavity

Ficarra G, Eversole LE: HIV-related tumors of the oral cavity. Crit Rev Oral Biol Med 5:159, 1994. (A discussion of risk conditions for squamous cell carcinoma, lymphoma, and Kaposi's sarcoma of the oral cavity.)

Iezzoni JC, et al: The role of Epstein-Barr virus in lymphoepithelioma-like carcinomas. Am J Clin Pathol 103:308, 1995. (A discussion of virus-induced neoplasms throughout the alimentary tract, including oral cavity squamous cell carcinoma and lymphoma-like lesions.)

Sciubba JJ: Oral leukoplakia. Crit Rev Oral Biol Med 6:147, 1995. (An up-to-date review of the molecular and potentially premalignant features of this worrisome oral cavity lesion.)

Simpson RH: Classification of salivary gland tumors—a brief histopathological review. Histol Histopathol 10:737, 1995. (A primer on the morphologic features of salivary gland tumors.)

Esophagus

Galmiche J-P, Janssens J: The pathophysiology of gastroesophageal reflux disease: an overview. Scand J Gastroenterol 30 (Suppl 211):7, 1995. (An examination of the underlying mechanisms of this very common condition.)

Haggitt RC: Barrett's esophagus, dysplasia, and adenocarcinoma. Hum Pathol 25:982, 1994. (A comparison of histological and molecular features of dysplasia in Barrett's esophagus.)

Hamilton SR: Reflux esophagitis and Barrett esophagus. Monogr Pathol 31:11, 1990. (A detailed definitive discussion of all aspects of reflux esophagitis and Barrett's esophagus.)

McCormick PA: Pathophysiology and prognosis of oesophageal varices. Scand J Gastroenterol 29 (Suppl 207):1, 1994. (A convincing discussion of the grave nature of this disease condition.)

Pera M, et al: Increasing incidence of adenocarcinoma of the esophagus and esophagogastric junction. Gastroenterology 104:510, 1993. (An examination of the epidemiology implicating Barrett's esophagus as an underlying risk condition.)

Reynolds JC, Parkman HP: Achalasia. Gastroenterol Clin North Am 18:223, 1989. (A comprehensive excellent review.)

Stemmermann G, et al: The molecular biology of esophageal and gastric cancer and their precursors: oncogenes, tumor suppressor genes, and growth factors. Hum Pathol 25:968, 1994. (A review focusing on the abnormalities of oncogenes, tumor suppressor genes, and growth factors commonly found in cancers of these two organs.)

Stomach

Appelman HD: Gastritis: terminology, etiology, and clinicopathological correlations: another biased view. Hum Pathol 25:1006, 1994. (An enlightened review of the many attempts to understand, and classify, chronic gastritis.)

Bjorkman DJ, Kimmey MB: Nonsteroidal anti-inflammatory drugs and gastrointestinal disease: pathophysiology, treatment and prevention. Dig Dis 13:199, 1995. (A review of the predominantly upper gastrointestinal tract disorders induced by these oft-used pharmaceuticals.)

Fuchs CS, Mayer RJ: Gastric carcinoma. N Engl J Med 333:32, 1995. (A review of epidemiology, pathology, and clinical features of gastric cancer.)

Gibaldi M: *Helicobacter pylori* and gastrointestinal disease. J Clin Pharmacol 35:647, 1995. (A review of the implication of *Helicobacter* as primary causal factor of gastritis, peptic ulcer disease, and possibly gastric carcinoma and lymphoma.)

Marshall BJ: *Helicobacter pylori* in peptic ulcer: have Koch's postulates been fulfilled. Ann Med 27:565, 1995. (*Helicobacter pylori* heralded as the cause of gastritis and peptic ulcer disease—is this true?)

McGowan CC, et al: *Helicobacter pylori* and gastric acid: biological and therapeutic implications. Gastroenterology 110:926, 1996. (An examination of the local physiologic effects on the gastric mucosa of *H. pylori* infection.)

Peddanna N: Genetics of gastric cancer. Anticancer Res 15:2055, 1995. (A description of the considerable recent progress in identifying the molecular events that may play a role in gastric carcinogenesis.)

Small and Large Intestines

Bachwich DR, et al: Cancer in inflammatory bowel disease. Med Clin North Am 6:1399, 1994. (A review of the cancer risks associated with inflammatory bowel disease.)

De la Chapelle A, Peltomaki P: Genetics of hereditary colon cancer. Annu Rev Genet 29:329, 1995. (Further analysis of this rapidly evolving area.)

Guerrant RL, et al: Diarrhea in developed and developing countries: magnitude, special settings, and etiologies. Rev Infect Dis 12 (Suppl 1):S41, 1990. (An excellent analysis of the various etiologies and their prevalence.)

Hermiston ML, Gordon JI: Inflammatory bowel disease and adenomas in mice expressing a dominant negative N-cadherin. Science 270:1203, 1995. (A study linking alterations in epithelial adhesion with both inflammatory bowel disease and the development of colorectal carcinoma.)

Isaacson PG: Gastrointestinal lymphoma. Hum Pathol 25:1020, 1994. (A review of the potential role of the mucosa-associated lymphoid tissue in the pathogenesis of gastrointestinal lymphoma.)

Levine JS: Intestinal ischemic disorders. Dig Dis 13:3, 1995. (A review of the clinical and pathophysiological features, particularly those of severe disease.)

Lynch HT, Smyrk T: Colorectal cancer, survival advantage, and hereditary nonpolyposis colorectal cancer. Gastroenterology 110:943, 1996. (An editorial addressing the genetics and epidemiology of a form of hereditary colorectal cancer.)

Manousos ON: Diverticular disease of the colon. Dig Dis 7:86, 1989. (A thorough review with good discussion of pathogenesis and clinical features.)

Podolsky DK: Inflammatory bowel disease. N Engl J Med 325:929, 1008, 1991. (The definitive summary of both Crohn's disease and ulcerative colitis, highlighting the similarities and differences.)

Potter JD, et al: Colon cancer: a review of the epidemiology. Epidemiol Rev 15:499, 1993. (A critical review of epidemiologic evidence for the many potential risk factors for colon cancer.)

Sartor RB: Insights into the pathogenesis of inflammatory bowel diseases provided by new rodent models of spontaneous colitis. Inflammatory Bowel Dis 1:64, 1995. (A detailed review of the important knockout mouse models of inflammatory bowel disease.)

Toribara NW, Sleisenger MH: Screening for colorectal cancer. N Engl J Med 332:861, 1995. (Discusses molecular carcinogenesis and clinical management issues.)

Appendix

Gray GF Jr, Wackym PA: Surgical pathology of the vermiform appendix. Pathol Annu 21:111, 1986. (A review of the essential pathology of the appendix.)

Young RH, et al: Mucinous tumors of the appendix associated with mucinous tumors of the ovary and pseudomyxoma peritonei: A clinicopathological analysis of 22 cases supporting an origin in the appendix. Am J Surg Pathol 15:415, 1991. (A definitive discussion of mucinous tumors of the appendix and peritoneum.)

16

The Liver and the Biliary Tract

JAMES M. CRAWFORD, MD, PhD

The contributions made by Dr. Mary F. Lipscomb to this chapter in the previous edition of *Basic Pathology* are gratefully acknowledged.

The Liver

The right upper quadrant of the abdomen is dominated by the liver and its companion biliary tree and gallbladder. These structures are considered together not only because of their anatomic proximity and interrelated functions but also because diseases affecting these organs may have overlapping features. Discussion of the liver dominates because the liver plays by far the greater role in normal physiology and is afflicted by a wider variety of diseases.

Residing at the crossroads between the digestive tract and the rest of the body, the liver has the enormous task of maintaining the body's metabolic homeostasis. This includes the processing of dietary amino acids, carbohydrates, lipids, and vitamins; synthesis of serum proteins; and detoxification and excretion into bile of endogenous waste products and pollutant xenobiotics. Hepatic disorders have far-reaching consequences, given the critical dependence of other organs on the metabolic function of the liver. Liver injury and its manifestations tend to follow characteristic patterns, which are discussed first before specific diseases are described.

GENERAL PRINCIPLES

The liver is vulnerable to a wide variety of metabolic, toxic, microbial, circulatory, and neoplastic insults. In some instances the disease process is primary to the liver. In others the hepatic involvement is secondary, often to some of the most common diseases in humans, such as cardiac decompensation, disseminated cancer, alcoholism, and extrahepatic infections. The functional reserve of the liver masks to some extent the clinical impact of early liver damage. However, with progression of diffuse disease or strategic disruption of bile flow, the consequences of deranged liver function become life threatening.

Hepatic Injury

From a morphologic standpoint, the liver is an inherently simple organ, with a limited repertoire of responses to injurious events. Regardless of cause, five general responses are seen. These processes, and the morphologic terms used to describe them, are summarized in the following brief overview.

INFLAMMATION. Injury to hepatocytes associated with an influx of acute or chronic inflammatory cells into the liver is termed **hepatitis**. Although hepatocyte necrosis may precede the onset of inflammation, the converse is also true. Attack of viable antigen-expressing liver cells by sensitized T cells is a common cause of liver damage. Inflammation may be limited to the site of leukocyte entry (portal tracts) or spill over into the parenchyma. When hepatocytes undergo necrosis, scavenger macrophages quickly engulf the dead cells, generating clumps of inflammatory cells in an otherwise normal parenchyma. Foreign bodies, organisms, and a variety of drugs may incite a granulomatous reaction.

DEGENERATION. Damage from toxic or immunologic insult may cause hepatocytes to take on a swollen, edematous appearance (**ballooning degeneration**) with irregularly clumped cytoplasm and large, clear spaces. Alternatively, retained biliary material may impart a diffuse, foamy, swollen appearance to the hepatocyte (**foamy degeneration**). Substances may accumulate in viable hepatocytes, including iron, copper, and retained biliary material. Accumulation of fat droplets within hepatocytes is known as **steatosis**. Multiple tiny droplets that do not displace the nucleus are known as **microvesicular steatosis** and appear in such conditions as alcoholic liver disease, Reye's syndrome, and acute fatty liver of pregnancy (a potentially fatal cause of hepatic failure in the third trimester of pregnancy). A single large droplet that displaces the nucleus, **macrovesicular steatosis,** may be seen in the alcoholic liver or in the livers of obese or diabetic individuals.

NECROSIS. Virtually any significant insult to the liver may cause hepatocyte necrosis. In ischemic necrosis, poorly stained mummified hepatocytes remain (**coagulative necrosis**). In necrosis that is toxic or immunologically mediated, isolated hepatocytes round up as shrunken, pyknotic, intensely eosinophilic **Councilman bodies**. This form of necrosis appears to be the consequence of **apoptosis**. Alternatively, hepatocytes may osmotically swell and rupture, so-called **hydropic degeneration** or **lytic necrosis.**

Necrosis frequently exhibits a zonal distribution.

■

Table 16–1. LABORATORY EVALUATION OF LIVER DISEASE

Test Category	Serum Measurement
Hepatocyte integrity	Cytosolic hepatocellular enzymes*
	Serum aspartate aminotransferase (AST)
	Serum alanine aminotransferase (ALT)
	Serum lactate dehydrogenase (LDH)
Biliary excretory function	Substances secreted in bile*
	Serum bilirubin
	Total: unconjugated plus conjugated
	Direct: conjugated only
	Delta: covalently linked to albumin
	Urine bilirubin
	Serum bile acids
	Plasma membrane enzymes*
	(from damage to bile canaliculus)
	Serum alkaline phosphatase
	Serum γ-glutamyl transpeptidase
	Serum 5′-nucleotidase
Hepatocyte function	Proteins secreted into the blood
	Serum albumin†
	*Prothrombin time**
	(factors V, VII, X, prothrombin, fibrinogen)
	Hepatocyte metabolism
	Serum ammonia*
	Aminopyrine breath test†
	(hepatic demethylation)
	Galactose elimination†
	(intravenous injection)

Most common tests are in italics.
* An elevation implicates liver disease.
† A decrease implicates liver disease.

This is most obvious with necrosis of hepatocytes immediately around the central vein (**centrilobular necrosis**), an injury that does not involve inflammation and is characteristic of ischemic injury and a number of drug and toxic reactions. Pure midzonal and periportal necrosis is rare. Instead, with most other causes of hepatic injury, a variable mixture of necrosis and inflammation is encountered. The hepatocyte necrosis may be limited to scattered cells within the hepatic lobules (**focal necrosis**) or to the interface between the periportal parenchyma and inflamed portal tracts (**piecemeal necrosis**). With more severe inflammatory injury, necrosis of contiguous hepatocytes may span adjacent lobules in a portal-to-portal, portal-to-central, or central-to-central fashion (**bridging necrosis**). Necrosis of entire lobules (**submassive necrosis**) or most of the liver (**massive necrosis**) is usually accompanied by hepatic failure. With disseminated candidal or bacterial infection, macroscopic abscesses may occur.

FIBROSIS. Fibrous tissue is formed in response to inflammation or direct toxic insult to the liver. Deposition of collagen has lasting consequences on hepatic patterns of blood flow and perfusion of hepatocytes. In the initial stages, fibrosis may develop within or around portal tracts or the central vein or may be deposited directly within the sinu-

soids. With time, fibrous strands link regions of the liver (portal-to-portal, portal-to-central, central-to-central), a process called **bridging fibrosis.**

Unlike all of the other lesions, which are reversible, **fibrosis is generally an irreversible consequence of hepatic damage.** The rare instances in which therapy may lead to regression of fibrosis include schistosomal infection of portal tracts and genetic hemochromatosis (see later).

CIRRHOSIS. With continuing fibrosis and parenchymal injury, the liver is subdivided into nodules of regenerating hepatocytes surrounded by scar tissue, termed **cirrhosis.** This end-stage form of liver disease is discussed later in this section.

The liver has enormous functional reserve, and regeneration occurs in all but the most fulminant of hepatic diseases. Thus, in a normal individual, surgical removal of 75% of the liver produces minimal hepatic impairment, and regeneration restores liver mass within a few weeks. When massive hepatocellular necrosis occurs and leaves the connective tissue framework intact, almost perfect restitution can occur.

The ebb and flow of hepatic injury may be imperceptible to the patient and detectable only by laboratory tests (Table 16–1). Alternatively, hepatic function may be so impaired as to be life threatening. The major clinical consequences of liver disease are listed in Table 16–2 and are discussed next.

Jaundice and Cholestasis

Hepatic bile formation serves two major functions. Bile constitutes the primary pathway for elimination of bilirubin,

■

Table 16–2. CLINICAL CONSEQUENCES OF LIVER DISEASE

Characteristic Signs	Hepatic dysfunction:
	Jaundice and cholestasis
	Hypoalbuminemia
	Hyperammonemia
	Hypoglycemia
	Fetor hepaticus
	Palmar erythema
	Spider angiomas
	Hypogonadism
	Gynecomastia
	Weight loss
	Muscle wasting
	Portal hypertension from cirrhosis:
	Ascites
	Splenomegaly
	Hemorrhoids
	Caput medusa—abdominal skin
Life-Threatening Complications	Hepatic failure
	Multiple organ failure
	Coagulopathy
	Hepatic encephalopathy
	Hepatorenal syndrome
	Portal hypertension from cirrhosis
	Esophageal varices, risk of rupture
	Malignancy with chronic disease
	Hepatocellular carcinoma

excess cholesterol, and xenobiotics that are insufficiently water soluble to be excreted into urine. Second, secreted bile salts and phospholipid molecules promote emulsification of dietary fat in the lumen of the gut. Because bile formation is one of the most sophisticated functions of the liver, it is also one of the most readily disrupted. Thus, *jaundice,* a yellow discoloration of skin and sclerae (icterus), occurs when systemic retention of bilirubin leads to elevated serum levels above 2.0 mg/dl, the normal in the adult being less than 1.2 mg/dl. *Cholestasis,* on the other hand, is defined as systemic retention of not only bilirubin but also other solutes eliminated in bile (particularly bile salts and cholesterol).

BILIRUBIN AND BILE ACIDS

Bilirubin is the end product of heme degradation (Fig. 16–1). Most of the daily production (0.2 to 0.3 gm) is derived from breakdown of senescent erythrocytes, with the remainder derived primarily from the turnover of hepatic hemoproteins and from premature destruction of newly formed erythrocytes in the bone marrow. The latter pathway is important in hematologic disorders associated with excessive intramedullary hemolysis of defective erythrocytes (ineffective erythropoiesis; Chapter 12). Whatever the source, heme oxygenase oxidizes heme to biliverdin, which is then reduced to bilirubin by biliverdin reductase. Bilirubin thus formed outside the liver in cells of the mononuclear phagocytic system (including the spleen) is released and bound to serum albumin. Hepatocellular processing of bilirubin involves (1) carrier-mediated uptake at the sinusoidal membrane, (2) cytosolic protein binding and delivery to the endoplasmic reticulum, (3) conjugation with one or two molecules of glucuronic acid by bilirubin uridine diphosphate-glucuronosyltransferase (UGT), and (4) excretion of the water-soluble, nontoxic bilirubin glucuronides into bile. Most bilirubin glucuronides are deconjugated by gut bacterial β-glucuronidases and degraded to colorless urobilinogens. The urobilinogens, and the residue of intact pigment, are largely excreted in feces. Approximately 20% of the urobilinogens are reabsorbed in the ileum and colon, returned to the liver, and promptly re-excreted into bile. The small amount escaping this enterohepatic circulation is excreted in urine.

The brilliant yellow color of bilirubin makes it an easily identified component of hepatic bile formation. However, bilirubin excretion is but a minor cog in the hepatic machinery that secretes 12 to 36 gm of bile acids into bile per day. Bile acids are carboxylated steroid molecules (derived from cho-

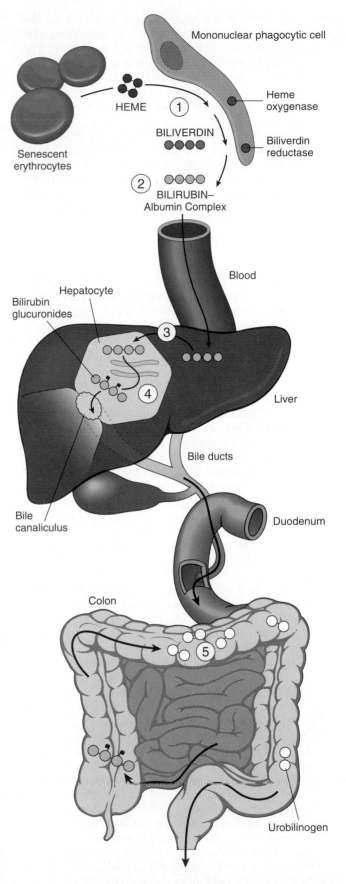

Figure 16–1   ■

Bilirubin metabolism and elimination. 1, Normal bilirubin production (0.2–0.3 gm/day) is derived primarily from the breakdown of senescent circulating erythrocytes, with a minor contribution from degradation of tissue heme-containing proteins. 2, Extrahepatic bilirubin is bound to serum albumin and delivered to the liver. 3, Hepatocellular uptake and (4) glucuronidation in the endoplasmic reticulum generates bilirubin mono- and diglucuronides, which are water soluble and readily excreted into bile. 5, Gut bacteria deconjugate the bilirubin and degrade it to colorless urobilinogens. The urobilinogens and the residue of intact pigments are excreted in the feces, with some reabsorption and re-excretion into bile.

lesterol) with supplemental hydroxyl groups and are the detergent molecules primarily responsible for promoting bile flow and the secretion of phospholipid and cholesterol. The primary human bile acids are cholic acid and chenodeoxycholic acid, which are secreted as taurine and glycine conjugates. Ten to 20% of secreted bile acids are deconjugated in the intestines by bacterial action. Virtually all conjugated and deconjugated bile acids are reabsorbed (especially in the ileum) and returned to the liver for uptake, reconjugation, and resecretion. Fecal loss of bile acids (0.2 to 0.6 gm/day) is matched by de novo hepatic synthesis of bile acids from cholesterol. The *enterohepatic circulation* of bile acids provides an efficient mechanism for maintaining a large endogenous pool of bile acids for digestive and excretory purposes.

PATHOPHYSIOLOGY OF JAUNDICE

Both unconjugated bilirubin and bilirubin glucuronides may accumulate systemically and deposit in tissues, giving rise to the yellow discoloration of jaundice. This is particularly evident in the yellowing of the sclerae (icterus). There are two important pathophysiologic differences between the two forms of bilirubin. *Unconjugated bilirubin is virtually insoluble in water at physiologic pH and is tightly complexed to serum albumin. This form cannot be excreted in the urine even when blood levels are high.* Normally, a very small amount of unconjugated bilirubin is present as an albumin-free anion in plasma. This fraction of unbound bilirubin may diffuse into tissues (particularly the brain in infants) and produce toxic injury. The unbound plasma fraction may increase in severe hemolytic disease or when protein-binding drugs displace bilirubin from albumin. Hence, hemolytic disease of the newborn (erythroblastosis fetalis) may lead to accumulation of unconjugated bilirubin in the brain, which can cause severe neurologic damage, referred to as *kernicterus* (Chapter 7). In contrast, *conjugated bilirubin is water soluble, nontoxic, and only loosely bound to albumin. Because of its solubility and weak association with albumin, excess conjugated bilirubin in plasma can be excreted in urine.* With prolonged conjugated hyperbilirubinemia, a portion of circulating pigment may become covalently bound to albumin (the delta fraction).

In the normal adult, serum bilirubin levels vary between 0.3 and 1.2 mg/dl and the rate of systemic bilirubin production is equal to the rates of hepatic uptake, conjugation, and biliary excretion. Jaundice becomes evident when the serum bilirubin levels rise above 2.0 to 2.5 mg/dl; levels as high as 30 to 40 mg/dl can occur with severe disease. Jaundice occurs when the equilibrium between bilirubin production and clearance is disturbed by one or more of the following mechanisms (Table 16–3): (1) excessive production of bilirubin, (2) reduced hepatocellular uptake, (3) impaired conjugation, (4) decreased hepatocellular excretion, and (5) impaired bile flow (both intra- and extrahepatic). The first three mechanisms produce unconjugated hyperbilirubinemia, and the latter two produce predominantly conjugated hyperbilirubinemia. More than one mechanism may operate to produce jaundice, especially in hepatitis, which may produce unconjugated and conjugated hyperbilirubinemia. In general, however, one mechanism predominates, so that knowledge of the predominant form of plasma bilirubin is of value in evaluating possible causes of hyperbilirubinemia.

Table 16–3. CAUSES OF JAUNDICE

Predominantly Unconjugated Hyperbilirubinemia
Excess production of bilirubin
 Hemolytic anemias
 Resorption of blood from internal hemorrhage
  (e.g., alimentary tract bleeding, hematomas)
 Ineffective erythropoiesis syndromes
  (e.g., pernicious anemia, thalassemia)
Reduced hepatic uptake
 Drug interference with membrane carrier systems
 Some cases of Gilbert syndrome
Impaired bilirubin conjugation
 Physiologic jaundice of the newborn
  (decreased UGT activity, decreased excretion)
 Breast milk jaundice (?inhibition of UGT activity)
 Genetic deficiency of bilirubin UGT activity
  (Crigler-Najjar syndromes types I and II)
 Gilbert syndrome (mixed etiologies)
 Diffuse hepatocellular disease
  (e.g., viral or drug-induced hepatitis, cirrhosis)
Predominantly Conjugated Hyperbilirubinemia
Decreased hepatic excretion of bilirubin glucuronides
 Deficiency in canalicular membrane transporters
  (Dubin-Johnson syndrome, Rotor's syndrome)
 Drug-induced canalicular membrane dysfunction
  (e.g., oral contraceptives, cyclosporine)
 Hepatocellular damage or toxicity
  (e.g., viral or drug-induced hepatitis, total parenteral nutrition,
  systemic infection)
Decreased intrahepatic bile flow
 Impaired bile flow through bile canaliculi
  (e.g., drug-induced microfilament dysfunction)
 Inflammatory destruction of intrahepatic bile ducts
  (e.g., primary biliary cirrhosis, primary sclerosing cholangitis,
  graft-versus-host disease, liver transplantation)
Extrahepatic biliary obstruction
 Gallstone obstruction of biliary tree
 Carcinomas of head of pancreas, extrahepatic bile ducts, ampulla
  of Vater
 Extrahepatic biliary atresia
 Biliary strictures and choledochal cysts
 Primary sclerosing cholangitis (extrahepatic)
 Liver fluke infestation

UGT, uridine diphosphate glucuronosyltransferase.

Of the various causes of jaundice listed in Table 16–3, the most common are hemolytic anemias (Chapter 12), hepatitis, and obstruction to the flow of bile (discussed later in this chapter). Physiologic jaundice of the newborn and jaundice resulting from inborn errors of metabolism merit brief consideration.

■ Because the hepatic machinery for conjugating and excreting bilirubin does not fully mature until about 2 weeks of age, almost every newborn develops transient and mild unconjugated hyperbilirubinemia, termed *neonatal jaundice* or *physiologic jaundice of the newborn*. Breast-fed infants tend to exhibit jaundice with greater frequency, possibly because of β-glucuronidases present in maternal milk.

■ *Crigler-Najjar syndrome type I* is a rare genetic condition in which there is a complete lack of the enzyme responsible for the conjugation of glucuronic acid to bilirubin (bilirubin UGT). This syndrome is invariably fatal, causing death within 18 months of birth secondary to brain damage (kernicterus).

■ *Crigler-Najjar syndrome type II* is a less severe, nonfatal disorder exhibiting a partial defect in bilirubin conjugation; the major consequence is extraordinarily yellow skin.

■ *Gilbert syndrome* is a relatively common, benign, somewhat heterogeneous inherited condition presenting with mild, fluctuating unconjugated hyperbilirubinemia. The primary cause is decreased hepatic levels of bilirubin UGT, although hepatic uptake may be impaired in some instances. Affecting up to 7% of the population, the hyperbilirubinemia may go undiscovered for years and *is not associated with functional derangements.*

■ *Dubin-Johnson syndrome* results from a hereditary defect in hepatocellular excretion of bilirubin glucuronides across the canalicular membrane. These patients exhibit conjugated hyperbilirubinemia, and the liver is darkly pigmented. Electron microscopy reveals coarse granules in hepatocellular lysosomes, which appear to be polymers of epinephrine metabolites.

■ *Rotor's syndrome* represents a form of asymptomatic conjugated hyperbilirubinemia with multiple defects in hepatocellular uptake and excretion of bilirubin pigments. The liver is not pigmented.

CHOLESTASIS

Cholestatic conditions, which result from hepatocellular dysfunction or intrahepatic or extrahepatic biliary obstruction, may also present as jaundice. Alternatively, *pruritus* may be a common presenting symptom, presumably related to the elevation in plasma bile acids and their deposition in peripheral tissues, particularly skin. *Skin xanthomas* (focal accumulations of cholesterol) sometimes appear, the result of hyperlipidemia and impaired excretion of cholesterol. A *characteristic laboratory finding is an elevated level of serum alkaline phosphatase,* an enzyme present in bile duct epithelium and in the canalicular membrane of hepatocytes. An isozyme is normally present in many other tissues such as bone, and so the increased levels must be verified as being hepatic in origin. Other manifestations of reduced bile flow relate to intestinal malabsorption, including inadequate absorption of the fat-soluble vitamins A, D, and K.

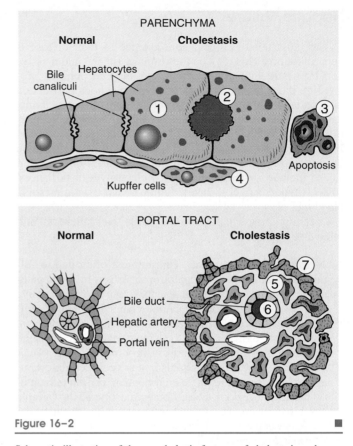

PARENCHYMA

Normal   Cholestasis

Bile canaliculi   Hepatocytes   ① ② ③ Apoptosis

Kupffer cells   ④

PORTAL TRACT

Normal   Cholestasis

Bile duct ⑤ ⑦
Hepatic artery ⑥
Portal vein

Figure 16–2   ■

Schematic illustration of the morphologic features of cholestasis and comparison with normal liver. In the parenchyma *(upper panel),* cholestatic hepatocytes (1) are enlarged with dilated canalicular spaces (2). Apoptotic cells (3) may be seen, and Kupffer cells (4) frequently contain regurgitated bile pigments. In the portal tracts of obstructed livers *(lower panel),* there is also bile duct proliferation (5), edema, bile pigment retention (6), and eventually neutrophilic inflammation *(not shown).* Surrounding hepatocytes (7) are swollen and undergoing toxic degeneration.

The morphologic features of cholestasis are similar for both nonobstructive and obstructive conditions. **Common to both forms is the accumulation of bile pigment within the hepatic parenchyma** (Fig. 16–2). Elongated green-brown plugs of bile are visible in dilated bile canaliculi. Rupture of canaliculi leads to extravasation of bile, which is quickly phagocytosed by Kupffer cells. Droplets of bile pigment also accumulate within hepatocytes, which can take on a wispy appearance (feathery or **foamy degeneration**). **Obstruction to the biliary tree, either intrahepatic or extrahepatic, induces distention of upstream bile ducts by bile.** The bile stasis and back-pressure induces proliferation of the duct epithelial cells and looping and redupli-

cation of ducts, termed **bile duct proliferation.** Associated portal tract findings include edema and periductal infiltrates of neutrophils. Prolonged obstructive cholestasis leads not only to foamy change of hepatocytes but also to focal destruction of the parenchyma, giving rise to **bile lakes** filled with cellular debris and pigment. **Unrelieved obstruction leads to portal tract fibrosis,** which initially extends into and subdivides the parenchyma with relative preservation of hepatic architecture. Ultimately, an end-stage bile-stained, cirrhotic liver is created (biliary cirrhosis, discussed later).

Because extrahepatic biliary obstruction is frequently amenable to surgical alleviation, correct and prompt diagnosis is imperative. In contrast, cholestasis due to diseases of the intrahepatic biliary tree or hepatocellular secretory failure (collectively termed *intrahepatic cholestasis*) cannot be benefited by surgery (short of transplantation), and the patient's condition may be worsened by an operative procedure. *There is thus some urgency in making a correct diagnosis of the cause of jaundice and cholestasis.*

Hepatic Failure

The most severe clinical consequence of liver disease is hepatic failure. This may be the result of sudden and massive hepatic destruction. More often, it is the end point of progressive damage to the liver, either by insidious destruction of hepatocytes or by repetitive discrete waves of parenchymal damage. Whatever the sequence, 80% to 90% of hepatic functional capacity must be eroded before hepatic failure ensues. In many cases, the balance is tipped toward decompensation by intercurrent diseases, which place demands on the liver. These include systemic infections, electrolyte disturbances, stress (major surgery, heart failure), and gastrointestinal bleeding.

The morphologic alterations that cause liver failure fall into three categories:

1. *Massive hepatic necrosis.* This is most often due to fulminant viral hepatitis (hepatotropic viruses or nonhepatotropic). Drugs and chemicals also may induce massive necrosis and include acetaminophen, halothane, antituberculosis drugs (rifampin, isoniazid), antidepressant monoamine oxidase inhibitors, industrial chemicals such as carbon tetrachloride, and mushroom poisoning (*Amanita phalloides*). The mechanism may be direct toxic damage to hepatocytes (e.g., acetaminophen, carbon tetrachloride, and mushroom toxins) but more often is a variable combination of toxicity and inflammation with immune-mediated hepatocyte destruction.
2. *Chronic liver disease.* This is the most common route to hepatic failure and is the end point of relentless chronic liver damage ending in cirrhosis. The many causes of cirrhosis are discussed later.
3. *Hepatic dysfunction without overt necrosis.* Hepatocytes may be viable but unable to perform normal metabolic function, as in Reye's syndrome, tetracycline toxicity, and acute fatty liver of pregnancy.

Clinical Features. Regardless of cause, the clinical signs of hepatic failure are much the same. *Jaundice* is an almost invariable finding. Impaired hepatic synthesis and secretion of albumin leads to *hypoalbuminemia,* which predisposes to peripheral edema. *Hyperammonemia* is attributable to defective hepatic urea cycle function. *Fetor hepaticus* is a characteristic body odor variously described as "musty" or "sweet and sour" and occurs occasionally. It is related to the formation of mercaptans by the action of gastrointestinal bacteria on the sulfur-containing amino acid methionine, and shunting of splanchnic blood from the portal into the systemic circulation (portosystemic shunting). Impaired estrogen metabolism and consequent hyperestrogenemia are the putative causes of *palmar erythema* (a reflection of local vasodilatation) and *spider angiomas* of the skin. Each angioma is a central, pulsating, dilated arteriole from which small vessels radiate. In the male, hyperestrogenemia also leads to *hypogonadism* and *gynecomastia.*

Hepatic failure is life threatening for a number of reasons. First, with severely impaired liver function, patients are highly susceptible to failure of multiple organ systems. Thus, respiratory failure with pneumonia and sepsis combine with renal failure to claim the lives of many patients with hepatic failure.

A *coagulopathy* develops, attributable to impaired hepatic synthesis of blood clotting factors II, VII, IX, and X. The resultant bleeding tendency may lead to massive gastrointestinal hemorrhage as well as petechial bleeding elsewhere. Intestinal absorption of blood places a metabolic load on the liver that worsens the severity of hepatic failure. The outlook of full-blown hepatic failure is grave: a rapid downhill course is usual, with death occurring within weeks to a few months in about 80%. A fortunate few can be tided over an acute episode until hepatocellular regeneration restores adequate hepatic function. Alternatively, liver transplantation may save the patient.

Two particular complications merit separate consideration, because they herald the most grave stages of hepatic failure.

HEPATIC ENCEPHALOPATHY

Hepatic encephalopathy is a feared complication of acute and chronic liver failure. Patients exhibit a spectrum of disturbances in consciousness, ranging from subtle behavioral abnormalities to marked confusion and stupor, to deep coma and death. These changes may progress over hours or days as, for example, in fulminant hepatic failure, or more insidiously in a patient with marginal hepatic function from chronic liver disease. Associated fluctuating neurologic signs include rigidity, hyperreflexia, nonspecific electroencephalographic changes, and, rarely, seizures. Particularly characteristic is *asterixis,* which is a pattern of nonrhythmic, rapid extension-flexion movements of the head and extremities, best seen when the arms are held in extension with dorsiflexed wrists.

Hepatic encephalopathy is regarded as a metabolic disorder of the central nervous system and neuromuscular system. In most instances, there are only minor morphologic changes in the brain, such as edema and an astrocytic reaction. Two physiologic factors appear to be important in the genesis of this disorder: (1) severe loss of hepatocellular function and (2) shunting of blood around the chronically diseased liver. The net result is exposure of the brain to an altered metabolic milieu, the specifics of which remain unclear. However, a key feature appears to be an elevated blood ammonia level, which impairs neuronal function and promotes generalized brain edema.

HEPATORENAL SYNDROME

Hepatorenal syndrome refers to the appearance of renal failure in patients with severe liver disease, in whom there are no intrinsic morphologic or functional causes for the renal failure. Excluded by this definition are concomitant damage to both organs, as may occur with carbon tetrachloride exposure, certain mycotoxins, and the copper toxicity of Wilson's disease. Also excluded are instances of advanced hepatic failure in which circulatory collapse leads to acute tubular necrosis and renal failure. Kidney function promptly improves if hepatic failure is reversed. Although the exact cause is unknown, evidence points to vasoconstriction with reduction of renal blood flow, particularly to the cortex. Onset of this syndrome is typically heralded by a drop in urine output, associated with rising blood urea nitrogen and creatinine values. *The ability to concentrate urine is retained, producing a hyperosmolar urine devoid of proteins and abnormal sediment that is sur-*

prisingly low in sodium (unlike renal tubular necrosis). The renal failure may hasten death in the patient with acute fulminant or advanced chronic hepatic disease. Alternatively, borderline renal insufficiency (serum creatinine of 2 to 3 mg/dl) may persist for weeks to months, as in cirrhotic patients whose ascites is refractory to diuretic therapy.

Cirrhosis

Cirrhosis is among the top 10 causes of death in the Western world. Although largely the result of alcohol abuse, other major contributors include chronic hepatitis, biliary disease, and iron overload. This end stage of chronic liver disease is defined by three characteristics:

1. *Bridging fibrous septa* in the form of delicate bands or broad scars replacing multiple adjacent lobules
2. *Parenchymal nodules* created by regeneration of encircled hepatocytes, varying from very small (<3 mm in diameter, micronodules) to large (several centimeters in diameter, macronodules)
3. Disruption of the architecture of the *entire liver*

The parenchymal injury and consequent fibrosis are diffuse, extending throughout the liver; focal injury with scarring does not constitute cirrhosis. Moreover, the fibrosis, once developed, is generally irreversible, although regression is observed in rare instances.

There is no satisfactory classification of cirrhosis save for specification of the presumed underlying etiology, which varies both geographically and socially. The following is the approximate frequency of etiologic categories in the Western world:

■ Alcoholic liver disease, 60% to 70%
■ Viral hepatitis, 10%
■ Biliary diseases, 5% to 10%
■ Genetic hemochromatosis, 5%
■ Wilson's disease, rare
■ α_1-Antitrypsin (ATT) deficiency, rare
■ Cryptogenic cirrhosis, 10% to 15%

Other infrequent types of cirrhosis are (1) the cirrhosis developing in infants and children with galactosemia or tyrosinosis; (2) liver destruction by a diffusely infiltrative cancer; (3) drug-induced cirrhosis, as with α-methyldopa; and (4) syphilis. Severe sclerosis can occur in the setting of cardiac disease (sometimes called cardiac cirrhosis, discussed later). After all the categories of cirrhosis of known causation have been excluded, a substantial number of cases remain, referred to as cryptogenic cirrhosis. The magnitude of this "wastebasket" speaks eloquently to the difficulties in discerning the many origins of cirrhosis. Once cirrhosis is established, it is extremely difficult to establish an etiologic diagnosis on histologic grounds alone.

Pathogenesis. The central pathogenetic process in cirrhosis is progressive fibrosis. In the normal liver, interstitial collagens (types I and III) are concentrated in portal tracts and around central veins, with occasional bundles in the parenchyma. A delicate reticulin framework of type IV collagen lies in the space between sinusoidal endothelial cells and hepatocytes (the space of Disse). In cirrhosis, types I and III collagen are deposited in all portions of the lobule, accompanied by alterations in the sinusoidal endothelial cells. The net result is severe disruption of blood flow and impaired diffusion of solutes between hepatocytes and plasma. In particular, the movement of proteins (e.g., albumin, clotting factors, lipoproteins) between hepatocytes and the plasma is markedly impaired.

The major source of excess collagen in cirrhosis appears to be the fat-storing stellate cell or Ito cell, which lies in the space of Disse. Although they normally function as vitamin A fat-storage cells, during the development of cirrhosis they become activated, loose their retinyl ester stores, and transform into myofibroblast-like cells. The stimuli for synthesis and deposition of collagen may come from several sources:

■ Chronic inflammation, with production of inflammatory cytokines such as tumor necrosis factor alpha (TNF-α) and beta (TNF-β) and interleukin 1
■ Cytokine production by injured endogenous cells (Kupffer cells, endothelial cells, hepatocytes, and bile duct epithelial cells)
■ Disruption of the extracellular matrix
■ Direct stimulation of stellate cells by toxins

Clinical Features. All forms of cirrhosis may be clinically silent. When symptomatic they lead to nonspecific manifestations: anorexia, weight loss, weakness, and, in advanced disease, frank debilitation. Incipient or overt hepatic failure may develop, usually precipitated by imposition of a metabolic load on the liver, as from systemic infection or a gastrointestinal hemorrhage. The ultimate mechanism of death in most patients with cirrhosis is (1) progressive liver failure, (2) a complication related to portal hypertension, or (3) the development of hepatocellular carcinoma.

PORTAL HYPERTENSION

Increased resistance to portal blood flow may develop in a variety of circumstances, which can be divided into prehepatic, intrahepatic, and posthepatic causes. The major prehepatic conditions are occlusive thrombosis and narrowing of the portal vein before it ramifies within the liver. Massive splenomegaly also may shunt excessive blood into the splenic vein. The major posthepatic causes are severe right-sided heart failure, constrictive pericarditis, and hepatic vein outflow obstruction. *The dominant intrahepatic cause is cirrhosis, accounting for most cases of portal hypertension.* Far less frequent are schistosomiasis, massive fatty change, diffuse granulomatous diseases such as sarcoidosis and miliary tuberculosis, and diseases affecting the portal microcirculation, exemplified by nodular regenerative hyperplasia (discussed later).

Portal hypertension in cirrhosis results from increased resistance to portal flow at the level of the sinusoids, and compression of central veins by perivenular fibrosis and expansile parenchymal nodules. Anastomoses between the arterial and portal systems in the fibrous bands also contribute to portal hypertension by imposing arterial pressure on the low-pressure portal venous system. The four major clinical consequences are (1) ascites; (2) the formation of portosystemic venous shunts; (3) congestive splenomegaly; and (4) hepatic encephalopathy (discussed earlier). The manifestations of portal hypertension in the setting of cirrhosis are illustrated in Figure 16–3, and described next.

Ascites. Ascites refers to the collection of excess fluid in the peritoneal cavity. It usually becomes clinically detectable when at least 500 ml has accumulated, but many liters may collect and cause massive abdominal distention. It is generally a serous fluid having up to 3 gm/dl of protein (largely albumin) as well as the same concentrations of solutes such as glucose, sodium, and potassium as in the blood. The fluid may contain a scant number of mesothelial cells and mononuclear leukocytes. Influx of neutrophils suggests secondary infection, whereas red cells point to possible disseminated intra-abdominal cancer. With long-standing ascites, seepage of peritoneal fluid through transdiaphragmatic lymphatics may produce hydrothorax, more often on the right side.

The pathogenesis of ascites is complex, involving one or more of the following mechanisms:

- Sinusoidal hypertension, altering Starling's forces and driving fluid into the space of Disse, which is then removed by hepatic lymphatics; this movement of fluid is also promoted by hypoalbuminemia.
- Percolation of hepatic lymph into the peritoneal cavity: normal thoracic duct lymph flow approximates 800 to 1000 ml/day. With cirrhosis, hepatic lymphatic flow may approach 20 L/day, exceeding thoracic duct capacity. Hepatic lymph is rich in proteins and low in triglycerides, which is reflected in the protein-rich ascitic fluid.
- Renal retention of sodium and water due to secondary hyperaldosteronism (Chapter 4), despite a total body sodium value greater than normal.

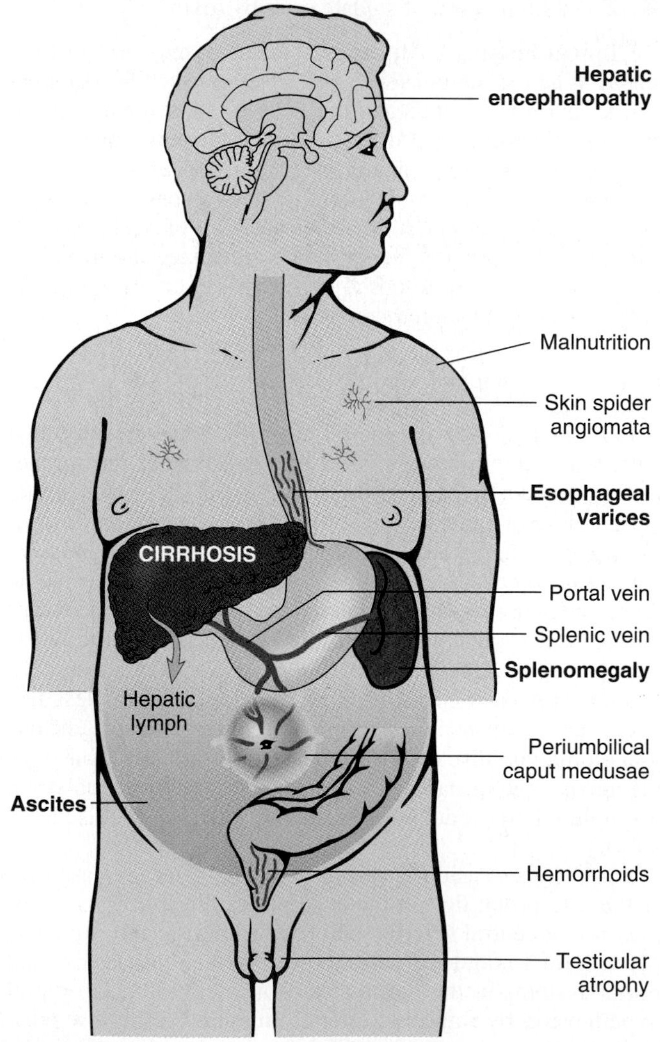
Hepatic encephalopathy
Malnutrition
Skin spider angiomata
Esophageal varices
CIRRHOSIS
Portal vein
Splenic vein
Splenomegaly
Hepatic lymph
Periumbilical caput medusae
Ascites
Hemorrhoids
Testicular atrophy

Figure 16–3

The major clinical consequences of portal hypertension in the setting of cirrhosis.

Portosystemic Shunts. With the rise in portal system pressure, bypasses develop wherever the systemic and portal circulation share capillary beds. Principal sites are veins around and within the rectum (manifest as hemorrhoids), the cardioesophageal junction (producing esophagogastric varices), the retroperitoneum, and the falciform ligament of the liver (involving periumbilical and abdominal wall collaterals). Although hemorrhoidal bleeding may occur, it is rarely massive or life threatening. Much more important are the esophagogastric varices that appear in about 65% of patients with advanced cirrhosis of the liver and cause massive hematemesis and death in about half of them. Abdominal wall collaterals appear as dilated subcutaneous veins extending from the umbilicus toward the rib margins (caput medusae) and constitute an important clinical hallmark of portal hypertension.

Splenomegaly. Long-standing congestion may cause congestive splenomegaly. The degree of enlargement varies widely (up to 1000 gm) and is not necessarily correlated with other features of portal hypertension. Massive splenomegaly may secondarily induce a variety of hematologic abnormalities attributable to hypersplenism (Chapter 12).

INFLAMMATORY DISORDERS

Inflammatory disorders of the liver dominate the clinical practice of hepatology. This in part is because virtually any insult to the liver can kill hepatocytes and recruit inflammatory cells, but also is because inflammatory diseases are frequently chronic and must be managed medically. Among inflammatory disorders, infection ranks supreme. The liver is almost inevitably involved in blood-borne infections, whether systemic or arising within the abdomen. Although discussed elsewhere, those in which the hepatic lesion is prominent include miliary tuberculosis, malaria, staphylococcal bacteremia, the salmonelloses, candidiasis, and amebiasis. The foremost primary hepatic infections are the viral hepatitides.

Viral Hepatitis

Systemic viral infections that can involve the liver include (1) infectious mononucleosis (Epstein-Barr virus), which may cause a mild hepatitis during the acute phase; (2) cytomegalovirus or herpesvirus infections, particularly in the newborn or immunosuppressed patient; and (3) yellow fever, which has been a major and serious cause of hepatitis in tropical countries. Infrequently in children and immunosuppressed patients, the liver is affected in the course of rubella, adenovirus, or enterovirus infections. However, unless otherwise specified, the term *viral hepatitis* is reserved for infection of the liver caused by a small (but growing) group of viruses having a particular affinity for the liver (Table 16–4). Because these viruses cause similar morphologic patterns of disease, the histologic changes in viral hepatitis are described together, after an introduction to the specific forms of viral hepatitis.

ETIOLOGIC AGENTS

Hepatitis A Virus (HAV). Hepatitis A, long known as "infectious hepatitis," is a benign, self-limited disease with an incubation period of 2 to 6 weeks. *HAV does not cause chronic hepatitis or a carrier state and only rarely causes fulminant hepatitis, and so the fatality rate associated with HAV is about 0.1%.* HAV occurs throughout the world and is endemic in countries with substandard hygiene and sanitation, so that most native populations have detectable anti-HAV by the age of 10 years. Clinical disease tends to be mild or asymptomatic and rare after childhood. In developed countries, the prevalence of seropositivity increases gradually with age, reaching 50% by age 50 years in the United States.

HAV is spread by ingestion of contaminated water and foods and is shed in the stool for 2 to 3 weeks before and 1 week after the onset of jaundice. Thus, close personal contact with an infected individual or fecal-oral contamination during this period accounts for most cases and explains the outbreaks in institutional settings such as schools and nurseries. Waterborne epidemics occur in developing countries where people live in overcrowded, unsanitary conditions. HAV is not shed in any significant quantities in saliva, urine, or semen. Among developed countries, sporadic infections may be contracted by the consumption of raw or steamed shellfish (oysters, mussels, clams), which concentrate the virus from sea water contaminated with human sewage. *Because HAV viremia is transient, blood-borne transmission of HAV occurs only rarely and, therefore, donated blood is not specifically screened for this virus.*

HAV is a small, nonenveloped, single-stranded RNA picornavirus. The virus itself does not appear to be cytotoxic to hepatocytes, and hence the liver injury seems to result from immunologically mediated damage of infected hepatocytes. As depicted in Figure 16–4, specific antibody against HAV of the IgM type appears in blood at the onset of symptoms, constituting a reliable marker of acute infection. Fecal shedding of the virus ends as the IgM titer rises. The IgM response declines in a few months, accompanied by the appearance of IgG anti-HAV. The latter persists for life, providing immunity against reinfection by all strains of HAV (hence the value of vaccination).

Hepatitis B Virus (HBV). HBV (the cause of "serum hepatitis") can produce (1) acute hepatitis, (2) chronic nonprogressive hepatitis, (3) progressive chronic disease ending in

Table 16–4.   THE HEPATITIS VIRUSES

	Hepatitis A Virus	Hepatitis B Virus	Hepatitis C Virus	Hepatitis D Virus	Hepatitis E Virus	Hepatitis G Virus
Year of Identification	1973	1965	1989	1977	1980	1995
Agent	27 nm icosahedral capsid, ssRNA	42 nm enveloped dsDNA	30–60 nm enveloped ssRNA	35 nm enveloped ssRNA; replication defective	32–34 nm unenveloped ssRNA	ssRNA virus
Classification	Picornavirus	Hepadnavirus	Flavivirus	Unknown	Caliciviridae	Flavivirus
Transmission	Fecal-oral	Parenteral; close personal contact	Parenteral; close personal contact	Parenteral; close personal contact	Water-borne	Parenteral
Incubation Period (Weeks)	2–6	4–26	2–26	4–7 in superinfection	2–8	Unknown
Fulminant Hepatitis	0.1%–0.4%	<1%	Rare	3%–4% in co-infection	0.3%–3%; 20% in pregnant women	Unknown
Carrier State	None	0.1%–1.0% of blood donors in United States and western world	0.2%–1.0% of blood donors in United States and western world	1%–10% in drug addicts and hemophiliacs	Unknown	1%–2% of blood donors in United States (estimated)
Chronic Hepatitis	None	5%–10% of acute infections	>50%	<5% co-infection, 80% superinfection	None	None
Hepatocellular Carcinoma	No	Yes	Yes	No increase above hepatitis B virus	Unknown, but unlikely	Unknown

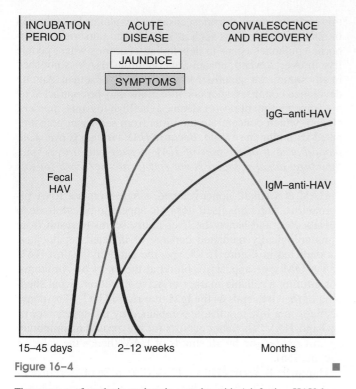

INCUBATION PERIOD | ACUTE DISEASE | CONVALESCENCE AND RECOVERY

JAUNDICE

SYMPTOMS

IgG–anti-HAV

Fecal HAV

IgM–anti-HAV

15–45 days | 2–12 weeks | Months

Figure 16–4 ■

The sequence of serologic markers in acute hepatitis A infection. HAV, hepatitis A virus.

cirrhosis, (4) fulminant hepatitis with massive liver necrosis, and (5) an asymptomatic carrier state, with or without progressive subclinical disease. HBV also plays an important role in the development of hepatocellular carcinoma. Figure 16–5 depicts the approximate frequencies of these outcomes.

Globally, liver disease caused by hepatitis B virus is an enormous problem with an estimated worldwide carrier rate of 300 million; in the United States alone there are 300,000 new infections per year. Unlike HAV, HBV remains in blood during the last stages of a prolonged incubation period (4 to 26 weeks) and during active episodes of acute and chronic hepatitis. It is also present in all physiologic and pathologic body fluids, with the exception of stool. HBV is a hardy virus and can withstand extremes of temperature and humidity. Thus, whereas blood and body fluids are the primary vehicles of transmission, virus may also be spread by contact with body secretions such as semen, saliva, sweat, tears, breast milk, and pathologic effusions. *Transfusion, blood products, dialysis, needle-stick accidents among health care workers, intravenous drug abuse, and homosexual activity constitute the primary risk categories for HBV infection.* In one third of patients the source of infection is unknown. In endemic regions such as Africa and Southeast Asia, spread from an infected mother to a newborn during birth (vertical transmission) is common. These neonatal infections often lead to the carrier state for life.

HBV is a member of the Hepadnaviridae, a group of DNA-containing viruses that cause hepatitis in multiple animal species. The genome of HBV is a partially double-stranded circular DNA molecule having 3200 nucleotides, which codes for the following:

■ A nucleocapsid "core" protein (HBcAg, hepatitis B core antigen) and a longer polypeptide transcript with a precore and core region, designated HBeAg (hepatitis B "e" antigen)
■ Envelope glycoprotein (HBsAg, hepatitis B surface antigen)
■ DNA polymerase
■ A protein from the X region, which acts as a transcriptional transactivator of host genes and may play a role in the causation of hepatocellular carcinoma

Infected hepatocytes can synthesize and secrete massive quantities of noninfective surface protein (HBsAg), which appears in cells and serum as spheres and tubules 22 nm in diameter.

After exposure to the virus, the long asymptomatic 4- to 26-week incubation period (mean, 6 to 8 weeks) is followed by acute disease lasting many weeks to months. The natural course of acute disease can be followed by serum markers (Fig. 16–6):

■ HBsAg appears before the onset of symptoms, peaks during overt disease, and then declines to undetectable levels in 3 to 6 months.
■ HBeAg, HBV-DNA, and DNA polymerase appear in serum soon after HBsAg, and all signify active viral replication. Persistence of HBeAg is an important indicator of continued viral replication, infectivity, and probable progression to chronic hepatitis.
■ IgM anti-HBc becomes detectable in serum shortly before the onset of symptoms, concurrent with the onset of elevated serum transaminase levels. Over months the IgM anti-HBc antibody is replaced by IgG anti-HBc.
■ The appearance of anti-HBe antibodies implies that an acute infection has peaked and is on the wane.
■ IgG anti-HBs does not rise until the acute disease is over and is usually not detectable for a few weeks to several months after the disappearance of HBsAg. Anti-HBs may persist for life, conferring protection; this is the basis for current vaccination strategies using noninfectious HBsAg.

HBV infections pass through two phases. During the *proliferative phase*, HBV-DNA is present in episomal form, with formation of complete virions and all associated antigens. Cell surface expression of viral HBsAg and HBcAg in association with MHC class I molecules leads to activation of cytotoxic CD8+ T lymphocytes. An *integrative phase* may follow, in which viral DNA may be incorporated into the host genome. With cessation of viral replication and the appearance of antiviral antibodies, infectivity ends and liver damage subsides. However, the risk of hepatocellular carcinoma persists.

Occasionally, infectious variant strains of hepatitis B virus emerge that are incapable of HBeAg expression. The loss of circulating HBeAg, and hence anti-HBe formation, is associated with fulminant hepatitis. A second ominous development is the appearance of vaccine-induced escape mutants, which replicate in the presence of vaccine-induced immunity.

There are several reasons to believe that HBV does not cause direct hepatocyte injury. Most important, many chronic carriers have virions in their hepatocytes with no evidence of cell injury. Hepatocyte damage is believed to result from damage to the virus-infected cells by CD8+ cytotoxic T cells.

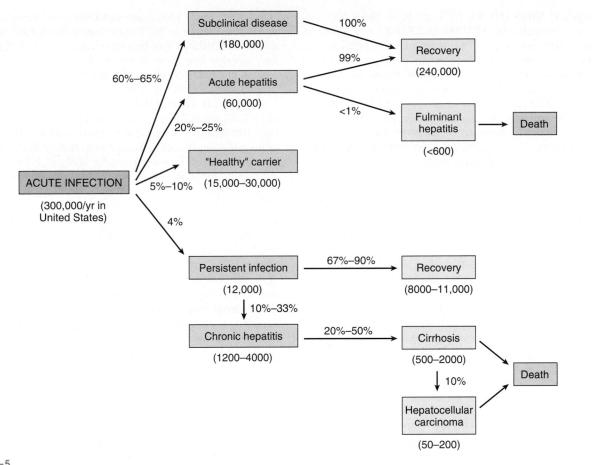

Figure 16-5

The potential outcomes of hepatitis B infection in adults, with their approximate annual frequencies in the United States. (Population estimates courtesy of John L. Gollan, MD, PhD, Brigham and Women's Hospital, Boston.)

Figure 16-6

The sequence of serologic markers in acute hepatitis B infection, showing resolution of active infection.

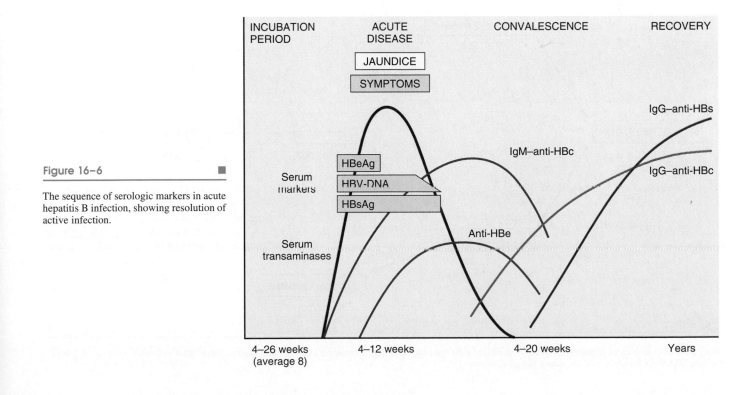

Hepatitis C Virus (HCV). HCV is also a major cause of liver disease worldwide; 150,000 to 170,000 new cases of HCV are estimated to occur annually in the United States. The major routes of transmission are inoculations and blood transfusions. Indeed, *HCV is believed to be the most important cause of transfusion-associated hepatitis, being responsible for 90% to 95% of cases.* Vertical transmission has been documented; transmission by sexual contact appears to be extremely low. Sporadic hepatitis of unknown source accounts for 40% of cases. *Unlike HBV, HCV has a high rate of progression to chronic disease and eventual cirrhosis, exceeding 50% (Fig. 16–7). Thus, HCV may in fact be the leading cause of chronic liver disease in the Western world.*

HCV occupies its own genus in the Flaviviridae and consists of a heterogeneous group of RNA virus strains. It is a small, enveloped, single-stranded RNA virus that is inherently unstable, and multiple types and subtypes have been documented (currently numbering more than 40). This variability has seriously hampered efforts to develop an HCV vaccine, particularly because *elevated titers of anti-HCV IgG occurring after active infection do not seem to confer effective immunity to subsequent HCV infection, either from reactivation of an endogenous strain or by infection with a new strain.*

The incubation period for HCV hepatitis ranges from 2 to 26 weeks, with a mean of 6 to 12 weeks. HCV RNA is detectable in blood for 1 to 3 weeks and is accompanied by elevations in serum transaminase levels. The clinical course of acute HCV hepatitis is usually milder than HBV hepatitis and is often asymptomatic. Although neutralizing anti-HCV antibodies develop within weeks to a few months, circulating HCV-RNA persists in a high percentage of patients. Hence, a characteristic feature of HCV infection is episodic elevations of serum transaminase levels, even in the absence of clinical symptoms, presumably reflecting recurrent bouts of hepato-

cellular necrosis. *Persistent infection and chronic hepatitis are the hallmarks of HCV infection in more than 50% of individuals.* Cirrhosis can be present at the time of diagnosis or may develop over 5 to 10 years. Alternatively, patients may have documented chronic HCV infection for decades, without progressing to cirrhosis. Fulminant hepatitis is rare.

Hepatitis D Virus (HDV). Also called hepatitis delta virus, HDV is a unique RNA virus that is replication defective, causing infection only when it is encapsulated by HBsAg. Thus, *although taxonomically distinct from HBV, HDV is absolutely dependent on HBV co-infection for multiplication.* Delta hepatitis thus arises in two settings (Fig. 16–8): (1) acute co-infection after exposure to serum containing both HDV and HBV and (2) superinfection of a chronic carrier of HBV with a new inoculum of HDV. In the first case, HBV infection must become established before HBsAg is available for development of complete HDV virions. Most co-infected individuals can clear the viruses and recover completely. Fulminant hepatitis, and rarely chronic hepatitis, may occur. The course is different in superinfected individuals. In most cases, there is an acceleration of hepatitis, most often to more severe chronic hepatitis, occurring 4 to 7 weeks later. The carrier may have been previously asymptomatic ("healthy") or may have already had underlying chronic hepatitis (Fig. 16–8).

Infection by HDV is worldwide, with prevalence rates of 20% to 40% in HBsAg carriers in Africa, the Middle East, and southern Italy. Surprisingly, HDV infection is uncommon in Southeast Asia and China. In the United States, HDV infection is largely restricted to drug addicts and hemophiliacs, who exhibit prevalence rates of 1% to 10%. Other high-risk groups for HBV are at low risk for HDV infection for unclear reasons.

HDV is a double-shelled particle that by electron microscopy resembles HBV. The external coat antigen of HBsAg

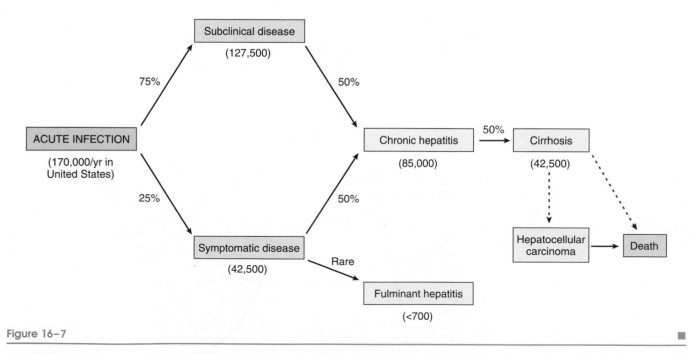

Figure 16–7

The potential outcomes of hepatitis C infection in adults, with their approximate frequencies in the United States. (Population estimates courtesy of John L. Gollan, MD, PhD, Brigham and Women's Hospital, Boston.)

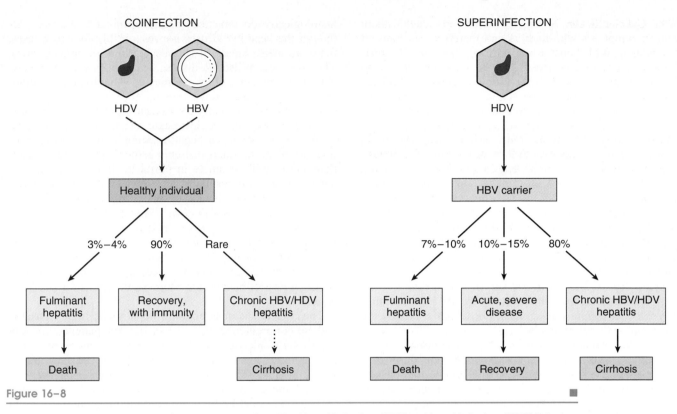

COINFECTION

SUPERINFECTION

HDV   HBV

HDV

Healthy individual

HBV carrier

3%–4%   90%   Rare

7%–10%   10%–15%   80%

Fulminant hepatitis   Recovery, with immunity   Chronic HBV/HDV hepatitis

Fulminant hepatitis   Acute, severe disease   Chronic HBV/HDV hepatitis

Death   Cirrhosis

Death   Recovery   Cirrhosis

Figure 16–8   ■

The differing clinical consequences of the two patterns of combined hepatitis D virus (HDV) and hepatitis B virus (HBV) infection.

surrounds an internal delta antigen (HDV Ag). Associated with HDV Ag is a small circular molecule of single-stranded RNA. Although insights into HDV-induced liver disease are few, HDV itself does not appear to be directly pathogenic; HBV appears to be critical for the pathologic effects of HDV.

HDV RNA and the HDV Ag are detectable in the blood and liver just before and in the early days of acute symptomatic disease. *IgM anti-HDV is the most reliable indicator of recent HDV exposure,* but its appearance is transient. Nevertheless, acute co-infection by HDV and HBV is best indicated by detection of IgM against both HDV Ag and HBcAg (denoting new infection with hepatitis B). With chronic delta hepatitis arising from HDV superinfection, HBsAg is present in serum, and anti-HDV antibodies (IgM and IgG) persist in low titer for months or longer.

Hepatitis E Virus (HEV). HEV hepatitis is an enterically transmitted, water-borne infection occurring primarily in young- to middle-aged adults; sporadic infection and overt illness in children are rare. Epidemics have been reported from Asia and the Indian subcontinent, sub-Saharan Africa, and Mexico. Sporadic infection seems to be uncommon and is seen mainly in travelers. *A characteristic feature of the infection is the high mortality rate among pregnant women, approaching 20%.* In most cases, the disease is self-limiting; HEV is not associated with chronic liver disease or persistent viremia. The average incubation period after exposure is 6 weeks (range, 2 to 8 weeks).

HEV is an unenveloped single-stranded RNA virus that is best characterized as a calicivirus. A specific antigen (HEV Ag) can be identified in the cytoplasm of hepatocytes during active infection. Virus can be detected in stool by immuno-electron microscopy, and serum anti-HEV and HEV-RNA are detectable.

Hepatitis G Virus. Epidemiologic studies have established that some cases of hepatitis are caused by infectious agents other than those listed earlier; these agents have tentatively been designated as "F" and "G." A viral agent bearing similarities to HCV has been cloned and has been designated hepatitis G virus. Transmission by transfusion has been documented, and HGV RNA has been found in patients with biopsy-proven cirrhosis. Information about this virus will surely accumulate rapidly in the coming years.

CLINICAL SYNDROMES

A number of clinical syndromes may develop after exposure to hepatitis viruses:

■ *Carrier state*: without apparent disease; or with subclinical chronic hepatitis
■ *Asymptomatic infection*: serologic evidence only
■ *Acute hepatitis*: anicteric or icteric
■ *Chronic hepatitis*: with or without progression to cirrhosis
■ *Fulminant hepatitis*: submassive to massive hepatic necrosis

Not all of the hepatotropic viruses provoke each of these clinical syndromes. With rare exception, HAV and HEV do not generate a carrier state or cause chronic hepatitis. Other infectious or noninfectious causes, particularly drugs and toxins, can lead to essentially identical syndromes. Therefore, serologic studies are critical for the diagnosis of viral hepatitis and the distinction between the various types.

The Carrier State. A "carrier" is an individual without manifest symptoms who harbors and therefore can transmit an organism. With hepatotropic viruses, there are (1) those who harbor one of the viruses but are suffering little or no adverse effects (a "healthy" carrier) and (2) those who have chronic liver damage but are essentially free of symptoms or disability. Both constitute reservoirs of infection. The carrier state is best characterized for HBV. Infection early in life, particularly through vertical transmission during childbirth, produces a carrier state 90% to 95% of the time. In contrast, only 1% to 10% of infections acquired in adulthood yield a carrier state. Individuals with impaired immunity are particularly likely to become carriers. The situation is less clear with HDV, although there is a well-defined low risk of post-transfusion hepatitis D, indicative of a carrier state in conjunction with HBV. HCV can clearly induce a carrier state, which is estimated to affect 0.2% to 0.6% of the general United States population.

Asymptomatic Infection. Not surprisingly, patients in this group are identified only incidentally on the basis of minimally elevated serum transaminases or after the fact by the presence of antiviral antibodies.

Acute Viral Hepatitis. Any one of the hepatotropic viruses can cause acute viral hepatitis. Whatever the agent, the disease is more or less the same and can be divided into four phases: (1) an incubation period, (2) a symptomatic preicteric phase, (3) a symptomatic icteric phase (with jaundice and scleral icterus), and (4) convalescence. The incubation period for the different viruses is provided in Table 16–4. Peak infectivity, attributed to the presence of circulating infectious viral particles, occurs during the last asymptomatic days of the incubation period and the early days of acute symptoms.

The preicteric phase is marked by nonspecific, constitutional symptoms. Malaise is followed in a few days by general fatigability, nausea, and loss of appetite. Weight loss, low-grade fever, headaches, muscle and joint aches, vomiting, and diarrhea are inconstant symptoms. About 10% of patients with acute hepatitis, most often those with hepatitis B, develop a serum sickness–like syndrome. This consists of fever, rash, and arthralgias, attributed to circulating immune complexes. The true origin of all these symptoms is suggested by elevated serum aminotransferase levels. Physical examination reveals a mildly enlarged, tender liver.

In some patients, the nonspecific symptoms are more severe, with higher fever, shaking chills, and headache, sometimes accompanied by right upper quadrant pain and tender liver enlargement. Surprisingly, as jaundice appears and these patients enter the icteric phase, other symptoms begin to abate. The jaundice is caused predominantly by conjugated hyperbilirubinemia and hence is accompanied by dark-colored urine related to the presence of conjugated bilirubin. The stools may become light colored, and the retention of bile salts may cause distressing skin itching (pruritus). An icteric phase is usual in adults (but not children) with HAV but is absent in about half the cases of HBV and most cases of HCV. In a few weeks to perhaps several months, the jaundice and most of the other systemic symptoms clear as convalescence begins.

Chronic Viral Hepatitis. *Chronic hepatitis* is defined as symptomatic, biochemical, or serologic evidence of continuing or relapsing hepatic disease for more than 6 months, with histologically documented inflammation and necrosis. Although the hepatitis viruses are responsible for most cases, there are many causes of chronic hepatitis (described later). They include Wilson's disease, α_1-antitrypsin deficiency, chronic alcoholism, drugs (isoniazid, α-methyldopa, methotrexate), and autoimmunity.

From 1968 to the early 1990s, chronic hepatitis was classified according to the histologic extent of inflammation. Thus, chronic persistent hepatitis denoted inflammation confined to the portal tracts. Chronic active hepatitis denoted inflammation spilling out from portal tracts into the adjacent parenchyma, with resultant hepatocyte necrosis. However, this subclassification is now obsolete, because *it has become clear that etiology rather than the histologic pattern is the single most important factor determining probability of developing progressive chronic hepatitis.* In particular, HCV is notorious for causing a chronic hepatitis evolving to cirrhosis in a high percentage of patients (see Fig. 16–7 and Table 16–4), regardless of histologic features at the time of initial evaluation.

The clinical features of chronic hepatitis are highly variable and are not predictive of outcome. In some patients, the only signs of chronic disease are persistent elevations of serum transaminase levels, hence the misleading designation of "transaminitis." The most common symptom is fatigue, and less commonly malaise, loss of appetite, and bouts of mild jaundice. Physical findings are few, the most common being spider angiomas, palmar erythema, mild hepatomegaly, hepatic tenderness, and mild splenomegaly. Laboratory studies may reveal prolongation of the prothrombin time and, in some instances, hyperglobulinemia, hyperbilirubinemia, and mild elevations in alkaline phosphatase levels. Occasionally in cases of HBV and HCV, circulating antibody-antigen complexes produce immune-complex disease, in the form of vasculitis (subcutaneous or visceral, Chapter 10) and glomerulonephritis (Chapter 14).

The clinical course is highly variable. Patients may experience spontaneous remission or may have indolent disease without progression for years. Conversely, some patients have rapidly progressive disease and develop cirrhosis within a few years. The major causes of death relate to cirrhosis, with liver failure and hepatic encephalopathy, or massive hematemesis from esophageal varices. Patients with long-standing HBV (particularly neonatal) or HCV infection are at a substantially increased risk for hepatocellular carcinoma.

The general morphologic features of viral hepatitis are listed in Table 16–5 and are depicted schematically in Fig. 16–9. Whereas the other viruses do not impart specific cytopathic changes, **HBV infection may generate "ground-glass" hepatocytes:** a finely granular, eosinophilic cytoplasm shown by electron microscopy to contain spheres and tubules of HBsAg. Other HBV-infected hepatocytes may have **"sanded" nuclei** due to abundant HBcAg, **indicating active viral replication.**

The morphologic changes in acute and chronic viral hepatitis are shared among the hepatotropic viruses and can be mimicked by drug reactions.

Table 16-5.   KEY MORPHOLOGIC FEATURES OF VIRAL HEPATITIS

Carrier State
Essentially normal liver biopsy
HBV: "ground-glass" hepatocytes, "sanded" nuclei
HCV: chronic hepatitis usually present histologically

Acute Hepatitis
Enlarged, reddened liver; greenish if cholestatic
Parenchymal changes:
    Hepatocyte injury: swelling (ballooning degeneration)
        Cholestasis: canalicular bile plugs
        HCV: fatty change of hepatocytes
    Hepatocyte necrosis: isolated cells or clusters
        Cytolysis (rupture) or apoptosis (shrinkage)
        If severe: bridging necrosis (portal-portal, central-central, portal-central)
        Lobular disarray: loss of normal architecture
    Regenerative changes: hepatocyte proliferation
    Sinusoidal cell reactive changes:
        Accumulation of phagocytosed cellular debris in Kupffer cells
        Influx of mononuclear cells into sinusoids
Portal tracts:
    Inflammation: predominantly mononuclear
    Inflammatory spillover into adjacent parenchyma, with hepatocyte necrosis

Chronic Hepatitis
Changes shared with acute hepatitis:
    Hepatocyte injury, necrosis, and regeneration
    Sinusoidal cell reactive changes
Portal tracts:
    Inflammation:
        Confined to portal tracts, *or*
        Spillover into adjacent parenchyma, with necrosis of hepatocytes, *or*
        Bridging inflammation and necrosis
    Fibrosis:
        Portal deposition, *or*
        Portal and periportal deposition, *or*
        Formation of bridging fibrous septa
    HCV: bile duct epithelial cell proliferation, lymphoid aggregate formation

Cirrhosis: the End-Stage Outcome

With acute hepatitis, hepatocyte injury takes the form of diffuse swelling (**ballooning degeneration**), so that the cytoplasm looks empty and contains only scattered wisps of cytoplasmic remnants. An inconstant finding is **cholestasis,** with bile plugs in canaliculi and brown pigmentation of hepatocytes. **Fatty change** is unusual except with HCV.

Two patterns of hepatocyte necrosis are seen. In the first, rupture of cell membranes leads to cytolysis. The necrotic cells appear to have "dropped out," with collapse of the collagen reticulin framework where the cells have disappeared; scavenger **macrophage aggregates** mark sites of dropout. The second pattern of cell death, **apoptosis,** is more distinctive. Apoptotic hepatocytes (Councilman bodies) shrink, become intensely eosinophilic, and have fragmented nuclei; effector T cells may still be present in the immediate vicinity. Apoptotic cells also are phagocytosed within

hours by macrophages, and hence may be difficult to find despite extensive apoptosis. In severe cases, confluent necrosis of hepatocytes may lead to **bridging necrosis** connecting portal-to-portal, central-to-central, or portal-to-central regions of adjacent lobules, signifying a more severe form of acute hepatitis. Hepatocyte swelling, necrosis, and regeneration produce compression of the vascular sinusoids and loss of the normal, more or less radial array of the parenchyma (so-called lobular disarray).

Inflammation is a characteristic and usually prominent feature of acute hepatitis. **Kupffer cells undergo hypertrophy and hyperplasia** and are often laden with lipofuscin pigment due to phagocytosis of hepatocellular debris. **The portal tracts are usually infiltrated with a mixture of inflammatory cells.** The inflammatory infiltrate may spill over into the parenchyma to cause necrosis of periportal hepatocytes. Although **periportal necrosis** can occur in both acute and chronic hepatitis, the term **piecemeal necrosis** has been used to describe this process in chronic hepatitis, engendering considerable confusion as to its prognostic significance. Etiology, not the presence or absence of piecemeal necrosis, is the most important indicator of the likelihood of progressive chronic disease. Finally, bile duct epithelia may become reactive and even proliferate, particularly in cases of HCV hepatitis, forming poorly defined ductular structures.

The histologic features of **chronic hepatitis** range from exceedingly mild to severe. Smoldering hepatocyte necrosis throughout the lobule may occur in all forms of chronic hepatitis. In the mildest forms, significant inflammation is limited to portal tracts and consists of lymphocytes, macrophages, occasional plasma cells, and rare neutrophils or eosinophils. **Lymphoid aggregates** in the portal tract are often seen in HCV infection. Liver architecture is usually well preserved. Continued **periportal necrosis** and **bridging necrosis** are harbingers of progressive liver damage. **The hallmark of irreversible liver damage is the deposition of fibrous tissue.** At first only portal tracts exhibit increased fibrosis, but with time **periportal fibrosis** occurs, followed by linking of fibrous septa between lobules (**bridging fibrosis**).

Continued loss of hepatocytes and fibrosis results in cirrhosis, with fibrous septa and hepatocyte regenerative nodules. This pattern of cirrhosis is characterized by irregularly sized nodules separated by variable but mostly broad scars (Fig. 16–10). Historically, this pattern of cirrhosis has been termed postnecrotic cirrhosis, but it should be noted that this term has been applied to all forms of cirrhosis in which the liver shows large irregular-sized nodules with broad scars, regardless of etiology. Hepatotoxins (carbon tetrachloride, mushroom poisoning), pharmaceutical agents

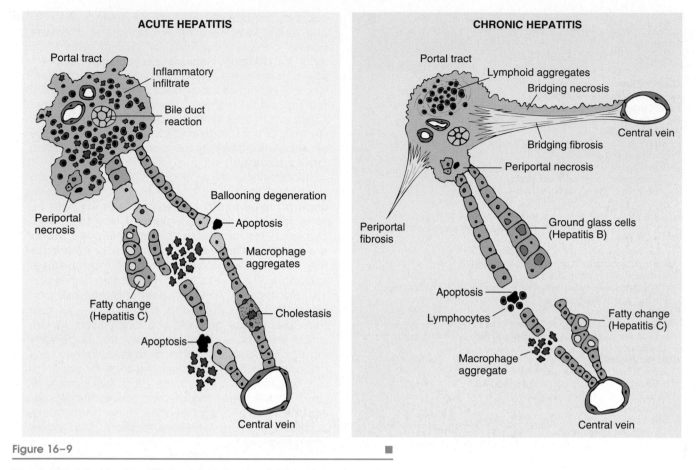

Figure 16–9 ■

Diagrammatic representation of the morphologic features of acute and chronic hepatitis.

(acetaminophen, α-methyldopa), and even alcohol (discussed later) may give rise to a nodular liver with fibrosis. In some cases that come to autopsy the inciting cause of the so-called postnecrotic cirrhosis cannot be determined at all (cryptogenic cirrhosis). It is thus best to avoid the use of the term postnecrotic cirrhosis because it is neither helpful in determining the basis of the liver injury nor related to any specific set of clinical circumstances.

Fulminant Hepatitis

Fulminant hepatic failure denotes hepatic insufficiency that progresses from onset of symptoms to hepatic encephalopathy within 2 to 3 weeks. A course extending up to 3 months is called subfulminant failure. Both patterns are fortunately uncommon. Viral hepatitis accounts for 50% to 65% of all cases: HBV is twice as frequent as HCV, with minor contributions from acute HDV-HBV, HAV, and herpesvirus. It is a serious complication of HEV infection in pregnant women (see Table 16–4). Various drugs and chemicals are responsible for 25% to 30% of cases, by acting as direct hepatotoxins or by evoking idiosyncratic inflammatory reactions. Principally implicated are acetaminophen (in suicidal doses), isoniazid, antidepressants (particularly monoamine oxidase inhibitors), halothane, methyldopa, and the mycotoxins of the mushroom *Amanita phalloides*. Other causes (discussed later) include obstruction of the hepatic veins, Wilson's disease, syndromes of microvesicular steatosis (e.g., acute fatty liver of pregnancy), massive malignant infiltration, reactivation of chronic hepa-

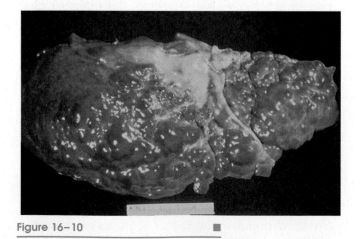

Figure 16–10 ■

Cirrhosis resulting from chronic viral hepatitis.

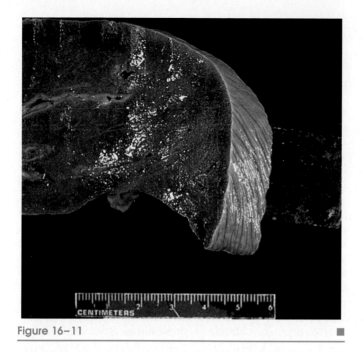

Figure 16–11 ■

Massive necrosis, cut section of liver. The liver is small (700 gm), bile stained, and soft in consistency. The capsule is wrinkled.

titis B or superinfection with HDV, autoimmune hepatitis, and hyperthermia (heat stroke).

All causative agents produce essentially identical morphologic changes that vary with the severity of the necrotizing process. With all, the distribution of liver destruction is extremely capricious: **the entire liver may be involved or only random areas.** With massive loss of substance, the liver may shrink to as little as 500 to 700 gm and become transformed into a limp, red organ covered by a wrinkled, too-large capsule. On transection (Fig. 16–11), necrotic areas have a muddy red, mushy appearance with blotchy bile staining. Microscopically, complete destruction of hepatocytes in contiguous lobules leaves only a collapsed reticulin framework and preserved portal tracts. There may be surprisingly little inflammatory reaction. Alternatively, with survival for several days there is a massive influx of inflammatory cells to begin the clean-up process (Fig. 16–12).

Patient survival for more than a week permits regeneration of surviving hepatocytes. If the parenchymal framework is preserved, regeneration is orderly and native liver architecture is restored in time. With more massive destruction of confluent lobules, regeneration is disorderly, yielding nodular masses of liver cells. Scarring may occur in patients with a protracted course of submassive or patchy necrosis, representing a route for developing so-called postnecrotic cirrhosis, as noted earlier.

Fulminant hepatic failure may present as jaundice, encephalopathy, and fetor hepaticus, as described previously. Notably absent on physical examination are stigmata of chronic liver disease (e.g., gynecomastia, spider angiomas). Life-threatening extrahepatic complications include coagulopathy with bleeding, cardiovascular instability, renal failure, adult respiratory distress syndrome, electrolyte and acid-base disturbances, and sepsis. Overall mortality ranges from 25% to 90% in the absence of liver transplantation.

Autoimmune Hepatitis

Autoimmune hepatitis is a syndrome of chronic hepatitis in patients with a heterogeneous set of immunologic abnormalities. The histologic features are indistinguishable from chronic viral hepatitis. This disease may run an indolent or severe course and typically responds dramatically to immunosuppressive therapy. Salient features include

- Female predominance (70%)
- The absence of serologic markers of a viral etiology
- Elevated serum IgG levels (>2.5 gm/dl)
- High titers of autoantibodies in 80% of cases, including antinuclear, anti–smooth muscle, and antimitochrondrial antibodies
- An increased frequency of HLA-B8 or HLA-DRw3

Other forms of autoimmune disease are present in up to 60% of patients, including rheumatoid arthritis, thyroiditis, Sjögren's syndrome, and ulcerative colitis. A subgroup of younger patients exhibits antibodies to liver/kidney microsome type 1, suggesting that two subtypes of autoimmune hepatitis exist.

Although autoimmune hepatitis presents with the entire spectrum of mild to severe chronic hepatitis, it is the symp-

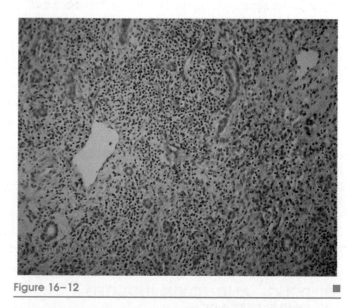

Figure 16–12 ■

Massive necrosis, microscopic section. The portal veins are closer together than normal owing to necrosis and collapse of the intervening parenchyma. The rudimentary ductal structures are the result of early hepatocyte regeneration. An infiltrate of chronic inflammatory cells is present.

tomatic patients who tend to present with established severe liver damage. The overall risk of cirrhosis is 5%. In these patients, death is largely a consequence of cirrhosis, as occurs in other types of chronic liver diseases.

Liver Abscesses

In developing countries, liver abscesses are common; most result from parasitic infections, such as amebic, echinococcal, and (less commonly) other protozoal and helminthic organisms. In developed countries, parasitic liver abscesses are distinctly uncommon, and many occur in immigrants. In the Western world, by contrast, bacterial or fungal abscesses are more common, representing a complication of an infection elsewhere. The organisms reach the liver through one of the following pathways: (1) ascending infection in the biliary tract (ascending cholangitis); (2) vascular seeding, either portal or arterial; (3) direct invasion of the liver from a nearby source; or (4) a penetrating injury. Debilitating disease with immune deficiency is a common setting; for example, extreme old age, immunosuppression, or cancer chemotherapy with marrow failure.

Pyogenic (bacterial) hepatic abscesses may occur as solitary or multiple lesions, ranging from millimeters to massive lesions many centimeters in diameter. Bacteremic spread through the arterial or portal system tends to produce multiple small abscesses, whereas direct extension and trauma usually cause solitary large abscesses. Biliary abscesses, which are usually multiple, may contain purulent material in adjacent bile ducts. Gross and microscopic features are those of any pyogenic abscess. Occasionally, fungi or parasites can be identified. On rare occasion, hepatic abscesses in the subdiaphragmatic region, particularly amebic ones, may extend into the thoracic cavity to produce empyema or a lung abscess.

Liver abscesses are associated with fever and, in many instances, with right upper quadrant pain and tender hepatomegaly. Jaundice is often the result of extrahepatic biliary obstruction. Although antibiotic therapy may control smaller lesions, surgical drainage is often necessary. Because diagnosis is frequently delayed, particularly in patients with serious coexistent disease, the mortality rate with large liver abscesses ranges from 30% to 90%. With early recognition and management, up to 80% of patients may survive.

DRUG- AND TOXIN-INDUCED LIVER DISEASE

As the major drug metabolizing and detoxifying organ in the body, the liver is subject to potential damage from an enormous array of therapeutic and environmental chemicals. Injury may result (1) from direct toxicity, (2) via hepatic conversion of a xenobiotic to an active toxin, or (3) through immune mechanisms, usually by the drug or a metabolite acting as a hapten to convert a cellular protein into an immunogen.

Principles of drug and toxic injury were discussed in Chapter 8. Here it suffices to recall that drug reactions may be classified as predictable (intrinsic) reactions or unpredictable (idiosyncratic) ones. Predictable drug reactions may occur in anyone who accumulates a sufficient dose. Unpredictable reactions depend on idiosyncrasies of the host, particularly the host's propensity to mount an immune response to the antigenic stimulus, and the rate at which the host metabolizes the agent. Major examples include chlorpromazine, an agent that causes cholestasis in those patients who are slow to metabolize it to an innocuous byproduct, and halothane, which can cause a fatal immune-mediated hepatitis in some patients exposed to this anesthetic on multiple occasions. A broad classification of offending agents is offered in Table 16–6. It should be noted that (1) the injury may be immediate or take weeks to months to develop and (2) it may take the form of overt hepatocyte necrosis, cholestasis, or insidious onset of liver dys-

■

Table 16–6. DRUG- AND TOXIN-INDUCED HEPATIC INJURY

Hepatocellular Damage

Microvesicular fatty change	Tetracycline, salicylates, yellow phosphorus, ethanol
Macrovesicular fatty change	Ethanol, methotrexate, amiodarone
Centrilobular necrosis	Bromobenzene, CCl_4, acetaminophen, halothane, rifampin
Diffuse or massive necrosis	Halothane, isoniazid, acetaminophen, α-methyldopa, trinitrotoluene, *Amanita phalloides* (mushroom) toxin
Hepatitis, acute and chronic	α-Methyldopa, isoniazid, nitrofurantoin, phenytoin, oxyphenisatin
Fibrosis-cirrhosis	Ethanol, methotrexate, amiodarone, most drugs that cause chronic hepatitis
Granuloma formation	Sulfonamides, α-methyldopa, quinidine, phenylbutazone, hydralazine, allopurinol
Cholestasis (with or without hepatocellular injury)	Chlorpromazine, anabolic steroids, erythromycin estolate, oral contraceptives, organic arsenicals

Vascular Disorders

Veno-occlusive disease	Cytotoxic drugs, pyrrolizidine alkaloids (bush tea)
Hepatic or portal vein thrombosis	Estrogens, including oral contraceptives, cytotoxic drugs
Peliosis hepatitis	Anabolic steroids, oral contraceptives, danazol

Hyperplasia and Neoplasia

Adenoma	Oral contraceptives
Hepatocellular carcinoma	Vinyl chloride, aflatoxin, Thorotrast
Cholangiocarcinoma	Thorotrast
Angiosarcoma	Vinyl chloride, inorganic arsenicals, Thorotrast

function. Most important, *drug-induced chronic hepatitis is clinically and histologically indistinguishable from chronic viral hepatitis, and hence serologic markers of viral infection are critical for making the distinction.* Among the agents listed in Table 16–6, predictable drug reactions are ascribed to acetaminophen (also called phenacetin), tetracycline, antineoplastic agents, *Amanita phalloides* toxin, carbon tetrachloride, and, to a certain extent, alcohol. Many others such as sulfonamides, α-methyldopa, and allopurinol cause idiosyncratic reactions.

A diagnosis of drug-induced liver disease may be made on the basis of a temporal association of liver damage with drug administration and, it is hoped, recovery on removal of the drug, combined with exclusion of other potential causes. Exposure to a toxin or therapeutic agent should always be included in the differential diagnosis of any form of liver disease.

Alcoholic Liver Disease

Excessive ethanol consumption is the leading cause of liver disease in most Western countries. The following statistics attest to the magnitude of the problem in the United States:

■ More than 10 million Americans are alcoholics.
■ Alcohol abuse causes 200,000 deaths annually, the fifth leading cause of death, many related to automobile accidents.
■ From 25% to 30% of hospitalized patients have problems related to alcohol abuse.

Chronic alcohol consumption has a variety of adverse effects, as pointed out in Chapter 8. Of great impact, however, are the three distinctive, albeit overlapping, forms of liver disease: (1) hepatic steatosis, (2) alcoholic hepatitis, and (3) cirrhosis, collectively referred to as alcoholic liver disease. Because the first two conditions may develop independently, they do not necessarily represent a continuum of changes. The morphology of the three forms of alcoholic liver disease is presented first, because this facilitates consideration of their pathogenesis. The various forms of alcoholic liver disease are depicted in Figure 16–13.

HEPATIC STEATOSIS (FATTY LIVER). After even moderate intake of alcohol, small (**microvesicular**) lipid droplets accumulate in hepatocytes. With chronic intake of alcohol, lipid accumulates to the point of creating large clear **macrovesicular** globules, compressing and displacing the nucleus to the periphery of the hepatocyte. This transformation is initially centrilobular, but in severe cases it may involve the entire lobule (Fig. 16–14). Macroscopically, the fatty liver of chronic alcoholism is large (up to 4 to 6 kg), soft, yellow, and greasy. Although there is little or no fibrosis at the outset, with continued alcohol intake fibrous tissue develops around the central veins and extends into the adjacent sinusoids. **Up to the time that fibrosis ap-**

pears, the fatty change is completely reversible if there is abstention from further intake of alcohol.

ALCOHOLIC HEPATITIS. This is characterized by the following:

■ **Hepatocyte swelling and necrosis.** Single or scattered foci of cells undergo swelling (ballooning) and necrosis. The swelling results from the accumulation of fat and water, as well as proteins that normally are exported.
■ **Mallory bodies.** Scattered hepatocytes accumulate tangled skeins of cytokeratin intermediate filaments and other proteins, visible as eosinophilic cytoplasmic inclusions in degenerating hepatocytes (Fig. 16–15). These inclusions are a characteristic but not specific feature of alcoholic liver disease, because they are also seen in primary biliary cirrhosis, Wilson's disease, chronic cholestatic syndromes, and hepatocellular tumors.
■ **Neutrophilic reaction.** Neutrophils permeate the lobule and accumulate around degenerating hepatocytes, particularly those containing Mallory bodies. Lymphocytes and macrophages also enter portal tracts and spill into the parenchyma.
■ **Fibrosis.** Alcoholic hepatitis is almost always accompanied by a brisk sinusoidal and perivenular fibrosis; occasionally periportal fibrosis may predominate, particularly with repeated bouts of heavy alcohol intake. In some cases there is cholestasis and mild deposition of hemosiderin (iron) in hepatocytes and Kupffer cells. Macroscopically, the liver is mottled red with bile-stained areas. Although the liver may be normal or increased in size, it often contains visible nodules and fibrosis, indicative of evolution to cirrhosis.

ALCOHOLIC CIRRHOSIS. The final and irreversible form of alcoholic liver disease usually evolves slowly and insidiously. At first the cirrhotic liver is yellow-tan, fatty, and enlarged, usually weighing over 2 kg. Over the span of years it is transformed into a brown, shrunken, nonfatty organ, sometimes weighing less than 1 kg. Arguably, cirrhosis may develop more rapidly in the setting of alcoholic hepatitis, within 1 to 2 years. Initially, the developing fibrous septa are delicate and extend through sinusoids from central vein to portal regions as well as from portal tract to portal tract. Regenerative activity of entrapped parenchymal hepatocytes generates fairly uniformly sized micronodules. With time, the nodularity becomes more prominent; scattered larger nodules create a "hobnail" appearance on the surface of the liver (Fig. 16–16). As fibrous septa dissect and surround nodules, the liver becomes more fibrotic, loses fat, and shrinks progressively. Parenchymal islands are engulfed by ever wider bands of fibrous tissue, and the liver is converted into a mixed micronodular and mac-

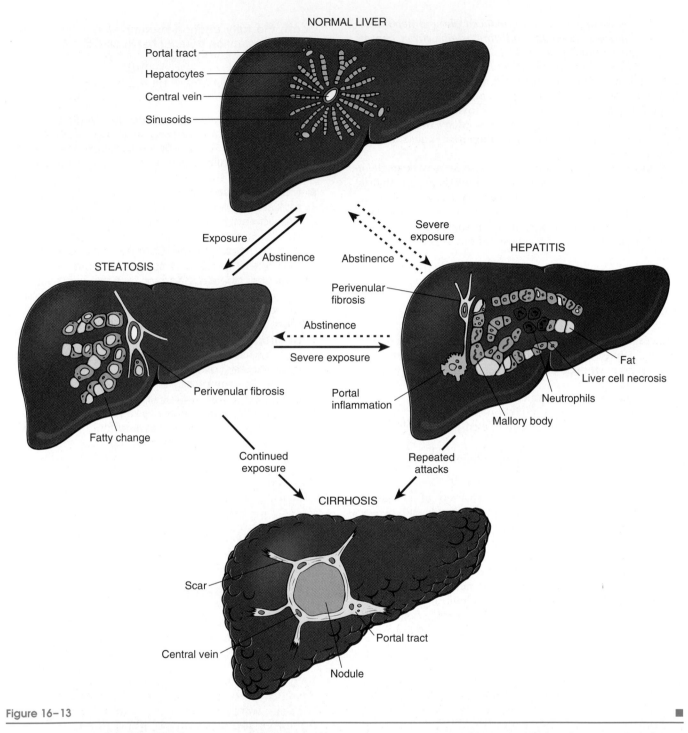

Figure 16-13

Alcoholic liver disease. The interrelationships among hepatic steatosis, hepatitis, and cirrhosis are shown, along with a depiction of key morphologic features at the microscopic level.

ronodular pattern (Fig. 16–17). Ischemic necrosis and fibrous obliteration of nodules eventually create broad expanses of tough, pale scar tissue (Laennec's cirrhosis). Bile stasis often develops; Mallory bodies are only rarely evident at this stage. Thus, **end-stage alcoholic cirrhosis comes to resemble, both macroscopically and micro-** **scopically, the cirrhosis developing from viral hepatitis and other causes.**

Pathogenesis of Alcoholic Liver Disease. Short-term ingestion of up to 80 gm of ethanol per day (eight beers or 7 ounces of 80-proof liquor) generally produces mild, reversible

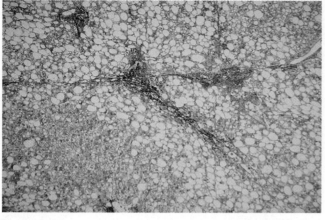

Figure 16–14 ■

Alcoholic liver disease: macrovesicular steatosis, involving most regions of the hepatic lobule. The intracytoplasmic fat is seen as clear vacuoles. Some early fibrosis *(stained blue)* is present. (Masson trichrome.)

hepatic changes, such as fatty liver. Daily ingestion of 160 gm or more of ethanol for 10 to 20 years is associated more consistently with severe injury; chronic intake of 80 to 160 gm/day is considered a borderline risk for severe injury. Only 10% to 15% of alcoholics, however, develop cirrhosis. For reasons that may relate to decreased gastric metabolism of ethanol and differences in body composition, women appear to be more susceptible to hepatic injury than men. Individual, possibly genetic, susceptibility must exist, but no reliable genetic markers of susceptibility have been identified. In addition, the relationship between hepatic steatosis and alcoholic hepatitis as precursors to cirrhosis, both causally and temporally, is not yet clear. Cirrhosis may develop without antecedent evidence of steatosis or alcoholic hepatitis. In the absence of a clear understanding of the pathogenetic factors influenc-

ing liver damage, no "safe" upper limit for alcohol consumption can be proposed (despite the current popularity of red wines for amelioration of coronary vascular disease).

The pharmacokinetics and metabolism of alcohol were examined in Chapter 8. Pertinent to this discussion are the detrimental effects of alcohol and its byproducts on hepatocellular function:

■ Hepatocellular steatosis results from (1) the shunting of normal substrates away from catabolism and toward lipid biosynthesis, owing to generation of excess reduced nicotinamide-adenine dinucleotide by the two major enzymes of alcohol metabolism, alcohol dehydrogenase and acetaldehyde dehydrogenase; (2) impaired assembly and secretion of lipoproteins; and (3) increased peripheral catabolism of fat.
■ Induction of cytochrome P-450 leads to augmented transformation of other drugs to toxic metabolites.
■ Free radicals are generated during oxidation of ethanol by the microsomal ethanol oxidizing system; the free radicals react with membranes and proteins.
■ Alcohol directly affects microtubular and mitochondrial function and membrane fluidity.
■ Acetaldehyde (the major intermediate metabolite of alcohol en route to acetate production) induces lipid peroxidation and acetaldehyde-protein adduct formation, further disrupting cytoskeletal and membrane function.
■ Alcohol induces an immunologic attack on hepatocytes that are antigenically altered by alcohol or acetaldehyde-induced alterations in hepatic proteins.

In addition, alcohol can become a major caloric source in the diet, displacing other nutrients and leading to malnutrition and vitamin deficiencies (such as thiamine and vitamin B_{12}) in the alcoholic. This is compounded by impaired digestive function, primarily related to chronic gastric and intestinal mucosal damage, and pancreatitis. Alcohol-induced stimulation of fibrosis is multifactorial and remains poorly under-

Figure 16–15 ■

Alcoholic hepatitis. *A,* The cluster of inflammatory cells marks the site of a necrotic hepatocyte. A Mallory body is present in a second hepatocyte *(arrow).* *B,* Eosinophilic Mallory bodies are seen in hepatocytes which are surrounded by fibrous tissue. (H & E.)

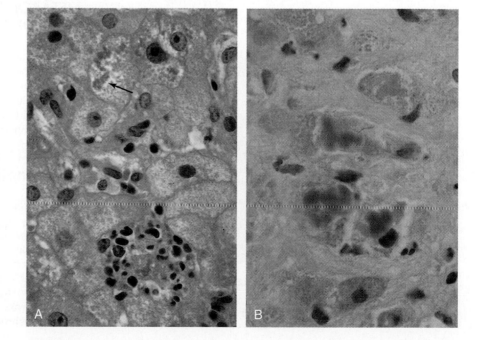

stood; possible mechanisms of hepatic fibrosis were discussed earlier in this chapter.

Clinical Features. *Hepatic steatosis* may become evident as hepatomegaly with mild elevation of serum bilirubin and alkaline phosphatase levels. Alternatively, there may be no clinical or biochemical evidence of liver disease. Severe hepatic compromise is unusual. Alcohol withdrawal and the provision of an adequate diet are sufficient treatment.

In contrast, *alcoholic hepatitis* tends to appear relatively acutely, usually after a bout of heavy drinking. Symptoms and laboratory abnormalities may be minimal or characteristic of fulminant hepatic failure. Between these two extremes are the nonspecific symptoms of malaise, anorexia, weight loss, upper abdominal discomfort, tender hepatomegaly, fever, and the laboratory findings of hyperbilirubinemia, elevated alkaline phosphatase, and often a neutrophilic leukocytosis. The outlook is unpredictable; each bout of hepatitis carries about a 10% to 20% risk of death. With repeated bouts, cirrhosis appears in about one third of patients within a few years; alcoholic hepatitis also may be superimposed on cirrhosis. With proper nutrition and total cessation of alcohol consumption, alcoholic hepatitis may clear slowly. However, in some patients the hepatitis persists despite abstinence and progresses to cirrhosis.

The manifestations of *alcoholic cirrhosis* are similar to other forms of cirrhosis, presented earlier. Commonly, the first signs of cirrhosis relate to complications of portal hypertension. The stigmata of cirrhosis (e.g., an abdomen grossly distended with ascites, wasted extremities, caput medusae) may be the presenting features. Alternatively, a patient may first present with life-threatening variceal hemorrhage, dying either as a result of exsanguination or the hepatic encephalopathy precipitated by the metabolism of excess blood in the gastrointestinal tract. In other cases, insidious onset of malaise, weakness, weight loss, and loss of appetite precede the appearance of jaundice, ascites, and peripheral edema. Laboratory findings reflect the developing hepatic compromise, with elevated serum transaminase levels, hyperbilirubinemia, variable elevation of alkaline phosphatase, hypoproteinemia

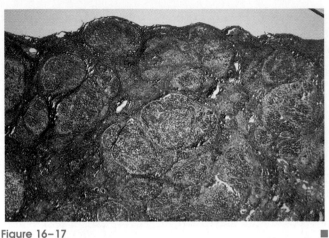

Figure 16–17 ■

Alcoholic cirrhosis. Nodules of varying sizes are entrapped in blue-staining fibrous tissue. (Masson trichrome.)

(globulins, albumin, and clotting factors), and anemia. Lastly, cirrhosis may be clinically silent, discovered only at autopsy or when stress such as infection or trauma tips the balance toward hepatic insufficiency.

The long-term outlook for alcoholics with liver disease is variable. Five-year survival approaches 90% in abstainers who are free of jaundice, ascites, or hematemesis but drops to 50% to 60% in those who continue to imbibe. In the end-stage alcoholic, the immediate causes of death are (1) hepatic failure, (2) a massive gastrointestinal hemorrhage, (3) an intercurrent infection (to which these patients are predisposed), (4) hepatorenal syndrome after a bout of alcoholic hepatitis, and (5) hepatocellular carcinoma in 3% to 6% of cases.

INBORN ERRORS OF METABOLISM AND PEDIATRIC LIVER DISEASE

A distinct group of liver diseases are attributable to inborn errors of metabolism, including hemochromatosis, Wilson's disease, and α_1-antitrypsin deficiency, which may present in children or in adults. An additional set of diseases appear in infancy, referred to as neonatal hepatitis, and represent a diverse group of inherited and acquired conditions.

Hemochromatosis

Hemochromatosis is characterized by the excessive accumulation of body iron, most of which is deposited in the parenchymal organs such as the liver and pancreas. Because humans do not have a major excretory pathway for iron, hemochromatosis results either from a genetic defect causing excessive iron absorption or as a consequence of parenteral administration of iron (usually in the form of transfusions). Genetic hemochromatosis, also called hereditary, primary, or idiopathic hemochromatosis, is an autosomal recessive dis-

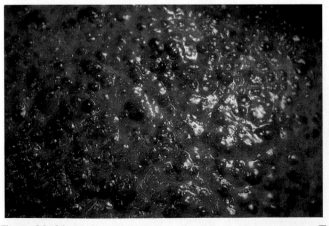

Figure 16–16 ■

Alcoholic cirrhosis showing the characteristic diffuse nodularity of the surface induced by the underlying fibrous scarring. The average nodule size is 3 mm in this close-up view. The greenish tint is due to bile stasis.

Table 16-7.   CLASSIFICATION OF IRON OVERLOAD

Genetic Hemochromatosis
Secondary Hemochromatosis
Parenteral iron overload
   Transfusions
      Long-term hemodialysis
      Aplastic anemia
      Sickle cell disease
      Myelodysplastic syndromes
      Leukemias
   Iron-dextran injections
Ineffective erythropoiesis with increased erythroid activity
   β-Thalassemia
   Sideroblastic anemia
   Pyruvate kinase deficiency
Increased oral intake of iron
   African iron overload (Bantu siderosis)
Congenital atransferrinemia
Chronic liver disease
   Chronic alcoholic liver disease
   Porphyria cutanea tarda

order. Acquired forms of hemochromatosis with known sources of excess iron are called secondary hemochromatosis (Table 16–7).

As discussed in Chapter 12, the total body iron pool ranges from 2 to 6 gm in normal adults; about 0.5 gm is stored in the liver, 98% of which is in hepatocytes. In genetic hemochromatosis, total iron accumulation may exceed 50 gm, over one third of which accumulates in the liver. The following features characterize this disease:

■ Fully developed cases exhibit (1) micronodular cirrhosis (all patients), (2) diabetes mellitus (75% to 80%), and (3) skin pigmentation (75% to 80%).
■ Iron accumulation is lifelong; symptoms usually first appear in the fifth to sixth decades of life.
■ The hemochromatosis gene, located on the short arm of chromosome 6 close to the HLA gene complex, has been recently cloned. This gene, called HLA-H, encodes a novel HLA class I–like molecule that in some uncharacterized manner influences iron absorption. HLA-H is in linkage disequilibrium with HLA-A3, thus accounting for the previously reported association with HLA-A3 and genetic hemochromatosis.
■ Males predominate (ratio of 5 to 7:1) with slightly earlier clinical presentation, partly because physiologic iron loss (menstruation, pregnancy) delays iron accumulation in women.

In white populations of northern European extraction, the gene frequency has been estimated at approximately 6%. The frequency of homozygosity is 0.45% (1 of every 220 persons), and heterozygosity is 11% (1 of every 9 persons), making genetic hemochromatosis one of the most common inborn errors of metabolism.

Pathogenesis. It may be recalled that the total body content of iron is tightly regulated, whereby the limited daily losses of iron are matched by gastrointestinal absorption. *In genetic hemochromatosis there seems to be a primary defect in the intestinal absorption of dietary iron, leading to net iron ac-*

cumulation of 0.5 to 1.0 gm/yr. The disease manifests itself typically after 20 gm of storage iron has accumulated. Excessive iron seems to be directly toxic to tissues by the following mechanisms: (1) lipid peroxidation by iron-catalyzed free radical reactions, (2) stimulation of collagen formation, and (3) direct interactions of iron with DNA, leading to lethal injury or predisposition to hepatocellular carcinoma. Whatever the actions of iron, they are reversible in cells not fatally injured, and removal of excess iron by therapy promotes recovery of tissue function.

The most common causes of secondary hemochromatosis are the anemias associated with ineffective erythropoiesis, discussed in Chapter 12. In these disorders, the excess iron may result not only from transfusions but also from increased absorption. Transfusions alone, as in sickle cell and aplastic anemias, lead to systemic hemosiderosis in which parenchymal organ injury tends to occur only in extreme cases. Alcoholic cirrhosis is often associated with a modest increase in stainable iron within liver cells. However, this may represent alcohol-induced redistribution of iron, because total body iron is not significantly increased. A rather unusual form of iron overload resembling genetic hemochromatosis occurs in sub-Saharan Africa, the result of ingesting large quantities of alcoholic beverage fermented in iron utensils (Bantu siderosis). Home-brewing in steel drums continues to this day.

The morphologic changes in genetic hemochromatosis are characterized principally by (1) the **deposition of hemosiderin** in the following organs (in decreasing order of severity): liver, pancreas, myocardium, pituitary, adrenal, thyroid and parathyroid glands, joints, and skin; (2) **cirrhosis;** and (3) **pancreatic fibrosis.** In the liver, iron becomes evident first as golden-yellow hemosiderin granules in the cytoplasm of periportal hepatocytes, which stain blue with the Prussian blue stain (Fig. 16–18). With increasing iron load, there is progressive involvement of the rest of the lobule, along with bile duct epithelium and Kupffer cell pigmentation.

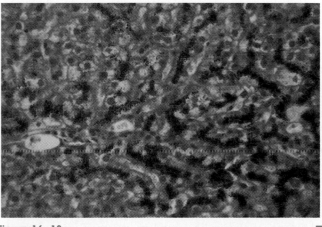

Figure 16–18   ■

Genetic hemochromatosis. Hepatocellular iron deposition is blue in this Prussian blue–stained histologic section. The parenchymal architecture is normal.

Iron is a direct hepatotoxin, and inflammation is characteristically absent. At this stage, the liver is typically slightly larger than normal, dense, and chocolate brown. Fibrous septa develop slowly, leading ultimately to a micronodular pattern of cirrhosis in an intensely pigmented liver.

In normal individuals the iron content of unfixed liver tissue is less than 1000 μg/gm dry weight. Adult patients with genetic hemochromatosis exhibit over 10,000 μg/gm dry weight of iron; hepatic iron concentrations in excess of 22,000 μg/gm dry weight are associated with the development of fibrosis and cirrhosis.

The **pancreas** becomes intensely pigmented, has diffuse interstitial fibrosis, and may exhibit some parenchymal atrophy. Hemosiderin is found both in the acinar and the islet cells and sometimes in the interstitial fibrous stroma. The **heart** is often enlarged and has hemosiderin granules within the myocardial fibers. The pigmentation may induce a striking brown coloration of the myocardium. A delicate interstitial fibrosis may appear. Although **skin** pigmentation is partially attributable to hemosiderin deposition in dermal macrophages and fibroblasts, most of the coloration results from increased epidermal melanin production. The combination of these pigments renders the skin slate-gray. With hemosiderin deposition in the **joint synovial linings,** an acute synovitis may develop. There is also excessive deposition of calcium pyrophosphate, which damages the articular cartilage and sometimes produces disabling polyarthritis, referred to as pseudogout. The **testes** may be small and atrophic but are usually not discolored.

Clinical Features. Genetic hemochromatosis is more often a disease of males and rarely becomes evident before age 40. The principal manifestations include hepatomegaly, abdominal pain, skin pigmentation (particularly in sun-exposed areas), deranged glucose homeostasis or frank diabetes mellitus due to destruction of pancreatic islets, cardiac dysfunction (arrhythmias, cardiomyopathy), and atypical arthritis. In some patients, the presenting complaint is hypogonadism (e.g., amenorrhea in the female and loss of libido and impotence in the male). It is thought that the hypogonadism is due to derangement in the hypothalamic-pituitary axis. The classic clinical triad of cirrhosis with hepatomegaly, skin pigmentation, and diabetes mellitus may not develop until late in the course of the disease. Death may result from cirrhosis or cardiac disease. A significant cause of death is hepatocellular carcinoma, because treatment for iron overload does not remove the risk for this aggressive neoplasm.

Fortunately, genetic hemochromatosis can be diagnosed long before irreversible tissue damage has occurred. Screening involves demonstration of very high levels of serum iron and ferritin, exclusion of secondary causes of iron overload, and liver biopsy if indicated. Also important is screening of family members of probands by biochemical studies and HLA typing. The recent discovery of the genetic hemochromatosis

gene may allow direct detection of carriers. The natural course of the disease can be substantially altered by a variety of interventions, mainly phlebotomy and the use of iron chelators to drain off the excess iron. Patients with genetic hemochromatosis diagnosed in the subclinical, precirrhotic stage and treated by regular phlebotomy have a normal life expectancy. Heterozygotes may exhibit a mild increase in iron absorption and accumulation but are not at risk for disease manifestations.

Wilson's Disease

This autosomal recessive disorder of copper metabolism is marked by the *accumulation of toxic levels of copper in many tissues and organs, principally the liver, brain, and eye.* The gene for Wilson's disease is on chromosome 13 and has a frequency of 1 : 200. The incidence of this disease is approximately 1 : 30,000; thus, it is much less common than genetic hemochromatosis.

Normal copper physiology involves (1) absorption of ingested copper (2 to 5 mg/day); (2) plasma transport complexed to albumin; (3) hepatocellular uptake, followed by incorporation into an α_2-globulin to form ceruloplasmin (a metallothionein); (4) secretion of ceruloplasmin into plasma, where it accounts for 90% to 95% of plasma copper; and (5) hepatic uptake of desialylated, senescent ceruloplasmin from the plasma, followed by lysosomal degradation and secretion of free copper into bile. In Wilson's disease, the initial steps of copper absorption and transport to the liver are normal. However, absorbed copper fails to enter the circulation in the form of ceruloplasmin and biliary excretion of copper is markedly diminished. Copper thus accumulates progressively in the liver, apparently causing toxic liver injury by (1) promoting the formation of free radicals, (2) binding to sulfhydryl groups of cellular proteins, and (3) displacing other metals in hepatic metalloenzymes. Usually by 5 years of age, non–ceruloplasmin-bound copper spills over into the circulation, causing hemolysis and pathologic changes at other sites, such as brain, cornea, kidneys, bones, joints, and parathyroids. Concomitantly, urinary excretion of copper becomes markedly increased. *The biochemical diagnosis of Wilson's disease is based on a decrease in serum ceruloplasmin, increase in hepatic copper content, and increased urinary excretion of copper.*

The liver often bears the brunt of injury in Wilson's disease, with hepatic changes ranging from relatively minor to massive damage. **Fatty change** may be mild to moderate, with vacuolated nuclei (glycogen or water) and occasional hepatocyte focal necrosis. An **acute hepatitis** can mimic acute viral hepatitis, save possibly for the accompanying fatty change. A **chronic hepatitis** resembles chronic hepatitis of either viral, drug, or alcoholic origin but may exhibit such distinguishing features as fatty change, vacuolated nuclei, and Mallory bodies. With progression of chronic hepatitis, **cirrhosis** develops. **Massive liver necrosis** is a rare manifestation that is indistinguishable from that caused by viruses or drugs. Excess copper deposition can often be demonstrated by special stains (e.g., rhodanine stain for copper, orcein stain for copper-associated protein). Because copper also accumulates in chronic obstructive cholestasis, and because histology cannot reliably distinguish Wilson's disease from viral- and drug-induced hepatitis, demonstration of hepatic copper content in excess of 250 μg/gm dry weight is most helpful for making a diagnosis.

In the **brain**, toxic injury primarily affects the basal ganglia, particularly the putamen, which demonstrates atrophy and even cavitation. Nearly all patients with neurologic involvement develop **eye lesions** called **Kayser-Fleischer rings** (green to brown deposits of copper in Desçemet's membrane in the limbus of the cornea)—hence the alternative designation of this condition as hepatolenticular degeneration.

Clinical Features. The age at onset and the clinical presentation of Wilson's disease are extremely variable, but the disorder rarely manifests before age 6 years. The most common presentation is acute or chronic liver disease. Neuropsychiatric manifestations, including mild behavioral changes, frank psychosis, or a Parkinson's disease–like syndrome, are the initial features in most of the remaining cases. Demonstration of Kayser-Fleischer rings or markedly elevated hepatic copper levels in a patient with a low serum ceruloplasmin level strongly favor the diagnosis. Early recognition and long-term copper chelation therapy (as with D-penicillamine) have dramatically altered the usual progressive downhill course. Patients with fulminant hepatitis and unmanageable cirrhosis require liver transplantation.

α_1-Antitrypsin Deficiency

α_1-Antitrypsin deficiency (AAT) is an autosomal recessive disorder marked by abnormally low serum levels of this protease inhibitor (Pi). The major function of AAT is the inhibition of proteases, particularly neutrophil elastase released at sites of inflammation. AAT deficiency leads to pulmonary emphysema, because a relative lack of this protein permits tissue-destructive enzymes to run amok (discussed in Chapter 13).

AAT is a small, 394–amino acid plasma glycoprotein synthesized predominantly by hepatocytes. The AAT gene, located on human chromosome 14, is very polymorphic, and at least 75 AAT forms have been identified. The most common allele is PiM, and the PiMM genotype occurs in 90% of individuals. Most allelic variants produce normal or mildly reduced levels of serum AAT. However, homozygotes for the Z allele (PiZZ genotype) have circulating AAT levels that are only 10% of normal levels.

The PiZ polypeptide contains a single amino acid substitution that results in misfolding of the nascent polypeptide in the hepatocyte endoplasmic reticulum. Because the mutant protein cannot be secreted by the hepatocyte, it accumulates in the endoplasmic reticulum and undergoes excessive lysosomal degradation. Curiously, all individuals with the PiZZ genotype accumulate AAT in the liver, but only 8% to 20% develop significant liver damage. Expression of alleles is autosomal codominant, and consequently PiMZ heterozygotes have intermediate plasma levels of AAT. The gene frequency of PiZ is 1.2% in the North American white population, yielding a PiZZ genotype frequency of approximately 1 : 7000.

> **Hepatocytes in AAT deficiency contain round-to-oval cytoplasmic globular inclusions of retained AAT, which are strongly positive in a periodic acid–Schiff diastase stain** (Fig. 16–19). By electron microscopy they lie within smooth, and sometimes rough, endoplasmic reticulum. Hepatic injury associated with PiZZ homozygosity may range from marked cholestasis with hepatocyte necrosis in newborns, to childhood cirrhosis, or to a smoldering chronic inflammatory hepatitis or cirrhosis that becomes apparent only late in life.

Clinical Course. Ten to 20% of newborns with AAT deficiency exhibit cholestasis. In older children, adolescents, and adults, presenting symptoms may be related to chronic hepatitis, cirrhosis, or pulmonary disease. The disease may remain silent until cirrhosis appears in middle to later life. Hepatocellular carcinoma develops in 2% to 3% of PiZZ adults, usually but not always in the setting of cirrhosis. The treatment, and cure, for the severe hepatic disease is orthotopic liver transplantation.

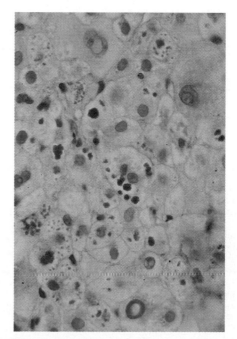

Figure 16–19 ■

α_1-Antitrypsin deficiency. Periodic acid–Schiff diastase stain of liver, highlighting the characteristic red cytoplasmic granules. (Courtesy of Dr. I. Wanless, Toronto Hospital.)

Neonatal Hepatitis

As mentioned earlier, mild transient elevations in serum unconjugated bilirubin are common in normal newborns. Prolonged conjugated hyperbilirubinemia in the newborn, termed *neonatal cholestasis*, affects approximately 1 in 2500 live births. The major conditions causing it are extrahepatic biliary atresia (EHBA), discussed later, and a variety of other disorders collectively referred to as *neonatal hepatitis*. Neonatal hepatitis is not a specific entity, nor are the disorders necessarily inflammatory. Instead, the finding of "neonatal cholestasis" should evoke a diligent search for recognizable toxic, metabolic, and infectious liver diseases. Some of the major causes are listed in Table 16–8, noting that this is an abbreviated version of an extensive list that contains many unusual infections and inherited diseases.

Clinical presentation of infants with any form of neonatal cholestasis is fairly stereotypical, with jaundice, dark urine, light or acholic stools, and hepatomegaly. Variable degrees of hepatic synthetic dysfunction may be present, such as hypoprothrombinemia. Despite the long list of disorders associated with neonatal cholestasis, most are quite rare. *"Idiopathic" neonatal hepatitis represents 50% to 60% of cases; about 20% are due to extrahepatic biliary atresia and 15% to AAT deficiency.* Differentiation of the two most common causes assumes great importance, because definitive treatment of biliary atresia requires surgical intervention, whereas surgery may adversely affect the clinical course of a child with idiopathic neonatal hepatitis. Fortunately, discrimination between neonatal hepatitis and biliary atresia can be made in about 90% of cases using clinical data and liver biopsy. Only in

■

Table 16–8. MAJOR CAUSES OF NEONATAL CHOLESTASIS

Bile duct obstruction
  Extrahepatic biliary atresia
Neonatal infection
  Cytomegalovirus
  Bacterial sepsis
  Urinary tract infection
  Syphilis
Toxic
  Drugs
  Parenteral nutrition
Metabolic diseases
  Amino acid
    Tyrosinemia
  Lipid
    Niemann-Pick disease
  Carbohydrate
    Galactosemia
  Bile acid metabolism
    Δ^4-3-oxosteroid 5β-reductase deficiency
  Miscellaneous
    α_1-Antitrypsin deficiency
    Cystic fibrosis
Miscellaneous
  Shock/hypoperfusion
  Indian childhood cirrhosis
  Alagille's syndrome (paucity of bile ducts)
Idiopathic neonatal hepatitis

extrahepatic biliary obstruction are there histologic features of biliary obstruction (described later).

Reye's Syndrome

Reye's syndrome is a rare disease characterized by fatty change in the liver and encephalopathy. The most severe forms are fatal. It primarily affects children younger than 4 years of age, typically developing 3 to 5 days after a viral illness. The onset is heralded by pernicious vomiting and is accompanied by irritability or lethargy and hepatomegaly. Serum bilirubin, ammonia, and aminotransferase levels are essentially normal at this time. Although most patients recover, about 25% progress to coma, accompanied by elevations in the serum levels of bilirubin, aminotransferases, and particularly ammonia. Death occurs due to progressive neurologic deterioration or liver failure. Survivors of more serious illness may be left with permanent neurologic impairments. Therapy is entirely symptomatic and supportive. The pathogenesis of Reye's syndrome is incompletely understood, but careful investigations are likely to reveal derangement of mitochondrial function, occurring alone or in combination with viral infection. Because Reye's syndrome has been associated with salicylate administration during viral illnesses, treatment of febrile illness in children with aspirin is now strongly discouraged. There is, however, no evidence that salicylates play a causal role in this disorder.

The key pathologic finding in the **liver** is microvesicular steatosis. Electron microscopy of hepatocellular mitochondria reveals pleomorphic enlargement and electron lucency of the matrices, with disruption of cristae and loss of dense bodies. In the **brain**, cerebral edema is usually present. Astrocytes are swollen and mitochondrial changes similar to those seen in the liver may develop. Inflammation is notably absent, as is any evidence of viral infection. **Skeletal muscles, kidneys,** and **heart** may also reveal microvesicular fatty change and mitochondrial alterations, although more subtle than those of the liver.

INTRAHEPATIC BILIARY TRACT DISEASE

Biliary tract disorders cannot always be divided into those that affect only the intrahepatic or extrahepatic portions, particularly because extrahepatic biliary disorders incite secondary changes within the liver. Accordingly, reference should be made to the subsequent section on the gallbladder and biliary tree, particularly biliary atresia, which affects both extrahepatic and intrahepatic bile ducts. In addition, hepatic bile ducts are frequently damaged as part of a more general liver disease, as in drug toxicity, viral hepatitis, and transplantation (both orthotopic liver transplantation and graft-versus-host disease after bone marrow transplantation). With these caveats, consideration will now be given to three disorders of intrahepatic bile ducts that culminate in cirrhosis, as summarized in Table 16–9.

Secondary Biliary Cirrhosis. Prolonged obstruction to the extrahepatic biliary tree results in profound damage to the liver itself. The most common cause of obstruction is extrahepatic cholelithiasis (gallstones, described later). Other obstructive conditions include biliary atresia, malignancies of the biliary tree and head of the pancreas, and strictures resulting from previous surgical procedures. The initial morphologic features of cholestasis were described earlier and are entirely reversible with correction of the obstruction. However, secondary inflammation resulting from biliary obstruction initiates periportal fibrogenesis, which eventually leads to scarring and nodule formation, generating secondary biliary cirrhosis. Subtotal obstruction may promote secondary bacterial infection of the biliary tree (ascending cholangitis), which further contributes to the damage. Enteric organisms such as coliforms and enterococci are common culprits.

Primary Biliary Cirrhosis. Primary biliary cirrhosis is a chronic, progressive, and often fatal cholestatic liver disease, characterized by the destruction of intrahepatic bile ducts, portal inflammation and scarring, and the eventual development of cirrhosis and liver failure. *The primary feature of this disease is a nonsuppurative, granulomatous destruction of medium-sized intrahepatic bile ducts;* cirrhosis appears only late in the course. This is primarily a disease of middle-aged women, with an age at onset between 20 and 80 years and peak incidence between 40 and 50 years of age. The onset is insidious, usually presenting as pruritus; jaundice develops late in the course. Over a period of two or more decades, the patients develop hepatic decompensation, including portal hypertension with variceal bleeding, and hepatic encephalopathy. For end-stage patients, liver transplantation offers the only hope for long-term survival.

Serum alkaline phosphatase and cholesterol levels are almost always elevated; hyperbilirubinemia is a late development and usually signifies incipient hepatic decompensation.

A striking feature of the disease is autoantibodies, especially antimitochondrial antibodies in over 90% of patients. Particularly characteristic of primary biliary cirrhosis are antibodies to mitochondrial pyruvate dehydrogenase. Associated extrahepatic conditions include sicca complex of dry eyes and mouth (Sjögren's syndrome), scleroderma, thyroiditis, rheumatoid arthritis, Raynaud's phenomenon, membranous glomerulonephritis, and celiac disease. Many lines of evidence suggest an autoimmune cause for primary biliary cirrhosis involving lymphocyte-mediated destruction of bile duct epithelial cells, but the inciting factors remain unclear.

Primary Sclerosing Cholangitis. *Primary sclerosing cholangitis is characterized by inflammation, obliterative fibrosis, and segmental dilation of the obstructed intrahepatic and extrahepatic bile ducts.* Endoscopic retrograde cholangiography demonstrates characteristic "beading" of the barium column in radiographs of the intrahepatic and extrahepatic biliary tree. This change is attributable to the irregular strictures and dilations of affected bile ducts. Primary sclerosing cholangitis is commonly seen in association with inflammatory bowel disease (Chapter 15), particularly chronic ulcerative colitis, which coexists in approximately 70% of patients. Conversely, the prevalence of primary sclerosing cholangitis in patients with ulcerative colitis is about 4%. The disorder tends to occur in the third through fifth decades, most often after development of inflammatory bowel disease. Males are affected more often in a ratio of 2 : 1.

Symptoms at presentation include progressive fatigue, pruritus, and jaundice. Asymptomatic patients may come to attention only on the basis of persistent elevation of serum alkaline phosphatase level. Unlike primary biliary cirrhosis, autoantibodies are present in less than 10% of patients. Severely afflicted patients exhibit symptoms associated with chronic liver disease, including weight loss, ascites, variceal bleeding, and encephalopathy. This disease also follows a protracted course over many years. There does appear to be an increased risk for cholangiocarcinoma in this patient population. The cause is unknown, but hypothesized mechanisms include exposure to gut-derived toxins, autoimmune immunologic attack, and ischemic damage to the end-arterial supply

■

Table 16–9.   DISTINGUISHING FEATURES OF THE MAJOR INTRAHEPATIC BILE DUCT DISORDERS

	Secondary Biliary Cirrhosis	Primary Biliary Cirrhosis	Primary Sclerosing Cholangitis
Etiology	Extrahepatic bile duct obstruction: biliary atresia, gallstones, stricture, carcinoma of pancreatic head	Possibly autoimmune; associated with other autoimmune conditions	Unknown, possibly autoimmune; 50%–70% of cases associated with inflammatory bowel disease
Sex Predilection	None	Female-to-male 10 : 1	Female-to-male 1 : 2
Symptoms and Signs	Pruritus, jaundice, malaise, dark urine, light stools, hepatosplenomegaly	Same as secondary biliary cirrhosis; insidious onset	Same as secondary biliary cirrhosis; insidious onset
Laboratory Findings	Conjugated hyperbilirubinemia, increased serum alkaline phosphatase, bile acids, cholesterol	Same as secondary biliary cirrhosis, plus elevated serum IgM and presence of autoantibodies, especially against mitochondrial pyruvate dehydrogenase	Same as secondary biliary cirrhosis, plus elevated serum IgM, hypergammaglobulinemia
Important Pathologic Findings Before Cirrhosis Develops	Prominent bile stasis in bile ducts, bile duct proliferation with surrounding neutrophils, portal tract edema	Dense lymphocytic infiltrate in portal tracts with granulomatous destruction of bile ducts	Periductal portal tract fibrosis, segmental stenosis of extrahepatic and intrahepatic bile ducts

of the biliary tree. As with primary biliary cirrhosis, liver transplantation is the definitive treatment.

In all three conditions (primary and secondary biliary cirrhosis and primary sclerosing cholangitis), the end-stage liver exhibits extraordinary yellow-green pigmentation, associated with marked icteric discoloration of body tissues and fluids. On cut surface, the liver is hard, with a finely granular appearance (Fig. 16–20). The histology of **secondary biliary cirrhosis** is characterized by coarse fibrous septa that subdivide the liver in a jigsaw-like pattern. Embedded in the septa are distended large and small bile ducts, which contain inspissated pigmented material. There is extensive proliferation of smaller bile ductules and edema (Fig. 16–21), particularly at the interface between septa (formerly portal tracts) and the parenchyma. The complication of bacterial infection incites a robust neutrophilic infiltration of bile ducts; severe pylephlebitis and cholangitic abscesses may develop.

In contrast to secondary biliary cirrhosis, interlobular bile ducts are absent in the end-stage of **primary biliary cirrhosis.** However, the morphology of this disease is most revealing in the precirrhotic stage. Interlobular bile ducts are destroyed by granulomatous inflammation (the **florid duct lesion**), accompanied by a dense portal tract infiltrate of lymphocytes, macrophages, plasma cells, and occasional eosinophils (Fig. 16–22). The obstruction to intrahepatic bile flow leads to upstream bile duct proliferation, inflammation and necrosis of the adjacent periportal hepatic parenchyma, and generalized cholestasis. Over years to

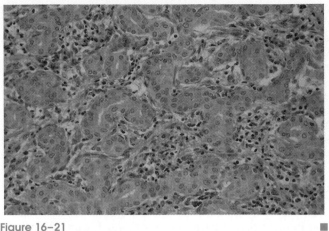

Figure 16–21 ■

Portal tract bile duct proliferation in the setting of biliary cirrhosis. A mixed inflammatory infiltrate is also present.

decades, relentless portal tract scarring and bridging fibrosis leads to cirrhosis.

The characteristic feature of **primary sclerosing cholangitis** is a fibrosing cholangitis of bile ducts. Specifically, affected portal tracts exhibit concentric periductal "onion-skin" fibrosis and a modest lymphocytic infiltrate (Fig. 16–23). Progressive atrophy of the bile duct epithelium leads to obliteration of the lumen, leaving behind a solid, cordlike fibrous scar. In between areas of progressive stricture, bile ducts become ectatic and inflamed, presumably the result of downstream obstruction.

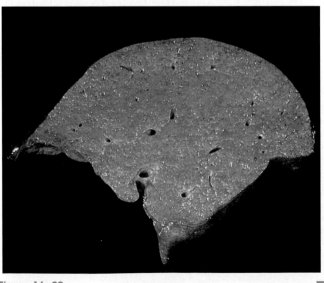

Figure 16–20 ■

Biliary cirrhosis. This sagittal section through the liver demonstrates the fine nodularity and bile staining of end-stage primary billiary cirrhosis.

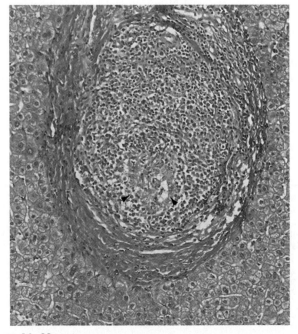

Figure 16–22 ■

Primary biliary cirrhosis. A portal tract is markedly expanded by an infiltrate of lymphocytes and plasma cells. The granulomatous reaction to a bile duct undergoing destruction (florid duct lesion) is highlighted by the arrowheads.

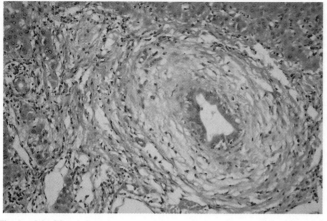

Figure 16–23

Primary sclerosing cholangitis. A bile duct undergoing degeneration is entrapped in a dense, "onion-skin" concentric scar.

As the disease progresses over years, the entire liver becomes markedly cholestatic and fibrotic. Ultimately, biliary cirrhosis develops, much like that seen with primary and secondary biliary cirrhosis.

CIRCULATORY DISORDERS

Given the enormous flow of blood through the liver, it is not surprising that circulatory disturbances have considerable impact on the liver. These disorders can be grouped according to whether blood flow into, through, or from the liver is impaired (Fig. 16–24).

Impaired Blood Flow Into the Liver

Hepatic Arterial Inflow. *Liver infarcts* are rare, thanks to the double blood supply to the liver. Nonetheless, thrombosis or compression of an intrahepatic branch of the hepatic artery by polyarteritis nodosa (Chapter 10), embolism, neoplasia, or sepsis may result in a localized infarct. Interruption of the main hepatic artery does not always produce ischemic necrosis of the organ, because retrograde arterial flow through accessory vessels and the portal venous supply may sustain the liver parenchyma. The one exception is hepatic artery thrombosis in the transplanted liver, which generally leads to loss of the organ.

Portal Vein Obstruction. Blockage of the portal vein may be insidious and well tolerated or may be a catastrophic and potentially lethal event; most cases fall somewhere in between. Occlusive disease of the portal vein or its major radicles typically produces abdominal pain and, in most instances, ascites and other manifestations of portal hypertension, principally esophageal varices that are prone to rupture. The ascites, when present, is often massive and intractable. Acute impairment of visceral blood flow leads to profound congestion and bowel infarction.

Extrahepatic portal vein obstruction may arise from the following:

■ Peritoneal sepsis (e.g., acute diverticulitis or appendicitis leading to pylephlebitis in the splanchnic circulation)

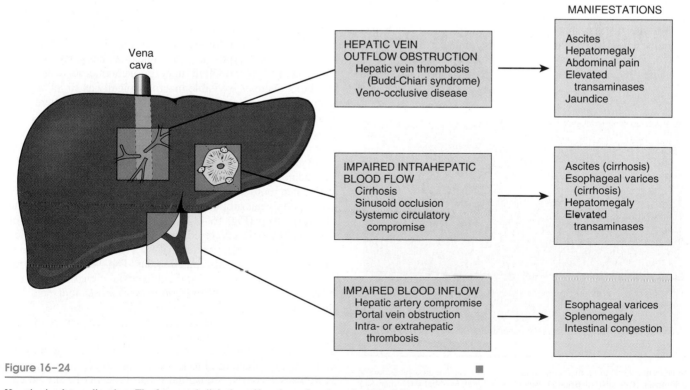

Figure 16–24

Hepatic circulatory disorders. The forms and clinical manifestations of compromised blood flow are contrasted.

- Lymphatic metastasis from abdominal cancers creating massive enlargement of hilar lymph nodes
- Pancreatitis that initiates splenic vein thrombosis that propagates into the portal vein
- Postsurgical thromboses after upper abdominal procedures
- Banti's syndrome, in which subclinical thrombosis of the portal vein (as from neonatal omphalitis or umbilical vein catheterization) produces a fibrotic, partially recanalized vascular channel presenting as splenomegaly or esophageal varices years after the occlusive event

Intrahepatic thrombosis of a portal vein radicle, when acute, does not cause ischemic infarction but instead results in a sharply demarcated area of red-blue discoloration (so-called infarct of Zahn). There is no necrosis, only hepatocellular atrophy and marked congestion in distended sinusoids. Vascular invasion by primary or secondary cancer in the liver can progressively occlude portal inflow to the liver; tongues of hepatocellular carcinoma can even occlude the main portal vein. Idiopathic portal hypertension is a chronic, generally bland condition of progressive portal tract sclerosis leading to impaired portal vein inflow. In those instances in which a cause can be identified, it may be myeloproliferative disorders with associated hypercoagulability, peritonitis, or exposure to arsenicals.

Impaired Blood Flow Through the Liver

The most common intrahepatic cause of portal blood flow obstruction is cirrhosis, as described earlier. In addition, physical occlusion of the sinusoids occurs in a small but important group of diseases. In sickle cell disease, the hepatic sinusoids may become packed with sickled erythrocytes, both free within the vascular space and erythrophagocytosed by Kupffer cells, leading to panlobular parenchymal necrosis. Disseminated intravascular coagulation may occlude sinusoids. This is usually inconsequential except for the periportal sinusoidal

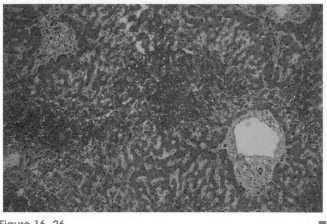

Figure 16–26 ■

Centrilobular hemorrhagic necrosis. The centrilobular region is suffused with red blood cells, and hepatocytes are not readily visible. Portal tracts and the periportal parenchyma are intact.

occlusion and parenchymal necrosis that may arise in pregnancy as part of eclampsia. Suffusion of blood under the capsule may precipitate a fatal intra-abdominal hemorrhage (Fig. 16–25).

Passive Congestion and Centrilobular Necrosis. These hepatic manifestations of systemic circulatory compromise are considered together because they represent a morphologic continuum. Both changes are commonly seen at autopsy, because there is an element of preterminal circulatory failure with virtually every death. Right-sided cardiac decompensation leads to passive congestion of the liver. The liver is slightly enlarged, tense, and cyanotic, with rounded edges. Microscopically, there is congestion of centrilobular sinusoids. With time, centrilobular hepatocytes become atrophic, resulting in markedly attenuated liver cell cords.

Left-sided cardiac failure or shock may lead to hepatic hypoperfusion and hypoxia. In this instance, hepatocytes in the central region of the lobule undergo ischemic necrosis. Centrilobular necrosis is visible macroscopically as slight depression of necrotic lobular centers. By microscopy there is a sharp demarcation of viable and necrotic hepatocytes as one progresses from the portal tract to the centrilobular region. The combination of hypoperfusion and retrograde congestion acts synergistically to generate a distinctive lesion, centrilobular hemorrhagic necrosis (Fig. 16–26). The liver takes on a variegated mottled appearance, reflecting hemorrhage and necrosis in the centrilobular regions, known traditionally as the "nutmeg" liver (Fig. 16–27). An uncommon complication of sustained chronic severe congestive heart failure is so-called cardiac sclerosis. The pattern of liver fibrosis is distinctive, inasmuch as it is mostly centrilobular. The damage rarely fulfills the accepted criteria for the diagnosis of cirrhosis, but the historically sanctified term *cardiac cirrhosis* cannot easily be dislodged.

In most instances, the only clinical evidence of centrilobular necrosis is mild to moderate transient elevation of serum aminotransaminase levels. The parenchymal damage may be sufficient to induce mild to moderate jaundice.

Peliosis Hepatis. Sinusoidal dilation occurs in any condition in which efflux of hepatic blood is impeded. Peliosis hep-

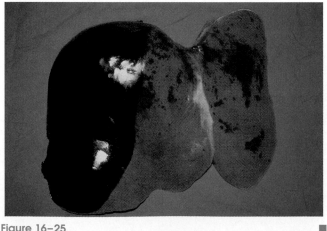

Figure 16–25 ■

Subcapsular hematoma dissecting under Glisson's capsule in a fatal case of eclampsia. (Courtesy of Brian D. Blackbourne, MD, Medical Examiner, San Diego, CA.)

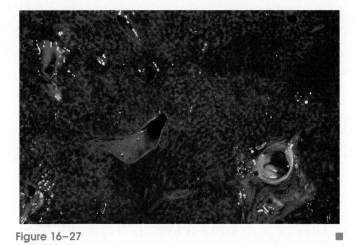

Figure 16-27   ■

Centrilobular hemorrhagic necrosis (nutmeg liver). The cut liver section, in which major blood vessels are visible, is notable for a variegated mottled red appearance, representing hemorrhage in the centrilobular regions of the parenchyma.

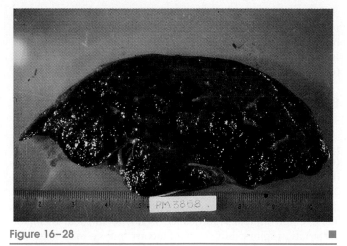

Figure 16-28   ■

Budd-Chiari syndrome. Thrombosis of the major hepatic veins has caused extreme blood retention in the liver.

atis is a rare condition in which the dilation is primary. It is most commonly associated with exposure to anabolic steroids, and rarely oral contraceptives and danazol. The pathogenesis is not known. Although clinical signs are generally absent even in advanced peliosis, potentially fatal intra-abdominal hemorrhage or hepatic failure may occur. Peliotic lesions usually disappear after cessation of drug treatment.

Hepatic Venous Outflow Obstruction

Hepatic Vein Thrombosis (Budd-Chiari Syndrome). The Budd-Chiari syndrome was originally used to describe acute and usually fatal thrombotic occlusion of the hepatic veins. The definition has now been expanded to include subacute and chronic occlusive syndromes, characterized by hepatomegaly, weight gain, ascites, and abdominal pain. Hepatic vein thrombosis is associated with (in order of frequency) polycythemia vera, pregnancy, the postpartum state, the use of oral contraceptives, paroxysmal nocturnal hemoglobinuria, and intra-abdominal cancers, particularly hepatocellular carcinoma. All these conditions produce thrombotic tendencies or, in the case of liver cancers, sluggish blood flow. About 30% of cases are idiopathic.

With acutely developing thrombosis of the major hepatic veins or inferior vena cava, the liver is swollen, is red-purple, and has a tense capsule (Fig. 16-28). Microscopically, the affected hepatic parenchyma reveals severe centrilobular congestion and necrosis. Centrilobular fibrosis develops in instances in which the thrombosis is more slowly developing. The major veins may contain totally occlusive fresh thrombi, subtotal occlusion, or, in chronic cases, organized adherent thrombi.

The mortality of untreated acute Budd-Chiari syndrome is high. Prompt surgical creation of a portosystemic venous shunt permits reverse flow through the portal vein and improves the prognosis considerably; direct dilation of caval obstruction may be possible during angiography. The chronic form of the syndrome is far less grave, and about half the patients are alive after 5 years.

Veno-Occlusive Disease. Originally described in Jamaican drinkers of pyrrolizidine alkaloid–containing bush tea, veno-occlusive disease now occurs primarily in the immediate weeks after bone marrow transplantation. The incidence may approach 25% in recipients of allogeneic marrow transplants, with mortality rates of over 30%. Small hepatic vein radicles are obliterated by varying amounts of subendothelial swelling and fine reticulated collagen. The presumed cause is toxic endothelial injury, as from chemotherapy and radiation therapy given before marrow transplantation. In acute disease, there is striking centrilobular congestion with hepatocellular necrosis. As the disease progresses, connective tissue is laid down in the lumen of the venule.

TUMORS AND TUMOR-LIKE CONDITIONS

The liver and lungs share the dubious distinction of being the visceral organs most often involved in the metastatic spread of cancers. Indeed, *the most common hepatic neoplasms are metastatic carcinomas,* with colon, lung, and breast heading the list as sites of the primary tumor. The incidence of primary hepatic malignancies varies with the local prevalence of risk factors, particularly HBV infection.

Hepatic masses come to attention for a variety of reasons. They may generate epigastric fullness and discomfort or be detected by routine physical examination. Radiographic studies for other indications may pick up incidental liver masses. Important in the differential diagnosis of hepatic masses are (1) whether there is underlying liver disease, especially cirrhosis, in which the risk for primary hepatocellular carcinoma is high, and (2) whether the mass is solitary or multiple. Nonmalignant conditions are more likely to occur as single lesions in livers without preexistent disease, although some lesions (e.g., cysts) may be multiple.

Benign Tumors

The most common benign lesions are cavernous hemangiomas, identical to those occurring in other parts of the body (Chapter 10). These well-circumscribed lesions consist of endothelial cell-lined vascular channels and intervening stroma. They appear as discrete red-blue, soft nodules, usually less than 2 cm in diameter, often directly beneath the capsule. Their chief clinical significance is not to mistake them for metastatic tumors; blind percutaneous biopsy may incur severe intra-abdominal bleeding.

Solitary or multiple benign hepatocellular nodules may develop in the liver in the absence of cirrhosis. Focal nodular hyperplasia appears as a well-demarcated but poorly encapsulated nodule with a central fibrous scar, ranging up to many centimeters in diameter. It is believed to represent nodular regeneration in response to local vascular injury and is not a neoplasm per se. Focal nodular hyperplasia occurs most frequently in young to middle-aged adults and does not appear to pose a risk for malignancy.

LIVER CELL ADENOMA

This benign neoplasm of hepatocytes tends to occur in young women who have used oral contraceptives, and it regresses on discontinuance of their use. These tumors are pale, yellow-tan, well-demarcated, and frequently bile-stained nodules, found anywhere in the hepatic substance but often beneath the capsule. They may reach 30 cm in diameter. Histologically, liver cell adenomas are composed of sheets and cords of cells that may resemble normal hepatocytes or have some variation in cell and nuclear size. Portal tracts are absent; instead, prominent arterial vessels and draining veins are distributed through the substance of the tumor. Liver cell adenomas are significant for two reasons: (1) when they present as an intrahepatic mass, they may be mistaken for the more ominous hepatocellular carcinoma; and (2) subcapsular adenomas have a tendency to rupture, particularly during pregnancy (under estrogenic stimulation), causing life-threatening intra-abdominal hemorrhage. They harbor hepatocellular carcinoma only rarely.

Primary Carcinoma of the Liver

Primary carcinomas of the liver are relatively uncommon in North America and Western Europe (0.5% to 2% of all cancers) but represent 20% to 40% of cancers in many other countries. Most arise from hepatocytes, and are termed *hepatocellular carcinoma (HCC)*. Much less common are carcinomas of bile duct origin, cholangiocarcinomas, or tumors that are a mixture of the two cell types. Two rare forms are mentioned only: the hepatoblastoma, an aggressive hepatocellular tumor of childhood, and highly malignant angiosarcoma, which resembles those occurring elsewhere (Chapter 10). Primary liver angiosarcoma is of interest because of its association with exposure to vinyl chloride, arsenic, or Thorotrast, with latency periods of up to several decades.

Epidemiology. There are striking differences in the frequency of HCC in different nations of the world, linked strongly to the prevalence of HBV infection. Annual incidence rates of 3 to 7 cases per 100,000 population in North and South America, north and central Europe, and Australia compare with intermediate rates of up to 20 cases per 100,000 in countries bordering the Mediterranean. The highest frequencies are found in Taiwan, Mozambique, and Southeast China, where annual incidence rates among males approach 150 per 100,000. A common feature of high-incidence areas is onset of the HBV carrier state in infancy, after vertical transmission from infected mothers. This chronic carrier state may confer a 200-fold increased risk for HCC by adulthood. In these regions, cirrhosis may be absent in up to half of HCC patients. In the Western world, where HBV carriers are not common, cirrhosis is present in 85% to 90% of cases of HCC, frequently arising from other chronic liver diseases.

There is a pronounced male preponderance throughout the world, on the order of 3:1 in low-incidence areas and up to 8:1 in high-incidence areas, related to the greater prevalence of HBV infection, alcoholism, and chronic liver disease among males. Within each area, blacks have attack rates approximately fourfold higher than whites. In high-incidence areas, HCC generally arises early in adult life (third to fifth decades), whereas in low-incidence areas it is most often encountered in the sixth and seventh decades.

Pathogenesis. Several factors relevant to the pathogenesis of HCC were discussed in Chapter 6. Only a few points deserve emphasis at this time.

Three major etiologic associations have been established: infection with HBV, hepatocarcinogens in food (primarily aflatoxins), and chronic liver disease.

■ Many factors, including age, sex, chemicals, viruses, hormones, alcohol, and nutrition, interact in the development of HCC. For example, the disease most likely to give rise to HCC is, in fact, the extremely rare hereditary tyrosinemia, in which almost 40% of patients develop this tumor despite adequate dietary control.

■ The exact pathogenesis of HCC may vary between high-incidence, HBV-prevalent populations versus low-incidence Western populations, in which other diseases (such as alcoholism and genetic hemochromatosis) are more common.

■ The development of cirrhosis appears to be an important, but not requisite, contributor to the emergence of HCC.

Extensive epidemiologic evidence links chronic HBV infection with liver cancer, and there is growing evidence implicating HCV infection. Molecular studies of HBV carcinogenesis reveal that the HBV genome does not contain any oncogenic sequences. Moreover, there is no selective site of integration of viral DNA into the host genome, precluding mutation or activation of a particular protooncogene. Rather, the following factors have been implicated:

■ Repeated cycles of cell death and regeneration, as with chronic hepatitis, are important in the pathogenesis of HBV (and HCV) associated liver cell cancers.

- The accumulation of mutations during continuous cycles of cell division may eventually transform some hepatocytes. Genomic instability is more likely in the presence of integrated HBV DNA, giving rise to chromosomal aberrations such as deletions, translocations, and duplications.
- Molecular analysis of tumor cells in HBV-infected individuals reveals that each case is clonal with respect to HBV DNA integration pattern, suggesting that viral integration precedes or accompanies a transforming event.
- The HBV genome encodes a regulatory element, the X-protein, that is a transacting transcriptional activator of many genes and is present in most tumors with integrated HBV DNA. It is conceivable that in liver cells infected with HBV, the X-protein disrupts normal growth control by activation of host cell protooncogenes.
- As with human papillomaviruses, recent studies suggest that certain HBV proteins bind to and inactivate the tumor suppressor gene *p53* (Chapter 6).

In certain regions of the world, such as China and South Africa, where HBV is endemic, there is also high exposure to dietary aflatoxins derived from the fungus *Aspergillus flavus*. These highly carcinogenic toxins are found in "moldy" grains and peanuts. Animal studies reveal that aflatoxin can bind covalently with cellular DNA and cause mutations in protooncogenes or tumor suppressor genes, particularly *p53*. However, carcinogenesis does not occur unless the liver is mitotically active, as is the case in chronic viral hepatitis with recurrent bouts of injury and regeneration.

None of the influences related to HCC has any bearing on the development of cholangiocarcinoma. The only recognized causal influences on this uncommon tumor are previous exposure to Thorotrast (formerly used in radiography of the biliary tract), invasion of the biliary tract by the liver fluke *Opisthorchis sinensis* and its close relatives, and primary sclerosing cholangitis. Most cholangiocarcinomas, however, arise without evidence of antecedent risk conditions.

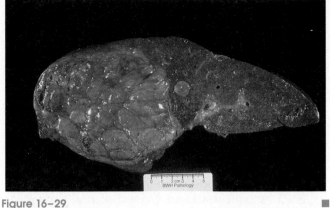

Figure 16–29   ■

Hepatocellular carcinoma, unifocal, massive type. A large neoplasm with extensive areas of necrosis has replaced most of the right hepatic lobe in this noncirrhotic liver. A satellite tumor nodule is directly adjacent.

Primary liver carcinoma, of which almost all are HCC, may appear grossly as (1) a **unifocal,** usually massive tumor (Fig. 16–29); (2) a **multifocal** malignancy, made of widely distributed nodules of variable size; or (3) a **diffusely infiltrative** cancer, permeating widely and sometimes involving the entire liver, blending imperceptibly into the cirrhotic liver background. In all variants, it may be difficult to distinguish large regenerative nodules of cirrhotic liver from nodules of neoplasm. Discrete masses are usually yellow white, punctuated sometimes by bile staining and areas of hemorrhage or necrosis. **All patterns of HCC have a strong propensity for invasion of vascular channels.** Extensive intrahepatic metastases ensue, and occasionally snakelike masses of tumor invade the portal vein (with occlusion of the portal circulation) or inferior vena cava, extending even into the right side of the heart.

Histologically, HCCs range from well-differenti-

ated lesions that reproduce hepatocytes arranged in cords or small nests (Fig. 16–30) to poorly differentiated lesions, often made up of large multinucleate anaplastic tumor giant cells. **In the better-differentiated variants, globules of bile may be found within the cytoplasm of cells and in pseudocanaliculi between cells.** Acidophilic hyaline inclusions within the cytoplasm may be present, resembling Mallory bodies. There is surprisingly scant stroma in most HCCs, explaining the soft consistency of these tumors.

A distinctive clinicopathologic variant of HCC is the **fibrolamellar carcinoma,** which occurs in young male and female adults (20 to 40 years of age) with equal incidence, has no association with cirrhosis or other risk factors, and has a distinctly better prognosis. It usually constitutes a single large, hard "scirrhous" tumor with fibrous

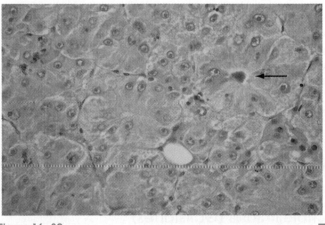

Figure 16–30   ■

Hepatocellular carcinoma. In this well-differentiated lesion, tumor cells are arranged in nests, sometimes with a central lumen, one of which contains bile *(arrow)*. Other tumor cells contain intracellular bile pigment.

bands coursing through it, vaguely resembling focal nodular hyperplasia. Histologically, it is composed of well-differentiated polygonal cells growing in nests or cords and separated by parallel lamellae of dense collagen bundles.

Cholangiocarcinomas appear as more or less well-differentiated adenocarcinomas, typically with an abundant fibrous stroma (desmoplasia), explaining their firm, gritty consistency. Most exhibit clearly defined glandular and tubular structures lined by somewhat anaplastic cuboidal-to-low columnar epithelial cells. **Bile pigment and hyaline inclusions are not found within the cells.**

HCC tends to remain confined to the liver until late in the course, at which time spread may occur to such extrahepatic sites as regional lymph nodes, lungs, bones, adrenal glands, and other sites. Cholangiocarcinoma has a greater propensity for extrahepatic spread to the same sites.

Clinical Features. Although primary carcinomas in the liver may present as silent hepatomegaly, they are often encountered in patients with cirrhosis of the liver who already have symptoms of the underlying disorder. In these patients, *rapid increase in liver size, sudden worsening of ascites, or*

the appearance of bloody ascites, fever, and pain calls attention to the development of a tumor. Laboratory studies are helpful but not diagnostic. Approximately 90% of patients have elevated serum levels of *α-fetoprotein.* Unfortunately, this tumor "marker" lacks specificity, because elevated levels are also encountered in other conditions, such as cirrhosis, massive liver necrosis, chronic hepatitis, normal pregnancy, fetal distress or death, fetal neural tube defects such as anencephaly and spina bifida (Chapter 23), and gonadal germ cell tumors (Chapter 18). *Very high levels, however (above 1000 ng/ml), are rarely encountered except in HCC.*

The natural history of primary liver cancer (HCC and cholangiocarcinoma) is grim. Death usually occurs within 6 months of diagnosis from (1) profound cachexia, (2) gastrointestinal or esophageal variceal bleeding, (3) liver failure with hepatic coma, or (4) rarely, rupture of the tumor with fatal hemorrhage. The only hope for cure is surgical resection, and even with complete liver extirpation (i.e., transplantation), tumors usually recur. In the fortunate patient, curative resection can be performed on a small tumor identified by ultrasonography, computed tomography, magnetic resonance imaging, or angiography. The only ray of light in this otherwise dismal scene is the possibility of significantly reducing the global mortality from HCC by immunization of high-risk populations against HBV, in whom infections are commonly acquired in early life.

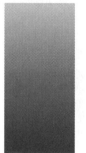

The Biliary Tract

Although disorders of the biliary tract do not garner the levels of attention given to other conditions, they are extremely common. Over 95% of biliary tract disease is directly attributable to cholelithiasis (gallstones) or the closely related cholecystitis (gallbladder inflammation). In the United States, the annual cost of managing cholelithiasis and its complications is $6 to $8 billion, representing 1% of the US health care budget.

DISORDERS OF THE GALLBLADDER

Cholelithiasis (Gallstones)

Gallstones afflict 10% to 20% of adult populations in developed countries, and pose a significant health burden, as these US statistics indicate:

■ Over 30 million patients are estimated to have gallstones, totaling 25 to 50 tons in weight!

■ About 1 million new patients annually are found to have gallstones, of whom half undergo surgery.

■ Overall surgical mortality for biliary tract surgery is somewhat less than 1%, with a morbidity of 7%.

Most gallstones (>80%) are "silent," in that most individuals remain free of biliary pain or stone complications. Indeed, gallstones may be silent passengers for decades. There are two main types of gallstones. In the West, about 80% are cholesterol stones, containing crystalline cholesterol monohydrate. The remainder are composed predominantly of bilirubin calcium salts and are designated pigment stones.

Pathogenesis and Risk Factors. Bile is the only significant pathway for elimination of excess cholesterol from the body, either as free cholesterol or as bile salts. Cholesterol is water insoluble and is rendered water soluble by aggregation with bile salts and lecithins cosecreted into bile. *When cholesterol* *concentrations exceed the solubilizing capacity of bile (supersaturation), cholesterol can no longer remain dispersed and nucleates into solid cholesterol monohydrate crystals.* Three conditions must therefore be met to permit the formation of cholesterol gallstones: (1) bile must be supersaturated with cholesterol, (2) nucleation must be kinetically favorable, and (3) cholesterol crystals must remain in the gallbladder long enough to aggregate into stones. Nucleation is promoted by microprecipitates of inorganic or organic calcium salts, serving as nucleation sites for cholesterol stones; a role for proteins in bile also has been proposed. Gallbladder stasis plays a key role in permitting stone formation and growth. As bile becomes more concentrated during storage in the gallbladder, cholesterol saturation of bile also may further increase.

Given the just-mentioned considerations, it is pertinent to examine the major risk factors for gallstones (Table 16–10). It should be noted, however, that 80% of patients with gallstones have no identifying risk factors other than age and gender.

■ *Age and gender.* The prevalence of gallstones increases throughout life. In the United States, less than 5% to 6% of the population younger than age 40 has stones, in contrast to 25% to 30% of those older than 80. The prevalence in white women is about twice as high as in men.

■ *Ethnic and geographic.* Cholesterol gallstone prevalence approaches 75% in Native American populations: the Pima, Hopi, and Navajos—whereas pigment stones are rare; the prevalence appears related to biliary cholesterol hypersecretion. Gallstones are more prevalent in industrialized societies and uncommon in underdeveloped or developing societies.

■ *Environment.* Estrogenic influences, including oral contraceptives and pregnancy, increase hepatic cholesterol uptake and synthesis, leading to excess biliary secretion of cholesterol. Obesity, rapid weight loss, and treatment with the hypocholesterolemic agent clofibrate are also strongly associated with increased biliary cholesterol secretion.

■ *Acquired disorders.* Any condition in which gallbladder motility is reduced predisposes to gallstones, such as pregnancy, rapid weight loss, and spinal cord injury. In most cases, however, gallbladder hypomotility is present without obvious cause.

■ *Heredity.* In addition to ethnicity, family history alone imparts increased risk, as do a variety of inborn errors of metabolism such as those associated with impaired bile salt synthesis and secretion.

Although the interplay of risk factors for pigment stones is less understood, it is clear that *the presence of unconjugated bilirubin in the biliary tree increases the likelihood of pigment stone formation, as would occur in hemolytic anemias.* Precipitation occurs primarily as insoluble calcium bilirubinate salts.

Cholesterol stones arise exclusively in the gallbladder and consist of 50% to 100% cholesterol. **Pure cholesterol stones** are pale yellow; increasing proportions of calcium carbonate, phosphates, and bilirubin impart gray-white to black discoloration (Fig. 16–31). They are ovoid and firm; they may be single but most often are multiple and have faceted surfaces, owing to apposition to one another. **Most cholesterol stones are radiolucent, although up to 20% may have sufficient calcium carbonate to render them radiopaque.**

Pigment stones may arise anywhere in the biliary tree and are trivially classified as black and as brown. In general, black pigment stones are found in sterile gallbladder bile and brown stones are found in infected intrahepatic or extrahepatic ducts. The stones contain calcium salts of unconjugated bilirubin and lesser amounts of other calcium salts, mucin glycoproteins, and cholesterol.

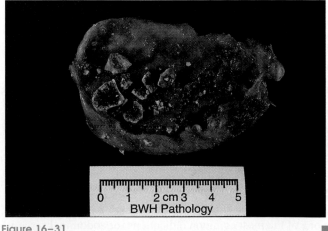

Figure 16–31   ■

Cholesterol gallstones. Mechanical manipulation during laparoscopic cholecystectomy has caused fragmentation of several cholesterol gallstones, revealing interiors that are pigmented because of entrapped bile pigments. The gallbladder mucosa is reddened and irregular as a result of coexistent acute and chronic cholecystitis.

■

Table 16–10.   RISK FACTORS FOR GALLSTONES

Cholesterol Stones
Demography: Northern Europe, North and South America, Native Americans, Mexican Americans
Advancing age
Female sex hormones
    Female gender
    Oral contraceptives
    Pregnancy
Obesity
Rapid weight reduction
Gallbladder stasis
Inborn disorders of bile acid metabolism
Hyperlipidemia syndromes
Pigment Stones
Demography: Asian more than Western, rural more than urban
Chronic hemolytic syndromes
Biliary infection
Gastrointestinal disorders: ileal disease (e.g., Crohn's disease), ileal resection or bypass, cystic fibrosis with pancreatic insufficiency

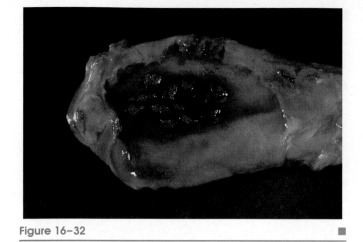

Figure 16–32 ■

Pigmented gallstones. Several faceted black gallstones are present in this otherwise unremarkable gallbladder from a patient with a mechanical mitral valve prosthesis, leading to chronic intravascular hemolysis.

Black stones are usually small and present in great number (Fig. 16–32) and crumble easily. Brown stones tend to be single or few in number and are soft with a greasy, soaplike consistency, owing to the presence of retained fatty acid salts. Because of calcium carbonates and phosphates, **50% to 75% of black stones are radiopaque.** Brown stones, which contain calcium soaps, are radiolucent.

Clinical Features. Gallstones may be present for decades before symptoms develop. Indeed, 70% to 80% of patients remain asymptomatic throughout life, the remainder becoming symptomatic at the rate of 1% to 3% per year. The symptoms are striking: biliary pain tends to be excruciating, either constant, or "colicky" (spasmodic) from an obstructed gallbladder or when small gallstones move downstream and lodge in the biliary tree. Inflammation of the gallbladder, in association with stones, also generates pain. More severe complications include empyema, perforation, fistulae, inflammation of the biliary tree, and obstructive cholestasis or pancreatitis. The larger the calculi, the less likely they are to enter the cystic or common ducts to produce obstruction—it is the very small stones, or "gravel," that are the more dangerous. Occasionally, a large stone may erode directly into an adjacent loop of small bowel, generating intestinal obstruction ("gallstone ileus").

Cholecystitis

Inflammation of the gallbladder may be acute, chronic, or acute superimposed on chronic and almost always occurs in association with gallstones. In the United States, cholecystitis is one of the most common indications for abdominal surgery. Its epidemiologic distribution closely parallels that of gallstones.

Acute Calculous Cholecystitis. Acute inflammation of a gallbladder that contains stones is termed acute calculous cholecystitis and is precipitated by obstruction of the gall-

bladder neck or cystic duct. It is the most common major complication of gallstones, and the most common reason for emergency cholecystectomy. Symptoms may appear with remarkable suddenness and constitute an acute surgical emergency. On the other hand, symptoms may be mild and resolve without medical intervention.

Acute calculous cholecystitis is initially the result of chemical irritation and inflammation of the gallbladder wall in the setting of obstruction to bile outflow. The action of phospholipases derived from the mucosa hydrolyzes biliary lecithin to lysolecithin, which is toxic to the mucosa. The normally protective glycoprotein mucous layer is disrupted, exposing the mucosal epithelium to the direct detergent action of bile salts. Prostaglandins released within the wall of the distended gallbladder contribute to mucosal and mural inflammation. Distention and increased intraluminal pressure may also compromise blood flow to the mucosa. These events occur in the absence of bacterial infection; only later in the course may bacterial contamination develop.

Acute Acalculous Cholecystitis. Between 5% and 12% of gallbladders removed for acute cholecystitis contain no gallstones. Most of these cases occur in seriously ill patients: (1) the postoperative state after major, nonbiliary surgery; (2) severe trauma (vehicular accidents, war injuries); (3) severe burns; (4) sepsis; and (5) the postpartum state. Multiple events are thought to contribute to acalculous cholecystitis, including dehydration, gallbladder stasis and sludging, vascular compromise, and ultimately bacterial contamination.

Chronic Cholecystitis. Chronic cholecystitis may be the sequel to repeated bouts of acute cholecystitis, but in most instances it develops without any history of acute attacks. Like acute cholecystitis it is almost always associated with gallstones. However, gallstones do not seem to play a direct role in the initiation of inflammation or the development of pain, particularly because chronic acalculous cholecystitis exhibits symptomatology and histology similar to the calculous form. Rather, supersaturation of bile predisposes to both chronic inflammation and, in most instances, stone formation. Microorganisms, usually *Escherichia coli* and enterococci, can be cultured from the bile in only about one third of cases. Unlike acute calculous cholecystitis, obstruction of gallbladder outflow is not a requisite. Nevertheless, the symptoms of calculous chronic cholecystitis are similar to the acute form and range from biliary colic to indolent right upper quadrant pain and epigastric distress. Because most gallbladders removed at elective surgery for gallstones exhibit features of chronic cholecystitis, one must conclude that biliary symptoms emerge after long-term coexistence of gallstones and low-grade inflammation.

In **acute cholecystitis,** the gallbladder is usually enlarged (twofold to threefold) and tense and assumes a bright red or blotchy, violaceous to green-black discoloration, imparted by subserosal hemorrhages. The serosal covering is frequently layered by fibrin and, in severe cases, by a suppurative exudate. In 90% of cases, stones are present, often obstructing the neck of the gallbladder or the cystic duct. The gallbladder lumen is filled with a cloudy or turbid bile that may contain fibrin, hemorrhage, and frank pus. When the contained exudate is virtually pure pus, the condition is referred to as **empyema of the gallbladder.** In mild cases, the gallbladder wall is thickened and edematous and hyperemic. In more severe cases the gallbladder is transformed into a green-black necrotic organ, termed **gangrenous cholecystitis.** Histologically, the inflammatory reactions are not distinctive and consist of the usual patterns of acute inflammation (i.e., edema, leukocytic infiltration, vascular congestion, frank abscess formation, or gangrenous necrosis).

The morphologic changes in **chronic cholecystitis** are extremely variable and sometimes minimal. The mere presence of stones within the gallbladder, even in the absence of acute inflammation, is often taken as sufficient justification for the diagnosis. The gallbladder may be contracted, of normal size, or enlarged. Mucosal ulcerations are infrequent; the submucosa and subserosa are often thickened due to fibrosis. In the absence of superimposed acute cholecystitis, mural lymphocytes are the only sentinels of inflammation.

Clinical Features. Cholecystitis has many faces. Acute calculous cholecystitis may barely achieve notice or may announce itself loudly, with severe, steady upper abdominal pain often radiating to the right shoulder. Sometimes, when stones are present in the gallbladder neck or in ducts, the pain is colicky. Fever, nausea, leukocytosis, and prostration are classic; the presence of conjugated hyperbilirubinemia suggests obstruction of the common bile duct. The right subcostal region is markedly tender and rigid, owing to spasm of the abdominal muscles; occasionally a tender, distended gallbladder can be palpated. Mild attacks usually subside spontaneously over 1 to 10 days; however, recurrence is common. Approximately 25% of symptomatic patients are sufficiently ill to require surgical intervention.

In contrast, symptoms arising from acute acalculous cholecystitis are usually obscured by the generally severe clinical condition of the patient. Diagnosis therefore rests on keeping this possibility in mind.

Chronic cholecystitis does not have the striking manifestations of the acute forms and is usually characterized by recurrent attacks of either steady or colicky epigastric or right upper quadrant pain. Nausea, vomiting, and intolerance for fatty foods are frequent accompaniments.

The diagnosis of both acute and chronic cholecystitis often rests on the detection of gallstones or dilation of the bile ducts by ultrasonography, computed tomography, or radionuclide imaging, typically accompanied by evidence of a thickened gallbladder wall. Attention to this disorder is important, because of the following complications:

■ Bacterial superinfection with cholangitis or sepsis
■ Gallbladder perforation and local abscess formation
■ Gallbladder rupture with diffuse peritonitis
■ Biliary enteric (cholecystenteric) fistula, with drainage of bile into adjacent organs, entry of air and bacteria into the biliary tree, and potentially gallstone-induced intestinal obstruction (ileus)
■ Aggravation of preexisting medical illness, with cardiac, pulmonary, renal, or liver decompensation

DISORDERS OF EXTRAHEPATIC BILE DUCTS

Choledocholithiasis and Ascending Cholangitis

These conditions are considered together, because they so frequently go hand in hand. *Choledocholithiasis* is the presence of stones within the biliary tree. In Western nations, almost all stones are derived from the gallbladder; in Asia, there is a much higher incidence of primary ductal and intrahepatic, usually pigmented, stone formation. Choledocholithiasis may not immediately obstruct major bile ducts; asymptomatic stones are found in about 10% of patients at the time of surgical cholecystectomy. Symptoms may develop owing to (1) biliary obstruction, (2) pancreatitis, (3) cholangitis, (4) hepatic abscess, (5) chronic liver disease with secondary biliary cirrhosis, or (6) acute calculous cholecystitis.

Cholangitis is the term used for acute inflammation of the wall of bile ducts, almost always due to bacterial infection of the normally sterile lumen. It can result from any lesion obstructing bile flow, most commonly choledocholithiasis. Uncommon causes include tumors, indwelling stents or catheters, acute pancreatitis, benign strictures, and rarely fungi, viruses, or parasites (cryptosporidiosis in acquired immunodeficiency disease). Bacteria most likely enter the biliary tract through the sphincter of Oddi, rather than by the hematogenous route. Ascending cholangitis refers to the fact that once bacteria are within the biliary tree they have a propensity to infect intrahepatic biliary radicals. The bacteria are usually enteric gram-negative aerobes such as *E. coli, Klebsiella, Clostridium, Bacteroides,* or *Enterobacter*; group D streptococci are also common, and two or more organisms are found in half the cases.

Cholangitis usually produces fever, chills, abdominal pain, and jaundice. The most severe form of cholangitis is suppurative cholangitis, in which purulent bile fills and distends bile ducts, with an attendant risk of liver abscess formation. Because sepsis rather than cholestasis is the dominant risk in cholangitic patients, prompt diagnosis and intervention are imperative.

Extrahepatic Biliary Atresia

The infant presenting with neonatal cholestasis has been discussed previously in the context of neonatal hepatitis. A major contributor to neonatal cholestasis is extrahepatic biliary atresia (EHBA), accounting for one third of infants with neonatal cholestasis and occurring in approximately 1 : 10,000 live births. *EHBA is defined as a complete obstruction of bile flow due to destruction or absence of all or part of the extrahepatic bile ducts.* EHBA is not a true atresia but rather is an acquired inflammatory disorder of unknown cause. It is the single most frequent cause of death from liver disease in early childhood and accounts for over half of the children referred for liver transplantation.

> The salient features of EHBA include (1) inflammation and fibrosing stricture of the hepatic or common bile ducts; (2) periductal inflammation of intrahepatic bile ducts, with progressive destruction of the intrahepatic biliary tree; (3) florid features of extrahepatic biliary obstruction on liver biopsy (i.e., marked bile duct proliferation, portal tract edema and fibrosis, and parenchymal cholestasis); and (4) periportal fibrosis and cirrhosis within 3 to 6 months of birth.

Clinical Course. Infants with EHBA present with neonatal cholestasis, as discussed earlier. They have normal birth weights and postnatal weight gain, a slight female preponderance, and the progression of initially normal stools to acholic stools as the disease evolves. Laboratory findings do not distinguish between EHBA and intrahepatic cholestasis, but a liver biopsy provides evidence of bile duct obstruction in 90% of cases. Liver transplantation remains the definitive treatment. Without surgical intervention, death usually occurs within 2 years of birth.

TUMORS

Carcinoma of the Gallbladder

Among cancers of the extrahepatic biliary tract, carcinoma of the gallbladder is much more prevalent than cancer arising in the ducts (2 to 4:1). It is the fifth most common cancer of the digestive tract, is slightly more common in women, and occurs most frequently in the seventh decade of life. Only rarely is it discovered at a resectable stage, and the mean 5-year survival has remained a dismal 1% for many years. Gallstones are present in 60% to 90% of cases. However, in Asia, where pyogenic and parasitic diseases of the biliary tree are more common, gallstones are less important. Presumably, gallbladders containing stones or infectious agents develop cancer as a result of recurrent trauma and chronic inflammation. The role of carcinogenic derivatives of bile acids is unclear.

> Cancers of the gallbladder assume either **infiltrating** or **fungating** patterns of growth. The infiltrating pattern is more common and usually appears as a poorly defined area of diffuse thickening and induration of the gallbladder wall that may cover several square centimeters or involve the entire gallbladder. These tumors are scirrhous and very firm. The fungating pattern grows into the lumen as an irregular, cauliflower mass, but at the same time it invades the underlying wall (Fig. 16–33).

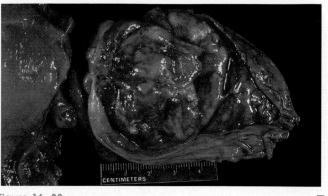

Figure 16–33 ■

Gallbladder adenocarcinoma. The opened gallbladder contains a large, fungating tumor that virtually fills the lumen.

> **Most carcinomas of the gallbladder are adenocarcinomas.** Some are papillary, and others are infiltrative and poorly differentiated to undifferentiated (Fig. 16–34). About 5% are squamous cell carcinomas or have adenosquamous differentiation. A minority are carcinoid tumors. By the time gallbladder cancers are discovered, **most have invaded the liver centrifugally** and many have extended to the cystic duct and adjacent bile ducts and portahepatic lymph nodes. The peritoneum, gastrointestinal tract, and lungs are less common sites of seeding.

Clinical Features. Preoperative diagnosis of carcinoma of the gallbladder is the exception, occurring in less than 20% of patients. Presenting symptoms are insidious and typically indistinguishable from those associated with cholelithiasis: abdominal pain, jaundice, anorexia, and nausea and vomiting. The fortunate patient develops early obstruction and acute cholecystitis before extension of the tumor into adjacent structures or undergoes cholecystectomy for coexistent sympto-

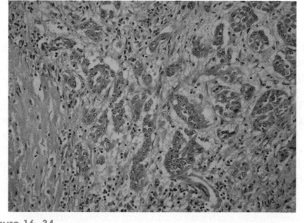

Figure 16–34 ■

Gallbladder adenocarcinoma. Malignant glandular structures are present within the gallbladder wall, which is fibrotic.

matic gallstones. Preoperative diagnosis rests largely on detection of gallstones along with abnormalities in the gallbladder wall documented by imaging studies.

Carcinoma of the Extrahepatic Bile Ducts, Including Ampulla of Vater

Carcinomas of the intrahepatic bile ducts (cholangiocarcinomas) present very much like hepatocellular carcinoma and were discussed previously. In contrast, cancers arising in the extrahepatic ducts are extremely insidious and generally produce painless, progressively deepening jaundice. They also occur in older individuals and, unlike cancers of the gallbladder, occur slightly more frequently in men. Attempts to relate gallstones to the genesis of these tumors have been unconvincing; gallstones are present in only about a third of cases. As with intrahepatic cholangiocarcinomas, risk is increased by biliary tree fluke infections (*Clonorchis sinensis*) in Asia or by preexisting primary sclerosing cholangitis or inflammatory bowel disease.

A subgroup of biliary tree carcinomas are those arising in the immediate vicinity of the ampulla of Vater. Tumors in this region also include pancreatic carcinoma and adenomas of the duodenal mucosa (discussed in Chapters 17 and 15, respectively). Collectively, these tumors are referred to as periampullary carcinomas, and all are treated by surgical resection.

Because partial or complete obstruction of bile ducts rapidly leads to jaundice, these tumors tend to be relatively small at the time of diagnosis. Most appear as firm, gray nodules within the bile duct wall; some may be diffusely infiltrative lesions, creating ill-defined thickening of the wall; others are papillary, polypoid lesions. **Most bile duct tumors are adenocarcinomas** that may or may not be mucin secreting. Uncommonly, squamous features are present. For the most part, an abundant fibrous stroma accompanies the epithelial proliferation.

Clinical Features. Symptoms arising from these neoplasms are generally the result of obstruction, namely, jaundice, decolorization of the stools, nausea and vomiting, and weight loss. Hepatomegaly is present in about 50% and a palpable gallbladder in about 25%. Associated changes are elevated levels of serum alkaline phosphatase and transaminases, bile-stained urine, and prolonged prothrombin time. Differ-

entiation of obstructive jaundice due to calculous disease or other benign conditions from neoplasia is a major clinical problem, particularly because the presence of stones does not preclude the existence of concomitant malignancy. Despite their small size, most ductal cancers are not surgically resectable at the time of diagnosis. Mean survival times range from 6 to 18 months, regardless of whether aggressive resections or palliative surgery are performed.

BIBLIOGRAPHY

Arcidi JM Jr, et al: Hepatic morphology in cardiac dysfunction: a clinicopathologic study of 1000 subjects at autopsy. Am J Pathol 104:159, 1981. (A good overview of hepatic outcome of chronic heart problems.)

Bhandari BN, Wright TL: Hepatitis C: an overview. Annu Rev Med 46:309, 1995. (A review of clinical features and disease pathogenesis in this rapidly changing field.)

Bloor JH, et al: Alcoholic liver disease: new concepts of pathogenesis and treatment. Adv Intern Med 39:49, 1994. (A definitive review of alcoholic liver disease.)

Carey MC: Pathogenesis of gallstones. Am J Surg 165:410, 1993. (One of many reviews by this author on the subject.)

Chisari FV, Ferrari C: Hepatitis B virus immunopathology. Springer Semin Immunopathol 17:261, 1995. (A discussion of the mechanisms of liver damage by hepatitis B virus.)

Desmet VJ, et al: Classification of chronic hepatitis: diagnosis, grading and staging. Hepatology 19:1513, 1994. (A modern view of the classification and pathology of chronic hepatitis.)

Feder JN, et al: A novel MHC class I–like gene is mutated in patients with hereditary hemochromatosis. Nat Genet 13:399, 1996. (The discovery of a gene that is mutated in genetic hemochromatosis.)

Gressner AM, Bachem MG: Molecular mechanisms of liver fibrogenesis—a homage to the role of activated fat-storing cells. Digestion 56:335, 1995. (A summary of recent studies of hepatic fibrogenesis, which is relevant to cirrhosis.)

Jones RS: Carcinoma of the gallbladder. Surg Clin North Am 70:1419, 1990. (A brief overview of pathogenesis, histology, diagnosis, and treatment and prognosis.)

Kaplan MM: Primary biliary cirrhosis. N Engl J Med 335:1570, 1996. (An excellent review that covers etiology, morphology, clinical features and treatment.)

Mousseau DD, Butterworth RF: Current theories on the pathogenesis of hepatic encephalopathy. Proc Soc Exp Biol Med 206:329, 1994. (A critical discussion of the causal roles of ammonia and altered neurotransmitters.)

Rapaport AM: The structural and functional units of the human liver (liver acinus). Microvasc Res 6:212, 1973. (Describes the functional anatomy of the microcirculatory unit of the liver: the lobule.)

Robinson WS: Molecular events in the pathogenesis of hepadnavirus-associated hepatocellular carcinoma. Annu Rev Med 45:297, 1994. (Examines putative nuclear events occurring in HBV-induced hepatocarcinogenesis.)

Stål P: Iron as a hepatotoxin. Dig Dis 13:205, 1995. (A review that is particularly relevant to genetic hemochromatosis.)

Yu M-W, Chen C-J: Hepatitis B and C viruses in the development of hepatocellular carcinoma. Crit Rev Oncol Hematol 17:71, 1994. (A review of epidemiologic studies implicating hepatitis viruses in hepatocellular carcinogenesis.)

17

The Pancreas

JAMES M. CRAWFORD, MD, PhD

As is well known, the pancreas is in reality two organs in one. Approximately 85% to 90% of the pancreas is an exocrine gland that secretes enzymes necessary for the digestion of food. The remaining 10% to 15% of the pancreatic substance is endocrine, consisting of the islets of Langerhans, which secrete insulin, glucagon, and a variety of other hormones. The most significant disorders of the exocrine pancreas are cystic fibrosis (Chapter 7), acute and chronic pancreatitis, and carcinoma. From the standpoints of both morbidity and mortality, diabetes mellitus (a disorder of the endocrine pancreas) overshadows all other pancreatic disorders.

EXOCRINE PANCREAS

The disorders of the exocrine pancreas are relatively uncommon in clinical practice but can be life-threatening, and therefore their recognition requires a high degree of suspicion. Only the three most common conditions are discussed. *Acute pancreatitis* may be subclinical or may produce a calamitous acute abdomen leading to death within a few days. *Chronic pancreatitis* is a cause of less severe abdominal pain, which, along with the attendant malabsorption, can be disabling. *Carcinoma of the pancreas* is a silent disease that comes to attention only after it is advanced and almost always beyond cure.

Pancreatitis

ACUTE PANCREATITIS

Inflammation of the pancreas, almost always associated with acinar cell injury, is termed pancreatitis. Clinically and histologically, pancreatitis occurs as a spectrum, both in duration and in severity. *Acute pancreatitis is characterized by the acute onset of abdominal pain resulting from enzymatic necrosis and inflammation of the pancreas.* Typically, there is an elevation of pancreatic enzymes in blood and urine. The release of pancreatic lipases causes fat necrosis in and about the pancreas; in the most severe form, there is damage to the vasculature with resulting hemorrhage into the parenchyma of this organ *(acute hemorrhagic pancreatitis).* Although by no means common, severe acute pancreatitis can be a life-threatening illness that demands quick diagnosis and prompt treatment.

The morphology of acute pancreatitis stems directly from the actions of activated pancreatic enzymes that are released into the pancreatic substance. The four basic alterations are: **(1) proteolytic destruction of pancreatic substance, (2) necrosis of blood vessels with subsequent interstitial hemorrhage, (3) necrosis of fat by lipolytic enzymes, and (4) an associated acute inflammatory reaction.** The extent and predominance of each of these alterations depend on the duration and severity of the process.

The most characteristic histologic lesions of acute pancreatitis are the focal areas of fat necrosis (Chapter 1) that occur in the stromal and peripancreatic fat and in fat deposits throughout the abdominal cavity (Fig. 17–1). These lesions consist of enzymatic destruction of fat cells, in which the vacuolated fat cells are transformed to shadowy outlines of cell membranes filled with pink, granular opaque precipitate. This granular material is derived from the hydrolysis of fat. The liberated glycerol is reabsorbed, and the released fatty acids combine with calcium to form insoluble salts that precipitate in situ. These deposits are evident as flocculent calcifications in abdominal radiographs, and they stain basophilic in routinely stained histologic sections.

The gross appearance of the most severe form of acute pancreatitis, **acute hemorrhagic pancreatitis**, is characterized by areas of blue-black hemorrhage interspersed with areas of gray-white necrotic softening, sprinkled with foci of yellow-white, chalky fat necrosis (Fig. 17–2). Foci of fat necrosis may also be found in any of the fat depots, such as the omentum and the mesentery of the bowel, and even outside the abdominal cavity, such as the subcutis. In addition, in most cases the peritoneal cavity contains a serous, slightly turbid, brown-tinged fluid in which globules of fat (derived from the action of enzymes on adipose tissue) can be identified. With time, this fluid may become secondarily infected to produce suppurative peritonitis.

A common sequela of acute pancreatitis is a **pancreatic pseudocyst**. Liquefied areas of necrotic pancreatic tissue are walled off by fibrous tissue to form a cystic space, which does not contain an epithelial lining. Drainage of pancreatic secretions into this space (from damaged pancreatic ducts) may lead to massive enlargement of the cyst over months to years.

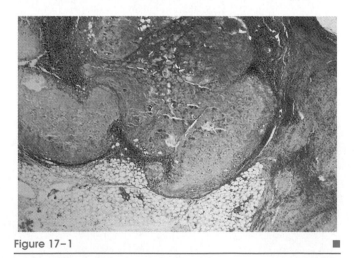

Figure 17–1 ■

Acute pancreatitis. The microscopic field shows an advancing region of fat necrosis *(upper left)*, impinging upon preserved adipose tissue *(lower left)* and with accompanying local hemorrhage *(right)*.

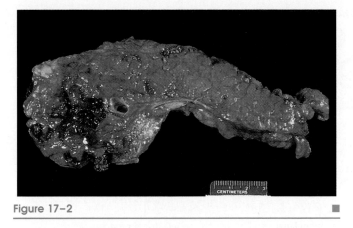

Figure 17–2   ■

Acute pancreatitis. The pancreas has been sectioned across to reveal dark areas of hemorrhage in the pancreatic substance, and a focal area of pale fat necrosis in the peripancreatic fat *(upper left).*

Etiology and Pathogenesis. A variety of predisposing conditions for acute pancreatitis have been identified and can be grouped into four major categories (Table 17–1). Most common are gallstones and alcoholism, which together are responsible for approximately 80% of the cases. The remaining specific causes are unusual, and 10% to 20% of cases of acute pancreatitis are without apparent predisposing influences.

The anatomic changes of acute pancreatitis strongly suggest autodigestion of the pancreatic substance by inappropriately activated pancreatic enzymes. The tissue lesions appear to be the consequence of proteolysis, lipolysis, and weakening of vessels. As is well known, pancreatic enzymes are present in the acini in the proenzyme form and have to be activated to fulfill their enzymatic potential. Among many possible activators, a major role is attributed to trypsin, which itself is synthesized as the proenzyme trypsinogen. Once trypsin is formed, it can activate other proenzymes such as prophospholipase and proelastase, which then take part in the process of autodigestion. The activated enzymes so generated cause

■

Table 17–1.   ETIOLOGIC FACTORS IN ACUTE PANCREATITIS

Metabolic
   Alcohol
   Hyperlipoproteinemia
   Hypercalcemia
   Drugs (e.g., thiazide diurectics)
   Genetic
Mechanical
   Gallstones
   Traumatic injury
   Perioperative injury
Vascular
   Shock
   Atheroembolism
   Polyarteritis nodosa
Infectious
   Mumps
   Coxsackievirus
   Mycoplasma pneumoniae

disintegration of fat cells and damage to the elastic fibers of blood vessels, respectively. In this manner, fat necrosis and rupture of blood vessels with ensuing hemorrhage can be explained. Trypsin also converts prekallikrein to its activated form, thus bringing into play the kinin system, and, by activation of Hageman factor, the clotting and complement systems as well. In this way, the inflammation and small-vessel thromboses (which may lead to congestion and rupture of already weakened vessels) are amplified. Thus, *activation of trypsinogen is an important triggering event in acute pancreatitis.*

The mechanisms by which pancreatic enzymes are activated are not entirely clear, but three possible factors have been considered: (1) pancreatic duct obstruction, (2) primary acinar cell injury, and (3) defective intracellular transport of proenzymes within acinar cells, leading to their inappropriate activation (Fig. 17–3).

1. *Pancreatic duct obstruction* is considered important in the pathogenesis of acute pancreatitis associated with gallstones. It may be recalled that the common bile duct is joined by the main pancreatic duct in 70% of normal persons. Obstruction of the common outflow channel, usually by a stone impacted in the ampulla of Vater, raises the intrapancreatic ductal pressure. In 75% to 80% of patients with cholelithiasis and pancreatitis, gallstones can be found in the ampulla or in the stools. The degree of pancreatic injury appears to be proportional to the duration of ampullary obstruction by an impacted gallstone. However, reflux of bile into the pancreas does not appear to occur, nor do duodenal juices appear to enter the pancreas through a dilated ampulla after passage of a stone. Rather, mechanical obstruction of the distal biliary tree alone appears to be sufficient to produce injury. First, obstruction causes interstitial edema, which is exacerbated by the stimulation of pancreatic secretions that occurs when the bile duct is obstructed. It is proposed that edema in turn causes impaired blood flow within the pancreatic substance, leading to ischemic injury of acinar cells. Mechanical obstruction also appears to cause deranged function of viable acinar cells (mechanism 3).

2. *Primary acinar cell injury* may lead to release of intracellular proenzymes and lysosomal hydrolases; the hydrolases cause aberrant activation of the enzymes (see below). This mechanism is most clearly involved in the pathogenesis of acute pancreatitis caused by certain viruses (mumps) and drugs, and after trauma. As noted above, pancreatic duct obstruction also may cause acinar injury.

3. *Defective intracellular transport of proenzymes within acinar cells* has been shown to occur both with pancreatic duct obstruction and alcohol exposure and in experimental animal models of metabolic pancreatic injury. In normal acinar cells, digestive enzymes and the lysosomal hydrolases are transported in separate pathways after being synthesized in the endoplasmic reticulum and packaged in the Golgi apparatus. The digestive enzymes make their way through zymogen granules to the apical cell surface, while lysosomal hydrolases are transported into the lysosomes. If acinar cells are injured, the pancreatic proenzymes may be delivered to an intracellular compartment containing lysosomal hydrolases, thereby permitting proenzyme activation.

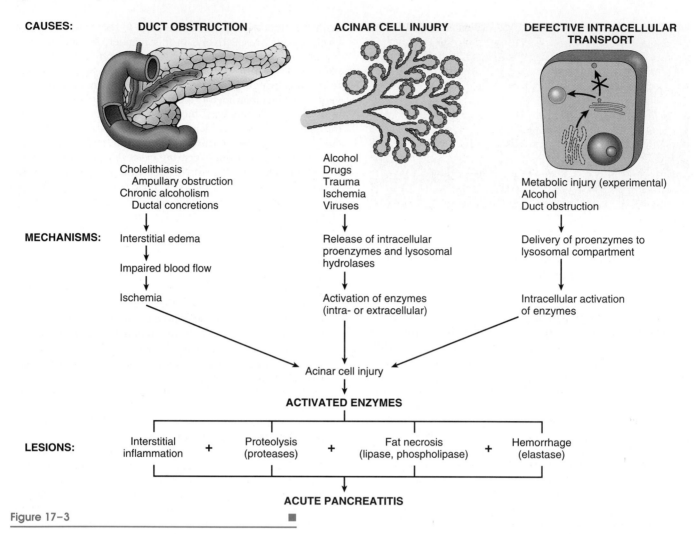

CAUSES:

DUCT OBSTRUCTION

Cholelithiasis
    Ampullary obstruction
Chronic alcoholism
    Ductal concretions

ACINAR CELL INJURY

Alcohol
Drugs
Trauma
Ischemia
Viruses

**DEFECTIVE INTRACELLULAR
TRANSPORT**

Metabolic injury (experimental)
Alcohol
Duct obstruction

MECHANISMS:

Interstitial edema
↓
Impaired blood flow
↓
Ischemia

Release of intracellular
proenzymes and lysosomal
hydrolases
↓
Activation of enzymes
(intra- or extracellular)

Delivery of proenzymes to
lysosomal compartment
↓
Intracellular activation
of enzymes

Acinar cell injury
↓
ACTIVATED ENZYMES

LESIONS:

Interstitial
inflammation   +   Proteolysis
(proteases)   +   Fat necrosis
(lipase, phospholipase)   +   Hemorrhage
(elastase)

↓
ACUTE PANCREATITIS

Figure 17–3 ■

Three proposed pathways in the pathogenesis of acute pancreatitis.

As mentioned previously, *alcoholism* is a strong predisposing factor for acute pancreatitis; however, the manner by which alcohol precipitates pancreatitis is not known. Transient increases in pancreatic exocrine secretion, contraction of the sphincter of Oddi, and direct toxic effects on acinar cells have all been postulated from experimental studies. Many authorities now think that most cases of alcoholic pancreatitis are sudden exacerbations of chronic disease presenting as de novo acute pancreatitis. According to this view, chronic alcohol ingestion causes secretion of protein-rich pancreatic fluid, leading to deposition of inspissated protein plugs and obstruction of small pancreatic ducts, followed by the train of events described above.

Clinical Features. *Abdominal pain* is the cardinal manifestation of acute pancreatitis. Its severity varies with the extent of pancreatic injury. It may be mild and tolerable, or severe and incapacitating. *Localization in the epigastrium with radiation to the back is characteristic.* Patients with extensive pancreatic necrosis and hemorrhage present with a medical emergency that must be differentiated from other causes of acute abdomen such as perforated peptic ulcer, acute cholecystitis, and infarction of the bowel. *Shock,* a common feature of acute pancreatitis, is caused not only by pancreatic hemorrhage but also by release of vasodilatory agents such as bradykinin and prostaglandins. An elevated serum level of amylase is a very important diagnostic finding. The amylase level rises within the first 12 hours and then often falls to normal within 48 to 72 hours. Although a variety of other diseases may produce elevation of this enzyme, including perforated peptic ulcer, carcinoma of the pancreas, intestinal obstruction, peritonitis, and indeed any disease that secondarily impinges on the pancreas, most of these conditions are associated with elevations of lesser degree. Serum lipase also is increased and remains elevated after serum amylase levels have returned to normal (7 to 10 days). *Used together, the serum amylase and lipase levels are highly sensitive and specific for acute pancreatitis.* Direct visualization of the enlarged, inflamed pancreas by high-resolution computed tomography (CT) is useful in the diagnosis of pancreatitis and its complications (e.g., pseudocysts). Hypocalcemia often develops, presumably because calcium is depleted as it binds with fatty acids in the abdomen. Jaundice, hyperglycemia, and glycosuria appear in fewer than half the patients.

The mortality rate with severe acute pancreatitis is high, about 20% to 40%. Death is usually caused by shock, secondary abdominal sepsis, or the adult respiratory distress syndrome. Patients who recover must be evaluated for gallstones; if these are present, cholecystectomy is indicated to prevent future acute attacks.

CHRONIC PANCREATITIS

Chronic pancreatitis is characterized by repeated bouts of mild to moderate pancreatic inflammation, with continued loss of pancreatic parenchyma and replacement by fibrous tissue. The chief distinction between acute and chronic pancreatitis is whether the pancreas is normal before a symptomatic attack or is already chronically damaged; this distinction may be impossible to apply in clinical settings. The disease is protean in its manifestations and most frequently affects middle-aged men, particularly alcoholics. Biliary tract disease plays a less important role in chronic pancreatitis than in the acute form of the disease, but hypercalcemia and hyperlipoproteinemia predispose to chronic pancreatitis. Almost half of the patients have no apparent predisposing influences.

The pathogenesis of chronic pancreatitis is obscure, and the distinction between the pathogenesis of acute and chronic pancreatitis remains blurred. Hypersecretion of protein from acinar cells in the absence of increased fluid secretion permits the precipitation of proteins that, when admixed with cellular debris, form ductal plugs. Such plugs are observed in all forms of chronic pancreatitis, but in alcoholics these plugs may enlarge to form laminar aggregates (stones) containing calcium carbonate precipitates. One proposal suggests that in alcoholics there is decreased secretion of an acinar protein that normally inhibits precipitation of calcium. With reduced concentrations of this so-called "lithostatine," calcification is favored, thus exacerbating small duct obstruction and atrophy of the draining pancreatic lobules. Alternatively, alcohol-induced oxidative stress may generate free radicals in acinar cells, leading to abnormal protein secretion, acinar cell necrosis, inflammation, and fibrosis. Protein-calorie malnutrition appears to play a role in the tropical pancreatitis of southeast Asia and parts of Africa, where alcohol consumption is extremely low.

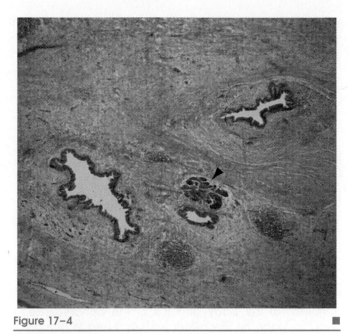

Figure 17-4   ■

Chronic pancreatitis. The exocrine pancreas has been replaced by fibrous tissue; ectatic intermediate-sized ducts and a small residuum of acinar tissue *(arrowhead)* remain.

In chronic pancreatitis, the pancreas is transformed into a densely fibrotic organ with extensive atrophy of the exocrine glands (Fig. 17-4), sometimes with remarkable sparing of the islets. A chronic inflammatory infiltrate around lobules and ducts is usually present, and there is variable obstruction of pancreatic ducts of all sizes by protein plugs. Grossly, the gland is hard, sometimes with extremely dilated ducts and visible calcified concretions. Pseudocysts similar to those described in acute pancreatitis may be present, either internal or external to the pancreatic substance.

Clinical Features. Chronic pancreatitis has many faces. It may present as repeated attacks of moderately severe abdominal pain, as recurrent attacks of mild pain, or as persistent abdominal and back pain. Yet again, the local disease may be entirely silent until pancreatic insufficiency and diabetes develop, the latter from associated destruction of islets. In still other instances, recurrent attacks of jaundice or vague attacks of indigestion may hint at pancreatic disease.

The diagnosis of chronic pancreatitis requires a high degree of suspicion. During an attack of abdominal pain, there may be mild elevations of serum amylase and serum lipase; after the disease has been present for a long time, the destruction of acinar cells may preclude such diagnostic clues. A very helpful finding is visualization of calcifications within the pancreas by CT and ultrasonography, assisted also by identification of pseudocyst formation. Other, more sophisticated techniques attempt to demonstrate inadequate pancreatic enzyme responses to such stimulants as secretin and cholecystokinin. The condition is more disabling than life-threatening. Severe pancreatic exocrine insufficiency and chronic malabsorption can develop, as can diabetes mellitus. Severe chronic pain may become the dominant problem.

Carcinoma of the Pancreas

The term carcinoma of the pancreas is meant to imply carcinoma arising in the exocrine portion of the gland. (The much less common islet tumors are discussed later.) Carcinoma of the pancreas is now the fifth most frequent cause of death from cancer in the United States, preceded only by lung, colon, breast, and prostate cancers. Moreover, its incidence has increased approximately threefold in the last 40 years. The peak incidence occurs between 60 and 80 years of age. Currently, 23,000 new patients are identified every year, of whom fewer than 600 are expected to survive 5 years. These figures are even more distressing when one considers that there are virtually no clues to the cause of pancreatic cancer. One consistent association has been noted: the incidence rates are several times higher in smokers than in nonsmokers.

Approximately 60% of the cancers of this organ arise in the head of the pancreas, 15% in the body, and 5% in the tail; in 20%, the tumor diffusely involves the entire gland. Virtually all of these lesions are adenocarcinomas arising from the ductal epithelium. Some may secrete mucin, and many have an abundant fibrous stroma. These desmoplastic lesions therefore appear as gritty, gray-white, hard masses. The tumor, in its early stages, infiltrates locally and eventually extends into adjacent structures.

With carcinoma of the head of the pancreas, the ampullary region is invaded, obstructing the outflow of bile (Fig. 17–5). Ulceration of the tumor into the duodenal mucosa may also occur. As a consequence of common bile duct obstruction, there is marked distention of the biliary tree in about half of the patients with carcinoma of the head of the pancreas. In marked contrast, **carcinomas of the body and tail of the pancreas do not impinge on the biliary tract and hence remain silent for some time. They may be quite large and widely disseminated by the time they are discovered**. They extend through the retroperitoneal spaces, infiltrate adjacent nerves, and occasionally invade the spleen, adrenals, vertebral column, transverse colon, and stomach. Peripancreatic, gastric, mesenteric, omental, and portohepatic nodes are frequently involved, and the liver is often enlarged owing to metastatic deposits. Distant metastases occur, principally to the lungs and bones.

Microscopically, there is no difference between carcinomas of the head of the pancreas and those of the body and tail of the pancreas. Most grow in more or less glandular patterns (Fig. 17–6);

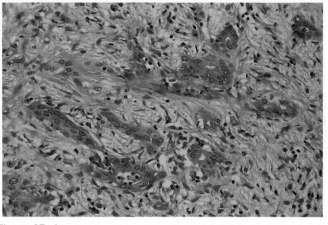

Figure 17–6 ■

Carcinoma of the pancreas. Poorly formed glands are present in densely fibrotic stroma within the pancreatic substance; some inflammatory cells are present.

they may be either mucinous or non–mucin secreting. In many cases, the glands are atypical, irregular, and small, and they are lined by anaplastic cuboidal to columnar epithelial cells. Other variants grow in a totally undifferentiated pattern. Perineural or intraneural invasion almost always is present in tumors that have extended into adjacent pancreatic tissues.

Clinical Features. From the preceding discussion, it should be evident that carcinomas in the pancreas usually remain silent until their extension impinges on some other structure. It is when they erode to the posterior wall of the abdomen and affect nerve fibers that pain appears. There has long been a prevalent misconception that carcinoma of the pancreas is a painless disease. Many large series have clearly documented that *pain is usually the first symptom*, although by the time pain appears these cancers are usually beyond cure. *Obstructive jaundice* is associated with most cases of carcinoma of the head of the pancreas but rarely draws attention to the invasive cancer soon enough. Spontaneously appearing phlebothrombosis, also called *migratory thrombophlebitis*, is sometimes seen with carcinoma of the pancreas, particularly those of the body and tail (Trousseau's sign). However, this syndrome is not pathognomonic for cancer in this organ (Chapter 6).

Because of the insidious nature of these lesions, there has long been a search for biochemical tests to indicate their presence. Levels of many enzymes and antigens (e.g., carcinoembryonic antigen, CA19-9 antigen) have been found to be elevated, but no single marker has proved to be specific for pancreatic cancer. Several imaging techniques, such as ultrasonography and CT, have great value in diagnosis; with these modalities, it is possible to perform percutaneous needle biopsy, obviating the need for exploratory laparotomy. Only 10% of patients survive the first year after diagnosis, and 2.5% survive for 5 years.

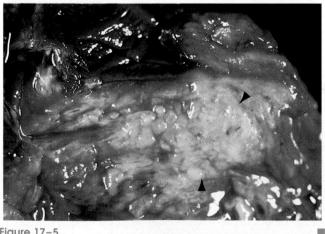

Figure 17–5 ■

Carcinoma of the pancreas. A cross-section through the head of the pancreas and adjacent common bile duct shows both an ill-defined tumorous mass in the pancreatic substance *(arrowheads)* and the green discoloration of the duct resulting from total obstruction of bile flow.

ENDOCRINE PANCREAS

The endocrine pancreas consists of about 1 million microscopic clusters of cells, the islets of Langerhans. There are several cell types in the islets of Langerhans that can be differentiated by their staining properties, by the ultrastructural morphology of their granules, and by their hormone content. Of these, the four most common cell types are the beta, alpha, delta, and PP (pancreatic polypeptide) cells. The *beta cells synthesize insulin and constitute 70% of the islet cell population. Alpha cells elaborate glucagon* and account for 5% to 20% of the islet. *Delta cells contain somatostatin,* which suppresses the release of glucagon and insulin. Delta cells make up 5% to 10% of the islet cell population. *PP cells* are found not only in the islets but also scattered within the exocrine part of the pancreas. Within the islets, they constitute 1% to 2% of all cells; their polypeptide exerts a number of gastrointestinal effects, such as stimulation of secretion of gastric and intestinal enzymes and inhibition of intestinal motility.

With this background, we can turn to the two main disorders of the islet cells, diabetes mellitus and islet cell tumors.

Diabetes Mellitus

Diabetes mellitus is a chronic disorder of carbohydrate, fat, and protein metabolism. A defective or deficient insulin secretory response, which translates into impaired carbohydrate (glucose) use, is a characteristic feature of diabetes mellitus, as is the resulting hyperglycemia.

CLASSIFICATION AND INCIDENCE

Diabetes mellitus represents a heterogeneous group of disorders that have hyperglycemia as a common feature. It may arise secondarily from any disease causing extensive destruction of pancreatic islets, such as pancreatitis, tumors, certain drugs, iron overload (hemochromatosis), certain acquired or genetic endocrinopathies, and surgical excision (Table 17–2). However, the most common and important forms of diabetes mellitus arise from primary disorders of the islet cell–insulin system. These can be divided into two major variants that differ in their patterns of inheritance, insulin responses, and origins (Table 17–3).

Table 17–2.   TYPES OF DIABETES MELLITUS

Primary (idiopathic)
  Type I (insulin-dependent diabetes mellitus)
  Type II (non–insulin-dependent diabetes mellitus)
Secondary
  Chronic pancreatitis
  Hormonal tumors (e.g., pheochromocytoma, pituitary tumors)
  Drugs (corticosteroids)
  Hemochromatosis
  Genetic disorders (e.g., lipodystrophy)
  Surgical (postpancreatectomy)

Table 17–3.   TYPE I VERSUS TYPE II DIABETES MELLITUS

	Type I	Type II
Clinical	Onset <20 years	Onset >30 years
	Normal weight	Obesity
	Decreased blood insulin	Normal or increased blood insulin
	Anti-islet cell antibodies	No anti-islet cell antibodies
	Ketoacidosis common	Ketoacidosis rare
Genetics	50% concordance in twins	60% to 80% concordance in twins
	HLA-D linked	No HLA association
Pathogenesis	Autoimmunity, immunopathologic mechanisms	Insulin resistance
	Severe insulin deficiency	Relative insulin deficiency
Islet Cells	Insulitis early	No insulitis
	Marked atrophy and fibrosis	Focal atrophy and amyloid deposits
	Severe beta-cell depletion	Mild beta-cell depletion

HLA, human leukocyte antigen.

- The first is *type I diabetes*, also called insulin-dependent diabetes mellitus and previously referred to as juvenile-onset diabetes. This variant accounts for 10% to 20% of all cases of primary diabetes.
- The remaining 80% to 90% of patients have the so-called *type II diabetes*, also called non–insulin-dependent diabetes mellitus and previously referred to as adult-onset diabetes.

It should be stressed that, although the two major types of diabetes have different pathogenetic mechanisms and metabolic characteristics, *the long-term complications in blood vessels, kidneys, eyes, and nerves occur in both types and are the major causes of morbidity and death from diabetes.*

Diabetes affects an estimated 13 million people in the United States. With an annual mortality rate of about 35,000, diabetes is the seventh leading cause of death in the United States. The lifetime risk of developing type II for the American adult population is estimated at 5% to 7%; for type I, the lifetime risk is about 0.5%. The prevalence of diabetes mellitus varies widely around the world and among racial and ethnic groups, probably as a reflection of genetic and environmental factors that have yet to be totally elucidated.

PATHOGENESIS

The two types are discussed separately, but first normal insulin metabolism is briefly reviewed, because many aspects of insulin release and action are important in the consideration of pathogenesis.

Normal Insulin Physiology

The insulin gene is expressed in the beta cells of the pancreatic islets, where insulin is synthesized and stored in gran-

ules before secretion. Release from beta cells occurs as a biphasic process involving two pools of insulin. A rise in the blood glucose level calls forth an immediate release of insulin, presumably that stored in the beta-cell granules. If the secretory stimulus persists, a delayed and protracted response follows, which involves active synthesis of insulin. *The most important stimulus that triggers insulin release is glucose, which also initiates insulin synthesis.* Glucose-induced alterations in intracellular metabolism, coupled with normal cholinergic input from the autonomic nervous system, promote beta-cell secretion of insulin. Other agents, including intestinal hormones and certain amino acids (leucine and arginine), as well as the sulfonylureas, stimulate insulin release but not insulin synthesis.

Insulin is a major anabolic hormone. It is necessary for (1) transmembrane transport of glucose and amino acids, (2) glycogen formation in the liver and skeletal muscles, (3) conversion of glucose to triglycerides, (4) nucleic acid synthesis, and (5) protein synthesis. Its principal metabolic function is to increase the rate of glucose transport into certain cells in the body. These are the striated muscle cells, including myocardial cells, fibroblasts, and fat cells, representing collectively about two thirds of the entire body weight.

Insulin interacts with its target cells by first binding to the insulin receptor; the number and function of these receptors are important in regulating the action of insulin. The insulin receptor is a tyrosine kinase that triggers a number of intracellular responses that affect metabolic pathways. *One of the important early effects of insulin involves translocation of glucose transport units (GLUTs) from the Golgi apparatus to the plasma membrane, which facilitates cellular uptake of glucose.* The several different forms of GLUTs differ in their tissue distribution, affinity for glucose, and sensitivity to insulin stimulation.

A singular feature of diabetes mellitus is impaired glucose tolerance. This is unmasked by an oral glucose tolerance test, in which blood glucose levels are sampled after overnight fasting, and then minutes to hours after an oral dose of glucose. In normal persons, blood glucose levels rise only modestly, and a brisk pancreatic insulin response ensures a return to normoglycemic levels within an hour. *In diabetic individuals and in those in a preclinical stage, blood glucose rises to abnormally high levels for a sustained period.* This may result from an absolute lack of pancreatic insulin release or from impaired target tissue response to insulin, or both.

Currently, the following criteria are utilized for the laboratory diagnosis of diabetes mellitus:

1. Fasting (overnight) venous plasma glucose concentrations ≥ 140 mg/dl on more than one occasion.
2. Following ingestion of 75 gm of glucose: (i) 2-hour venous plasma glucose concentration ≥ 200 mg/dl and (ii) at least one plasma glucose value ≥ 200 mg/dl during the 2-hour test.

Pathogenesis of Type I Diabetes Mellitus

This form of diabetes results from a severe, absolute lack of insulin caused by a reduction in the beta-cell mass. Type I diabetes usually develops in childhood, becoming manifest and severe at puberty. Patients depend on insulin for survival; hence the term *insulin-dependent diabetes mellitus.* Without

insulin, they develop serious metabolic complications such as acute ketoacidosis and coma.

Three interlocking mechanisms are responsible for the islet cell destruction: genetic susceptibility, autoimmunity, and an environmental insult. A postulated sequence of events involving these three mechanisms is shown in Figure 17–7: (1) it is thought that genetic susceptibility linked to specific alleles of the class II major histocompatibility complex predisposes certain persons to the development of autoimmunity against beta cells of the islets; (2) the autoimmune reaction either develops spontaneously or, more likely, is triggered by (3) an environmental event that alters beta cells, rendering them immunogenic. Overt diabetes appears after most of the beta cells have been destroyed (Fig. 17–8). With this overview, we can discuss each of the pathogenetic influences separately.

Genetic Susceptibility. Type I diabetes mellitus occurs most frequently in persons of Northern European descent. The disease is much less common among other racial groups, including blacks, Native Americans, and Asians. Diabetes can aggregate in families; however, the precise mode of inheritance of susceptibility genes remains unknown. About 6% of children of first-order relatives with type I diabetes develop the disease. Among identical twins, the concordance rate (i.e., both twins affected) is only 40%, indicating that both genetic and environmental factors must play an important role.

At least one of the susceptibility genes for type I diabetes

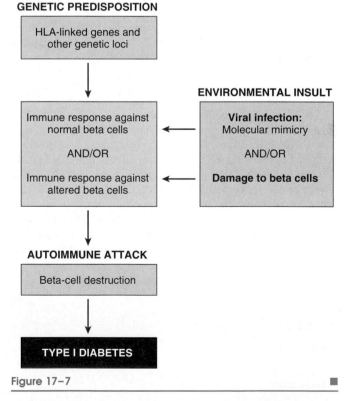

Figure 17–7 ■

Possible pathways of beta-cell destruction leading to type I (insulin-dependent) diabetes mellitus. An environmental insult, possibly viral infection, is thought to provoke autoimmune attack of beta cells in genetically susceptible individuals. Environmental insults may involve molecular mimicry, in which a viral antigen evokes autoimmune attack against a cross-reactive beta-cell antigen, or may cause direct damage to beta cells and thus evoke an immune response against altered beta-cell antigens.

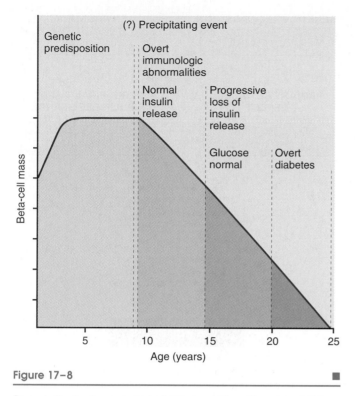

Figure 17–8 ■

Stages in the development of type I diabetes mellitus. The stages of diabetes are listed from left to right; hypothetical beta-cell mass is plotted against age. (From Eisenbarth GE: Type I diabetes—a chronic autoimmune disease. N Engl J Med 314:1360, 1986. Reprinted by permission of *The New England Journal of Medicine.* Copyright 1986, Massachusetts Medical Society.)

resides in the region that encodes the class II antigens of the major histocompatibility complex on chromosome 6 (HLA-D). The HLA-D region contains three classes of genes—DP, DQ, and DR—that are highly polymorphic (Chapter 5). About 95% of Caucasian patients with type I diabetes have either HLA-DR3 or HLA-DR4 alleles, or both, whereas in the general population the prevalence of these antigens is only 45%. There is an even stronger association with certain HLA-DQ alleles that are probably in linkage disequilibrium (i.e., coinherited) with HLA-DR genes. In the DQ locus, HLA-DQβ peptide chains with amino acid differences in the region close to the antigen-binding cleft of the molecule seem to affect the risk for type I diabetes in Caucasians.

The mechanisms by which HLA-DR or -DQ genes influence susceptibility to type I diabetes are not clear. It is well known that T lymphocytes can recognize an antigen only after the peptide fragment of the antigen binds to the HLA class II molecule on the surface of the antigen-presenting cell, enabling presentation to the T-cell receptor (Chapter 5). It is possible that genetic variations in the HLA class II molecule may alter their recognition by the T-cell receptor or may modify the presentation of the antigen because of variations in the antigen-binding cleft. Thus, *class II HLA genes may affect the degree of immune responsiveness to a pancreatic beta-cell autoantigen, or a beta-cell autoantigen may be presented in a manner that promotes an abnormal immunologic reaction.*

In addition to the established influence of HLA-linked genes, human genome analysis has revealed about 20 independent chromosomal regions associated with predisposition to the disease. Identification of these genes will be a major emphasis in coming years.

Autoimmunity. Although the clinical onset of type I diabetes mellitus is abrupt, this disease in fact results from a chronic autoimmune attack against beta cells that usually exists for years before disease onset (Fig. 17–8). The classic manifestations of the disease (hyperglycemia and ketosis) occur late, after more than 90% of the beta cells have been destroyed. Several observations merit comment.

■ A lymphocyte-rich inflammatory infiltrate, often intense (*insulitis*), is frequently observed in the islets of patients early in the course of clinically manifest disease. The infiltrate consists mostly of CD8 T lymphocytes, with variable numbers of CD4 T lymphocytes and macrophages. Furthermore, CD4 T lymphocytes from diseased animals can transfer diabetes to normal animals, thus establishing the primacy of T cell–mediated autoimmunity in type I diabetes.

■ Islet beta cells are selectively destroyed, with preservation of other cell types.

■ The insulitis is associated with expression of class II HLA molecules on the beta cells. Normal beta cells do not possess cell surface class II molecules. This aberrant expression of HLA molecules is most likely induced by locally produced cytokines (e.g., interferon-γ) derived from activated T cells.

■ About 70% to 80% of patients with type I diabetes have islet cell antibodies when tested within a year after diagnosis. Among the intracellular antigens against which autoantibodies react are glutamic acid decarboxylase (GAD) and several other cytoplasmic proteins. Whether these and other autoantibodies participate in causing damage to the beta cells or are formed against sequestered antigens released by T cell–mediated injury is not entirely settled. It is intriguing, however, to note that autoantibodies against GAD can be detected long before the onset of clinical symptoms, and similar antibodies are found in mouse models of spontaneous diabetes. These mice also have T cells reactive for GAD.

■ Asymptomatic relatives of patients with type I diabetes (who are at increased risk) develop islet cell autoantibodies months to years before they manifest overt diabetes.

■ Approximately 10% of persons who have type I diabetes also have other organ-specific autoimmune disorders such as Graves' disease, Addison's disease, thyroiditis, or pernicious anemia.

To summarize, *overwhelming evidence implicates autoimmunity and immune-mediated injury as causes of beta-cell loss in type I diabetes.* Indeed, immunosuppressive therapies have been shown to ameliorate type I diabetes in experimental animals and in children with the disease.

Environmental Factors. Assuming that a genetic susceptibility predisposes to autoimmune destruction of islet cells, what triggers the autoimmune reaction? *One proposal is an immune response against a viral protein that shares an amino acid sequence with a beta-cell protein (molecular mimicry).* As mentioned, autoantibodies and T cells reactive to GAD are often present in patients with type I diabetes; surprisingly, this protein shares amino acid sequences with a coxsackievirus protein.

Alternatively, an environmental insult could trigger auto-immunity by damaging the beta cell. Epidemiologic observations suggest the action of viruses. Seasonal trends that often correspond to the prevalence of common viral infections have been noted in the diagnosis of new cases. In addition to coxsackievirus B, implicated viral infections include mumps, measles, rubella, and infectious mononucleosis. Although many viruses are beta cell tropic, direct virus-induced injury is rarely severe enough to cause diabetes mellitus. The most likely scenario is that viruses cause mild beta-cell injury, which is followed by an autoimmune reaction against altered beta cells in persons with HLA-linked susceptibility.

To summarize, *it is proposed that type I diabetes is a rare outcome of some relatively common viral infection, delayed by the long latency period necessary for progressive autoimmune loss of beta cells to occur and dependent on the modifying effects of the genetic background, particularly that of HLA class II molecules.*

Pathogenesis of Type II Diabetes Mellitus

Much less is known about the pathogenesis of type II diabetes, despite its being by far the more common type. *There is no evidence that autoimmune mechanisms are involved.* Life style clearly plays a role, as will become evident when obesity is considered. Nevertheless, *genetic factors are even more important than in type I diabetes.* Among identical twins, the concordance rate is 60% to 80%. In first-degree relatives with type II diabetes (and in nonidentical twins), the risk of developing disease is 20% to 40%, compared with 5% to 7% in the population at large. Unlike type I diabetes, the disease is not linked to any HLA genes. Rather, epidemiologic studies indicate that *type II diabetes appears to result from a collection of multiple genetic defects,* each contributing its own predisposing risk and each modified by environmental factors. Most of the hypothesized defects remain unidentified.

The two metabolic defects that characterize type II diabetes are a derangement in beta-cell secretion of insulin and an inability of peripheral tissues to respond to insulin (insulin resistance) (Fig. 17–9). The primacy of the secretory defect, in comparison with insulin resistance, is a matter of continuing debate.

Deranged Beta-Cell Secretion of Insulin. In populations at risk for development of type II diabetes (i.e., relatives of patients), a modest hyperinsulinemia may be observed, attributed to beta-cell hyperresponsiveness to physiologic elevations in blood glucose. With the development of overt disease, the pattern of insulin secretion exhibits a subtle change. Early in the course of type II diabetes, insulin secretion appears to be normal and plasma insulin levels are not reduced. However, the normal pulsatile, oscillating pattern of insulin secretion is lost, and the rapid first phase of insulin secretion triggered by glucose is obtunded. Collectively, these and other observations suggest derangements in beta-cell responses to hyperglycemia early in type II diabetes, rather than deficiencies in insulin synthesis per se.

However, later in the course of the disease, a mild to moderate deficiency of insulin is present, which is less severe than that of type I diabetes. The cause of the insulin deficiency in type II diabetes is not entirely clear, but irreversible beta-cell damage appears to be present. Unlike type I diabetes, there is no evidence for viral or immune-mediated injury to the islet

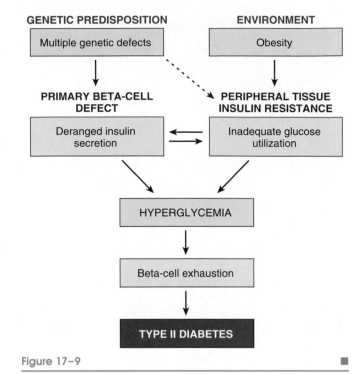

Figure 17–9 ■

Pathogenesis of type II diabetes mellitus. Genetic predisposition and environmental influences converge to cause hyperglycemia and overt diabetes. The primacy of deranged beta-cell insulin secretion and peripheral insulin resistance is not established; in patients with clinical disease, both defects can be demonstrated.

cells. According to one view, all the somatic cells of diabetics, including pancreatic beta cells, are genetically vulnerable to injury, leading to accelerated cell turnover and premature aging, and ultimately to a modest reduction in beta-cell mass. Chronic hyperglycemia, by causing persistent beta-cell stimulation, may contribute by exhaustion of beta-cell function.

Insulin Resistance. Although insulin deficiency is present late in the course of type II diabetes, it is not of sufficient magnitude to explain the metabolic disturbances. Rather, the evidence suggests that *insulin resistance is a major factor in the development of type II diabetes.*

At the outset, it should be noted that insulin resistance is a complex phenomenon that is not restricted to the diabetes syndrome. In both obesity and pregnancy, insulin sensitivity of target tissues decreases (even in the absence of diabetes), and serum levels of insulin may be elevated to compensate for insulin resistance. Thus, either obesity or pregnancy may unmask subclinical type II diabetes by increasing the insulin resistance to a degree that cannot be compensated by increased production of insulin.

The cellular and molecular basis of insulin resistance is not entirely clear. There is a decrease in the number of insulin receptors, and, more important, the postreceptor signaling by insulin is impaired. As discussed previously, binding of insulin to its receptors leads to translocation of glucose transport units (GLUTs) to the cell membrane, which in turn facilitates uptake of glucose. It is widely suspected that reduced synthesis and translocation of GLUTs in muscle and fat cells underlies insulin resistance in obesity as well as in type II diabetes. Other postreceptor signaling defects also have been described. *From a physiologic standpoint, insulin resistance, regardless of its mechanism, results in (1) the inability of circulating insulin to properly direct the disposition of glucose (and other metabolic fuels); (2) a more persistent hyperglycemia; and therefore (3) more prolonged stimulation of the pancreatic beta cells.*

Obesity. Regardless of which initiating event is proposed for type II diabetes, obesity is an extremely important environmental influence. Approximately 80% of type II diabetics are obese. As noted previously, nondiabetic obese individuals exhibit insulin resistance and hyperinsulinemia. However, when obese patients with type II diabetes are compared with weight-matched nondiabetics, it appears that the insulin levels of obese diabetics are below those observed in obese nondiabetics, suggesting a relative insulin deficiency. Fortunately, in many obese diabetics, especially early in the course of the disease, weight loss (and physical exercise) can reverse impaired glucose tolerance. Although obesity is emphasized as a factor in insulin resistance, such resistance is also encountered in nonobese patients with type II diabetes.

Amylin. Current interest is also focused on the role of amylin in the pathogenesis of type II diabetes. This protein is normally produced by the beta cells, copackaged with insulin, and cosecreted with insulin in response to food ingestion. In patients with type II diabetes, amylin tends to accumulate in the sinusoidal space outside the beta cells, in close contact with their cell membranes, eventually acquiring the tinctorial characteristics of amyloid. It is unknown whether amylin deposition contributes to the disturbance in glucose sensing by beta cells that is noted early in the course of type II diabetes or whether it is instead a result of disordered beta-cell function.

To summarize, type II diabetes is a complex, multifactorial disorder involving both impaired insulin release and end-organ insensitivity. Insulin resistance, frequently associated with obesity, produces excessive stress on beta cells, which may fail in the face of sustained need for a state of hyperinsulinism. A genetic factor is definitely involved, but how it fits into this puzzle remains unclear.

Pathogenesis of the Complications of Diabetes

The morbidity associated with long-standing diabetes of either type results from complications such as *microangiopathy, retinopathy, nephropathy, and neuropathy.* The basis of these chronic long-term complications is the subject of a great deal of research. *Most of the available experimental and clinical evidence suggests that the complications of diabetes result from metabolic derangements, mainly hyperglycemia.* The most telling evidence comes from the finding that kidneys, when transplanted into diabetics from nondiabetic donors, develop the lesions of diabetic nephropathy within 3 to 5 years after transplantation. Conversely, kidneys with lesions of diabetic nephropathy demonstrate a reversal of the lesion when transplanted into normal recipients. Finally, multicenter studies clearly show delayed progression of diabetic complications by strict control of the hyperglycemia.

Many mechanisms linking hyperglycemia to the complications of long-standing diabetes have been explored. Currently, two such mechanisms are considered important.

1. Nonenzymatic glycosylation is the process by which glu-

cose chemically attaches to free amino groups of proteins without the aid of enzymes. The degree of nonenzymatic glycosylation is directly related to the level of blood glucose. Indeed, the measurement of glycosylated hemoglobin (HbA_{1c}) levels in blood is a useful adjunct in the management of diabetes mellitus, because it provides an index of the average blood glucose levels over the 120-day life span of erythrocytes. The early glycosylation products on collagen and other long-lived proteins in interstitial tissues and blood vessel walls undergo a slow series of chemical rearrangements to form *irreversible advanced glycosylation end products (AGEs),* which accumulate over the lifetime of the vessel wall. AGEs have a number of chemical and biologic properties that are potentially pathogenic.

■ *AGE formation on proteins such as collagen causes cross-links between polypeptides; this in turn may trap nonglycosylated plasma and interstitial proteins.* Trapping of circulating low-density lipoprotein (LDL), for example, retards its efflux from the vessel wall and promotes the deposition of cholesterol in the intima, thus accelerating atherogenesis (Chapter 10). AGEs may also affect the structure and function of capillaries, including those of the renal glomeruli, which develop thickened basement membranes and become leaky.

■ *AGEs bind to receptors on many cell types*—endothelium, monocytes, macrophages, lymphocytes, and mesangial cells. Binding induces a variety of biologic activities, including monocyte emigration, release of cytokines and growth factors from macrophages, increased endothelial permeability, and enhanced proliferation of fibroblasts and smooth muscle cells and synthesis of extracellular matrix. All these effects can potentially contribute to diabetic complications.

2. Intracellular hyperglycemia with disturbances in polyol pathways is the second major mechanism proposed for complications related to hyperglycemia. In some tissues that do not require insulin for glucose transport (e.g., nerves, lens, kidney, blood vessels), hyperglycemia leads to an increase in intracellular glucose, which is then metabolized by aldose reductase to *sorbitol,* a polyol, and eventually to fructose. These changes have several untoward effects. *The accumulated sorbitol and fructose lead to increased intracellular osmolarity and influx of water, and, eventually, to osmotic cell injury.* In the lens, osmotically imbibed water causes swelling and opacity. *Sorbitol accumulation also impairs ion pumps and is believed to promote injury of Schwann cells and pericytes of retinal capillaries, with resultant peripheral neuropathy and retinal microaneurysms.* In keeping with this hypothesis, experimental inhibition of aldose reductase is capable of ameliorating the development of cataracts and neuropathy.

MORPHOLOGY OF DIABETES MELLITUS AND ITS LATE COMPLICATIONS. Pathologic findings in the pancreas are variable and not necessarily dramatic. Rather, the important morphologic changes in diabetes are related to its many late systemic complications, because they are the major causes of morbidity and mortality. There is extreme variability among patients in the time of onset of these complications, their severity, and the particular organ or organs involved. In those with tight control of diabetes, the onset may be delayed. In most patients, however, after 10 to 15 years, morphologic changes are likely to be found in arteries (atherosclerosis), the basement membranes of small vessels (microangiopathy), kidneys (diabetic nephropathy), retina (retinopathy), nerves (neuropathy), and other tissues. These changes are seen in both types of diabetes. A schematic overview is provided in Figure 17–10.

PANCREAS. Lesions in the pancreas are inconstant and rarely of diagnostic value. Distinctive changes are more commonly associated with type I than with type II diabetes. One or more of the following alterations may be present.

■ **Reduction in the number and size of islets.** This is most often seen in type I diabetes, particularly with rapidly advancing disease. Most of the islets are small, inconspicuous, and not easily detected.

■ **Leukocytic infiltration of the islets** (insulitis), principally composed of T lymphocytes, is observed in type I diabetes. This may be seen at the time of clinical presentation, and presumably has been present for some time before the onset of overt disease. The distribution of insulitis may be strikingly uneven. Eosinophilic infiltrates may also be found, particularly in diabetic infants who fail to survive the immediate postnatal period.

■ By electron microscopy, **beta-cell degranulation** may be observed, reflecting depletion of stored insulin in already damaged beta cells. This is more commonly seen in patients with newly diagnosed type I diabetes, when some beta cells are still present.

■ **In type II diabetes, there may be a subtle reduction in islet cell mass**, which is demonstrated only by special morphometric studies.

■ **Amyloid replacement of islets in type II diabetes** appears as deposits of pink, amorphous material beginning in and around capillaries and between cells. At advanced stages, the islets may be virtually obliterated (Fig. 17–11), and fibrosis also may be observed. This change is often seen in long-standing cases of type II diabetes. As mentioned earlier, the amyloid in this instance is composed of amylin fibrils derived from the beta cells. Similar lesions may be found in elderly nondiabetics, apparently as part of normal aging.

■ **An increase in the number and size of islets is especially characteristic of nondiabetic newborns of diabetic mothers.** Presumably, fetal islets undergo hyperplasia in response to the maternal hyperglycemia.

VASCULAR SYSTEM. Diabetes exacts a heavy toll on the vascular system. Vessels of all sizes are affected, from the aorta down to the smallest arterioles and capillaries. **The aorta and large- and medium-sized arteries suffer from accelerated severe atherosclerosis.** Except for its greater severity and earlier age of onset, atherosclerosis in diabetics is indistinguishable from that in nondiabetics (Chapter 10). **Myocardial infarction, caused by atherosclerosis of the coronary arteries, is the most common cause of death in diabetics.** Significantly, it is almost as common in diabetic females as in diabetic males. In contrast, myocardial infarction is uncommon in nondiabetic females of reproductive age. **Gangrene of the lower extremities**, as a result of advanced vascular disease, is about 100 times more common in diabetics than in the general population. The larger renal arteries are also subject to severe atherosclerosis, but the most damaging effect of diabetes on the kidneys is exerted at the level of the glomeruli and the microcirculation (see later discussion).

Hyaline arteriolosclerosis, the vascular lesion associated with hypertension (Chapter 10), is both more prevalent and more severe in diabetics than in nondiabetics, but it is not specific for diabetes and may be seen in elderly nondiabetics without hypertension. It takes the form of an amorphous, hyaline thickening of the wall of the arterioles, which causes narrowing of the lumen (Fig. 17–12). In the diabetic it is related not only to the duration of disease but also to the level of blood pressure. The cause and nature of this vascular change are still uncertain. Although at one time it was attributed to hypertension, so common among diabetics, it can also be seen in diabetics who do not have hypertension. The hyaline material consists of plasma proteins and basement membrane material. As noted earlier, it is presumed that the plasma proteins penetrate into the abnormally permeable walls of the arterioles and are trapped.

The pathogenesis of accelerated atherosclerosis is not well understood, and in all likelihood multiple factors are involved. About one third to one half of patients have elevated blood lipid levels, known to predispose to atherosclerosis, but the remainder also have an increased predisposition to atherosclerosis. Qualitative changes in the lipoproteins, brought about by excessive nonenzymatic glycosylation, may affect their turnover and tissue deposition. Low levels of high-density lipoproteins (HDLs) have been demonstrated in patients with type II diabetes. Because HDL is a "protective molecule" against atherosclerosis (Chapter 10), this could contribute to increased susceptibility to atherosclerosis. Diabetics have increased platelet adhesiveness to the vessel wall, possibly owing to increased thromboxane A_2 synthesis and reduced prostacyclin. In addition to all these factors, diabetics tend to have

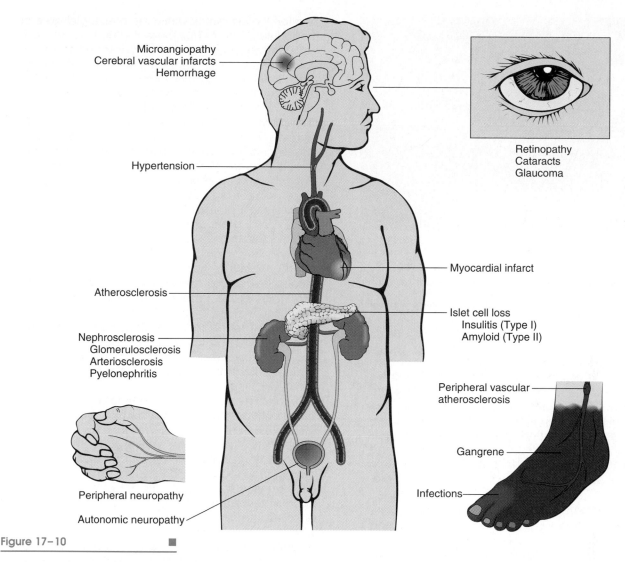

Figure 17–10 ■

The long-term complications of diabetes.

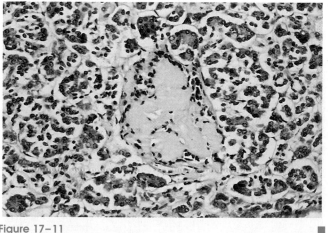

Figure 17–11 ■

Amyloidosis of a pancreatic islet in a 65-year-old man with diabetes of 25 years' duration. (H & E.)

an increased incidence of hypertension, which is a well-known risk factor for atherosclerosis (Chapter 10).

DIABETIC MICROANGIOPATHY. One of the most consistent morphologic features of diabetes is **diffuse thickening of basement membranes**. The thickening is most evident in the capillaries of the skin, skeletal muscles, retinas, renal glomeruli, and renal medullae. However, it may also be seen in such nonvascular structures as renal tubules, Bowman's capsule, peripheral nerves, and placenta. By light microscopy, the normal basal lamina consists of a relatively uniform layer of extracellular material that separates parenchymal or endothelial cells from the surrounding connective tissue stroma. In diabetics, this single layer is widened and sometimes replaced by concentric layers of

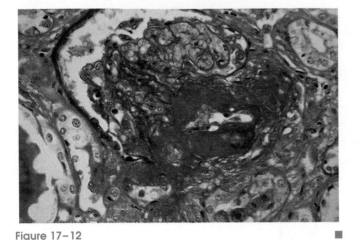

Figure 17–12 ■

Hyaline arteriolosclerosis. Note a markedly thickened, tortuous afferent arteriole in the kidney. The amorphous nature of the thickened vascular wall is evident. (Periodic acid–Schiff stain.) (Courtesy of Dr. M.A. Venkatachalam, Department of Pathology, University of Texas Health Science Center at San Antonio, TX.)

hyaline material composed predominantly of type IV collagen. **Despite the increase in the thickness of basement membranes, diabetic capillaries are more leaky than normal to plasma proteins. The microangiopathy underlies the development of diabetic nephropathy and some forms of neuropathy.** An indistinguishable microangiopathy can be found in aged nondiabetic patients, but rarely to the extent seen in patients with long-standing diabetes.

DIABETIC NEPHROPATHY. The kidneys are prime targets of diabetes, and renal failure is second only to myocardial infarction as a cause of death from this disease. **Three important lesions are encountered: (1) glomerular lesions; (2) renal vascular lesions, principally arteriolosclerosis; and (3) pyelonephritis, including necrotizing papillitis.**

The most important glomerular lesions are capillary basement membrane thickening, diffuse glomerulosclerosis, and nodular glomerulosclerosis (Kimmelstiel-Wilson lesion). **The glomerular capillary basement membranes are thickened throughout their entire length.** This change can be detected by electron microscopy within a few years of the onset of diabetes, sometimes without any associated change in renal function.

Diffuse glomerulosclerosis consists of a diffuse increase in mesangial matrix along with mesangial cell proliferation and is always associated with basement membrane thickening. It is found in most patients with disease of more than 10 years' duration. After glomerulosclerosis becomes marked, patients manifest the nephrotic syndrome (Chapter 14), characterized by proteinuria, hypoalbuminemia, and edema.

Nodular glomerulosclerosis describes a glomerular lesion made distinctive by ball-like deposits of a laminated matrix within the mesangial core of the lobule (Fig. 17–13). These nodules tend to develop in the periphery of the glomerulus, and because they arise within the mesangium, they push the glomerular capillary loops even more to the periphery. Often these capillary loops create halos about the nodule. This distinctive change has been called the Kimmelstiel-Wilson lesion, after the pioneers who described it. Nodular glomerulosclerosis occurs irregularly throughout the kidney and affects random glomeruli as well as random lobules within a glomerulus. In advanced disease, many nodules are present within a single glomerulus, and most glomeruli become involved. The deposits are positive on periodic acid–Schiff staining and contain mucopolysaccharides, lipids, and fibrils as well as collagen fibers, as do the matrix deposits of diffuse glomerulosclerosis.

Because tubules are perfused by vessels arising from glomerular efferent arterioles, advanced glomerulosclerosis is associated with tubular ischemia and interstitial fibrosis. In addition, patients with uncontrolled glycosuria may reabsorb glucose and store it as glycogen in the tubular epithelium. This change does not affect tubular function.

Renal atherosclerosis and arteriolosclerosis constitute only one part of the systemic involvement of blood vessels in diabetics. The kidney is one of the most frequently and most severely affected organs; however, the changes in the arteries and arterioles are similar to those found throughout the body. **Hyaline arteriolosclerosis affects not only the afferent but also the efferent arteriole.** Such efferent arteriolosclerosis is rarely if ever encountered in persons who do not have diabetes.

Pyelonephritis is an acute or chronic inflammation of the kidneys that usually begins in the interstitial tissue and then spreads to affect the tubules and, in extreme cases, the glomeruli. Both the acute and chronic forms of this disease occur in

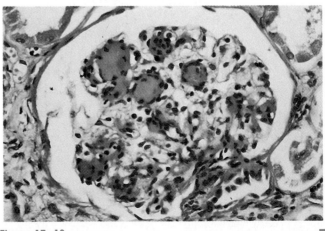

Figure 17–13 ■

Nodular glomerulosclerosis in a patient who had had diabetes for 17 years.

nondiabetics as well as in diabetics; they are described more fully in Chapter 14. However, these inflammatory disorders are more common in diabetics than in the general population, and, once affected, diabetics tend to have more severe involvement. One special pattern of acute pyelonephritis, **necrotizing papillitis**, is much more prevalent in diabetics than in nondiabetics. As the term implies, necrotizing papillitis is an acute necrosis of the renal papillae, described in Chapter 14. Although this lesion is not limited to diabetics, they are particularly prone to develop it, owing to the combination of ischemia resulting from microangiopathy and increased susceptibility to bacterial infection.

The sclerotic lesions of the glomeruli destroy renal function and constitute potentially fatal forms of diabetic nephropathy. Nodular glomerulosclerosis is encountered in perhaps 10% to 35% of diabetics and is a major cause of morbidity and mortality. As with diffuse glomerulosclerosis, the appearance is related to the duration of the disease but conditioned by the genetic background. Unlike the diffuse form, which may also be seen in association with old age and hypertension, the nodular form of glomerulosclerosis, for all practical purposes, implicates diabetes. Both the diffuse and the nodular forms of glomerulosclerosis induce sufficient ischemia to cause overall fine scarring of the kidneys, marked by a finely granular cortical surface (Fig. 17–14).

DIABETIC OCULAR COMPLICATIONS. Visual impairment, sometimes even total blindness, is one of

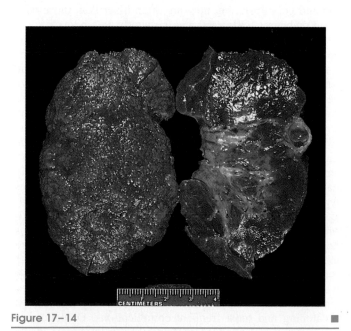

Figure 17–14

Nephrosclerosis in a patient with long-standing diabetes. The kidney has been bisected to demonstrate both diffuse granular transformation of the surface *(left)* and marked thinning of the cortical tissue *(right).* Additional features include some irregular depressions, the result of pyelonephritis, and an incidental cortical cyst *(far right).*

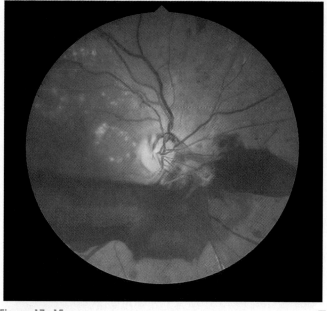

Figure 17–15

Diabetic retinopathy. A view of the fundus shows large areas of preretinal hemorrhage below the optic disc; pale dots represent exudates in the left side. Neovascularization is present on the right side of the optic disc. (Courtesy of Dr. Rajiv Anand, Texas Retina Associates, Dallas, TX.)

the more feared consequences of long-standing diabetes. This disease is the fourth leading cause of acquired blindness in the United States. **The ocular involvement may take the form of retinopathy, cataract formation, or glaucoma.** Retinopathy, the most common pattern, consists of a constellation of changes that together are considered by many ophthalmologists to be virtually diagnostic of the disease. **The lesion in the retina takes two forms: nonproliferative (background) retinopathy and proliferative retinopathy.**

Nonproliferative retinopathy includes intraretinal or preretinal hemorrhages, retinal exudates, microaneurysms, venous dilations, edema, and, most importantly, thickening of the retinal capillaries (microangiopathy). The retinal exudates can be either "soft" (microinfarcts) or "hard" (deposits of plasma proteins and lipids) (Fig. 17–15). The microaneurysms are discrete saccular dilations of retinal choroidal capillaries that appear through the ophthalmoscope as small red dots. Dilations tend to occur at focal points of weakening, resulting from loss of pericytes. Retinal edema presumably results from excessive capillary permeability. Underlying all these changes is the microangiopathy, which is thought to lead to loss of capillary pericytes and hence to focal weakening of capillary structure.

The so-called proliferative retinopathy is a process of neovascularization and fibrosis. This lesion can lead to serious consequences, including blindness, especially if it involves the macula. Vitreous hemorrhages can result from rupture of the newly formed capillaries; the resultant organization of the hemorrhage can pull the retina off its substratum (retinal detachment).

DIABETIC NEUROPATHY. The central and peripheral nervous systems are not spared by diabetes. The most frequent pattern of involvement is a peripheral, symmetric neuropathy of the lower extremities that affects both motor and sensory function but particularly the latter. Other forms include autonomic neuropathy, which produces disturbances in bowel and bladder function and sometimes sexual impotence, and diabetic mononeuropathy, which may manifest as sudden footdrop, wristdrop, or isolated cranial nerve palsies. The neurologic changes may be caused by microangiopathy and increased permeability of the capillaries that supply the nerves as well as by direct axonal damage due to alterations in sorbitol metabolism (discussed earlier).

The brain, along with the rest of the body, develops widespread microangiopathy. Such microcirculatory lesions may lead to generalized neuronal degeneration. There is in addition a predisposition to cerebrovascular infarcts and brain hemorrhages, perhaps related to the hypertension and atherosclerosis often seen in diabetics. Degenerative changes have also been observed in the spinal cord. None of the neurologic disorders, including the peripheral neuropathy, are specific for this disease.

Clinical Features. It is difficult to sketch with brevity the diverse clinical presentations of diabetes mellitus. Only a few characteristic patterns are presented.

Type I diabetes, which begins by age 20 years in most patients, is dominated by polyuria, polydipsia, polyphagia, and ketoacidosis—all resulting from metabolic derangements. Because insulin is a major anabolic hormone in the body, *a deficiency of insulin affects not only glucose metabolism but also fat and protein metabolism.* With insulin deficiency, the assimilation of glucose into muscle and adipose tissue is sharply diminished or abolished. Not only does storage of glycogen in liver and muscle cease, but also reserves are depleted by glycogenolysis. Severe fasting hyperglycemia and glycosuria ensue. The glycosuria induces an osmotic diuresis and thus *polyuria,* causing a profound loss of water and electrolytes (Na^+, K^+, Mg^{++}, PO_4^-) (Fig. 17–16). The obligatory renal water loss, combined with the hyperosmolarity resulting from the increased levels of glucose in the blood, tends to deplete intracellular water, triggering the osmoreceptors of the thirst centers of the brain. In this manner, intense thirst (*polydipsia*) appears. With a deficiency of insulin, the scales swing from insulin-promoted anabolism to catabolism of proteins and fats. Proteolysis follows, and the gluconeogenic amino acids are removed by the liver and used as building blocks for glucose. The catabolism of proteins and fats tends to induce a negative energy balance, which in turn leads to increasing appetite (*polyphagia*), thus completing the classic

triad of diabetes: polyuria, polydipsia, and polyphagia. Despite the increased appetite, catabolic effects prevail, resulting in weight loss and muscle weakness. The combination of polyphagia and weight loss is paradoxical and should always raise the suspicion of diabetes (or possibly thyrotoxicosis, Chapter 20).

In patients with type I diabetes, glucose intolerance is of the unstable or brittle type, in that the blood glucose level is quite sensitive to administered insulin, deviations from normal dietary intake, unusual physical activity, infection, or other forms of stress. Inadequate fluid intake or vomiting can rapidly lead to significant disturbances in fluid and electrolyte balance. Therefore, these patients are vulnerable, on the one hand, to *hypoglycemic episodes* and, on the other, to *ketoacidosis. This complication occurs almost exclusively in type I diabetes and is the result of severe insulin deficiency coupled with absolute or relative increases of glucagon* (Fig. 17–16). The insulin deficiency causes excessive breakdown of adipose stores, resulting in increased levels of free fatty acids. Oxidation of free fatty acids within the liver through acetyl coenzyme A produces ketone bodies (acetoacetic acid and β-hydroxybutyric acid). *Glucagon* accelerates such fatty acid oxidation. The rate at which ketone bodies are formed may exceed the rate at which acetoacetic acid and β-hydroxybutyric acid can be utilized by muscles and other tissues, thus leading to ketonemia and ketonuria. If the urinary excretion of ketones is compromised by dehydration, the plasma hydrogen ion concentration increases and systemic metabolic ketoacidosis results. Release of ketogenic amino acids by protein catabolism aggravates the ketotic state. As discussed later, diabetics have increased susceptibility to infections. Because the stress of infection increases insulin requirements, infections often precipitate diabetic ketoacidosis.

Patients with type II diabetes may also present with polyuria and polydipsia, but they are often older than those with type I diabetes (>40 years) and frequently are obese. In some cases, medical attention is sought because of unexplained weakness or weight loss. Frequently, however, the diagnosis is made by routine blood or urine testing in asymptomatic persons. Although patients with type II diabetes also have metabolic derangements, these are easier to control and less severe. In the decompensated state, these patients develop *hyperosmolar nonketotic coma,* a syndrome engendered by the severe dehydration resulting from sustained hyperglycemic diuresis in patients who do not drink enough water to compensate for urinary losses. Typically, the patient is an elderly diabetic, disabled by a stroke or an infection that increases hyperglycemia, who has limited mobility and therefore inadequate water intake. The absence of ketoacidosis and its symptoms (nausea, vomiting, respiratory difficulties) often delays the seeking of medical attention in these patients until severe dehydration and coma occur.

In both forms of long-standing diabetes, atherosclerotic events such as myocardial infarction, cerebrovascular accidents, gangrene of the leg, and renal insufficiency are the most threatening and most frequent complications. Diabetics are also plagued by enhanced susceptibility to infections of the skin and to tuberculosis, pneumonia, and pyelonephritis. Such infections cause the deaths of about 5% of diabetics. The basis for this susceptibility is probably multifactorial; impaired leu-

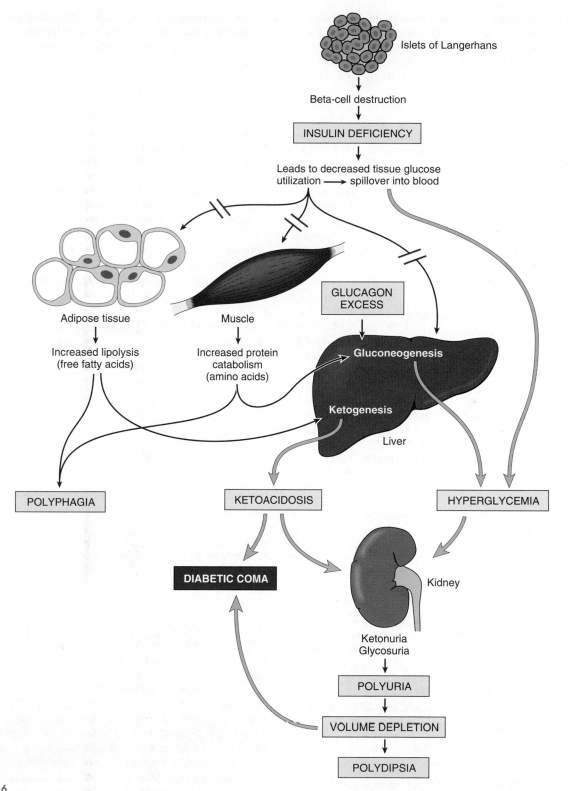

Figure 17–16

Sequence of metabolic derangements in type I diabetes mellitus. An absolute insulin deficiency leads to a catabolic state, eventuating in ketoacidosis and severe volume depletion. These cause sufficient central nervous system compromise to cause coma, and eventual death if left untreated.

kocyte function and poor blood supply secondary to vascular disease are involved. A trivial infection in a toe may be the first event in a long succession of complications (gangrene, bacteremia, and pneumonia) that ultimately lead to death.

Patients with type I diabetes are more likely to die from their disease than those with type II diabetes. The causes of death are myocardial infarction, renal failure, cerebrovascular disease, atherosclerotic heart disease, and infections, followed by a large number of other complications more common in the diabetic than in the nondiabetic (e.g., gangrene of an extremity). Hypoglycemia and ketoacidosis are uncommon causes of death today.

As mentioned at the outset, this disease continues to be one of the top 10 "killers" in the United States. It is hoped that islet cell transplantation, which is still in the experimental stage, will lead to a cure for diabetes mellitus. Until then, strict glycemic control offers the only hope for preventing the deadly complications of diabetes.

Islet Cell Tumors

Tumors of pancreatic islet cells are rare in comparison with tumors of the exocrine pancreas. Islet cell tumors may be embedded in the substance of the pancreas, or they may arise in the immediate peripancreatic tissues. They resemble in appearance their counterparts, carcinoid tumors, found elsewhere in the alimentary tract (Chapter 15). Although both share a common neuroendocrine origin, islet cell tumors have a propensity to elaborate pancreatic hormones. However, some islet cell tumors are totally nonfunctional. Among the many distinctive clinical syndromes associated with tumors of the islet cells, only three are sufficiently common to merit description: (1) hyperinsulinism, (2) hypergastrinemia and the Zollinger-Ellison syndrome, and (3) multiple endocrine neoplasia. The last of these is characterized by the occurrence of tumors in several endocrine glands and is described in Chapter 20.

HYPERINSULINISM (INSULINOMAS)

Certain islet cell tumors secrete insulin and therefore cause hypoglycemia. Patients with these tumors present with neuropsychiatric symptoms such as nervousness, confusion, and sometimes stupor. The hypoglycemic attacks are precipitated by fasting or exercise and are promptly relieved by glucose administration or by eating. The critical laboratory findings are hypoglycemia and high circulating levels of insulin. The islet cell tumors giving rise to such symptoms are called *insulinomas*.

Insulinomas are most often found within the pancreas and usually are benign. Most are solitary lesions, although multiple tumors or tumors ectopic to the pancreas may be encountered. Bona fide carcinomas, comprising only about 10% of cases, are diagnosed on the basis of local invasion and distant metastases. Solitary tumors are usually small (often <2 cm in diameter), and are encapsulated,

pale to red-brown nodules located anywhere in the pancreas (Fig. 17–17). Histologically, these benign tumors look remarkably like giant islets, with preservation of the regular cords of normally oriented cells. Not even the malignant lesions present much evidence of anaplasia, and they may be deceptively encapsulated. By immunocytochemistry, insulin can be localized in the tumor cells. Under the electron microscope, neoplastic beta cells, like their normal counterparts, display distinctive, round granules that contain polygonal or rectangular dense crystals separated from the enclosing membrane by a distinct halo. It should be cautioned that granules may be present in the absence of clinically significant hormone activity.

Diffuse hyperplasia of the islets may be encountered in newborn infants of diabetic mothers. Prolonged exposure to maternal hyperglycemia seems to underlie the development of this lesion.

There are many other causes of hypoglycemia besides islet cell tumors. The differential diagnosis of this uncommon metabolic abnormality includes such conditions as insulin sensitivity, diffuse liver disease, inherited glycogenoses, and ectopic formation of insulin by certain retroperitoneal fibromas and fibrosarcomas. Factitious hypoglycemia resulting from self-injection of insulin must also be kept in mind.

ZOLLINGER-ELLISON SYNDROME (GASTRINOMAS)

Marked hypersecretion of gastrin usually has its origin in gastrin-producing tumors (*gastrinomas*), which are just as likely to arise in the duodenum and peripancreatic tissues as in the pancreas. Zollinger and Ellison first called attention to the association of pancreatic islet cell lesions with hypersecretion of gastric acid and severe peptic ulceration. Ulcers are

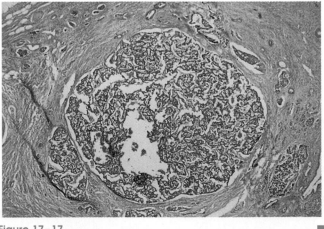

Figure 17–17 ■

Pancreatic islet cell tumor less than 1 cm in diameter in a focal area of pancreatic fibrosis. Despite the small size of the tumor, clinical hypoglycemia was present.

present in 90% to 95% of patients; the ratio of duodenal to gastric ulcers is 6:1 (Chapter 15).

> Gastrinomas may arise in the pancreas, the peripancreatic region, or the wall of the duodenum. More than half of gastrin-producing tumors are locally invasive or already have metastasized at the time of diagnosis. In some instances, multiple gastrin-producing tumors are encountered in patients who have other endocrine tumors, thus conforming to multiple endocrine neoplasia I (Chapter 20). Like insulin-secreting tumors of the pancreas, gastrin-producing tumors are histologically bland and rarely exhibit marked anaplasia.

In the classic case of the Zollinger-Ellison syndrome, hypergastrinemia stimulates extreme gastric acid secretion, which in turn causes peptic ulceration. The duodenal and gastric ulcers, sometimes multiple, are identical to those found in the general population; they differ only in their intractability to usual modalities of therapy. In addition, ulcers may also occur in unusual locations such as the jejunum; whenever intractable jejunal ulcers are found, the Zollinger-Ellison syndrome should be considered. More than 50% of the patients have diarrhea, and in 30% it is the presenting symptom.

Treatment of the Zollinger-Ellison syndrome involves control of gastric acid secretion by use of histamine (H$_2$) receptor blockers and excision of the neoplasm. Total resection of the neoplasm eliminates the syndrome. Patients with hepatic metastases have a significantly shortened life expectancy, with progressive tumor growth leading to liver failure usually within 10 years.

BIBLIOGRAPHY

Exocrine Pancreas

Blackstone MO: Hypothesis: vascular compromise is the central pathogenic mechanism for acute hemorrhagic pancreatitis. Perspect Biol Med 39:57, 1995. (A brief discussion of the potential role of ischemia in damaging pancreatic acinar cells.)

Müller-Höcker J: Pathomorphology and morphological diagnosis of exocrine pancreatic carcinomas. Diagn Oncol 3:133, 1993. (A thorough review of the pathology of pancreatic carcinoma.)

Steer ML: Recent insights into the etiology and pathogenesis of acute biliary pancreatitis. Am J Radiol 164:811, 1995. (A brief review of the role of gallstones in causing pancreatitis.)

Steer ML, et al: Chronic pancreatitis. N Engl J Med 332:1482, 1995. (A balanced overview of clinical and pathogenic aspects of chronic pancreatitis.)

Endocrine Pancreas

Atkinson MA, Maclaren NK: The pathogenesis of insulin-dependent diabetes mellitus. N Engl J Med 331;1428, 1994. (A review of the genetics and autoimmune basis of type I diabetes mellitus.)

Bach JF: Insulin-dependent diabetes mellitus as an autoimmune disease. Endocr Rev 15:516, 1994. (A thorough examination of the autoimmune arm of diabetes pathogenesis.)

Capella C, et al: Revised classification of neuroendocrine tumours of the lung, pancreas and gut. Virchows Arch 425:547, 1995. (A brief but sensible overview of current concepts regarding the pathobiology of the neuroendocrine system.)

Ghosh S, Schork NJ: Genetic analysis of NIDDM: the study of quantitative traits. Diabetes 45:1, 1996. (A critical examination of genetics and epidemiology in type II diabetes mellitus.)

Kahn CR: Insulin action, diabetogenes, and the cause of type II diabetes. Diabetes 43:1066, 1994. (A detailed review of molecular insights into insulin action and pathobiology.)

Polonsky KS, et al: Non–insulin-dependent diabetes mellitus: a genetically programmed failure of the beta cell to compensate for insulin resistance. N Engl J Med 334:777, 1996. (An examination of the interplay between pathophysiology and genetics in type II diabetes mellitus.)

Solimena M, DeCamililli P: Coxsackie-viruses and diabetes. Nat Med 1:25, 1995. (A concise discussion of the role of Coxsackie virus and molecular mimicry with glutamic acid decarboxylase in the pathogenesis of type I diabetes.)

Sacks DB: Amylin: a glucoregulatory hormone involved in the pathogenesis of diabetes mellitus? Clin Chem 42:494, 1996. (A brief editorial discussing this protein, which is elaborated by the beta cell.)

Yoon J-W: A new look at viruses in Type I diabetes. Diabetes Metab Rev 11:83, 1995. (An extensive review of both human and animal studies implicating viruses in the pathogenesis of type I diabetes mellitus.)

18

The Male Genital System

DENNIS K. BURNS, MD

Disorders of the male genital system include a variety of malformations, inflammatory conditions, and neoplasms involving the penis and scrotum, prostate, and testicles. In this chapter, the major anatomic subdivisions of the male genital system are considered individually, because many of the diseases discussed tend to involve the various organs in a fairly selective fashion. The major exception to this anatomic grouping is the discussion of sexually transmitted diseases (STDs), which are described separately because of their frequent multisystem involvement. Because of many similarities in their presentations in both sexes, the manifestations of STDs in females are also considered in this chapter.

PENIS

The penis may be affected by many congenital and acquired disorders. Only the most common malformations, inflammatory conditions, and neoplasms are considered here. Of the inflammatory disorders affecting the penis, a significant number represent STDs, which are discussed later in the chapter.

Malformations

The most common malformations of the penis include abnormalities in the location of the distal urethral orifice, termed *hypospadias* and *epispadias*. *Hypospadias*, the more common of the two lesions, designates an abnormal opening of the urethra along the ventral aspect of the penis. The urethral orifice, which may lie anywhere along the shaft of the penis, is sometimes constricted, resulting in urinary tract obstruction and an increased risk of urinary tract infections. The abnormality occurs in approximately 1 in 300 live male births and may be associated with other genital anomalies, including inguinal hernias and undescended testes. The term *epispadias* indicates the presence of the urethral orifice on the dorsal aspect of the penis. Like hypospadias, epispadias may produce lower urinary tract obstruction; in other cases, the condition may result in urinary incontinence.

Inflammatory Lesions

A significant number of inflammatory conditions of the penis are caused by STDs. Local inflammatory processes unrelated to STDs may also involve the penis. In addition, a number of other systemic inflammatory diseases may, on occasion, produce penile lesions.

The terms *balanitis* and *balanoposthitis* refer to local inflammation of the glans penis, or of the glans penis and the overlying prepuce, respectively. Most cases occur as a consequence of poor local hygiene in uncircumcised males, with accumulations of desquamated epithelial cells, sweat, and debris, termed *smegma*, acting as a local irritant. In such cases, the distal penis is typically red, swollen, and tender; a purulent discharge may be present. *Phimosis* represents a condition in which the prepuce cannot be retracted easily over the glans penis. Although phimosis may occur as a congenital anomaly, most cases are acquired from scarring of the prepuce secondary to previous episodes of balanoposthitis. Regardless of its origin, most cases of phimosis are accompanied by evidence of ongoing distal penile inflammation. When a stenotic prepuce is forcibly retracted over the glans penis, the circulation to the glans may be compromised, with resultant congestion, swelling, and pain of the distal penis, a condition known as *paraphimosis*. Urinary retention may develop in severe cases.

Fungi may infect the skin of the penis and scrotum, because growth of fungi is favored by warm, moist conditions at this site and poor local hygiene. *Genital candidiasis* may occur in otherwise normal individuals, but it is particularly common in patients with diabetes mellitus. Candidiasis typically presents as an erosive, painful, intensely pruritic lesion involving the glans penis, scrotum, and adjacent intertriginous areas. Scrapings or biopsies of the lesions yield characteristic budding yeast forms and pseudohyphae within the superficial epidermis.

Neoplasms

Most neoplasms of the penis originate from squamous epithelium. Squamous cell carcinomas of the penis are relatively uncommon, accounting for about 0.25% of all cancers in males in the United States. Most cases occur in uncircumcised patients older than 40 years of age. A number of factors have been implicated in the pathogenesis of squamous cell carcinoma of the penis, including poor hygiene with resultant exposure to potential carcinogens in smegma and infection with certain subtypes of human papillomavirus (HPV), particularly types 16 and 18. Exposure to environmental irritants, such as coal tar and soot, has long been recognized as an important factor in the development of squamous carcinomas of the scrotum but has not been implicated in the development of penile cancer. As with squamous cell carcinomas at other sites, carcinomas of the penis are generally preceded by the presence of malignant cells confined to the epidermis, termed *carcinoma in situ*.

Bowen's disease is one of the more common forms of carcinoma in situ at this site, where it appears grossly as a solitary, plaque-like lesion on the shaft of the penis. Histologic examination reveals morphologically malignant cells within the epidermis with no invasion of the underlying stroma (Fig. 18–1). Bowen's disease is not unique to the penis but may also occur on other mucosal surfaces, including the vulva and oral mucosa. Its major clinical importance lies in the potential for transformation to invasive squamous cell carcinoma, a complication estimated to occur in 10% of cases. Bowen's disease has also been associated with an increased incidence of visceral malignancies. Other variants of carcinoma in situ include *erythroplasia of Queyrat*, which occurs as an erythematous patch on the glans penis, and *Bowenoid papulosis,* a premalignant, venerally transmitted viral lesion involving the penile shaft.

Squamous cell carcinoma of the penis appears as a gray, crusted, papular lesion, most commonly on the glans penis or prepuce. In many cases, the carcinoma infiltrates the underlying connective tissue to produce an indurated, ulcerated lesion with irregular margins (Fig. 18–2). In other cases, particularly the so-called *verrucous carcinomas,* the tumor may

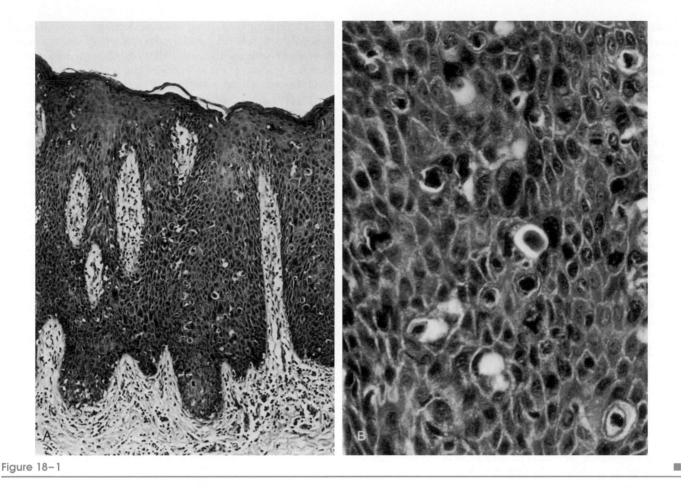

Figure 18–1

Bowen's disease (carcinoma in situ) of the penis *A,* Low-power photomicrograph demonstrating intact basement membrane. *B,* Higher magnification demonstrating cellular atypia, with occasional mitoses and a lack of normal maturation. (Courtesy of Dr. Jag Bhawan, Boston University School of Medicine, Boston.)

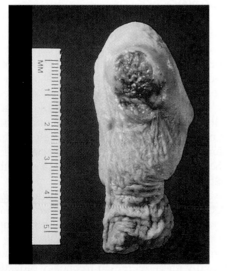

Figure 18–2

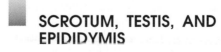

Carcinoma of the penis. The glans penis is deformed by a firm, ulcerated, infiltrative mass. (Courtesy of Dr. Kyle Molberg, Department of Pathology, University of Texas Southwestern Medical Center, Dallas, TX.)

grow in a predominantly papillary pattern. The histologic appearance is usually that of an invasive squamous cell carcinoma with ragged, infiltrating margins, indistinguishable from squamous carcinomas in other sites. Verrucous carcinomas are characterized by less striking cytologic atypia and bulbous, rounded, deep margins. Most cases of squamous cell carcinoma of the penis are indolent, locally infiltrative lesions. Regional metastases are present in the inguinal lymph nodes in approximately 25% of patients at the time of diagnosis. Distant metastases are relatively uncommon. The overall 5-year survival rate averages 70%.

SCROTUM, TESTIS, AND EPIDIDYMIS

The skin of the scrotum may be affected by a number of inflammatory processes, including local fungal infections and systemic dermatoses. Neoplasms of the scrotal sac are unusual. *Squamous cell carcinoma,* the most common of these, is of historical interest in that it represents the first human malignancy associated with environmental factors, dating from Pott's observation of a high incidence of the disease in chimney sweeps. A number of disorders unrelated to the testes and epididymis may also present with scrotal enlargement. *Hydrocele*, the most common cause of scrotal enlargement, represents accumulations of serous fluid within the tunica vaginalis. It may be a response to neighboring infections or tumors, or it may be idiopathic. Accumulations of blood or lymphatic fluid within the tunica vaginalis, termed *hematoceles* and *chyloceles*, respectively, may also cause testicular enlargement. In extreme cases of lymphatic obstruction, caused for example by filariasis, the scrotum and the lower extremities may enlarge to grotesque proportions, a lesion termed *elephantiasis*.

The more important disorders of the scrotum involve the testes and their adnexal structures. Testicular diseases may be congenital, inflammatory, or neoplastic. They may manifest themselves in a variety of ways, including infertility, atrophy, enlargement, and local pain. The distinctions among many of these conditions on the basis of physical examination, particularly among those associated with testicular enlargement, can be exceedingly difficult.

Cryptorchidism and Testicular Atrophy

Cryptorchidism represents *failure of testicular descent* into the scrotum. Normally, the testes descend from the coelomic cavity into the pelvis by the third month of gestation, and through the inguinal canals into the scrotum during the last 2 months of intrauterine life. The diagnosis of cryptorchidism is difficult to establish with certainty before 1 year of age, because complete descent into the scrotum is not invariably present at birth. A number of factors, including hormonal abnormalities, intrinsic testicular abnormalities, and mechanical problems (e.g., obstruction of the inguinal canal), may interfere with this normal descent, resulting in malpositioning of the gonad anywhere along its migration pathway. Cryptorchidism is present in about 0.7% to 0.8% of the male population.

> Cryptorchidism involves the right testis somewhat more commonly than the left. In 25% of cases, the condition is bilateral. The cryptorchid testis may be of normal size early in life, although some degree of atrophy is usually present by the time of puberty. Microscopic evidence of tubular atrophy is evident by 5 to 6 years of age, and hyalinization is present by the time of puberty. Loss of tubules is usually accompanied by hyperplasia of interstitial (Leydig) cells. Similar histologic changes may be caused by a number of other conditions, including chronic ischemia, trauma, radiation, antineoplastic chemotherapy, and conditions associated with chronic elevation of female sex hormones, as may occur in cirrhosis.

Not surprisingly, bilateral cryptorchidism causes sterility. Unilateral cryptorchidism may be associated with atrophy of the contralateral descended gonad and therefore may also lead to sterility. In addition to infertility, failure of descent is also associated with an increased risk of *testicular malignancy*. Surgical placement of the undescended testis into the scrotum (orchiopexy) before puberty may decrease the likelihood of atrophy but does not guarantee fertility. In addition, orchiopexy does not diminish the risk of subsequent neoplasia.

Inflammatory Lesions

Inflammatory lesions of the testicle are more common in the epididymis than in the testis proper. Some of the more important inflammatory diseases of the testicle are associated with venereal disease and are discussed later in this chapter. Other causes of testicular inflammation include nonspecific epididymitis and orchitis, mumps, and tuberculosis. *Nonspecific epididymitis and orchitis* usually begins as a primary urinary tract infection with secondary ascending infection of the testicle through the vas deferens or lymphatics of the spermatic cord. The involved testis is typically swollen and tender and contains a predominantly neutrophilic inflammatory infiltrate. Orchitis complicates *mumps infection* in roughly 20% of adult males but rarely in children. The affected testis is edematous and congested and contains a predominantly lymphoplasmacytic inflammatory infiltrate. Severe cases may be associated with considerable loss of seminiferous epithelium with resultant tubular atrophy, fibrosis, and sterility. A number of conditions, including infections and autoimmune injury, are associated with a granulomatous inflammatory reaction in the testis. Of these, *tuberculosis* is the most common. It generally begins as an epididymitis, with secondary involvement of the testis. The histologic changes include a granulomatous inflammatory reaction and caseous necrosis, identical to that seen in active tuberculosis in other sites.

Testicular Neoplasms

Testicular neoplasms are the most important cause of firm, painless enlargement of the testis. Such neoplasms occur in roughly 2 per 100,000 males, with a peak incidence in the 15- to 34-year-old age group. Tumors of the testis represent a heterogeneous group of neoplasms, 95% of which arise from germ cells. Virtually all are malignant. Neoplasms derived from Sertoli or Leydig cells (or both) are uncommon and are more often benign than are those of germ cell origin. The non-germ cell tumors may come to attention because of their ability to synthesize and secrete steroid hormones, with resultant endocrine abnormalities.

The cause of testicular neoplasms remains unknown. As noted previously, *cryptorchidism is associated with a 10- to 40-fold increase in the risk of neoplasia* in the undescended testis. Syndromes characterized by *testicular dysgenesis*, including testicular feminization and Klinefelter syndrome, are also associated with an increased frequency of testicular cancer. The risk of neoplasia is increased in siblings of patients with testicular cancers, suggesting that genetic factors may also play a role. Testicular tumors are more common in whites than in blacks.

Classification and Histogenesis. A number of different classification schemes have been proposed for testicular neoplasms, based on the histologic features of the tumors and on differing theories about their histogenesis. The World Health Organization (WHO) classification is the most widely used in the United States. In this schema, germ cell tumors of the testis are divided into two broad categories, based on whether they contain a single histologic pattern (40% of cases) or multiple histologic patterns (60% of cases). This classification is based on the view that germ cell tumors of the testis arise from primitive cells that may either differentiate along gonadal lines to produce *seminomas* or transform into a totipotential cell population, giving rise to *nonseminomatous germ cell tumors.* Such totipotential cells may remain largely undifferentiated to form *embryonal carcinomas,* may differentiate along extraembryonic lines to form *yolk sac tumors* and *choriocarcinomas,* or may differentiate along somatic cell lines to produce *teratomas.* This proposed histogenesis is supported by the high frequency of mixed histologic patterns among nonseminomatous germ cell tumors, the most common of which is the so-called *teratocarcinoma,* containing a mixture of teratoma and embryonal carcinoma. The histologic variants of testicular germ cell neoplasms are listed in Table 18–1. The morphology of the more common forms is presented below, along with a discussion of some of their more salient clinical features.

Seminomas, or germinomas, account for about 30% of testicular germ cell neoplasms. They are histologically identical to ovarian dysgerminomas. Seminomas are large, soft, well-demarcated, usually homogeneous, gray-white tumors that bulge from the cut surface of the affected testis (Fig. 18–3). The neoplasms are typically confined to the testis by an intact tunica albuginea. Large tumors may contain foci of coagulation necrosis, but usually there is no hemorrhage. The presence of hemorrhage should prompt careful scrutiny for an associated nonseminomatous germ cell component to the tumor. Microscopically, seminomas are

■

Table 18–1. SIMPLIFIED CLASSIFICATION OF TESTICULAR GERM CELL TUMORS

Tumors with one histologic pattern
  Seminoma
  Embryonal carcinoma
  Yolk sac tumor
  Choriocarcinoma
  Teratomas
    Mature
    Immature
    With malignant transformation of somatic elements

Miscellaneous rare variants

Tumors with more than one histologic pattern
  Embryonal carcinoma plus teratoma (teratocarcinoma)
  Choriocarcinoma and other types
  Other combinations

composed of large **cells with distinct cell borders, clear, glycogen-rich cytoplasm, and round nuclei with conspicuous nucleoli** (Fig. 18–4). The cells are often arrayed in small lobules with intervening fibrous septa. A lymphocytic infiltrate is usually present and may, on occasion, overshadow the neoplastic cells. A granulomatous inflammatory reaction may also be present. In a minority of cases, syncytiotrophoblast-like giant cells containing human chorionic gonadotropin (hCG) may be seen; they are presumably the source of the elevated serum hCG levels that may be encountered in some patients with pure seminoma.

Embryonal carcinomas are ill-defined, invasive masses containing foci of hemorrhage and necrosis (Fig. 18–5). The primary lesions may be small, even in the setting of systemic metastases. Larger lesions may invade the epididymis and spermatic cord. The constituent cells are **large and primitive looking, with basophilic cytoplasm, indistinct cell borders, and large nuclei with prominent nucleoli.** The neoplastic cells may be arrayed in undifferentiated, solid sheets or may, in other cases, contain glandular structures and irregular papillae (Fig. 18–6). Other patterns of germ cell neoplasia (e.g., yolk sac carcinoma, teratoma, choriocarcinoma) may be admixed with the embryonal areas.

Yolk sac tumors are the most common primary testicular neoplasm in children younger than 3 years of age. In adults, yolk sac tumors are most often seen admixed with embryonal carcinoma. In the histogenetic scheme noted previously, yolk sac tumors represent **endodermal sinus** differentiation of totipotential neoplastic cells. Grossly, these tumors are typically large and may be well-demarcated. Histologic examination discloses low cuboidal to columnar epithelial cells forming sheets, glands, papillae, and microcysts, often associated with eosinophilic hyaline globules. A distinctive feature is the presence of structures resembling primitive glomeruli, the so-called **Schiller-Duvall bodies.** α-Fetoprotein can be demonstrated within the cytoplasm of the neoplastic cells by immunohistochemical techniques.

Choriocarcinomas represent differentiation of pluripotent neoplastic germ cells along **trophoblastic** lines. Grossly, the primary tumors are often small, nonpalpable lesions, even if there are extensive systemic metastases. Microscopically, choriocarcinomas are composed of sheets of small cuboidal cells irregularly intermingled with large, eosinophilic syncytial cells containing multiple dark, pleomorphic nuclei; these represent **cytotrophoblastic** and **syncytiotrophoblastic** differentiation, respectively (Fig. 18–7). Well-formed placental villi are not seen. The hormone hCG can be identified with appropriate immunohistochemical staining, particularly within the cytoplasm of the syncytiotrophoblastic elements.

Teratomas represent differentiation of neoplastic

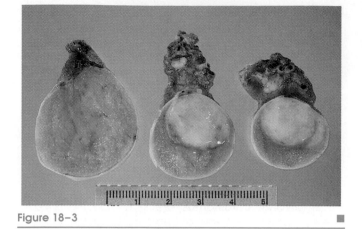

Figure 18-3 ■

Seminoma of the testis appears as a fairly well circumscribed, pale, fleshy, homogeneous mass.

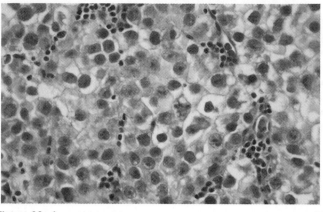

Figure 18-4 ■

Seminoma of the testis. Microscopic examination reveals large cells with distinct cell borders, pale nuclei, prominent nucleoli, and a sparse lymphocytic infiltrate.

germ cells along **somatic** cell lines. Teratomas are firm masses that on cut surface often contain cysts and recognizable areas of cartilage. Histologically, three major variants of pure teratoma are recognized. **Mature teratomas** contain fully differentiated tissues from one or more germ cell layers (e.g., neural tissue, cartilage, adipose tissue, bone, epithelium) in a haphazard array (Fig. 18-8). **Immature teratomas,** in contrast, contain immature somatic elements reminiscent of those in developing fetal tissue. **Teratomas with malignant transformation** are characterized by the development of frank malignancy in preexisting teratomatous elements, usually in the form of a squamous cell carcinoma or adenocarcinoma. Most cases of malignant teratomas occur

in adults; pure teratomas in prepubertal males are usually benign. As with other forms of germ cell neoplasia, testicular teratomas in adults are often associated with the presence of other germ cell elements. All testicular teratomas in adults therefore should be regarded as malignant neoplasms.

Mixed germ cell tumors, as noted, account for approximately 60% of all testicular germ cell neoplasms. Combinations of any of the described patterns may occur in mixed tumors, the most common of which is a combination of teratoma and embryonal carcinoma, sometimes termed **teratocarcinoma.** This should not be confused with malignant transformation of somatic elements in a mature teratoma.

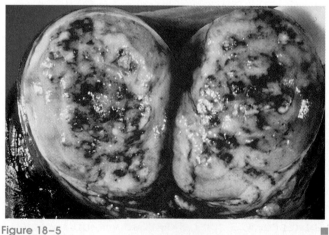

Figure 18-5 ■

Embryonal carcinoma. In contrast to the seminoma illustrated in Figure 18-3, the embryonal carcinoma is a bulky, hemorrhagic mass. (Courtesy of Dr. Kyle Molberg, Department of Pathology, University of Texas Southwestern Medical Center, Dallas, TX.)

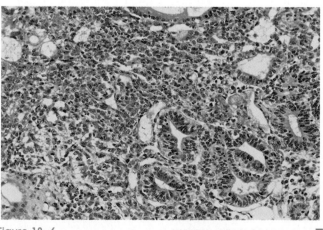

Figure 18-6 ■

Embryonal carcinoma. Microscopic examination reveals primitive hyperchromatic cells that form sheets and occasional glands. (Courtesy of Dr. Trace Worrell, Department of Pathology, University of Texas Southwestern Medical Center, Dallas, TX.)

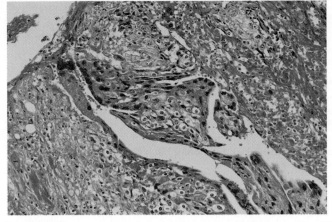

Figure 18-7   ■

Choriocarcinoma. The tumor contains both cytotrophoblastic elements, with clear cytoplasm and central nuclei, and syncytiotrophoblastic cells, with multiple nuclei and abundant eosinophilic cytoplasm. Such cells elaborate human chorionic gonadotropin, which is detectable in the serum. (Courtesy of Dr. Trace Worrell, Department of Pathology, University of Texas Southwestern Medical Center, Dallas, TX.)

Clinical Features. Patients with testicular germ cell neoplasms present most frequently with *painless enlargement of the testis.* However, some tumors, especially nonseminomatous germ cell neoplasms, may have widespread metastases at diagnosis, in the absence of a palpable testicular lesion. *Seminomas often remain confined to the testis* for prolonged intervals and may reach considerable size before diagnosis.

Metastases are most commonly encountered in the iliac and para-aortic lymph nodes, particularly in the upper lumbar region. Hematogenous metastases are unusual. In contrast, *nonseminomatous germ cell neoplasms tend to metastasize earlier,* by both lymphatic and hematogenous routes. Hematogenous metastases are most common in the liver and lungs. Metastatic lesions may be histologically identical to the primary testicular tumor, or they may contain other germ cell elements. Testicular germ cell neoplasms are staged by a variety of imaging techniques and studies of tumor markers as follows:

Stage I: Tumor confined to the testis
Stage II: Metastases confined to retroperitoneal nodes below the level of the diaphragm
Stage III: Metastases beyond retroperitoneal lymph nodes

Assay of *tumor markers* secreted by tumor cells is important in the clinical evaluation of germ cell neoplasms. hCG, produced by neoplastic syncytiotrophoblastic cells, is always elevated in patients with choriocarcinoma. As noted, other germ cell tumors, including seminoma, may also contain syncytiotrophoblastic cells without cytotrophoblastic elements and hence may elaborate hCG. Approximately 10% of seminomas elaborate hCG. Alpha-fetoprotein (AFP) is a glycoprotein normally synthesized by the fetal yolk sac and several other fetal tissues. Nonseminomatous germ cell tumors containing elements of yolk sac (endodermal sinus) often produce AFP; in contrast to hCG, the presence of AFP is a reliable indicator of the presence of a nonseminomatous component to the germ cell neoplasm, because yolk sac elements are not found in seminomas. Because mixed patterns are common,

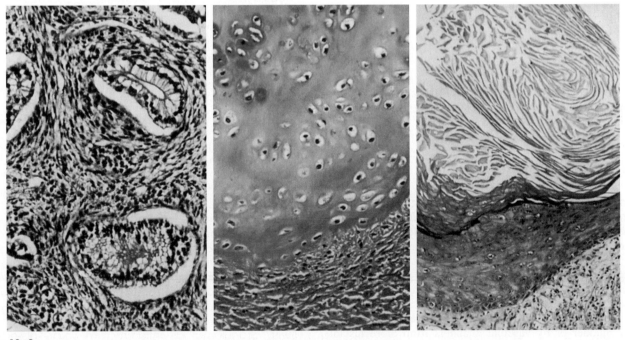

Figure 18-8   ■

Teratoma. Testicular teratomas contain mature cells from endodermal, mesodermal, and ectodermal lines. Pictured here are three different fields from the same tumor containing glandular (endodermal), cartilaginous (mesodermal), and squamous epithelial (ectodermal) elements. (Courtesy of Dr. Fred Silva, Department of Pathology, University of Texas Southwestern Medical Center, Dallas, TX.)

Table 18–2. SUMMARY OF TESTICULAR TUMORS

Tumor	Peak Age (yr)	Morphology	Tumor Markers
Seminoma	40–50	Sheets of uniform polygonal cells with cleared cytoplasm; lymphocytes in the stroma	~10% have elevated hCG
Embryonal carcinoma	20–30	Poorly differentiated, pleomorphic cells in cords, sheets, or papillary formation; most contain some yolk sac and choriocarcinoma cells	90% have elevated hCG or AFP or both
Yolk sac tumor	3	Poorly differentiated endothelium-like, cuboidal, or columnar cells	100% have elevated AFP
Choriocarcinoma (pure)	20–30	Cytotrophoblast and syncytiotrophoblast without villus formation	100% have elevated hCG
Teratoma	All ages	Tissues from all three germ-cell layers with varying degrees of differentiation	50% have elevated hCG or AFP or both
Mixed tumor	15–30	Variable, depending on mixture; commonly teratoma and embryonal carcinoma	90% have elevated hCG and AFP

most nonseminomatous tumors have elevations of both hCG and AFP. In addition to their role in the primary diagnosis of testicular germ cell tumors, serial determinations of hCG and AFP are useful for monitoring patients for persistent or recurrent tumor after therapy.

The treatment of testicular germ cell neoplasms is determined by both the histologic pattern of the tumor and the stage of disease at the time of diagnosis. Seminomas are exquisitely radiosensitive, and they also respond well to chemotherapy. The prognosis of many nonseminomatous germ cell tumors has improved dramatically with the introduction of platinum-based chemotherapy regimens. Table 18–2 summarizes salient features of testicular tumors.

PROSTATE

The most important categories of prostatic disease are inflammatory lesions (prostatitis), nodular hyperplasia, and carcinoma.

Prostatitis

Prostatitis, or clinically apparent inflammation of the prostate, may be acute or chronic. The classification of prostatitis is based on a combination of clinical features, microscopic examination, and culture of fractionated urine specimens obtained before and after prostatic massage. *Acute bacterial prostatitis* is caused by the same organisms associated with other acute urinary tract infections, particularly *Escherichia coli* and other gram-negative rods. In these cases, organisms may reach the prostate by direct extension from the urethra or urinary bladder or by vascular channels from more distant sites. *Chronic prostatitis* may follow obvious episodes of acute prostatitis, or it may develop insidiously, without previous episodes of acute infection. In some cases of chronic prostatitis, bacteria similar to those responsible for acute bacterial prostatitis can be isolated. Such cases are designated as *chronic bacterial prostatitis*. In other instances, the presence of an increased number of leukocytes in prostatic secretions attests to prostatic inflammation, but bacteriologic findings are negative. Such cases, termed *chronic abacterial prostatitis*, or prostatodynia, account for most cases of chronic prostatitis. A number of nonbacterial agents implicated in the pathogenesis of nongonococcal urethritis, including *Chlamydia trachomatis* and *Ureaplasma urealyticum*, have also been suggested as possible causes of chronic abacterial prostatitis.

MORPHOLOGY. Acute prostatitis is characterized by the presence of an acute, neutrophilic inflammatory infiltrate, congestion, and stromal edema. Neutrophils are initially most conspicuous within the prostatic glands. With progression the glandular epithelium is destroyed resulting in the formation of microabscesses. Grossly visible abscesses are uncommon but may develop with extensive tissue destruction, as may occur in diabetic patients.

The histologic features of **chronic prostatitis** are nonspecific in most cases and include a variable amount of lymphoid infiltrate, evidence of glandular injury, and, frequently, concomitant acute inflammatory changes. With advancing age, isolated lymphoid aggregates occur commonly and are not, by themselves, sufficient for a diagnosis of chronic prostatitis. Evidence of tissue destruction and fibroblastic proliferation, along with the presence of other inflammatory cells, such as neutrophils, is required. **Granulomatous inflammation** may be encountered in the prostate in patients with systemic inflammatory processes associated with granulomatous inflammation (e.g., disseminated tuberculosis, sarcoidosis, fungal infections). It may also occur as a nonspecific reaction to inspissated prostatic secretions.

The clinical manifestations of prostatitis include *dysuria, urinary frequency, lower back pain,* and poorly localized pelvic pain. The prostate may be enlarged and tender, particularly in acute prostatitis, in which local symptoms are often accompanied by fever and leukocytosis. Chronic prostatitis, even if asymptomatic, may serve as a reservoir for organisms capable of causing urinary tract infections. Chronic bacterial prostatitis, therefore, is one of the most important causes of recurrent urinary tract infection in males.

Nodular Hyperplasia of the Prostate

The normal prostate consists of glandular and stromal elements surrounding the urethra. Recent studies have suggested that the prostatic parenchyma can be divided into several anatomically and biologically distinct regions, including peripheral, central, transitional, and periurethral zones (Fig. 18–9). The types of proliferative lesions are different in each region. For example, most *hyperplastic* lesions arise in the so-called transitional and periurethral zones of the prostate, while most *carcinomas* arise in the peripheral zones.

Nodular hyperplasia, also termed *glandular and stromal hyperplasia*, is an extremely common abnormality of the prostate. It is present in approximately 20% of males by 40 years of age. Its frequency rises progressively with age, reaching

90% by the eighth decade. Prostatic hyperplasia is characterized by proliferation of both epithelial and stromal elements, with resultant enlargement of the gland and, in some cases, urinary obstruction. Benign prostatic hypertrophy, or BPH, a time-honored synonym for nodular hyperplasia of the prostate, is both redundant and a misnomer, because all hypertrophies are benign, and the fundamental lesion is a hyperplasia rather than a hypertrophy.

The cause of nodular hyperplasia remains incompletely understood, although current evidence indicates that *both androgens and estrogens play a synergistic role in its development.* It is clear that an intact testis is necessary for the development of nodular hyperplasia. Nodular hyperplasia does not occur in males castrated before the onset of puberty, in keeping with a central role for androgens in its pathogenesis. Dihydroxytestosterone (DHT), an androgen derived from testosterone through the action of 5α-reductase, appears to be the major hormonal stimulus for glandular and stromal proliferation. This forms the basis for the current use of 5α-reductase inhibitors in the treatment of symptomatic nodular hyperplasia. Paradoxically, however, nodular hyperplasia of the prostate becomes clinically manifest in older males, at a time when testosterone levels are either stable or have begun to decline. Moreover, the administration of testosterone does not exacerbate preexisting nodular hyperplasia. These observations suggest that factors other than androgenic activity must also be considered in the pathogenesis of this condition. Experimental work suggests that age-related increases in estrogen levels may contribute to the development of nodular hyperplasia, by increasing the expression of DHT receptors on prostatic parenchymal cells and thereby enhancing the effects of DHT.

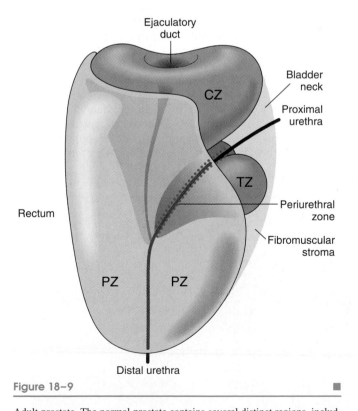

Figure 18–9 ■

Adult prostate. The normal prostate contains several distinct regions, including a central zone (CZ), a peripheral zone (PZ), a transitional zone (TZ), and a periurethral zone. Most carcinomas arise from the peripheral glands of the organ and are often palpable during digital examination of the rectum. Nodular hyperplasia, in contrast, arises from more centrally situated glands and is more likely to produce urinary obstruction early on than is carcinoma.

MORPHOLOGY. As noted, nodular hyperplasia arises most commonly in the periurethral glands of the prostate, particularly from those that lie above the verumontanum. The affected prostate is enlarged, with weights in excess of 200 gm reported in severe cases. The cut surface contains multiple, fairly well circumscribed nodules, which bulge from the cut surface (Fig. 18–10). This nodularity may be present throughout the prostate, but it is **usually most pronounced in the inner (transitional and periurethral) region.** The nodules may have a solid appearance, or may contain cystic spaces, the latter corresponding to dilated glandular elements seen in histologic sections. The urethra is usually compressed by the hyperplastic nodules, often to a slit-like orifice. In some cases, hyperplastic glandular and stromal elements lying just under the epithelium of the proximal prostatic urethra may project into the bladder lumen as a pedunculated mass, resulting in a ball-valve type of urethral obstruction.

Microscopically, the hyperplastic nodules are composed of varying proportions of proliferating glandular elements and fibromuscular stroma. The hyperplastic glands are lined by tall, columnar epithelial cells and a peripheral layer of flattened

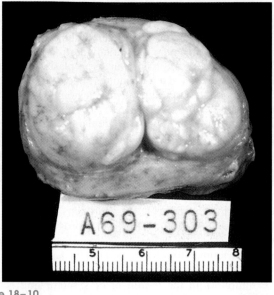

Figure 18-10 ■

Nodular hyperplasia of the prostate. Well-defined nodules bulge from the cut surface. The proximity of the nodules to the urethra accounts for the urinary obstruction associated with this lesion.

basal cells; crowding of the proliferating epithelium results in the formation of papillary projections in some glands (Fig. 18-11). The glandular lumina often contain inspissated, proteinaceous secretory material, termed corpora amylacea. The glands are surrounded by proliferating stromal elements; although it is scanty in some cases, stroma is always present between the hyperplastic glands, in contrast to carcinomas (discussed later). Other nodules are composed predominantly of spindle-shaped stromal cells and connective tissue. Recent studies suggest that predominantly glandular or stromal hyperplasias respond best to different

forms of medical treatment. Areas of necrosis, which are fairly common in advanced cases of nodular hyperplasia, are frequently accompanied by areas of squamous metaplasia in adjacent glands.

Clinical Features. Clinical manifestations of prostatic hyperplasia occur in only about 10% of men with the disease. Because nodular hyperplasia preferentially involves the inner (periurethral) portions of the prostate, its most common manifestations are those of *lower urinary tract obstruction.* These include difficulty in starting the stream of urine (hesitancy) and intermittent interruption of the urinary stream while voiding. In some patients complete urinary obstruction may occur, with resultant painful distention of the bladder and, on occasion, hydronephrosis (Chapter 14). Symptoms of obstruction are frequently accompanied by urinary urgency, frequency, and nocturia, all indicative of bladder irritation. The combination of residual urine in the bladder and chronic obstruction increases the risk of urinary tract infections.

Carcinoma of the Prostate

Carcinoma of the prostate is the most common visceral cancer in males, ranking as the second most common cause of cancer-related deaths in men older than 50 years of age, after carcinoma of the lung. It is predominantly a disease of older males, with a peak incidence between the ages of 65 and 75 years. Latent cancers of the prostate are even more common than those that are clinically apparent, with an overall frequency of more than 50% in men older than 80 years of age.

Although the cause of carcinoma of the prostate remains unknown, clinical and experimental observations suggest that hormonal, genetic, and environmental factors may all play a role in its pathogenesis. Cancer of the prostate does not develop in males castrated before puberty, suggesting that *androgens* probably play some part in its development. A hormonal influence is further suggested by the fact that the

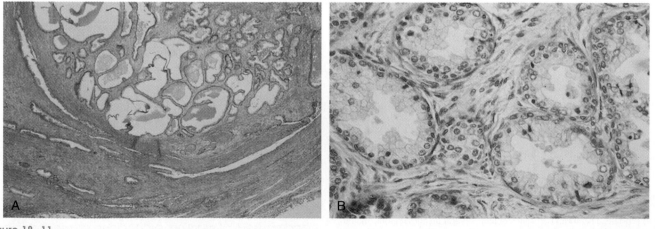

Figure 18-11 ■

Photomicrograph of nodular hyperplasia. *A,* Low-power photograph demonstrates a well-demarcated nodule at the top of the field, populated by hyperplastic glands. *B,* Higher power demonstrates the morphology of the hyperplastic glands, with a characteristic inner columnar and outer cuboidal cell layer. In other cases of nodular hyperplasia the nodularity is caused predominantly by stromal, rather than glandular, proliferation.

growth of many carcinomas of the prostate can be inhibited by orchiectomy or by the administration of estrogens such as diethylstilbestrol. As in the case of nodular hyperplasia of the prostate, however, the role played by hormones in the pathogenesis of carcinoma of the prostate is not fully understood.

Genetic factors have also been implicated, based on the increased risk of disease among first-degree relatives of patients with prostate cancer. Symptomatic carcinoma of the prostate is more common and occurs at an earlier age in American blacks than in whites, Asians, or Hispanics. Whether such racial differences occur as a consequence of genetic factors, environmental factors, or some combination of the two remains unknown. However, the frequency of *incidental* prostatic cancers is comparable in all races, suggesting that race plays a more important role in the growth of established lesions than in the initial development of carcinoma. A possible role for *environmental factors* is suggested by the increased frequency of prostatic carcinoma in certain industrial settings and by significant geographic differences in the incidence of the disease. Carcinoma of the prostate is particularly common in the Scandinavian countries and relatively uncommon in Japan and certain other Asian countries. Males emigrating from low-risk to high-risk areas maintain their low risk of prostate cancer; the risk of disease is intermediate in subsequent generations, in keeping with environmental influence on the development of this disease.

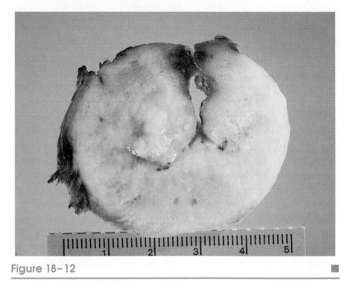

Figure 18–12   ■

Adenocarcinoma of the prostate. The parenchyma contains a poorly defined, pale, infiltrative tumor, in contrast to the well-demarcated nodules seen in nodular hyperplasia. Compare with Figure 18–10.

MORPHOLOGY. Approximately 70% of the carcinomas of the prostate arise in the outer (peripheral) glands and hence may be palpable by rectal digital examination. Because of the peripheral location, prostate cancer is less likely to cause urethral obstruction in its initial stages than is nodular hyperplasia. Early lesions typically appear as ill-defined masses just beneath the capsule of the prostate. On cut surface, foci of carcinoma appear as firm, gray-white to yellow lesions that infiltrate the adjacent gland with ill-defined margins (Fig. 18–12). Metastases to regional pelvic lymph nodes may occur early. Locally advanced cancers often infiltrate the seminal vesicles and periurethral zones of the prostate and may invade the adjacent soft tissues and the wall of the urinary bladder. Denonvilliers' fascia, the connective tissue layer separating the lower genitourinary structures from the rectum, usually prevents growth of the tumor posteriorly. Invasion of the rectum therefore is fairly uncommon.

Microscopically, most prostatic carcinomas are **adenocarcinomas** exhibiting variable degrees of differentiation. The better differentiated lesions are composed of small glands that infiltrate the adjacent stroma in an irregular, haphazard fashion. In contrast to normal and hyperplastic prostate, the glands in carcinomas are not encircled by collagen or stromal cells but rather lie "back to back" and appear to dissect sharply though the native stroma (Fig. 18–13). The neoplastic glands are lined by a single layer of cuboidal cells with con-

spicuous nucleoli; the basal cell layer seen in normal or hyperplastic glands is absent. With increasing degrees of anaplasia, irregular, ragged glandular structures, papillary or cribriform epithelial structures, and, in extreme cases, sheets of poorly differentiated cells are noted.

A number of histologic grading schemes have been proposed for carcinoma of the prostate. They are based on features such as the degree of glandular differentiation, the architecture of the neoplastic glands, nuclear anaplasia, and mitotic activity. Despite the potential difficulties associated with incomplete sampling in biopsy material

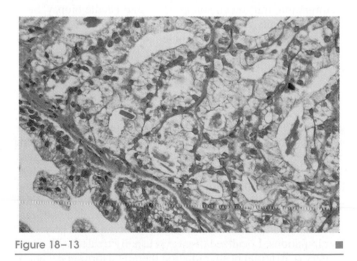

Figure 18–13   ■

Photomicrograph of well-differentiated adenocarcinoma of the prostate demonstrating crowded, "back-to-back" glands lined by a single layer of cuboidal cells. Glandular differentiation is much less obvious in some higher-grade lesions. (Courtesy of Dr. Kyle Molberg, Department of Pathology, University of Texas Southwestern Medical Center, Dallas, TX.)

and the subjectivity inherent in histologic evaluation, histologic grade has proved to correlate reasonably well with both the anatomic stage of prostatic carcinoma (discussed below) and the prognosis.

Clinical Features. Carcinomas of the prostate are often clinically silent, particularly during their early stages. Approximately 20% of localized carcinomas are discovered retrospectively, during histologic examination of prostate tissue removed for nodular hyperplasia. In autopsy studies, the incidence approaches 60% in men older than 80 years of age. Because most cancers begin in the peripheral regions of the prostate, they may be discovered during routine digital rectal examination. More extensive disease may produce signs and symptoms of "prostatism," including local discomfort and evidence of lower urinary tract obstruction similar to that encountered in patients with nodular hyperplasia. Physical examination in such cases typically reveals evidence of locally advanced disease, in the form of a hard, fixed prostate. More aggressive carcinomas of the prostate may first come to clinical attention because of the presence of metastases. Regrettably, this is not an uncommon mode of presentation. Bone metastases, particularly to the axial skeleton, are common in prostatic carcinoma and may cause either osteolytic (destructive) or, more commonly, osteoblastic (bone-producing) lesions. *The presence of osteoblastic metastases in males is virtually diagnostic of advanced prostatic carcinoma.*

Assay of serum levels of *prostate-specific antigen* (PSA) has gained widespread use in the diagnosis of early carcinomas. PSA is produced by both normal and neoplastic prostatic epithelium, and its level may be elevated (>4 ng/ml) in conditions such as nodular hyperplasia, prostatitis, as well as in carcinomas. Because there is an overlap in serum PSA levels among patients with nodular hyperplasia and those with carcinomas, PSA is of limited value as an isolated screening test. Its diagnostic value is enhanced considerably when it is used in conjunction with other procedures, such as digital rectal examination, transrectal sonography, and needle biopsy. Several refinements in the interpretation of PSA values are currently being tested. These include rate of change of PSA values with time (PSA velocity), and the ratio between the serum PSA value and volume of the prostate gland (PSA density).

Anatomic staging of the extent of disease plays an important role in the evaluation and treatment of prostatic carcinoma. Prostate cancer is staged by clinical examination, surgical exploration, radiographic imaging techniques, and, in some systems, levels of tumor markers. One staging system commonly used in the United States is summarized in Figure 18–14. The anatomic extent of disease, along with the histologic grade of the lesion, influences the therapy of prostate cancer and correlates well with prognosis. Depending on the grade and stage, carcinoma of the prostate is treated with various combinations of surgery, radiation therapy, and hormonal manipulations. Localized disease is usually treated with either surgery or external beam radiation therapy. Hormonal therapy plays a central role in the treatment of advanced carcinomas. Specifically, most prostate cancers are androgen-sensitive and are inhibited to some degree by androgen ablation. Surgical or pharmacologic castration, estrogens, and androgen recep-

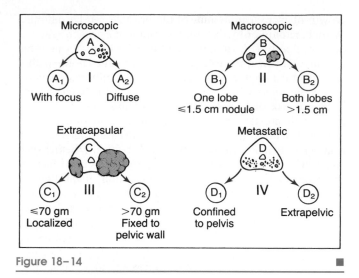

Figure 18–14 ■

Staging system for carcinoma of the prostate. Stage A: microscopic, non-palpable tumor (A_1, tumor is low grade and involves less than 5% of tissue sampled; A_2, tumor is high grade and/or involves more than 5% of tissue sampled). Stage B: palpable tumor (B_1, ≤1.5 cm in diameter; B_2, >1.5 cm in diameter, or several palpable nodules in both lobes). Stage C: extracapsular extension present (C_1, not fixed to pelvic wall; C_2, fixed to pelvic wall). Stage D: metastatic disease (D_1, metastases in less than three pelvic nodes; D_2, more extensive nodal metastases, or extrapelvic metastases). The tumor, node, and metastasis (TNM) staging is indicated by roman numerals I to IV. (Redrawn and adapted with permission from Gittes RF: Carcinoma of the prostate. N Engl J Med 324:240, 1991. Reprinted by permission of *The New England Journal of Medicine.* Copyright 1991, Massachusetts Medical Society.)

tor–blocking agents have all been used to control the growth of disseminated lesions. Serial evaluation of serum levels of PSA has proved to be a valuable method by which to monitor patients for recurrent or progressive disease. The prognosis for patients with limited-stage disease is favorable: more than 90% of patients with stage A or B lesions survive 10 years or longer. The outlook for patients with disseminated disease remains poor, with 10-year survival rates in this group ranging from 10% to 40%.

SEXUALLY TRANSMITTED DISEASES (STDs)

Venereal diseases, or STDs, have complicated human existence for centuries. Although the origins of many of the STDs remain shrouded in antiquity, ancient literature is replete with descriptions of maladies highly suggestive of venereal disease. By the twentieth century, the clinicopathologic characteristics of the classic venereal diseases—syphilis, gonorrhea, chancroid, lymphogranuloma venereum, and granuloma inguinale—were reasonably well defined. With the discovery of antibiotics and the development of aggressive public health programs, there was a sense of optimism, if not complacency, that control of the traditional venereal diseases was a realistic goal. STDs have continued to evolve in an unpredictable fashion, however. With the changing social mores of the late twentieth century, the incidence of STDs has increased, a problem compounded further by the emergence of strains of sexually transmitted pathogens that are resistant to multiple antibiotics. In addition to the problems posed by the persistence of these traditional venereal diseases, the spectrum of STDs has also broadened dramatically in recent years, with the emergence of new entities, such as human immunodeficiency virus (HIV) infection, and the recognition of venereal spread of pathogens historically transmitted by other means, such as hepatitis B virus and *Entamoeba histolytica*. The disorders currently regarded as STDs are listed in Table 18–3. A number of these entities, such as HIV infection, hepatitis B, and *E. histolytica*, are discussed in other chapters. Our comments here focus on some of the more important of these entities that are not conveniently addressed in other areas of this book.

Syphilis

Syphilis, or lues, is a chronic venereal infection caused by the spirochete *Treponema pallidum*. First recognized in epidemic form in sixteenth-century Europe as the Great Pox, syphilis has remained an endemic infection in all parts of the world. Although penicillin and public health programs resulted in a gratifying reduction in cases of syphilis from the late 1940s until the late 1970s, a significant resurgence of cases of both primary and secondary syphilis has been documented over the past two decades. In the 1990s, in particular, significant increases in the incidence of syphilis have occurred in both urban and rural areas, particularly in the southeastern part of the United States. Many of these new cases of syphilis have been associated with heterosexual contact, and, as a consequence, there has been an increase in the incidence of cases of congenital syphilis.

T. pallidum is a fastidious spirochete whose only natural hosts are humans. The usual source of infection is an active cutaneous or mucosal lesion in a patient in the early (primary or secondary) stages of syphilis. The organism is transmitted from such lesions during sexual intercourse across minute breaks in the skin or mucous membranes of the uninfected partner. In cases of congenital syphilis, *T. pallidum* is transmitted across the placenta from mother to fetus, particularly during the early stages of maternal infection. Once introduced into the body, the organisms are rapidly disseminated to distant sites by lymphatics and the bloodstream, even before the appearance of lesions at the primary inoculation site. Approximately 2 to 6 weeks after the initial infection, a primary lesion, termed a *chancre*, appears at the point of entry. Systemic dissemination of organisms continues during this period,

Table 18–3.　CLASSIFICATION OF IMPORTANT SEXUALLY TRANSMITTED DISEASES

Pathogens	Disease or Syndrome and Population Principally Affected		
	Males	Both	Females
Viruses			
Herpes simplex virus		Primary and recurrent herpes, neonatal herpes	
Hepatitis B virus	Hepatitis		
Human papillomavirus	Cancer of penis (?)	Condyloma acuminatum	Cervical dysplasia and cancer, vulvar cancer
Human immunodeficiency virus		Acquired immunodeficiency syndrome	
Chlamydiae			
Chlamydia trachomatis	Urethritis, epididymitis, proctitis	Lymphogranuloma venereum	Urethral syndrome, cervicitis, bartholinitis, salpingitis and sequelae
Mycoplasmas			
Ureaplasma urealyticum	Urethritis		
Bacteria			
Neisseria gonorrhoeae	Epididymitis, prostatitis, urethral stricture	Urethritis, proctitis, pharyngitis, disseminated gonococcal infection	Cervicitis, endometritis, bartholinitis, salpingitis and sequelae (infertility, ectopic pregnancy, recurrent salpingitis)
Treponema pallidum		Syphilis	
Haemophilus ducreyi		Chancroid	
Calymmatobacterium granulomatis		Granuloma inguinale (donovanosis)	
Shigella	*Enterocolitis		
Campylobacter	*Enterocolitis		
Protozoa			
Trichomonas vaginalis	Urethritis, balanitis		Vaginitis
Entamoeba histolytica	*Amebiasis		
Giardia lamblia	*Giardiasis		

* Most important in homosexual populations.
Modified and updated from Krieger JN: Biology of sexually transmitted diseases. Urol Clin North Am 11:15, 1984.

while the host mounts an antibody response. Two types of antibodies are formed: nontreponemal antibodies and antibodies to specific treponemal antigens. As discussed in detail later, detection of these antibodies plays an important part in the diagnosis of syphilis. This acquired immunity, however, fails to eradicate spirochetes introduced during the primary inoculation.

The chancre of primary syphilis resolves spontaneously over a period of 4 to 6 weeks and is followed in a significant number of patients by the development of *secondary syphilis*. The manifestations of secondary syphilis, discussed in more detail later, include generalized lymphadenopathy and variable mucocutaneous lesions and reflect the presence of organisms disseminated throughout the body during the primary phase of the disease. *The mucocutaneous lesions of both primary and secondary syphilis are teeming with spirochetes and are highly infectious.* Like the chancre, the lesions of secondary syphilis resolve even without specific antimicrobial therapy, at which point patients are said to be in *early latent phase syphilis*. Mucocutaneous lesions may recur during this phase of the disease.

After a period of several years, patients with untreated syphilis enter into an asymptomatic, *late latent* phase of the illness. In about one third of cases, subsequent symptomatic lesions may develop over the next 10 to 20 years. This late symptomatic phase, or *tertiary syphilis*, is marked by the development of lesions in the cardiovascular system, central nervous system, or, less frequently, other organs. Spirochetes are much more difficult to demonstrate during the later stages of disease, and patients with late latent or tertiary syphilis are much less likely to be infectious than are those in the primary or secondary stages of disease.

MORPHOLOGY. The macroscopic lesions of syphilis vary with the stage of disease and are discussed later. The fundamental microscopic lesion of syphilis is a **proliferative endarteritis** and an accompanying **inflammatory infiltrate rich in plasma cells.** The treponemes cause endothelial hypertrophy and proliferation, with subsequent intimal fibrosis and narrowing of the vessel lumen. Local ischemia caused by the vascular changes undoubtedly accounts for some of the local cell loss and fibrosis seen in syphilis, although other factors, including delayed hypersensitivity, also appear to contribute to parenchymal injury. Spirochetes are readily demonstrable in histologic sections of early lesions with the use of standard silver stains (e.g., Warthin-Starry stains). There is no evidence that the organisms cause direct toxic injury to the host tissues. Large areas of parenchymal damage in tertiary syphilis result in the formation of a so-called **gumma,** an irregular, firm mass of necrotic tissue surrounded by resilient connective tissue. Microscopically, the gumma contains a central zone of coagulation necrosis, surrounded by a mixed inflammatory infiltrate composed of lymphocytes, plasma cells, activated macrophages (epithelioid

cells), and occasional giant cells and a peripheral zone of dense fibrous tissue.

PRIMARY SYPHILIS

This stage is characterized by the presence of a chancre at the site of initial inoculation. *The chancre of syphilis is characteristically indurated and has been referred to in the past as a "hard chancre"* to distinguish it from the "soft chancre" of chancroid (discussed later). The primary chancre in males is usually on the penis. In females, multiple chancres may be present, usually in the vagina or on the uterine cervix. The chancre begins as a small, firm papule, which gradually enlarges to produce a painless ulcer with well-defined, indurated margins and a "clean," moist base (Fig. 18–15). Spirochetes are readily demonstrable in material scraped from the ulcer base using darkfield microscopy (Fig. 18–16). Regional lymph nodes are often slightly enlarged and firm, but painless. Histologic examination of the ulcer reveals a loss of the overlying epidermis, with epidermal hyperplasia at its periphery. The underlying dermis contains the usual *lymphocytic and plasmacytic inflammatory infiltrate and proliferative vascular changes* as described previously. Even without therapy, the primary chancre resolves over a period of several weeks to form a subtle scar. *Serologic tests for syphilis are often negative during the early stages of primary syphilis* and therefore must always be complemented by darkfield microscopy if primary syphilis is suspected.

SECONDARY SYPHILIS

Within approximately 2 months of resolution of the chancre, the lesions of secondary syphilis occur. The manifestations of secondary syphilis are varied but typically include a combination of *generalized lymph node enlargement* and a variety of *mucocutaneous lesions*. Skin lesions are usually symmetrically distributed and may be maculopapular, scaly, or pustular. *Involvement of the palms of the hands and soles of the feet is common.* In moist skin areas, such as the anogenital region, inner thighs, and axillae, broad-based, elevated lesions termed *condyloma lata* may occur. Superficial mucosal lesions resembling condyloma lata can occur anywhere, but they are particularly common in the oral cavity, pharynx, and external genitalia. Histologic examination of mucocutaneous lesions during the secondary phase of the disease reveals the characteristic *proliferative endarteritis,* accompanied by a *lymphoplasmacytic inflammatory infiltrate.* Spirochetes are easily demonstrable within the mucocutaneous lesions, and they are therefore contagious. Lymph node enlargement is most common in the neck and inguinal areas. Biopsy of enlarged nodes reveals nonspecific hyperplasia of germinal centers accompanied by increased numbers of plasma cells or, less commonly, granulomas or neutrophils. Less common manifestations of secondary syphilis include hepatitis, renal disease, eye disease (iritis), and gastrointestinal abnormalities. The mucocutaneous lesions of secondary syphilis resolve over a period of several weeks, at which point the patient enters the early latent phase of the disease, which lasts approximately 1 year. Lesions may recur at any time during the early latent phase, during which the disease may still be

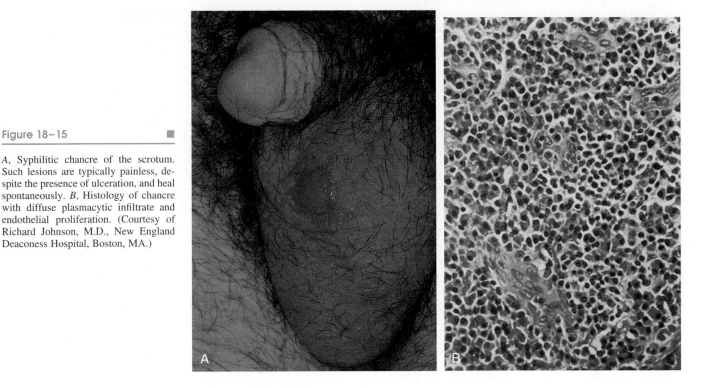

Figure 18–15   ■

A, Syphilitic chancre of the scrotum. Such lesions are typically painless, despite the presence of ulceration, and heal spontaneously. *B,* Histology of chancre with diffuse plasmacytic infiltrate and endothelial proliferation. (Courtesy of Richard Johnson, M.D., New England Deaconess Hospital, Boston, MA.)

spread. *Both nontreponemal and antitreponemal antibody tests are strongly positive in virtually all cases of secondary syphilis.*

TERTIARY SYPHILIS

Tertiary syphilis develops in approximately one third of untreated patients, usually after a latent period of 5 years or more. This phase of syphilis is divided into three major categories: cardiovascular syphilis, neurosyphilis, and so-called

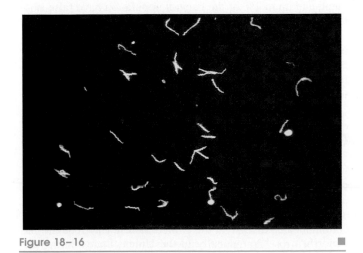

Figure 18–16   ■

Treponema pallidum (darkfield microscopy) showing several spirochetes in scrapings from the base of the chancre. (Courtesy of Dr. Paul Southern, Department of Pathology, University of Texas Southwestern Medical School, Dallas, TX.)

benign tertiary syphilis. The various forms may occur singly or in combination in a given patient. *Nontreponemal antibody tests may revert to negative during the tertiary phase, although antitreponemal antibody tests remain positive.*

Cardiovascular syphilis, in the form of *syphilitic aortitis,* accounts for more than 80% of cases of tertiary disease; it is much more common in men than in women. Briefly, the disease is fundamentally an endarteritis of the vasa vasorum of the proximal aorta. Microvascular disease results in scarring of the media of the proximal aortic wall, with consequent loss of elasticity. The aortic disease is characterized by slowly progressive dilation of the aortic root and arch, with resultant aortic insufficiency and saccular aneurysms of the proximal aorta. In some cases there is narrowing of the coronary artery ostia due to subintimal scarring with secondary myocardial ischemia. The morphologic and clinical features of syphilitic aortitis are discussed in greater detail with diseases of the blood vessels (Chapter 10).

Neurosyphilis accounts for only about 10% of cases of tertiary syphilis. Variants of neurosyphilis include chronic meningovascular disease, tabes dorsalis, and a generalized brain parenchymal disease termed general paresis. They are discussed in detail in Chapter 23.

A third, relatively uncommon, form of tertiary syphilis is the so-called benign tertiary syphilis, characterized by the development of gummas in various sites. These lesions are probably related to the development of delayed hypersensitivity. *Gummas occur most commonly in bone, skin, and the mucous membranes of the upper airway and mouth,* although any organ may be affected. Skeletal involvement characteristically causes local pain, tenderness, swelling, and, sometimes pathologic fractures. Involvement of skin and mucous membranes may produce nodular lesions, or, in exceptional cases, destructive, ulcerative lesions that mimic malignant neoplasms. *Spirochetes are rarely demonstrable within the lesions.* Once common, gummas have become exceedingly rare thanks to the development of effective antibiotics such as penicillin.

CONGENITAL SYPHILIS

T. pallidum may be transmitted across the placenta from an infected mother to the fetus at any time during pregnancy. The likelihood of maternal transmission is greatest during the early (primary and secondary) stages of disease, when spirochetes are most numerous. In contrast, congenital syphilis is rare if maternal syphilis has been present for more than 5 years. Pregnancy may actually cause a remission of signs and symptoms of syphilis in an infected mother, particularly when the mother is infected near the onset of pregnancy. Because the manifestations of maternal disease may be subtle, routine serologic testing for syphilis is mandatory in all pregnancies. The stigmata of congenital syphilis typically do not develop until after the fourth month of pregnancy, suggesting that the morphologic changes depend to some extent on the development of an immunologic response in the fetus. In the absence of treatment, up to 40% of infected infants die in utero, typically after the fourth month.

Manifestations of *congenital syphilis* include stillbirth, infantile syphilis, and late (tardive) congenital syphilis. Among infants who are stillborn, the most common manifestations are *hepatomegaly, bone abnormalities, pancreatic fibrosis, and pneumonitis.* The enlarged liver contains foci of extramedullary hematopoiesis and a mononuclear inflammatory infiltrate in the portal areas. Pancreatitis is common and may be severe. Changes in the bones include inflammation and disruption of the osteochondral junction in long bones and, on occasion, bone resorption and fibrosis of the flat bones of the skull. The lungs may be firm and pale, owing to the presence of inflammatory cells and fibrosis in the alveolar septa (pneumonia alba). Spirochetes are readily demonstrable in tissue sections.

Infantile syphilis refers to congenital syphilis in liveborn infants that is clinically manifest at birth or within the first few months of life. Affected infants present with chronic rhinitis (snuffles) and subsequently develop a desquamating skin rash or other mucocutaneous lesions similar to those seen in secondary syphilis in adults. Visceral and skeletal changes resembling those seen in stillborn infants may also be present.

Late, or tardive, congenital syphilis refers to cases of untreated congenital syphilis of more than 2 years' duration. Classic manifestations include Hutchinson's triad: notched central incisors, interstitial keratitis with blindness, and deafness due to eighth cranial nerve injury. Other changes include a saber shin deformity caused by chronic inflammation of the periosteum of the tibia, deformed molar teeth ("mulberry" molars), chronic meningitis, chorioretinitis, and gummas of the nasal bone and cartilage with a resultant "saddle nose" deformity.

In cases of congenital syphilis, the placenta is enlarged, pale, and edematous. Microscopy reveals proliferative endarteritis involving the fetal vessels, a mononuclear inflammatory reaction (villitis), and villous immaturity. Spirochetes are demonstrable with the use of the appropriate special stains.

SEROLOGIC TESTS FOR SYPHILIS

Serologic tests for syphilis include both nontreponemal antibody tests and antitreponemal antibody tests. Nontreponemal tests measure antibody to cardiolipin, an antigen that is present in both host tissues and the treponemal cell wall. These antibodies are detected by the rapid plasma reagin (RPR) and Venereal Disease Research Laboratory (VDRL) tests. Nontreponemal antibody tests begin to become positive after 1 to 2 weeks of infection and are usually positive by 4 to 6 weeks. Titers of these antibodies usually fall after successful treatment. The VDRL and RPR, widely used as screening tests for syphilis, are also used to monitor the results of therapy. They may be negative, however, in the late latent or tertiary phases of the disease. Nontreponemal antibodies may persist in some patients even after successful treatment. Two additional points about nontreponemal antibody tests deserve emphasis:

- *Nontreponemal antibody tests are often negative during the early stages of disease,* even in the presence of a primary chancre. Hence, darkfield microscopy should always be performed in the evaluation of a suspected chancre, even if serologic tests for syphilis are negative.
- Up to 15% of positive VDRL tests represent *biologic false-positives.* These false-positive tests, which may be acute (transient) or chronic (persistent), increase in frequency with age. Conditions associated with false-positive VDRL results include certain acute infections, collagen vascular diseases (e.g., SLE), drug addiction, pregnancy, hypergammaglobulinemia of any cause, and lepromatous leprosy.

Treponemal antibody tests include the fluorescent treponemal antibody absorption test (FTA-Abs) and the microhemagglutination assay for *Treponema pallidum* antibodies (MHATP). These tests also become positive within 4 to 6 weeks after an infection, but, unlike nontreponemal antibody tests, they remain positive indefinitely, even after successful treatment. They are not recommended as primary screening tests, because they are significantly more expensive than nontreponemal tests; furthermore, they remain positive after treatment, and up to 2% of the general population have false-positive test results.

It should be noted that serologic response may be delayed or sometimes absent in patients with syphilis with coexistent HIV disease. However, in most cases, these tests remain useful for the diagnosis and management of syphilis in patients with the acquired immunodeficiency syndrome.

Gonorrhea

Gonorrhea is a sexually transmitted infection of the lower genitourinary tract caused by *Neisseria gonorrhoeae.* With the exception of chlamydial infection of the genitourinary tract, discussed later, gonorrhea is the most common reportable communicable disease in the United States. The frequency of gonorrhea rose dramatically in the United States during the 1960s and early 1970s and reached a peak in 1975, when the incidence approached 500 per 100,000 in the general population. Since then, its incidence has declined, but with more than 1 million new cases reported annually in the United

States it still remains a major public health problem. The gravity of gonococcal infections has increased further by the emergence of strains of *N. gonorrhoeae* that are resistant to multiple antibiotics.

Humans are the only natural reservoir for *N. gonorrhoeae*. The organism is highly fastidious, and spread of infection requires direct contact with the mucosa of an infected person, usually during sexual intercourse. There is no evidence that gonorrhea is transmitted by contact with toilet seats or other fomites. The bacteria initially attach to mucosal epithelium, particularly of the columnar or transitional type, using a variety of membrane-associated adhesion molecules and structures termed *pili* (Chapter 9). Such attachment prevents the organism from being washed away by body fluids such as urine or endocervical mucus. The organism then penetrates through the epithelial cells and invades the deeper tissues of the host.

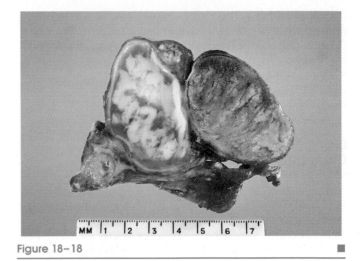

Figure 18–18 ■

Acute epididymitis caused by gonococcal infection. The epididymis is replaced by an abscess. Normal testis is seen on the right.

MORPHOLOGY. *N. gonorrhoeae* provokes an intense, suppurative inflammatory reaction. In males, this is manifested most often as a **purulent urethral discharge,** associated with an edematous, congested urethral meatus. Gram-negative diplococci, many within the cytoplasm of neutrophils, are readily identified in Gram stains of the purulent exudate (Fig. 18–17). Ascending infection results in the development of acute prostatitis, epididymitis (Fig. 18–18), and, sometimes, orchitis. Abscesses may complicate severe cases. Urethral and endocervical exudates tend to be less conspicuous in females, although acute inflammation of adjacent structures, such as Bartholin's glands, is fairly common. Ascending infection involving the uterus, fallopian tubes, and ovaries results in acute salpingitis, sometimes complicated by tubo-ovar-

ian abscesses (see Fig. 19–15 in Chapter 19). The acute inflammatory process is followed by the development of granulation tissue and scarring, with resultant strictures and other permanent deformities of the involved structures.

Clinical Features. In most infected males, gonorrhea is manifested by the presence of *dysuria, urinary frequency, and a mucopurulent urethral exudate* within 2 to 7 days of the time of initial infection. Treatment with appropriate antimicrobial therapy results in eradication of the organism and prompt resolution of symptoms. Untreated infections may ascend to involve prostate, seminal vesicles, epididymis, and testis. Neglected cases may be complicated by chronic urethral stricture and, in more advanced cases, by permanent sterility. Untreated men may also become chronic carriers of *N. gonorrhoeae.*

Among female patients, initial infection may be asymptomatic or associated with *dysuria, lower pelvic pain, and vaginal discharge.* Untreated cases may be complicated by ascending infection, leading to acute inflammation of the fallopian tubes (salpingitis) and ovaries. Chronic scarring of the fallopian tubes may occur, with resultant infertility and an increased risk of ectopic pregnancy. Gonococcal infection of the upper genital tract may spread to the peritoneal cavity, where the exudate may extend up the right paracolic gutter to the dome of the liver, resulting in gonococcal perihepatitis. Resolution of inflammation in such cases may result in the formation of so-called "violin string" adhesions between the dome of the liver and the adjacent diaphragm.

Other sites of primary infection, more commonly encountered in male homosexuals than in heterosexuals, include the oropharynx and the anorectal area, with resultant acute pharyngitis and proctitis, respectively.

Disseminated infection is much less common than local infection, occurring in 0.5% to 3% of cases of gonorrhea. Manifestations include tenosynovitis and arthritis, pustular or hemorrhagic skin lesions, endocarditis, and, rarely, meningitis.

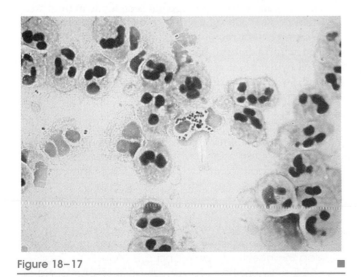

Figure 18–17 ■

Neisseria gonorrhoeae. Gram stain of urethral discharge, demonstrating characteristic gram-negative, intracellular diplococci. (Courtesy of Dr. Rita Gander, Department of Pathology, University of Texas Southwestern Medical School, Dallas, TX.)

Gonococcal *infection may be transmitted to infants* during passage through the birth canal. The affected neonate may develop purulent infection of the eyes (ophthalmia neonatorum), an important cause of blindness in the past. The routine administration of antibiotic ointment to the eyes of newborn infants has resulted in a marked reduction in the incidence of this disorder.

Nongonococcal Urethritis and Cervicitis

Nongonococcal urethritis and cervicitis are the most common forms of STDs today. A variety of organisms have been implicated in the pathogenesis of nongonococcal urethritis and cervicitis, including *C. trachomatis, Trichomonas vaginalis, U. urealyticum,* and *Mycoplasma hominis.* Most cases appear to be caused by *C. trachomatis,* an obligate intracellular parasite. *C. trachomatis* infections may be associated with a spectrum of clinical features that are virtually indistinguishable from those caused by *N. gonorrhoeae.* Thus, the patients may develop epididymitis, prostatitis, pelvic inflammatory disease, pharyngitis, conjunctivitis, perihepatic inflammation, and, among people engaging in anal intercourse, proctitis. *C. trachomatis* also causes lymphogranuloma venereum, discussed in greater detail in a subsequent section. The serotypes responsible for lymphogranuloma venereum are different from those causing chlamydial urethritis or cervicitis.

The morphologic and clinical features of chlamydial infection, with the exception of lymphogranuloma venereum, are virtually identical to those of gonorrhea. The primary infection is characterized by a *mucopurulent discharge containing a predominance of neutrophils.* Organisms are not visible in gram-stained sections. In contrast to the gonococcus, *C. trachomatis* cannot be isolated with the use of conventional culture media. *C. trachomatis* infection should therefore be considered in any patient with culture-negative urethritis or cervicitis. It should also be considered in patients with gonorrhea whose symptoms persist or recur after eradication of *N. gonorrhoeae.* Other manifestations of chlamydial infection include a reactive arthritis, predominantly in patients who are HLA-B27 positive. These patients, said to have Reiter's syndrome, typically present with combination of urethritis, conjunctivitis, arthritis, and generalized mucocutaneous lesions (Chapter 6).

Chancroid (Soft Chancre)

Chancroid, sometimes termed the "third" venereal disease, is an acute, ulcerative, infection caused by *Hemophilus ducreyi,* a small, gram-negative coccobacillus. The disease is most common in tropical and subtropical areas and is more prevalent in lower socioeconomic groups, particularly among men who have regular contact with prostitutes. *Chancroid is one of the most common causes of genital ulcers in Africa and southeast Asia,* where it probably serves as an important cofactor in the transmission of HIV-1 infection. The incidence of chancroid has been increasing in the United States since the 1980s.

MORPHOLOGY. Four to 7 days after inoculation, the patient develops a tender, erythematous papule involving the external genitalia. In males, the primary lesion is usually on the penis; in females, most lesions occur in the vagina or periurethral area. Over the course of several days, the surface of the primary lesion erodes to produce an irregular ulcer, which is more apt to be painful in males than in females. In contrast to the primary chancre of syphilis, the ulcer of chancroid is not indurated, and multiple lesions may be present. The base of the ulcer is covered by shaggy, yellow-gray exudate. The regional lymph nodes, particularly in the inguinal region, become enlarged and tender in about 50% of cases within 1 to 2 weeks of the primary inoculation. In untreated cases, the inflamed and enlarged nodes (buboes) may erode the overlying skin to produce chronic draining ulcers.

Microscopically, the ulcer of chancroid contains a superficial zone of neutrophilic debris and fibrin, with an underlying zone of granulation tissue containing areas of necrosis and thrombosed vessels. A dense, lymphoplasmacytic inflammatory infiltrate is present beneath the layer of granulation tissue. Gram-negative coccobacillary organisms are demonstrable in Gram stains but may be obscured by the mixed bacterial growth invariably present at the ulcer base. Usually, *H. ducreyi* can be cultured from the ulcer.

Granuloma Inguinale

Granuloma inguinale is a chronic inflammatory disease caused by *Calymmatobacterium donovani,* a small, encapsulated, gram-negative rod. This disease is uncommon in the United States and western Europe but is endemic in rural areas in certain tropical and subtropical regions. When it occurs in urban settings, transmission of *C. donovani* is typically associated with sexual promiscuity. Untreated cases are characterized by the development of extensive scarring, often associated with lymphatic obstruction and lymphedema (elephantiasis) of the external genitalia.

MORPHOLOGY. Granuloma inguinale begins as a raised, papular lesion involving the moist, stratified squamous epithelium of the genitalia. The lesion eventually ulcerates and is accompanied by the development of abundant granulation tissue, manifested grossly as a protuberant, soft, painless mass. As the lesion enlarges, its borders become raised and indurated. Disfiguring scars may develop in untreated cases and are sometimes associated with urethral, vulvar, or anal strictures. Regional lymph nodes typically are spared or show only nonspecific reactive changes, in contrast to chancroid.

Microscopic examination of active lesions reveals marked epithelial hyperplasia at the borders of the ulcer, sometimes mimicking carcinoma (*pseudoepitheliomatous hyperplasia*). A mixture of neutrophils and mononuclear inflammatory cells is present at the base of the ulcer and beneath the surrounding epithelium. The organisms are demonstrable in Giemsa-stained smears of the exudate as minute coccobacilli within vacuoles in macrophages (Donovan's bodies). Silver stains (e.g., the Warthin-Starry stain) may also be used to demonstrate the organism.

Lymphogranuloma Venereum

Lymphogranuloma venereum (LGV) is a chronic, ulcerative disease caused by certain strains of *C. trachomatis*, which are distinct from those causing the more common nongonococcal urethritis or cervicitis discussed previously. It is a sporadic disease in the United States and western Europe but is endemic in parts of Asia, Africa, the Caribbean region, and South America. As in the case of granuloma inguinale, sporadic cases of LGV appear to be associated most often with sexual promiscuity.

MORPHOLOGY. The patient with LGV may present with nonspecific urethritis, papular or ulcerative lesions involving the lower genitalia, regional adenopathy, or an anorectal syndrome. The lesions contain a **mixed granulomatous and neutrophilic inflammatory response,** with a variable number of chlamydial inclusions in the cytoplasm of epithelial cells or inflammatory cells. Regional lymphadenopathy is common, usually occurring within 30 days of the time of infection. Lymph node involvement is characterized by a granulomatous inflammatory reaction associated with irregularly shaped foci of necrosis and neutrophilic infiltration (stellate abscesses). With time, the inflammatory reaction is dominated by nonspecific chronic inflammatory infiltrates and extensive fibrosis. The latter, in turn, may cause local lymphatic obstruction with lymphedema and strictures. Rectal strictures are particularly common in women. In active lesions, the diagnosis of LGV may be made by demonstration of the organism in biopsy sections or smears of exudate. In more chronic cases, the diagnosis rests with the demonstration of antibodies to the appropriate chlamydial serotypes in the patient's serum.

Trichomoniasis

Trichomonas vaginalis is a sexually transmitted protozooan that is a frequent cause of vaginitis. The trophozoite form adheres to, and causes superficial lesions of, the mucosa. In females, *T. vaginalis* infection is often associated with loss of acid-producing Döderlein bacilli. It may be asymptomatic, but frequently causes itching and a profuse watery vaginal discharge. Urethral colonization may cause urinary frequency and dysuria. *T. vaginalis* infection is usually asymptomatic in males but in some cases may present as nongonococcal urethritis.

Genital Herpes Simplex

Genital herpes infection, or herpes genitalis, affects an estimated 30 million people in the United States and accounts for about 5% of all visits to STD clinics. Most cases are caused by *herpes simplex virus (HSV) type 2,* although HSV type 1 accounts for a significant number of infections as well. Genital HSV infection may occur in any sexually active population. As with other STDs, the risk of infection is directly related to the number of sexual contacts. HSV is transmitted when virus comes into contact with a mucosal surface or broken skin of a susceptible host. Such transmission requires direct contact with an infected person, because the virus is readily inactivated at room temperature, particularly if dried.

MORPHOLOGY. The initial lesions of genital HSV infection are painful, erythematous vesicles on the mucosa or skin of the lower genitalia and adjacent extragenital sites. The anorectal area is a particularly common site of primary infection among homosexual males. Histologic changes include the presence of intraepithelial vesicles accompanied by necrotic cellular debris, neutrophils, and cells harboring characteristic intranuclear viral inclusions. The classic **Cowdry type A inclusion** appears as a light purple, homogeneous intranuclear structure surrounded by a clear halo. Infected cells commonly fuse to form multinucleated syncytia. The inclusions readily stain with antibodies to HSV, permitting a rapid, specific diagnosis of HSV infection in histologic sections or smears.

The manifestations of HSV infection vary considerably, depending on whether the infection is primary or recurrent. Among patients experiencing their first episode, locally painful vesicular lesions are often accompanied by dysuria, urethral discharge, local lymph node enlargement and tenderness, and systemic manifestations, such as fever, muscle aches, and headache. HSV is actively shed during this period, and it continues to be shed until the mucosal lesions have completely healed. Signs and symptoms may last for several weeks during the primary phase of disease. Episodes of recurrent disease are common during the first several years after the primary infection, but they tend to be milder and of shorter duration than the primary episode. As with primary infection, HSV is shed while active lesions are present.

Among immunocompetent adults, herpes genitalis is generally not life-threatening. However, HSV does pose a major threat to immunosuppressed patients, in whom fatal, disseminated disease may develop. *Neonatal herpes infection* occurs in about half of infants delivered vaginally to mothers suffering from either primary or recurrent genital HSV infection. The viral infection is acquired during passage through the birth canal. Its incidence has risen in parallel with the rise in genital HSV infection. The manifestations of neonatal herpes, which typically develop during the second week of life, include skin rash, encephalitis, pneumonitis, and hepatic necrosis. Approximately 60% of affected infants die of the disease, with significant morbidity occurring in about half of the survivors (see also Chapter 7).

Human Papillomavirus Infection

HPV is the cause of a number of squamous proliferations in the genital tract, including condyloma acuminata, some precancerous lesions, and some carcinomas. *Condyloma acuminata*, also known as venereal warts, are caused by HPV types 6 and 11. They occur on the penis as well as on the female genitalia. They should not be confused with the condyloma lata seen in secondary syphilis. Genital HPV infection may be transmitted to neonates during vaginal delivery. These infants may subsequently develop recurrent and potentially life-threatening papillomas of the upper respiratory tract.

MORPHOLOGY. In males, condyloma acuminata usually occur on the coronal sulcus or inner surface of the prepuce, where they range from small, sessile lesions to large, papillary proliferations measuring several centimeters in diameter. In females, they commonly occur on the vulva. The microscopic appearance is that of an exuberant proliferation of stratified squamous epithelium supported by fibrovascular papillae. The more superficial epithelial cells contain irregular, hyperchromatic nuclei surrounded by a characteristic clear perinuclear halo, a change referred to as **koilocytosis** (see Figs. 19–2 and 19–3 in Chapter 19).

In addition to HSV and HPV, other important viral infections that are sexually transmitted include HIV-1 and HIV-2, cytomegalovirus, and hepatitis B virus, all discussed in detail elsewhere.

BIBLIOGRAPHY

Bunting PS: A guide to the interpretation of serum prostate specific antigen levels. Clin Biochem 28:221, 1995. (A review of the structure and metabolism of PSA, reference ranges, and the effects of various clinical manipulations on PSA levels.)

Cook LS, et al: Clinical presentation of genital warts among circumcised and uncircumcised heterosexual men attending an urban STD clinic. Genitourin Med 69:262, 1993. (A review of the clinical presentation of human papillomavirus infection in an urban male population.)

Cupp MR, Oesterling JE: Prostate-speciifc antigen, digital rectal examination, and transrectal ultrasonography: their roles in diagnosing early prostate cancer. Mayo Clin Proc 68:297, 1993. (Guidelines for the use of these modalities in a cost-effective manner.)

Garnick MB, Fair WR: Prostate cancer: emerging concepts. Part I. Ann Intern Med 125:118, 1996. (A review of the refinements in the interpretation of PSA values in the diagnosis of prostate cancer.)

Goldmeier D, Hay P: A review and update of adult syphilis, with particular reference to its treatment. Int J STD AIDS 4:70, 1993. (A review of the diagnostic value of selected serologic tests for syphilis and recent recommendations for antimicrobial therapy.)

Grigor KM, Skakkebaek NE: Pathogenesis and cell biology of germ cell neoplasia: general discussion. Eur Urol 23:46, 1993. (A brief discussion of the malignant transformation of germ cells and progression of in situ lesions.)

Humphry PA, Walther PJ: Adenocarcinoma of the prostate. Part II: Tissue prognosticators. Am J Clin Pathol 100:256, 1993. (A review of the relation between the histologic characteristics of prostate cancer in biopsy material and patient prognosis.)

Kirkby RS: The clinical assessment of benign prostatic hyperplasia. Cancer 70 (Suppl 1):284, 1992. (A review of techniques used in the clinical evaluation of patients with nodular hyperplasia, including comments about the role of prostate-specific antigen determinations.)

Mandegar M, Schaff EA: Is the clinical spectrum of gonorrhea changing? J Adolesc Health 17:123, 1995. (A review of the epidemiology and clinical presentation of gonorrhea in an inner city health care program.)

Mostofi FK, et al: Pathology of carcinoma of the prostate. Cancer 70 (Suppl 1):235, 1992. (A thorough review of the pathology of carcinoma of the prostate by one of the leading authorities in the field, with additional comments on the pathology of precursor lesions, therapeutic effects, and the relation between histology and prognosis.)

Nandwani R, Evans DT: Are you sure it's syphilis? A review of false positive serology. Int J STD AIDS 6:241, 1995. (A review of some of the important pitfalls in the serologic diagnosis of syphilis, including a discussion of biologic false-positive tests.)

Rawstron SA, et al: Maternal and congenital syphilis in Brooklyn, New York: epidemiology, transmission, and diagnosis. Am J Dis Child 147:727, 1993. (A review of some of the more recent epidemiologic trends and clinical features of congenital syphilis in a major metropolitan center.)

Roehrborn CG, et al: Variability of repeated serum prostate specific antigen (PSA) measurements within less than 90 days in a well-defined patient population. Urology 47:59, 1996. (A study discussing the potential problems associated with a single determination of PSA.)

Ulbright TM: Germ cell neoplasms of the testis. Am J Surg Pathol 17:1075, 1993. (A comprehensive review of pathology, classification and precursor lesions of germ cell neoplasms of the testis.)

van der Sluiss JJ: Laboratory techniques in the diagnosis of syphilis: a review. Genitourin Med 68:413, 1992. (A concise review of serologic tests for syphilis.)

Vohra S, Badlani G: Balanitis and balanoposthitis. Urol Clin North Am 19: 143, 1992. (A review of the clinical features and treatment of these entities.)

Walsh PC: Treatment of benign prostatic hyperplasia. N Engl J Med 335: 586, 1996. (An excellent and important editorial that relates the treatment of prostatic hyperplasia to predominant glandular or stromal proliferation. It suggests that BPH is heterogeneous, both histologically and clinically.)

19

Female Genital System and Breast

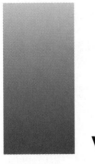

Vulva

Clinically significant diseases of the vulva do not loom large in gynecologic practice. Only the uncommon carcinomas are life threatening. Far more frequent are the inflammatory disorders (vulvitis), which are more uncomfortable than serious. Only a few other conditions need to be mentioned here: non-neoplastic epithelial disorders (discussed later); the painful Bartholin cysts due to obstruction of the excretory ducts of the glands; and imperforate hymen in children, impounding secretions and later menstrual flow.

VULVITIS

The moist hair-bearing skin and delicate membrane of the vulva are vulnerable to many nonspecific microbe-induced inflammations and dermatologic disorders. Intense itching (pruritus) and subsequent scratching often exacerbate the primary

condition. There are also many specific forms of vulval infection related to the sexually transmitted diseases. Most were discussed in Chapter 18. The four most important of these infectious agents in North America are human papillomavirus (HPV), producing condylomata acuminata and vulvar intra-epithelial neoplasia (both discussed in some detail later); herpes genitalis (herpes simplex virus [HSV]), causing a vesicular eruption; gonococcal suppurative infection of the vulvovaginal glands; and syphilis, with its primary chancre at the site of inoculation.

NON-NEOPLASTIC EPITHELIAL DISORDERS (VULVAL DYSTROPHIES)

The epithelium of the vulvar mucosa may undergo atrophic thinning or hyperplastic thickening. For want of a better term, these alterations were collectively referred to as dystrophies but are now simply referred to as non-neoplastic epithelial disorders (NNEDs) to differentiate them from the premalignant lesions discussed later. There are two forms of NNED: lichen sclerosus and squamous hyperplasia. Both may coexist in different areas in the same patient, and both may appear macroscopically as depigmented white lesions, referred to as leukoplakia. Similar white patches or plaques are also seen with (1) vitiligo (loss of pigment) of the skin, (2) a variety of benign dermatoses such as psoriasis and lichen planus (Chapter 22), (3) carcinoma in situ, (4) Paget's disease (described later), and (5) invasive carcinoma. Thus, leukoplakia is merely a descriptive term that gives no indication of its underlying nature. Only biopsy and microscopic examinations can differentiate among these similar-looking lesions.

Lichen Sclerosus

This lesion is characterized by thinning of the epidermis and disappearance of rete pegs, accompanied by superficial hyperkeratosis and dermal fibrosis with a scant perivascular, mononuclear inflammatory cell infiltrate (Fig. 19–1). The lesions appear clinically as smooth, white plaques or papules that in time may extend and coalesce. The surface is smoothed out and sometimes parchment-like. When the entire vulva is affected, the labia become somewhat atrophic and stiffened and the vaginal orifice is constricted. It occurs in all age groups but is most common in postmenopausal women. It may also be encountered elsewhere on the skin. The pathogenesis is uncertain, but some autoimmune reaction is suspected based on the increased frequency of other autoimmune disorders in these women and the demonstration of activated T cells in the subepithelial inflammatory infiltrate. About 1% to 4% of these women have in time developed cancerous changes.

Squamous Hyperplasia

Previously called "hyperplastic dystrophy," this disorder is marked by epithelial thickening with significant surface hyperkeratosis. It appears clinically as an area of leukoplakia. The epithelium may show increased mitotic activity in both the basal and prickle cell layer. Leukocytic infiltration of the dermis is sometimes pronounced. The hyperplastic epithelial changes show no atypia (Fig. 19–1). No increased predisposition to cancer is generally held to be the case, but suspiciously, squamous hyperplasia is often present at the margins of established cancer of the vulva.

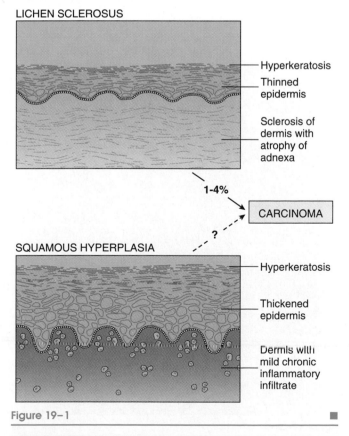

LICHEN SCLEROSUS
- Hyperkeratosis
- Thinned epidermis
- Sclerosis of dermis with atrophy of adnexa

1-4%

CARCINOMA

?

SQUAMOUS HYPERPLASIA
- Hyperkeratosis
- Thickened epidermis
- Dermis with mild chronic inflammatory infiltrate

Figure 19–1   ■

Schematic comparison of lichen sclerosus and squamous hyperplasia of the vulvar mucosa with approximate indications of the risk of carcinomatous transformation.

■ TUMORS

Condylomas

Condylomas are essentially anogenital warts, but in the moist environment of the vulva they tend to be large. Most fall into two distinctive biologic forms, but rarer types also exist. *Condylomata lata,* rarely seen today, are flat, moist, minimally elevated lesions that occur in secondary syphilis (Chapter 18). The more common *condylomata acuminata* may be papillary and distinctly elevated or somewhat flat and rugose. They occur anywhere on the anogenital surface, sometimes singly but more often in multiple sites. On the vulva they range from a few millimeters to many centimeters in diameter and are red-pink to pink-brown (Fig. 19–2). The histologic appearance of these lesions was described earlier (Chapter 18), but particularly significant is the characteristic cellular morphology, namely, perinuclear cytoplasmic vacuolization with nuclear angular pleomorphism—koilocytosis (Fig. 19–3). Such cells are considered to be hallmarks of HPV infection. Indeed, there is a strong association with at least two types (6 and 11) of HPV, closely related to the virus that causes common warts. The HPV can be transmitted venereally; identical lesions occur in men on the penis and around the anus. Vulvar condylomas are not precancerous but may coexist with foci of intraepithelial neoplasia in the vulva and cervix. As discussed later (p 605), the types of HPV isolated from the cancers differ from those most often found in condylomas.

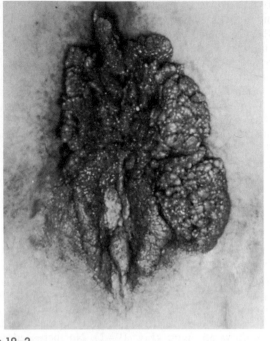

Figure 19–2 ■

Numerous condylomas of the vulva, almost obscuring the labia minora. (Courtesy of Dr. Arthur Hertig.)

Carcinoma of the Vulva and Vulvar Intraepithelial Neoplasia

Carcinoma of the vulva represents about 3% of all genital tract cancers in women, occurring mostly in women over the age of 60. However, there has been a dramatic increase in the frequency of this form of cancer as well as vulvar intraepithelial neoplasia (VIN) in the past few decades, principally among younger women (40 to 60 years of age). In all age groups, approximately 90% of these tumors are squamous cell carcinomas; the remainder are adenocarcinomas, melanomas, or basal cell carcinomas.

Many findings suggest that there are two biologic forms of vulvar carcinoma. The most common is seen in the relatively younger patients, particularly in cigarette smokers. HPV, especially types 16 and 18 and less frequently other types, is present in 75% to 90% of cases, and in many cases there is coexisting vaginal or cervical carcinoma or carcinoma in situ or condylomata acuminata, suggesting a common causal agent, probably HPV. Often in these patients, in situ cancerous changes confined to the epithelium, so-called VIN, precede the development of the overt cancer, in the past referred to as Bowen's disease. The VIN may consist of only relatively mild dysplastic/anaplastic changes graded VIN I, or with increasing dysplasia may be graded VIN II or VIN III (carcinoma in situ). In many instances the VIN has preceded by many years the development of the vulvar cancer. It may be found in multiple, apparently separate foci or may coexist with an invasive lesion. Whether VIN is always destined to become an invasive cancer remains unclear, but there is good evidence that at least in some individuals, the VIN has been present for many years, perhaps decades. Whether genetic, immunologic, or environ-

mental influences (e.g., cigarette smoking or superinfection with new strains of HPV) determine the course is unclear. The other subgroup of vulvar carcinoma occurs in older women. It is not associated with HPV but is often preceded by years of non-neoplastic epithelial changes, principally lichen sclerosus. In some instances, atypical epithelial changes meriting the diagnosis of VIN have preceded the appearance of the overt neoplasm. Regression is infrequent in this group.

VIN and early vulvar carcinomas appear as areas of leukoplakia caused by epithelial thickening involving any region of the vulva or adjacent skin. In about one quarter of cases the changes are melanin pigmented. In the course of time, these areas are transformed into overt **exophytic** or ulcerative **endophytic tumors.** HPV-positive tumors are more often multifocal and appear warty or condylomatous.

Histologically, HPV-positive neoplasms tend to be poorly differentiated squamous cell carcinoma, whereas the HPV negative lesions, which are usually unifocal, tend to show well-differentiated keratinizing squamous cells. Although all patterns tend to remain confined to their site of origin for a few years, ultimately, direct invasion with involvement of regional nodes and lymphohematogenous spread occurs. The risk of such spread is

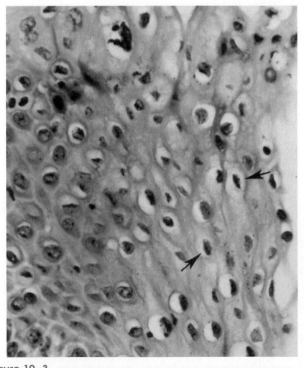

Figure 19–3 ■

High-power detail of koilocytes with cytoplasmic clearing and striking angulated nuclear pleomorphism *(arrows).*

correlated with the size of the tumor and the depth of invasion.

Patients with a tumor less than 2 cm in diameter have about a 75% 5-year survival after radical excision, whereas only 10% of those with larger lesions survive 10 years.

Extramammary Paget's Disease

Paget's disease of the vulva, like that of the breast, is essentially a form of intraepithelial carcinoma rendered distinctive by scattered single cells and small clusters of recognizable carcinomatous cells. These are set off from the surrounding more or less normal epithelium by cleared halos of periodic acid–Schiff (PAS)-positive mucopolysaccharide secreted by the cancerous cells (Fig. 19–4). The isolated intraepithelial cancer cells are believed to arise from aberrant differentiation of epithelial progenitors, but in a few instances there is an accompanying subepithelial or submucosal small tumor arising in an adnexal structure. These microscopic changes usually appear clinically as solitary or multiple well-demarcated geographic foci of red-crusted inflammatory-looking areas, usually on the labia majora and easily mistaken for a form of dermatitis. When the Paget cells are confined to the epithelium, the lesion may persist for years or even decades without evidence of invasion. However, in some instances, particularly when there is an associated appendageal tumor, the Paget cells extend into the skin appendages, invade locally, and ultimately metastasize more widely to distant sites, usually within the first 2 to 5 years.

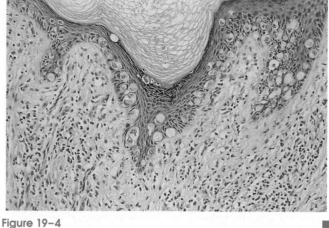

Figure 19–4 ■

Paget's disease of the vulva, with scattered large, clear tumor cells within the squamous epithelium.

Melanoma of the Vulva

These highly aggressive neoplasms account for less than 3% to 5% of all vulvar cancers and so can be discussed briefly. In the early stages the melanoma cells may be dispersed within the epidermis and thus create a microscopic pattern resembling Paget's disease. However, because the melanoma cells are not enclosed within a halo of mucopolysaccharide, they can be distinguished from Paget cells. The histologic characteristics are those of melanomas elsewhere and so are not discussed here (Chapter 22). The prognosis is related to depth of invasion, as it is in extravulvar melanomas, but overall the invasive lesions are treacherous neoplasms that are often fatal.

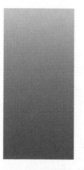

Vagina

The vagina in adults is seldom the site of primary disease. More often, it is secondarily involved in the spread of cancer or infections arising in close proximity (e.g., cervix, vulva, bladder, rectum). The only primary disorders that merit brief comment are a few congenital anomalies, vaginitis, and primary tumors.

Congenital anomalies of the vagina are fortunately uncommon entities such as total absence of the vagina, a septate or double vagina (usually associated with a septate cervix and, sometimes, uterus), and congenital small lateral Gartner's duct cysts arising from persistent embryonic remnants.

VAGINITIS

Vaginitis is a relatively common clinical problem that is usually transient, is not serious, and is responsible for producing a vaginal discharge (leukorrhea). A large variety of organisms have been implicated at one time or another, including bacteria, fungi, and parasites. Many represent normal commensals that become pathogenic in predisposed individuals such as diabetics; with systemic antibiotic therapy that disrupts the normal microbial flora; after abortion or pregnancy; in elderly persons with compromised immune function; and, of course, in patients with AIDS. Other implicated agents are sexually transmitted. In adults, primary gonorrheal infection of the vagina is uncommon. However, it may occur in a newborn infant born to an infected mother. The only other two organisms worthy of specific mention, because they are frequent offenders, are *Candida albicans* and *Trichomonas vaginalis.* Candidal (monilial) vaginitis produces a curdy-white discharge. This organism is present in about 5% of normal adults, and so the appearance of symptomatic infection must involve predisposing influences, or sexual transmission of a new, more aggressive strain. Biopsies, which are rarely obtained, reveal only superficial, nonspecific submucosal inflammation. *T. vaginalis,* which is also a frequent offender, produces a watery, copious gray-green discharge in which parasites can be identified microscopically in fresh specimens. However, *Trichomonas* can be identified in about 10% of asymptomatic women, and so active infection usually represents a sexually transmitted new strain (Chapter 18). The inflammatory reaction is confined to the superficial squamous mucosa without invasion of the underlying tissue.

Nonspecific atrophic vaginitis may be encountered in postmenopausal women with preexisting atrophy and thinning of the squamous vaginal mucosa.

VAGINAL INTRAEPITHELIAL NEOPLASIA AND SQUAMOUS CELL CARCINOMA

These are extremely uncommon lesions that usually occur in women over the age of 60. A preexisting or concurrent carcinoma of the cervix or vulva is sometimes present. How often HPV is implicated in the development of these neoplasms is not well known, but the concurrence of neoplasms in other sites in the female genital tract strongly suggests a common, probably viral, effect. Of particular interest is vaginal clear cell adenocarcinoma, usually encountered in girls in their late teens whose mothers took diethylstilbestrol during pregnancy. Sometimes these cancers do not appear until the third or fourth decade of life. The overall risk is 1 per 1000 or less of those exposed in utero. In about one third of instances, these cancers arise in the cervix. Much more frequently, perhaps in one third of the population at risk, small glandular or microcystic inclusions appear in the vaginal mucosa: vaginal adenosis. These benign lesions appear as red granular foci and are lined by mucus-secreting or ciliated columnar cells. It is from such inclusions that the rare clear cell adenocarcinoma arises.

SARCOMA BOTRYOIDES

Sarcoma botryoides (embryonal rhabdomyosarcoma), producing soft polypoid masses, is another fortunately rare form of primary vaginal cancer usually encountered in infants and children under the age of 5 years. It may occur in other sites, such as the urinary bladder and bile ducts. These lesions are described in more detail in Chapter 21.

Cervix

The cervix lives a troubled life: it must serve as a barrier to the ingress of air and the microflora of the normal vaginal tract, yet must permit the escape of menstrual flow and sustain the mild buffeting of intercourse and the trauma of childbirth. No small wonder it is often the seat of disease. Fortunately, most cervical lesions are relatively banal inflammations (cervicitis), but this is also the site of one of the most common cancers in women: squamous cell carcinoma.

CERVICITIS

Before considering these inflammatory lesions, we must digress to differentiate true inflammatory cervicitis from so-called "erosions." During development, the columnar mucus-secreting epithelium of the endocervix meets the squamous epithelial covering of the exocervix at the external os; thus, the entire "exposed" cervix is covered by squamous epithelium. The endocervical columnar epithelium is not visible to the naked eye or colposcopically. In time, in most young women, there is down-growth of the columnar epithelium below the exocervical os—ectropion, and thus the squamocolumnar junction comes to lie below the exocervix. This "exposed" mucus-secreting columnar epithelium may appear reddened and moist and is mistakenly called cervical "erosion," but in actual fact it is the result of normal changes in adult women. Remodeling occurs continuously with regrowth of the squamous epithelium up to the original external os. The area replaced by the squamous epithelium is known as the *transformation zone* (Fig. 19–5). Frequently, overgrowth of the regenerating squamous epithelium blocks the orifices of endocervical glands in the transformation zone to produce small *nabothian cysts* lined by columnar mucus-secreting epithelium. Thus, "erosions" are normal developmental changes and are to be differentiated from true cervicitis. Nonetheless, in the transformation zone, there may be a mild banal inflammatory infiltrate resulting, possibly, from changes in the vaginal pH or the ever-present microflora of the vagina.

Inflammations of the cervix are extremely common and are associated with a mucopurulent to purulent vaginal discharge. Cytologic examination of the discharge reveals white cells and inflammatory atypia of shed epithelial cells, as well as possible microorganisms. These inflammations have been variously subdivided into noninfectious and infectious cervicitis. Since microorganisms are invariably present in the vagina, with or without associated inflammatory changes on cytologic examination, it is difficult to differentiate noninfectious from infectious cervicitis. Often present are indigenous and, for the most part, incidental vaginal aerobes and anaerobes, streptococci, staphylococci, enterococci, and *Escherichia coli.* Much more important are *Chlamydia trachomatis, Ureaplasma urealyticum, Trichomonas vaginalis, Candida* species, *Neisseria gonorrhoeae,* herpes simplex II (genitalis), and one or more types of HPV. Many of these microorganisms are transmitted sexually, and so the cervicitis represents a sexually transmitted disease (STD). Among these pathogens, *C. trachomatis* is by far the most common and accounts for up to 40% of cases of cervicitis encountered in STD clinics, thus being far more common than gonorrhea. Herpetic infections of the cervix are noteworthy because this organism may be transmitted to the infant during passage through the birth canal, sometimes resulting in a serious, sometimes fatal, systemic herpetic infection (Chapter 7).

Nonspecific cervicitis may be either **acute** or **chronic.** Excluding gonococcal infection, which causes a specific form of acute disease, the rela-

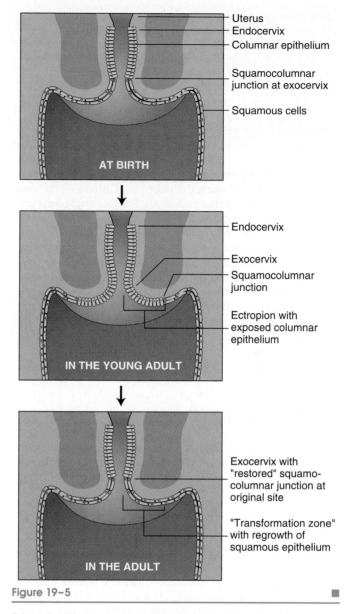

Uterus
Endocervix
Columnar epithelium

Squamocolumnar junction at exocervix

Squamous cells

AT BIRTH

↓

Endocervix

Exocervix
Squamocolumnar junction

Ectropion with exposed columnar epithelium

IN THE YOUNG ADULT

↓

Exocervix with "restored" squamocolumnar junction at original site

"Transformation zone" with regrowth of squamous epithelium

IN THE ADULT

Figure 19–5   ■

Schematic of the development of the cervical transformation zone.

tively uncommon **acute nonspecific** form is limited to postpartum women and is usually caused by staphylococci or streptococci. The chronic form is the nearly ubiquitous entity usually referred to by the unqualified term *nonspecific cervicitis.*

Grossly, chronic cervicitis appears as a reddening, swelling, and granularity around the margins of the external cervical os. Histologically, the infiltration is largely mononuclear. Inflammatory obstruction of the cervical glands may yield **nabothian cysts.**

The cervical epithelium may show hyperplasia and reactive atypia, characterized by epithelial disorganization and nuclear alterations, not to be confused with the changes of dysplasia. In the course of these changes, the epithelial cells are depleted of their normal content of glycogen and so may yield falsely positive Schiller reactions (failure to take up applied iodinate solution—characteristic of glycogen depleted cells in cancers). The herpesvirus may produce ulcerations with characteristic intranuclear inclusions in the cells at the margins of the ulcers. *C. trachomatis* is typically associated with numerous plasma cells in the inflammatory infiltrate.

Cervicitis commonly comes to attention on routine examination or because of marked leukorrhea. Culture of the discharge must be interpreted cautiously because organisms are virtually always present. Only the identification of known pathogens is helpful. When the lesion is severe, differentiation from carcinoma may be difficult even with colposcopy and may require a biopsy. Cervicitis per se is not a precancerous lesion, but the secondary epithelial dysplastic changes may constitute a favorable subsoil for carcinogenic influences such as HPV. Severe cervicitis may lead also to sterility through deformation and exudative blocking of the cervical os, while simultaneously producing an unfavorable environment for sperm.

TUMORS OF THE CERVIX

Cervical carcinoma, despite dramatic improvements in early diagnosis and treatment, continues to be one of the major causes of cancer-related deaths in women, particularly in the developing world. The only other "tumor" meriting mention is the endocervical polyp.

Endocervical Polyp

Although these lesions constitute tumors insofar as they may protrude as polypoid masses (sometimes through the exocervix), they may in reality be inflammatory in origin. They range up to a few centimeters in diameter; are soft and yielding to palpation; and are covered by a smooth, glistening surface with underlying cystically dilated spaces filled with mucinous secretion. The surface epithelium and lining of the underlying cysts are composed of the same mucus-secreting columnar cells that line the endocervical canal. The stroma is edematous and may contain scattered mononuclear cells. Superimposed chronic inflammation may lead to squamous metaplasia of the covering epithelium and ulcerations. These lesions may bleed and thus cause some concern, but they have no malignant potential.

Cervical Intraepithelial Neoplasia and Squamous Cell Carcinoma

Cervical carcinoma was once the most frequent form of cancer in women around the world. Only 50 years ago it occupied this same unenviable position in the United States, but the widespread use of Papanicolaou (cytologic) screening of women has dramatically lowered the incidence of invasive tumors to about 15,000 new cases annually and the mortality to about 5000 (1996 estimate), making cervical cancer now eighth in the roster of cancer-killers. By contrast, the incidence of precursor cervical intraepithelial carcinoma has increased (this being in part attributable to better case finding) to its present level of over 50,000 cases annually. This growing divergence is a testament to detection of precursor lesions by the Pap smear at an early stage, permitting discovery of these lesions when curative treatment is possible. Few women know the name Papanicolaou (fewer yet can spell it) to which they may well owe their lives.

It is important to emphasize here that most (perhaps all) invasive cervical squamous cell carcinomas arise from precursor epithelial changes referred to as cervical intraepithelial neoplasia (CIN). However, not all cases of CIN progress to invasive cancer, and indeed may persist without change or regress, as will be pointed out.

CERVICAL INTRAEPITHELIAL NEOPLASIA (CIN), SQUAMOUS INTRAEPITHELIAL LESION (SIL)

Cytologic examination can detect CIN (SIL) long before any abnormality can be seen grossly. The follow-up of such women has made it clear that precancerous epithelial changes may precede the development of an overt cancer by many years, perhaps as long as 20 years. However, as noted above, only a fraction of cases of CIN progress to invasive carcinoma. The precancerous changes referred to as CIN begin with minimal atypia, becoming more marked over time in some women, with the eventual development of an overt carcinoma. By time-honored precedent, the early changes have been referred to as dysplasia, but in time they may convert to anaplastic changes on the way to becoming a carcinoma in situ and, in some instances, an invasive carcinoma. The severity and extent of the cellular atypia has been graded as follows:

■ CIN I: Mild dysplasia
■ CIN II: Moderate dysplasia
■ CIN III: Severe dysplasia and carcinoma in situ

Because of difficulties in segregating one grade from another, it has been recommended that they simply be divided into low-grade and high-grade squamsus intraepithelial lesions. The low-grade lesions correspond to CIN I or flat condylomas (described later) and the high-grade lesions to CIN II or III. Progression from a lower grade to a higher grade is not inevitable. Although studies vary, with CIN I the likelihood of regression is about 50% to 60%; of persistence, 30%; and of progression to CIN III, 20%. Only 1% to 5% become invasive. With CIN III the likelihood of regression is only 33% and of progression 6% to 74% (in various studies). It is evident that the higher the grade of CIN, the greater is the likelihood of progression, but it should be noted that many instances of even the higher-grade lesions do not progress to cancer.

Epidemiology and Pathogenesis. The peak age incidence of CIN is about 30 years, whereas that of invasive carcinoma is about 45 years. It is evident that precancerous changes take many years, perhaps decades, to evolve into overt carcinomas.

Prominent risk factors for the development of CIN and invasive carcinoma are

- Early age at first intercourse
- Multiple sexual partners
- A male partner with multiple previous sexual partners

Many other risk factors can be related to these three, including the higher incidence in lower socioeconomic groups, the rarity among virgins, and the association with multiple pregnancies. They point strongly to the likelihood of sexual transmission of a causative agent, in this case HPV. Indeed, HPV can be detected in 85% to 90% of precancerous lesions and invasive neoplasms, and more specifically, certain high-risk types in order of frequency: 16, 18, 31, and 33. By contrast, condylomas, which you recall are benign lesions, are associated with infection by low-risk types, i.e., 6, 11, 42, and 44 (Fig. 19–6). In these lesions the viral DNA does not integrate into the host genome, remaining in the free episomal form. By contrast, HPV types 16 and 18 possess genes that, after integration into the cellular genome, encode proteins that block or inactivate tumor suppressor genes p53 and Rb in target epithelial cells, and thus permit their uncontrolled proliferation (Chapter 6). Although many women harbor these viruses, only a few develop cancer, and moreover, in about 10% to 15% of cervical carcinomas, no HPV can be found. Thus, other influences must be involved, such as other carcinogens or cocarcinogens, genetic factors, altered immunity in the host, and (in some poorly understood manner) cigarette smoking.

> The cervical epithelial changes encompassed within the term *CIN* begin with mild dysplasia (Grade I CIN). At this stage cellular atypicality is minimal, and it affects the lower third or fourth of the epithelium. Such changes may be seen in the usual cervical epithelium or in flat epithelium marked by koilocytotic changes (sometimes called **flat condyloma**). Koilocytosis, as you will recall from the discussion of condylomata accuminata on page 599, constitutes nuclear angulation surrounded by perinuclear vacuolization produced by a viral cytopathic effect, in this case HPV. Koilocytic changes are found mostly in the upper layers of the epithelium. With progression to CIN II, the dysplasia becomes more severe, affecting the lower half of the epithelium. It is associated with some variation in cell and nuclear size and with normal-looking mitoses above the basal layer. Such changes are designated moderate dysplasia. The superficial layer of cells is still well differentiated, but in some cases shows the koilocytotic changes described. The next step in progression is severe dysplasia (grade III CIN) marked by greater variation in cell and nuclear size, disorderly orientation of the cells, and normal or abnormal mitoses; these changes affect virtually all layers of the epithelium. Differentiation of surface cells and koilocytotic changes have usually disappeared (Fig. 19–7 and 19–8). In time, such changes become more atypical and may extend into the endocervical glands, but **the alterations are confined to the epithelial layer and its glands**. It is apparent that these changes constitute **carcinoma in situ**. The next stage, if it is to appear, is invasive cancer. However, as previously emphasized, there is no inevitability to this progression nor to the development of an invasive carcinoma.

Cellular atypicalities usually first appear near the squamocolumnar junction in the "transformation zone." The likelihood of progression to higher grades is correlated with the severity of the changes when first discovered and to the presence of high-risk types of HPV such as 16 or 18. However, viral isolation and typing does not predict the course; moreover, in 10% to 15% of cases, no HPV can be identified. These findings make it clear that something more than viral action is probably involved in the evolution of an invasive squamous cell carcinoma. Only careful follow-up with repeated colposcopic examinations, possibly combined with the acetic acid test (when dilute acetic acid is applied to the exocervix, areas of abnormal epithelial hyperplasia or neoplasia appear paler than the normal mucosa), and repeated Pap smears, followed when necessary by biopsy, will determine the nature and gravity of the changes. Overall, about 1% to 5% of low-grade CIN lesions eventually progress to invasive cancer, whereas with

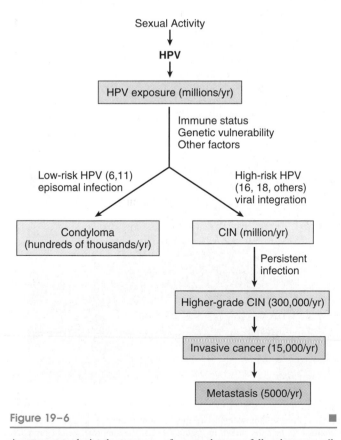

Figure 19–6 ■

An attempt to depict the sequence of events that may follow human papillomavirus (HPV) infection. CIN, cervical intraepithelial neoplasia.

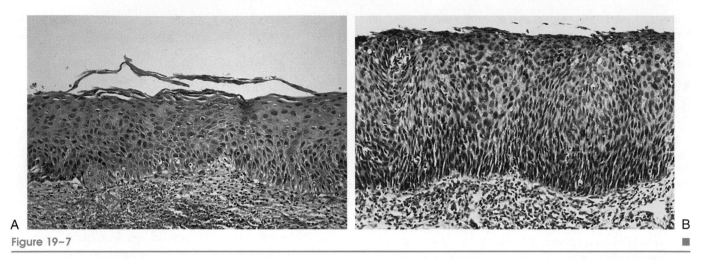

Figure 19–7 ■

A, The mildly dysplastic epithelial changes of CIN I (low-grade SIL) affecting the lower layers of epithelium. Most cells reveal more or less usual maturation. *B,* The more marked atypical changes of CIN III (high-grade SIL) with total loss of maturation. The dysplasia affects the entire thickness of the epithelium.

high-grade lesions the percentage has been reported variously as 6% to 74%.

INVASIVE CARCINOMA OF THE CERVIX

The importance of cervical cancer as a cause of morbidity and mortality around the world, in both developing and developed countries, has already been emphasized. About 80% to 95% of these cancers are squamous cell carcinoma, which generally evolve from precursor CIN. The remainder are adenocarcinomas or variants thereof. The squamous cell lesions are appearing in increasingly younger women, now with a peak incidence at about 45 years, some 10 to 15 years later than their precursors. In some individuals with particularly aggressive intraepithelial changes, the time interval may be considerably shorter, whereas in other women, CIN precur-

sors may persist for life. Many factors, both constitutional and acquired, modify the course. Careful follow-up and repeat biopsies are the only reliable way to monitor the course of the disease. Recall, CIN I and even CIN II may regress, as noted earlier.

Invasive carcinoma takes one of three distinct macroscopic forms. The most frequent is a **fungating** tumor that begins as a nodular thickening of the epithelium and eventually develops into a cauliflower-like mass projecting above the surrounding mucosa, sometimes completely encircling the external os (Fig. 19–9). The second is an **ulcerative** form, characterized by sloughing of the central surface of the tumor. The least frequent variety is **infiltrative,** which tends to grow down-

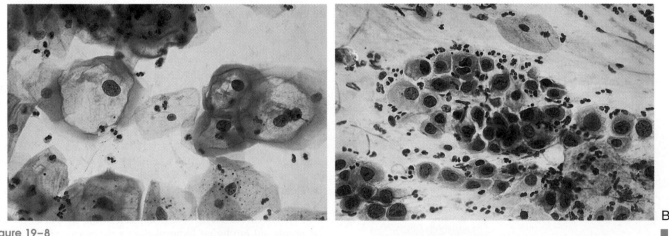

Figure 19–8 ■

A, Cytologic smear from a CIN I or low-grade SIL. To the left of center is a normal mature squamous cell. Grouped around it are the atypical cells with enlarged hyperchromatic nuclei and less cytoplasm, hence they are smaller. *B,* In contrast to the cells shown in Figure 19–8*A,* the abnormal cells from CIN III or high-grade SIL are smaller, have less cytoplasm with large atypical nuclei, and have a corresponding increase in the nuclear-cystoplasmic ratio. Note the normal squamous cell at the top. (Courtesy of Dr. Edmund Cibas, Department of Pathology, Brigham & Women's Hospital, Boston.)

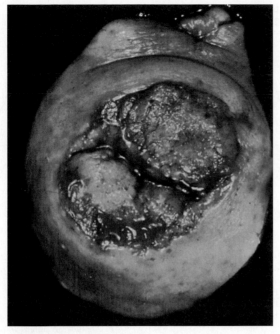

Figure 19–9   ■

Carcinoma of the cervix, well advanced.

ward into the underlying stroma. With time, these forms tend to merge as they infiltrate the underlying tissue, obliterate the external os, grow upward into the endocervical canal and lower uterine segment, and eventually extend into and through the wall of the fundus into the broad ligaments. Advanced lesions may extend into the rectum or base of the urinary bladder, sometimes to obstruct one or both ureters. In due course there is involvement of lymph nodes or distant metastases. Distant metastases, when present, usually target the lungs, bones, and liver.

The histologic character of carcinomas of the cervix is that of a typical **squamous cell carcinoma** of varying differentiation from keratinizing to poorly differentiated. A small minority of cervical cancers are **adenocarcinomas,** presumably arising in endocervical glands or mixed squamous adeno- forms, and are termed **adenosquamous carcinomas.**

Both a grading system, based on the degree of cellular differentiation, and a staging system, based on tumor spread, have been devised. Grades I to III refer to progressively less well differentiated lesions. The details of the currently used staging system are beyond our needs. In brief, the system recognizes stage 0 (carcinoma in situ) and then stages 1 to 4, based on whether the carcinoma is strictly confined to the cervix (stage 1) or has extended beyond the cervix, ultimately to reach stage 4, marked by extension beyond the uterus into the pelvis and by involvement of adjacent organs or metastatic dissemination.

Clinical Course. Carcinoma in situ is usually asymptomatic, except possibly for the presence of some leukorrhea, which is more often related to concurrent cervicitis or vaginitis. The cervix may still appear normal to the naked eye, but colposcopy and the application of dilute acetic acid, discussed above, may disclose an abnormal area. When invasive carcinoma appears, usually in the fifth or sixth decade of life, it is often associated with irregular vaginal bleeding, leukorrhea, painful coitus, and dysuria. Biopsy is always necessary to confirm the cytologic findings and to evaluate the depth of penetration of the lesion.

The mortality from this form of cancer is more often related to its local effects (i.e., obstruction of the ureters or penetration into the bladder or rectum) than to distant metastases. Death from this disease is a particularly lamentable tragedy because at least a decade elapses between the in situ and the invasive stages, providing ample opportunity for early diagnosis. Neither is there any need for hasty, ill-considered treatment; if the interpretation of a biopsy is in doubt, there is time to permit the lesion to declare itself.

The outlook with this disease, assuming appropriate management, depends largely on the stage when it is first discovered, as the following data on 5-year survival indicate: stage 0, 100%, stage 1, 85% to 90%; stage 2, 70% to 75%; stage 3, 35%; stage 4, 10%.

Body of Uterus

The corpus with its endometrium is the principal seat of female reproductive tract disease. Many disorders of this organ are common, often chronic and recurrent, and sometimes disastrous. Only the more frequent and significant ones are considered here.

ENDOMETRITIS

The endometrium is relatively resistant to infections. Acute reactions are virtually limited to bacterial infections that arise after parturition or miscarriage. Retained products of conception are the usual predisposing influence. The inflammatory response is chiefly limited to the interstitium and is entirely nonspecific. Removal of the retained gestational fragments by curettage is followed by prompt remission of the infection. Chronic endometritis occurs in the following settings: (1) in association with chronic gonorrheal pelvic disease; (2) in tuberculosis, either from miliary spread or (more commonly) from drainage of tuberculous salpingitis; (3) in postpartal or postabortal endometrial cavities, usually due to retained gestational tissue; (4) in patients with intrauterine contraceptive devices (IUDs); and (5) spontaneously, without apparent cause, in 15% of patients. Histologically, chronic endometritis is manifested by the irregular proliferation of endometrial glands and the presence of chronic inflammatory cells: plasma cells, macrophages, and lymphocytes in the endometrial stroma.

ADENOMYOSIS

Adenomyosis refers to the growth of the basal layer of the endometrium down into the myometrium. Nests of endometrial stroma or glands, or both, are found well down in the myometrium between the muscle bundles. In the fortuitous microscopic section, continuity between these nests and the overlying endometrium can be established. The uterine wall often becomes thickened owing to the presence of endometrial tissue and a reactive hypertrophy of the myometrium. Cyclic bleeding into the penetrating nests, producing hemosiderin pigmentation, is extremely unusual because the stratum basalis of the endometrium, from which the penetrations arise, is nonfunctional. Marked involvement may produce menorrhagia, dysmenorrhea, and pelvic pain before the onset of menstruation.

ENDOMETRIOSIS

Endometriosis is a far more important clinical condition than adenomyosis; it often causes infertility, dysmenorrhea, pelvic pain, and other problems. The condition is marked by the appearance of foci of more or less recognizable endometrial tissue in the pelvis (ovaries, pouch of Douglas, uterine ligaments, tubes, and rectovaginal septum), less frequently in more remote sites of the peritoneal cavity and about the umbilicus. Uncommonly, the lymph nodes, lungs, and even heart or bone are involved. Three possibilities (not mutually exclusive) have been invoked to explain the origin of these dispersed lesions (Fig. 19–10). First, the *regurgitation theory* proposes menstrual backflow through the fallopian tubes and subsequent implantation. Indeed, menstrual endometrium is

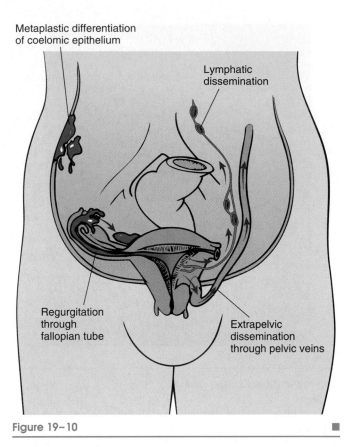

Figure 19–10 ■

The potential origins of endometrial implants.

viable and survives when injected into the anterior abdominal wall; however, this theory cannot explain lesions in the lymph nodes or lungs, for example. Second, the *metaplastic theory* proposes endometrial differentiation of coelomic epithelium, which in the last analysis is the origin of the endometrium itself. This theory, too, cannot explain endometriotic lesions in the lungs or lymph nodes. Third, the *vascular* or *lymphatic dissemination theory* has been invoked to explain extrapelvic or intranodal implants. Conceivably, all pathways are valid in individual instances.

In contrast to adenomyosis, **endometriosis almost always contains functioning endometrium, which undergoes cyclic bleeding.** Because blood collects in these aberrant foci, they usually appear grossly as red-blue to yellow-brown nodules or implants. They vary in size from microscopic to 1 to 2 cm in diameter and lie on or just under the affected serosal surface. Often, individual lesions coalesce to form larger masses. When the ovaries are involved, the lesions may form large, blood-filled cysts that are transformed into so-called **chocolate cysts** as the blood ages (Fig. 19–11). Seepage and organization of the blood leads to widespread fibrosis, adherence of pelvic structures, sealing of the tubal fimbriated ends, and distortion of the oviducts and ovaries. The histo-

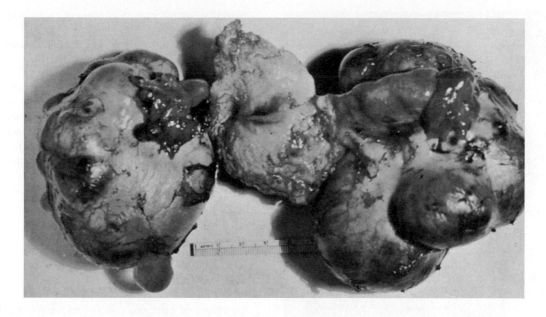

Figure 19–11 ■

Endometriosis. The ovaries are converted into enlarged, irregular masses by large "chocolate cysts." (Courtesy of Dr. Arthur Hertig.)

logic diagnosis at all sites depends on finding within the lesions two of the following three features: endometrial glands, stroma, and hemosiderin pigment.

The clinical manifestations of endometriosis depend on the distribution of the lesions. Extensive scarring of the oviducts and ovaries often produces discomfort in the lower quadrant and eventually causes sterility. Pain on defecation reflects rectal wall involvement, and dyspareunia (painful intercourse) and dysuria reflect involvement of the uterine and bladder serosa, respectively. In almost all cases, there is severe dysmenorrhea and pelvic pain as a result of intrapelvic bleeding and periuterine adhesions.

DYSFUNCTIONAL UTERINE BLEEDING AND ENDOMETRIAL HYPERPLASIA

By far the most common problem for which women seek medical attention is some disturbance in menstrual function: menorrhagia (profuse or prolonged bleeding at the time of the period), metrorrhagia (irregular bleeding between the periods), or ovulatory (intermenstrual) bleeding. Common causes include polyps, leiomyomas, endometrial carcinoma, cervical carcinoma, endometritis, endometriosis, and (of interest here) dysfunctional uterine bleeding and endometrial hyperplasia.

Dysfunctional Uterine Bleeding

Abnormal bleeding in the absence of a well-defined organic lesion in the uterus is called dysfunctional uterine bleeding.

The probable cause of abnormal uterine bleeding, dysfunctional and organic (related to a well-defined lesion), depends somewhat on the age of the patient (Table 19–1).

The various causes of dysfunctional bleeding can be segregated into three functional groups:

■ *Failure of ovulation.* Anovulatory cycles are very common at both ends of reproductive life; with any dysfunction of the hypothalamic-pituitary axis, adrenal or thyroid; with a functioning ovarian lesion producing an excess of estrogen; with malnutrition, obesity, or debilitating disease; and with severe physical or emotional stress. In many instances the basis for the failure of ovulation is mysterious, but,

■

Table 19–1. CAUSES OF ABNORMAL UTERINE BLEEDING BY AGE GROUP

Age Group	Cause(s)
Prepuberty	Precocious puberty (hypothalamic, pituitary, or ovarian origin)
Adolescence	Anovulatory cycle
Reproductive age	Complications of pregnancy (abortion, trophoblastic disease, ectopic pregnancy)
	Organic lesions (leiomyoma, adenomyosis, polyps, endometrial hyperplasia, carcinoma)
	Anovulatory cycle
	Ovulatory dysfunctional bleeding (e.g., inadequate luteal phase)
Perimenopause	Anovulatory cycle
	Irregular shedding
	Organic lesions (carcinoma, hyperplasia, polyps)
Postmenopause	Organic lesions (carcinoma, hyperplasia, polyps)
	Endometrial atrophy

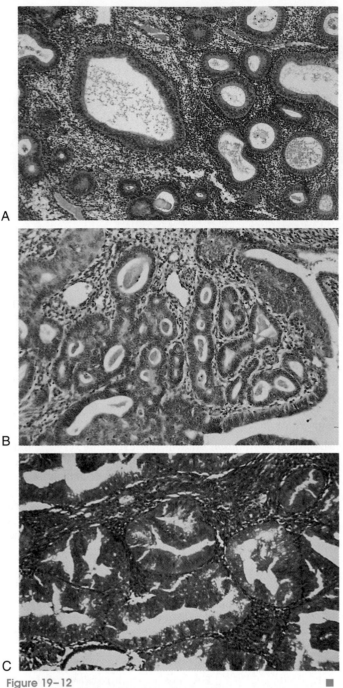

A

B

C

Figure 19–12 ■

A, Simple (cystic, mild) hyperplasia with dilatation of glands. B, Complex hyperplasia of a nest of closely packed glands. C, Atypical endometrial hyperplasia with crowding of glands, unfolding of tall columnar cells, and some loss of polarity.

whatever the basis, it leads to an excess of estrogen relative to progesterone. Thus, the endometrium goes through a proliferative phase that is not followed by the normal secretory phase. The endometrial glands may develop mild cystic changes, or in other places may appear disorderly with a relative scarcity of stroma, which requires progesterone for its support. The poorly supported endometrium

partially collapses, with rupture of spiral arteries, accounting for the bleeding.

■ *Inadequate luteal phase.* The corpus luteum may fail to mature normally or may regress prematurely, leading to a relative lack of progesterone. The endometrium under these circumstances reveals delay in the development of the secretory changes expected at the date of biopsy.

■ *Contraceptive-induced bleeding.* Oral contraceptives at one time contained sufficient amounts of usually synthetic estrogens and progestin to induce a variety of endometrial responses, depending on the particular steroids being employed and the dosage. A common factor was a discrepancy between a lush, decidua-like stroma and inactive, nonsecretory glands. The newer "mini" pills in current use have corrected these abnormalities.

Endometrial Hyperplasia

An excess of estrogen relative to progestin, if sufficiently prolonged or marked, will induce endometrial hyperplasia ranging from simple hyperplasia to complex hyperplasia, and possibly to atypical hyperplasia (Fig. 19–12). These three categories represent a continuum based on the level and duration of the estrogen excess. Not surprisingly, in time the endometrial hyperplasia may give rise to carcinoma of the endometrium, the risk being dependent on the severity of the hyperplastic changes and associated cellular atypia.

Any basis for estrogen excess may lead to hyperplasia. Failure of ovulation, such as is seen around the menopause; prolonged administration of estrogenic steroids without counterbalancing progestin; estrogen-producing ovarian lesions such as polycystic ovaries (including Stein-Leventhal syndrome); cortical stromal hyperplasia; and granulosa–theca cell tumors of the ovary are all potential backgrounds.

As has been indicated, endometrial hyperplasia, particularly the more severe forms, not only calls attention to some underlying basis for the abnormal endometrial changes, but also causes excessive and irregular uterine bleeding. Even more important, atypical hyperplasia incurs a 20% to 25% risk of progressing to adenocarcinoma of the endometrium. It is evident that when atypical hyperplasia is discovered, it must be carefully evaluated for the possible presence of a focus of cancer, and must be monitored over time by repeated endometrial biopsy to evaluate its course.

TUMORS OF THE ENDOMETRIUM AND MYOMETRIUM

The most common neoplasms are endometrial polyps, leiomyomas, and endometrial carcinomas. In addition, exotic mesodermal tumors are encountered, such as stromal sarcoma botryoides (also encountered in the vagina). All tend to produce bleeding from the uterus as the earliest manifestation.

Endometrial Polyps

These are sessile, usually hemispheric (rarely pedunculated) lesions 0.5 to 3 cm in diameter. Larger polyps may project from the endometrial mucosa into the uterine cavity. On histologic examination, they are seen to be covered with columnar cells; some have an adenomatous stroma with essentially normal endometrial architecture, but more often they have cystically dilated glands similar to those seen with cystic hyperplasia. Recently, it has been noted that the stromal cells in many, perhaps most, endometrial polyps are monoclonal and have a cytogenetic rearrangement at 6p21, making it clear that the stromal cells are the neoplastic component of the polyp.

Although endometrial polyps may occur at any age, they develop more commonly at the time of menopause. Their clinical significance lies in the production of abnormal uterine bleeding and, more important, the risk (however rare) of giving rise to a cancer.

Leiomyoma and Leiomyosarcoma

Benign tumors that arise from the smooth muscle cells in the myometrium are properly termed *leiomyomas,* but perhaps because they are firm, or for some other illogical reason, they are more often referred to as *fibroids.* They are the most common benign tumor in females and are found in 30% to 50% of women during reproductive life. Genetic influences are involved, because these tumors are considerably more frequent in blacks than in whites. Estrogens and possibly oral contraceptives stimulate their growth; conversely, they shrink in size postmenopausally. These tumors are clearly monoclonal and nonrandom chromosomal abnormalities have been found in about 40% of tumors, but it should be noted that 60% are karyotypically normal.

Macroscopically, these tumors are typically sharply circumscribed, firm gray-white masses with a characteristic whorled cut surface. They may occur singly, but most often multiple tumors are scattered within the uterus, ranging in size from small seedlings to massive neoplasms that dwarf the size of the uterus (Fig. 19–13). Some are embedded within the myometrium (intramural), whereas others may lie directly beneath the endometrium (submucosal) or directly beneath the serosa (subserosal). The latter may develop attenuated stalks and even become attached to surrounding organs, from which they develop a blood supply and then free themselves from the uterus to become "parasitic" leiomyomas. Larger neoplasms may develop foci of ischemic necrosis with areas of hemorrhage and cystic softening, and after menopause they may become densely collagenous and even calcified. Histologically, the tumors are characterized by whorling bundles of smooth muscle cells duplicating the histology of the normal myometrium. Foci of fibrosis, calcification, ischemic necrosis, cystic degeneration, and hemorrhage may be present.

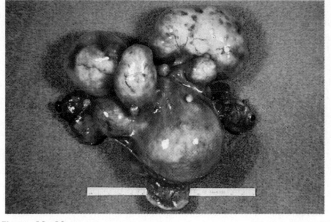

Figure 19–13 ■

Multiple leiomyomas of the uterus. Several large, almost pedunculated tumors protrude from the dome of the fundus. The lower uterine segment and cervix are below *(on top of the rule).* (Courtesy of Dr. Kyle Molberg, Department of Pathology, University of Texas Southwestern Medical School, Dallas, TX.)

Leiomyomas of the uterus may be entirely asymptomatic and be discovered only on routine pelvic examination or post mortem. The most frequent manifestation, when present, is menorrhagia, with or without metrorrhagia. Large masses may become palpable to the patient in the pelvic region or produce a dragging sensation. Whether these benign tumors ever become transformed into sarcomas is highly questionable, and indeed this may never occur.

Leiomyosarcomas arise directly from the mesenchymal cells of myometrium, not from preexisting leiomyomas. They are almost always solitary tumors, in contradistinction to the frequently multiple leiomyomas.

Grossly, leiomyosarcomas develop in several distinct patterns: as bulky masses infiltrating the uterine wall; as polypoid lesions projecting into the uterine cavity; or as deceptively discrete tumors that masquerade as large, benign leiomyomas. Histologically, they present a wide range of differentiation, from those that closely resemble leiomyoma to wildly anaplastic tumors. With this range in morphology, it is understandable that some well-differentiated tumors lie at the interface between benign and malignant, and sometimes these are designated *leiomyoblastomas* (a euphemism to say "we don't know whether to call it benign or malignant"). The diagnostic features of leiomyosarcoma include relatively frequent mitoses, with or without cellular atypia, or less numerous mitoses with cellular atypia.

Recurrence after removal is common with these cancers, and many metastasize widely, yielding about a 40% 5-year survival rate. Understandably, the more anaplastic tumors have a poorer outlook than the better-differentiated lesions.

Endometrial Carcinoma

In the United States and many other Western countries, endometrial carcinoma is the most frequent cancer of the female genital tract. Some years ago, it was much less common than cervical cancer. However, early detection of CIN by periodic cytologic examinations, and its appropriate treatment, have dramatically reduced the incidence of invasive cervical cancer.

Epidemiology and Pathogenesis. This form of cancer appears most frequently between the ages of 55 and 65 and is distinctly uncommon under 40 years of age. A constellation of well-defined risk factors has long been noted:

■ Obesity: increased synthesis of estrogens in fat depots from adrenal and ovarian precursors
■ Diabetes
■ Hypertension
■ Infertility: women tend to be single and nulliparous, and they often have nonovulatory cycles.

Some of these risk factors point to *increased estrogen stimulation,* and indeed it is well recognized that prolonged estrogen replacement therapy, depending on duration and dosage, increases the risk of this form of cancer, as do ovarian estrogen-secreting tumors. Many of these risk factors are the same as those for endometrial hyperplasia, and *endometrial carcinoma frequently arises on a background of endometrial hyperplasia.* Similarly, breast carcinoma occurs in women with endometrial cancer (and vice versa) more frequently than by chance alone. The great preponderance of endometrial carcinomas arise in the setting just described. However, a significant subset (approximately 20%) of cancers do not appear to be associated with hyperestrinism or preexisting hyperplasia. On average, these cancers arise at a later stage in life, are more poorly differentiated, and have a poorer prognosis.

> **MORPHOLOGY.** Endometrial carcinomas assume one of two macroscopic appearances: either they **infiltrate,** causing diffuse thickening of the affected uterine wall, or they assume an **exophytic form** (Fig. 19–14). In both cases, they eventually fill the endometrial cavity with firm to soft, partially necrotic tumor tissue, and in time they extend through the myometrial wall to the serosa and thence by direct extension to periuterine structures. Late in the course, there is metastasis to regional lymph nodes, and later still to distant organs.
>
> Most of these tumors are adenocarcinomas with well-defined gland patterns resembling the endometrial glands from which they arose. These are sometimes referred to as **endometrioid carcinomas.** However, less well differentiated tumors may fail to produce glandular patterns, growing as solid sheets of cells with nuclear atypia and mitotic activity.
>
> Some of the better-differentiated carcinomas contain foci of squamous differentiation, designated **adenocarcinoma with squamous metaplasia** or **adenoacanthoma.** In such lesions the squamous elements are quite well differentiated. However, occasional tumors may show an area of squamous growth that is frankly malignant, giving rise to the term **adenosquamous carcinoma.** There are still other specialized histologic patterns, such as papillary serous carcinomas and clear cell carcinomas, that we need not delve into.
>
> Like most cancers, endometrial carcinoma is graded according to cellular differentiation and staged according to the extent of the disease at diagnosis. The grades are G1 to G3, from well differentiated to undifferentiated. The following staging system is most widely used: stage I, confined to the uterine corpus; stage II, involvement of corpus and cervix; stage III, extension outside of the uterus but not outside the true pelvis; stage IV, extension beyond stage III.

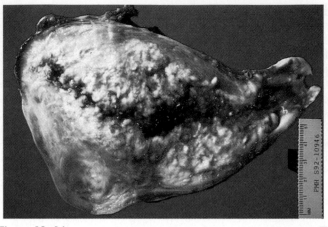

Figure 19–14 ■

Endometrial carcinoma projecting into the uterine cavity and infiltrating the myometrium. The uterine cavity is almost obliterated. (The cervix is on the right.) (Courtesy of Dr. Kyle Molberg, Department of Pathology, University of Texas Southwestern Medical School, Dallas, TX.)

Clinical Course. The first clinical indications of endometrial carcinoma are usually marked leukorrhea and irregular bleeding, raising a red flag in a postmenopausal woman. This reflects erosion and ulceration of the endometrial surface. With progression, the uterus may be palpably enlarged, and in time it becomes fixed to surrounding structures by extension of the cancer beyond the uterus. Fortunately, these are usually late-metastasizing neoplasms, but dissemination eventually occurs, with involvement of regional nodes and more distant sites. With therapy, stage I carcinoma is associated with a 90% 5-year survival rate; this rate drops to 30% to 50% in stage II and to less than 20% in stages III and IV.

Fallopian Tubes

The fallopian tubes should be treasured organs to the pathology student because they are so seldom the site of primary disease. Their most common afflictions are inflammation, almost always as part of pelvic inflammatory disease. Much less often they are affected by ectopic (tubal) pregnancy (p 620), followed in order of frequency by endometriosis (p 608) and the rare primary tumors. Only a few comments on salpingitis and tumors are necessary.

Inflammations of the tube are almost always bacterial in origin. With the declining incidence of gonorrhea, nongonococcal organisms, such as *Chlamydia, Mycoplasma hominis,* coliforms, and (in the postpartum setting) streptococci and staphylococci, are now the major offenders. The morphologic changes produced by gonococci conform to those already described (Chapter 18). Nongonococcal infections differ somewhat, inasmuch as they are more invasive, penetrating the wall of the tubes and thus tending more often to give rise to blood-borne infections and seeding of the meninges, joint spaces, and sometimes the heart valves. Rarely, tuberculous salpingitis is encountered, almost always in combination with involvement of the endometrium. All forms of salpingitis may produce fever, lower abdominal or pelvic pain, and pelvic masses when the tubes become distended with either exudate or, later, burned-out inflammatory debris and secretions (Fig. 19–15). Even more serious is the potential for obstruction of the tubal lumina, which sometimes produces permanent sterility.

Primary adenocarcinomas may arise in the tubes. They are curiosities that are not usually discovered until they spread. In time they may cause death.

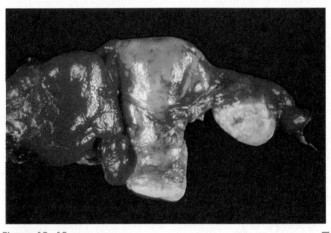

Figure 19–15   ■

Pelvic inflammatory disease, asymmetric albeit bilateral. One side has a large inflammatory mass totally obscuring the tube and ovary. The other is less involved, but the tube is widely adherent to the still recognizable ovary.

Ovaries

The ovaries are infrequently the primary site of any disease except, notably, neoplasms. Indeed, carcinomas of the ovaries account for more deaths than do cancers of the cervix and uterine corpus together. In 1996 they caused about 14,800 deaths in the United States. It is less their frequency than their lethality (because of their silent growth) that makes them so evil. Non-neoplastic cysts are commonplace but generally are not serious problems. Primary inflammations of the ovary are rarities, but salpingitis of the tubes frequently causes a periovarian reaction called *salpingo-oophoritis.* As discussed earlier, the ovary is frequently secondarily affected in endometriosis. Only the non-neoplastic cysts and neoplasms merit further consideration here.

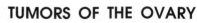

FOLLICLE AND LUTEAL CYSTS

Follicle and luteal cysts in the ovaries are so commonplace as almost to constitute physiologic variants. These innocuous lesions originate in unruptured graafian follicles or in follicles that have ruptured and immediately sealed. Such cysts are often multiple and develop immediately subjacent to the serosal covering of the ovary. Usually they are small—1 to 1.5 cm in diameter—and are filled with clear serous fluid. Occasionally, they achieve diameters of 4 to 5 cm and may thus become palpable masses and indeed produce pelvic pain. When small, they are lined by granulosa lining cells or luteal cells, but as the fluid accumulates, pressure may cause atrophy of these cells. Sometimes, these cysts rupture, producing intraperitoneal bleeding and acute abdominal symptoms.

POLYCYSTIC OVARIES

Oligomenorrhea, hirsutism, infertility, and sometimes obesity may appear in young women, usually postmenarchal girls, secondary to excessive production of estrogens and androgens (mostly the latter) by multiple cystic follicles in the ovaries. This condition is also called *polycystic ovaries,* or *Stein-Leventhal syndrome.*

> The ovaries are usually twice normal in size, are gray-white with a smooth outer cortex, and are studded with subcortical cysts 0.5 to 1.5 cm in diameter. Histologically, there is a thickened fibrosed outer tunica, sometimes referred to as *cortical stromal fibrosis,* beneath which are innumerable cysts lined by granulosa cells with a hypertrophic and hyperplastic luteinized theca interna. There is a conspicuous absence of corpora lutea.

The principal biochemical abnormalities in most patients are excessive production of androgens, high levels of luteinizing hormone (LH), and low levels of follicle-stimulating hormone (FSH). The origins of these changes are poorly understood, but it is proposed that the ovaries in this condition elaborate excess androgens, which are converted in peripheral fatty depots to estrone, and these, through the hypothalamus, inhibit the secretion of FSH by the pituitary. The basis of excess ovarian androgen secretion is mysterious.

TUMORS OF THE OVARY

Tumors of the ovary make up an amazing diversity of pathologic entities. This diversity is attributable to the three cell types that make up the normal ovary: the multipotential sur-

face (coelomic) covering epithelium, the totipotential germ cells, and the multipotential sex cord–stromal cells. Each of these cell types gives rise to a variety of tumors, as indicated in Figure 19–16.

It is evident that neoplasms of surface epithelial origin account for the great majority of all primary ovarian tumors, and in their malignant forms account for almost 90% of all ovarian cancers. These epithelial tumors are then the "big bananas" that require most attention. Germ cell and sex cord–stromal cell tumors are much less frequent and, although they constitute 15% to 20% of all ovarian tumors, are collectively responsible for less than 10% of cancers of the ovary.

Pathogenesis. There has been a recent explosion of information about the potential genetic origins of ovarian cancers. Unfortunately, the results of the many studies are not consistent, and so only some general comments will be made here. Cytogenetic abnormalities have been observed in some ovarian cancers, including trisomy 12 and a diversity of chromosome losses, deletions, and translocations involving other chromosomes. The large variety of these alterations suggests that they may be secondary events incurred in the oncogenic process. Other findings have been overexpression of *myc, c-erbB2,* and epidermal growth factor receptor, possibly as late events in oncogenesis. There are, in addition, familial syndromes based on inherited germ line mutations; for example, those affecting the p53 tumor suppressor gene in the Li-Fraumeni syndrome with a predisposition to breast, ovarian, and other forms of cancer; and the Lynch syndrome II, with a familial predisposition to ovarian, endometrial, and colonic cancer. Collectively, these familial syndromes account for no more than 3% to 5% of all ovarian cancers. Recently, mutations in a presumed tumor suppressor gene, BRCA-1, on chromosome 17q21 have been identified in some familial cases (discussed in more detail in Chapter 6 and on p. 630). Inheritance of this gene predisposes to the development of breast and ovarian cancer and at a younger age than is the case with nonfamilial cancers. The role of BRCA-1 in sporadic ovarian cancers has not yet been established. However, hormonal influences must also exist, because pregnancy and the use of oral contraceptives lower the risk. With these few introductory comments, we can turn to the morphology of some of the neoplasms; the clinical correlation for all brings up the rear.

SURFACE EPITHELIAL-STROMAL TUMORS

These neoplasms are derived from the coelomic epithelium. They can be strictly epithelial (e.g., serous, mucinous tumors) or can have a distinct stromal component (cystadenofibroma, Brenner tumor). Although it is traditional to divide neoplasms into benign and malignant categories, the surface epithelial tumors also have an intermediate, borderline category currently referred to as *tumors of low malignant potential.* These appear to be low-grade cancers with limited invasive potential. Thus, they have a better prognosis than their uglier cousins, as will be evident.

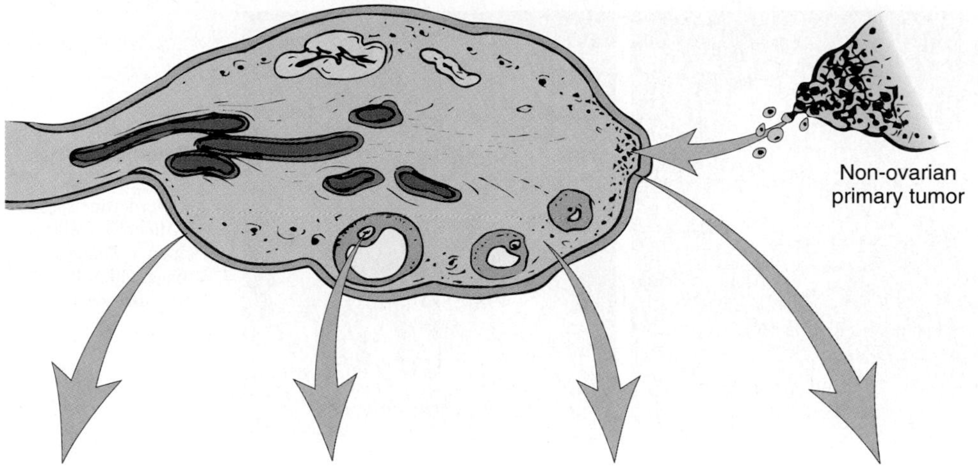

Figure 19–16   ■

Derivation of various ovarian neoplasms and some data on their frequency and age distribution.

ORIGIN	SURFACE EPITHELIAL CELLS (Surface epithelial–stromal cell tumors)	GERM CELL	SEX CORD–STROMA	METASTASIS TO OVARIES
Overall frequency	65%-70%	15%-20%	5%-10%	5%
Proportion of malignant ovarian tumors	90%	3%-5%	2%-3%	5%
Age group affected	20+ years	0-25+ years	All ages	Variable
Types	• Serous tumor • Mucinous tumor • Endometrioid tumor • Clear cell tumor • Brenner tumor • Cystadenofibroma	• Teratoma • Dysgerminoma • Endodermal sinus tumor • Choriocarcinoma	• Fibroma • Granulosa–theca cell tumor • Sertoli–Leydig cell tumor	

Serous Tumors

These most frequent of the ovarian tumors are usually encountered between ages 30 and 40 years. Although they may be solid, they are usually cystic, so they are commonly known as *cystadenomas* or *cystadenocarcinomas*. About 60% are benign, 15% of low malignant potential, and 25% malignant. Combined borderline and malignant lesions are the most common malignant ovarian tumors and account for about 60% of all ovarian cancers.

Grossly, serous tumors may be small (5 to 10 cm) in diameter, but most are large, spherical to ovoid, cystic structures, up to 30 to 40 cm in diameter. **About 25% of the benign forms are bilateral.** In the benign form, the serosal covering is smooth and glistening. In contrast, the covering of the cystadenocarcinoma shows nodular irregularities, which represent penetration of the tumor to or through the serosa. On transection, the small cystic tumor may reveal a single cavity, but larger ones are usually divided by multiple septa into a multiloculated mass (Fig. 19–17). The cystic spaces are usu-

ally filled with a clear serous fluid, although a considerable amount of mucus may also be present. Jutting into the cystic cavities are polypoid or papillary projections, which become more marked in malignant tumors (Fig. 19–17).

Histologically, the benign tumors are characterized by a single layer of tall columnar epithelium that lines the cyst or cysts. The cells are in part ciliated and in part dome-shaped secretory cells. **Psammoma bodies** (concentrically laminated concretions) are common in the tips of papillae. When frank carcinoma develops, anaplasia of the lining cells appears, as does invasion of the stroma. Papillary formations are complex and multilayered, with invasion of the axial fibrous tissue by nests or totally undifferentiated sheets of malignant cells. Between these clearly benign and obviously malignant forms are the **tumors of low malignant potential,** with obvious epithelial anaplasia and little stromal invasion. In thinned areas of the cyst wall, these borderline lesions may penetrate into the peritoneal cavity and implant on other structures. The overt carcinomas tend to spread contiguously within the pelvis and by seeding the

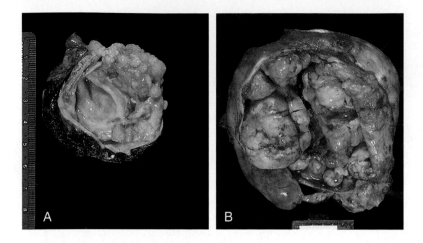

Figure 19–17 ■

A, Borderline serous cystadenoma opened to display a cyst cavity lined by delicate papillary tumor growths. *B*, Cystadenocarcinoma. The cyst is opened to reveal a large, bulky tumor mass. (Courtesy of Dr. Christopher Crum, Brigham & Women's Hospital, Boston.)

frequently associated ascitic fluid. These dispersed cells may implant throughout the peritoneal cavity. Spread to regional lymph nodes is frequent, but distant lymphatic and hematogenous metastases are infrequent.

The prognosis for the patient with clearly invasive serous cystadenocarcinoma after surgery, sometimes followed by radiation and chemotherapy, is poor and depends heavily on the stage of the disease at the time of diagnosis. If the tumor appears to be confined to the ovary, the frankly carcinomatous lesions yield about a 70% 5-year survival, whereas those of low malignant potential demonstrate about 100% survival. With cancers that have penetrated the capsule, the 10-year survival rate is only 13%. In contrast, for cancers of low malignant potential with capsular penetration, the overall 10-year survival rate is about 80%, but almost 40% of such patients eventually die of their tumors.

Mucinous Tumors

These are in most respects analogous to the serous tumors, differing essentially in that the epithelium consists of mucin-secreting cells similar to those of the endocervical mucosa. These tumors occur in patients in the same age range as those with serous tumors, but mucinous lesions are considerably less likely to be malignant, accounting for about 10% of all ovarian cancers. Eighty per cent of these tumors are benign and 10% are of low malignant potential; the remainder are malignant *(cystadenocarcinomas)*.

Only about 5% of benign and 20% of malignant tumors are bilateral, a much lower incidence than for their serous counterparts. On gross examination, they may be indistinguishable from serous tumors except by the mucinous nature of the cystic contents. However, **they are more likely to be larger and multilocular, and papillary formations are less common. (Unlike their serous counter-**

parts, psammoma bodies are not found within the tips of the papillae). Prominent papillation, serosal penetration, and solidified areas point to malignancy.

Histologically, these mucinous tumors are identified by the apical vacuolation of the tall columnar epithelial cells and by the absence of cilia. Two histologic types have been recently distinguished: **endocervix-like** (müllerian) and **intestine-type,** depending on the resemblance to endocervical or colonic epithelium, respectively (Fig. 19–18). Malignant lesions are identified by the presence of stromal invasion. Metastasis or rupture of mucinous

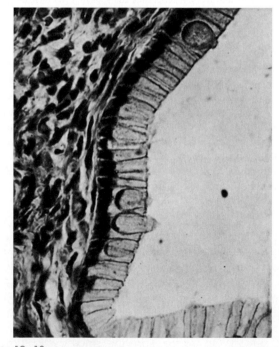

Figure 19–18 ■

Histologic detail of classic nonciliated, mucin-secreting, columnar lining epithelium of a mucinous cystadenoma of the ovary. (Courtesy of Dr. Arthur Hertig.)

cystadenocarcinomas may give rise to **pseudo-myxoma peritonei.** The peritoneal cavity becomes filled with glairy mucinous material resembling the cystic contents of the tumor. Multiple tumor implants are found on all the serosal surfaces, and the abdominal viscera become matted together. This form of pseudomyxoma peritonei is analogous to that encountered with rupture of a carcinomatous mucocele of the appendix (Chapter 15). Pseudomyxoma peritonei can also occur with tumors of low malignant potential.

The prognosis of mucinous cystadenocarcinoma is better than that for the serous counterpart. The overall 10-year survival rate is about 35%. Mucinous tumors of low malignant potential are associated with an 85% 10-year survival rate.

Endometrioid Tumors

These tumors may be solid or cystic, but sometimes they develop as a mass projecting from the wall of an endometriotic cyst filled with chocolate-colored fluid. Microscopically, they are distinguished by the formation of tubular glands, similar to those of the endometrium, within the linings of cystic spaces. Although benign and borderline forms exist, endometrioid tumors are usually malignant. They are bilateral in about 30% of cases, and 15% to 30% of patients with these ovarian tumors have a concomitant endometrial carcinoma.

When these tumors are relatively well differentiated, there is a 62% 5-year survival rate; with the more aggressive carcinomas, it is 23%.

Cystadenofibroma

The cystadenofibroma is essentially a variant of the serous cystadenoma in which there is more pronounced proliferation of the fibrous stroma that underlies the columnar lining epithelium. These benign tumors are usually small and multilocular. The epithelial lining is usually quite regular. Carcinomatous transformation is rare.

Brenner Tumor

The Brenner tumor is an uncommon ovarian, solid, usually unilateral tumor consisting of an abundant stroma containing nests of transitional epithelium resembling that of the urinary tract. Occasionally, the nests are cystic and are lined by columnar mucus-secreting cells. Brenner tumors are generally smoothly encapsulated and gray-white on transection and range from a few centimeters to 20 cm in diameter. These tumors may arise from the surface epithelium or from urogenital epithelium trapped within the germinal ridge. Rarely, they are formed as nodules within the wall of a mucinous cystadenoma. Although most are benign, both malignant and borderline tumors have been described.

OTHER OVARIAN TUMORS

Many other types of tumors of germ cell or sex cord–stromal origin also arise in the ovary, but only the teratomas of germ cell origin are sufficiently common to merit description. Table 19–2 presents some salient features of a few other neoplasms of germ cell and sex cord origin.

Teratomas

These neoplasms of germ cell origin constitute about 15% to 20% of ovarian tumors. They display the distressing behavior of arising in the first two decades of life, and the younger the patient, the greater is the likelihood of malignancy. However, over 90% of these germ cell neoplasms are benign cystic mature teratomas. The immature malignant variant is rare.

Benign (Mature) Cystic Teratomas. Almost all of these neoplasms are marked by ectodermal differentiation of the totipotential germ cells. Usually there is the formation of a cyst lined by recognizable epidermis replete with adnexal appendages; hence, the common designation *dermoid cysts.* Most are discovered in young women as ovarian masses, or are found incidentally on abdominal radiographs or scans because they contain foci of calcification produced by contained teeth. About 90% are unilateral, more often on the right. Rarely do these cystic masses exceed 10 cm in diameter. On transection they are often filled with sebaceous secretion and matted hair that, when removed, reveal a hair-bearing epidermal lining (Fig. 19–19). Sometimes, there is a nodular projection from which teeth protrude. Children take note, the teeth are unbrushed and may be carious! Occasionally, foci of bone, cartilage, nests of bronchial or gastrointestinal epithelium, and other recognizable lines of development are also present.

For unknown reasons, these neoplasms sometimes produce infertility. But more seriously, in about 1% of cases there is malignant transformation of one of the tissue elements, usually taking the form of a squamous cell carcinoma. Also, for unknown reasons, these tumors are prone to undergo torsion (10% to 15% of cases), producing an acute surgical emergency.

Immature Malignant Teratomas. These neoplasms are found early in life, the mean age being 18. They differ strikingly from benign mature teratomas insofar as they are often bulky, are predominantly solid or near-solid on transection, and are punctuated here and there by areas of necrosis; uncommonly, one of the cystic foci may contain sebaceous secretion, hair, and other features similar to those in the mature teratoma. Microscopically, the distinguishing feature is a variety of mature or barely recognizable areas of differentiation toward cartilage, bone, muscle, nerve, and other structures. Particularly ominous are the foci of neuroepithelial differentiation, because most such lesions are aggressive and metastasize widely. Immature teratomas are both graded and staged in an effort to predict their future. Those of grade I, stage I can often be cured with appropriate therapy, whereas the opposite end of the spectrum carries a much graver outlook.

Table 19-2. SELECTED OVARIAN NEOPLASMS

	Selected Peak Incidence	Usual Location	Morphologic Features	Behavior
Germ Cell Origin				
Dysgerminoma	2nd–3rd decades Occur with gonadal dysgenesis	80%–90% unilateral	Counterpart of testicular seminoma. Solid large to small gray masses. Sheets or cords of large cleared cells separated by scant fibrous strands. Stroma may contain lymphocytes and occasional granuloma.	All malignant but only one third aggressive and spread; all radiosensitive with 80% cure.
Choriocarcinoma	First three decades of life	Unilateral	Identical to placental tumor. Often small, hemorrhagic focus with two types, epithelium cytotrophoblast and syncytiotrophoblast.	Metastasizes early and widely. Primary focus may disintegrate, leaving only "mets." In contrast to placental tumors, ovarian primaries are resistant to chemotherapy.
Sex Cord Tumors				
Granulosa-theca cell	Most postmenopausal but at any age	Unilateral	May be tiny or large, gray to yellow (with cystic spaces). Composed of mixture of cuboidal granulosa cells in cords, sheets, or strands and spindled or plump lipid-laden theca cells. Granulosal elements may recapitulate ovarian follicle (Call-Exner bodies).	May elaborate large amounts of estrogen (from thecal elements) and so may promote endometrial or breast carcinoma. Granulosal element may be malignant (5%–25%).
Thecoma-fibroma	Any age	Unilateral	Solid gray fibrous cells to yellow (lipid-laden) plump thecal cells.	Most hormonally inactive. Few elaborate estrogens. About 40%, for obscure reasons, produce ascites and hydrothorax (Meigs syndrome). Rarely malignant.
Sertoli-Leydig cell	All ages	Unilateral	Usually small, gray to yellow-brown and solid. Recaps development of testis with tubules, or cords and plump pink Sertoli cells.	Many masculinizing or defeminizing. Uncommonly malignant.
Metastases to Ovary	Older ages	Mostly bilateral	Usually solid-gray white masses up to 20 cm in diameter. Anaplastic tumor cells, cords, glands, dispersed through fibrous background. Cells may be "signet-ring" mucin-secreting.	Primaries are breast, lung and principally gastrointestinal tract (Krukenberg tumors).

Specialized Teratomas. These curiosities are mentioned only because they tend to evoke "I don't believe it" reactions. Struma ovarii is composed entirely of mature thyroid tissue that, interestingly, may hyperfunction and produce hyperthyroidism. These tumors appear as small, solid, unilateral brown ovarian masses. Equally incongruous is the ovarian carcinoid, which in rare instances has produced the carcinoid syndrome! If you live long enough, you may come across a combined struma ovarii and carcinoid in the same ovary. More seriously, one of these elements may become malignant.

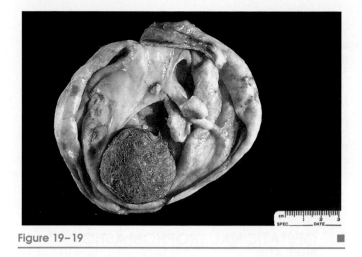

Figure 19–19   ■

Opened mature cystic teratoma (dermoid cyst) of the ovary. Hair *(bottom)* and a mixture of tissues are evident. (Courtesy of Dr. Christopher Crum, Brigham and Women's Hospital, Boston.)

Clinical Correlations for All Ovarian Tumors

All ovarian neoplasms pose formidable clinical challenges, because they produce no symptoms or signs until they are well advanced. Among the almost 27,000 new cases reported in the United States in 1996, more than half proved fatal because of this silent growth and extension beyond the point of cure. The clinical presentation of all ovarian tumors is remarkably similar despite their great morphologic diversity, except for the functioning neoplasms that have hormonal effects. Ovarian tumors of surface cell origin are usually asymptomatic until they become large enough to cause local pressure symptoms (e.g., pain, gastrointestinal complaints, urinary frequency). Indeed, about 30% of all ovarian neoplasms are discovered incidentally on routine gynecologic examination. Larger masses, notably the common epithelial tumors, may cause an increase in abdominal girth. Smaller masses, particularly dermoid cysts, sometimes become twisted on their pedicles (torsion), producing severe abdominal pain and an acute abdomen. Fibromas and malignant serous tumors often cause ascites, the latter being due to metastatic seeding of the peritoneal cavity, so that tumor cells can be identified in the ascitic fluid. Mucinous cancers may literally fill the abdominal cavity with a gelatinous neoplastic mass (pseudomyxoma peritonei). Functioning ovarian tumors often come to attention because of the endocrinopathies they induce.

Unfortunately, methods of treatment remain unsatisfactory, as proved by the only modest increase of survival that has been achieved since the mid-1970s. Thus, ovarian cancers rank fourth in the number of cancer deaths behind those of the lung, breast, and large intestine. Screening detection methods are being developed, but to this point they are of only limited value in discovering ovarian cancers while they are still curable. Among the many markers being explored, elevated serum levels of CA125 have been reported in 50% to 80% of women with ovarian cancer. However, this is undetectable in early-stage disease, and, moreover, may be spuriously elevated in a variety of benign conditions, as well as nonovarian cancers. So the search for markers and improved cure rates continues.

Diseases of Pregnancy

Diseases of pregnancy and pathologic conditions of the placenta are important causes of intrauterine or perinatal death, premature birth, congenital malformations, intrauterine growth retardation, maternal death, and a great deal of morbidity for both mother and child. Here we shall discuss only a limited number of disorders in which knowledge of the morphologic lesions contributes to an understanding of the clinical problem.

PLACENTAL INFLAMMATIONS AND INFECTIONS

Infections reach the placenta by two pathways: (1) ascending infection through the birth canal and (2) hematogenous (transplacental) infection.

Ascending infections are by far the most common; in most instances, they are bacterial and are associated with premature birth and premature rupture of the membranes. The chorioamnion shows leukocytic polymorphonuclear infiltration associated with edema and congestion of the vessels (acute chorioamnionitis). When the infection extends beyond the membranes, it may involve the umbilical cord and placental villi and cause acute vasculitis of the cord. Ascending infections are caused by mycoplasmas, *Candida,* and the numerous bacteria of the vaginal flora. Uncommonly, placental infections may arise by the *hematogenous spread* of bacteria and other organisms; histologically, the villi are most often affected (villitis). Syphilis, tuberculosis, listeriosis, toxoplasmosis, and various viruses (rubella, cytomegalovirus, herpes simplex) can all cause placental villitis. Transplacental infections can affect the fetus and give rise to the so-called TORCH complex discussed in Chapter 7.

ECTOPIC PREGNANCY

Ectopic pregnancy is implantation of the fertilized ovum in any site other than the normal uterine location. The condition occurs in as many as 1% of pregnancies. In more than 90% of these cases, implantation is in the oviducts (tubal pregnancy); other sites include the ovaries, the abdominal cavity, and the intrauterine portion of the oviducts (interstitial pregnancy). Any hindrance that retards passage of the ovum along its course through the oviducts to the uterus predisposes to an ectopic pregnancy. In about half of the cases, such obstruction is based on chronic inflammatory changes in the oviduct, although intrauterine tumors and endometriosis may also hamper passage of the ovum. In approximately 50% of tubal pregnancies, no anatomic cause can be demonstrated. Ovarian pregnancies probably result from those rare instances of fertilization of the ovum within its follicle just at the time of rupture. Gestation within the abdominal cavity occurs when the fertilized egg drops out of the fimbriated end of the oviduct and implants on the peritoneum.

In all sites, ectopic pregnancies are characterized by fairly normal early development of the embryo, with the formation of placental tissue, the amniotic sac, and decidual changes. An abdominal pregnancy is occasionally carried to term. With tubal pregnancies, however, the invading placenta eventually burrows through the wall of the oviduct, causing **intratubal hematoma (hematosalpinx), intraperitoneal hemorrhage,** or both. The tube is usually locally distended up to 3 to 4 cm by a contained mass of freshly clotted blood in which may be seen bits of gray placental tissue and fetal parts. The histologic diagnosis depends on the visualization of placental villi or, rarely, of the embryo. Less commonly, poor attachment of the placenta to the tubal wall results in death of the embryo, with spontaneous proteolysis and absorption of the products of conception.

Until rupture occurs, an ectopic pregnancy may be indistinguishable from a normal one, with cessation of menstruation and elevation of serum and urinary placental hormones. Under the influence of these hormones, the endometrium (in about 50% of cases) undergoes the characteristic hypersecretory and decidual changes. *However, the absence of elevated gonadotropin levels does not exclude this diagnosis, because poor attachment with necrosis of the placenta is common.* Rupture of an ectopic pregnancy may be catastrophic, with the sudden onset of intense abdominal pain and signs of an acute abdomen, often followed by shock. Prompt surgical intervention is necessary.

GESTATIONAL TROPHOBLASTIC DISEASE

Traditionally, the gestational trophoblastic tumors have been divided into three overlapping morphologic categories: *hydatidiform mole, invasive mole,* and *choriocarcinoma.* They range in level of aggressiveness from the hydatidiform moles, most of which are benign, to the highly malignant choriocarcinomas. All elaborate human chorionic gonadotropin (hCG), which can be detected in the circulating blood and urine at titers considerably higher than those found during normal pregnancy, the titers progressively rising from hydatidiform mole to invasive mole to choriocarcinoma. In addition to aiding diagnosis, the fall or (alternatively) rise in the level of the hormone in the blood or urine can be used to monitor the effectiveness of treatment. Clinicians therefore prefer the term *gestational trophoblastic disease,* because the response to therapy as judged by the hormone titers is significantly more important than any arbitrary anatomic segregation of one lesion from another. Nonetheless, it is necessary to understand their individual characteristics to appreciate the spectrum of lesions.

Hydatidiform Mole: Complete and Partial

The typical hydatidiform mole is a voluminous mass of swollen, sometimes cystically dilated, chorionic villi, appearing grossly as grapelike structures. The swollen villi are covered by varying amounts of banal to highly atypical chorionic epithelium. Two distinctive subtypes of moles have been characterized: *complete* and *partial* moles. The complete hydatidiform mole does not permit embryogenesis and therefore never contains fetal parts. All of the chorionic villi are abnormal, and the chronic epithelial cells are diploid (46,XX or, uncommonly, 46,XY). The partial hydatidiform mole is compatible with early embryo formation and therefore contains fetal parts, has some normal chorionic villi, and is almost always triploid (e.g., 69,XXY, Table 19–3). The two patterns result from abnormal fertilization; in a complete mole an empty egg is fertilized by two spermatozoa (or a diploid sperm), yielding the diploid karyotype, while in a partial mole a normal egg is fertilized by two spermatozoa (or a diploid sperm), resulting in the triploid karyotype.

Table 19-3. FEATURES OF COMPLETE VERSUS PARTIAL HYDATIDIFORM MOLE

Feature	Complete Mole	Partial Mole
Karyotype	46,XX (46,XY)	Triploid (69,XXY)
Villous edema	All villi	Some villi
Trophoblast proliferation	Diffuse; circumferential	Focal; slight
Atypia	Often present	Absent
Serum hCG	Elevated	Less elevated
hCG in tissue	++++	+
Behavior	2% choriocarcinoma	Rare choriocarcinoma

The incidence of complete hydatidiform moles is about 1 to 1.5 per 2000 pregnancies in the United States and other Western countries. For unknown reasons, there is a much higher incidence in Asian countries. They are much more common before age 20 and after age 40. They usually present clinically with painless vaginal bleeding, on average 12 to 14 weeks after conception. When the condition is discovered early by ultrasonography, the uterus may or may not be "too large for dates," but no fetal parts or heart sounds are present. Elevated levels of hCG are present in maternal blood and urine, and ultrasonography provides the positive diagnosis.

When the condition is discovered, usually in the fourth month of gestation, the uterine cavity is filled with a delicate, friable mass of thin-walled, translucent cystic structures (Fig. 19–20). Fetal

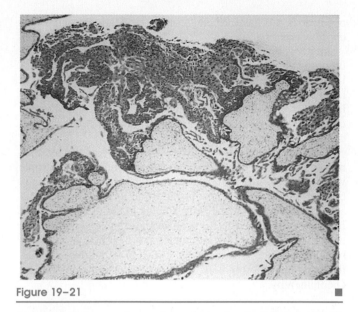

Figure 19–21

A microscopic close-up of a complete mole showing distended hydropic villi (*below*) and proliferation of the chorionic epithelium (*above*). (Courtesy of Dr. Kyle Molberg, Department of Pathology, University of Texas Southwestern Medical School, Dallas, TX.)

parts are rarely seen in complete moles but are common in partial moles. Microscopically, the **complete mole** shows hydropic swelling of chorionic villi and virtual absence of vascularization of villi. The central substance of the villi is a loose, myxomatous, edematous stroma. The chorionic epithelium almost always shows some degree of proliferation of both cytotrophoblast and syncytial trophoblast (Fig. 19–21). The proliferation may be mild, but in many cases there is striking circumferential hyperplasia. Histologic grading to predict this clinical outcome of moles has been supplanted by careful following of hCG levels. In **partial moles** the villous edema involves only some of the villi, and the trophoblastic proliferation is focal and slight.

Overall, 80% to 90% of moles remain benign after thorough curettage; 10% of complete moles become invasive, but not more than 2% to 3% give rise to choriocarcinoma. Partial moles rarely give rise to choriocarcinomas. With complete moles, monitoring the postcurettage blood and urine levels of hCG, particularly the more definitive beta subunit of the hormone, permits detection of incomplete removal or a more ominous complication and leads to the institution of appropriate therapy, including in some cases chemotherapy, which is almost always curative.

Invasive Mole

Biologically, an invasive mole is intermediate between a benign mole and choriocarcinoma. It is more invasive locally,

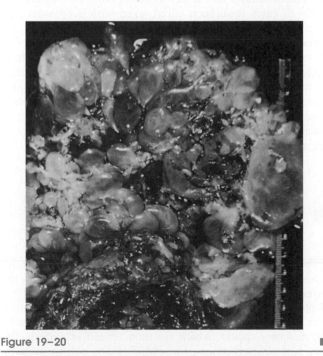

Figure 19–20

Hydatidiform mole evacuated from the uterus. The "bunch-of-grapes" appearance of the lesion is readily apparent.

but it does not have the aggressive metastatic potential of a choriocarcinoma.

An invasive mole retains hydropic villi, which penetrate the uterine wall deeply, possibly causing rupture and sometimes life-threatening hemorrhage. Local spread to the broad ligament and vagina may also occur. Microscopically, the epithelium of the villi is marked by hyperplastic and atypical changes, with proliferation of both cuboidal and syncytial components.

Although the marked invasiveness of this lesion makes removal technically difficult, metastases do not occur. Hydropic villi may embolize to distant organs, such as lungs or brain, but these emboli do not constitute true metastases and may actually regress spontaneously. Owing to the greater depth of invasion of the myometrium, an invasive mole is usually not removed completely by curettage, and therefore hCG levels remain elevated. This alerts the clinician to the need for further treatment. Fortunately, in most cases, cure is possible by chemotherapy.

Choriocarcinoma

This very aggressive malignant tumor arises either from gestational chorionic epithelium or, less frequently, from totipotential cells within the gonads or elsewhere. Choriocarcinomas are rare in the Western hemisphere, and in the United States occur in about 1 in 30,000 pregnancies. They are much more common in Asian and African countries, reaching a frequency of 1 in 2000 pregnancies. The risk is somewhat greater before age 20 and is significantly elevated after age 40. In about 50% of cases, choriocarcinomas follow a complete hydatidiform mole but only rarely a partial mole. About 25% arise after an abortion, and most of the remainder occur in a previously normal pregnancy. Stated in another way, the more abnormal the conception, the greater is the risk of developing gestational choriocarcinoma. Most cases are discovered by the appearance of a bloody, brownish discharge accompanied by a rising titer of hCG, particularly the beta subunit, in blood and urine, and the absence of marked uterine enlargement, such as would be anticipated with a mole. In general, the titers are much higher than those associated with a mole. In those instances that follow abortion or pregnancy, the fact that maternal age influences the frequency of this neoplasm suggests origin from an abnormal ovum rather than retained chorionic epithelium.

Choriocarcinomas usually appear as very hemorrhagic, necrotic masses within the uterus. Sometimes the necrosis is so complete as to make anatomic diagnosis difficult because there is deceptively little recognizable viable neoplasm. Indeed, the primary lesion may self-destruct, and only the metastases tell the story. Very early, the tumor insinuates itself into the myometrium and into vessels. **In contrast to the case with hydatidiform moles and invasive moles, chronic villi are not formed; instead, the tumor is purely epithelial, composed of anaplastic cuboidal cytotrophoblast and syncytiotrophoblast** (Fig. 19–22).

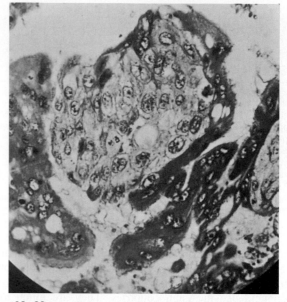

Figure 19–22 ■

High-power detail of choriocarcinoma illustrating the two types of epithelial cells: cytotrophoblast and synctiotrophoblast. (Courtesy of Dr. Arthur Hertig.)

By the time most neoplasms are discovered, there is usually widespread dissemination via the blood, most often to the lungs (50%), vagina (30% to 40%), brain, liver, and kidneys. Lymphatic invasion is uncommon.

Despite the extreme aggressiveness of these neoplasms, which made them nearly uniformly fatal in the past, present-day chemotherapy has achieved remarkable results. Nearly 100% of cases have been cured, even with neoplasms that have spread beyond the pelvis and vagina and into the lungs. Equally remarkable are reports of healthy infants born later to these survivors. By contrast, there is relatively poor response to chemotherapy in choriocarcinomas that arise in the gonads (ovary or testis). This striking difference in prognosis may be related to the presence of paternal antigens on placental choriocarcinomas, but not on gonadal lesions. Conceivably, a maternal immune response against the foreign (paternal) antigens helps by acting as an adjunct to chemotherapy.

PREECLAMPSIA/ECLAMPSIA (TOXEMIA OF PREGNANCY)

The development of hypertension, accompanied by proteinuria and edema in the third trimester of pregnancy, is referred to as *preeclampsia*. This syndrome occurs in 5% to 10% of pregnancies, particularly with first pregnancies in women over 35 years of age. In those severely affected, convulsive seizures may appear, which are then termed *eclampsia*. By long historical precedent, preeclampsia and eclampsia have been referred to as *toxemia of pregnancy*. No blood-borne toxin has ever been identified, however, and so the historically sanctified term (still in use) is clearly a misnomer. Full-blown eclampsia may lead to disseminated intravascular coagulation (DIC), with all of its attendant widespread ischemic organ injuries, and so eclampsia is potentially fatal. However, recognition and treatment of preeclampsia has now made eclampsia and, particularly, fatal eclampsia rare.

The triggering events initiating these syndromes are unknown, but a basic feature underlying all cases is inadequate maternal blood flow to the placenta secondary to inadequate dilation of the spiral arteries of the uteroplacental bed. In the third trimester of normal pregnancy, the musculoelastic walls of the spiral arteries are replaced by a fibrinous material, permitting them to dilate into wide vascular sinusoids. In preeclampsia and eclampsia the musculoelastic walls are retained and the channels remain narrow. The basis of these vascular abnormalities remains unknown, but a number of consequences ensue:

■ Placental hypoperfusion with an increased predisposition to the development of infarcts
■ Reduced elaboration by the trophoblast of vasodilators: PGI_2, PGE_2, and nitric oxide, which in normal pregnancies oppose the effects of renin-angiotensin—hence the hypertension of preeclampsia and eclampsia
■ Production by the ischemic placenta of thromboplastic substances such as tissue factor and thromboxane, which probably account for the development of DIC

The morphologic changes of preeclampsia/eclampsia are variable and depend somewhat on the severity of the toxemic state.

Placental changes are most consistent. They include the following:

■ Infarcts, which are a feature of normal pregnancy, are much more numerous in about one third of patients with severe preeclampsia/eclampsia. They may, however, be absent.

■ Retroplacental hemorrhages occur in up to 15% of patients.
■ Placental villi reveal the changes of premature aging with villous edema, hypovascularity, and increased production of syncytial epithelial knots.
■ Prominent in well-advanced eclampsia is **acute atherosis** in the spiral arteries, characterized by thickening and fibrinoid necrosis of the vessel wall with focal accumulations of lipid-containing macrophages. Necrosis of these cells releases lipid, which is followed by the accumulation of lymphocytes and macrophages within and about the vessels. Such lesions accentuate the placental ischemia.

Multiorgan changes may be present, reflecting the development of DIC, which is discussed more fully in Chapter 12. Only major findings are considered here. The kidneys are variably affected, depending on the severity of the DIC. Basically, the changes consist of fibrin thrombi within the glomerular capillaries, accompanied by endothelial swelling and possibly mesangial hyperplasia. Focal glomerulitis may ensue. When numerous glomeruli are affected, blood flow to the cortex is reduced, possibly resulting in renocortical necrosis, which when bilateral may be fatal. Microvascular thrombi are also found in the brain, pituitary, heart, and elsewhere, having the potential of producing focal ischemic lesions sometimes accompanied by microhemorrhages.

Clinically, preeclampsia appears insidiously in the 24th to 25th weeks of gestation, with the development of edema, proteinuria, and rising blood pressure. Should the condition evolve into eclampsia, renal function is impaired, the blood pressure mounts, and convulsions may appear. Prompt therapy early in the course aborts the organ changes, with clearance of all abnormalities promptly after delivery or cesarean section.

Breast

Lesions of the female breast are much more common than lesions of the male breast, which is remarkably seldom affected. These lesions usually take the form of palpable, sometimes painful, nodules or masses. Fortunately, most are innocent, but as is well known, breast cancer was the foremost cause of cancer deaths in women in the United States until 1986, when it was supplanted by carcinoma of the lung. The following discussion deals largely with lesions of the female breast. The conditions to be described should be considered in terms of their possible confusion clinically with a malig-

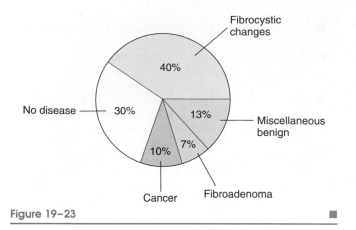

Figure 19–23

Representation of the findings in a series of women seeking evaluation of apparent breast "lumps."

nancy. This problem is most acute with fibrocystic change, because it is the most common cause of breast "lumps" and because of the continuing controversy about the association of particular variants with breast carcinoma. However, a significant proportion of women have sufficient irregularity of the "normal" breast tissue to cause them to seek clinical attention (Fig. 19–23).

Before we turn to the extremely common fibrocystic change, several relatively minor lesions should be mentioned. *Supernumerary nipples or breasts* may be found along the embryonic ridge (milk line). Besides being merely curiosities, these congenital anomalies are subject to the same diseases that affect the definitive breasts. *Congenital inversion of the nipple* is of significance because similar changes may be produced by an underlying cancer, and, moreover, the inversion may thwart nursing. *Galactocele* is a cystic dilation of an obstructed duct that arises during lactation. Besides being painful "lumps," the cysts may rupture to incite a local inflammatory reaction, which may yield a persistent focus of induration causing some concern years later.

FIBROCYSTIC CHANGES

This designation is applied to a miscellany of changes in the female breast that range from those that are entirely innocuous to patterns associated with an increased risk of breast carcinoma. The only unifying feature is that all of these alterations—stromal fibrosis, concurrent stromal and epithelial hyperplasia (often inducing micro- or macrocysts), various patterns of banal epithelial hyperplasia, and the more serious atypical hyperplasia—produce palpable "lumps." It is widely accepted that *this range of changes is the consequence of an exaggeration and distortion of the cyclic breast changes that occur normally in the menstrual cycle.* Estrogenic therapy and oral contraceptives (OCs) do not appear to increase the incidence of these alterations; indeed, OCs may *decrease* the risk.

In past years, these breast alterations were called *fibrocystic disease;* however, physicians have expressed much dissatisfaction with this term. Most of the changes encompassed

within the diagnosis of fibrocystic disease have little clinical significance except that they cause nodularity; only a small minority represent forms of epithelial hyperplasia that are clinically important. Thus, the term *fibrocystic changes* is preferred, since it does not stigmatize the subject with "a disease." Despite this semantic controversy, the "lumps" produced by the various patterns of fibrocystic change must all be distinguished from cancer, and the distinction between the trivial variants and the not so trivial ones can be made by examination of fine-needle aspiration material, or more definitively by biopsy and histologic evaluation. In a somewhat arbitrary manner, the alterations are here subdivided into nonproliferative and proliferative patterns. The nonproliferative lesions include cysts and/or fibrosis *without* epithelial cell hyperplasia, known as *simple fibrocystic change.* The proliferative lesions include a range of banal to atypical duct or ductular epithelial cell hyperplasias and *sclerosing adenosis.* All tend to arise during reproductive life but may persist after the menopause. The various changes, particularly the nonproliferative ones, are so common, being found at autopsy in 60% to 80% of women, that they almost constitute physiologic deviations.

Nonproliferative Change

CYSTS AND FIBROSIS

Nonproliferative change is the most common type of alteration, characterized by an increase in fibrous stroma associated with dilation of ducts and formation of cysts of various sizes.

> Grossly, a single large cyst may form within one breast, but the disorder is usually multifocal and often bilateral. The involved areas show ill-defined, diffusely increased density and discrete nodularities. The cysts vary from smaller than 1 cm to 5 cm in diameter. Unopened, they are brown to blue **(blue dome cysts)** and are filled with serous, turbid fluid (Fig. 19–24). The secretory products within the cysts may calcify to appear as microcalcifications in mammograms. Histologically, in smaller cysts, the epithelium is more cuboidal to columnar and is sometimes multilayered in focal areas. In larger cysts, it may be flattened or even totally atrophic (Fig. 19–25). Occasionally, mild epithelial proliferation leads to piled-up masses or small papillary excrescences. Frequently, cysts are lined by large polygonal cells that have an abundant granular, eosinophilic cytoplasm, with small, round, deeply chromatic nuclei, so-called **apocrine metaplasia;** this is virtually always benign.

The stroma surrounding all forms of cysts is usually compressed fibrous tissue, having lost its normal delicate, myxomatous appearance. A stromal lymphocytic infiltrate is common in this and all other variants of fibrocystic change.

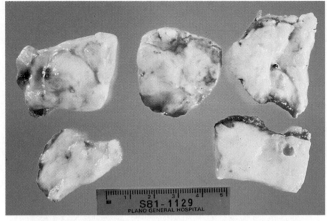

Figure 19–24 ■

Several biopsies of fibrocystic change of the breast. The scattered, poorly demarcated white areas represent foci of fibrosis. The biopsy at the lower right reveals a transected empty cyst; those on the left have unopened "blue-dome" cysts. (Courtesy of Dr. Kyle Molberg, Department of Pathology, University of Texas Southwestern Medical School, Dallas, TX.)

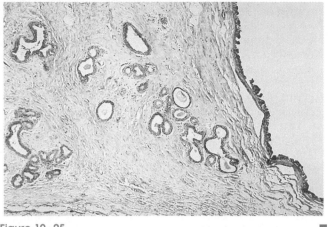

Figure 19–25 ■

Microscopic detail of fibrocystic change of the breast revealing dilation of ducts producing microcysts and, at right, the wall of a large cyst with visible lining epithelial cells. (Courtesy of Dr. Kyle Molberg, Department of Pathology, University of Texas Southwestern Medical School, Dallas, TX.)

Proliferative Change

EPITHELIAL HYPERPLASIA

The terms *epithelial hyperplasia* and *proliferative fibrocystic change* encompass a range of proliferative lesions within the ductules, the terminal ducts, and sometimes the lobules of the breast. Some of the epithelial hyperplasias are mild and orderly and carry little risk of carcinoma, but at the other end of the spectrum are the more florid atypical hyperplasias that carry a significantly greater risk, commensurate with the se-

verity and atypicality of the changes. The epithelial hyperplasias are often accompanied by other histologic variants of fibrocystic change, but nonetheless they are the "cutting edge" of the histologic changes.

The gross appearance of epithelial hyperplasia is not distinctive and is often dominated by coexisting fibrous or cystic changes. Histologically, there is an almost infinite spectrum of proliferative alterations (Fig. 19–26). The ducts, ductules, or lobules

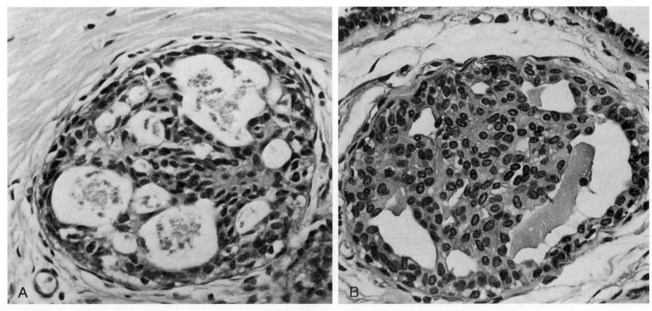

Figure 19–26 ■

A, Moderate duct epithelial hyperplasia. Note that the cells fill part of the duct lumen. *B,* More florid duct epithelial hyperplasia, with irregular lumina at the periphery, so-called *fenestrations.* (Courtesy of Dr. Noel Weidner.)

may be filled with orderly cuboidal cells, within which small gland patterns can be discerned (so-called **fenestrations**). Sometimes the proliferating epithelium projects in multiple small papillary excrescences into the ductal lumen (**ductal papillomatosis**). The degree of hyperplasia, manifested in part by the number of layers of intraductal epithelial proliferation, can be mild, moderate, or severe.

In some instances the hyperplastic cells are more multilayered and disorderly and vary in nuclear and cell size and shape with nuclear hyperchromasia; in short, they have changes approaching those of carcinoma in situ (described later). Such irregular hyperplasia is called **atypical**. The line separating the epithelial hyperplasias without atypia from atypical hyperplasia is poorly defined, just like the line distinguishing between atypical hyperplasia and carcinoma in situ, but these distinctions are important, as will soon become clear.

Atypical lobular hyperplasia is the term used to describe hyperplasias of the terminal ducts and ductules (acini). Cytologically, the atypical cells resemble those of carcinoma in situ, but they do not fill or distend more than 50% of the terminal duct units. Atypical lobular hyperplasia is associated with an increased risk of invasive carcinoma.

Epithelial hyperplasia per se does not often produce a clinically discrete breast mass. Occasionally it produces microcalcifications on mammography, raising doubts about cancer. Such nodularity as may be present usually relates to other concurrent variants of fibrocystic change; however, florid papillomatosis may be associated with a serous or serosanguineous nipple discharge.

SCLEROSING ADENOSIS

This variant is less common than cysts and hyperplasia, but it is significant because its clinical and morphologic features may be deceptively similar to those of carcinoma. There is in this lesion marked intralobular fibrosis and proliferation of small ductules and acini.

Grossly, the lesion has a hard, rubbery consistency, similar to that of breast cancer. Histologically, sclerosing adenosis is characterized by proliferation of lining epithelial cells and myoepithelial cells in small ducts and ductules, yielding masses of small gland patterns within a fibrous stroma (Fig. 19–27). Aggregated glands or proliferating ductules may be virtually back to back, with single or multiple layers of cells in contact with one another (**adenosis**). Always associated with the adenosis is marked stromal fibrosis, which may compress and distort the proliferating epithelium; hence, the designation *sclerosing adenosis*. **This overgrowth of fibrous tissue may completely compress the lumina**

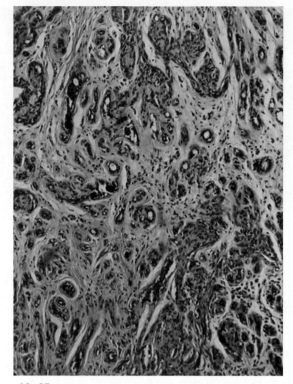

Figure 19–27 ■

Sclerosing adenosis of the breast. The epithelial hyperplasia has produced the nests of cells, which appear quite disorderly. The overgrowth of fibrous tissue enmeshes and partially obliterates many of the epithelial nests, creating a pattern very similar to the infiltrative growth of a cancer.

of the acini and ducts, so that they appear as solid cords of cells. This pattern may then be difficult to distinguish histologically from an invasive scirrhous carcinoma. Helpful in suggesting a benign diagnosis is the presence of double layers of epithelium and the identification of myoepithelial elements.

Although sclerosing adenosis is sometimes difficult to differentiate clinically and histologically from carcinoma, it is associated with only a minimally increased risk of progression to carcinoma.

Relationship of Fibrocystic Changes to Breast Carcinoma

Here we enter a stormy arena filled with claims and counterclaims. Only some reasonably supportable summary statements are possible. Clinically, although certain features of fibrocystic change tend to distinguish it from cancer, the only certain way of making this distinction is biopsy and histologic examination. With respect to the relationship of the various patterns of fibrocystic change to cancer, the following statements currently represent the best-informed opinion (Fig. 19–28):

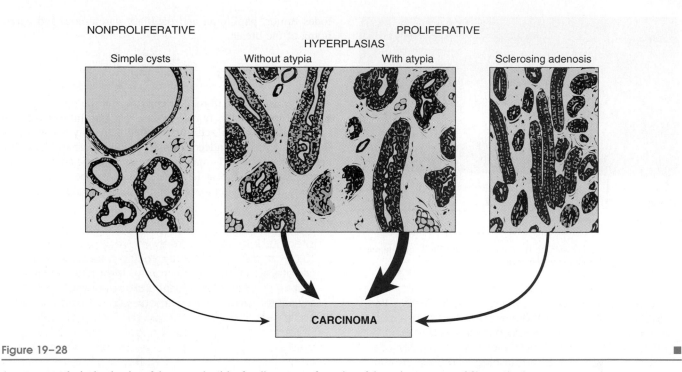

NONPROLIFERATIVE   PROLIFERATIVE

HYPERPLASIAS

Simple cysts   Without atypia   With atypia   Sclerosing adenosis

CARCINOMA

Figure 19–28   ■

An attempt to depict by the size of the arrow the risk of malignant transformation of the various patterns of fibrocystic change.

■ *Minimal or no increased risk of breast carcinoma:* fibrosis, cystic changes (micro- or macroscopic), apocrine metaplasia, sclerosing adenosis, mild hyperplasia.

■ *Slightly increased risk (1.5 to 2 times):* moderate to florid hyperplasia, ductal papillomatosis.

■ *Significantly increased risk (5 times):* atypical hyperplasia, ductular or lobular with duct involvement.

■ Proliferative lesions may be multifocal, and the risk of subsequent carcinoma extends to both breasts.

■ *A family history of breast cancer increases the risk in all categories* (e.g., to about tenfold with atypical hyperplasia).

Only about 5% of biopsy specimens exhibit atypical epithelial hyperplasia. Thus, most women who have lumps related to fibrocystic change can be reassured that there is little or no increased predisposition to cancer. The need to differentiate among the many variants, and the grounds for dissatisfaction with the unqualified terms *fibrocystic changes* or, even worse, *fibrocystic disease,* are apparent. The risks inherent in the various patterns are shown in Figure 19–28.

INFLAMMATIONS

Inflammations of the breast are uncommon, and during the acute stages usually cause pain and tenderness in the involved areas. Included in this category are several forms of mastitis and traumatic fat necrosis, none of which is associated with increased risk of cancer.

Acute mastitis develops when bacteria gain access to the breast tissue through the ducts; when there is inspissation of

secretions; through fissures in the nipples, which usually develop during the early weeks of nursing; or from various forms of dermatitis involving the nipple.

Staphylococcal infections induce single or multiple abscesses accompanied by the typical clinical acute inflammatory changes when they are near the surface. They are usually small, but when sufficiently large they may leave in the course of healing residual foci of scarring that are palpable as localized areas of induration. **Streptococcal infections generally spread throughout the entire breast, causing pain, marked swelling, and breast tenderness.** Resolution of these infections rarely leaves residual areas of induration.

Mammary duct ectasia (*periductal* or *plasma cell mastitis*) is a nonbacterial inflammation of the breast associated with inspissation of breast secretions in the main excretory ducts. Ductal dilation with ductal rupture leads to reactive changes in the surrounding breast substance. It is an uncommon condition, usually encountered in women in their forties and fifties who have borne children.

Usually the inflammatory changes are confined to an area drained by one or several of the major excretory ducts of the nipple. There is increased firmness of the tissue, and on cross-section dilated ropy ducts are apparent from which thick, cheesy

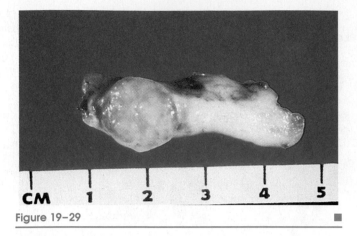

Figure 19–29 ■

Fibroadenoma of the breast. The tan-colored encapsulated small tumor is sharply demarcated from the whiter breast tissue.

secretions can be extruded. Histologically, the ducts are filled by granular debris, sometimes containing leukocytes, principally lipid-laden macrophages. The lining epithelium is generally destroyed. **The most distinguishing features are the prominence of the lymphocytic and plasma cell infiltration and occasional granulomas in the periductal stroma.**

Mammary duct ectasia is of principal importance because it leads to induration of the breast substance and, more significantly, to retraction of the skin or nipple, mimicking the changes caused by some carcinomas.

Traumatic fat necrosis is an uncommon and innocuous lesion that is significant only because it produces a mass. Most, but not all, patients report some antecedent trauma to the breast.

During the early stage, the lesion is small, often tender, rarely more than 2 cm in diameter, and sharply localized. It consists of a central focus of necrotic fat cells surrounded by neutrophils and lipid-filled macrophages, which is later enclosed by fibrous tissue and mononuclear leukocytes. Eventually, the focus is replaced by scar tissue, or the debris becomes encysted within the scar. Calcifications may develop in either the scar or cyst wall.

■ TUMORS OF THE BREAST

Tumors are the most important lesions of the female breast. Although they may arise from either connective tissue or epithelial structures, it is the latter that give rise to the common breast neoplasms. Here we will describe fibroadenoma, phyl-

lodes tumor, papilloma and papillary carcinoma, and carcinoma of the breast.

Fibroadenoma

The encapsulated fibroadenoma is by far the most common benign tumor of the female breast. An absolute or relative increase in estrogen activity is thought to play a role in its development, and indeed similar lesions, perhaps less discretely encapsulated, may appear with fibrocystic changes (fibroadenosis). Fibroadenomas usually appear in young women; the peak incidence is in the third decade of life.

The fibroadenoma occurs as a discrete, encapsulated, usually solitary, freely movable nodule, 1 to 10 cm in diameter. Rarely, multiple tumors are encountered and, equally rarely, they may exceed 10 cm in diameter **(giant fibroadenoma).** Whatever their size, they are encapsulated and usually easily "shelled out." Grossly, all are firm, with a uniform tan-white color on cut section, punctuated by softer yellow-pink specks representing the glandular areas (Fig. 19–29). Histologically, there is a loose fibroblastic stroma containing ductlike, epithelium-lined spaces of various forms and sizes. These ductlike or glandular spaces are lined with single or multiple layers of cells that are regular and have a well-defined, intact basement membrane. Although in some lesions the ductal spaces are open, round to oval, and fairly regular **(pericanalicular fibroadenoma),** others are compressed by extensive proliferation of the stroma, so that on cross-section they appear as slits or irregular, star-shaped structures **(intracanalicular fibroadenoma)** (Fig. 19–30).

Clinically, fibroadenomas usually present as solitary, discrete, movable masses. They may enlarge late in the menstrual

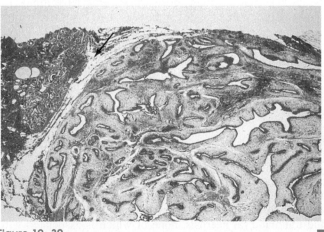

Figure 19–30 ■

Low-power microscopic view of a fibroadenoma of the breast showing the discrete margins *(arrow)* and the intracanalicular and pericanalicular patterns.

cycle and during pregnancy. Postmenopausally, they may regress and calcify. Cytogenetic studies reveal that the stromal cells are monoclonal and so represent the neoplastic element of these tumors. The basis of ductal proliferation is not clear. They almost never become malignant.

Phyllodes Tumor

These tumors are much less common than fibroadenomas and are thought to arise from the intralobular stroma, not from preexisting fibroadenomas. They may be small (3 to 4 cm in diameter), but most grow to large, possibly massive size, distending the breast. Some become lobulated and cystic; because on gross section they exhibit leaflike clefts and slits, they have been designated phyllodes (Greek for leaflike) tumors. In the past they had the tongue-tangling name "cystosarcoma phyllodes," an unfortunate term because these tumors are usually benign, although some become malignant. The most ominous change is the appearance of increased stromal cellularity with anaplasia and high mitotic activity, accompanied by rapid increase in size, usually with invasion of adjacent breast tissue by malignant stroma. Most of these tumors remain localized and are cured by excision; malignant lesions may recur, but they also tend to remain localized. Only the most malignant, about 15% of cases, metastasize to distant sites.

Intraductal Papilloma

This is a neoplastic papillary growth within a duct. Most lesions are solitary, found within the principal lactiferous ducts or sinuses. They present clinically as a result of (1) the appearance of serous or bloody nipple discharge, (2) the presence of a small subareolar tumor a few millimeters in diameter, or (3) rarely, nipple retraction.

> The tumors are usually solitary and less than 1 cm in diameter, consisting of delicate, branching growths within a dilated duct or cyst. Histologically, they are composed of multiple papillae, each having a connective tissue axis covered by cuboidal or cylindrical epithelial cells that are frequently double layered, the outer epithelial layer overlying a myoepithelial layer.

In some cases there are multiple papillomas in several ducts or intraductal papillomatosis. These lesions sometimes become malignant, whereas the solitary papilloma almost always remains benign. Similarly, papillary carcinoma must be excluded; it lacks a myoepithelial component and shows severe cytologic atypia and abnormal mitotic figures.

Carcinoma

No cancer is more feared by women than carcinoma of the breast, and for good reason. In the United States it is estimated by the American Cancer Society that in 1996 over 185,000 new breast cancers were discovered in women and they caused 44,500 deaths, making this scourge second only to lung cancer as a cause of cancer death. The data make clear that despite advances in diagnosis and treatment, almost one third of women who develop these neoplasms will die of the disease. For unknown reasons (possibly related in some part to better case finding), there has been an increase in the incidence of breast cancer throughout the world. In the United States the increase was holding steady at about 2% a year, when it started to climb in 1980 to 3% to 4% a year. Fortunately, the rate has now plateaued at about 107 cases per 100,000 women. Understandably, then, there has been intense study of the possible origins of this form of cancer and of means to diagnose it early enough to permit cure.

Epidemiology and Risk Factors. A large number of risk factors have been identified that modify a woman's likelihood of developing this form of cancer. They are briefly listed in Table 19–4, which divides them into well-established and less well-established groups and indicates where possible the relative risk imposed by each. Comments about some of the more important risk factors follow.

Geographic Variations. There are surprising differences among countries in the incidence rates and mortality rates

■

Table 19–4. BREAST CANCER RISK FACTORS

Factor	Relative Risk
Well-Established Influences	
Geographic factors	Varies in different areas
Age	Increases after age 30 yr
Family History	
First-degree relative with breast cancer	1.2–3.0
Premenopausal	3.1
Premenopausal and bilateral	8.5–9.0
Postmenopausal	1.5
Postmenopausal and bilateral	4.0–5.4
Menstrual History	
Age at menarche <12 yr	1.3
Age at menopause >55 yr	1.5–2.0
Pregnancy	
First live birth from ages 25–29 yr	1.5
First live birth after age 30 yr	1.9
First live birth after age 35 yr	2.0–3.0
Nulliparous	3.0
Benign Breast Disease	
Proliferative disease	1.9
Proliferative disease with atypical hyperplasia	4.4
Lobular carcinoma in situ	6.9–12.0
Less Well-Established Influences	
Exogenous estrogens	
Oral contraceptives	
Obesity	
High-fat diet	
Alcohol consumption	
Cigarette smoking	

Extensively modified from Bilimoria MM, Morrow M: The women at increased risk for breast cancer: evaluation and management strategies. CA: Cancer J Clin 46: 263, 1995.

from breast cancer. The risk for this form of neoplasia is significantly higher in North America and northern Europe than in Asia and Africa. For example, the incidence and mortality rates are five times higher in the United States than in Japan. These differences appear to be environmental rather than genetic in origin, because migrants from low-incidence locales to high-incidence areas tend to acquire the rates of their adoptive countries, and vice versa. Diet, reproductive patterns, and nursing habits are thought to be involved.

Age. Breast cancer is uncommon under age 30. Thereafter, the risk steadily increases throughout life, but after the menopause the upward slope of the curve almost plateaus.

Genetics and Family History. About 5% to 10% of breast cancers are thought to be related to specific inherited mutations. Germ line mutations in the tumor suppressor gene p53 underlie patients with the Li-Fraumeni syndrome (Chapter 6), with its predisposition to a variety of cancers, including breast carcinomas. In this syndrome *the breast cancers appear in women under 40 years of age and are more often bilateral than in the population at large.* Overall, this particular mutation accounts for not more than 1% of all breast cancers. Another gene associated with a familial disposition to breast cancer is the relatively recently discovered BRCA-1 gene on chromosome 17q21. Germ line mutations of this gene are thought to underlie the great majority of cases that have an inherited predisposition to both breast and ovarian cancer. It has been calculated that with a mutation of BRCA-1, the woman has a 50% chance of developing a breast cancer by age 50 and an 80% chance by age 65. A second breast cancer gene, called BRCA-2 and located on chromosome 13q12-13, has recently been discovered. It is believed to be responsible for 10% to 15% of familial breast cancer. Both are thought to be tumor suppressor genes. The function of BRCA-1 is unclear. According to some this gene encodes a growth inhibitory protein secreted by cells; others believe that the BRCA-1 protein remains within the nucleus, where it exerts its function by binding to other nuclear proteins. Specific identification of BRCA-1 and 2 is not yet widely available in clinical laboratories, and there is much debate about the ethical issues surrounding such testing.

Prolonged exposure to endogenous estrogens, particularly in the early decades of life, appears to represent a major risk factor. Thus, the early onset of menstrual cycles, a late menopause, delayed childbearing, nulliparity, and lowered cumulative months of lactation all increase the risk of breast cancer, because all prolong the lifetime exposure to the estrogenic peaks of the menstrual cycle.

Preexisting proliferative breast disease, especially with atypical hyperplasia, constitutes a significant risk factor, as already emphasized in the discussion of fibrocystic change.

In addition to the well-established predisposing influences mentioned above, there are many other less well-established risk factors. In approximate descending order of importance, they include the following:

■ *Prolonged exposure to exogenous estrogens* postmenopausally, known as estrogen replacement therapy (ERT). On the one hand, ERT is acknowledged to prevent or at least delay the onset of osteoporosis and protect against heart disease and stroke; on the other hand, it is considered by many authors to increase the risk of breast cancer. There is no consensus yet about the magnitude of the increased risk, if it exists at all, but the weight of evidence favors a relative risk of 1.5 to 1.8 after more than 5 years of use of ERT, with no clear evidence that the combined use of estrogen and progestin reduces this risk. However, very recent studies indicate that when all the pros and cons are balanced, the cardiovascular benefits far outweigh the possible adverse effects of ERT in terms of overall longevity.

■ *Oral contraceptives* have also been suspected of increasing the risk of breast cancer. Although once again the evidence is contradictory, the newer formulations of balanced low doses of combined estrogens and progestins impose only a slightly increased risk, especially in nulliparous women under the age of 25 years.

■ *Many other less well-established risk factors,* such as obesity, alcohol consumption, cigarette smoking, and a high-fat diet, have been implicated in favoring the development of breast cancer on the basis of population studies, but the evidence is at best inferential.

Pathogenesis. As is the case with all cancers, the cause of breast cancer remains unknown. However, three sets of influences appear to be important: (1) genetic changes, (2) hormonal influences, and (3) environmental factors.

Genetic changes, in addition to those producing the well-established familial syndromes mentioned earlier, have been implicated in the genesis of this form of neoplasia. As with most other cancers, mutations affecting protooncogenes and tumor suppressor genes in breast epithelium contribute to the oncogenic transformation process. Among the best characterized is overexpression of the c-*erbB*2 protooncogene, which has been found to be amplified in up to 30% of breast cancers. This gene is a member of the epidermal growth factor receptor family, and its overexpression is associated with a poor prognosis in patients with lymph node–positive breast cancer. Analogously, amplification of c-*ras* and c-*myc* genes has also been reported in some human breast cancers. Mutations of the well-known suppressor genes Rb and p53 may also be present. Most likely, multiple acquired mutations are involved in the sequential transformation of a normal epithelial cell into a cancerous cell.

Hormonal influences, particularly estrogens, clearly play some role, as already noted. In addition, there is the evidence of an increased risk of breast cancer in patients with estrogen-producing ovarian tumors. Estrogens stimulate the production of growth factors by normal breast epithelial cells and by cancer cells. It is hypothesized the estrogen and progesterone receptors normally present in breast epithelium, and often present in breast cancer cells, may interact with growth promoters, such as transforming growth factor α (related to epithelial growth factor [EGF]), platelet-derived growth factor, and fibroblast growth factor elaborated by human breast cancer cells, to create an autocrine mechanism of tumor development.

Environmental influences such as those previously mentioned—obesity, high-fat diet, cigarette smoking, and alcohol consumption—appear to participate on the basis of statistical studies, but direct evidence is lacking. Nonetheless, the migrant studies mentioned earlier cannot be dismissed.

MORPHOLOGY. Cancer of the breast affects the left breast slightly more often than the right. In about 4% of patients there are bilateral primary tumors or sequential lesions in the same breast. The locations of the tumors within the breast are as follows:

	%
Upper outer quadrant	50
Central portion	20
Lower outer quadrant	10
Upper inner quadrant	10
Lower inner quadrant	10

Most cancers (90%) arise in the ductal epithelium, and the small remainder in the lobular epithelium. Unless otherwise specified, the term *breast carcinoma* implies ductal origin. Both ductal and lobular cancers are further divided into those that have not penetrated the limiting basement membrane (noninvasive) and those that have (invasive). Thus, the chief forms of carcinoma of the breast can be classified as follows:

A. Noninvasive
   1. Intraductal carcinoma
   2. Intraductal carcinoma with Paget's disease
   3. Lobular carcinoma in situ
B. Invasive (infiltrating)
   1a. Invasive ductal carcinoma not otherwise specified
   1b. Invasive ductal carcinoma with Paget's disease
   2. Invasive lobular carcinoma
   3. Medullary carcinoma
   4. Colloid carcinoma (mucinous carcinoma)
   5. Tubular carcinoma
   6. Other rare types

Of these, invasive ductal carcinoma is by far the most common. Because it usually has an abundant fibrous stroma, it is also referred to as *scirrhous carcinoma.* Comments on the more common types follow.

NONINVASIVE (IN SITU) CARCINOMA. There are two types of noninvasive breast carcinoma: intraductal and lobular carcinoma in situ.

Intraductal carcinoma is much more common than lobular carcinoma in situ, and indeed with the advent of mammography and the ability to detect linear arrays of microcalcifications seen with the former, intraductal carcinoma now represents 20% to 25% of all breast carcinomas. At the time of discovery, there may or not be a clinically palpable mass, but sometimes there are ropy cords that are palpable and from which cheesy necrotic tumor tissue can be extruded with slight pressure when the ducts are transected (hence the name **comedocarcinoma**). Histologically, the ducts may be more or less filled with masses of anaplastic tumor cells, creating small glandular spaces **(cribriform pattern).** In some lesions, ducts are filled with solid masses of cells, sometimes with central areas of necrosis that often calcify (hence the microcalcifications). Rarely, the tumor cells grow in papillary formations, and, equally rarely, the anaplastic cancer cells extend into the epidermis of the nipple and areola region to produce Paget's disease of the nipple (described later). However, whatever the distribution of cancer, and whatever the histologic pattern, by definition the tumor cells do not penetrate the basement membranes of the ducts, and so remain noninvasive and in situ. However, in up to 40% of high-grade comedocarcinomas, invasion will occur in time.

Lobular carcinoma in situ is a distinctive form of breast cancer that arises in the terminal ducts and ductules (acini). Typically, these structures become distended with loosely cohesive anaplastic tumor cells, which have often undergone necrosis in the center of the ductule. Such changes can be found in association with fibrocystic change and may be admixed with intraductal carcinoma or be present in the vicinity of invasive carcinoma. The carcinomatous lesions are frequently multifocal and bilateral, complicating the approach to treatment. When monitored for long periods, about one third of such lesions will be followed by invasive carcinoma in the same or contralateral breast. Interestingly, many of these subsequent carcinomas are ductal in origin, making lobular carcinoma in situ a marker of invasive cancer.

INVASIVE (INFILTRATING) CARCINOMA. The morphology of the various tumor patterns is presented first, followed by the clinical features of all.

Invasive ductal carcinoma not otherwise specified is the most common form of breast cancer, accounting for about 70% of all carcinomas of the breast. Clinically, it is a deceptively delimited mass, rarely over 3 to 4 cm in diameter, of stony hard consistency; hence, the commonly used designation **scirrhous carcinoma.** On cut section the tumor is infiltrative and retracted below the surrounding fibrous fatty tissue; it has a gritty texture that produces a grating sound when scraped with a knife (Fig. 19-31). Foci of chalky white necrosis and sometimes calcification are often evident on the cut surface. Extension of the growth may cause dimpling of the skin, retraction of the nipple, or fixation to the chest wall. Histologically, the lesion is composed principally of dense, fibrous stroma, in which are found scattered nests or cords of tumor cells (Fig. 19-32). These are round to polygonal, are compressed, and contain fairly uniform, small, dark nuclei with remarkably few mitotic figures. At the margins of the tumor the neoplastic cells can be seen infiltrating the surrounding tissue (Fig. 19-33), frequently invading

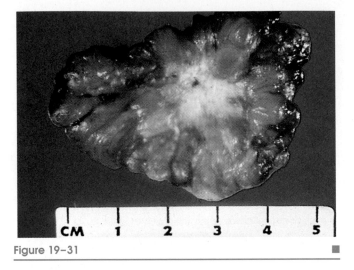

Figure 19-31 ■

A cut section of an invasive ductal carcinoma of the breast. The lesion is retracted, infiltrating the surrounding breast substance, and would be stony hard on palpation.

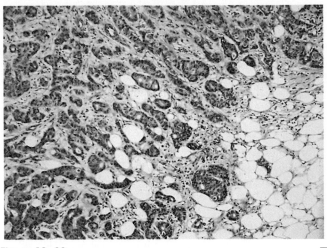

Figure 19-33 ■

The margin of a cancer of the breast revealing tumorous infiltration of the adjacent fatty tissue *(at right)*.

perivascular and perineurial spaces as well as blood vessels.

Paget's disease of the breast is an unusual form of ductal breast cancer that affects women in a slightly older age group than those who experience the usual invasive ductal carcinoma. It begins as a typical intraductal carcinoma involving the main excretory ducts, but it then extends to infiltrate the skin of the nipple and areola. There may or may not be a palpable mass in the breast. The involved areolar and periareolar skin is frequently fissured, ulcerated, and oozing, with an accompanying inflammatory hyperemia and edema. Superimposed bacterial infections are common. The histologic hallmark of this tumor is the invasion of the epidermis by pathognomonic neoplastic cells termed **Paget cells**. These are

scattered, singly or clustered, and are large, hyperchromatic cells having pleomorphic nuclei surrounded by a clear halo, which represents the intracellular accumulation of mucopolysaccharides (Fig. 19-34). In other respects, the morphology of Paget's disease is similar to that of an intraductal carcinoma, which may or may not be invasive. The prognosis depends on the extent of the ductal carcinoma and does not appear to be worsened by the skin extension.

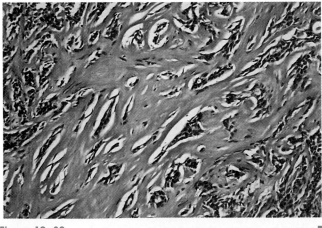

Figure 19-32 ■

Microscopic view of so-called *scirrhous carcinoma* of the breast reveals the dense collagenous background in which are scattered cords and nests of tumor cells.

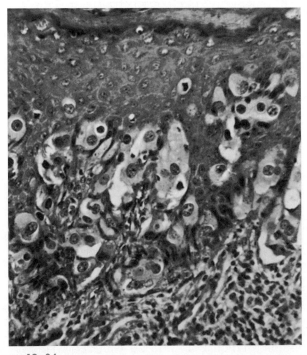

Figure 19-34 ■

Paget's disease of the breast. Paget's cells dot the epithelium.

Medullary carcinoma represents about 1% of breast cancers. The morphology of these tumors contrasts sharply with that of the usual breast carcinoma. They tend to be large (up to 10 cm), soft, and fleshy rather than stony hard. Histologically, unlike scirrhous carcinoma, medullary carcinoma has a scant stroma. The tumor cells grow in large, irregular sheets of undifferentiated polygonal to spindled cells, although occasionally well-differentiated gland formations are present. There is usually moderate to marked lymphocytic infiltration between the tumor cells, particularly in the margins of the tumor mass. This feature is presumed to represent a host response to the tumor, and correspondingly, these tumors have a distinctly better prognosis than the usual infiltrating breast carcinoma.

Colloid (mucinous) carcinoma is even more uncommon than medullary carcinoma. It is characterized by the production of mucin, intracellularly and extracellularly. These lesions are extremely soft, bulky, gray-blue masses. Histologically, mucus-containing tumor cells may form glands filled with mucin, or small clusters of tumor cells may be scattered in a large lake of basophilic mucin. The prognosis of these variants is better than that of the usual infiltrative neoplasm.

INFILTRATING LOBULAR CARCINOMA. Infiltrating lobular carcinoma is poorly circumscribed and usually rubbery in consistency, but sometimes the lesion is hard and scirrhous. It often does not create a palpable discrete mass. Histologically, in the classic form, strands of tumor cells, often one cell in width, are loosely dispersed in a fibrous stroma (Fig. 19–35). In most cases the tumor cells are small and uniform, with little pleomorphism. Occasionally, they surround cancerous or normal-appearing acini or ducts, creating a so-called "bull's eye" pattern, which is considered characteristic. Not uncommonly, the tumors have histologic features of both ductal and lobular patterns. It is therefore difficult to determine the precise incidence of infiltrating lobular carcinoma. Most studies report that they account for about 5% of breast carcinomas. These tumors are especially important because of their high incidence of bilaterality (about 20%), which mandates a careful clinical and histologic evaluation (by biopsy) of the contralateral breast.

Features Common to All Invasive Cancers

In all the forms of breast cancer discussed previously, progression of the disease leads to certain local morphologic features. These include a tendency to become adherent to the pectoral muscles or deep fascia of the chest wall, with consequent *fixation* of the lesion, as well as adherence to the overlying skin, with *retraction* or *dimpling* of the skin or nipple. The latter is an important sign, because it may be the first indication of a lesion, observed by the patient herself during self-examination. Involvement of the lymphatic pathways may cause localized *lymphedema*. In these cases the skin becomes thickened around exaggerated hair follicles, a change known as *peau d'orange* (orange peel). Sometimes, particularly in pregnancy, the tumor spreads so rapidly that it excites an acute inflammatory reaction with swelling, redness, and tenderness. This picture has been referred to as *inflammatory carcinoma*. The advent of mammography as a diagnostic tool has called attention to the frequency of microcalcifications in breast carcinoma. Although certain variants (e.g., intraductal carcinoma) infrequently have such calcifications, they are common in the usual infiltrative scirrhous lesion, so that overall they are found in 60% to 80% of breast cancers. They may

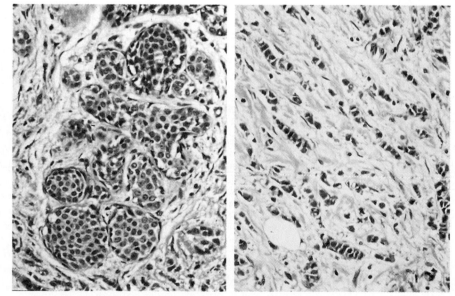

Figure 19–35   ■

Lobular carcinoma. *Left,* the terminal ducts and ductules of the breast are distended with tumor cells (lobular carcinoma in situ). *Right,* strands of tumor cells are infiltrating the fibrous pink stroma. (Courtesy of Dr. Kyle Molberg, Department of Pathology, University of Texas Southwestern Medical School, Dallas, TX.)

also be present in the epithelial proliferation of fibrocystic changes.

Spread eventually occurs through lymphatic and hematogenous channels. Nodal metastases are present in about two thirds of cases at the time of diagnosis. Outer quadrant and centrally located lesions typically spread first to the axillary nodes. Those in the inner quadrants often involve the lymph nodes along the internal mammary arteries. The supraclavicular nodes are sometimes the primary site of spread, but they may become involved only after the axillary and internal mammary nodes are affected. More distant dissemination eventually ensues, with metastatic involvement of almost any organ or tissue in the body. Favored locations are the lungs, skeleton, liver, and adrenals and (less commonly) the brain, spleen, and pituitary. However, no site is exempt. *Metastases may appear many years after apparent therapeutic control of the primary lesion, sometimes 15 years later.* Nevertheless, with each passing year the scene brightens. Breast cancer is an ugly lesion for many reasons, not the least being its potential to reappear so many years later.

Grading and Staging. These neoplasms have been graded on the basis of their level of anaplasia (grades I to III) and have been divided into three categories based on their biologic aggressiveness:

■ *Nonmetastasizing:* intraductal carcinoma without stromal invasion; in situ lobular carcinoma
■ *Uncommonly metastasizing:* colloid carcinoma; medullary carcinoma with lymphocytic infiltration
■ *Moderately to aggressively metastasizing:* all other types

In addition, there are other staging systems; regrettably, too many are currently in use. All attempt to create stages based on the size of the primary lesion, the possible presence of nodal metastases, and the possibility of distant dissemination. One system widely used is shown in Table 19–5.

■

Table 19–5.	AMERICAN JOINT COMMITTEE ON CANCER STAGING OF BREAST CARCINOMA
Stage Tis	In situ cancer (in situ lobular, pure intraductal, and Paget's disease of the nipple without palpable tumor)
Stage I	Tumor 2 cm or less in greatest diameter and without evidence of regional or distant spread
Stage II	Tumor more than 2 cm but not more than 5 cm in greatest dimension, with regional lymph node involvement but without distant spread
Stage III (A)	Tumor of up to and more than 5 cm in diameter with or without homolateral regional (local) spread that may or may not be fixed, but without distant spread
Stage III (B)	Tumor of up to and more than 5 cm in diameter with homolateral metastatic supraclavicular and infraclavicular nodes
Stage IV	Tumor of any size with or without regional spread but with evidence of distant metastases

From Beahrs OH: Staging of cancer of the breast as a guide to therapy. Cancer 53:592, 1984.

Clinical Course. Breast cancer is often discovered by the patient or her physician as a deceptively discrete, solitary, painless, and movable mass. At this time the lesion is typically less than 4 cm in diameter, although, as mentioned, involvement of the regional lymph nodes (most often axillary) is already present in about two thirds of patients. With increasing frequency, an occult lesion is detected by a routine mammogram. Admittedly, "mammos" incur increased costs and worry produced by questionable findings (calcifications are also seen with fibrocystic changes). Nonetheless, there is currently an apparent consensus for mammography being performed every 1 or 2 years beginning at about age 40 unless there is a family history of cancer or a history of atypical hyperplastic fibrocystic change, in which case screening should begin earlier and be performed more frequently. This technique is well established as a valuable diagnostic tool in the differentiation of cancerous from benign breast masses.

The prognosis of breast cancer is influenced by many factors. Obvious poor prognostic signs include extensive edema or multiple nodules in the skin of the breast, fixation to the chest wall, spread to internal mammary or supraclavicular lymph nodes, inflammatory carcinoma, and, of course, distant metastases. In early breast cancer, when these signs are not apparent, prognosis is affected by the following variables:

1. *The size of the primary tumor.* Tumors smaller than 2 cm are associated with favorable prognosis.
2. *Lymph node involvement and the number of lymph nodes involved by metastases.* With no axillary lymph node involvement the 5-year survival rate is close to 80%. The disease-free survival rate falls off to 21% in the presence of four or more involved nodes.
3. *The histologic type and grade of tumor.* The 30-year survival rate for various types is as follows: intraductal carcinoma, 74%; papillary carcinoma, 65%; medullary carcinoma, 58%; colloid, 58%; infiltrating lobular, 34%; and infiltrating ductal, 29%.
4. *The presence or absence of estrogen and progesterone receptors.* The number of estrogen receptors in breast cancer cells can be large or moderate, or there may be none; it is proportional to the degree of cell differentiation, which in turn is roughly proportional to the responsiveness of the tumor to antiestrogen therapy by oophorectomy or tamoxifen. The highest response rates to such therapy are seen in patients with tumors that contain both estrogen and progesterone receptors, but the correlation is not perfect. Some tumors with receptors fail to respond, and, conversely, some tumors lacking receptors do respond.
5. *The proliferative rate and the degree of aneuploidy* (increased and scattered DNA values), as measured by flow cytometry. The larger the fraction of cells scattered outside the modal peaks of DNA histograms, the poorer is the outcome.
6. *Overexpression resulting from amplification of c-erbB2 predicts a poor outcome.* However, recent studies have questioned the prognostic value of c-*erbB*2 overexpression in patients with lymph node negative breast cancer.
7. *Abundant growth of new vessels within and about the tumor (angiogenesis)* is correlated with an increased likelihood of metastases.

However, despite all of these prognostic indicators, it is impossible in the individual case to foresee the outcome. Sadly, only time tells the story. The overall 5-year survival rate for stage I cancer is 80%; for stage II, 65%; for stage III, 40%; and for stage IV, 10%. It should be noted that recurrence may appear late, even after 10 years, but with each passing year free of disease the prognosis improves. Overall, the 10-year survival rate for breast cancers is still no more than 50%.

MALE BREAST

The rudimentary male breast is relatively free from pathologic involvement. Only two disorders occur with sufficient frequency to merit consideration: *gynecomastia* and *carcinoma.*

Gynecomastia

As in females, male breasts are subject to hormonal influences, but they are considerably less sensitive than female breasts. Nonetheless, enlargement of the male breast, or gynecomastia, may occur in response to absolute or relative estrogen excesses. Gynecomastia, then, is the male analog of fibrocystic change in the female. The most important cause of such hyperestrinism in the male is cirrhosis of the liver, with consequent inability of the liver to metabolize estrogens. Other causes include Klinefelter syndrome, estrogen-secreting tumors, estrogen therapy, and occasionally digitalis therapy. Physiologic gynecomastia often occurs in puberty and in extreme old age.

The morphologic features of gynecomastia are similar to those of intraductal hyperplasia. Grossly, a button-like, subareolar swelling develops, usually in both breasts but occasionally in only one.

Carcinoma

This is a rare occurrence, with a frequency ratio to breast cancer in the female of 1 : 125. It occurs in advanced age. Because of the scant amount of breast substance in the male, the tumor rapidly infiltrates the overlying skin and underlying thoracic wall. Both morphologically and biologically, these tumors resemble invasive carcinomas in the female. Surprisingly, considering the size of the male breast, almost half have spread to regional nodes and more distant sites by the time they are discovered.

REFERENCES

Bilimoria MM, Morrow M: The woman at increased risk for breast cancer; evaluation and management strategies. CA: Cancer J Clin 45:263, 1995.

Haefner HK, et al: Vulvar intraepithelial neoplasia: age, morphologic phenotype, papillomavirus DNA, and coexisting invasive carcinoma. Hum Pathol 26:147, 1995.

Herbst AL: The epidemiology of ovarian carcinoma and the current status of tumor markers to detect disease. Am J Obstet Gynecol 170:1099, 1994.

Kurman RJ, Trimble CL: The behavior of serous tumors of low malignant potential; are they ever malignant? Int J Gynecol Pathol 12:120, 1995.

Kurman RJ, et al: The behavior of endometrial hyperplasia. A long term study of untreated hyperplasia in 170 patients. Cancer 56:403, 1995.

Lipworth L: Epidemiology of breast cancer. Eur J Cancer Prev 4:7, 1995.

Monk BJ, et al: Prognostic significance of human papillomavirus DNA in vulvar carcinoma. Obstet Gynecol 85:709, 1995.

Ostor AG: Natural history of cervical intraepithelial neoplasia, a critical review. Int J Gynecol Pathol 12:186, 1993.

Pejovic T: Genetic changes in ovarian cancer. Ann Med 27:73, 1995.

Rose PG: Medical progress: endometrial carcinoma. N Engl J Med 335:640, 1996. (An excellent review.)

Weidner N: Prognostic factors in breast carcinoma. Curr Opin Obstet Gynecol 7:4, 1995.

Wooster R, et al: Localization of a breast cancer susceptibility gene BRCA-2 to chromosome 13q12-13. Science 265:2088, 1994.

Wu LC, et al: Identification of a RING protein that can interact in vivo with BRCA-1 gene product. Nat Genet 14:430, 1996. (Evidence that BRCA-1 exerts its action by binding to certain other nuclear proteins.)

20

The Endocrine System

DENNIS K. BURNS, MD
VINAY KUMAR, MD

The endocrine system consists of a highly integrated and widely distributed group of organs whose purpose is to maintain a state of metabolic equilibrium, or homeostasis, between the various organs of the body. To accomplish this, the endocrine glands secrete a variety of chemical messengers, or hormones, that regulate the activity of various organs. Increased activity of the target tissue, in turn, typically down-regulates the activity of the gland secreting the stimulating hormone, a process known as *feedback inhibition* (Fig. 20–1). Hormones transported to their target organs via the bloodstream are referred to as "endocrine" hormones. They include a number of steroid hormones, peptides, and amines that modify the activity of cells and tissues throughout the body.

A number of processes may disturb the normal activity of the endocrine system, including impaired synthesis or release of hormones, abnormal interactions between hormones and their target tissues, and abnormal responses of target organs to their hormones. Endocrine diseases can be broadly classified as (1) diseases of *under-* or *overproduction of hormones* and their resultant biochemical and clinical consequences and (2) diseases associated with the development of *mass lesions.* Such lesions may be nonfunctional, or they may be associated with over- or underproduction of hormones. As will become apparent, a proper understanding of endocrine diseases requires a careful integration of morphologic findings with biochemical measurements of the levels of hormones, their regulators, and other metabolites.

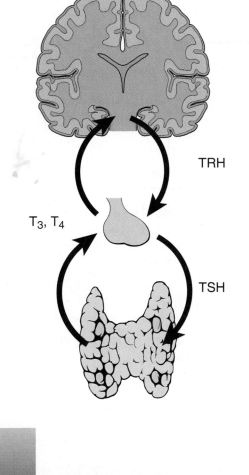

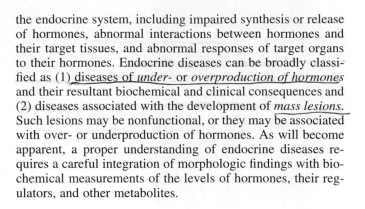

Figure 20–1 ■

Diagram of the relationships among the hypothalamus, the anterior pituitary, and a peripheral endocrine gland, exemplified here by the thyroid gland. Secretion of thyroid hormones (T_3 and T_4) is controlled by trophic factors secreted by both the hypothalamus and the anterior pituitary. Decreased levels of T_3 and T_4 stimulate the release of thyroid-releasing hormone (TRH) from the hypothalamus and thyroid-stimulating hormone (TSH) from the anterior pituitary, causing T_3 and T_4 levels to rise. Elevated T_3 and T_4 levels in turn suppress the secretion of both TRH and TSH. These interactions constitute a negative-feedback loop. (Modified from an original sketch by Dr. Ronald A. DeLellis, New England Medical Center, Boston.)

Pituitary

The pituitary gland is a small, bean-shaped structure that lies at the base of the brain within the confines of the sella turcica. It is intimately related to the hypothalamus, with which it is connected by both a "stalk," composed of axons extending from the hypothalamus, and a rich venous plexus. Along with the hypothalamus, the pituitary plays a central role in the regulation of most of the other endocrine glands. The pituitary is composed of two morphologically and function-

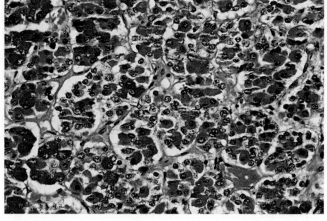

Figure 20-2   ■

Photomicrograph of normal anterior pituitary. The gland is populated by several distinct cell populations containing a variety of stimulating (trophic) hormones. Each of the hormones has different staining characteristics, resulting in a mixture of cell types in routine histologic preparations.

ally distinct components: the anterior lobe (adenohypophysis) and the posterior lobe (neurohypophysis). Diseases of the pituitary, accordingly, can be divided into those that primarily affect the anterior lobe and those that predominantly affect the posterior lobe.

The *anterior pituitary,* or *adenohypophysis,* is composed of epithelial cells derived embryologically from the developing oral cavity. In routine histologic sections, a colorful array of cells containing basophilic cytoplasm, eosinophilic cytoplasm, or poorly-staining cytoplasm ("chromophobic") cells is present (Fig. 20-2). Detailed studies employing electron microscopy and immunocytochemistry have demonstrated that the staining properties of these cells are related to the presence of various trophic hormones within their cytoplasm; these are released into the circulation in response to various *releasing factors* secreted by the hypothalamus.

Diseases of the anterior pituitary may come to clinical attention owing to increased or decreased secretion of trophic hormones, designated hyperpituitarism or hypopituitarism, respectively. In most cases, *hyperpituitarism* is caused by a functional adenoma within the anterior lobe. *Hypopituitarism* may be caused by a variety of destructive processes, including ischemic injury, radiation, inflammatory reactions, and nonfunctioning neoplasms. In addition to endocrine abnormalities, diseases of the anterior pituitary may also be manifested by *local mass effects,* including radiographic evidence of enlargement of the sella turcica, visual field abnormalities due to encroachment of mass lesions on the visual pathways, and evidence of increased intracranial pressure.

HYPERPITUITARISM AND PITUITARY ADENOMAS

In most cases, excess production of anterior pituitary hormones is caused by the presence of an adenoma arising in the

anterior lobe. Other, less common causes are hyperplasias and carcinomas of the anterior pituitary, secretion of hormones by nonpituitary tumors, and certain hypothalamic disorders. As discussed later, pituitary adenomas may be nonfunctional and may also cause hypopituitarism as they encroach upon and destroy adjacent native anterior pituitary parenchyma. Functional pituitary adenomas are usually composed of a single cell type and produce a single predominant hormone. Exceptions to this occur. Some pituitary adenomas are composed of a single cell type but secrete more than one hormone (e.g., growth hormone [GH] and prolactin), and occasionally adenomas contain more than one cell population. The various types of anterior pituitary adenomas and their relative frequencies are listed in Table 20-1.

Pituitary adenomas account for roughly 10% of intracranial neoplasms that come to clinical attention and are discovered incidentally in up to 25% of routine autopsies. They are usually found in adults, with a peak incidence from the fourth to the sixth decades. Most pituitary adenomas occur as isolated lesions. In about 3% of cases, however, adenomas are associated with *multiple endocrine neoplasia, type I* (discussed later). Pituitary adenomas are designated, somewhat arbitrarily, *macroadenomas* if they exceed 1 cm in diameter and *microadenomas* if less than 1 cm. Nonfunctional adenomas are likely to present at a later stage than those associated with obvious endocrine abnormalities and are therefore more likely to be macroadenomas.

> **MORPHOLOGY.** The usual pituitary adenoma is a well-circumscribed, soft lesion that may, in the case of smaller tumors, be confined by the sella turcica. Larger lesions typically extend superiorly through the sellar diaphragm into the suprasellar region, where they often compress the optic chiasm and adjacent structures (Fig. 20-3). As these adenomas expand, they frequently erode the sella turcica and anterior clinoid processes. They may also extend locally into the cavernous and sphenoid sinuses. In up to 30% of cases the adenomas are grossly nonencapsulated and infiltrate adjacent bone, dura, and (uncommonly) brain. Such lesions are designated *invasive* adenomas.

■

Table 20-1.   PITUITARY ADENOMAS

Type	Frequency (%)
Prolactin cell adenoma	20-30
Growth hormone cell adenomas	5
Mixed GH-prolactin adenomas	5
ACTH cell adenomas	10-15
Gonadotroph cell adenomas	10-15
Null cell adenomas	20
TSH cell adenomas	1
Other pleurihormonal adenomas	15

Modified from Burger PC, et al: Pituitary neoplasia. In Burger, PC (ed): Surgical Pathology of the Nervous System and its Coverings, 3rd ed. New York, Churchill Livingstone, 1991.

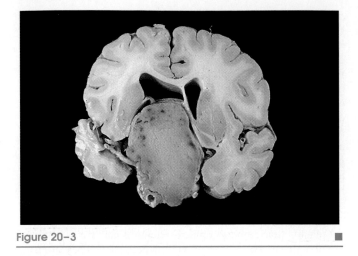

Figure 20–3 ■

Gross view of a pituitary adenoma. This massive, nonfunctional adenoma has grown far beyond the confines of the sella turcica and has distorted the overlying brain. Nonfunctional adenomas tend to be larger at the time of diagnosis than those that secrete a hormone.

Foci of hemorrhage and/or necrosis are common in larger adenomas. On occasion, acute hemorrhage into an adenoma is associated with clinical evidence of rapid enlargement of the lesion, a situation sometimes termed *pituitary apoplexy.*

Microscopically, pituitary adenomas are composed of relatively uniform, polygonal cells arrayed in sheets, cords, or papillae. Supporting connective tissue, or reticulin, is sparse, accounting for the soft, gelatinous consistency of many lesions. The nuclei of the neoplastic cells may be uniform or pleomorphic. Mitotic activity is usually scanty. The cytoplasm of the constituent cells may be acidophilic, basophilic, or chromophobic, depending on the type and amount of secretory product within the cell, but it is fairly uniform throughout the neoplasm. **This cellular monomorphism and the absence of a significant reticulin network distinguish pituitary adenomas from nonneoplastic anterior pituitary parenchyma** (Fig. 20–4). The functional status of the adenoma cannot be reliably predicted from its histologic appearance.

Clinical Features. The signs and symptoms of pituitary adenomas include hormonal abnormalities and mass effects. The endocrine abnormalities associated with the secretion of excessive quantities of anterior pituitary hormones are discussed below with the specific variants of pituitary adenoma. *Local mass effects* may be encountered in any type of pituitary tumor. Among the earliest changes referable to mass effect are *radiographic abnormalities of the sella turcica*, including sellar expansion, bony erosion, and disruption of the diaphragma sellae. Because of the close proximity of the optic nerves and chiasm to the sella, expanding pituitary lesions

often compress decussating fibers in the optic chiasm. This gives rise to *visual field abnormalities,* classically in the form of defects in the lateral (temporal) visual fields—a so-called *bitemporal hemianopsia.* In addition, a variety of other visual field abnormalities may be caused by asymmetric growth of many tumors. As in the case of any expanding intracranial mass, pituitary adenomas may produce signs and symptoms of *elevated intracranial pressure*, including headache, nausea, and vomiting. Finally, expanding pituitary adenomas may compress the adjacent non-neoplastic anterior pituitary sufficiently to compromise its function, resulting in *hypopituitarism.* As noted previously, acute hemorrhage into an adenoma is sometimes associated with a rapid increase in local mass effects.

pituitary apoplexy - hemmorage into adenoma

Prolactinomas

Prolactinomas are the most common type of hyperfunctioning pituitary adenoma. They range from small microadenomas to large, expansile tumors associated with considerable mass effect. Microscopically, most prolactinomas are composed of chromophobic or weakly acidophilic cells. Prolactin is demonstrable within the cytoplasm of the neoplastic cells by immunohistochemical techniques.

Hyperprolactinemia causes amenorrhea, galactorrhea, loss of libido, and infertility. Because many of the manifestations of hyperprolactinemia (e.g., amenorrhea) are more obvious in premenopausal females than in males or postmenopausal females, prolactinomas are usually diagnosed at an earlier stage in females of reproductive age than in other patients. In contrast, hormonal manifestations may be quite subtle in men and older women, in whom the tumors may reach considerable size before coming to clinical attention. Hyperprolactinemia may be caused by conditions other than prolactin-secreting pituitary adenomas, including pregnancy, high-dose estrogen therapy, renal failure, hypothyroidism, hypothalamic lesions,

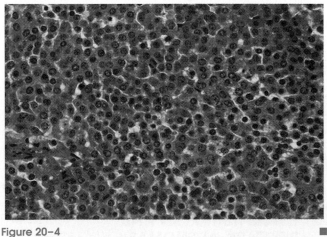

Figure 20–4 ■

Photomicrograph of pituitary adenoma. The monomorphism of these cells contrasts markedly with the mixture of cells seen in the normal anterior pituitary in Figure 20–2. Note also the absence of reticulin network.

and dopamine-inhibiting drugs (e.g., reserpine). In addition, any mass in the suprasellar compartment may disturb the normal inhibitory influence of the hypothalamus on prolactin secretion, resulting in hyperprolactinemia, the so-called *stalk effect*. It should be kept in mind, therefore, that *mild* elevations of serum prolactin (<200 μg/L) in a patient with a pituitary adenoma do not necessarily indicate a prolactin-secreting neoplasm. Prolactinomas are treated with bromocriptine, a dopamine receptor agonist, which causes shrinkage of the neoplasm in most cases.

Growth Hormone (Somatotroph Cell) Adenomas

Growth hormone–secreting neoplasms, including those that secrete a mixture of growth hormone and other hormones (e.g., prolactin), are the second most common type of functional pituitary adenoma. Because the clinical manifestations of excessive GH may be subtle, somatotroph cell adenomas may be quite large by the time they come to clinical attention. Microscopically, GH-producing adenomas are composed of densely or sparsely granulated cells, which appear acidophilic or chromophobic in routine sections. Immunocytochemical stains demonstrate GH within the cytoplasm of the neoplastic cells. Small amounts of immunoreactive prolactin are often present as well.

If a GH-secreting adenoma occurs before the epiphyses close, as in the case of prepubertal children, excessive levels of GH result in the development of *gigantism*. This is characterized by a generalized increase in body size, with disproportionately long arms and legs. If elevated levels of GH persist, or present, after closure of the epiphyses, patients develop *acromegaly*, in which growth is most conspicuous in soft tissues, skin, and viscera and in the bones of the face, hands, and feet. Enlargement of the jaw results in its protrusion (prognathism), with broadening of the lower face and separation of the teeth. The hands and feet are enlarged, with broad, sausage-like fingers. In practice, most cases of gigantism are also accompanied by evidence of acromegaly. GH excess is also associated with a number of other disturbances, including abnormal glucose tolerance and diabetes mellitus, generalized muscle weakness, hypertension, arthritis, osteoporosis, and congestive heart failure. Prolactin is demonstrable in a number of GH-producing adenomas and in some cases may be released in sufficient quantities to produce signs and symptoms of hyperprolactinemia.

Corticotroph Cell Adenomas

Most corticotroph adenomas are small (microadenomas) at the time of diagnosis, although some tumors may be quite large. These adenomas are basophilic or chromophobic and stain positively with periodic acid–Schiff (PAS) stains owing to the presence of carbohydrates in the adrenocorticotropic hormone (ACTH) precursor molecule. As in the case of other pituitary hormones, the secretory granules can be detected by

immunocytochemical methods. Under the electron microscope they appear as membrane-bound, electron-dense granules averaging 300 nm in diameter.

Corticotroph adenomas may be clinically silent or may cause *hypercortisolism* (also known as *Cushing's syndrome*) because of the stimulatory effect of ACTH on the adrenal cortex. Cushing's syndrome, discussed in more detail later with diseases of the adrenal gland, may be caused by a wide variety of conditions in addition to ACTH-producing pituitary neoplasms. When the hypercortisolism is due to excessive production of ACTH by the pituitary, the process is designated *Cushing's disease*. Large, clinically aggressive corticotroph adenomas may develop in patients after surgical removal of the adrenal glands for treatment of Cushing's syndrome. This condition, known as *Nelson's syndrome*, occurs in most cases because of a loss of the inhibitory effect of adrenal corticosteroids on a preexisting corticotroph microadenoma. Because the adrenals are absent in patients with Nelson's syndrome, hypercortisolism does not develop. Instead, patients present with the mass effects of the pituitary tumor. In addition, there may be hyperpigmentation due to the stimulatory effect of the ACTH precursor molecule on melanocytes.

Other Anterior Pituitary Neoplasms

A significant number of pituitary adenomas produce no demonstrable hormonal product and are designated *null cell adenomas*. Such nonfunctional tumors account for approximately 20% of all pituitary adenomas. The tumors either are chromophobic or contain cells with granular, eosinophilic cytoplasm. In contrast to hormonally active acidophilic tumors, the granular cytoplasmic staining in such cases is due, in large part, to the presence of numerous mitochondria. Electron microscopy in such cases reveals only scant secretory granules. Null cell adenomas typically present because of mass effect. They may also compromise the residual anterior pituitary sufficiently to produce *hypopituitarism*.

Gonadotroph (luteinizing hormone [LH]– and follicle-stimulating hormone [FSH]–producing) adenomas comprise 10% to 15% of pituitary adenomas. These adenomas are diagnosed most commonly in middle-aged men and women. They may cause decreased libido in men but often produce no obvious endocrine abnormalities. The neoplasms are basophilic or chromophobic and may reach large size before they are diagnosed.

Thyrotroph (thyroid-stimulating hormone [TSH]–producing) adenomas are rare, accounting for about 1% of all pituitary adenomas. Thyrotroph adenomas are chromophobic or basophilic and are a rare cause of hyperthyroidism.

Pituitary adenomas may elaborate more than one hormone. As noted, somatotroph adenomas commonly contain immunoreactive prolactin. In some neoplasms, designated *mixed adenomas*, more than one cell population is present. In other cases, a single cell type is apparently capable of synthesizing more than one hormone.

Pituitary carcinomas are exceedingly rare. This diagnosis is made only if the tumors have metastasized.

HYPOPITUITARISM

Hypofunction of the anterior pituitary may occur with loss or absence of 75% or more of the anterior pituitary parenchyma. This may be congenital or may result from a wide range of acquired abnormalities that are intrinsic to the pituitary. Less frequently, disorders that interfere with the delivery of pituitary hormone–releasing factors from the hypothalamus, such as hypothalamic tumors, may also cause hypofunction of the anterior pituitary. Hypopituitarism of hypothalamic origin is usually accompanied by evidence of posterior pituitary dysfunction in the form of diabetes insipidus (discussed below). Most cases of anterior pituitary hypofunction are caused by

■ Nonsecretory pituitary adenomas
■ Ischemic necrosis of the pituitary
■ Ablation of the pituitary by surgery or radiation

Other, less common causes of anterior pituitary hypofunction include the empty sella syndrome, inflammatory lesions, trauma, and metastatic neoplasms involving the pituitary.

Nonsecretory pituitary adenomas may compress and compromise the anterior pituitary sufficiently to result in hypopituitarism. This may occur as a consequence of gradual enlargement of the adenoma or after abrupt enlargement of the tumor due to acute hemorrhage (pituitary apoplexy).

Ischemic necrosis of the anterior pituitary is an important cause of pituitary insufficiency. In general, the anterior pituitary tolerates ischemic insults fairly well; loss of up to half of the anterior pituitary parenchyma is without clinical consequences. However, with destruction of larger amounts of the anterior pituitary (e.g., 75% or more), signs and symptoms of hypopituitarism develop. *Sheehan's syndrome,* or postpartum necrosis of the anterior pituitary, is the most common form of clinically significant ischemic necrosis of the anterior pituitary. During pregnancy, the anterior pituitary enlarges considerably, largely because of an increase in the size and number of prolactin-secreting cells. However, this physiologic enlargement of the gland is not accompanied by an increase in blood supply from the low-pressure portal venous system. The enlarged gland is thus especially vulnerable to ischemic injury in patients who develop significant hemorrhage and hypotension during the peripartum period. The posterior pituitary, because it receives its blood directly from arterial branches, is much less susceptible to ischemic injury in this setting and is therefore usually not affected. Clinically significant pituitary necrosis may also be encountered in conditions other than pregnancy, including disseminated intravascular coagulation, sickle cell anemia, elevated intracranial pressure, traumatic injury, and shock of any origin. The residual gland is shrunken and scarred (Fig. 20–5).

An "empty sella" can result from any condition that destroys part or all of the pituitary gland. The term *empty sella syndrome* designates the presence of an enlarged, empty sella turcica caused by chronic herniation of the subarachnoid space into the sella turcica. In these patients a defect in the diaphragma sellae allows the arachnoid mater and cerebrospinal fluid to herniate into the sella, with resultant expansion of the

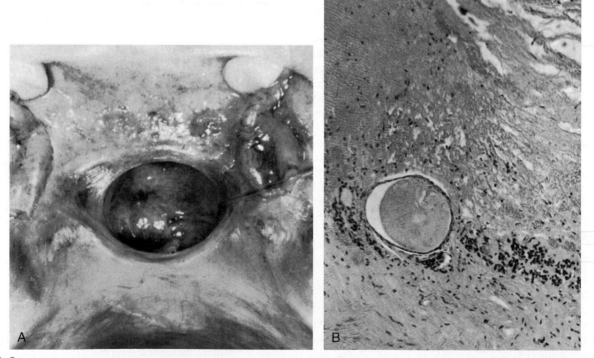

Figure 20–5 ■

A, View of the sella turcica in a patient dying of chronic pituitary insufficiency. A tiny nubbin of residual pituitary can be seen protruding from the posterior wall of the sella *(below)*. *B,* Photomicrograph of the residual anterior pituitary illustrated in *A*. Most of the gland has been replaced by the dense fibrous tissue, save for a few residual cells.

sella and compression of the pituitary. Classically, affected patients are obese women with a history of multiple pregnancies. The empty sella syndrome may be associated with visual field deficits and sometimes with endocrine abnormalities, most commonly hyperprolactinemia due to interruption of inhibitory hypothalamic influences ("stalk effect"). It is rarely associated with generalized hypopituitarism because sufficient functioning parenchyma is preserved.

The clinical manifestations of anterior pituitary hypofunction typically develop slowly. They are related to a hypofunction of the adrenal cortices, thyroid, and gonads. Specific manifestations of hypoadrenalism and hypothyroidism are discussed later in this chapter. Additional manifestations of hypopituitarism include pallor, due to a loss of melanocyte-stimulating hormone; atrophy of the gonads and genitalia with resultant amenorrhea, impotence, and loss of libido; and loss of pubic and axillary hair.

POSTERIOR PITUITARY SYNDROMES

The posterior pituitary, or neurohypophysis, is composed of modified glial cells (termed *pituicytes*) and axonal processes extending from nerve cell bodies in the supraoptic and paraventricular nuclei of the hypothalamus. The hypothalamic neurons produce two peptides: antidiuretic hormone (ADH) and oxytocin. They are stored in axon terminals in the neurohypophysis and released into the circulation in response to appropriate stimuli. Oxytocin stimulates the contraction of smooth muscle in the pregnant uterus and that which surrounds the lactiferous ducts of the mammary glands. Abnormal oxytocin synthesis and release has not been associated with significant clinical abnormalities. The clinically important posterior pituitary syndromes involve ADH. They include

diabetes insipidus and *secretion of inappropriately high levels of ADH*.

ADH is a nonapeptide hormone synthesized predominantly in the supraoptic nucleus. In response to a number of different stimuli, including increased plasma oncotic pressure, left atrial distention, exercise, and certain emotional states, ADH is released from axon terminals in the neurohypophysis into the general circulation. The hormone acts on the collecting tubules of the kidney to promote the resorption of free water. ADH deficiency causes *diabetes insipidus,* a condition characterized by excessive urination (polyuria) due to an inability of the kidney to properly resorb water from the urine. Diabetes insipidus can result from a number of processes, including head trauma, neoplasms and inflammatory disorders of the hypothalamus and pituitary, and surgical procedures involving the hypothalamus or pituitary. The condition sometimes arises spontaneously, in the absence of an underlying disorder. The clinical manifestations include the excretion of large volumes of dilute urine with an inappropriately low specific gravity. Serum sodium and osmolality are increased owing to excessive renal loss of free water, resulting in thirst and polydipsia. Patients who can drink water can generally compensate for urinary losses; patients who are obtunded, bedridden, or otherwise limited in their ability to obtain water may develop life-threatening dehydration.

In the *syndrome of inappropriate ADH (SIADH)* secretion, ADH excess is caused by a number of extracranial and intracranial disorders. It causes resorption of excessive amounts of free water, with resultant hyponatremia. The most common causes of SIADH include the secretion of ectopic ADH by malignant neoplasms (particularly small cell carcinomas of the lung), non-neoplastic diseases of the lung, and local injury to the hypothalamus and/or neurohypophysis. The clinical manifestations of SIADH are dominated by hyponatremia, cerebral edema, and resultant neurologic dysfunction. Although total body water is increased, blood volume remains normal and peripheral edema does not develop.

— made by small cell carcinomas paraneoplastically

Thyroid

The thyroid gland is a bilobed structure below and anterior to the larynx. The gland develops from an evagination of the developing pharyngeal epithelium that descends to its normal position in the anterior neck. This pattern of descent explains the occasional presence of thyroid tissue in atypical locations, such as the base of the tongue. The thyroid is composed of roughly spherical follicles, lined by low cuboidal-to-columnar epithelium, and filled with thyroglobulin-rich colloid. In re-

sponse to TSH released by thyrotrophs in the anterior pituitary, the follicular epithelial cells of the thyroid pinocytize colloid and ultimately convert thyroglobulin into *thyroxine* (T_4) and lesser amounts of *triiodothyronine* (T_3). T_4 and T_3 are released into the systemic circulation, where they are reversibly bound to circulating plasma proteins for transport to peripheral tissues. The unbound T_3 and T_4 interact with intracellular receptors, to ultimately up-regulate carbohydrate and

$TRH \rightarrow TSH \rightarrow T_3 / T_4$

lipid catabolism and stimulate protein synthesis in a wide range of cells. The net effect of these processes is an increase in the *basal metabolic rate*. The thyroid gland also contains a population of parafollicular cells, or "C" cells, that synthesize and secrete the hormone calcitonin. This hormone promotes absorption of calcium by the skeletal system and inhibits resorption of bone by osteoclasts. Diseases of the thyroid include conditions associated with excessive release of thyroid hormones (hyperthyroidism), those associated with thyroid hormone deficiency (hypothyroidism), and mass lesions of the thyroid. We will first consider the general features of hyperthyroidism and hypothyroidism, and then discuss specific diseases of the thyroid.

HYPERTHYROIDISM

Thyrotoxicosis is a hypermetabolic state caused by elevated circulating levels of free T_3 and T_4. Because it is caused most commonly by hyperfunction of the thyroid gland, it is often referred to as hyperthyroidism. However, in certain conditions (e.g., some types of thyroiditis) the oversupply is related to excessive release of preformed thyroid hormone and not hyperfunction of the gland. *Thus, strictly speaking, hyperthyroidism is only one (albeit the most common) category of thyrotoxicosis.* Keeping this in mind, we will follow the common practice of using thyrotoxicosis and hyperthyroidism interchangeably. The terms *primary* and *secondary* hyperthyroidism are sometimes used to designate hyperthyroidism arising from an intrinsic thyroid abnormality, and that arising from disorders outside of the thyroid, such as a TSH-secreting pituitary tumor. The latter is uncommon. The most common causes of hyperthyroidism are

■ *Diffuse hyperplasia* of the thyroid associated with Graves' disease
■ The ingestion of excess *exogenous thyroid hormone* (administered for hypothyroidism)
■ Hyperfunctional *multinodular goiter*
■ Hyperfunctional *adenoma* of the thyroid

Less common causes of hyperthyroidism include certain forms of thyroiditis, TSH-secreting pituitary adenomas, and the secretion of excessive amounts of thyroid hormone by ectopic thyroid arising in ovarian teratomas *(struma ovarii)*.

The clinical manifestations of thyrotoxicosis include changes referable to the *hypermetabolic state* induced by excess thyroid hormone, as well as those related to *overactivity of the sympathetic nervous system*. Excessive levels of thyroid hormone result in an increase in the basal metabolic rate. Stimulation of the gut results in hypermotility, malabsorption, and diarrhea. Overactivity of the sympathetic nervous system produces nervousness, tremor, tachycardia, palpitations, hyperreflexia, and irritability. Congestive heart failure may develop, particularly in elderly patients with preexisting cardiac disease. A wide, staring gaze and lid lag are present owing to sympathetic overstimulation of the levator palpebrae superioris (Fig. 20–6). The skin of thyrotoxic patients tends to be soft, warm, and flushed; excessive sweating and heat intolerance are common. Increased sympathetic activity and hy-

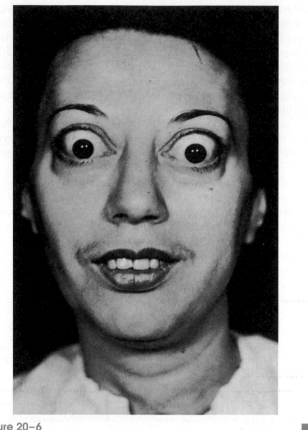

Figure 20–6 ■

Patient with hyperthyroidism. A wide-eyed, staring gaze, caused by overactivity of the sympathetic nervous system, is one of the features of this disorder. In Graves' disease, one of the most important causes of hyperthyroidism, accumulation of loose connective tissue behind the eyeballs also adds to the protuberant appearance of the eyes.

permetabolism result in weight loss despite increased appetite.

The term *thyroid storm* is used to designate the abrupt onset of severe hyperthyroidism. This condition occurs most commonly in patients with underlying Graves' disease (discussed below), probably resulting from an acute elevation in catecholamine levels, as might be encountered during stress. Thyroid storm is a medical emergency: a significant number of untreated patients die of cardiac arrhythmias.

The diagnosis of hyperthyroidism is based on clinical features and laboratory data. *The measurement of serum TSH concentration, in conjunction with measurement of unbound ("free") T_4, provides the most useful screening tests in cases of suspected hyperthyroidism.* Free T_4 levels are typically increased. TSH levels are exquisitely sensitive to free T_4 levels and are therefore suppressed to very low levels in patients with primary hyperthyroidism (i.e., hyperthyroidism due to intrinsic thyroid disease). However, TSH levels are not a reliable indicator of thyroid function in patients with thyrotoxicosis caused by hypothalamic or primary pituitary disease (e.g., TSH-secreting pituitary adenomas). In an occasional patient, hyperthyroidism results predominantly from increased circulating levels of T_3 (T_3 toxicosis). In these cases, free T_4 levels may be decreased, and direct measurement of serum T_3

loss of lateral eye brows - Greenfrau's Sign

may be useful. Measurement of TSH levels after injection of thyroid-releasing hormone (TRH stimulation test) is used to evaluate cases of suspected hyperthyroidism with equivocal changes in the baseline serum TSH level. A normal rise in TSH after injection of TRH excludes secondary hyperthyroidism. Measurement of radioactive iodine uptake provides an additional direct indication of the level of activity within the thyroid gland.

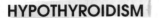

HYPOTHYROIDISM

Hypothyroidism is caused by any structural or functional derangement that interferes with the production of adequate levels of thyroid hormone. As in the case of hyperthyroidism, this disorder is sometimes divided into primary and secondary categories, depending on whether the hypothyroidism arises from an intrinsic abnormality in the thyroid or results from hypothalamic or pituitary disease. Primary hypothyroidism accounts for most cases of hypothyroidism. The most common causes include *ablation of the thyroid* by surgery or radiation therapy, *Hashimoto's thyroiditis*, and *primary idiopathic hypothyroidism.*

The clinical manifestations of hypothyroidism include cretinism and myxedema. *Cretinism* refers to hypothyroidism developing in infancy or early childhood. In the past, this disorder was fairly common in areas of the world where dietary iodine deficiency is endemic, including the Himalayas, inland China, Africa, and other mountainous areas. It has now become much less frequent because of the widespread supplementation of foods with iodine. On rare occasions, cretinism may also result from inborn errors in metabolism (e.g., enzyme deficiencies) that interfere with the biosynthesis of normal levels of thyroid hormone (sporadic cretinism). Clinical features of cretinism include impaired development of the skeletal system and central nervous system, with severe mental retardation, short stature, coarse facial features, a protruding tongue, and umbilical hernia. The severity of the mental impairment in cretinism appears to be directly influenced by the time at which thyroid deficiency occurs in utero. Normally, maternal hormones, including T_3 and T_4, cross the placenta and are critical to fetal brain development. If there is maternal thyroid deficiency before the development of the fetal thyroid gland, mental retardation is severe. In contrast, reduction in maternal thyroid hormones later in pregnancy, after the fetal thyroid has developed, allows normal brain development.

Hypothyroidism developing in older children and adults results in a condition known as *myxedema.* Myxedema, or Gull's disease, was first linked with thyroid dysfunction in 1873 by Sir William Gull in a paper addressing the development of a "cretinoid state" in adults. Manifestations of myxedema include generalized apathy and mental sluggishness that, in the early stages of disease, may mimic depression. Patients with myxedema are listless, cold intolerant, and often obese. Mucopolysaccharide-rich edema accumulates in skin *(chin)* subcutaneous tissue, and a number of visceral sites, with resultant broadening and coarsening of facial features, enlargement of the tongue, and deepening of the voice. Bowel mo-

do tests on all kids

tility is decreased, resulting in constipation. Pericardial effusions are common; in later stages the heart is enlarged, and heart failure may supervene.

Laboratory evaluation plays a vital role in the diagnosis of suspected hypothyroidism because of the nonspecific nature of symptoms. Assay of the serum TSH level is the most sensitive screening test for this disorder. The *TSH level is increased* in primary hypothyroidism due to a loss of feedback inhibition of TRH and TSH production by the hypothalamus and pituitary, respectively. The TSH level is not increased in patients with hypothyroidism due to primary hypothalamic or pituitary disease. *T_4 levels are decreased* in patients with hypothyroidism of any origin.

GRAVES' DISEASE

In 1835, Robert Graves reported on his observations of a disease characterized by "violent and long continued palpitations in females" associated with enlargement of the thyroid gland. *Graves' disease is the most common cause of endogenous hyperthyroidism.* It is characterized by a triad of manifestations, including *thyrotoxicosis* due to hyperfunctional, diffuse enlargement of the thyroid present in all cases; an infiltrative ophthalmopathy with resultant *exophthalmos* noted in up to 40% of patients; and, in a minority of cases, a localized, infiltrative dermopathy sometimes designated *pretibial myxedema.* Graves' disease occurs primarily in younger adults, with a peak incidence between the ages of 20 and 40. Women are affected up to seven times more frequently than men. An increased incidence of Graves' disease occurs among family members of affected patients, with a 50% concordance among identical twins. The occurrence of this disorder is strongly associated with the inheritance of human leukocyte antigen (HLA)-DR3.

Pathogenesis. Graves' disease is an autoimmune disorder in which a variety of autoantibodies may be present in the serum. These include antibodies to the TSH receptor, microsomes, thyroglobulin, and thyroid hormones (T_3 and T_4). At least some of these autoantibodies appear to play a direct role in the pathogenesis of Graves' disease by stimulating thyroid epithelial cell activity. One such antibody, termed *thyroid-stimulating immunoglobulin (TSI),* binds to the TSH receptor to stimulate adenylate cyclase activity, with resultant increased release of thyroid hormones. Another class of antibodies, also directed against the TSH receptor, has been implicated in the proliferation of thyroid follicular epithelium (thyroid growth-stimulating immunoglobulins, or TGI). Still other antibodies, termed *TSH-binding inhibitor immunoglobulins (TBIIs),* prevent TSH from binding normally to its receptor on thyroid epithelial cells. In so doing, some forms of TBII mimic the action of TSH, resulting in the stimulation of thyroid epithelial cell activity, while other forms may actually *inhibit* thyroid cell function. It is likely that autoantibodies also play a role in the development of the infiltrative ophthalmopathy and dermopathy characteristic of Graves' disease. Possibly the ocular muscles and TSH receptor share some cross-reactive epitopes. A defect in suppressor T-cell function that permits the development of organ-specific (in this case, thyroid-specific) antibodies likely plays a role in the development of the autoantibodies responsible for Graves' disease. The factors that trigger the autoimmune reaction remain unclear.

Autoimmune disorders of the thyroid span a spectrum in which Graves' disease characterized by hyperfunction of the thyroid lies at one extreme and Hashimoto's disease manifesting as hypothyroidism occupies the other end. Antibodies against thyroidal antigens are common to both, but their specific epitopes are different and hence their functional consequences differ. In both disorders the frequency of other autoimmune diseases such as systemic lupus erythematosus, pernicious anemia, type I diabetes, and Addison's disease is increased.

MORPHOLOGY. In the typical case the thyroid gland is diffusely enlarged because of the presence of **diffuse hypertrophy and hyperplasia** of thyroid follicular epithelial cells. The gland is usually smooth and soft, and its capsule is intact. Microscopically, the follicular epithelial cells in untreated cases are tall, columnar, and more crowded than usual. This crowding often results in the formation of small papillae, which project into the follicular lumen (Fig. 20–7). Such papillae lack fibrovascular cores, in contrast to those of papillary carcinoma (discussed later). The colloid within the follicular lumen is pale, with scalloped margins. Lymphoid aggregates consisting of autoreactive B cells are usually present within the interstitium. Preoperative therapy alters the morphology of the thyroid in Graves' disease. Treatment with the antithyroid drug propylthiouracil, for example, exaggerates the epithelial hypertrophy and hyperplasia by stimulating TSH secretion. On the other hand, preoperative administration of iodine causes involution of the epithelium and the accumulation of colloid by blocking thyroglobulin secretion.

Changes in extrathyroidal tissues include generalized lymphoid hyperplasia. The heart may be hypertrophied and ischemic changes may be present, particularly in patients with preexisting coronary artery disease. In patients with ophthalmopathy, the tissues of the orbit are edematous owing to the presence of hydrophilic mucopolysaccharides. In addition, there is infiltration by lymphocytes. Orbital muscles are edematous initially but may undergo fibrosis late in the course of the disease. The dermopathy, if present, is characterized by thickening of the dermis due to deposition of mucopolysaccharides and lymphocyte infiltration.

Clinical Features. The clinical manifestations of Graves' disease include those common to all forms of thyrotoxicosis (discussed earlier), as well as those associated uniquely with Graves' disease: *diffuse hyperplasia of the thyroid, ophthalmopathy, and dermopathy.* The degree of thyrotoxicosis varies from case to case and may sometimes be less conspicuous than other manifestations of the disease. Diffuse enlargement of the thyroid is present in all cases of Graves' disease. The thyroid enlargement is usually smooth and symmetric, but may be asymmetric. Increased flow of blood through the hyperactive gland often produces an audible bruit. The ophthalmopathy of Graves' disease, when present, is caused by a combination of the sympathetic overactivity that accompanies thyrotoxicosis and the deposition of mucopolysaccharide-rich connective tissue behind the eyeball. Sympathetic overactivity produces a characteristic wide, staring gaze and lid lag. Infiltration of the orbit by increased amounts of connective tissue causes the eyes to protrude abnormally (exophthalmos). The extraocular muscles are often weak. The proptosis may persist or progress despite successful treatment of the thyrotoxicosis, sometimes resulting in corneal injury. The dermopathy, sometimes designated *pretibial myxedema,* is present in a minority of cases. It is manifested most typically by localized areas of thickening and hyperpigmentation of the skin over the anterior aspect of the feet and lower legs. Laboratory findings in Graves' disease include elevated free T_4 and T_3 levels and depressed TSH levels. Because of ongoing stimulation of the thyroid follicles by thyroid-stimulating immunoglobulins, radioactive iodine uptake is increased and radioiodine scans show a *diffuse uptake* of iodine.

DIFFUSE NONTOXIC GOITER AND MULTINODULAR GOITER

Goiter, or simple enlargement of the thyroid, is the most common thyroid disease. The disorder is endemic in certain areas of the world and may also occur sporadically. Whether sporadic or endemic, *the presence of goiter reflects impaired synthesis of thyroid hormone,* most often due to dietary iodine

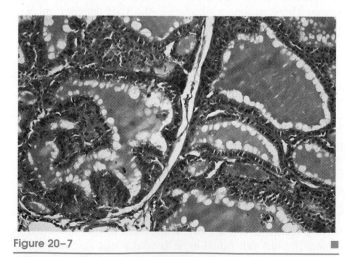

Figure 20–7 ■

Photomicrograph of a diffusely hyperplastic gland in a case of Graves' disease. The follicles are lined by tall, columnar epithelium. The crowded, enlarged epithelial cells project into the lumina of the follicles. These cells actively resorb the colloid in the centers of the follicles, resulting in the "scalloped" appearance of the edges of the colloid.

deficiency. Impairment of thyroid hormone synthesis leads to a compensatory rise in the serum TSH level, which in turn causes hypertrophy and hyperplasia of thyroid follicular cells and, ultimately, gross enlargement of the thyroid gland.

Endemic goiter occurs in geographic areas where the soil, water, and food supply contain low levels of iodine. The term *endemic* is used when goiters are present in more than 10% of the population in a given region. Such conditions are particularly common in mountainous areas of the world, including the Himalayas and the Andes. With increasing dietary iodine supplementation, the frequency and severity of endemic goiter have declined significantly. *Sporadic goiter* occurs less commonly than endemic goiter. The condition is more common in females than in males, with a peak incidence in puberty or young adult life, when there is an increased physiologic demand for thyroxine. Sporadic goiter may be caused by a number of conditions, including the ingestion of substances that interfere with thyroid hormone synthesis at some level, such as excessive calcium and vegetables belonging to the *Brassica* and Cruciferae groups (e.g., cabbage, cauliflower, Brussels sprouts, and turnips). In other instances, goiter may result from hereditary enzymatic defects that interfere with thyroid hormone synthesis. In most cases, however, the cause of sporadic goiter is not apparent.

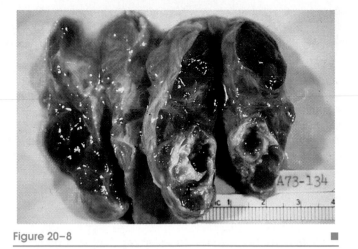

Figure 20–8   ■

Gross view of nodular goiter. The gland is coarsely nodular and contains areas of fibrosis and cystic change.

MORPHOLOGY. The pathogenesis of goiter involves hypertrophy and hyperplasia of thyroid follicular cells by elevated levels of TSH. In most cases, such changes result initially in diffuse, symmetric enlargement of the gland **(diffuse nontoxic goiter).** The follicles are lined by crowded columnar cells, which may pile up and form projections similar to those seen in Graves' disease. If dietary iodine subsequently increases, or if the demands for thyroid hormone decrease, the stimulated follicular epithelium involutes to form an enlarged, colloid-rich gland **(colloid goiter).** The cut surface of the thyroid in such cases is usually brown, somewhat glassy, and translucent. Microscopically, the follicular epithelium may be hyperplastic in the early stages of disease, or flattened and cuboidal during periods of involution. Colloid is abundant during the latter periods. With time, recurrent episodes of stimulation and involution combine to produce a more irregular enlargement of the thyroid, termed **nodular,** or **multinodular, goiter.** The basis of nodule formation is not clear. It may be related to differential ability of normal thyroid epithelial cells to replicate in response to TSH. Conceivably, this variation in cell growth potential can cause nodule formation with cyclical and long-term exposure to increased levels of TSH.

Multinodular goiters are multilobulated, asymmetrically enlarged glands, which may reach massive size (Fig. 20–8). On the cut surface, irregular nodules containing variable amounts of brown, gelatinous colloid are present. Regressive changes are quite common, particularly in older lesions,

and include areas of fibrosis, hemorrhage, calcification, and cystic change. The microscopic appearance includes colloid-rich follicles lined by flattened, inactive epithelium and areas of follicular epithelial hypertrophy and hyperplasia, accompanied by the regressive changes noted previously.

Clinical Features. The dominant clinical features of goiter are those caused by the mass effects of the enlarged gland. In addition to the obvious cosmetic effects of a large neck mass, goiters may also cause airway obstruction, dysphagia, and compression of large vessels in the neck and upper thorax. In a significant minority of patients, a hyperfunctioning nodule may develop within the goiter, resulting in *hyperthyroidism.* This condition, known as *Plummer's syndrome*, is not accompanied by the infiltrative ophthalmopathy and dermopathy of Graves' disease. Less commonly, goiter may be associated with clinical evidence of *hypothyroidism.* Goiters are also of clinical significance because of their ability to mask or to mimic neoplastic diseases arising in the thyroid.

THYROIDITIS

Inflammation of the thyroid gland, or thyroiditis, can occur in a number of different settings. Sometimes the thyroid gland may be the site of specific infections, such as tuberculosis, and may contain granulomatous lesions identical to those associated with this disease in sites outside the thyroid gland. Such infectious disorders are fairly uncommon in the thyroid. We will focus our attention in this section on some of the more common types of thyroiditis, including nonspecific lymphocytic thyroiditis, Hashimoto's thyroiditis, and subacute (granulomatous) thyroiditis.

Nonspecific Lymphocytic Thyroiditis

This form of thyroiditis is most often diagnosed as an incidental lesion in euthyroid patients. The condition is more common in females than in males. Although it may occur at any age, it is most often seen in middle-aged adults. Whether nonspecific lymphocytic thyroiditis represents a specific entity or a nonspecific reaction to more than one initiating agent is unclear. The association with the HLA-DR5 antigen in a significant number of patients suggests that, as in the cases of Graves' disease and Hashimoto's thyroiditis, autoimmune factors may play a role in its development.

MORPHOLOGY. Except for possible mild symmetric enlargement, the thyroid appears normal on gross inspection. Microscopic examination of the gland reveals a multifocal inflammatory infiltrate composed predominantly of small lymphocytes. Plasma cells and germinal centers are not conspicuous and, when present, suggest the diagnosis of Hashimoto's disease (discussed below).

Clinical Features. As noted, many cases of nonspecific lymphocytic thyroiditis represent incidental morphologic findings in patients with no clear history of thyroid disease. A minority of cases are associated with clinical evidence of thyrotoxicosis, which may be severe. The hyperthyroidism in such cases results from injury to follicles, with subsequent release of thyroid hormone. It is transient, usually abating within several months. Infiltrative ophthalmopathy and other manifestations of Graves' disease are not present. Laboratory findings during periods of thyrotoxicosis include elevated levels of T_4 and T_3 and depressed levels of TSH. In contrast to Graves' disease, in which radioactive iodine uptake is increased, the radioactive iodine uptake is consistently decreased in thyrotoxicosis associated with thyroiditis.

Hashimoto's Thyroiditis

Hashimoto's disease is an autoimmune inflammatory disorder of the thyroid. It begins with the activation of thyroid-specific CD4+ T cells that induce formation of CD8+ cytotoxic T cells and autoantibodies. Many of the same antibodies present in the sera of patients with Graves' disease are also present in patients with Hashimoto's disease. However, in Hashimoto's disease the anti-TSH receptor antibodies block the action of TSH, thus accounting for hypothyroidism. As in the case of Graves' disease, the frequency of other autoimmune disorders such as systemic lupus erythematosus and rheumatoid arthritis is also increased in patients with Hashimoto's disease. Most cases of Hashimoto's thyroiditis are associated with HLA-DR5; a minority characterized by severe thyroid atrophy are linked to HLA-DR3, suggesting that two different mechanisms may play a role in the development of this disorder. Hashimoto's disease is most prevalent between 45 and 65 years of age, and is more common in females than

in males, with a female predominance of 10:1 to 20:1. This disorder accounts for a significant number of cases of spontaneous hypothyroidism, but it may also be associated with transient hyperthyroidism.

MORPHOLOGY. Grossly, the thyroid is usually diffusely and symmetrically enlarged, although more localized enlargement may be seen in some cases. The capsule is intact, and the gland is well demarcated from adjacent structures. The cut surface is pale, gray-tan, firm, and somewhat friable. Microscopic examination discloses widespread infiltration of the parenchyma by a **mononuclear inflammatory infiltrate** containing small lymphocytes, plasma cells, and well-developed **germinal centers** (Fig. 20–9). The thyroid follicles are small and are lined in many areas by epithelial cells distinguished by the presence of abundant eosinophilic, granular cytoplasm, termed **Hürthle**, or **oxyphil**, cells. Interstitial connective tissue is increased and may be abundant. The fibrosis does not extend beyond the capsule of the gland. Less commonly, the thyroid is small and atrophic as a result of more extensive fibrosis.

Clinical Features. Hashimoto's thyroiditis presents as painless enlargement of the thyroid, usually associated with some degree of hypothyroidism. The enlargement of the gland is usually symmetric and diffuse, but in some cases it may be sufficiently localized to raise the suspicion of a neoplasm. Hypothyroidism usually develops gradually, but it may be preceded by transient thyrotoxicosis ("hashitoxicosis") caused by disruption of thyroid follicles, with secondary release of thyroid hormones. During this phase, free T_4 and T_3 levels are increased, TSH is decreased, and radioactive iodine uptake is diminished. As hypothyroidism supervenes, T_4 and T_3 levels

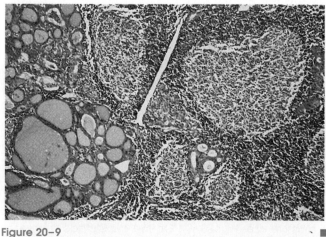

Figure 20–9 ■

Photomicrograph of Hashimoto's thyroiditis. The thyroid parenchyma contains a dense lymphocytic infiltrate with germinal centers. Residual thyroid follicles lined by deeply eosinophilic Hürthle cells are also seen.

progressively decline, accompanied by a compensatory rise in TSH. Patients with Hashimoto's disease are at increased risk for the development of B-cell lymphomas.

Subacute (Granulomatous) Thyroiditis

Subacute thyroiditis, also known as granulomatous thyroiditis or de Quervain's thyroiditis, is much less common than Hashimoto's disease. This disorder is most common between the ages of 30 and 50 and, like other forms of thyroiditis, occurs more frequently in women than in men. The cause of subacute thyroiditis is unknown. It is often preceded by an upper respiratory infection, suggesting the possibility of *viral* origin.

> **MORPHOLOGY.** The gland may be unilaterally or bilaterally enlarged and firm, with an intact capsule. Histologically, there is extensive infiltration of the thyroid by a neutrophilic inflammatory infiltrate, accompanied by scattered lymphocytes, plasma cells, and macrophages. Thyroid follicles are disrupted, with resultant extrusion of colloid. This in turn provokes a granulomatous inflammatory reaction, with exuberant giant cell formation.

Clinical Features. The onset of this form of thyroiditis is often acute, characterized by pain in the neck (particularly when swallowing), fever, malaise, and variable enlargement of the thyroid. Transient hyperthyroidism may occur, as in other cases of thyroiditis, owing to disruption of thyroid follicles and release of excessive thyroid hormone. Thyroid function tests are similar to those encountered in thyrotoxicosis associated with other forms of thyroiditis. The leukocyte count and erythrocyte sedimentation rate are increased. The condition is typically self-limited, with most patients returning to a euthyroid state within 6 to 8 weeks.

Other, less common forms of thyroiditis include acute bacterial thyroiditis associated with infection by streptococci, staphylococci, and other pyogenic organisms, and thyroiditis caused by hematogenous seeding of *Mycobacterium tuberculosis* or fungi. Riedel's thyroiditis is a rare disorder of unknown etiology, characterized by extensive fibrosis involving the thyroid and contiguous neck structures. It may be associated with idiopathic fibrosis in other sites in the body, such as the retroperitoneum.

NEOPLASMS OF THE THYROID

The thyroid gland gives rise to a variety of neoplasms, ranging from circumscribed, benign adenomas to highly aggressive, anaplastic carcinomas. From a clinical standpoint, the possibility of neoplastic disease is of major concern in patients who present with thyroid nodules. Fortunately, the over-

whelming majority of solitary nodules of the thyroid prove to be benign lesions, either follicular adenomas or localized, non-neoplastic conditions (e.g., nodular hyperplasia, simple cysts, or foci of thyroiditis). Carcinomas of the thyroid, in contrast, are uncommon, accounting for well under 1% of solitary thyroid nodules. Several clinical criteria provide a clue to the nature of a given thyroid nodule:

- Solitary nodules, in general, are more likely to be neoplastic than are multiple nodules.
- Nodules that take up radioactive iodine in imaging studies ("hot" nodules) are more likely to be benign than malignant.
- Nodules in younger patients are more likely to be neoplastic than are those in older patients.
- Nodules in males are more likely to be neoplastic than are those in females.

Such statistics and general trends, however, are of little significance in the evaluation of a given patient, in whom the timely recognition of a malignancy, however uncommon, can be lifesaving. Ultimately, it is the morphologic evaluation of a given thyroid nodule, in the form of fine-needle aspiration biopsy and histologic study of surgically resected thyroid parenchyma, that provides the most definitive information about its nature. In the following sections, we will consider the major thyroid neoplasms, including adenomas and carcinoma in its various forms.

Adenomas

Adenomas of the thyroid are benign neoplasms derived from follicular epithelium. As in the case of all thyroid neoplasms, follicular adenomas are usually solitary. Clinically and morphologically, they may be difficult to distinguish, on the one hand, from foci of follicular hyperplasia, or, on the other hand, from the less common follicular carcinomas.

> **MORPHOLOGY.** The typical thyroid adenoma is a solitary, spherical, encapsulated lesion that is well demarcated from the surrounding thyroid parenchyma (Fig. 20–10). In freshly resected specimens, the adenoma bulges from the cut surface and compresses the adjacent thyroid. The color ranges from gray-white to red-brown, depending on the cellularity and colloid content of the tumor. Areas of hemorrhage, fibrosis, calcification, and cystic change similar to those encountered in multinodular goiters are common, particularly within larger lesions. Microscopically, the constituent cells often form normal-appearing follicles that contain colloid (Fig. 20–11). Various histologic subtypes of adenomas are recognized on the basis of the degree of follicle formation and the colloid content of the follicles (e.g., trabecular, microfollicular, macrofollicular), but these subdivisions are of no biologic significance. Papillary change is not a typical feature of adenomas and, if present, should raise the suspicion of an encapsulated

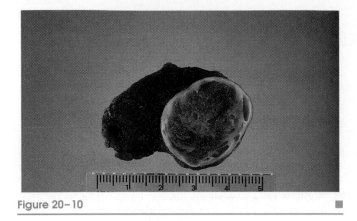

Figure 20–10 ■

Follicular adenoma of the thyroid. A solitary, well-circumscribed nodule is seen.

papillary carcinoma (discussed below). The neoplastic cells are demarcated from the adjacent parenchyma by a well-defined, intact capsule. Careful evaluation of the integrity of the capsule is important in distinguishing follicular adenomas from well-differentiated follicular carcinomas.

Clinical Features. Most adenomas of the thyroid present as a painless mass, often discovered during a routine physical examination. Larger masses may produce local symptoms such as difficulty in swallowing. In a minority of cases, adenomas may be hyperfunctional, producing signs and symptoms of hyperthyroidism. After injection of radioactive iodine, most adenomas take up iodine less avidly than does normal thyroid parenchyma. On radionuclide scanning, therefore, adenomas appear as "cold" nodules relative to the adjacent normal thyroid gland. The occasional hyperfunctional adenoma, however, will appear as a "warm" or "hot" nodule in the scan. Up to 10% of "cold" nodules eventually prove to be malig-

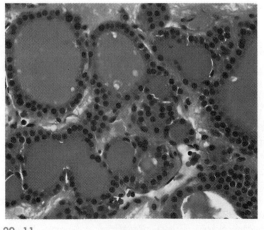

Figure 20–11 ■

Photomicrograph of follicular adenoma. Well-differentiated follicles resemble normal thyroid parenchyma.

nant. By contrast, malignancy is rare in "hot" nodules. Additional techniques used in the preoperative evaluation of suspected adenomas are ultrasonography and fine-needle aspiration biopsy. The definitive diagnosis of adenomas, however, is based on careful histologic examination of the resected specimen. Current evidence suggests that thyroid carcinomas arise de novo and that malignant transformation of adenomas does not occur.

Carcinomas

Carcinomas of the thyroid are relatively uncommon in the United States, being responsible for less than 1% of cancer-related deaths. Most cases occur in adults, although some forms, particularly papillary carcinomas, may present in childhood. A female predominance has been noted among patients developing thyroid carcinoma in the early and middle adult years, probably related to the expression of estrogen receptors on neoplastic thyroid epithelium. In contrast, cases presenting in childhood and late adult life are distributed equally among males and females. Most thyroid carcinomas are well-differentiated lesions. The major subtypes of thyroid carcinoma and their relative frequencies are

■ Papillary carcinoma (75% to 85% of cases)
■ Follicular carcinoma (10% to 20% of cases)
■ Medullary carcinoma (5% of cases)
■ Anaplastic carcinomas (<5% of cases)

Because of the unique clinical and biologic features associated with each variant of thyroid carcinoma, these subtypes will be described separately, after discussion of pathogenesis.

Pathogenesis. Exposure to ionizing radiation, particularly during the first two decades of life, has emerged as one of the most important factors predisposing to the development of thyroid cancer. In the past, radiation therapy was liberally employed in the treatment of a number of head and neck lesions in infants and children, including reactive tonsillar enlargement, acne, and tinea capitis. Up to 9% of people receiving such treatment during childhood subsequently developed thyroid malignancies, usually several decades after exposure. The incidence of carcinoma of the thyroid is substantially higher, in addition, among atomic bomb survivors in Japan and in those exposed to ionizing radiation after the Chernobyl nuclear plant disaster. Certain thyroid diseases, namely, Hashimoto's thyroiditis and nodular goiter, have also been suggested as predisposing factors in some cases. As noted previously, there is little evidence that follicular adenomas progress to carcinoma. The activation of certain protooncogenes appears to play a role in the development of some thyroid carcinomas, for example, the so-called PTC oncogene in cases of papillary carcinoma, and the RET protooncogene in some medullary carcinomas. The RET protooncogene is a growth factor receptor (Chapter 6). Recent studies indicate that the PTC oncogene is also related to the RET gene. It is formed when the RET gene is displaced by rearrangements from its normal location, and is overexpressed under the influence of other, adjacent genes at the new location.

PAPILLARY CARCINOMA

Papillary carcinomas represent the most common form of thyroid cancer (80% of all cases). They may occur at any age and account for the vast majority of thyroid carcinomas associated with previous exposure to ionizing radiation.

MORPHOLOGY. Papillary carcinomas may present as solitary or multifocal lesions within the thyroid. In some cases, they may be well circumscribed and even encapsulated; in other instances, they infiltrate the adjacent parenchyma with ill-defined margins. The lesions may contain areas of fibrosis and calcification and are often cystic. On the cut surface, they may appear granular and may sometimes contain grossly discernible papillary foci. The definitive diagnosis of papillary carcinoma can be made only after microscopic examination. As currently used, the diagnosis of papillary carcinoma is based on nuclear features rather than a papillary architecture. The nuclei of papillary carcinoma cells contain very finely dispersed chromatin, which imparts an **optically clear** appearance, giving rise to the designation "ground-glass" or "Orphan Annie" nuclei (Fig. 20–12). In addition, invaginations of the cytoplasm may in cross-sections give the appearance of intranuclear inclusions. A **papillary architecture** is present in many cases, although some tumors are composed predominantly or exclusively of follicles. The latter still behave biologically as papillary lesions if they have the nuclear features described. When present, the papillae of papillary carcinoma differ from those seen in areas of hyperplasia. Unlike hyperplastic papillary lesions, the neoplastic papillae have dense fibrovascular cores. Concentrically calcified structures termed **psammoma bodies** are often present within the lesion. Foci of lymphatic permeation by tumor are often present, but invasion of blood vessels is relatively uncommon, particularly in smaller lesions. Metastases to adjacent cervical lymph nodes are estimated to occur in about half of cases.

Clinical Features. Papillary carcinomas present most often as a mass in the neck, either within the thyroid or in a cervical lymph node. The presence of isolated cervical nodal metastases, interestingly, does not appear to have a significant influence on the generally good prognosis of these lesions. In a minority of patients, hematogenous metastases are present at the time of diagnosis, most commonly in the lung. Most papillary carcinomas are indolent lesions, with 10-year survival rates of up to 85%. In general, the prognosis is less favorable among elderly patients, patients with invasion of extrathyroidal tissues, and patients with distant metastases.

FOLLICULAR CARCINOMA

Follicular carcinomas are the second most common form of thyroid cancer (15% of all cases). They usually present at an older age than do papillary carcinomas, with a peak incidence in the middle adult years. The incidence of follicular carcinoma is increased in areas of dietary iodine deficiency, suggesting that, in some cases, nodular goiter may predispose to the development of the neoplasm. There is no compelling evidence that follicular carcinomas arise from preexisting adenomas.

MORPHOLOGY. Follicular carcinomas may be grossly infiltrative or well circumscribed. Sharply demarcated lesions may be impossible to distinguish from follicular adenomas on gross examination. Larger lesions may infiltrate well beyond the thyroid capsule into the soft tissues of the neck. Microscopically, most follicular carcinomas are composed of fairly uniform cells forming small follicles, reminiscent of normal thyroid. In other cases, follicular differentiation may be less apparent. Occasional tumors are dominated by cells with abundant granular, eosinophilic cytoplasm (Hürthle cells). Extensive invasion of adjacent thyroid parenchyma makes the diagnosis of carcinoma obvious in some cases. In other cases, however, invasion may be limited to microscopic foci of capsular and/or vascular invasion. Such lesions may require extensive histologic sampling before they can be distinguished from follicular adenomas. As mentioned earlier, follicular lesions in which the nuclear features are typical of papillary carcinomas should be regarded as papillary cancers.

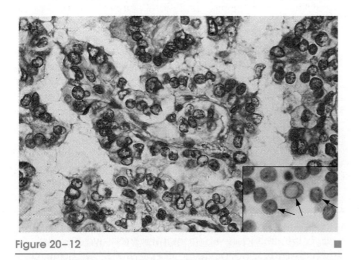

Figure 20–12

Papillary carcinoma of the thyroid. This particular example contains well-formed papillae lined by cells with characteristic empty-appearing nuclei, sometimes termed "Orphan Annie eye" nuclei. Inset shows cells obtained by fine-needle aspiration of a papillary carcinoma. Characteristic intranuclear inclusions (*arrows*) are visible in cytologic preparations. (Courtesy of Dr. Edmund Cibas, Brigham and Women's Hospital, Boston.)

Clinical Features. Follicular carcinomas present most frequently as solitary "cold" thyroid nodules. In rare cases, they _painless_ may be hyperfunctional. These neoplasms tend to metastasize via the bloodstream to the lungs, bone, and liver. Regional nodal metastases are uncommon, in contrast to papillary carcinomas. Follicular carcinomas are treated with surgical excision. Well-differentiated metastases may take up radioactive iodine, which can be used to identify, and ablate, such lesions. Because better-differentiated lesions may be stimulated by TSH, patients are usually treated with thyroid hormone after surgery in order to suppress endogenous TSH.

MEDULLARY CARCINOMA

Medullary carcinomas of the thyroid are neuroendocrine neoplasms derived from the parafollicular cells, or C cells, of the thyroid. Like normal C cells, medullary carcinomas secrete calcitonin, the measurement of which plays an important role in the diagnosis and postoperative follow-up of patients. In some cases the tumor cells elaborate other polypeptide hormones such as carcinoembryonic antigen, somatostatin, serotonin, and vasoactive intestinal peptide (VIP). Medullary carcinomas arise sporadically in about 80% of cases. The remainder occur in the setting of multiple endocrine neoplasia (MEN) syndrome IIa or IIb, or as familial tumors without an associated MEN syndrome. Germ line mutations in the RET protooncogene appear to play an important role in the development of medullary carcinomas associated with the MEN IIa and IIb syndromes. More recently, RET protooncogene mutations have also been identified in some sporadic cases. Sporadic medullary carcinomas, as well as some familial tumors, occur in adults, with a peak incidence in the fifth to sixth decades. Cases associated with MEN II, in contrast, occur in younger patients and may even arise in children.

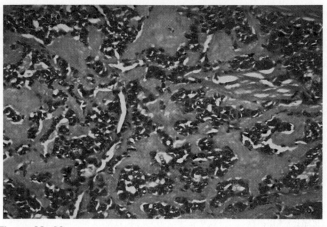

Figure 20–13 ■

Medullary carcinoma of the thyroid. These tumors typically contain amyloid, visible here as homogeneous extracellular material, derived from calcitonin molecules secreted by the neoplastic cells.

with mass effects such as dysphagia or hoarseness. In some instances the initial manifestations are caused by the secretion of a peptide hormone (e.g., diarrhea due to the secretion of VIP). Screening of relatives for elevated calcitonin levels or RET mutations permits early detection of tumors in familial cases. Sporadic medullary carcinomas, and those arising in patients with MEN IIb, are aggressive lesions, with a propensity to metastasize via the bloodstream, and 5-year survival rates of about 50%. Familial medullary carcinomas not associated with MEN, in contrast, are often fairly indolent lesions.

> **MORPHOLOGY.** Medullary carcinomas may arise as a solitary nodule or may present as multiple lesions involving both lobes of the thyroid. **Multicentricity** is particularly common in familial cases. Larger lesions often contain areas of necrosis and hemorrhage and may extend through the capsule of the thyroid. Microscopically, medullary carcinomas are composed of polygonal to spindle-shaped cells, which may form nests, trabeculae, and even follicles. Small, more anaplastic cells are present in some tumors and may be the predominant cell type. Acellular **amyloid deposits,** derived from altered calcitonin molecules, are present in the adjacent stroma in many cases (Fig. 20–13). Calcitonin is readily demonstrable within the cytoplasm of the tumor cells by immunohistochemical methods. Electron microscopy reveals variable numbers of intracytoplasmic membrane-bound electron-dense granules. Areas of **C-cell hyperplasia** are present in the surrounding thyroid parenchyma in many familial cases but are usually absent in sporadic lesions.

Clinical Features. Sporadic cases of medullary carcinoma present most often as a mass in the neck, sometimes associated

ANAPLASTIC CARCINOMA

Anaplastic carcinomas of the thyroid are among the most aggressive human neoplasms. They occur predominantly in elderly patients, particularly in areas of endemic goiter.

> **MORPHOLOGY.** Anaplastic carcinomas present as bulky masses that typically grow rapidly beyond the thyroid capsule into adjacent neck structures. Microscopically, these neoplasms are composed of highly anaplastic cells, which may take the form of large, pleomorphic giant cells; spindle cells with a sarcomatous appearance; or cells with a vaguely squamous appearance. Some tumors are composed of small anaplastic cells resembling those seen in small cell carcinomas arising in other sites. A significant number of such small cell tumors ultimately prove to be medullary carcinomas (discussed previously). Small cell carcinomas must also be distinguished from malignant lymphomas, which may also occur in the thyroid but have a much better prognosis. Foci of papillary or follicular differentiation may be present in some tumors, suggesting origin from a better-differentiated carcinoma.

Clinical Features. Anaplastic carcinomas grow with wild abandon despite therapy. Metastases to distant sites are common, but in most cases death occurs in less than 1 year as a result of aggressive local growth and compromise of vital structures in the neck.

Parathyroid Glands

The parathyroid glands are derived from the developing pharyngeal pouches that also give rise to the thymus. They normally lie in close proximity to the upper and lower poles of each thyroid lobe, but they may be found anywhere along the pathway of descent of the pharyngeal pouches, including the carotid sheath, the thymus, and elsewhere in the anterior mediastinum. *In contrast to several other endocrine glands, the activity of the parathyroids is controlled by the level of free (ionized) calcium in the bloodstream rather than by trophic hormones secreted by the hypothalamus and pituitary.* Normally, decreased levels of free calcium stimulate the synthesis and secretion of parathyroid hormone (PTH), which in turn

- Activates osteoclasts, thereby mobilizing calcium from bone
- Increases the renal tubular reabsorption of calcium
- Increases the conversion of vitamin D to its active dihydroxy form in the kidneys
- Increases urinary phosphate excretion
- Augments gastrointestinal calcium absorption

The net result of these activities is an increase in the level of free calcium, which in turn inhibits further PTH secretion. Abnormalities of the parathyroids include both hyperfunction and hypofunction. *Tumors of the parathyroid glands, unlike thyroid tumors, usually come to attention because of excessive secretion of PTH rather than mass effects.*

HYPERPARATHYROIDISM

Hyperparathyroidism occurs in two major forms, *primary* and *secondary,* and (less commonly) *tertiary* hyperparathyroidism. The first condition represents an autonomous, spontaneous overproduction of PTH, while the latter two conditions typically occur as secondary phenomena in patients with chronic renal insufficiency.

Primary Hyperparathyroidism

Primary hyperparathyroidism is one of the most common endocrine disorders and is an important cause of hypercalcemia. This condition is usually caused by a parathyroid *adenoma* or by *primary hyperplasia* of the glands. On rare occasions (less than 1% of cases), it is caused by a carcinoma of the parathyroids. Primary hyperparathyroidism is typically a disease of adults and is more common in women than in men. It may occur either sporadically or in association with one of the MEN syndromes. The elevated levels of PTH produce a number of changes, including excessive bone resorption, renal disease, and, of course, hypercalcemia.

MORPHOLOGY. The morphologic changes seen in primary hyperparathyroidism include those in the parathyroid glands, as well as those in other organs affected by elevated levels of calcium. In most cases the parathyroids harbor a solitary **adenoma,** which, like the normal parathyroids, may lie in close proximity to the thyroid gland or in an ectopic site (e.g., the mediastinum). The typical parathyroid adenoma is a well-circumscribed, soft, tan nodule, invested by a delicate capsule (Fig. 20–14). Unlike primary hyperplasia, the remaining glands are usually normal in size or somewhat shrunken owing to feedback inhibition by elevations in serum calcium. Microscopically, parathyroid adenomas are often composed predominantly of fairly uniform, polygonal "chief" cells with small, centrally placed nuclei. In most cases, at least a few nests of larger cells containing eosinophilic granular cytoplasm (oxyphil cells), or cells with more abundant clear cytoplasm, are also present. Follicles reminiscent of those seen in the thyroid are present in some cases. Mitotic figures are rare. A rim of compressed, non-neoplastic parathyroid tissue is often visible at the edge of the adenoma (Fig. 20–14). In contrast to the nor-

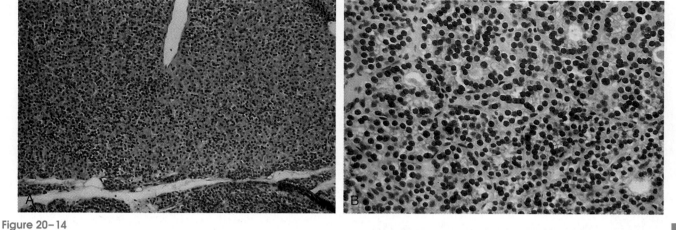

Figure 20–14

A, Solitary chief cell parathyroid adenoma (low-power view) revealing clear delineation from the residual gland below. *B,* High-power detail of chief cell parathyroid adenoma. There is slight variation in nuclear size and tendency to follicular formation, but no anaplasia.

mal parathyroid parenchyma, adipose tissue is inconspicuous within the adenoma.

Primary hyperplasia may occur sporadically or as a component of MEN syndrome I or IIa. In all of these settings there is variable enlargement of all parathyroids. In some cases, however, enlargement may be grossly apparent in only one or two glands, rendering the distinction between hyperplasia and adenoma difficult. Microscopically, the most common pattern seen is that of chief cell hyperplasia, which may involve the glands in a diffuse or multinodular pattern. Less commonly, the constituent cells contain abundant clear cytoplasm, a condition designated *water–clear cell hyperplasia.* As in the case of adenomas, stromal fat is inconspicuous within the foci of hyperplasia.

Parathyroid carcinomas may be fairly circumscribed lesions that are difficult to distinguish from adenomas. The tumor cells may be variable in shape or size but are usually remarkably uniform. They may be arrayed in trabeculae or form nodules, and are often separated by dense fibrous stroma. Because the usual cytologic features of malignancy are often absent, definitive diagnosis requires evidence of invasion or metastases.

Morphologic changes in other organs deserving special mention are found in the skeleton and kidneys. **Skeletal changes** include prominence of osteoclasts, which in turn erode bone matrix and mobilize calcium salts, particularly in the metaphyses of long tubular bones. Bone resorption is accompanied by increased osteoblastic activity and the formation of new bone trabeculae. In many cases the resultant bone contains widely spaced, delicate trabeculae reminiscent of those seen in osteoporosis. In more severe cases the cortex is grossly thinned, and the marrow contains increased amounts of fibrous tissue accompanied by foci of hemorrhage and cyst formation (osteitis fibrosa cystica). Aggregates of osteoclasts, reactive giant cells, and hemorrhagic debris occasionally form masses that may be mistaken for neoplasms ("brown tumors" of hyperparathyroidism). PTH-induced hypercalcemia favors the formation of **urinary tract stones** (nephrolithiasis), as well as calcification of the renal interstitium and tubules (nephrocalcinosis). Metastatic calcification secondary to hypercalcemia may also be seen in other sites, including the stomach, lungs, myocardium, and blood vessels.

Clinical Features. *The most common manifestation of primary hyperparathyroidism is an increase in the level of serum ionized calcium.* It should be noted that other conditions (Table 20–2) also produce hypercalcemia. Malignancy, in particular, is the most common cause of clinically significant hypercalcemia in adults and must be excluded by appropriate clinical and laboratory investigations in patients with suspected hyperparathyroidism. In patients with primary hyperparathyroidism, serum PTH levels are inappropriately elevated for the level of serum calcium, whereas PTH levels are low to undetectable in hypercalcemia due to nonparathyroid diseases. In patients with hypercalcemia due to secretion of PTH-related protein (PTHrP) by certain nonparathyroid tumors, radioimmunoassays specific for PTH and PTHrP can distinguish between the two molecules. Other laboratory alterations referable to PTH excess include hypophosphatemia and increased urinary excretion of both calcium and phosphate. Secondary renal disease may lead to phosphate retention with normalization of serum phosphate levels.

Primary hyperparathyroidism has been traditionally associated with a constellation of symptoms that included "painful bones, renal stones, abdominal groans, and psychic moans." Pain, secondary to fractures of bones weakened by osteoporosis or osteitis fibrosa cystica, and renal stones, with attendant pain and obstructive uropathy, were at one time prominent presenting manifestations of primary hyperparathyroidism. Because serum calcium levels are routinely assessed in the work-up of most patients who need blood tests for unrelated

Table 20-2. CAUSES OF HYPERCALCEMIA

Primary hyperparathyroidism
Malignancy, with or without bone metastases
Other endocrine disorders
    Hyperthyroidism
    Pheochromocytoma
    Vipoma
Vitamin D toxicity
Granulomatous diseases
    Sarcoidosis
    Tuberculosis
    Histoplasmosis
    Coccidioidomycosis
    Leprosy
Lymphomas, with ectopic production of 1,25-dihydroxyvitamin D
Drugs
    Thiazide diuretics
    Lithium
    Estrogens/antiestrogens
    Milk alkali syndrome
    Vitamin A, vitamin D toxicity
Immobilization
Acute and chronic renal disease

Modified from Petti GH: Hyperparathyroidism. Otolaryngol Clin North Am 23: 339, 1990.

conditions, clinically silent hyperparathyroidism is detected early. Hence, many of the classic clinical manifestations, particularly those referable to bone and renal disease, are seen much less frequently. Additional signs and symptoms that may be encountered in hyperparathyroidism include

- Gastrointestinal disturbances, including constipation, nausea, peptic ulcers, pancreatitis, and gallstones
- Central nervous system alterations, including depression, lethargy, and seizures
- Neuromuscular abnormalities, including weakness and hypotonia
- Polyuria and secondary polydipsia

Although some of these alterations, for example, polyuria and muscle weakness, are clearly related to hypercalcemia, the pathogenesis of many of the other manifestations of the disorder remains poorly understood.

Secondary Hyperparathyroidism

Secondary hyperparathyroidism is caused by any condition associated with a chronic depression in the serum calcium level, because low serum calcium leads to compensatory overactivity of the parathyroids. *Renal failure is by far the most common cause of secondary hyperparathyroidism*, although a number of other diseases, including inadequate dietary intake of calcium, steatorrhea, and vitamin D deficiency, may also cause this disorder. The mechanisms by which chronic renal failure induces secondary hyperparathyroidism are complex and not fully understood. Chronic renal insufficiency is associated with decreased phosphate excretion, which in turn results in hyperphosphatemia. The elevated serum phosphate levels directly depress serum calcium levels and thereby stim-

ulate parathyroid gland activity. In addition, loss of renal substances reduces the availability of α_1-hydroxylase necessary for the synthesis of the active form of vitamin D, which in turn reduces intestinal absorption of calcium (Chapter 8).

MORPHOLOGY. The parathyroid glands in secondary hyperparathyroidism are hyperplastic. As in the case of primary hyperplasia, the degree of glandular enlargement is not necessarily symmetric. Microscopically, the hyperplastic glands contain an increased number of chief cells, or cells with more abundant, clear cytoplasm (*water-clear cells*), in a diffuse or multinodular distribution. Fat cells are decreased in number. **Bone changes** similar to those seen in primary hyperparathyroidism may also be present. **Metastatic calcification** may be seen in many tissues, including lungs, heart, stomach, and blood vessels.

Clinical Features. The clinical manifestations of secondary hyperparathyroidism are usually dominated by those related to chronic renal failure. Bone abnormalities (renal osteodystrophy) and other changes associated with PTH excess are, in general, less severe than those seen in primary hyperparathyroidism. Serum calcium levels remain near normal due to the compensatory increase in PTH secretion. The metastatic calcification of blood vessels (resulting from hyperphosphatemia) may occasionally result in significant ischemic damage to skin and other organs, a process sometimes referred to as *calciphylaxis*. In a minority of patients, parathyroid activity may become autonomous and excessive, with resultant hypercalcemia, a process sometimes termed *tertiary hyperparathyroidism*. Parathyroidectomy may be necessary to control the hyperparathyroidism in such patients.

■ HYPOPARATHYROIDISM

Hypoparathyroidism is far less common than hyperparathyroidism. This disorder may be caused by surgical ablation of the thyroid, or by primary (idiopathic) atrophy of the glands. Certain developmental abnormalities, such as thymic aplasia (DiGeorge's syndrome), are also associated with hypoparathyroidism. Idiopathic primary hypoparathyroidism most likely represents an autoimmune disease. In some cases, this disorder is familial and associated with other endocrine abnormalities and autoimmune disorders. Chronic mucocutaneous candidiasis is sometimes encountered in these patients, suggesting an underlying defect in T-cell function. The major clinical manifestations of hypoparathyroidism are referable to hypocalcemia and include *tingling, neuromuscular irritability with Chvostek's and Trousseau's signs, carpopedal spasm,* and, on occasion, *seizures.* Morphologic changes are generally inconspicuous but may include cataracts, calcification of the cerebral basal ganglia, dental abnormalities, osteosclerosis, and osteomalacia.

Adrenal Cortex

Diseases of the adrenal cortex include those associated with cortical hyperfunction and hypofunction. In addition, a variety of mass lesions may occur in the adrenal cortex that may be nonfunctional or associated with cortical hyperfunction.

ADRENOCORTICAL HYPERFUNCTION (HYPERADRENALISM)

The adrenal cortex synthesizes and secretes steroid hormones, which fall into three major categories: glucocorticoids, exemplified by cortisol; mineralocorticoids, exemplified by aldosterone; and adrenocortical androgens. Hyperfunction of the adrenal cortex produces three major categories of clinical syndromes referable to excessive hormone levels. These include *Cushing's syndrome*, *hyperaldosteronism*, and a number of *virilizing syndromes*. Because of the overlapping functions of some of the adrenal steroid hormones the clinical features of these syndromes may also overlap.

Hypercortisolism (Cushing's Syndrome)

This disorder is caused by any condition that produces an elevation in glucocorticoid levels. *In clinical practice, most cases of Cushing's syndrome are caused by the administration of exogenous glucocorticoids.* The remaining cases are endogenous and caused by one of the following:

■ Primary hypothalamic-pituitary diseases associated with hypersecretion of ACTH
■ Primary adrenocortical hyperplasia or neoplasia
■ The secretion of ectopic ACTH by nonendocrine neoplasms (Fig. 20–15)

Primary hypothalamic-pituitary disease associated with oversecretion of ACTH, also known as *Cushing's disease*, accounts for more than half of the cases of spontaneous, endogenous Cushing's syndrome. The disease occurs most frequently during the third to fourth decades of life and affects women about five times more frequently than men. In most of these patients the pituitary gland contains a small *ACTH-producing adenoma* that does not produce mass effects in the brain. The responsible adenoma may be composed of either basophilic or chromophobe cells. In most of the remaining patients, the anterior pituitary contains areas of *corticotroph cell hyperplasia* without a discrete adenoma. In at least some patients the pituitary abnormality appears to result from excessive stimulation of ACTH release by the hypothalamus. The adrenal glands in patients with Cushing's disease are characterized by variable degrees of nodular cortical hyperplasia (discussed below), caused by elevated levels of ACTH. The cortical hyperplasia, in turn, is responsible for the hypercortisolism.

Primary adrenocortical neoplasms and hyperplasia account for between 15% and 30% of cases of endogenous Cushing's syndrome. This variant of Cushing's syndrome is also sometimes designated *adrenal Cushing's syndrome* or, because the adrenals function autonomously, *ACTH-independent Cushing's syndrome*. In most cases, adrenal Cushing's syndrome is caused by an adrenocortical neoplasm, which may be benign (adenoma) or malignant (carcinoma). Primary hyperplasia of the adrenal cortices is less common and its cause is poorly understood. It may be inherited as an autosomal dominant trait.

Secretion of ectopic ACTH by nonendocrine tumors accounts for most of the remaining cases of endogenous Cushing's syndrome. In most cases the responsible tumor is a *small cell carcinoma of the lung,* although other neoplasms, including *carcinoid tumors, medullary carcinomas of the thyroid, and islet cell tumors of the pancreas,* have also been associated with the syndrome. In addition to tumors that elaborate ectopic ACTH, an occasional neoplasm produces ectopic corticotropin-releasing factor, which in turn causes ACTH secretion and hypercortisolism. As with Cushing's syndrome associated with hypothalamic-pituitary disease, nodular cortical hyperplasia is present in the adrenals.

MORPHOLOGY. The morphology of the **adrenal glands** depends on the cause of the hypercortisolism. In patients in whom the syndrome results from **exogenous** glucocorticoids, **suppression of endogenous ACTH results in bilateral atrophy of the adrenal cortices,** due to a lack of stimulation of the zonae fasciculata and reticularis by ACTH. The zona glomerulosa is of normal thickness in such cases, because this portion of the cortex functions independently of ACTH. In cases of **endogenous** hypercortisolism, in contrast, the adrenals are either hyperplastic or contain a cortical neoplasm.

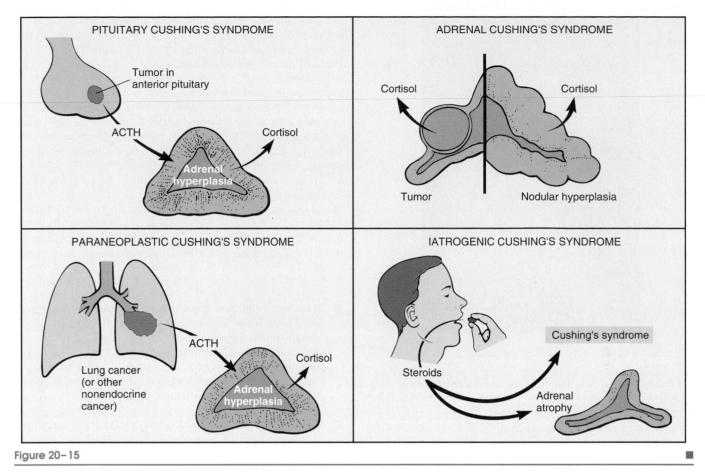

Figure 20–15   ■

Schematic representation of the various forms of Cushing's syndrome, illustrating the three endogenous forms as well as the more common exogenous (iatrogenic) form. ACTH, adrenocorticotropic hormone.

In Cushing's syndrome caused by increased ACTH secretion by either the pituitary or an ectopic source (e.g., a small cell carcinoma of the lung), **stimulation of the adrenal glands causes bilateral hyperplasia.** The adrenal cortices in such cases are diffusely thickened and yellow, owing to an increase in the size and number of lipid-rich cells in the zonae fasciculata and reticularis (Fig. 20–16). Some degree of nodularity is common and may be pronounced (nodular hyperplasia). The zona glomerulosa may be atrophic. An additional, rare form of hyperplasia is a familial condition associated with prominent lipofuscin deposits in the cells of the zona fasciculata and resultant brown-black discoloration of the adrenals. **Primary adrenocortical neoplasms** causing Cushing's syndrome may be benign or malignant. Adrenocortical adenomas are encapsulated, expansile, yellow tumors, usually composed of lipid-rich cells similar to those encountered in the normal zona fasciculata (Fig. 20–17). Their morphology is identical to that of nonfunctional adenomas and of adenomas associated with hyperaldosteronism (discussed below). The adjacent adrenal cortex and that of the contralateral adrenal gland are atrophic, owing to suppression of endogenous ACTH by high cortisol levels. Carcinomas associated with Cushing's syndrome tend to be larger than adenomas. Their morphology is identical to that of nonfunctional adrenocortical carcinomas, discussed below.

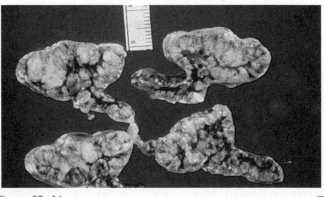

Figure 20–16   ■

Adrenocortical hyperplasia. The adrenal cortex is yellow, thickened, and multinodular owing to hypertrophy and hyperplasia of the lipid-rich zonae fasciculata and reticularis.

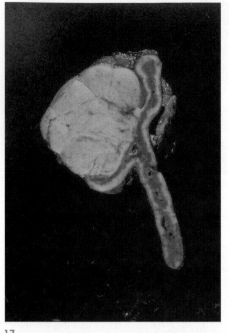

Figure 20–17 ■

Adrenocortical adenoma. The adenoma is distinguished from nodular hyperplasia by its solitary, circumscribed nature. The functional status of an adrenocortical adenoma cannot be predicted from its gross or microscopic appearance.

The **pituitary gland** shows changes in all forms of Cushing's syndrome. The most common alteration, resulting from high levels of endogenous or exogenous glucocorticoids, is termed **Crooke's hyaline change.** In this condition, the normal granular, basophilic cytoplasm of the ACTH-producing cells in the anterior pituitary is replaced by homogeneous, lightly basophilic material; this change is caused by the accumulation of intermediate cytokeratin filaments in their cytoplasm. In patients with Cushing's syndrome of hypothalamic-pituitary origin **(Cushing's disease),** the pituitary usually contains either an **ACTH-secreting pituitary adenoma** or foci of **ACTH-cell hyperplasia.**

Clinical Features. Cushing's syndrome usually develops gradually and, like many other endocrine abnormalities, may be quite subtle in its early stages. Early manifestations include *hypertension* and *weight gain.* With time, the more characteristic centripetal distribution of adipose tissue becomes apparent, with resultant *truncal obesity,* "moon" facies, and accumulation of fat in the posterior neck and back ("buffalo hump"). Hypercortisolism causes selective atrophy of fast-twitch (type II) myofibers, with resultant *decreased muscle mass* and proximal limb weakness. Glucocorticoids induce gluconeogenesis and inhibit the uptake of glucose by cells, with resultant *hyperglycemia, glucosuria,* and *polydipsia.* The

catabolic effects on proteins cause loss of collagen and resorption of bones. Thus, the skin is thin, fragile, and easily bruised; *cutaneous striae* are particularly common in the abdominal area. Bone resorption results in the development of *osteoporosis,* with consequent backache and increased susceptibility to fractures. Because glucocorticoids suppress the immune response, patients with Cushing's syndrome are also at increased risk for a variety of infections. Additional manifestations include *hirsutism* and *menstrual abnormalities,* as well as a number of *mental disturbances,* including mood swings, depression, and frank psychosis.

The laboratory diagnosis of Cushing's syndrome is based on (1) the 24-hour urinary free cortisol level, which is always increased; and (2) loss of the normal diurnal pattern of cortisol secretion. Localization of the cause of Cushing's syndrome depends on the level of serum ACTH and measurement of urinary steroid excretion after administration of dexamethasone.

■ In the most common form, pituitary Cushing's syndrome, ACTH levels are elevated and cannot be suppressed by administration of a low dose of dexamethasone. Hence, there is no reduction in urinary excretion of 17-hydroxycorticosteroids. However, the pituitary responds to a higher dose of injected dexamethasone by a reduction in ACTH secretion that is reflected by suppression of urinary steroid excretion.

■ With ectopic ACTH secretion, the ACTH level is elevated as expected, but its secretion is completely insensitive to low or high doses of exogenously administered dexamethasone.

■ When Cushing's syndrome is caused by an adrenal tumor, the ACTH level is very low because of feedback inhibition of the pituitary. As with ectopic ACTH secretion, both low- and high-dose dexamethasone fail to suppress cortisol production and excretion.

Hyperaldosteronism

Excessive levels of aldosterone cause *sodium retention and potassium excretion, with resultant hypertension and hypokalemia.* Hyperaldosteronism may be primary, or it may be secondary to an extra-adrenal cause. In *secondary hyperaldosteronism,* aldosterone release occurs in response to activation of the renin-angiotensin system. It is characterized by *increased levels of plasma renin* and is encountered in conditions such as congestive heart failure, decreased renal perfusion (e.g., arteriolar nephrosclerosis, renal artery stenosis), hypoalbuminemia, and pregnancy (due to estrogen-induced increases in plasma renin substrate). *Primary hyperaldosteronism,* in contrast, indicates a primary, autonomous overproduction of aldosterone, with resultant suppression of the renin-angiotensin system, and *decreased plasma renin activity.* Primary hyperaldosteronism is caused either by an aldosterone-producing adrenocortical neoplasm, usually an adenoma, or by primary adrenocortical hyperplasia.

MORPHOLOGY. In roughly 80% of cases, primary hyperaldosteronism is caused by an **aldosterone-secreting adenoma** in one adrenal gland, a condition referred to as **Conn's syndrome.** In most cases, the adenomas are solitary, although multiple adenomas may be present in an occasional patient. In contrast to cortical adenomas associated with Cushing's syndrome, those associated with hyperaldosteronism do not usually suppress ACTH secretion. Therefore the adjacent adrenal cortex, and that of the contralateral gland, are not atrophic. Morphologically the adenomas that cause primary hyperaldosteronism are indistinguishable from other functional or nonfunctional adrenocortical adenomas. In about 15% of cases, primary hyperaldosteronism is caused by **primary adrenocortical hyperplasia,** also termed **idiopathic hyperaldosteronism.** In most of these latter cases, the adrenal cortex is either diffusely or irregularly hyperplastic, owing to proliferation of the cells in the zona glomerulosa.

Clinical Features. The clinical manifestations of primary hyperaldosteronism are those of hypertension and hypokalemia. Serum renin, as mentioned above, is low. Conn's syndrome occurs most frequently in middle adult life and is more common in females than in males (2:1). Although aldosterone-producing adenomas account for less than 1% of cases of hypertension, it is important to recognize them, because they cause a surgically correctable form of hypertension. Primary adrenal hyperplasia associated with hyperaldosteronism occurs more often in children and young adults than in older adults; it is managed with medical therapy.

Adrenogenital Syndromes

Virilization may be caused by a number of diseases, including primary gonadal disorders, and several primary adrenal disorders. The latter include adrenocortical neoplasms and an uncommon group of disorders collectively designated *congenital adrenal hyperplasia.* Adrenocortical neoplasms associated with virilization are more likely to be carcinomas than adenomas. They are morphologically identical to other functional or nonfunctional cortical neoplasms and will not be discussed further. Congenital adrenal hyperplasias represent a group of autosomal recessive disorders, each characterized by a hereditary defect in an enzyme involved in cortisol biosynthesis. In these conditions, decreased cortisol production results in a compensatory increase in ACTH secretion, with resultant adrenal hyperplasia, as well as increased production of cortisol precursor steroids, a number of which have androgenic (virilizing) activity (Fig. 20–18). *The most common enzymatic defect in congenital adrenal hyperplasia is 21-hydroxylase deficiency,* which accounts for approximately 95% of cases. Several clinical variants of

21-hydroxylase deficiency exist, each resulting from a different mutation in the 21-hydroxylase gene on chromosome 6.

MORPHOLOGY. In all cases of congenital adrenal hyperplasia, the adrenals are bilaterally hyperplastic, reflecting a sustained elevation of ACTH. The adrenal cortex is thickened and nodular, populated by lipid-rich cells indistinguishable from those seen in other forms of cortical hyperplasia. Hyperplasia of corticotroph (ACTH-producing) cells is present in the anterior pituitary.

Clinical Features. The clinical manifestations of congenital adrenal hyperplasia are determined by the specific enzyme deficiency and include *abnormalities related to androgen excess or deficiency, sodium metabolism, and (in severe cases) glucocorticoid deficiency.* Depending on the nature and severity of the enzymatic defect, the onset of clinical symptoms may occur in the perinatal period, later childhood, or (less commonly) adulthood.

The biochemical consequences of 21-hydroxylase deficiency are illustrated in Figure 20–18. In this form, *excessive androgenic activity* causes signs of masculinization in females, ranging from clitoral hypertrophy and pseudohermaphroditism in infants, to oligomenorrhea, hirsutism, and acne in postpubertal females. In males, androgen excess is associated with enlargement of the external genitalia and other evidence of precocious puberty in prepubertal patients, and oligospermia in older individuals. *Androgen deficiency* may be encountered in some forms of congenital adrenal hyperplasia (e.g., 17-hydroxylase deficiency), manifested by a lack of development of secondary sexual characteristics in females and by pseudohermaphroditism in males. In some forms of congenital adrenal hyperplasia the accumulated intermediary steroids have mineralocorticoid activity, with resultant *sodium retention* and hypertension. In other cases, however, including about one third of patients with 21-hydroxylase deficiency, the enzymatic defect produces mineralocorticoid deficiency, with resultant *sodium wasting.* Cortisol deficiency places individuals with congenital adrenal hyperplasia at risk for *acute adrenal insufficiency* (discussed below).

Patients with congenital adrenal hyperplasia are treated with exogenous glucocorticoids, which, in addition to providing adequate levels of glucocorticoids, also suppress ACTH levels and thus decrease the excessive synthesis of the steroid hormones responsible for many of the clinical abnormalities.

ADRENAL INSUFFICIENCY

Adrenal insufficiency, or adrenocortical hypofunction, may occur in a number of different clinical situations. As in the case of adrenal hyperfunction, adrenal insufficiency may reflect either primary adrenal disease (primary hypoadrenalism)

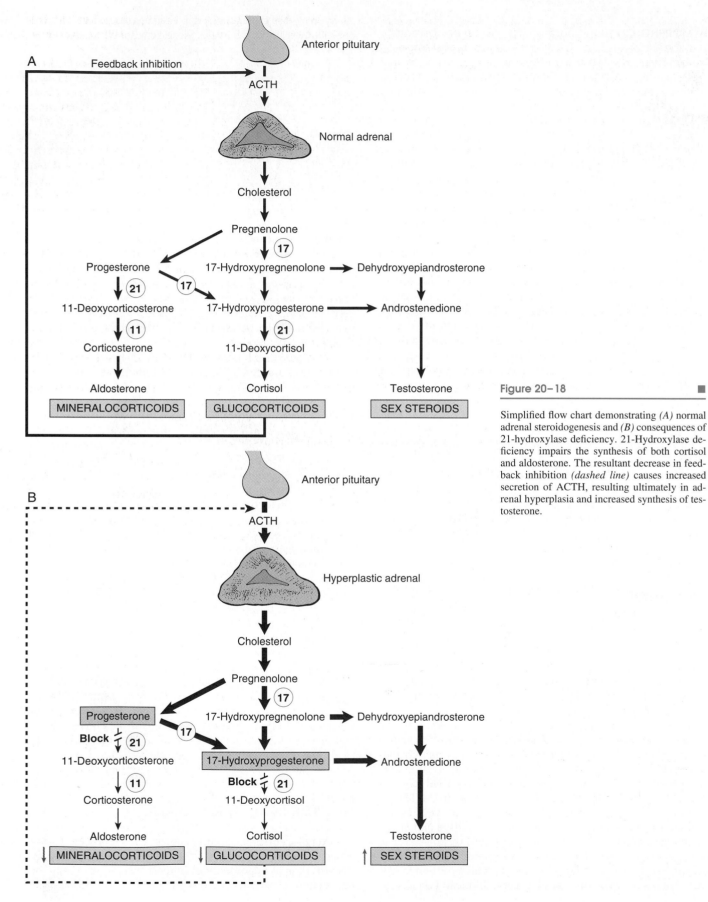

Figure 20–18 ■

Simplified flow chart demonstrating *(A)* normal adrenal steroidogenesis and *(B)* consequences of 21-hydroxylase deficiency. 21-Hydroxylase deficiency impairs the synthesis of both cortisol and aldosterone. The resultant decrease in feedback inhibition *(dashed line)* causes increased secretion of ACTH, resulting ultimately in adrenal hyperplasia and increased synthesis of testosterone.

or decreased stimulation of the adrenals due to a deficiency of ACTH (secondary hypoadrenalism). *Secondary hypoadrenalism* may be encountered in any of the disorders associated with hypopituitarism, such as Sheehan's syndrome, nonfunctional pituitary adenomas, and lesions involving the hypothalamus and suprasellar region. *Primary hypoadrenalism* may be further subdivided into chronic primary adrenal insufficiency, also known as Addison's disease, and acute primary adrenal insufficiency.

Chronic Adrenocortical Insufficiency (Addison's Disease)

In a paper published in 1855, Thomas Addison described a group of patients suffering from a constellation of symptoms, including "general languor and debility, remarkable feebleness of the heart's action . . . and a peculiar change in the color of the skin" associated with disease of the "suprarenal capsules" or, in more current terminology, the adrenal glands. Addison's disease, or chronic adrenocortical insufficiency, is an uncommon disorder resulting from progressive destruction of the adrenal cortex. In general, clinical manifestations of adrenocortical insufficiency do not appear until at least 90% of the adrenal cortex has been compromised. The causes of chronic adrenocortical insufficiency are listed in Table 20–3.

Autoimmune adrenalitis accounts for 60% to 70% of cases of Addison's disease. It may occur as a sporadic or familial disorder. In about half of the patients the autoimmune disease is apparently restricted to the adrenal glands; in the remaining patients, other autoimmune diseases, such as Hashimoto's disease, pernicious anemia, type I diabetes mellitus, and idiopathic hypoparathyroidism, coexist. The term *polyglandular syndromes* has been used to designate the various combinations of organ involvement that may be encountered. The frequency of autoimmune adrenalitis is increased in association with certain histocompatibility antigens, particularly HLA-B8 and -DR3. As with other autoimmune endocrine disorders, the factors that initiate autoimmunity remain unknown.

Infections, particularly tuberculosis and those produced by fungi, may also cause primary chronic adrenocortical insufficiency. Tuberculous adrenalitis, which once accounted for up to 90% of cases of Addison's disease, has become less common with the advent of antituberculous chemotherapy. However, with the resurgence of tuberculosis in many urban centers, this cause of adrenal deficiency must be borne in mind. When present, tuberculous adrenalitis is almost always associated with active infection in other sites, particularly the lungs and genitourinary tract. Among fungi, disseminated infections caused by *Histoplasma capsulatum* and *Coccidioides immitis* may also result in chronic adrenocortical insufficiency.

Metastatic neoplasms involving the adrenals are another potential cause of adrenal insufficiency. The adrenals are a fairly common site for metastases in patients with disseminated carcinomas. Although adrenal function is preserved in most such patients, the metastatic growths sometimes destroy sufficient adrenal cortex to produce a degree of adrenal insufficiency. Carcinomas of the lung and breast are the source of a majority of metastases in the adrenals, although many other neoplasms, including gastrointestinal carcinomas, malignant melanomas, and hematopoietic neoplasms, may also metastasize to the organ.

MORPHOLOGY. The appearance of the adrenal glands varies with the cause of the adrenocortical insufficiency. In cases of hypoadrenalism secondary to hypothalamic or pituitary disease **(secondary hypoadrenalism),** the adrenals are reduced to small, flattened structures that usually retain their yellow color owing to a small amount of residual lipid. A uniform, thin rim of atrophic, yellow cortex surrounds a central, intact medulla. Histologically, there is atrophy of cortical cells with loss of cytoplasmic lipid, particularly in the zonae fasciculata and reticularis. **Primary autoimmune adrenalitis** is characterized by irregularly shrunken glands, which may be exceedingly difficult to identify within the suprarenal adipose tissue. Histologically, the cortex contains only scattered residual cortical cells in a collapsed network of connective tissue. A variable lymphoid infiltrate is present in the cortex and may extend into the subjacent medulla. The medulla is otherwise preserved. In cases of **tuberculosis and fungal disease,** the adrenal architecture is effaced by a granulomatous inflammatory reaction identical to that encountered in other sites of infection. Demonstration of the responsible organism may require the use of special stains. When hypoadrenalism is caused by **metastatic carcinoma,** the adrenals are enlarged and their normal architecture is obscured by the infiltrating neoplasm.

■

Table 20–3.   CAUSES OF ADRENAL INSUFFICIENCY

Acute
Waterhouse-Friderichsen syndrome
Sudden withdrawal of long-term steroid therapy
Stress in patients with underlying chronic adrenal insufficiency

Chronic
Major contributors
  Autoimmune adrenalitis
  Tuberculosis
  Metastatic disease
Minor contributors
  Systemic amyloidosis
  Fungal infections
  Hemochromatosis
  Sarcoidosis

Clinical Features. The onset of chronic adrenocortical insufficiency is usually insidious. The initial manifestations often include progressive weakness and easy fatigability, which may be dismissed as nonspecific complaints. *Gastrointestinal disturbances* are common and include anorexia, nausea, vomiting, weight loss, and diarrhea. In patients with primary adrenal disease, increased levels of ACTH precursor hormone stimulate melanocytes, with resultant *hyperpigmentation* of the skin and mucosal surfaces. The face, axillae, nipples, areolae, and perineum are particularly common sites of hyperpigmentation. By contrast, hyperpigmentation is not seen in patients with adrenocortical insufficiency caused by primary pituitary or hypothalamic disease. Decreased mineralocorticoid activity in patients with primary adrenal insufficiency results in potassium retention and sodium loss, with consequent *hyperkalemia, hyponatremia, volume depletion,* and *hypotension.* The heart is often smaller than normal, presumably because of chronic hypovolemia. Hypoglycemia may occasionally occur as a result of glucocorticoid deficiency and impaired gluconeogenesis. Stresses such as infections, trauma, or surgical procedures in such patients may precipitate an acute adrenal crisis, manifested by intractable vomiting, abdominal pain, hypotension, coma, and vascular collapse. Death follows rapidly unless corticosteroids are replaced immediately.

Acute Adrenocortical Insufficiency

Acute adrenocortical insufficiency occurs most commonly in the clinical settings listed in Table 20–3. As noted above, patients with chronic adrenocortical insufficiency may develop an acute crisis following any stress that taxes their limited physiologic reserves. In patients maintained on exogenous corticosteroids, rapid withdrawal of steroids or failure to increase steroid doses in response to an acute stress may precipitate a similar adrenal crisis, owing to the inability of the atrophic adrenals to produce glucocorticoid hormones. *Massive adrenal hemorrhage* may destroy the adrenal cortex sufficiently to cause acute adrenocortical insufficiency. This condition may occur in newborns secondary to birth trauma, in patients maintained on anticoagulant therapy, in postoperative patients who develop disseminated intravascular coagulation, during pregnancy, and in patients suffering from overwhelming sepsis (Waterhouse-Friderichsen syndrome). This catastrophic syndrome is classically associated with *Neisseria meningitidis* septicemia but can also be caused by other organisms, including *Pseudomonas* species, pneumococci, and *Haemophilus influenzae.* The pathogenesis of the Waterhouse-Friderichsen syndrome remains unclear, but it likely involves endotoxin-induced vascular injury with associated disseminated intravascular coagulation.

ADRENOCORTICAL NEOPLASMS

It should be evident from the discussion of adrenocortical hyperfunction that functional adrenal neoplasms may be responsible for any of the various forms of hyperadrenalism. However, not all adrenocortical neoplasms elaborate steroid hormones. Determination of whether a cortical neoplasm is functional or not is based on clinical evaluation and measurement of the hormone or its metabolites in the laboratory. In other words, *functional and nonfunctional adrenocortical neoplasms cannot be distinguished on the basis of morphologic features.*

Adrenocortical adenomas were described in the earlier discussions of Cushing's syndrome and hyperaldosteronism. Most cortical adenomas are nonfunctional tumors, and are usually encountered as incidental lesions at the time of autopsy. Whether functional or nonfunctional, the typical cortical adenoma is a well-circumscribed, nodular lesion that expands the adrenal or, in some cases, lies immediately outside the adrenal capsule. On cut surface, adenomas are usually yellow to yellow-brown, owing to the presence of lipid within the neoplastic cells. As a general rule, they are small in size, averaging 1 to 2 cm in diameter; in some cases, they may be difficult to distinguish from foci of nodular hyperplasia. Microscopically, adenomas are composed of cells similar to those populating the normal adrenal cortex. The nuclei tend to be small, although some degree of pleomorphism may be encountered even in benign lesions. The cytoplasm of the neoplastic cells ranges from eosinophilic to vacuolated, depending on their lipid content. Mitotic activity is generally inconspicuous.

Adrenocortical carcinomas are rare neoplasms that may occur at any age, including childhood. They are more likely to be functional than are adenomas and are therefore often associated with virilism or other clinical manifestations of hyperadrenalism. In most cases, adrenocortical carcinomas are large, invasive lesions that efface the native adrenal gland. The less common, smaller, and better-circumscribed lesions may be difficult to distinguish from an adenoma. On cut surface, adrenocortical carcinomas are typically variegated, poorly demarcated lesions containing areas of necrosis, hemorrhage, and cystic change. Invasion of contiguous structures, including the adrenal vein and inferior vena cava, is common. Microscopically, adrenocortical carcinomas may be composed of well-differentiated cells resembling those seen in cortical adenomas or bizarre, pleomorphic cells, which may be difficult to distinguish from those of an undifferentiated carcinoma metastatic to the adrenal. Adrenal carcinomas invade locally and metastasize via lymphatics and the bloodstream, with a median patient survival of about 2 years.

Adrenal Medulla

The adrenal medulla is embryologically, functionally, and structurally distinct from the adrenal cortex. It is populated by cells derived from the neural crest, termed *chromaffin* cells, and their supporting (sustentacular) cells. The chromaffin cells, so named because of their brown-black color after exposure to potassium dichromate, synthesize and secrete catecholamines in response to signals from preganglionic nerve fibers in the sympathetic nervous system. Similar collections of cells are distributed throughout the body in the extra-adrenal paraganglion system. The most important diseases of the adrenal medulla are neoplasms, which include both neuronal neoplasms (including neuroblastomas and more mature ganglion cell tumors) and neoplasms composed of chromaffin cells (pheochromocytomas).

PHEOCHROMOCYTOMA

Pheochromocytomas are neoplasms composed of chromaffin cells, which, like their non-neoplastic counterparts, synthesize and release catecholamines and, in some cases, other peptide hormones. Similar neoplasms may also occur in extra-adrenal sites, such as the organ of Zuckerkandl and the carotid body, where they are usually called *paragangliomas* rather than pheochromocytomas. These tumors are of special importance because, although uncommon, they (like aldosterone-secreting adenomas) give rise to a surgically correctable form of hypertension. Most of these neoplasms arise sporadically. In about 10% of cases, pheochromocytomas arise in association with one of several familial syndromes. These include the MEN syndromes (described later), type I neurofibromatosis (Chapters 7 and 23), von Hippel-Lindau disease (Chapters 6 and 23), and Sturge-Weber syndrome (Chapter 23). *About 10% of the adrenal pheochromocytomas are biologically malignant*, although the associated hypertension represents a serious and potentially lethal complication of even "benign" tumors. Frank malignancy is somewhat more common in tumors arising in extra-adrenal sites.

MORPHOLOGY. Pheochromocytomas range from small, circumscribed lesions confined to the adrenal (Fig. 20–19) to large, hemorrhagic masses weighing several kilograms. In most sporadic cases the pheochromocytomas are unilateral. In about ·

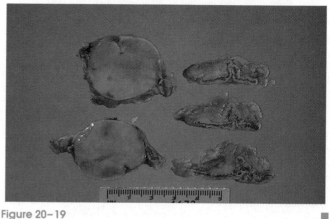

Figure 20–19 ■

Pheochromocytoma. A large bisected tumor affecting an adrenal gland is shown on the left. On the right, three slices of a normal adrenal gland are shown for comparison.

10% of cases, however, particularly when associated with a familial syndrome, they are multicentric and/or bilateral. On cut surface, smaller pheochromocytomas are yellow-tan, well-defined lesions that compress the adjacent adrenal. Larger lesions tend to be hemorrhagic, necrotic, and cystic and typically efface the adrenal gland. Incubation of the fresh tissue with potassium dichromate solutions turns the tumor a dark brown color, as noted previously.

Microscopically, pheochromocytomas are composed of polygonal to spindle-shaped chromaffin cells and their supporting cells, compartmentalized into small nests, or "Zellballen," by a rich vascular network (Fig. 20–20). The cytoplasm of the neoplastic cells often has a finely granular appearance, highlighted by a variety of silver stains, owing to the presence of granules containing catecholamines. Electron microscopy reveals variable numbers of membrane-bound, electron-dense granules, representing catecholamines and sometimes other peptides. The nuclei of the neoplastic cells are often quite pleomorphic. Both capsular and vascular invasion may be encountered in benign lesions. **The diagnosis of malignancy in pheochromocytomas is therefore based**

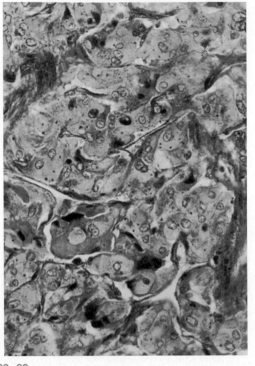

Figure 20–20 ■

Photomicrograph of pheochromocytoma, demonstrating characteristic nests of cells ("Zellballen") with abundant cytoplasm. Granules containing catecholamine are not visible in this preparation.

exclusively on the presence of metastases. These may involve regional lymph nodes, as well as more distant sites, including liver, lung, and bone.

Clinical Features. The dominant clinical manifestation of pheochromocytoma is *hypertension.* Classically, this is described as an abrupt, precipitous elevation in blood pressure, associated with tachycardia, palpitations, headache, sweating, tremor, and a sense of apprehension. Such episodes may also be associated with pain in the abdomen or chest, nausea, and vomiting. In practice, *isolated, paroxysmal episodes of hypertension occur in less than half of patients* with pheochromocytoma. In about two thirds of patients the hypertension occurs in the form of a chronic, sustained elevation in blood pressure, although an element of labile hypertension is often present as well. Whether sustained or episodic, the hypertension is associated with an increased risk of myocardial ischemia, heart failure, renal injury, and cerebrovascular accidents. Sudden death may occur, probably secondary to catecholamine-induced myocardial instability and ventricular arrhythmias. In some cases, pheochromocytomas secrete other hormones such as ACTH and somatostatin and may therefore be associated with clinical features related to the secretion of these and other peptide hormones. The laboratory diagnosis of pheochromocytoma is based on demonstration of *increased urinary excretion of free catecholamines and their metabolites, such as vanillylmandelic acid (VMA) and metanephrines.* Isolated benign pheochromocytomas are treated with surgical excision, after pre- and intraoperative medication of patients with adrenergic-blocking agents. Multifocal lesions may require long-term medical treatment for hypertension.

NEUROBLASTOMA AND OTHER NEURONAL NEOPLASMS

Neuroblastoma is the most common extracranial solid tumor of childhood. These neoplasms occur most commonly during the first 5 years of life and may arise during infancy. Neuroblastomas may occur anywhere in the sympathetic nervous system and occasionally within the brain, but they are most common in the abdomen; most cases arise in either the adrenal medulla or the retroperitoneal sympathetic ganglia. Most neuroblastomas are sporadic, although familial cases also occur. These tumors are discussed in Chapter 7, along with other pediatric neoplasms.

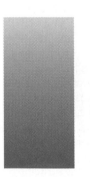

Multiple Endocrine Neoplasia Syndromes

The MEN syndromes are a group of familial diseases associated with neoplasms and/or hyperplasia of various endocrine organs. The disorders are inherited as an autosomal dominant trait. Their salient features are summarized in Table 20–4.

MEN I, or *Wermer's syndrome,* is characterized by abnormalities involving the *parathyroids, pancreas,* and *pituitary glands* (the "3 Ps"). The defect has been linked to a putative tumor suppressor gene on chromosome 11 (11q13). Hyperparathyroidism is the most common manifestation of MEN I.

Table 20–4. MEN SYNDROMES

	MEN I (Wermer's Syndrome)	MEN II or IIa (Sipple's Syndrome)	MEN IIb or III
Pituitary	Adenomas		
Parathyroid	Hyperplasia^{+++} Adenomas$^+$	Hyperplasia$^+$	
Pancreatic islets	Hyperplasia$^+$ Adenomas^{++} Carcinoma^{+++}		
Adrenal	Cortical hyperplasia^{++}	Pheochromocytoma^{++}	Pheochromocytoma^{+++}
Thyroid	C-cell hyperplasia$^{\pm}$	Medullary carcinoma^{+++}	Medullary carcinoma^{++}
Extraendocrine changes			Mucocutaneous ganglioneuromas Marfanoid habitus
Mutant gene locus	11q13	10q11.2 (*RET*)	10q11.2 (*RET*)

Relative frequency: +, uncommon; +++, common.

Parathyroid abnormalities include both hyperplasia and adenomas. The pancreatic lesions are the next most common. They include islet cell tumors, which may secrete a wide range of peptide hormones, including insulin, glucagon, gastrin, somatostatin, and vasoactive intestinal peptide. The dominant clinical manifestations are usually defined by the peptide hormone and include such abnormalities as recurrent hypoglycemia in insulinomas and recurrent peptic ulcers in patients with gastrin-secreting neoplasms (Zollinger-Ellison syndrome). The pancreatic islet cell tumors are often multiple and may be benign or malignant. Pituitary adenomas of any type may be encountered but are usually a less prominent feature than are abnormalities referable to the parathyroid and pancreas.

MEN II, also known as *MEN IIa* or *Sipple's syndrome*, is best remembered as the *pheochromocytoma–medullary carcinoma syndrome*. MEN II is clinically and genetically distinct from MEN I and has been convincingly linked to germ line mutations in the RET protooncogene on chromosome 10. Medullary carcinomas of the thyroid occur in 100% of patients. They are usually multifocal, virtually always associated with foci of C-cell hyperplasia. As noted in the earlier discussion of medullary carcinoma of the thyroid, the lesions in patients with MEN II are usually aggressive. The pheochromocytomas associated with MEN II are often bilateral and may arise in extra-adrenal sites. As in the case of pheochromocytomas in general, they may be benign or malignant.

MEN IIb, also known as *MEN III*, bears many clinical similarities to MEN IIa. Recent evidence indicates that it is a genetically distinct syndrome involving mutations in the RET protooncogene that are different from those associated with MEN IIa. In addition to medullary carcinomas and pheochromocytomas, MEN IIb is also accompanied by neuromas and/or ganglioneuromas involving the skin, oral mucosa, eyes, respiratory tract, and gastrointestinal tract. These additional characteristics distinguish MEN IIb from MEN IIa.

BIBLIOGRAPHY

Bilezikian JP: Etiologies and therapy of hypercalcemia. Endocrinol Metab Clin North Am 18:389, 1989. (A concise, useful review of hypercalcemia and its causes.)

Bravo EL, Gifford RW Jr: Pheochromocytoma. Endocrinol Metab Clin North Am 22:329, 1993. (A comprehensive review of the clinical aspects of this neoplasm.)

Brown RS: Immunoglobulins affecting thyroid growth: A continuing controversy. J Clin Endocrinol Metab 80:1506, 1995. (A short editorial on the pathogenesis of Graves' disease.)

Dawson DB, Jialal I: Multiple endocrine neoplasia. Diagn Endocrinol Metabol 14:281, 1996. (A lucid review of the clinical features and genetic basis of various MEN syndromes.)

Dayan CM, Daniels GH: Chronic autoimmune thyroiditis. N Engl J Med 335:99, 1996. (An excellent review that covers immunologic and clinical features.)

Eng CE: The *RET* proto-oncogene in multiple endocrine neoplasia type 2 and Hirschsprung's disease. N Engl J Med 335:943, 1996. (A concise discussion of RET mutations in MEN II.)

Feliciano DV: Everything you wanted to know about Graves' disease. Am J Surg 164:404, 1992. (A good clinical review.)

Gagel RF, et al: Changing concepts in the pathogenesis and management of thyroid carcinoma. CA 46:261, 1996. (An excellent review of the clinical and molecular aspects of thyroid cancer.)

Ikeda K, Ogata E: Humoral hypercalcemia of malignancy: some enigmas on the clinical features. J Cell Biochem 57:384, 1995. (A comprehensive discussion of the similarities and differences between hypercalcemia resulting from parathyroid hormone–related peptides secreted by malignant neoplasms, and primary hyperparathyroidism.)

Kovacs K: The pathology of Cushing's disease. J Steroid Biochem Mol Biol 45:179, 1993. (A concise review of the pathology of the pituitary gland in patients with Cushing's syndrome of hypothalamic-pituitary origin.)

Kovacs K, Horvath E: Pathology of pituitary tumors. Endocrinol Metab Clin North Am 16:529, 1987. (An authoritative review of the pathology of the pituitary, with emphasis on pituitary adenomas.)

LiVolsi VA: The pathology of autoimmune thyroid disease: a review. Thyroid 4:333, 1994. (A review of the morphologic features of autoimmune thyroid disease, including Graves' disease and various forms of chronic thyroiditis.)

Studer H, Derwahl M: Mechanisms of nonneoplastic endocrine hyperplasia—a changing concept: a review focused on the thyroid gland. Endocr Rev 16:411, 1995. (A review of hyperplasias of the thyroid, with a discussion of the differences and similarities between endocrine organ hyperplasia and neoplasia.)

Tomer Y, Davies TF: Infection, thyroid disease, and autoimmunity. Endocr Rev 14:107, 1993. (A review of the relationship between documented autoimmune thyroid diseases, including Graves' disease and Hashimoto's thyroiditis, and infectious agents.)

Tsigos C, Chrousos GP: Differential diagnosis and management of Cushing's syndrome. Annu Rev Med 47:443, 1996. (The title aptly describes this review.)

Vasen HF, Vermey A: Hereditary medullary thyroid carcinoma. Cancer Detect Prev 19:143, 1995. (A review of the diagnosis and prognosis of this neoplasm, including a discussion of screening methods for the detection of familial cases.)

Yanovski JA, Cutler GB Jr: Glucocorticoid action and the clinical features of Cushing's syndrome. Endocrinol Metab Clin North Am 23:487, 1995. (A discussion of the clinical features of Cushing's syndrome. This issue of the monograph also has several other articles on various aspects of Cushing's syndrome.)

21

The Musculoskeletal System

DENNIS K. BURNS, MD
VINAY KUMAR, MD

The musculoskeletal system imparts form and movement to the human body. The term *musculoskeletal disease* embraces a large number of conditions ranging from localized, benign lesions of the bone such as the osteochondroma, to generalized, life-threatening disorders such as muscular dystrophy.

In this chapter we will first consider some of the more common conditions affecting the bones and joints, followed by a discussion of selected non-neoplastic diseases of skeletal muscle. We will conclude with a few brief comments about tumors arising within skeletal muscle and other soft tissues.

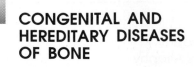

Diseases of Bone

The human skeleton is a complex system, well adapted to providing structural support, translating the activity of skeletal muscles into movement, and providing a protected environment for delicate internal organs. In addition, the skeleton houses the body's blood-forming (hematopoietic) elements and serves as the major reservoir of calcium and a number of other vital minerals. Disorders of the marrow are discussed in Chapter 12 and will not be repeated here. In this chapter we will consider those disorders of bone that do not originate within the hematopoietic tissues.

CONGENITAL AND HEREDITARY DISEASES OF BONE

Congenital diseases of bone include structural anomalies that may arise as isolated lesions or as components of a more complex syndrome. Some of the most common congenital structural lesions include aplasia (e.g., congenital absence of a digit or rib), the formation of extra bones (e.g., supernumerary digits or ribs), and abnormal fusion of bones (e.g., premature closure of the cranial sutures or congenital fusion of the ribs). Other hereditary conditions interfere with bone growth and/or maintenance of a normal osteoid matrix. These include achondroplasia and other forms of dwarfism, and osteogenesis imperfecta. In addition, a number of hereditary metabolic disorders, such as Hurler syndrome, may affect the bone matrix as well as other organs. These are discussed briefly with other genetic disorders in Chapter 7.

Achondroplasia. Achondroplasia is an hereditary disorder characterized by impaired maturation of cartilage in the developing growth plate. It is a major cause of *dwarfism* and is the most common of the congenital disorders of the growth plate (osteochondrodysplasias). Although it is an autosomal dominant disorder, only 20% of patients present with a family history; the remaining 80% of cases seem to arise from a spontaneous new mutation. Achondroplasia is most commonly encountered as a nonlethal heterozygous condition. Homozygous individuals are seen only rarely, because abnormal development of the chest cavity leads to death from respiratory failure soon after birth. The specific genetic abnormality responsible for achondroplasia remains unknown. Achondroplasia affects all bones, which are formed from cartilage. In heterozygotes, the most conspicuous changes are marked, disproportionate shortening of the proximal extremities, bowing of the legs, and a lordotic (sway-backed) posture. The cartilaginous growth plates contain hypoplastic or disorganized aggregates of chondrocytes instead of the long, orderly columns normally seen at this site.

Osteogenesis Imperfecta. *Osteogenesis imperfecta (OI), or "brittle bone disease," is a group of hereditary conditions characterized by abnormal development of type I collagen.* Type I collagen is present in many different tissues, including skin, joints, and eyes, and it is a major component of normal osteoid. A number of different genetic defects have been shown to interfere with the normal synthesis of type I collagen. OI is therefore not a single disease, but rather a spectrum of disorders of varying severity united by the common feature of *abnormal collagen synthesis and resultant bone fragility.* Four major forms of OI have been identified; most variants are inherited as autosomal dominants. As explained in Chapter 7, a single mutant allele prevents normal assembly of collagen owing to a dominant negative effect. Autosomal recessive forms are less common. Recognition of the various subtypes of OI is important for genetic counseling of affected families.

Whatever the subtype, OI is characterized by the presence of *multiple bone fractures.* In the more severe forms of the disease, bone fragility causes multiple fractures and fetal demise in utero or shortly after birth. In other variants fractures may not appear until childhood and do not appreciably shorten life. Other tissues containing type I collagen are also affected in OI, resulting in abnormal dentition; hearing loss; and a blue appearance to the sclera, caused by decreased scleral collagen.

OSTEOPOROSIS AND ACQUIRED METABOLIC DISEASES

Many nutritional and endocrine disorders affect the skeletal system. Nutritional deficiencies causing bone disease include deficiencies of vitamin C (scurvy) and vitamin D (rickets and osteomalacia). Both of these are discussed with other nutritional diseases in Chapter 8. Hyperparathyroidism, discussed in Chapter 20, also causes significant skeletal changes, which will be briefly reviewed in this section. The major focus of our discussion here is osteoporosis, a leading form of metabolic bone disease in the Western world.

Osteoporosis

Osteoporosis is a disorder in which a reduction of bone mass and the associated structural changes lead to increased bone fragility. The condition may be localized (as in disuse osteoporosis developing in a chronically immobilized extrem-

ity), or it may involve the entire skeletal system. Generalized osteoporosis may occur as a primary disorder, or it may be secondary to a wide range of conditions, listed in Table 21–1. When the term *osteoporosis* is used without qualification, it usually refers to the primary senile and postmenopausal forms of the disease. Primary osteoporosis is an extremely common condition that affects more than 15 million people in the United States. The medical care of these patients costs nearly $1 billion annually. *Senile osteoporosis* occurs in adults of both sexes and increases in severity with age. *Postmenopausal osteoporosis,* as indicated by its designation, affects women after menopause. It is by far the more common form and is an important cause of fractures in older women.

Pathogenesis. Although the pathogenesis of primary osteoporosis has remained frustratingly elusive, intensive investigations in the recent past have greatly increased our understanding of this disorder. It now appears that osteoporosis is not a single disease, but rather a group of disorders with a

■

Table 21–1. CATEGORIES OF GENERALIZED OSTEOPOROSIS

Primary
  Postmenopausal
  Senile
  Idiopathic juvenile
  Idiopathic middle adulthood
Secondary
  Endocrine Disorders
    Hyperparathyroidism
    Hyperthyroidism
    Hypothyroidism
    Hypogonadism
    Acromegaly
    Cushing's syndrome
    Prolactinoma
    Diabetes, type I
    Addison's disease
  Neoplasia
    Multiple myeloma
    Carcinomatosis
    Mast cell disease
  Gastrointestinal
    Malnutrition
    Malabsorption
    Subtotal gastrectomy
    Hepatic insufficiency
    Vitamin C, D deficiencies
  Rheumatologic Disease
  Drugs
    Anticoagulants
    Chemotherapy
    Corticosteroids
    Anticonvulsants
    Lithium
    Alcohol
  Miscellaneous
    Osteogenesis imperfecta
    Immobilization
    Pulmonary disease
    Chronic obstructive pulmonary disease
    Homocystinuria
    Gaucher disease
    Anemia

common morphologic expression: namely, a decrease in total bone mass and density. Some of the major factors related to the development of osteoporosis are summarized below.

Normally, the bone mass increases steadily during infancy and childhood, reaching a peak in the young adult years. *The total bone mass is an important determinant of the subsequent risk of osteoporosis.* It is determined in large part by genetic factors, although external factors, including physical activity, diet, and hormonal status, also play a role. Men achieve a higher bone density than do women, and blacks have greater peak bone mass than do whites. Hence, white females are the most vulnerable to osteoporosis and its attendant complications.

Age-related changes in bone density occur in all individuals and clearly contribute to the development of osteoporosis in both sexes. Bone is a dynamic tissue, and even in adults it undergoes continuous remodeling. This is characterized by alternating periods of bone resorption and new bone formation. Maximum bone density is reached during the third decade of life. Thereafter, it gradually declines. The rate of bone loss averages about 0.7% per year, although the rates vary considerably from one bone to another, with the greatest losses generally occurring in the spine and femoral necks. Hence, these are common sites of fractures in individuals with osteoporosis. The age-related loss of bone mass appears to be caused in large part by an *age-related decrease in osteoblastic activity.* Beyond the third decade, with each bone remodeling cycle, new bone formation does not quite compensate for bone loss, resulting in a gradual attrition of bones.

Hormonal factors play a significant role in the development of osteoporosis, especially in postmenopausal women. The administration of estrogen to postmenopausal women reduces bone loss and is associated with a decrease in the incidence of fractures. The effects of estrogen on bones appear to be mediated, at least in part, by regulation of cytokines that affect the bone. Decreased estrogen levels are associated with increased production of interleukin 1 (IL-1) by monocytes, which in turn stimulates increased production of interleukin 6 (IL-6) by osteoblasts. The latter recruits and activates osteoclasts, thus causing increased resorption of bone. Recent evidence suggests that estrogen deficiency may also lead to decreased synthesis of cytokines and growth factors that promote bone formation. Thus, *estrogen deficiency may cause bone loss by increasing bone loss as well as by decreasing bone synthesis.* Testosterone deficiency is present in about one third of men with senile osteoporosis. It also appears to contribute to increased bone turnover through local effects on cytokine production. However, this effect is not of the same magnitude as that caused by a lack of estrogen.

Genetic factors are another important piece in the osteoporosis puzzle. As noted previously, the maximum bone density that an individual reaches is determined, in large part, by genetic influences. Although many of the genetic factors responsible for normal bone development remain to be identified, one determinant of maximum bone density appears to be the vitamin D receptor (VDR) molecule. Certain variants of the VDR gene are associated with a lower maximum bone density, presumably because they impair the bone-forming effects of vitamin D. In one study of postmenopausal women, the genetic component in the pathogenesis of osteoporosis could be attributed largely to polymorphisms of VDR gene.

Mechanical factors, particularly weight bearing, are important stimuli for normal remodeling of bone, and reduced physical activity is associated with accelerated bone loss. This is demonstrated most dramatically by bone loss in paralyzed or immobilized extremities. The generally sedentary life style of many older adults undoubtedly contributes to the progression of osteoporosis.

The role of diet, including calcium and vitamin D intake, in the development, prevention, and treatment of osteoporosis remains incompletely understood. A person's maximum bone density is determined in part by the total dietary calcium intake, particularly before puberty. It appears that dietary calcium intake in adolescent females is considerably less than that in males of comparable age, and this may be one factor that predisposes women to the development of osteoporosis later in life.

To summarize, osteoporosis is a multifactorial disorder. Age-related bone loss, due in large part to reduced bone formation, is common to all forms of primary generalized osteoporosis. This loss is compounded in postmenopausal women by an increased resorption of bone, as well as by further reduction in bone synthesis brought about by declining levels of estrogen. Thus, both reduced bone formation and increased bone loss occur in osteoporosis. Although both of these factors play a role in most cases of osteoporosis, their relative contributions to bone loss may vary depending on age, sex, nutritional status, and genetic influences.

MORPHOLOGY. The hallmark of osteoporosis is a loss of bone, which tends to be **most conspicuous in parts of the skeleton containing abundant trabecular bone.** The bony trabeculae are thinner and more widely separated than usual, resulting in an increased susceptibility to fractures (Fig. 21–1). In postmenopausal osteoporosis, the bone loss is often particularly severe in the vertebral bodies, which may fracture and collapse. Similar bone loss is common in other weight-bearing bones, such as the femoral necks, another common site for fractures. The major microscopic changes are thinning of the trabeculae and widening of Haversian canals. Osteoclastic activity is present but is not dramatically increased. The mineral content of the remaining bone is normal, and thus there is no alteration in the ratio of minerals to protein matrix.

Clinical Features. In its early stages, osteoporosis is asymptomatic. Reliable diagnosis in such patients generally requires sophisticated radiographic measurements of bone density. In the later stages of the disease, decreased bone density becomes evident in routine radiographs, and the individual becomes prone to skeletal fractures, particularly involving the vertebral bodies, pelvis, femur, and other weight-bearing bones. Because the treatment of such fractures often requires long periods of immobilization in elderly patients, complications such as pneumonia and pulmonary thromboembolism are common and are a major cause of death.

The treatment of osteoporosis has been the subject of vigorous study. Estrogen supplementation has been shown to sig-

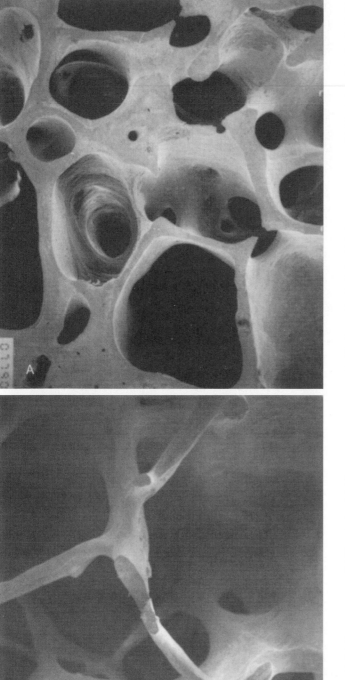

Figure 21–1 ■

Scanning electron micrograph of normal bone *(A)* and a bone with osteoporosis *(B)*. Note the thinning and wide separation of the trabeculae in the osteoporotic bone. (From Dempster DW, et al: A simple method for correlative light and scanning electron microscopy of human iliac crest bone biopsies. J Bone Miner Res 1:15, 1986.)

nificantly reduce the rate of bone and calcium loss in postmenopausal women, but it does not appear to reverse the established structural changes in the bone. Adequate dietary calcium intake before the age of 30 appears to reduce the risk of osteoporosis later in life, presumably by increasing peak bone denisty. Calcium supplementation later in life may cause a modest reduction in the rate of bone loss. Other, newer, therapeutic maneuvers include the administration of calcitonin, which has been shown to increase bone mass in some patients, and the administration of fluoride supplements.

Rickets and Osteomalacia

Both rickets and osteomalacia are manifestations of vitamin D deficiency (Chapter 8). It is important to recall that the fundamental change in these diseases is defective mineralization of bone, accompanied by an increase in nonmineralized osteoid. This is in contrast to osteoporosis, in which, although total bone mass is decreased, the mineral content of the remaining bone is normal.

In rickets, the defective mineralization involves the developing bones in children. Osteomalacia represents defective mineralization of bone that has completed its normal development. These disorders are detailed in Chapter 8.

Bone Diseases Associated With Hyperparathyroidism

As noted in the discussion of endocrine disorders in Chapter 20, parathyroid hormone (PTH) plays a central role in calcium homeostasis. The effects of PTH include the following:

■ Osteoclast activation, with increased bone resorption and calcium mobilization
■ Increased resorption of calcium by the renal tubules
■ Increased synthesis of active vitamin D, $1,25\text{-}(OH)_2D$, by the kidneys, which in turn enhances calcium absorption from the gut

The net effect of these activities is to raise the level of serum calcium, which, under normal circumstances, inhibits further PTH synthesis and release. Excessive levels of PTH, whether they result from autonomous secretion (primary hyperparathyroidism) or underlying renal disease (secondary hyperparathyroidism), cause significant skeletal changes related to abnormal osteoclastic activity. While the bone changes seen in primary hyperparathyroidism are caused exclusively by the effects of PTH, additional factors contribute to the development of bone disease in secondary hyperparathyroidism associated with renal failure. In chronic renal insufficiency, the loss of renal tissue leads to defective synthesis of $1,25\text{-}(OH)_2D$. Hyperphosphatemia also suppresses the activity of renal α_1-hydroxylase, further impairing the synthesis of active vitamin D. The resultant decrease in calcium absorption from the gut superimposes changes related to osteomalacia. Additional factors implicated in the development of bone disease in chronic renal failure include metabolic acidosis and aluminum deposition in bone.

> **MORPHOLOGY.** The hallmark of PTH excess is **increased osteoclastic activity, with bone resorption.** Cortical and, to a lesser extent, trabecular bone is lost and replaced by loose connective tissue. Bone resorption is especially pronounced in the subperiosteal regions and produces characteristic radiographic changes, best seen along the radial aspect of the middle phalanges of the second and third fingers. Microscopically, excessive osteoclastic activity is manifested by the presence of **increased numbers of osteoclasts and accompanying erosion of bone surfaces.** The marrow space contains increased amounts of loose fibrovascular tissue. Hemosiderin deposits are present, reflecting episodes of hemorrhage resulting from fractures of the weakened bone. In some instances collections of osteocytes and fibroblasts form a distinct mass, termed a **"brown tumor" of hyperparathyroidism.** Cystic change is common in such lesions, which may be confused with primary bone neoplasms, particularly giant cell tumor of bone (discussed later).

OSTEOMYELITIS

Osteomyelitis designates inflammation of the bone and marrow cavity. Although a number of different agents may cause bone inflammation, by convention, the use of the term *osteomyelitis* is restricted to lesions caused by infectious agents. Osteomyelitis may be an acute or chronic, debilitating illness. Although any microorganism can cause osteomyelitis, the most common etiologic agents are pyogenic bacteria and *Mycobacterium tuberculosis.*

Pyogenic Osteomyelitis

Most cases of acute purulent osteomyelitis are caused by bacteria. The offending organisms reach the bone by one of three routes: (1) hematogenous dissemination, (2) direct extension from a focus of acute infection in the adjacent joint or soft tissue, or (3) traumatic implantation after compound fractures or orthopedic surgical procedures. In most patients osteomyelitis is hematogenous in origin. In many cases the infection arises in a previously healthy individual without a known primary infection, while in other cases the source of infection is more obvious. *Staphylococcus aureus* is the most common causative organism. Other common pathogens include pneumococci and gram-negative rods. *Escherichia coli* and group B streptococci are important causes of acute osteomyelitis in neonates. *Salmonella* is an especially common pathogen responsible for osteomyelitis in patients with sickle cell disease. Mixed bacterial infections, including anaerobes, are frequent offenders in patients who develop osteomyelitis after bone trauma. The metaphyseal plate is the most common site of infection in children, while any area of the bone may

be involved in adults. In up to 50% of cases of pyogenic osteomyelitis, the causative organisms cannot be isolated because of previous antibiotic therapy, inadequate sampling for culture, or suboptimal culture methods.

> **MORPHOLOGY.** **Acute osteomyelitis** is characterized by an intense, neutrophilic inflammatory infiltrate at the site of bacterial invasion. The involved bone becomes necrotic within a matter of days owing to compression of vascular spaces by increased pressure in the marrow cavity and high concentrations of enzymes and other toxins released during the acute inflammatory reaction. The infection spreads through the cortical bone and may reach the periosteum, sometimes creating a subperiosteal abscess. Such abscesses are particularly common in children, in whom the periosteum is more loosely anchored to the cortical bone than it is in adults. From the subperiosteal area, the infection may spread into adjacent soft tissues to create draining sinuses, or it may track along the surface of the bone for a considerable distance. Detachment of the periosteum in such cases may disrupt the blood supply to bone, resulting in even more extensive ischemic necrosis of the bone. In infants, the existence of loose periosteal attachments and connections between the vessels in the metaphysis and epiphysis allows the infection to spread to the epiphysis and joint capsule. Extension of infection to the joints is less common in adults, because the periosteum is quite firmly attached to the articular margins.
>
> **Chronic osteomyelitis** develops as a sequela of acute infection. Over time, an influx of chronic inflammatory cells into the focus of osteomyelitis initiates a repair reaction that includes osteoclast activation, fibroblastic proliferation, and new bone formation. Residual necrotic bone, termed the **sequestrum,** may be resorbed by osteoclastic activity. Larger sequestra are eventually surrounded by a rim of reactive bone, termed the **involucrum** (Fig. 21–2). When a well-defined rim of sclerotic bone surrounds a residual abscess, the lesion is sometimes designated a **Brodie's abscess.** Viable organisms may persist in the sequestered area for years after the original infection. Chronic osteomyelitis may be complicated by the development of draining sinuses that open on the overlying skin.

Clinical Features. In its initial stages, pyogenic osteomyelitis causes systemic manifestations similar to those seen in any other acute infection, including fever, malaise, and leukocytosis. Local signs and symptoms of bone inflammation may be subtle and easily missed, particularly in infants and young children. Conversely, local pain, swelling, and redness may occur in some adults in the absence of systemic complaints. Although radiographic studies play an important role in the diagnosis of acute osteomyelitis, bone changes may not

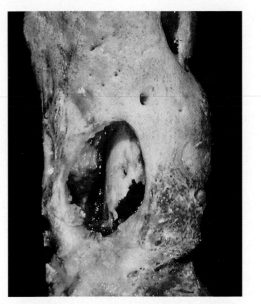

Figure 21–2

Resected femur from a patient with chronic osteomyelitis. Necrotic bone (the sequestrum) is visible in the center of a draining sinus tract, surrounded by a rim of new bone (the involucrum).

be visible on routine radiographs for more than a week after the onset of systemic manifestations. During this period significant bone destruction may occur. Radionuclide scans (e.g., gallium scans) are helpful in locating the site of infection early in the course of osteomyelitis. Infections of the bone demand vigorous and prolonged antimicrobial therapy and, if necessary, surgical debridement. Chronic osteomyelitis may supervene despite aggressive therapy in some cases, but it is particularly likely to develop when the diagnosis of osteomyelitis has been delayed or when the course of antibiotic therapy has been too brief. Complications of osteomyelitis include pathologic fractures, bacteremia, and endocarditis. Much less common complications are reactive systemic amyoidosis (Chapter 5) and squamous cell carcinomas within chronic sinus tracts.

Tuberculous Osteomyelitis

Mycobacterial infection of bone has long been a problem in developing countries of the world and, with the resurgence of tuberculosis, it is becoming an increasingly important disease in industrialized countries as well. Bone infection complicates an estimated 1% to 3% of cases of pulmonary tuberculosis. The organisms usually reach the bone through the bloodstream, although direct spread from a contiguous focus of infection (e.g., from mediastinal nodes to the vertebrae) may also occur. With hematogenous spread, *long bones and vertebrae are favored sites of localization.* The lesions are often solitary, but they may be multicentric, particularly in patients with an underlying immunodeficiency (e.g., acquired immunodeficiency syndrome [AIDS]). Because the tubercle bacillus requires fairly high concentrations of oxygen, the synovium, with its higher oxygen pressures, is a common site of

initial infection. The infection spreads to the adjacent epiphysis, where it causes a typical granulomatous inflammatory reaction with caseous necrosis and extensive bone destruction. *Tuberculosis of the vertebral bodies, or Pott's disease, is an important form of tuberculous osteomyelitis.* Infection at this site causes vertebral deformity and collapse, with secondary neurologic deficits. Extension of the infection to the adjacent soft tissues is fairly common in tuberculosis of the spine and often manifests as a so-called "cold abscess" in the psoas muscle.

PAGET'S DISEASE (OSTEITIS DEFORMANS)

Paget's disease of bone, first described in 1882 by the British surgeon Sir James Paget, is a peculiar disorder characterized by episodes of localized, frenzied osteoclastic activity and bone resorption, followed by exuberant bone formation. The end result of these intermittent processes is skeletal deformity caused by the accumulation of excessive amounts of architecturally abnormal, unstable bone. There are three phases in the development of Paget's disease: (1) an initial phase of osteoclastic activity, hypervascularity, and bone loss, followed by (2) a phase of mixed osteoclastic and osteoblastic proliferation, which gradually evolves into (3) a late, "osteosclerotic" phase, characterized by formation of dense, mineralized bone with minimal cellular activity. Paget's disease is uncommon before the age of 40, but its incidence increases steadily after that time. Males are affected slightly more often than females. In addition to causing bone deformities and related symptoms, Paget's disease is also an important predisposing factor in the development of osteogenic sarcoma in older patients.

Pathogenesis. When first described, Paget's disease was thought to be an inflammatory condition, a concept embodied in the synonym *osteitis deformans.* Although the idea that Paget's disease is inflammatory in origin remained out of favor for many decades, current evidence suggests that Paget's disease may in fact have an infectious etiology. Paramyxovirus-like particles and antigens have been identified within osteoclasts obtained from patients with Paget's disease. More recently, nucleic acid sequences of the canine distemper virus, a paramyxovirus related to the agent responsible for measles in humans, have been identified within lesions of Paget's disease. It is hypothesized that Paget's disease is a slow viral infection and that a paramyxovirus or a related agent induces the synthesis of IL-6 in infected cells, which in turn causes abnormal recruitment and activation of osteoclasts, thereby causing pathologic bone resorption. The subsequent osteoblastic activity may be a reaction to osteolysis.

MORPHOLOGY. Paget's disease may present with a solitary lesion (monostotic) or may be multifocal (polyostatic). The lesions are solitary in only 10% of cases. Although any bone may be affected, the spine, skull, and pelvic bones are especially common sites of involvement in patients with multifocal disease. The appearance of the individual lesions varies considerably, depending on their age. As noted, three basic morphologic phases have been described (Fig. 21–3). In the **primary (osteolytic) phase** of the disease, there is focal replacement of the marrow by loose, highly vascular connective tissue. The bony trabeculae are lined by huge multinucleated osteoclasts that cause extensive resorption of bone. In the next stage, osteoblastic proliferation is superimposed, resulting in a **mixed phase,** characterized by concomitant

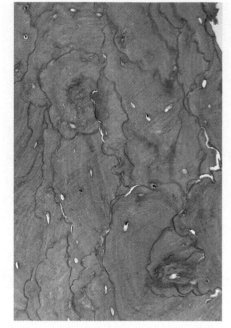

Figure 21–4 ■

Photomicrograph of Paget's disease demonstrating characteristic "mosaic" lines between areas of new bone formation.

bone resorption and new bone formation. Finally, the osteoclastic activity subsides, but irregular bone deposition continues in the so-called **osteosclerotic phase.** The new bone lacks the lamellar architecture of normal bone and is referred to as **woven bone.** Progressive deposition of new bone ultimately results in substantial thickening of both the cortical and trabecular bone. Because the bone formation occurs in an erratic pattern, areas of new bone are juxtaposed in a random mosaic pattern, giving the appearance of a jigsaw puzzle (Fig. 21–4). **This mosaic pattern of bone deposition is virtually pathognomonic of Paget's disease.** Although abnormally dense, the bone is weaker than usual and is subject to mechanical deformity and fracture.

Clinical Features. Paget's disease of bone is usually asymptomatic, discovered as an incidental radiographic finding. Sometimes it comes to attention because of an unexpected elevation in serum alkaline phosphatase in routine blood tests. In some patients, the early hypervascular bone lesions cause warmth of the overlying skin and subcutaneous tissue. In patients with extensive disease, hypervascularity may cause an increase in cardiac output; in exceptional cases, high-output congestive heart failure may develop as a complication of this hypervascular state. In the proliferative phase, common symptoms include headache, enlargement of the head, visual disturbances, and deafness, all caused by deformity of the bones of the skull and impingement on cranial nerves. Back pain is common and may be associated with disabling vertebral fractures and spinal nerve root compression. The long bones of the legs are often deformed because of the inability of the

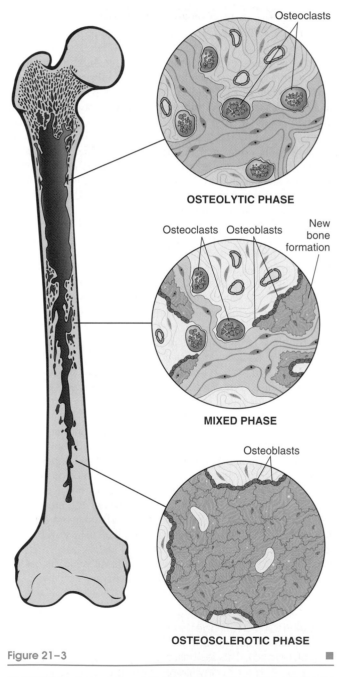

OSTEOLYTIC PHASE

MIXED PHASE

OSTEOSCLEROTIC PHASE

Figure 21–3 ■

Diagrammatic representation of Paget's disease of bone demonstrating the three phases in the evolution of the disease.

pagetoid bone to adequately accommodate the mechanical stresses associated with weight bearing. Transverse fractures of the brittle long bones have been likened to breakage of chalk, giving rise to the term *chalkstick fracture*. Laboratory evaluation discloses elevated levels of serum alkaline phosphatase, reflecting increased osteoblastic activity. Serum calcium and phosphate levels are typically normal, although urinary calcium excretion may be increased during the lytic phase of the disease.

The development of a sarcoma in association with the osteoblastic lesions of Paget's disease is a dreaded but fortunately uncommon complication, occurring in an estimated 1% of patients. The sarcomas are usually of the osteogenic type, although other histologic variants may also occur. They may develop in patients with either monostotic or polyostotic disease, and in the latter they may be multicentric. Their distribution generally parallels that of the Paget's lesions, with the exception of the vertebral bodies, which rarely harbor sarcomas. Even with aggressive multimodality therapy, the prognosis of patients who develop secondary osteosarcomas is poor.

BONE TUMORS

Primary bone tumors are considerably less common than are metastatic lesions. The most common primary sites for bone metastases, in descending order of frequency, are the prostate, breast, lung, kidney, gastrointestinal tract, and thyroid. Metastases may be destructive (osteolytic) or associated with reactive new bone formation (osteoblastic). It is common for both patterns to be present in a given lesion, although in some tumors, as exemplified by carcinoma of the prostate, osteoblastic activity dominates. The distinction between metastatic and primary bone tumors is straightforward in most cases but may be difficult in patients who present with a solitary lesion without a history of a primary tumor in another site.

The relative infrequency and great diversity of primary bone tumors combine to make them a diagnostic challenge. As a group, primary bone tumors occur at all ages and may arise in any part of the body. However, certain types of tumors target particular age groups and anatomic sites, and the recognition of these patterns is very helpful in arriving at a proper diagnosis. Most osteogenic sarcomas, for example, occur in adolescents and are especially common around the knee joint, a site of rapid bone growth during normal development. Diagnosis of bone tumors requires careful integration of the clinical history and radiographic appearance with the gross and microscopic features of the tumor. The salient features of the most common primary bone tumors, excluding multiple myeloma and other hematopoietic tumors, are listed in Table 21–2. Comments about some of the more common bone tumors follow.

Table 21–2. TUMORS OF BONE

Tumor Type	Common Locations	Age (yr)	Morphology
Bone-Forming—Benign			
Osteoma	Facial bones, skull	40–50	Exophytic growths attached to bone surface; histologically resemble normal bone
Osteoid osteoma	Metaphysis of femur and tibia	10–20	Cortical tumors, characterized by pain; histologically interlacing trabeculae of woven bone
Osteoblastoma	Vertebral column	10–20	Arise in vertebral transverse and spinous processes; histologically similar to osteoid osteoma
Bone-Forming—Malignant			
Primary osteosarcoma	Metaphysis of distal femur, proximal tibia and humerus	10–20	Grow outward, lifting periosteum, and inward to the medullary cavity; microscopically malignant cells form osteoid; cartilage may also be present
Secondary osteosarcoma	Femur, humerus, pelvis	>40	Complication of polyostotic Paget's disease; histologically similar to primary osteosarcoma
Cartilaginous Tumors—Benign			
Osteochondroma	Metaphysis of long tubular bones	10–30	Bony excrescence with a cartilagenous cap; may be solitary or multiple and hereditary
Chondroma	Small bones of hand and feet	30–50	Well-circumscribed single tumors resembling normal cartilage; arise within medullary cavity of bone; uncommonly multiple and hereditary
Cartilaginous Tumor—Malignant			
Chondrosarcoma	Bones of shoulder, pelvis, proximal femur, and ribs	40–60	Arise within medullary cavity and erode cortex; microscopically well-differentiated cartilage-like or anaplastic
Miscellaneous			
Giant cell tumor	Epiphysis of long bone	20–40	Lytic lesions that erode cortex; microscopically contain osteoclast-like giant cells and round- to spindle-shaped mononuclear cells; majority are benign
Ewing's tumor	Diaphysis and metaphysis	10–20	Arise in medullary cavity; microscopically, sheets of small round cells that contain glycogen; aggressive neoplasm

Bone-Forming Tumors

These neoplasms are characterized by the production of osteoid by the tumor cells. This type of intrinsic osteoid formation must be distinguished from bone formation in osteoblastic metastases, in which the osteoid is produced by reactive osteoblasts rather than neoplastic cells. In some primary bone-forming tumors, other mesenchymal elements, such as cartilage, may also be present. Given the origin of several elements of bone from common mesenchymal stem cells, such admixtures are not entirely surprising.

OSTEOMA

Osteomas are benign lesions of bone that in many cases represent developmental aberrations or reactive growths rather than true neoplasms. They are most commonly encountered in the head and neck, including the paranasal sinuses, but may occur in other sites as well. Osteomas present as localized, usually solitary, hard, exophytic growths attached to the surface of the bone. Histologically, they are composed of a bland mixture of woven and lamellar bone, which may be difficult to distinguish from normal bone. Although they may cause local mechanical problems and cosmetic deformities, they are not invasive and do not undergo malignant transformation.

OSTEOID OSTEOMA AND OSTEOBLASTOMA

Osteoid osteomas and osteoblastomas are benign neoplasms that have very similar histologic features. They are distinguished primarily by their size, site of origin, and certain radiographic features. *Osteoid osteomas* arise most often in the proximal femur and tibia during the second to third decades of life. They occur more commonly in males than in females. By definition, they are less than 2 cm in greatest dimension, whereas osteoblastomas are larger. Local pain, an almost universal complaint, can usually be relieved by aspirin. *Osteoblastomas* arise most often in the vertebral column, although they may occur in other sites as well. Like osteomas, they occur most often during the second to third decades, and they affect males more often than females. They may also cause pain, which is often more difficult to localize than the pain associated with osteoid osteomas. Local excision is the treatment of choice for most lesions; incompletely resected lesions may recur.

Radiographically, these neoplasms present as well-circumscribed lesions, which usually involve the cortex and rarely the medullary cavity of bone. The central area of the tumor, termed the **nidus,** is characteristically radiolucent but may become mineralized and sclerotic. A rim of sclerotic bone is present at the edge of both types of tumors; however, it is much more conspicuous in osteoid osteomas. Microscopically, both neoplasms are composed of interlacing trabeculae of woven bone surrounded by osteoblasts. The intervening stroma is made up of loose, vascular connective tissue instead of normal marrow elements and contains a variable number of giant cells.

OSTEOSARCOMA (OSTEOGENIC SARCOMA)

Osteosarcomas are malignant mesenchymal neoplasms in which the neoplastic cells produce osteoid. Excluding multiple myeloma, a tumor of B cells (Chapter 12), osteosarcoma is the most common primary malignant tumor of bone. Once a universally fatal disease, recent therapeutic advances have dramatically improved the outlook for these neoplasms. Several different variants of osteosarcoma exist; these can be distinguished from one another by clinical presentation; radiographic findings; histology; and, most importantly, prognosis. In the simplest classification scheme, osteosarcomas can be divided into primary forms, which arise de novo, and secondary forms, which arise as a complication of a known underlying process, such as Paget's disease of bone or a history of radiation exposure.

A number of different forms of primary osteosarcoma have been recognized. These include the "conventional" form, which accounts for about three fourths of the cases, and several less common variants. Conventional osteosarcomas *occur most often during the second decade of life.* Although they may arise anywhere in the body, *the most common site of origin is the area around the knee, specifically the distal femur and proximal tibia.* Males are affected more often than are females. Although the cause of most primary osteosarcomas remains unknown, as with other malignant neoplasms, mutations appear to be important in their pathogenesis. Mutations in the *p53* tumor suppressor gene, in particular, are present in many sporadic osteosarcomas. Germ line mutations in the retinoblastoma gene predispose patients to develop hereditary retinoblastomas as well as osteosarcomas.

MORPHOLOGY. The typical osteosarcoma presents as a large, ill-defined lesion in the metaphyseal region of the involved bone (Fig. 21–5). It characteristically destroys the cortex and frequently extends inwards into the marrow cavity and outwards into adjacent soft tissues. The tumor often elevates the periosteum to produce the so-called *Codman's triangle* on radiographs, which is formed by the angle between the elevated periosteum and the surface of the involved bone. Invasion of the epiphyseal plate is uncommon. Microscopically, **the hallmark of osteosarcoma is the formation of osteoid by malignant mesenchymal cells** (Fig. 21–6). This is seen in the form of islands of primitive bony trabeculae hugged by a rim of malignant osteoblasts. The amount of osteoid varies considerably in different tumors, but it must be present for the diagnosis of osteosarcoma to be made. Other mesenchymal elements, particularly cartilage, may also be present, sometimes in large amounts. The neoplastic mesenchymal cells in between osteoid and cartilage elements may be spindle shaped and uniform or quite pleomorphic, with bizarre, hyperchromatic nuclei and frequent mitotic figures. Giant cells, sometimes mistaken for osteoclasts, are often present.

Clinical Features. Osteosarcomas present as progressively enlarging, often painful masses that may come to attention because of a fracture of the involved bone. Although the combination of clinical and radiographic features may strongly suggest the diagnosis, histologic confirmation is necessary in all cases. Conventional osteosarcomas are aggressive lesions that metastasize via the bloodstream early in their course. Lung is a common site of metastases. Approximately 20% of patients have detectable pulmonary spread at the time of diagnosis; many more have occult metastases that raise their ugly heads later in the course of the disease. However, advances in surgical techniques, combined with radiation therapy and chemotherapy for metastases, have greatly improved the prognosis for patients with these tumors.

Secondary osteosarcomas occur in an older age group than do primary conventional osteosarcomas. They most commonly develop in the setting of Paget's disease or previous radiation exposure and rarely in patients with fibrous dysplasia and chronic osteomyelitis. Secondary osteosarcomas are highly aggressive neoplasms, which respond less favorably to current therapies than do conventional osteosarcomas. Other forms of osteosarcoma include the so-called parosteal, periosteal, telangiectatic, and small cell variants. A discussion of

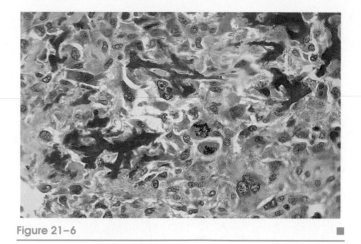

Figure 21–6   ■

Photomicrograph of osteosarcoma. Pleomorphic, mitotically active mesenchymal cells are producing dark-staining (calcified) osteoid, an essential feature of this tumor.

these less common lesions can be found in references included at the end of the chapter.

Cartilaginous Tumors

Like the bone-forming tumors of the skeleton, cartilaginous tumors span a spectrum of lesions ranging from benign, self-limited growths to highly aggressive malignancies. The more common types will be discussed here.

OSTEOCHONDROMA

Osteochondromas, sometimes called *exostoses,* are benign proliferations composed of mature bone and a cartilaginous cap. They are fairly common, comprising about one third of all benign tumors of the bone. Like some osteomas, osteochondromas probably represent malformations rather than true neoplasms. In keeping with this, they tend to stop growing once the normal growth of the skeleton is completed. Osteochondromas occur most often as solitary, sporadic lesions, but they may be multiple in a rare familial disorder termed *multiple hereditary exostosis.* Most osteochondromas are asymptomatic, but some may cause troubling cosmetic deformities. They usually arise from the metaphysis near the growth plate of long tubular bones and present as broad-based, bony excrescences, firmly anchored to the cortex of the adjacent bone. A cap of hyaline cartilage is present (Fig. 21–7), which, in young subjects, contains a growth plate similar to that seen in the normal epiphysis. The growth plate usually disappears once epiphyseal closure has occurred in other sites. Most follow a benign course. Rare instances of sarcomatous transformation have been documented, predominantly in patients with familial disease.

CHONDROMA (ENCHONDROMA)

Chondromas are benign lesions composed of mature hyaline cartilage that occur most often in the small bones of the hands and feet. Although most common in the third to fifth

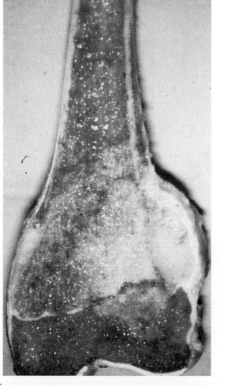

Figure 21–5   ■

Osteosarcoma originating in the metaphyseal region. The tumor has grown through the cortex and elevated the periosteum.

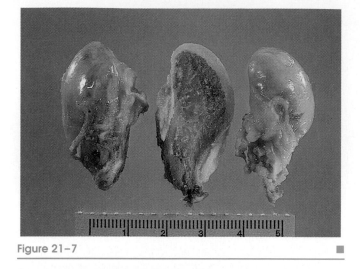

Figure 21–7   ■

Osteochondroma. Note the glistening cartilaginous cap, characteristic of this tumor.

MORPHOLOGY. The typical chondrosarcoma arises within the medullary cavity of the bone to form an expansile, glistening mass that frequently erodes the cortex (Fig. 21–8). Occasional lesions arise on the surface of the bone. Microscopically, chondrosarcomas vary greatly in appearance. The well-differentiated lesions may be quite innocuous looking, with only minimal cytologic atypia and are sometimes difficult to distinguish from non-neoplastic cartilage. At the other extreme, they may be composed of highly pleomorphic chondroblasts with frequent mitotic figures. Multinucleate cells are present, as are two or more chondroblasts lying within a lacuna. About 10% of low-grade chondrosarcomas transform into a high-grade sarcoma and are referred to as "dedifferentiated chondrosarcomas." The sarcomatous element may be an osteosarcoma or a fibrosarcoma.

decades of life, they may occur at any age and may be solitary or multiple. Several syndromes are associated with multiple chondromas: *Ollier's disease* is characterized by multiple chondromas preferentially involving one side of the body, and *Maffucci's syndrome* is characterized by multiple chondromas associated with benign vascular tumors (angiomas) of the soft tissues.

Chondromas are well-circumscribed lesions that usually arise within the medullary cavity of the bone (hence the term *enchondroma*). Less commonly, they may occur on the surface of the bone. Microscopically, they are composed of mature, hypocellular hyaline cartilage and normal-looking chondrocytes. Solitary chondromas are almost always innocuous. In contrast, chondrosarcomas develop in about one third of patients with multiple chondroma syndromes.

CHONDROSARCOMA

Chondrosarcomas are malignant neoplasms *populated by mesenchymal cells that produce a cartilaginous matrix.* Males are affected about twice as frequently as females. Among malignant nonhematopoietic tumors of bone, they are second only to osteosarcoma in frequency. Unlike cartilage-forming osteosarcomas the neoplastic cells in chrondrosarcomas do not form osteoid. Furthermore, as compared to osteosarcomas chondrosarcomas occur in older patients, with a peak incidence in the sixth decade. Their distribution also differs from that of osteosarcomas. They arise in central portions of the skeleton; common sites of origin include the shoulder area, pelvis, proximal femur, and ribs, although these tumors may occur anywhere. Most chondrosarcomas arise de novo, although some occur in patients with multiple enchondromas or, more rarely, osteochondromas. As in the case of osteosarcomas, several different variants of chondrosarcoma have been described, all with particular clinical and morphologic characteristics.

Clinical Features. Chondrosarcomas present most often as progressively enlarging, sometimes painful masses involving the central portions of the skeleton. Their rate of growth and ultimate behavior are closely correlated with histologic grade, with poorly differentiated lesions behaving in a more aggressive fashion than better differentiated tumors. Chondrosarcomas metastasize via the hematogenous route, most often to the lungs.

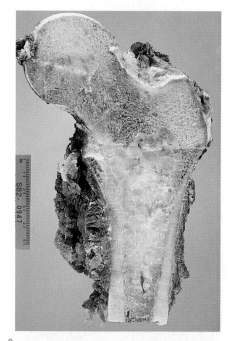

Figure 21–8   ■

Chondrosarcoma. Cartilage formation by the neoplasm causes the glistening, gray-blue appearance visible on the cut surface. The tumor has infiltrated the medullary cavity and invaded the overlying cortex.

Other Tumors and Tumor-Like Conditions of Bone

GIANT CELL TUMOR OF BONE

Giant cell tumor of bone, also known as *osteoclastoma,* is a neoplasm that contains large numbers of osteoclast-like giant cells admixed with mononuclear cells. They are fairly common tumors, comprising 20% of all benign tumors of the bone. *Most cases arise in the epiphyses of long bones, particularly the distal femur, proximal tibia, proximal humerus, and distal radius.* They occur most often between the ages of 20 and 40, with a slight female predominance. The histogenesis of giant cell tumors is incompletely understood. Current opinion suggests that the giant cell component is likely a reactive cell population derived from macrophages and that only the accompanying mononuclear cells are neoplastic.

MORPHOLOGY. Giant cell tumors present as radiolucent lesions involving the end of a long bone or, less commonly, another bone such as the sacrum. These tumors are almost always solitary. Longstanding tumors erode the cortex of the bone and may extend through the overlying periosteum. Grossly, the typical giant cell tumor has a dark-brown appearance owing to abundant vascularity. Areas of necrosis and cystic change are sometimes present. Histologically, they are composed of two major cell populations. The most conspicuous elements are usually large **multinucleated giant cells** that closely resemble osteoclasts (Fig. 21–9). These cells appear to be derived from fusion of monocytes and are thought to be a reactive, rather than neoplastic, component of the tumor. The proliferating neoplastic component is made up of round- to spindle-shaped **mononuclear cells.** This cell population contains a variable number of mitotic figures but usually has a fairly benign appearance. On rare occasions malignancy may develop, either de novo or in a previously treated giant cell tumor. In such cases it is the mononuclear cells, rather than the giant cells, that develop anaplastic features.

Clinical Features. Giant cell tumors usually present with local pain, which, because of the proximity of the tumors to joints, may be mistaken for arthritis. Biopsy is usually necessary to establish the diagnosis. It should be noted that a wide variety of bone disorders may contain multinucleated giant cells and that their presence alone is not diagnostic of a giant cell tumor of bone. Multicentricity is exceedingly uncommon in giant cell tumors and, when present, should raise suspicion of hyperparathyroidism, in which the presence of multinucleate osteoclasts creates a more than passing resemblance to giant cell tumors. The behavior of these neoplasms is somewhat unpredictable. Although they are histologically benign, recurrences are common after simple curettage. Sarcomatous transformation is rare but, as noted, may occur de novo or in a previously benign tumor treated with radiation therapy. On occasion, a histologically benign giant cell tumor may metastasize, usually to the lung.

EWING'S SARCOMA

Ewing's sarcoma is a primitive malignant neoplasm of bone and soft tissues that occurs predominantly in children and adolescents, with a peak incidence in the second decade of life. *It is a common malignancy of bone in children, second only to osteosarcoma.* Overall, it is the third most common malignant bone tumor, exceeded only by osteosarcoma and chondrosarcoma. The histogenesis of Ewing's sarcoma remained a mystery until recently. It has now been demonstrated that most cases possess a t(11;22) (q24;q12) chromosomal translocation identical to that seen in primitive neuroectodermal tumors (PNETs) of bone and soft tissue. This translocation involves the Ewing's sarcoma gene at 22q12. This similarity has led some observers to believe that Ewing's sarcoma represents a type of undifferentiated neuroectodermal malignancy. Whatever its histogenesis, Ewing's sarcoma is a highly aggressive neoplasm that must be differentiated from other pediatric tumors composed of "small blue cells" (Chapter 7).

MORPHOLOGY. Ewing's sarcoma arises within the medullary cavity of the affected bone to produce a soft, expansile mass. **The femur, tibia, and pelvis are favored sites of origin,** although the tumor can arise in other bones and, on occasion, in the soft tissues. It occurs most often in the diaphysis, but spread to other parts is not uncommon. The tumor usually extends beyond the medullary cavity into the cortical bone and periosteum, where it may produce lamellae of reactive bone in an onion-skin pattern. Microscopically, Ewing's sarcoma is composed of **sheets of primitive cells with small, fairly uniform nuclei and only scant cytoplasm.** The cytoplasm of the tumor cells contains glyco-

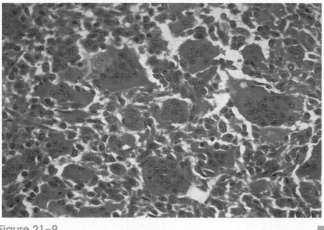

Figure 21–9

Photomicrograph of giant cell tumor of bone. Numerous osteoclast-like giant cells admixed with neoplastic mononuclear cells are visible.

gen, a feature readily demonstrated in periodic acid–Schiff (PAS) stains or by electron microscopy. The neoplasm may be associated with reactive bone formation in the medullary cavity, but the neoplastic cells do not produce osteoid. Immunohistochemical studies may be required to distinguish Ewing's sarcoma from other small blue cell tumors such as neuroblastoma, rhabdomyosarcoma, and malignant lymphoma.

Clinical Features. Ewing's sarcoma classically presents with pain, often accompanied by local inflammation. Fever is fairly common and may initially suggest the possibility of an inflammatory lesion. The diagnosis requires biopsy, with demonstration of the characteristic morphologic and cytogenetic features of the tumor. It is important that Ewing's sarcoma be distinguished from other small blue cell tumors, because each type requires a different therapy. Recent advances in treatment have significantly improved the outlook for patients with this sarcoma, with the 5-year survival rate close to 75%.

FIBROUS DYSPLASIA

Fibrous dysplasia is an uncommon, benign, tumor-like lesion of bone in which the normal trabecular bone is replaced by proliferating fibrous tissue and disorderly islands of malformed bone. It occurs in three forms: (1) involving a single bone (monostotic fibrous dysplasia); (2) involving multiple, but not all, bones (polyostotic fibrous dysplasia); and (3) polyostotic disease with endocrine abnormalities. The pathogenesis of fibrous dysplasia is unclear. It appears to be a developmental defect in bone formation. Overexpression of the c-*fos* protooncogene and somatic mutations in the gene coding for a stimulatory nucleotide binding protein have been recently described in the polyostitic form of the disease and may play some role in its pathogenesis.

Monostotic fibrous dysplasia is the most common form of the disease, accounting for about 70% of all cases. It usually arises during adolescence and becomes quiescent after bone growth is complete. The most common sites of involvement are the ribs, femur, tibia, bones of the jaw, and calvarium, although other bones may be affected. Although most cases are asymptomatic, in some the lesion may come to attention because of fractures or local deformity of the bone.

Polyostotic fibrous dysplasia limited to bone accounts for about 25% of cases of fibrous dysplasia. It appears at a slightly earlier age than the monostotic form of the disease and can continue to cause problems during adulthood. Craniofacial involvement is common and, when present, may cause significant facial deformity. Involvement of the pelvis, femur, and shoulder girdle is also common and may cause debilitating deformities and pathologic fractures.

Polyostotic fibrous dysplasia associated with endocrine abnormalities, the least common of the fibrous dysplasias, accounts for approximately 3% of all cases. It occurs most often in females. Affected individuals develop unilateral bone lesions, café-au-lait spots on the same side of the body, and

precocious puberty. This constellation of clinical features is referred to as the *McCune-Albright syndrome.* Other endocrine abnormalities, including hyperthyroidism and Cushing's syndrome, may also develop in patients with this syndrome. More recently, fibrous dysplasia has been described in association with neurofibromatosis type 1 (von Recklinghausen disease).

MORPHOLOGY. The lesions of fibrous dysplasia are circumscribed and radiolucent. They are usually surrounded by a thin margin of sclerotic bone. Histologically, foci of fibrous dysplasia contain proliferating fibroblasts and abundant collagen, surrounding small, erratically distributed islands of woven bone (Fig. 21–10). Cartilaginous elements may be present but are usually only a minor component of the proliferation.

Clinical Features. The clinical features depend on the extent of skeletal involvement. Monostatic lesions may be asymptomatic. Pathologic fractures and bone deformity may occur in any type of fibrous dysplasia, but they are a much greater problem for patients with polyostotic disease. They may require curettage and bone grafting. Sarcomas are a very rare complication of fibrous dysplasia, usually encountered in patients who have received radiation therapy for their disease.

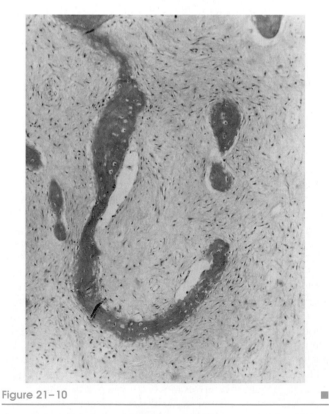

Figure 21–10 ■

Photomicrograph of fibrous dysplasia demonstrating slender bone trabeculae of woven bone surrounded by dense fibrous tissue.

Diseases of the Joints

The joints are subject to a wide variety of disorders, including degenerative changes, infections, autoimmune diseases, metabolic derangements, and neoplasms. In this section we will confine our comments to the most common forms of arthritis, such as degenerative joint disease, infectious arthritis, and gout. Rheumatoid arthritis, another important and potentially devastating disease of the joints, is discussed in detail in Chapter 5.

OSTEOARTHRITIS

Osteoarthritis, also termed *degenerative joint disease,* is the most common disorder of the joints. It is a very frequent, if not inevitable, part of aging and is an important cause of physical disability in individuals over the age of 65. *The fundamental feature of osteoarthritis is degeneration of the articular cartilage;* the structural changes that follow in the underlying bone are secondary. In most cases it arises without obvious predisposing factors and hence is called *primary.* In contrast, *secondary osteoarthritis* refers to degenerative changes developing in a previously deformed joint, or joint degeneration that occurs in the context of certain metabolic disorders, such as hemochromatosis or diabetes mellitus. The suffix *-itis,* commonly used to refer to inflammatory disorders, is misleading, because osteoarthritis is not primarily an inflammation of joints. Inflammation occurs secondarily; however, it may play a role in disease progression.

Pathogenesis. As mentioned earlier, articular cartilage is the major target of degenerative changes in osteoarthritis. Normal articular cartilage is strategically located at the end of bones to perform two functions: (1) bathed in synovial fluid, it ensures virtually friction-free movements within the joint; and (2) in weight-bearing joints, it spreads the load across the joint surface in a manner that allows the underlying bones to absorb shock and weight without being crushed. These functions require the cartilage to be elastic (i.e., to regain normal architecture after being compressed) and for it to have unusually high tensile strength. These attributes are provided by the two major components of the cartilage: a special type of collagen (type II) and proteoglycans, both secreted by chondrocytes. As is the case with adult bones, articular cartilage is not static; it undergoes turnover in which "worn out" matrix components are degraded and replaced. This balance is maintained by chondrocytes, which not only synthesize the matrix, but also secrete matrix-degrading enzymes. Thus, the health of the chondrocytes and their ability to maintain the essential properties of the cartilage matrix determine joint integrity. In osteoarthritis, this process is disturbed by a variety of influences.

Perhaps most important are *aging and mechanical effects.* Although osteoarthritis is not exclusively a "wear-and-tear" process, there is little doubt that mechanical stresses on the joint play a major role in its development. Evidence for this includes the increasing frequency of osteoarthritis with advancing age; its occurrence in weight-bearing joints; and an increase in the frequency of the disease in conditions that predispose the joints to abnormal mechanical stresses, such as obesity and previous joint deformity.

Osteoarthritis is accompanied by significant changes in both the composition and the mechanical properties of cartilage. Early in the course of the disease, the degenerating cartilage contains increased water and a decreased concentration of proteoglycans compared to healthy cartilage. In addition, there appears to be a weakening of the collagen network. These changes tend to reduce the tensile strength and the resilience of the articular cartilage. In response to these regressive changes, chondrocytes in the deeper layers proliferate and attempt to "repair" the damage by producing new collagen and proteoglycans. At the outset, the reparative activities are able to keep pace with the deterioration of cartilage. Eventually, however, the chondrocytes become "exhausted," and there appears to be a shift in the factors produced by them. They begin to secrete IL-1, which in turn activates the production of proteolytic enzymes, such as collagenases, by other chondrocytes. How this switch to chondrolysis occurs is not clear, but it is suspected that with persistent injury, changes in the biomechanical properties of the cartilage or changes in the underlying bone alter the function of chondrocytes.

MORPHOLOGY. The earliest structural changes in osteoarthritis include enlargement and disorganization of the chondrocytes in the superficial part of the articular cartilage. This is accompanied by changes in the cartilaginous matrix, including **fibrillation and splitting** at the articular surface (Fig. 21–11). Fissures gradually extend through the full thickness of the cartilage and into the subchondral bone. **Portions of the articular cartilage are eventually completely eroded** (Fig. 21–12), and the surface of the exposed subchondral bone becomes thickened and polished to an ivory-like consistency (**eburnation**) (Fig. 21–12). Fragments of cartilage and bone are often dislodged to form free-floating "joint mice" in the joint cavity. Synovial fluid may leak through defects in the residual cartilage and underlying bone to form **cysts** within the bone. The underlying trabecular bone becomes sclerotic in response to the increased pressure on the surface. Additional bone proliferation occurs at the margins of the joints to produce bony excrescences, termed **osteophytes.** As the joint begins to lose its integrity, there is trauma to the synovial membrane, which develops nonspecific inflammation. Compared with rheumatoid arthritis, the changes in the synovium are not as pronounced, nor do they occur as early.

Clinical Features. Signs and symptoms of osteoarthritis develop very gradually and usually affect only one or a few joints. The *joints commonly involved include the hips, knee, lower lumbar and cervical vertebrae, proximal and distal interphalangeal joints of the fingers, first carpometacarpal joints, and first tarsometatarsal joints.* Most individuals with primary osteoarthritis are asymptomatic until after the age of 50, although those with the secondary form of the disease may develop problems much earlier. Common complaints include joint stiffness and deep, aching pain, particularly in the morning. Repeated use of the joint tends to aggravate the pain. Crepitus, a crackling sound caused by exposed surfaces of bone rubbing against each other, is often present in severe cases. Some degree of joint swelling is common, and small effusions may develop. Heberden's nodes, small osteophytes on the distal interphalangeal joints, are most often encountered in women with primary osteoarthritis. With time, significant joint deformity may supervene, but unlike rheumatoid arthritis, fusion of the joint does not occur. In the differential diagnosis, rheumatoid arthritis features prominently (Chapter 5). The important morphologic features of these two disorders are illustrated in Figure 21–13.

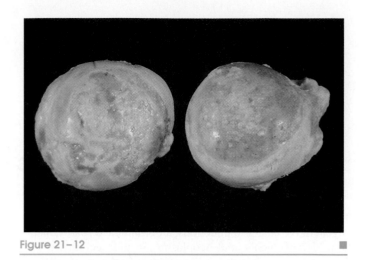

Figure 21–12 ■

Osteoarthritis in two femoral heads. *Left,* marked erosion of the articular cartilage; very little shiny cartilage remains. *Right,* a more advanced case, in which all cartilage is lost. Rubbing of the underlying bone has given it a polished, eburnated appearance. (Courtesy of Jim Richardson, DVM, PhD, Department of Pathology, University of Texas Southwestern Medical School, Dallas, TX.)

GOUT

Gout is a disorder caused by the tissue accumulation of excessive amounts of uric acid, an end product of purine metabolism. It is marked by recurrent episodes of acute arthritis, sometimes accompanied by the formation of large crystalline aggregates termed *tophi,* chronic joint deformity, and renal injury. All of these result from precipitation of monosodium urate crystals from supersaturated body fluids into the tissues. Although an elevated level of uric acid is an essential component of gout, not all individuals with hyperuricemia develop gout, indicating that factors in addition to hyperuricemia must play some role in the pathogenesis of the disorder. Gout is traditionally divided into primary and secondary forms, accounting for about 90% and 10% of cases, respectively. The term *primary gout* is used to designate cases in which the basic cause is unknown or, less commonly, when the cause is an inborn metabolic abnormality characterized primarily by hyperuricemia and gout. In the remaining cases, termed *secondary gout,* the cause of the hyperuricemia is known, but gout is not the main or dominant clinical disorder. The major categories of gout are listed in Table 21–3.

Pathogenesis. Elevation of the level of serum uric acid may result from overproduction or reduced excretion of uric acid, or from both. To understand the mechanisms underlying disturbances in uric acid production or excretion, a brief review of normal uric acid synthesis and excretion is warranted. Uric acid is the end product of purine metabolism. Increased synthesis of uric acid, a common feature of primary gout, results from some abnormality in the production of purine nucleotides. The synthesis of purine nucleotides occurs along two pathways, referred to as the *de novo* and *salvage pathways* (Fig. 21–14):

■ The de novo pathway involves synthesis of purines and then uric acid from nonpurine precursors. The starting sub-

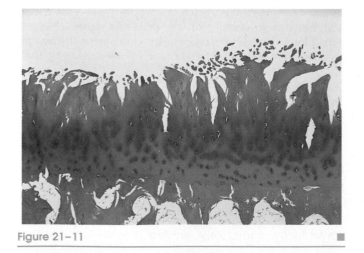

Figure 21–11 ■

Photomicrograph of osteoarthritis demonstrating characteristic splitting of the articular cartilage.

RHEUMATOID ARTHRITIS   OSTEOARTHRITIS

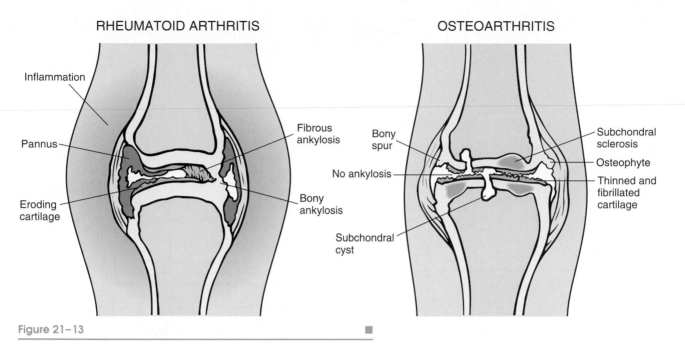

Figure 21–13   ■

Comparison of the morphologic features of rheumatoid arthritis and osteoarthritis.

strate for this pathway is ribose-5-phosphate, which is converted through a series of intermediates into purine nucleotides (inosinic acid, guanylic acid, and adenylic acid). This pathway is controlled by a complex array of regulatory mechanisms. Particularly important for our discussion are (1) the negative (feedback) regulation of the enzyme amidophosphoribosyl transferase (amido-PRT) and 5-phosphoribosyl-1-pyrophospate (PRPP) synthetase by purine nucleotides, and (2) the activation of amido-PRT by its substrate, PRPP.

■ The salvage pathway represents a mechanism by which free purine bases, derived from catabolism of purine nucleotides, breakdown of nucleic acids, and dietary intake, are utilized for the synthesis of purine nucleotides. This occurs in a single-step reaction whereby free purine bases (hypoxanthine, guanine, and adenine) condense with PRPP to form the purine nucleotide precursors of uric acid (inosinic acid, guanylic acid, and adenylic acid, respectively). These reactions are catalyzed by two transferases: hypoxanthine guanine phosphoribosyl transferase (HGPRT) and adenine phosphoribosyl transferase (APRT).

Circulating uric acid is freely filtered by the glomerulus and virtually completely resorbed in the proximal tubules of the kidney. A small fraction of the resorbed urate is subsequently secreted by the distal nephron and excreted in the urine.

As stated earlier, hyperuricemia may be caused by overproduction or underexcretion of uric acid, or by some combination of the two processes. *Most cases of gout are characterized by a primary overproduction of uric acid, with or without excessive excretion of uric acid; in most such cases, the cause of the overproduction is unknown.* Less commonly, uric acid is produced at normal rates, and hyperuricemia occurs because of decreased excretion of urate by the kidneys. Although the cause of excessive uric acid biosynthesis is unknown in most cases, rare patients with known enzyme defects have provided valuable information on the regulation of uric acid biosynthesis. This is illustrated by patients with an inherited deficiency of the enzyme HGPRT.

Complete lack of HGPRT gives rise to the *Lesch-Nyhan syndrome.* This X-linked genetic condition, seen only in males, is characterized by excretion of excessive amounts of

Table 21–3.   CLASSIFICATION OF GOUT

Clinical Category	Metabolic Defect
Primary Gout (90% of cases)	

Enzyme defects unknown (85% to 90% of primary gout)	Overproduction of uric acid
	  Normal excretion (majority)
	  Increased excretion (minority)
	Underexcretion of uric acid with normal production

Known enzyme defects (e.g., partial HGPRT deficiency [rare])	Overproduction of uric acid
Secondary Gout (10% of cases)	
Associated with increased nucleic acid turnover (e.g., leukemias)	Overproduction of uric acid with increased urinary excretion
Chronic renal disease	Reduced excretion of uric acid with normal production
Inborn errors of metabolism (e.g., complete HGPRT deficiency [Lesch-Nyhan syndrome])	Overproduction of uric acid with increased urinary excretion

HGPRT, hypoxanthine guanine phosphoribosyl transferase.

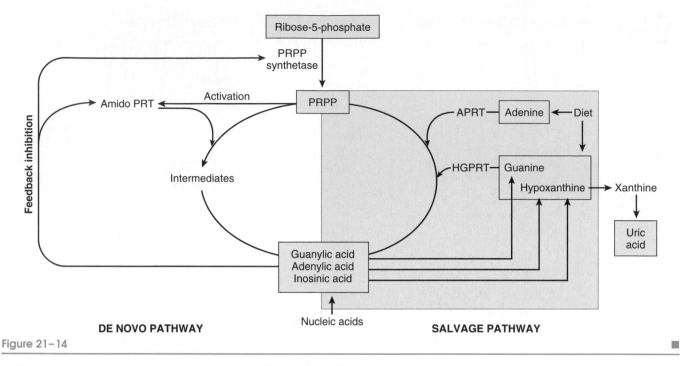

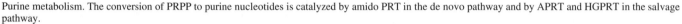

Figure 21–14 ■

Purine metabolism. The conversion of PRPP to purine nucleotides is catalyzed by amido PRT in the de novo pathway and by APRT and HGPRT in the salvage pathway.

uric acid, severe neurologic disease with mental retardation, and self-mutilation. Because there is an almost complete lack of HGPRT, the synthesis of purine nucleotides by the salvage pathway is blocked. This has two effects: an accumulation of PRPP, a key substrate for the de novo pathway, and increased activity of the enzyme amido-PRT, a result of the dual effect of allosteric activation brought about by PRPP and reduced feedback inhibition owing to a reduction in purine nucleotides. Both of these have the effect of augmenting purine biosynthesis by the de novo pathway, resulting eventually in excess production of the end product, uric acid. It should be noted that typical gouty arthritis is neither common nor a prominent clinical feature, and hence the Lesch-Nyhan syndrome is considered an example of secondary gout.

Less severe deficiencies of this enzyme (known as *partial HGPRT deficiency,* see Table 21–3) may occur, and these patients present clinically with severe gouty arthritis, beginning in adolescence, that is associated in some cases with mild neurologic disease.

In secondary gout, the hyperuricemia may be caused by either increased urate production (e.g., rapid cell lysis during treatment of lymphoma or leukemia) or decreased excretion (chronic renal insufficiency), or some combination of the two. Reduced renal excretion may also be caused by drugs such as thiazide diuretics, presumably because of their effects on tubular transport of uric acid.

Whatever the cause, increased levels of uric acid in the blood and other body fluids (e.g., synovium) lead to the precipitation of monosodium urate crystals. Precipitation of the crystals in turn triggers a chain of events that culminate in joint injury (Fig. 21–15). The released crystals are chemotactic and also activate complement, with the generation of C3a and C5a leading to accumulation of neutrophils and macro-phages in the joints and synovial membranes. Phagocytosis of crystals induces release of toxic free radicals and leukotrienes, particularly leukotriene B_4 (LTB_4). Death of the neutrophils releases destructive lysosomal enzymes. Macrophages also participate in joint injury. Following ingestion of urate crystals, they secrete a variety of proinflammatory mediators like IL-1, IL-6, IL-8, and TNF-α. These on one hand intensify the inflammatory response, and on the other hand activate synoviocytes and cartilage cells to release proteases (e.g., collagenase) that cause tissue injury. Activation of Hageman factor pours fuel onto the fire. Thus comes about an acute arthritis, which typically remits (days to weeks), even when untreated.

MORPHOLOGY. The major morphologic manifestations of gout are acute arthritis, chronic tophaceous arthritis and soft tissue tophi, and gouty nephropathy.

The primary morphologic change in **acute arthritis** is the deposition of **monosodium urate crystals** in the synovial tissues. These appear as pale, elongated, needle-like structures in synovial fluid aspirates and tissue sections. The crystals are accompanied by a predominantly neutrophilic inflammatory infiltrate, local congestion, and edema.

Chronic tophaceous arthritis develops after recurrent episodes of urate deposition and acute arthritis. Large, irregular deposits of chalky white sodium urate known as **tophi** are deposited on

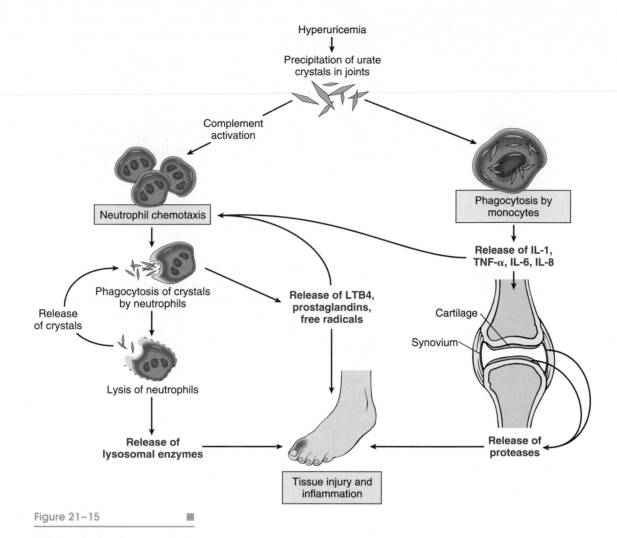

Figure 21–15   ■

Pathogenesis of acute gouty arthritis.

the articular cartilage and adjacent joint capsule. At these sites they provoke a chronic granulomatous inflammatory reaction. Thus, the tophus is seen in tissues as a mass of amorphous or crystalline urates surrounded by macrophages, lymphocytes, and fibroblasts. Large foreign body–type giant cells are wrapped around the urate crystals and are often very prominent (Fig. 21–16). Persistent chronic inflammation ultimately leads to fibrosis of the synovium and erosion of the articular cartilage. This may be followed by fusion of the joint (ankylosis). Tophi may also form in other sites, such as tendons, bursae and other soft tissues, and, on occasion, in the heart and other organs. Large subcutaneous tophi may ulcerate.

Gouty nephropathy includes several different lesions. In patients with marked hyperuricemia and hyperuricaciduria, uric acid crystals may precipitate within and obstruct the renal tubules. This is a particularly important complication in patients with myeloproliferative disorders. These patients

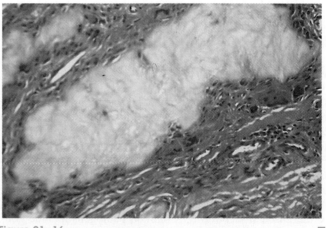

Figure 21–16   ■

Photomicrograph of a gouty tophus. An aggregate of urate crystals is surrounded by reactive fibroblasts, mononuclear inflammatory cells, and giant cells.

excrete large amounts of uric acid at the initiation of chemotherapy, when massive cell and nuclear lysis occurs. In most other cases, over time, urate crystals may form within the interstitium of the medulla and may, in neglected cases, form visible tophi. Patients with gout may also develop uric acid renal stones, which may be complicated by obstructive uropathy and pyelonephritis. In advanced cases, the kidneys are shrunken and scarred owing to a combination of tubular atrophy, obstructive uropathy, and recurrent episodes of pyelonephritis.

Clinical Features. Gout is more common in men than in women and does not usually cause symptoms before the age of 30. Four stages have been described in the evolution of gout, namely (1) asymptomatic hyperuricemia, (2) acute gouty arthritis, (3) "intercritical" gout, and (4) chronic tophaceous gout. Acute gouty arthritis is manifested by local pain, which often involves a single joint in the early stages of the disease but may subsequently become polyarticular. Although any joint may be involved, the following joints, in order of frequency, are affected: great toe (90% of patients), instep, ankle, heel, and wrist. In most cases the pain is abrupt and intense. The initial acute attacks usually resolve completely and are followed by an asymptomatic interval (intercritical gout). In the absence of treatment, recurrent episodes of arthritis involve increasing numbers of joints and eventually lead to permanent joint deformity. In severe cases, chronic tophi may cause significant additional soft tissue deformity. Curiously, the tophi themselves are usually painless, despite the tendency of advanced lesions to ulcerate. Acute urate nephropathy may cause acute renal failure; more chronic disease is associated with recurrent episodes of pyelonephritis and, eventually, chronic renal failure.

INFECTIOUS ARTHRITIS

Acute Suppurative Arthritis

Virtually every infectious agent has been implicated at one time or another as a cause of arthritis. The most common forms of infectious arthritis are those caused by bacteria. Infection of the joints may occur during episodes of bacteremia, via traumatic implantation, or from direct spread of an infection from the adjacent bone or soft tissues. Bacterial arthritis can occur in previously healthy individuals. However, immunodeficiency, joint trauma, or intravenous drug abuse leads to increased susceptibility. Common pathogens include gonococci, staphylococci, streptococci, *Haemophilus influenzae*, and gram-negative rods. Those individuals with a deficiency of certain complement proteins (C5, C6, C7) are particularly susceptible to dissemination of gonococci, and hence gonococcal arthritis (Chapter 18). *Salmonella* is a particularly important cause of acute bacterial arthritis in patients with sickle cell disease.

The usual reaction to infection is an acute suppurative arthritis, manifested by local pain, fever, and an intense neutrophilic inflammatory reaction within the joint and periarticular tissues. Aspiration of the joint space in such cases typically yields pus; the offending organisms may be visible in gram-stained smears of the exudate. Prompt diagnosis and treatment are necessary if permanent joint damage is to be avoided.

Lyme Disease

Lyme disease—named for the Connecticut town where, in the mid-1970s, there was an epidemic of arthritis associated with skin erythema—is caused by the spirochete *Borrelia burgdorferi*. Lyme disease is transmitted from rodents to people by tiny, hard deer ticks (*Ixodes dammini, Ixodes ricinus*, and others); it is the major arthropod-borne disease in the United States and is also frequent in Europe and Japan. Thus, Lyme disease has added another burden to the outdoor enthusiast, who is already plagued by poison ivy, contaminated water, and unpredictable weather.

As in another major spirochetal disease, syphilis, clinical disease caused by Lyme spirochetes involves multiple organ systems and is usually divided into three stages. In *stage 1* (Fig. 21–17), *Borrelia* spirochetes multiply at the site of the tick bite and cause an expanding area of redness, often with an indurated or pale center. This skin lesion, called *erythema chronicum migrans*, may be accompanied by fever and lymphadenopathy but usually disappears in a few weeks' time. In *stage 2,* the *early disseminated stage,* spirochetes spread hematogenously and cause secondary annular skin le-

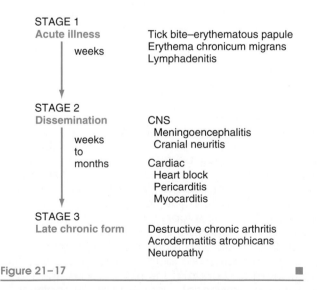

Figure 21–17 ■

The three stages and corresponding clinical features of Lyme disease.

sions, lymphadenopathy, migratory joint and muscle pain, cardiac arrhythmias, and meningitis, often with cranial nerve involvement. In untreated patients, antibodies develop that are useful for serodiagnosis of *Borrelia* infection. Some spirochetes, however, escape host antibody and T-cell responses by sequestering themselves in the central nervous system or as intracellular forms within endothelial cells. In *stage 3,* the *late disseminated stage,* which occurs 2 or 3 years after the initial bite, Lyme *Borrelia* organisms cause a chronic arthritis, sometimes with severe damage to large joints, and an encephalitis that varies from mild to debilitating. Joint involvement is the most common manifestation of disseminated infection and eventually develops in 80% of patients. Lyme arthritis typically affects large joints such as the knee, shoulder, and elbow, but any joint may be involved.

MORPHOLOGY. Skin lesions caused by *B. burgdorferi* are characterized by edema and a lymphocytic–plasma cell infiltrate. In early Lyme arthritis, the synovium resembles that of early rheumatoid arthritis, with villous hypertrophy, lining cell hyperplasia, and abundant lymphocytes and plasma cells in the subsynovium. A distinctive feature of Lyme arthritis is an arteritis, with onion-skin–like lesions resembling those seen in hypertension (Chapter 10). In late Lyme disease, there may be extensive erosion of the cartilage in large joints. In Lyme meningitis, the cerebrospinal fluid is hypercellular, shows a marked lymphoplasmacytic pleocytosis, and contains antispirochete immunoglobulins.

Diseases of Skeletal Muscle

The skeletal muscles are an elegant assembly of contractile proteins and their supporting membranes and organelles. Muscle development and normal activity are dependent on and closely integrated with the central and peripheral nervous systems, which together contribute to the *motor unit.* A motor unit is composed of a motor neuron in the brain stem or spinal cord; the peripheral axon emanating from the motor neuron; the neuromuscular junction; and finally, the skeletal muscle fiber. Two major subpopulations of skeletal muscle fibers exist—namely, type I, or "slow-twitch," fibers and type II, or "fast-twitch," fibers. Whether a fiber is type I or type II is determined by the spinal motor neuron responsible for innervating the fiber. These fibers can be distinguished by special stains for specific enzymes. Diseases of the skeletal muscle may affect any portion of the motor unit. These include primary disorders of the motor neuron or its axon, abnormalities of the neuromuscular junction, and a host of primary abnormalities of the skeletal muscle itself (myopathies). For the purposes of this discussion, we will divide skeletal muscle diseases into (1) those disorders that produce predominantly myofiber atrophy, including neurogenic atrophy and type II myofiber atrophy; (2) disorders of the neuromuscular junction (exemplified by myasthenia gravis); and (3) selected primary myopathies, including inflammatory myopathies and the muscular dystrophies.

MUSCLE ATROPHY

Although virtually any skeletal muscle disease can be associated with myofiber atrophy, here we will consider those disorders in which myofiber atrophy is the predominant, and sometimes the only, abnormality. The two most common causes of simple skeletal muscle atrophy are neurogenic atrophy and type II myofiber atrophy.

Neurogenic Atrophy

As mentioned in the introductory comments, skeletal muscle development and function are dependent on intact connections with lower motor neurons in the central nervous system (CNS). If deprived of their normal innervation, skeletal muscle fibers undergo progressive atrophy. Diseases involving the spinal motor neuron or the axons from that motor neuron produce similar morphologic changes in the affected skeletal muscle.

MORPHOLOGY. Under the microscope, denervated myofibers appear sharply **angular and**

atrophic. Both fast-twitch and slow-twitch fibers are involved. In many cases the atrophic fibers lie in small clusters, a pattern termed **small group atrophy.** The activities of certain enzymes are also altered in denervated fibers. These include increased activity of certain oxidative enzymes and esterases, which are readily demonstrated by staining for the enzyme in tissue sections (Fig. 21–18). Demonstration of these abnormalities permits a distinction between denervation atrophy and other forms of muscle atrophy. If an injured nerve regenerates and re-establishes contact with skeletal muscle fibers, fiber size may return to normal. As a given axon regenerates, however, its sprouts tend to innervate contiguous fibers, resulting in back-to-back aggregation of muscle fibers of the same histochemical type. This loss of randomness, termed **fiber type grouping,** is readily demonstrable in enzyme histochemical preparations and may be the only clue to the presence of a previous episode of denervation.

Clinical Features. The most consistent clinical manifestation of denervation atrophy is muscle weakness. This may vary from mild, localized weakness to severe, generalized weakness with respiratory compromise. Infantile spinal muscular atrophy is an important cause of generalized hypotonia in the neonate and is sometimes termed the *"floppy infant" syndrome.*

Type II Myofiber Atrophy

This pattern of muscle fiber atrophy is one of the most common abnormalities encountered in skeletal muscle. Type

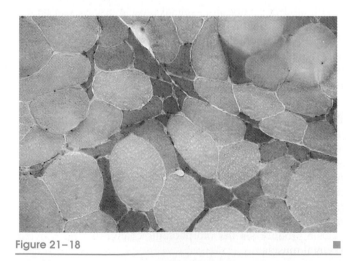

Figure 21–18 ■

Photomicrograph of skeletal muscle demonstrating neurogenic atrophy. The denervated cells are angular and atrophic, and they express increased esterase activity, manifested in this section as a red-orange reaction product (esterase stain).

II atrophy is seen in patients who develop disuse atrophy when bedridden or otherwise immobilized. It is also commonly seen in patients receiving glucocorticoids and in patients with endogenous hypercortisolism of any cause.

With routine histology, type II muscle fiber atrophy may be difficult to distinguish from denervation atrophy, especially in older children and adults. Like denervated fibers, the atrophic type II fibers appear angular and atrophic, although the group atrophy seen in some cases of denervation is absent. With special stains for enzymes, the detection of atrophy involving only the fast-twitch (type II) fibers is a reliable indication of this from denervation atrophy. Type II atrophy is typically associated with some degree of muscle weakness and may be suspected in patients who develop muscle atrophy under certain clinical conditions, such as Cushing's syndrome or prolonged immobilization of some part of the body.

MYASTHENIA GRAVIS

Myasthenia gravis is an acquired autoimmune disorder of neuromuscular transmission characterized by muscle weakness. The disease may present at any age and affects females somewhat more frequently than males. However, males are more commonly affected in late adult life. The evidence that myasthenia gravis is immunologically mediated is substantial. Antibodies to the acetylcholine receptor (AChR) on skeletal muscle fibers are demonstrable in nearly 90% of patients with the disorder and appear to play a direct role in the pathogenesis of this disease. The antibodies either injure the AChR or inhibit the binding of acetylcholine molecules to the receptor. Using appropriate stains, both immunoglobulin and various complement components are demonstrable at the neuromuscular junction. Additional observations supporting an immunologic basis for myasthenia gravis include an association between this disease and other autoimmune disorders, such as systemic lupus erythematosus, rheumatoid arthritis, and Sjögren's syndrome. Thymic abnormalities are also quite common in myasthenia gravis. About two thirds of patients have hyperplasia of the thymus, and thymomas are present in 15% to 20% of patients. The relative roles played by thymic abnormalities and humoral abnormalities in the pathogenesis of myasthenia gravis are incompletely understood.

MORPHOLOGY. Myasthenia gravis is associated with minimal morphologic changes in skeletal muscle, despite the presence of profound weakness. The muscle may be normal in routine histologic sections, although a mild degree of type II myofiber atrophy may occur secondary to generalized weakness and resulting muscle disuse. Scattered **collections of lymphocytes,** sometimes designated **lymphorrhages,** may also be present in the connective tissue. Electron microscopy demonstrates simplification of the neuromuscular junction.

Clinical Features. As the name *myasthenia* suggests, the clinical manifestations of myasthenia gravis are dominated by muscle weakness. The onset of this disease is typically insidious, but it may be abrupt. The muscle weakness usually becomes more pronounced with repeated contraction or stimulation and is therefore often worse during the latter part of the day than in the early morning. The most common sites of initial involvement are the *muscles of the eyelids* and the *muscles controlling eye movement,* manifested by drooping of the eyelids (ptosis) and double vision. Involvement of other facial and neck muscles commonly causes difficulty in chewing food and holding the head upright. The speech frequently assumes a nasal quality, particularly with prolonged attempts at conversation. The course of myasthenia gravis is slowly progressive, with involvement of other muscle groups. *Respiratory muscle involvement* may result in respiratory failure in untreated cases. It should be noted that the degree of muscle weakness varies considerably among patients, and it is not related to the titer of anti-AChR antibodies. Regardless of the specific thymic pathology, most patients show clinical improvement after thymectomy.

INFLAMMATORY MYOPATHIES

Inflammation of the skeletal muscles can occur in a number of different settings, including infections, autoimmune disorders, and some muscular dystrophies. The idiopathic inflammatory myopathies account for most cases of significant inflammation. These disorders, which include polymyositis, dermatomyositis, and inclusion body myositis, are generally regarded as autoimmune diseases of skeletal muscle and are discussed with other immunologic disorders in Chapter 5. They may occur as isolated diseases or in association with other autoimmune diseases, such as systemic lupus erythematosus.

Other important causes of skeletal muscle inflammation include infections, particularly parasitic diseases such as toxoplasmosis, cysticercosis, and trichinosis. Of these, the most well known is trichinosis, a disease caused by the ingestion of inadequately cooked meat infected with *Trichinella spiralis* cysts. The offending meat is most often pork, although other animals may also harbor the parasite. When infected meat is ingested by humans, the cyst wall is digested, and the *Trichinella* larvae attach to the wall of the duodenum or jejunum. The larvae mature and produce additional larvae, which then migrate from the gut into the general circulation. Once in the bloodstream, the parasites may spread to a number of different sites, including the lungs; central nervous system; heart; and ultimately, skeletal muscle. Within the skeletal muscle, the young larvae enlarge and encapsulate, provoking a variable host inflammatory reaction. The cysts may begin to calcify within a matter of months or, alternatively, may remain viable for several years. Clinical manifestations of trichinosis are referable to sites of parasite localization and include gastrointestinal disturbances; pneumonitis; altered mental status; and, in exceptional cases, myocardial failure. Skeletal muscle disease

is manifested by muscle pain and weakness, often associated with facial edema.

Other pathogens may also infect skeletal muscles. A number of viruses have been implicated in the development of myositis in humans, including influenza viruses, coxsackieviruses, and human immunodeficiency virus (HIV). The manifestations of viral myositis range from nonspecific muscle aches to fulminant muscle necrosis with myoglobinuria and renal failure. Bacterial myositis is rare in the United States but is an important form of inflammatory muscle disease in tropical areas of the world.

MUSCULAR DYSTROPHIES

The muscular dystrophies are a heterogeneous group of inherited diseases characterized by spontaneous, progressive degeneration of skeletal muscle fibers. In the past the diagnosis and classification of muscular dystrophies were based solely on the clinical features and patterns of inheritance of the disease. Recent work has shed considerable light on the molecular basis and pathogenesis of many of the muscular dystrophies, and hence it is possible to describe them as specific genetic disorders. Of the various muscular dystrophies, the two most common forms—Duchenne muscular dystrophy and the closely related Becker muscular dystrophy—are described here.

Duchenne and Becker Muscular Dystrophy

Duchenne muscular dystrophy (DMD) is an X-linked hereditary disease caused by the absence of a structural protein termed dystrophin. This disorder occurs in one of every 3500 live male births. The dystrophin gene is located on the short arm of the X chromosome (Xp21), where it spans an estimated 2400 kilobases (about 1% of the total X chromosome), making it one of the largest in the human genome. It is the enormous size of this gene that most likely renders it particularly vulnerable to deletions and other types of mutations. Dystrophin is a large protein that is expressed in a wide variety of tissues, including muscles of all types, brain, and peripheral nerves. In skeletal and cardiac muscles, dystrophin attaches portions of the sarcomere (the I and M bands) to the cell membrane, thus playing an important role in the structural and functional integrity of the myocyte. Absence or abnormalities of the dystrophin molecule are associated with impaired contractile activity and a variety of other derangements in both skeletal and cardiac muscles.

Becker muscular dystrophy (BMD) is another form of X-linked muscular dystrophy related to a mutation in the dystrophin gene. In contrast to DMD, however, dystrophin is present, but in an abnormal form. Accordingly, the resultant muscle abnormalities and clinical manifestations tend to be less severe than those of DMD.

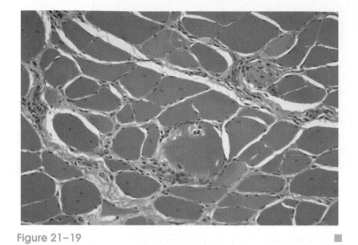

Figure 21–19 ■

Muscular dystrophy. The muscle fibers vary considerably in size and shape. Interstitial connective tissue is increased.

MORPHOLOGY. The histologic features of DMD and BMD are similar and include **marked variation in muscle fiber size,** caused by concomitant hypertrophy and atrophy of the myofibers. Many of the residual muscle fibers exhibit a range of **degenerative changes,** including fiber splitting and necrosis, while other fibers show evidence of **regeneration,** including sarcoplasmic basophilia, nuclear enlargement, and nucleolar prominence. **Connective tissue is increased** throughout the muscle (Fig. 21–19). The definitive diagnosis is based on the demonstration of **abnormal staining**

for dystrophin in immunohistochemical preparations (Fig. 21–20) or by Western blot analysis of skeletal muscle. In the late stages of the disease, extensive fiber loss and adipose tissue infiltration are present in most muscle groups. Changes that may occur in cardiac muscle in either DMD or BMD include variable degrees of fiber hypertrophy and interstitial fibrosis.

Clinical Features. As would be expected in an X-linked disorder, most of the affected patients with either DMD or BMD are males. Affected females are rare. The cardinal manifestation of both of these disorders is muscle weakness, which initially is most pronounced in the proximal muscles. Early manifestations include a generalized clumsiness, followed by weakness in the pelvic and shoulder girdles. Some muscle enlargement may be present in the early phases of the disease, particularly in the calf muscles. This is inevitably followed by the development of muscle atrophy.

In DMD, signs and symptoms begin by about the age of 5 and progress inexorably over the next several years to leave most patients wheelchair-bound by their teens. Most patients die in their 20s, usually as a result of progressive respiratory failure or pneumonia. The course may also be complicated by cardiac abnormalities, including congestive heart failure and cardiac arrhythmias.

The manifestations of BMD are variable but in general occur later and are more slowly progressive than those of DMD. Some patients may present with cardiac abnormalities even before skeletal muscle weakness is recognized. Patients with milder forms of the disease may remain ambulatory well into adult life.

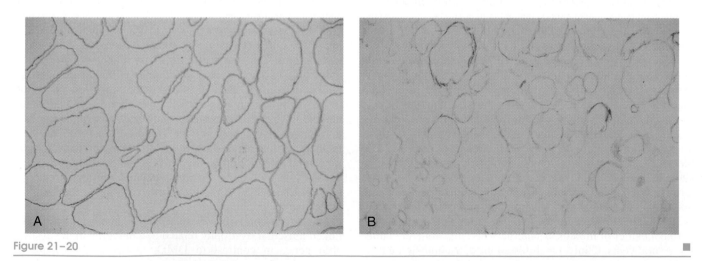

Figure 21–20 ■

A, Photomicrograph demonstrating normal, uniform distribution of dystrophin in the skeletal muscle membrane from a patient suffering from a myopathy not related to an abnormality in dystrophin. B, In contrast, in a patient with Becker-type muscular dystrophy, dystrophin staining is weak and irregularly distributed. In a patient with Duchenne muscular dystrophy, staining would be completely absent.

Soft Tissue Tumors

By convention, the term *soft tissue* is used to describe any nonepithelial tissue other than bone, cartilage, the brain and its coverings, hematopoietic cells, and lymphoid tissues. Soft tissue tumors are generally classified on the basis of the tissue type that they recapitulate, including fat, fibrous tissue, muscle, and neurovascular tissue. In some soft tissue neoplasms, however, no corresponding normal mesenchymal counterpart is known.

Soft tissue tumors may occur at any age. Most are benign lesions that are discovered incidentally or come to attention because of local mass effects. Less common are soft tissue sarcomas, characterized by aggressive local growth and widespread metastases. Occupying an intermediate position are neoplasms that may grow in a locally aggressive fashion and thus threaten a person's health, but usually do not metastasize. Malignant soft tissue neoplasms are fortunately uncommon, accounting for less than 2% of all malignancies. They are, however, the fourth most common type of malignancy in children, after hematopoietic neoplasms, neural tumors, and Wilms' tumor.

The outlook for patients with soft tissue tumors is influenced by several factors. The distinction between benign and malignant lesions is straightforward in most cases but may be exceedingly difficult in others. The degree of differentiation, reflected by the histologic grade, and the size and anatomic extent, expressed by the stage, influence the biologic behavior of malignant soft tissue tumors. In addition, the histologic type also affects the aggressiveness of the tumor. For example, certain sarcomas, such as childhood rhabdomyosarcomas, respond favorably to multimodality therapy, whereas others, such as the synovial sarcomas, seem unresponsive even to aggressive therapy. A classification of soft tissue tumors and tumor-like conditions is presented in Table 21–4. Only the more common forms will be described here.

TUMORS OF ADIPOSE TISSUE

Lipoma

Lipomas are the most common soft tissue tumors. They may arise anywhere in the body but are encountered most often in the subcutaneous tissues of adults. Most lipomas are solitary, sporadic lesions. Rare familial cases are associated with the presence of multiple lipomas. Most lipomas present

■

Table 21–4. SOFT TISSUE TUMORS

Tumors of Adipose Tissue
  Lipomas
  Liposarcoma
Tumors and Tumor-Like Lesions of Fibrous Tissue
  Nodular fasciitis
  Fibromatoses
    Superficial fibromatoses
    Deep fibromatoses
  Fibrosarcoma
Fibrohistiocytic Tumors
  Fibrous histiocytoma
  Dermatofibrosarcoma protuberans
  Malignant fibrous histiocytoma
Tumors of Skeletal Muscle
  Rhabdomyoma
  Rhabdomyosarcoma
Tumors of Smooth Muscle
  Leiomyoma
  Leiomyosarcoma
  Smooth muscle tumors of uncertain malignant potential
Vascular Tumors
  Hemangioma
  Lymphangioma
  Hemangioendothelioma
  Hemangiopericytoma
  Angiosarcoma
Peripheral Nerve Tumors
  Neurofibroma
  Schwannoma
  Malignant peripheral nerve sheath tumors
Tumors of Uncertain Histogenesis
  Granular cell tumor
  Synovial sarcoma
  Alveolar soft part sarcoma
  Epithelioid sarcoma

as slowly enlarging masses that seldom cause the patient difficulty. One histologic variant, the angiolipoma, may present with local pain. Complete excision is usually curative.

MORPHOLOGY. The typical lipoma is a soft, yellow mass. Superficial lesions tend to be well circumscribed, although more deeply situated lesions (e.g., intramuscular lipomas) may be less well demarcated. Microscopically, most lipomas are composed of mature adipose tissue that is indistinguishable from normal fat. Several less common histologic variants also occur, including those containing fibrous tissue (fibrolipoma), large numbers of blood vessels (angiolipoma), smooth muscle (myolipoma), and bone marrow (myelolipoma). One additional variant is the angiomyolipoma, containing a mixture of adipose tissue, smooth muscle, and blood vessels. Angiomyolipomas occur most commonly in the kidneys of patients with tuberous sclerosis and probably represent hamartomas rather than true neoplasms.

Liposarcoma

Liposarcomas are malignant neoplasms of adipocytes. They usually occur in adults, with a peak incidence in the fifth to sixth decades, and are one of the most common soft tissue malignancies in this age group. In contrast to lipomas, most liposarcomas arise in the deep soft tissues or in visceral sites. The lower extremities and abdomen are particularly common sites of origin. A t(12;16) chromosomal translocation has been identified in one variant of liposarcoma (myxoid liposarcoma).

MORPHOLOGY. Liposarcomas usually present as relatively well-circumscribed lesions. A number of different histologic subtypes are recognized, including two low-grade variants (the **well-differentiated liposarcoma** and the **myxoid liposarcoma)** and two high-grade, aggressive variants (the **round cell liposarcoma** and the rare **pleomorphic liposarcoma).** Some of the better-differentiated lesions may be difficult to distinguish histologically from lipomas, while at the other extreme, very poorly differentiated tumors may be difficult to distinguish from other high-grade malignancies.

The evolution and prognosis of liposarcomas is greatly influenced by the histologic subtype of the lesion. Well-differentiated and myxoid variants tend to grow in a fairly indolent fashion and have a more favorable prognosis than do the more aggressive round cell and pleomorphic variants.

TUMORS AND TUMOR-LIKE LESIONS OF FIBROUS TISSUE

Fibrous tissue proliferations are a heterogenous and perplexing group of lesions. Some, such as nodular fasciitis, are not true tumors but are reactive, self-limited proliferations, whereas others such as fibromatoses are characterized by persistent local growth that may defy surgical excision. Yet others are highly malignant fibrosarcomas that not only tend to recur locally, but also can metastasize. The histologic distinction between these various forms requires considerable skill and experience.

Nodular Fasciitis

Nodular fasciitis is a self-limited, reactive fibroblastic proliferation that may be mistaken for a sarcoma. The lesion is most common in young adults, in whom it presents as a rapidly enlarging, sometimes painful mass of several weeks' duration. Nodular fasciitis may arise in any part of the body but is most common in the upper extremities and trunk. In about 10% to 15% of cases, there is a history of local trauma at the site of the lesion. Simple excision is curative in most cases.

MORPHOLOGY. Grossly, nodular fasciitis presents as an unencapsulated lesion in the subcutaneous tissue, muscle, or deep fascia, usually measuring less than 3 cm in diameter. Many lesions, particularly those arising in more superficial locations, are quite well circumscribed. Microscopically, nodular fasciitis is composed of plump, immature-appearing fibroblastic cells with bland, open nuclei and prominent nucleoli (Fig. 21–21). The fibroblasts are often arrayed in small fascicles in a loose, myxoid matrix. Mitotic figures are usually present, but abnormal mitoses are not seen.

Fibromatoses

The fibromatoses are a group of fibroblastic proliferations distinguished by their tendency to grow in an infiltrative fashion and, in many cases, to recur after surgical excision. While some growths are locally aggressive, unlike fibrosarcomas, they do not metastasize. The fibromatoses are divided into two major clincopathologic groups: the superficial fibromatoses and the deep fibromatoses. The *superficial fibromatoses,* which include such entities as palmar fibromatosis (Dupuytren's contacture) and penile fibromatosis (Peyronie's disease), arise in the superficial fascia and tend to be more innocuous than their deep-seated cousins. They are more

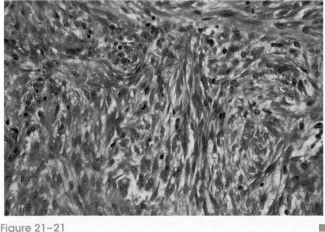

Figure 21–21 ■

Nodular fasciitis. The high cellularity of the lesions evident in this photomicrograph causes them to be confused with a sarcoma in some cases.

bothersome than serious. Because of their abundant collagen content, they give rise to deforming contractures in the palms or soles. The *deep fibromatoses* include the so-called desmoid tumors that arise in the abdomen and muscles of the trunk and extremities. Compared with the superficial lesions, they are characterized by a greater tendency to recur and to grow in a locally aggressive manner.

> **MORPHOLOGY.** The appearance of the fibromatoses varies considerably, depending on the site. Some lesions present as well-defined nodules, while others appear as grossly infiltrative masses without an obvious margin. Microscopically, the fibromatoses are composed of proliferating, sometimes plump fibroblasts that have a fairly uniform appearance. Some lesions may be quite cellular, particularly early in their evolution, while others, especially the superficial fibromatoses, contain abundant dense collagen.

Fibrosarcomas

Fibrosarcomas are malignant neoplasms composed of fibroblasts. Most cases occur in adults, in whom favored sites of origin include the deep tissues of the thigh, knee, and trunk. Fibrosarcomas have no specific clinical features that allow them to be distinguished from other soft tissue tumors. As a rule, they tend to grow slowly, and they have usually been present for several years by the time they are diagnosed. As with other types of sarcomas, fibrosarcomas often recur locally after excision and may metastasize, usually by the hematogeneous route to the lungs.

> **MORPHOLOGY.** Fibrosarcomas are solitary lesions that may be grossly infiltrative or deceptively circumscribed. Histologically, the typical fibrosarcoma is composed of interlacing fascicles of fibroblasts, sometimes arrayed in a herringbone pattern. Nuclear atypia and mitotic activity are present but may be mild in some cases. Extreme degrees of pleomorphism are not a typical feature of these neoplasms.

■ FIBROHISTIOCYTIC TUMORS

Fibrohistiocytic tumors are composed of a mixture of fibroblasts and phagocytic, lipid-laden cells with a histiocytic appearance. Like the fibroblastic tumors, the fibrohistiocytic group spans a broad range of histologic patterns and biologic behavior, from self-limited, benign lesions to high-grade sarcomas. Other lesions occupy an intermediate position; they recur locally but seldom metastasize.

Fibrous Histiocytoma

Fibrous histiocytomas are benign lesions that present as a well-defined, mobile nodule in the dermis or subcutaneous tissue. Most cases occur in adults. A number of histologic patterns may be encountered, including proliferations dominated by bland, interlacing spindle cells and lesions rich in foamy, lipid-rich cells with a histiocytic morphology. The borders of the lesions tend to be infiltrative, but extensive local invasion does not occur. They are cured by simple excision.

Dermatofibrosarcoma Protuberans

This neoplasm occupies an intermediate position between the benign fibrohistiocytic tumors and malignant fibrous histiocytoma. It presents as a slowly growing, nodular lesion involving the dermis and subcutaneous tissue. Most patients are adults. The tumors are infiltrative and often recur after local excision. In exceptional cases, metastases may develop. Microscopically, dermatofibrosarcoma protuberans is composed of plump, fibroblastic cells arrayed in a "storiform" pattern. Mitotic activity is sparse, and there is little cytologic atypia.

Malignant Fibrous Histiocytoma

Malignant fibrous histiocytoma (MFH) is the most common soft tissue sarcoma in adults. Most occur in older adults between the ages of 50 and 70. It is also the most common type of postirradiation sarcoma. MFHs tend to arise in the deep muscular tissues of the extremities or in the retroperitoneal area. Most are highly aggressive tumors that often recur locally and metastasize in about 50% of patients.

> **MORPHOLOGY.** These tumors are usually gray-white, encapsulated masses that appear deceptively circumscribed, despite their infiltrative growth at the microscopic level. Retroperitoneal tumors may reach a very large size before coming to clinical attention. Microscopically, several different subtypes of MFH are recognized. The most common of these is the so-called storiform-pleomorphic variant, populated by cytologically atypical spindle cells arrayed in whorls, sometimes admixed with bizarre, histiocyte-like cells (Fig. 21–22). Other forms of MFH include the more vascular angiomatoid variant, inflammatory MFH, and myxoid MFH. The angiomatoid variant tends to occur in younger patients.

■ NEOPLASMS OF SKELETAL MUSCLE

Neoplasms of skeletal muscle include rhabdomyoma and its malignant counterpart, rhabodmyosarcoma. The rhabdo-

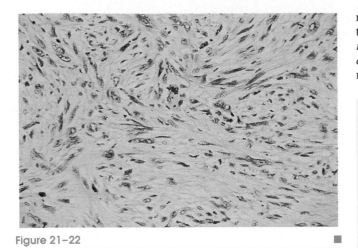

Figure 21–22 ■

Photomicrograph of malignant fibrous histiocytoma showing the characteristic high cellularity, atypical spindle cells, and mitotic activity. There are no histiocytic cells in this field.

myoma is an uncommon tumor. At least one form, the cardiac rhabdomyoma associated with tuberous sclerosis, probably represents a hamartoma rather than a true neoplasm (Chapter 11).

Rhabdomyosarcoma

Rhabdomyosarcoma is a malignant mesenchymal neoplasm that exhibits skeletal muscle differentiation. In contrast to the soft tissue sarcomas discussed previously, *rhabdomyosarcoma is predominantly a neoplasm of infancy, childhood, and adolescence,* with a peak incidence in the first decade of life. It is the most common form of soft tissue sarcoma in the pediatric population. Several different but sometimes overlapping histologic variants exist, the most common of which is the *embryonal rhabdomyosarcoma.* They arise most frequently in the head and neck area, genitourinary tract, and

retroperitoneum. Occasional tumors originate in the extremities. Other, less common histologic patterns include *alveolar rhabodmyosarcoma* and the rare *pleomorphic rhabdomyosarcoma;* many of the latter probably represent variants of MFH rather than true skeletal muscle neoplasms.

MORPHOLOGY. The gross appearance of rhabdomyosarcomas is variable. Some tumors, particularly those arising near the mucosal surfaces of the lower genitourinary tract and in the head and neck, may present as soft, gelatinous, grape-like masses, designated **sarcoma botryoides.** In other cases the pattern may be that of a poorly defined, infiltrating mass. Microscopically, the **embryonal variants,** including sarcoma botryoides, are composed of small, primitive cells, some of which contain eosinophilic "straplike" cell processes. Such strap cells are evidence of myoblastic differentiation. The malignant cells tend to cluster immediately beneath mucosal surfaces, a configuration known as a **cambium layer.** In the absence of telltale features of myoblastic differentiation, these tumors are very difficult to distinguish from other small round cell tumors of childhood. The diagnosis of rhabdomyosarcoma is based on the demonstration of skeletal muscle differentiation, either in the form of sarcomeres under the electron microscope or by the demonstration of muscle-associated antigens such as desmin in immunocytochemical preparations (Fig. 21–23). In the **alveolar pattern,** neoplastic rhabdomyoblasts are supported by fibrous septa to form spaces somewhat suggestive of alveolar spaces in the lung. **Pleomorphic variants,** as the name implies, are populated by highly pleomorphic malignant cells, including bizarre neoplastic giant cells. As has been noted, many such cases likely represent variants of MFH rather than rhabdomyosarcomas.

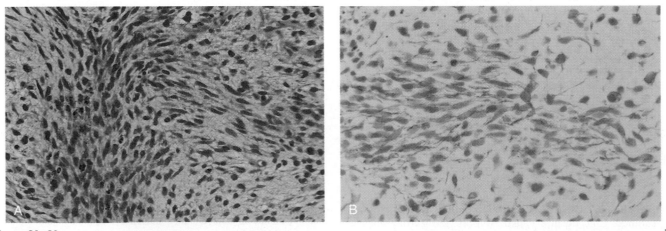

Figure 21–23 ■

Rhabdomyosarcoma. *A,* The rhabdomyoblasts are round or spindle shaped, some cells having elongated cytoplasm. *B,* Immunohistochemical staining reveals desmin (brown reaction product) confirming the presence of rhabdomyoblasts. (Courtesy of Jorgé Albores-Saavedra, MD, Department of Pathology, University of Texas Southwestern Medical School, Dallas, TX.)

SMOOTH MUSCLE TUMORS

Benign smooth muscle tumors, or leiomyomas, are common, well-circumscribed neoplasms encountered most frequently in the uterus, although they may arise from smooth muscle cells anywhere in the body. They are discussed in detail with other tumors of the uterus in Chapter 19. Malignant smooth muscle tumors, designated *leiomyosarcomas,* occur most often in the uterus and gastrointestinal tracts, although they may arise in virtually any area of the body. Most arise de novo, rather than in a preexisting leiomyoma. They are distinguished from leiomyomas by the infiltrative growth; greater cellularity and pleomorphism; and most importantly, greater mitotic activity.

MISCELLANEOUS NEOPLASMS

As noted in the introductory comments to this section, soft tissue tumors also include vascular neoplasms and peripheral nerve sheath tumors, which are discussed in Chapters 10 and 23, respectively. An additional group of soft tissue neoplasms includes a small number of sarcomas of uncertain histogenesis. These include the alveolar soft part sarcoma, synovial sarcoma, and epithelioid sarcoma. Only synovial sarcoma is sufficiently common to warrant a brief description here.

Synovial Sarcoma

This tumor accounts for 10% of all soft tissue sarcomas. The first point to be emphasized is that despite its name, synovial sarcoma does not arise from synovial cells; rather, it derives from mesenchymal cells about joint cavities, and sometimes in sites totally removed from joints.

MORPHOLOGY. Synovial sarcomas range from quite small, deceptively circumscribed lesions to infiltrative sarcomatous masses. Histologically, they are characterized by a biphasic pattern that has an epithelial component forming glands, interspersed in a spindle cell pattern replicating fibroblast-like sheets. (Fig. 21–24). Less commonly, the synovial sarcoma may be monophasic and composed entirely of epithelial elements that resemble a carcinoma or, alternatively, of spindle cells, which make synovial sarcoma difficult to distinguish from other sarcomas. Immunocytochemical demonstration of keratin and epithelial membrane antigen are helpful in diagnosis, but more definitive is demonstration of the (X;18)(p11.2;q11.2) chromosomal translocation.

BIBLIOGRAPHY

Brazel US: Osteoporosis: Taking a fresh look. Hosp Pract 31:59, 1996. (A concise discussion of pathogenesis, clinical features, and management.)

Brown RH: Dystrophin-associated proteins and the muscular dystrophies: a glossary. Brain Pathol 6:19, 1996. (A very informative, concise summary of dystrophin and related proteins in various forms of muscular dystrophy.)

Dijkgraaf LC, et al: The structure, biochemistry, and metabolism of osteoarthritic cartilage: a review of the literature. J Oral Maxillofac Surg 53: 1182, 1995. (An informative review of the role played by various cytokines and other mediators in the pathogenesis of osteoarthritis.)

Gallacher SJ: Paget's disease of bone. Curr Opin Rheumatol 5:351, 1993. (A concise summary of current ideas about the pathogenesis of this disorder, including a discussion of the possible role played by viruses in its pathogenesis.)

Greenspan A: Benign bone-forming lesions: osteoma, osteoid osteoma, and osteoblastoma. Clinical, imaging, pathologic, and differential considerations. Skeletal Radiol 22:485, 1993. (A brief review of the clinical presentations and morphologic features of this group of lesions.)

Hadjipavlou A, et al: Malignant transformation in Paget's disease of bone. Cancer 70:2802, 1992. (A review of the incidence, clinical features, and pathology of malignancies complicating Paget's disease in four large Canadian hospitals.)

Ho G Jr: Bacterial arthritis. Curr Opin Rheumatol 4:509, 1992. (A concise summary of septic arthritis in adults, including comments about causative organisms, predisposing conditions, and experimental models.)

Johnston CC, Slemada CW: Pathogenesis of osteoporosis. Bone 17(2S):19S, 1995. (A review of the factors responsible for osteoporosis and associated fractures.)

Kretschmar CS: Ewing's sarcoma and the "peanut" tumors. N Engl J Med 331:294, 1994. (A well-written editorial on an article in the same issue, describing the relationship of Ewing's tumor to other small round cell tumors of children.)

Manolagas SC, Jilka RL: Bone marrow, cytokines, and bone remodeling: emerging insights into the pathophysiology of osteoporosis. N Engl J Med 332:305,1995. (A scholarly review of the factors that influence bone mass.)

Papac RJ: Bone marrow metastases. A review. Cancer 74:2403, 1994. (A concise review of the clinical and morphologic aspects of bone marrow

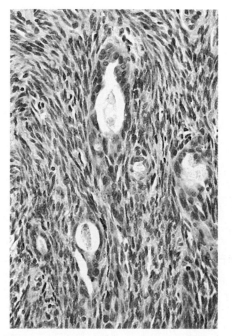

Figure 21–24   ■

Photomicrograph of synovial sarcoma showing the classic biphasic pattern composed of epithelial cells forming glands, with intervening spindle cells.

metastases, including a discussion of the most common tumors giving rise to such lesions.)

Parisien M, et al: Bone disease in primary hyperparathyroidism. Endocrinol Metab Clin North Am 1:19, 1990. (A concise but thorough review of the pathogenesis and morphology of this condition.)

Snaith ML: ABC of rheumatology. Gout, hyperuricemia, and crystal arthritis. BMJ 310:521, 1995. (A short but lucid commentary.)

Sutton RAL, Cameron EC: Renal osteodystrophy: pathophysiology. Semin Nephrol 12:91, 1992. (A comprehensive review of the biochemical and cellular events responsible for bone disease in chronic renal failure.)

Turkeltaub RA: Gout and mechanisms of crystal-induced inflammation. Curr Opin Rheumatol 5:510, 1993. (An informative discussion of potential mechanisms of urate deposition and subsequent inflammatory events in gout.)

Unni KK, Dahlin DC: Osteosarcoma: pathology and classification. Semin Roentgenol 24:43, 1989. (A short review of the various subtypes of this important malignancy.)

Weinberger A: Gout, uric acid metabolism, and crystal-induced inflammation. Curr Opin Rheumatol 7:359, 1995. (A good discussion of the pathways of inflammation in gouty arthritis.)

22

The Skin

GEORGE F. MURPHY, MD

Disorders affecting the skin are extremely common and range from the relatively innocuous viral warts to life-threatening malignant melanomas. It is estimated that each year approximately 30% of people in the United States develop a skin problem. Fully 10% of outpatient visits are related to a skin disorder, and more than half of these come to the attention of primary care providers such as internists, pediatricians, and family practitioners. While most of the cutaneous disorders are intrinsic to the skin, many skin lesions are external manifestations of a systemic disease, such as systemic lupus erythematosus and acquired immunodeficiency syndrome (AIDS) (e.g., Kaposi's sarcoma). Thus, skin provides an important window for the recognition of systemic disorders that are likely to be encountered by virtually every practitioner of medicine.

The structure of skin is well known to every student of medicine. However, what is not widely appreciated is that skin is not merely a passive, protective mantle. Because skin is in constant contact with the environment, it is bathed with microbial and nonmicrobial antigens. These antigens are processed by bone marrow–derived epidermal Langerhans cells that have dendritic morphology and escape casual inspection of the epidermis under the microscope. Langerhans cells possess all the attributes of antigen-presenting cells and they communicate with the immune system by migrating to regional lymph nodes. Even the dull and uninteresting looking squamous cells (keratinocytes) participate in maintaining the delicate homeostasis in skin by secreting a plethora of cytokines. These soluble messengers not only regulate interactions among the epidermal cells but also diffuse down and influence the dermal microenvironment. Thus, skin, simple in structure, is a complex organ in which precisely regulated cellular and molecular events govern the body's response to the external environment. With this broad overview of skin as a dynamic organ, we can proceed to describe disorders of the skin. The focus in this chapter is on those diseases that are common and that are generally localized to or originate in the skin. Cutaneous manifestations of many systemic disorders are covered elsewhere in the text, along with discussions of specific diseases.

Diseases of the skin are often perplexing to students (and nonspecialists) because dermatologists and dermatopathologists use a vocabulary that is not commonly used in describing lesions in other tissues. Thus, we begin our discussion by providing a glossary of commonly used terminology.

MACROSCOPIC TERMS

Macule: Circumscribed area of any size characterized by its flatness and usually distinguished from surrounding skin by its coloration.

Papule: Elevated solid area 5 mm or less across.

Nodule: Elevated solid area more than 5 mm across.

Plaque: Elevated flat-topped area, usually more than 5 mm across.

Vesicle: Fluid-filled raised area 5 mm or less across.

Bulla: Fluid-filled raised area more than 5 mm across; a large vesicle.

Blister: Common term used for vesicle or bulla.

Pustule: Discrete, pus-filled raised area.

Scale: Dry, horny, platelike excrescence; usually the result of imperfect cornification.

Lichenification: Thickened and rough skin characterized by prominent skin markings; usually the result of repeated rubbing in susceptible persons.

Excoriation: A traumatic lesion characterized by breakage of the epidermis, causing a raw linear area (i.e., a deep scratch). Such lesions are often self-induced.

MICROSCOPIC TERMS

Hyperkeratosis: Hyperplasia of the stratum corneum often associated with a qualitative abnormality of the keratin.

Parakeratosis: Mode(s) of keratinization characterized by retention of the nuclei in the stratum corneum. On mucous membranes, parakeratosis is normal.

Acanthosis: Epidermal hyperplasia.

Dyskeratosis: Abnormal keratinization occurring prematurely within individual cells or groups of cells below the stratum granulosum.

Acantholysis: Loss of intercellular connections resulting in loss of cohesion between keratinocytes.

Papillomatosis: Hyperplasia of the papillary dermis with elongation and/or widening of the dermal papillae.

Lentiginous: Refers to a linear pattern of melanocyte proliferation within the epidermal basal cell layer; lentiginous melanocytic hyperplasia can occur as a reactive change or as part of a neoplasm of melanocytes.

Spongiosis: Intercellular edema of the epidermis.

ACUTE INFLAMMATORY DERMATOSES

Literally thousands of specific inflammatory dermatoses exist. In general, acute lesions last from days to weeks and are characterized by inflammation (often marked by mononuclear cells, rather than neutrophils), edema, and (in some instances) epidermal, vascular, or subcutaneous injury. The lesions discussed here are selected as examples of the more commonly encountered dermatoses within this category.

Urticaria

Urticaria (hives) is a common disorder of the skin characterized by *localized mast cell degranulation and resultant der-*

mal microvascular hyperpermeability, culminating in pruritic edematous plaques called wheals.

Clinically, urticaria most often occurs between the ages of 20 and 40 years, although all age groups are susceptible. Individual lesions develop and fade within hours (usually less than 24 hours), and episodes may last for days or persist for months. Lesions vary from small, pruritic papules to large edematous plaques. Sites of predilection for urticarial eruptions include any area exposed to pressure, such as the trunk, distal extremities, and ears.

> **MORPHOLOGY.** The histologic features of urticaria may be so subtle that many biopsy specimens at first resemble normal skin. Usually there is a very sparse superficial perivenular infiltrate consisting of mononuclear cells and rare neutrophils. Eosinophils may be present, often in the midreticular dermis. Collagen bundles are more widely spaced than in normal skin, a result of superficial dermal edema fluid that does not stain in routinely prepared tissue.
>
> In most cases, urticaria results from antigen-induced release of vasoactive mediators from mast cell granules via sensitization with specific IgE antibodies (type I hypersensitivity, Chapter 5). This **IgE-dependent** degranulation can follow exposure to a number of antigens (pollens, foods, drugs, insect venom). **IgE-independent** urticaria may result from substances that directly incite the degranulation of mast cells, such as opiates and certain antibiotics. Hereditary angioneurotic edema is the result of an inherited deficiency of C1 esterase inhibitor that results in uncontrolled activation of the early components of the complement system (Chapter 5).

Acute Eczematous Dermatitis

Eczema is a clinical term that embraces a number of pathogenetically different conditions. All are characterized by red, *papulovesicular, oozing, and crusted lesions* at an early stage that with persistence develop into raised, *scaling plaques.* Clinical differences permit classification of eczematous dermatitis into the following categories: (1) allergic contact dermatitis, (2) atopic dermatitis, (3) drug-related eczematous dermatitis, (4) photoeczematous dermatitis, and (5) primary irritant dermatitis (Table 22–1).

The most obvious example of acute eczematous dermatitis is an acute contact reaction to poison ivy, characterized by pruritic, edematous, oozing plaques, often containing small and large blisters (vesicles and bullae) (Fig. 22–1A). With time, persistent lesions become less "wet" (fail to ooze or form vesicles) and become progressively scaly (hyperkeratotic) as the epidermis thickens (acanthosis).

> **MORPHOLOGY. Spongiosis—the accumulation of edema fluid within the epidermis—**characterizes acute eczematous dermatitis, hence the synonym "spongiotic dermatitis." Whereas in urticaria edema is localized to the perivascular spaces of the superficial dermis, in spongiotic dermatitis edema seeps into the intercellular spaces of the epidermis, splaying apart keratinocytes. Intercellular bridges become prominent, giving a "spongy" appearance to the epidermis (Fig. 22–1B). These epidermal changes are accompanied by a superficial, perivascular, lymphocytic infiltrate associated with papillary dermal edema and mast cell degranulation. In cases resulting from drug exposure, eosinophils may also be present.

Table 22–1. CLASSIFICATION OF ECZEMATOUS DERMATITIS

Type	Cause or Pathogenesis	Histology*	Clinical Features
Contact Dermatitis	Topically applied chemicals Pathogenesis: delayed hypersensitivity	Spongiotic dermatitis	Marked itching, burning, or both; requires antecedent exposure
Atopic Dermatitis	Unknown, may be heritable	Spongiotic dermatitis	Erythematous plaques in flexural areas; family history of eczema, hay fever, or asthma
Drug-Related Eczematous Dermatitis	Systemically administered antigens or haptens (e.g., penicillin)	Spongiotic dermatitis; eosinophils often present in infiltrate; deeper infiltrate	Eruption occurs with administration of drug; remits when drug is discontinued
Photoeczematous Eruption	Ultraviolet light	Spongiotic dermatitis; deeper infiltrate	Occurs on sun-exposed skin; phototesting may help in diagnosis
Primary Irritant Dermatitis	Repeated trauma (rubbing)	Spongiotic dermatitis in early stages; epidermal hyperplasia in late stages	Localized to site of trauma

* All types, with time, may develop chronic changes.

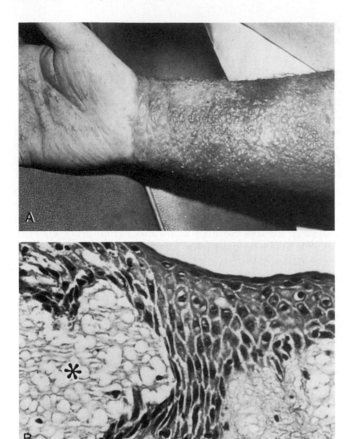

Figure 22–1

Eczematous dermatitis. *A,* In acute allergic contact dermatitis, numerous vesicles appear at the site of antigen exposure (in this case, laundry detergent). *B,* Histologically, intercellular edema produces widened intercellular spaces within the epidermis, eventually resulting in small, fluid-filled intraepidermal vesicles (*).

Spongiotic dermatitis due to contact hypersensitivity (e.g., poison ivy dermatitis) is mediated by sensitized T cells (type IV hypersensitivity, Chapter 5). After initial exposure, antigens derived from poison ivy are processed by epidermal Langerhans cells, leading ultimately to sensitization of T cells. These CD4+ cells, upon re-exposure to the antigen, release cytokines that recruit additional inflammatory cells and also mediate the epidermal change.

Erythema Multiforme

Erythema multiforme is an uncommon, self-limited disorder that appears to be a *hypersensitivity response to certain infections and drugs.* It is associated with the following conditions: (1) infectious disorders (e.g., herpes simplex, *Mycoplasma* infections, histoplasmosis, coccidioidomycosis, typhoid, and leprosy); (2) administration of certain drugs (sulfonamides, pencillin, barbiturates, salicylates, hydantoins, and antimalarials); (3) malignancy (carcinomas and lymphomas); and (4) collagen vascular diseases (lupus erythematosus, dermatomyositis, and periarteritis nodosa).

Clinically, patients present with an *array of "multiform"*

lesions, including macules, papules, vesicles, and bullae, as well as the characteristic target lesion consisting of a red macule or papule with a pale vesicular or eroded center (Fig. 22–2A, inset). An extensive and symptomatic febrile form of the disease, more common in children, is called the Stevens-Johnson syndrome. It is marked by erosions and crusting of the mucosal surfaces of the lips, conjunctiva, oral cavity, urethra, and anogenital region. Another variant, termed *toxic epidermal necrolysis*, results in diffuse necrosis and sloughing of cutaneous and mucosal epithelial surfaces, producing a clinical situation analogous to an extensive burn.

MORPHOLOGY. Histologically, early lesions show a superficial perivascular, lymphocytic infiltrate associated with dermal edema and margination of lymphocytes along the dermoepidermal junction, where they are intimately associated with degenerating and necrotic keratinocytes. With time, discrete and confluent zones of epidermal necrosis occur, with concomitant blister formation (Fig. 22–2A and *B*).

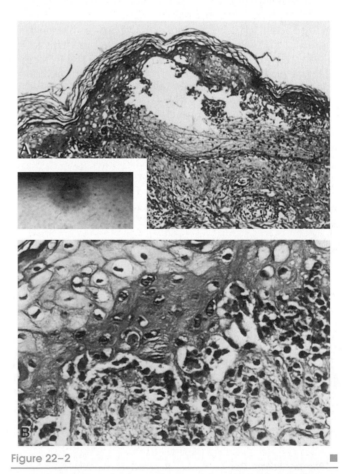

Figure 22–2

Erythema multiforme. *A,* A central blister and zone of epidermal necrosis correlates with a target-like clinical lesion *(inset)* surrounded by macular erythema. *B,* Higher magnification of a biopsy specimen from the erythematous edge shows numerous lymphocytes in intimate contact with degenerating basal epidermal cells.

The lesions of erythema multiforme are caused, in all likelihood, by cytotoxic CD8+ T cells.

CHRONIC INFLAMMATORY DERMATOSES

This category focuses on those persistent inflammatory dermatoses that exhibit their most characteristic clinical and histologic features over many months to years. Unlike the normal cutaneous surface, the skin surface in some chronic inflammatory dermatoses is roughened as a result of excessive or abnormal scale formation and shedding (desquamation). Included in this category, but not described here, are cutaneous lesions of systemic lupus erythematosus (Chapter 5).

Psoriasis

Psoriasis is a common chronic inflammatory dermatosis affecting 1% to 2% of people in the United States. It is sometimes associated with arthritis, myopathy, enteropathy, spondylitic heart disease, and AIDS.

Clinically, psoriasis most frequently affects the skin of the elbows, knees, scalp, lumbosacral areas, intergluteal cleft, and glans penis. *The most typical lesion is a well-demarcated, pink to salmon-colored plaque covered by loosely adherent scales that are characteristically silver-white in color* (Fig. 22–3). Nail changes occur in 30% of cases of psoriasis and consist of yellow-brown discoloration (often likened to an oil slick), with pitting, separation of the nail plate from the underlying bed (onycholysis), thickening, and crumbling. In the rare variant called pustular psoriasis, multiple small pustules form on erythematous plaques.

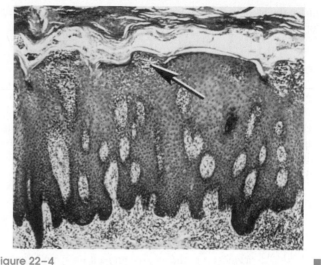

Figure 22–4   ■

Psoriasis. Histologically, established lesions demonstrate marked epidermal hyperplasia, parakeratotic scale, and (importantly) minute microabscesses of neutrophils *(arrow)* within the superficial epidermal layers.

MORPHOLOGY. There is increased epidermal cell turnover resulting in marked epidermal thickening (acanthosis), with regular downward elongation of the rete ridges (Fig. 22–4). **The stratum granulosum is thinned or absent, and extensive overlying parakeratotic scale is seen.** Typical of psoriatic plaques is the thinning of the portion of the epidermal cell layer that overlies the tips of dermal papillae (suprapapillary plates) and dilated, tortuous blood vessels within these papillae. These blood vessels bleed readily when the plaque is lifted, giving rise to multiple minute bleeding points **(Auspitz's sign).** Neutrophils form small aggregates within slightly spongiotic foci of the superficial epidermis **(spongiform pustules)** and within the parakeratotic stratum corneum **(Munro's microabscesses).**

The pathogenesis of psoriasis is not clear. An increased incidence of disease in association with certain HLA types suggests a genetic predisposition to disease development. It has been postulated that psoriasis may result from a complement-mediated reaction localized to the stratum corneum. According to this hypothesis, exogenous or endogenous damage to the stratum corneum of certain individuals results in the unmasking of stratum corneum antigens. These antigens elicit the formation of specific autoantibodies, which bind to the stratum corneum, fix complement, and activate the complement cascade. This in turn leads to neutrophil recruitment and activation. The inflammatory process also seems to release proliferative factors for the underlying keratinocytes, resulting in increased epidermal turnover. Another recently considered possibility is that the primary defect in psoriasis resides in the superficial dermal microvessels. The capillary endothelium is unusually sensitive to cytokine-mediated induction of adhe-

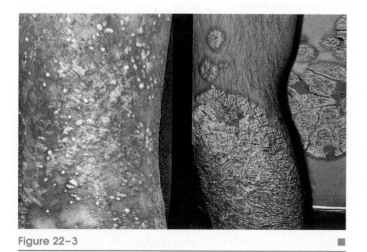

Figure 22–3   ■

Clinical evolution of psoriasis. Early, eruptive, and pustular lesions may be dominated by signs of inflammation and erythema *(left panel)*. Established, chronic lesions demonstrate erythema surmounted by characteristic silver-white scale *(right panel)*. Rarely, the early inflammatory phase predominates throughout the course of the disease (pustular psoriasis).

sion molecules, with subsequent enhanced recruitment of neutrophils.

Lichen Planus

"Pruritic, purple, polygonal papules" are the presenting signs of this disorder of skin and mucous membranes. Lichen planus is self-limiting and generally resolves spontaneously 1 to 2 years after onset, often leaving zones of postinflammatory hyperpigmentation. Oral lesions may persist for years.

Cutaneous lesions consist of *itchy, violaceous, flat-topped papules, which may coalesce focally to form plaques.* These papules are often highlighted by white dots or lines, called *Wickham's striae* (Fig. 22–5A). Multiple lesions are characteristic and are symmetrically distributed, particularly on the extremities, often about the wrists and elbows, and on the glans penis. In 70% of cases, oral lesions are present as white, reticulated, or netlike areas involving the mucosa.

> **MORPHOLOGY.** Lichen planus is characterized histologically by a dense, continuous infiltrate of lymphocytes along the dermoepidermal junction (Fig. 22–5B). The lymphocytes are intimately associated with basal keratinocytes, which show degeneration, necrosis, and a resemblance in size and contour to more mature cells of the stratum spinosum (squamatization). This pattern of inflammation causes the dermoepidermal interface to assume an angulated zigzag contour ("sawtoothing"). Anucleate, necrotic basal cells may become incorporated into the inflamed papillary dermis, where they are referred to as **colloid** or **Civatte bodies.** Although these changes bear some similarities to those in erythema multiforme (discussed above), lichen planus shows changes of chronicity: epidermal hyperplasia (or rarely atrophy) and thickening of the granular cell layer and stratum corneum (hypergranulosis and hyperkeratosis, respectively).

The precise pathogenesis of lichen planus is not known. It is plausible that release of antigens at the levels of the basal cell layer and the dermoepidermal junction may elicit a cell-mediated immune response in this disorder.

BLISTERING (BULLOUS) DISEASES

Although vesicles and bullae (blisters) occur as a secondary phenomenon in a number of unrelated conditions (e.g., herpesvirus infection, spongiotic dermatitis), there is a group of disorders in which blisters are the primary and most distinctive features. Blisters can occur at multiple levels within the skin, and assessment of these levels is essential to an accurate histologic diagnosis.

Pemphigus

Pemphigus is a rare *autoimmune blistering disorder resulting from loss of the integrity of normal intercellular attachments within the epidermis and mucosal epithelium.* Most individuals who develop pemphigus are in the fourth to sixth decades of life, and men and women are affected equally. There are four clinical and pathologic variants: (1) pemphigus vulgaris, (2) pemphigus vegetans, (3) pemphigus foliaceus, and (4) pemphigus erythematosus.

Pemphigus vulgaris, by far the most common type (accounting for over 80% of cases worldwide), involves mucosa and skin, especially on the scalp, face, axilla, groin, trunk, and points of pressure. The primary lesions are very superficial vesicles and bullae that rupture easily, leaving shallow erosions covered with dried serum and crust. *Pemphigus vegetans* is a rare form that usually presents not with blisters but with large, moist, verrucous (wartlike), vegetating plaques studded

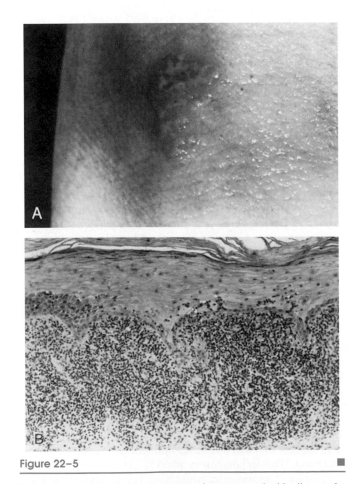

Figure 22–5 ■

Lichen planus. *A,* A small erythematous plaque, covered with oil to render the stratum corneum translucent, shows characteristic Wickham's striae. *B,* Biopsy of this lesion demonstrates the bandlike infiltrate of lymphocytes at the dermoepidermal junction and pointed rete ridges ("saw-toothing").

with pustules on the groin, axilla, and flexural surfaces. *Pemphigus foliaceus*, a more benign form of pemphigus, occurs in an epidemic form in South America, and there are isolated cases in other countries. Bullae are confined to skin, with only rare involvement of mucous membranes. They are so superficial that only zones of erythema and crusting, sites of previous blister rupture, are detected. *Pemphigus erythematosus* is considered a localized, less severe form of pemphigus foliaceus that may selectively involve the malar area of the face in a lupus erythematosus–like fashion.

> **MORPHOLOGY.** The common histologic denominator in all forms of pemphigus is **acantholysis.** This term implies dissolution, or lysis, of the intercellular adhesion sites within a squamous epithelial surface. Detached from their moorings, acantholytic cells become rounded. In pemphigus vulgaris and pemphigus vegetans, acantholysis selectively involves the layer of cells immediately above the basal cell layer, giving rise to the **suprabasal acantholytic blister** characteristic of pemphigus vulgaris (Fig. 22–6). In pemphigus foliaceus, acantholysis selectively involves the superficial epidermis at the level of the stratum granulosum. Variable superficial dermal infiltration by lymphocytes, histiocytes, and eosinophils accompanies all forms of pemphigus.

Pemphigus is caused by a type II hypersensitivity reaction (Chapter 5). Sera from patients with pemphigus contain pathogenic IgG antibodies to intercellular cement substance (desmogleins) of skin and mucous membranes. Lesional sites show a characteristic netlike pattern of intercellular IgG deposits by direct immunofluorescence localized to sites of developed or incipient acantholysis (Fig. 22–7).

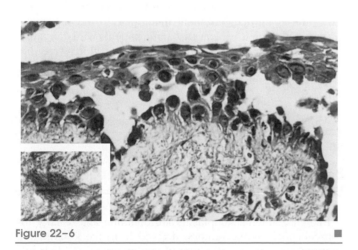

Figure 22–6 ■

Pemphigus vulgaris. Suprabasal acantholysis results in an intraepidermal blister in which rounded (acantholytic) epidermal cells are identified. Dissolution of intercellular cement substance of keratinocyte attachment plaques (desmosomes) *(inset)* results in acantholysis in this disorder.

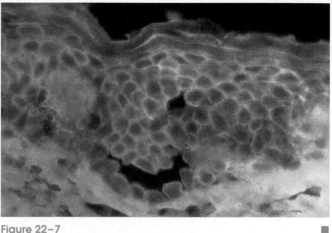

Figure 22–7 ■

Pemphigus vulgaris, direct immunofluorescence. There is deposition of immunoglobulin along the plasma membranes of epidermal keratinocytes in a fishnet-like pattern. Also note the early suprabasal separation due to loss of cell-cell adhesion (acantholysis).

Bullous Pemphigoid

Generally affecting elderly individuals, bullous pemphigoid shows a wide range of clinical presentations, with localized to generalized cutaneous lesions and involvement of mucosal surfaces.

Clinically, *lesions are tense bullae, filled with clear fluid, on normal or erythematous skin* (Fig. 22–8A). The bullae do not rupture as easily as the blisters seen in pemphigus and, if uncomplicated by infection, heal without scarring. Sites of occurrence include the inner aspects of the thighs, flexor surfaces of the forearms, axillae, groin, and lower abdomen. Oral involvement is present in up to one third of patients.

> **MORPHOLOGY.** Bullous pemphigoid is characterized by a **subepidermal, nonacantholytic** blister. Early lesions show a perivascular infiltrate of lymphocytes and variable numbers of eosinophils, occasional neutrophils, superficial dermal edema, and associated basal cell layer vacuolization. The vacuolated basal cell layer eventually gives rise to a fluid-filled blister (Fig. 22–8B).

The immunopathology of bullous pemphigoid features *linear* deposition of immunoglobulin and complement in the basement membrane zone. Ultrastructural studies have shown that circulating antibody reacts with an antigen that extends into the narrow clear zone (lamina lucida) of the epidermal basement membrane that separates the underlying lamina densa from the plasma membrane of the basal cells (Fig. 22–8C). Reactivity also occurs in the basal cell–basement membrane attachment plaques (hemidesmosomes) where most of the bullous pemphigoid antigen is actually located. It is likely

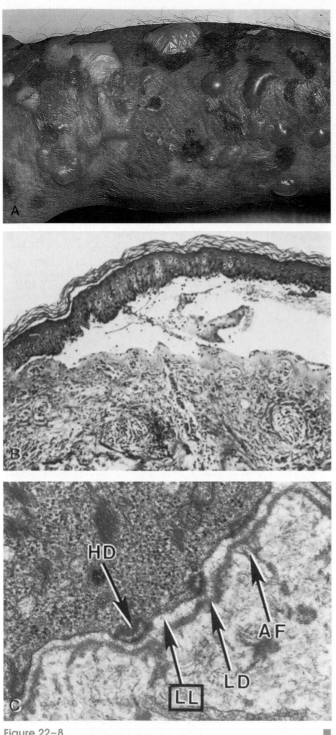

Figure 22–8

Bullous pemphigoid. Clinical bullae *(A)* result from basal cell layer vacuolization, producing a subepidermal blister *(B). C,* Bullous pemphigoid antigen is located primarily in the hemidesmosomes from where it extends into the lamina lucida (LL) of the basement membrane. HD, hemidesmosome; LD, lamina densa; AF, anchoring fibrils.

that the generation of autoantibodies to this hemidesmosome component results in the fixation of complement and subsequent tissue injury at this site via locally recruited neutrophils and eosinophils. Like pemphigus vulgaris, bullous pemphi-

goid is also caused by a type II hypersensitivity reaction, but the target antigens are different in the two conditions.

Dermatitis Herpetiformis

Dermatitis herpetiformis is a rare and fascinating entity, characterized by *urticaria and vesicles.* Males tend to be affected more frequently than females, and the age of onset is often in the third and fourth decades. In some cases it occurs in association with celiac disease and responds to a gluten-free diet (Chapter 15).

The urticarial plaques and vesicles of dermatitis herpetiformis are extremely *pruritic.* They characteristically occur bilaterally and symmetrically, involving preferentially the extensor surfaces, elbows, knees, upper back, and buttocks. *Vesicles are frequently grouped,* as are those of true herpesvirus; hence, the name "herpetiform."

MORPHOLOGY. In the early stages of the disease, fibrin and neutrophils accumulate selectively at the **tips of dermal papillae,** forming small microabscesses (Fig. 22–9*A*). The basal cells overlying these microabscesses show vacuolization and minute zones of dermoepidermal separation (microscopic blisters). In time, these zones coalesce to form a true **subepidermal blister.** Eosinophils may occur in the infiltrates of older lesions. By direct immunofluorescence, dermatitis herpetiformis shows granular deposits of **IgA** selectively localized in the tips of dermal papillae, where they are deposited on anchoring fibrils (Fig. 22–9*B*).

The association of dermatitis herpetiformis with celiac disease was mentioned earlier. It seems that some genetically predisposed individuals develop IgA and IgG antibodies to dietary gluten (derived from wheat). These antibodies cross-react with reticulin, a component of the anchoring fibrils that tether the epidermal basement membrane to the superficial dermis. Although it is clear that some patients with dermatitis herpetiformis and enteropathy respond to a gluten-free diet (as with celiac disease), the immunopathogenesis of the disease remains to be fully clarified.

 TUMORS

Benign and Premalignant Epithelial Lesions

Benign epithelial neoplasms are common and usually inconsequential. These tumors, derived from the keratinizing stratified squamous epithelium of the epidermis and hair follicles (keratinocytes) and the ductular epithelium of cutaneous glands, may recapitulate the cell layers from which they arise. The overwhelming majority do not undergo malignant transformation; only some, such as those in actinic keratosis, have

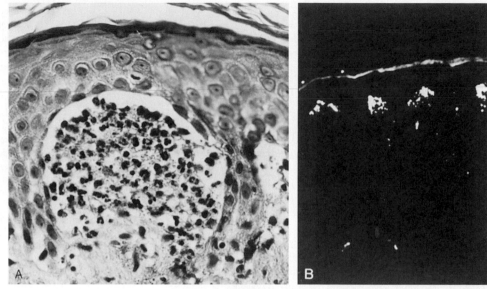

Figure 22–9

Dermatitis herpetiformis. *A,* Neutrophilic microabscess selectively involving the dermal papilla. *B,* Direct immunofluorescence demonstrates granular IgA deposits within four adjacent dermal papillae. These deposits are specifically localized to the anchoring fibrils.

malignant potential. In the ensuing discussion, some common epidermal lesions are described. Tumors arising from hair follicles and other appendages are too infrequent to merit further consideration here.

SEBORRHEIC KERATOSIS

These common epidermal tumors occur most frequently in middle-aged or older individuals. They arise spontaneously and may become particularly numerous on the trunk, although the extremities, head, and neck may also be involved.

Clinically, seborrheic keratoses appear as *round, flat, coin-like plaques that vary in diameter from millimeters to several centimeters* (Fig. 22–10A). They are uniformly tan to dark brown in color and usually show a velvety to granular surface.

> **MORPHOLOGY.** Histologically, these neoplasms are exophytic and are demarcated sharply from the adjacent epidermis (Fig. 22–10B). They are composed of sheets of small cells that most resemble basal cells of the normal epidermis. Variable melanin pigmentation is present within these basaloid cells, accounting for the brown coloration seen clinically that may mimic melanoma. Exuberant keratin production (hyperkeratosis) occurs at the surface of seborrheic keratoses, and the presence of small keratin-filled cysts (horn cysts) and downgrowths of keratin into the main tumor mass (pseudo-horn cysts) are characteristic features.

Seborrheic keratosis is an indolent but benign condition that is readily treated by excision and rarely, if ever, progresses to squamous cell carcinoma. The explosive onset of hundreds of lesions may occur as a *paraneoplastic syndrome* in some cases. Patients with this presentation may harbor inter-

nal malignancies that produce growth factors that stimulate epidermal proliferation.

KERATOACANTHOMA

Keratoacanthoma is a rapidly developing neoplasm that clinically and histologically may mimic well-differentiated squamous cell carcinoma (see later discussion), but it heals spontaneously without treatment. Men are affected more often than women, and lesions most frequently affect sun-exposed skin of whites over 50 years of age.

Clinically, keratoacanthomas appear as *flesh-colored, dome-shaped nodules with a central, keratin-filled plug,* imparting a crater-like topography. Lesions range in size from 1 cm to several centimeters across and have a predilection for the cheeks, nose, ears, and dorsa of the hands.

> **MORPHOLOGY.** Histologically, keratoacanthomas are characterized by a central, keratin-filled crater, surrounded by proliferating epithelial cells that extend upward in a liplike fashion over the sides of the crater and downward into the dermis as irregular tongues (Fig. 22–11A). This epithelium is composed of enlarged cells showing evidence of reactive cytologic atypia. These cells have a characteristically "glassy" eosinophilic cytoplasm (Fig. 22–11B) and produce keratin abruptly (without the development of an intervening granular cell layer).

VERRUCAE (WARTS)

Verrucae are common lesions of children and adolescents, although they may be encountered at any age. They are caused by human papillomaviruses (HPVs). Transmission of disease

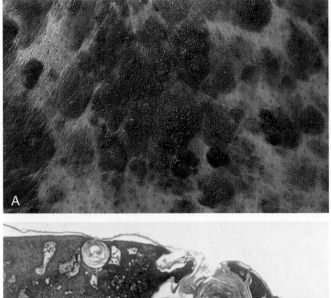

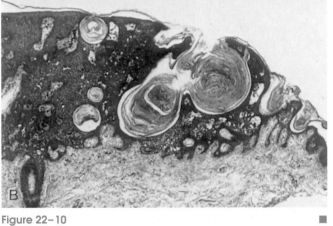

Figure 22-10 ■

Seborrheic keratoses. Multiple coalescent, coinlike pigmented lesions on the back *(A)* are composed of well-demarcated, orderly proliferations of basaloid cells forming small, keratin-filled cysts *(B)*.

usually involves direct contact between individuals or auto-inoculation. Verrucae are generally self-limiting, regressing spontaneously within 6 months to 2 years.

Warts can be classified into several types on the basis of their morphology and location. In addition, each type of wart is caused by a different HPV type. *Verruca vulgaris* is the most common type of wart. These lesions occur anywhere but are found most frequently on the hands, particularly on the dorsal surfaces and periungual areas, where they appear as gray-white to tan, flat to convex, 0.1- to 1-cm papules with a rough, pebble-like surface (Fig. 22-12A). *Verruca plana,* or *flat wart,* is common on the face or the dorsal surfaces of the hands. These warts are slightly elevated, flat, smooth, tan papules that are generally smaller than those of verruca vulgaris. *Verruca plantaris* and *verruca palmaris* occur on the soles and palms, respectively. Rough, scaly lesions may reach 1 to 2 cm in diameter, coalesce, and be confused with ordinary calluses. *Condyloma acuminatum (venereal wart)* occurs on the penis, female genitalia, urethra, perianal areas, and rectum. These lesions appear as soft, tan, cauliflower-like masses that sometimes reach many centimeters in diameter (Chapter 19).

MORPHOLOGY. Histologic features common to verrucae include epidermal hyperplasia that is often undulant in character (so-called verrucous or papillomatous epidermal hyperplasia, Fig. 22-12B) and cytoplasmic vacuolization (koilocytosis) that preferentially involves the more superficial epidermal layers, producing halos of pallor surrounding infected nuclei (see Fig. 19-3). Infected cells may also demonstrate prominent and apparently condensed keratohyaline granules and jagged eosinophilic intracytoplasmic keratin aggregates as a result of viral cytopathic effects.

As mentioned above, verrucae are caused by HPV, the virus associated with preneoplastic and invasive cancers of the anogenital region (Chapters 6 and 19). However, in contrast to

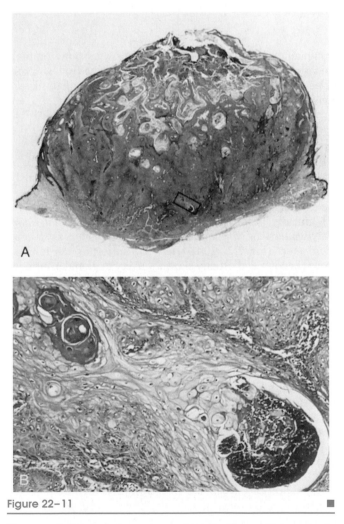

Figure 22-11 ■

Keratoacanthoma. *A,* At lower power, the crater-like architecture may be appreciated. *B,* Higher-power view of the small rectangle in *A*. These tumors are composed of large, glassy squamous cells that form islands of keratin *(upper left)*. The dark mass in the lower right corner is a characteristic aggregate of neutrophils within the tumor.

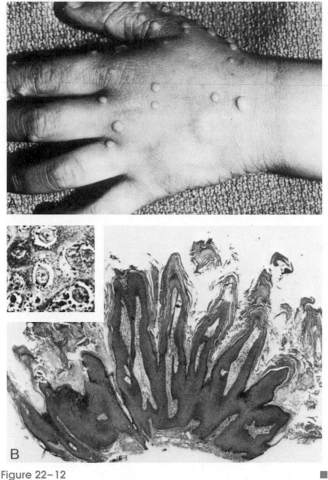

Figure 22–12

Verrucae. *A,* Multiple papules with rough, pebble-like surfaces are present. *B,* Histologically, such lesions show papillomatous epidermal hyperplasia and cytopathic alterations that include nuclear pallor and prominent keratohyaline granules *(inset).* (See also Fig. 19–3.)

HPV-associated carcinomas, warts are caused by distinct HPV types that do not have the potential for causing malignant transformation in normal individuals.

ACTINIC KERATOSIS

Before the development of overt malignancy of the epidermis, a series of progressively dysplastic changes occur, a phenomenon analogous to the atypia that precedes carcinoma of the squamous mucosa of the uterine cervix (Chapter 19). Because this dysplasia is usually the result of chronic exposure to sunlight and is associated with build-up of excess keratin, these lesions are called actinic keratoses.

Lesions of actinic keratosis are usually *less than 1 cm in diameter; are tan-brown, red, or skin colored; and have a rough, sandpaper-like consistency.* Some lesions may produce so much keratin that a "cutaneous horn" develops (Fig. 22–13A, inset). As would be expected, skin sites commonly involved by sun exposure (face, arms, dorsum of the hands) are most frequently affected.

MORPHOLOGY. Cytologic atypia is seen in the lowermost layers of the epidermis and may be associated with hyperplasia of basal cells (Fig. 22–13A and B), or with early atrophy that results in diffuse thinning of the epidermal surface of the lesion. The dermis contains thickened, blue-gray elastic fibers (elastosis), a probable result of abnormal dermal elastic fiber synthesis by sun-damaged fibroblasts within the superficial dermis. The stratum corneum is thickened and, unlike normal skin, nuclei in the cells in this layer are often retained (a pattern termed "parakeratosis").

Whether all actinic keratoses would result in skin cancer (usually squamous cell carcinoma), if given enough time, is conjectural. Indeed, it is likely that many lesions regress or remain stable during a normal life span. However, enough do become malignant to warrant local eradication of these precursor lesions.

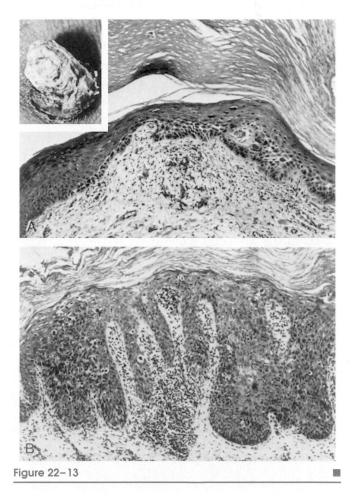

Figure 22–13

A, Actinic keratosis. Basal cell layer atypia (affecting the right side of epidermis) is associated with marked hyperkeratosis and parakeratosis that may result in the clinical appearance of a horn *(inset). B,* Progression to full-thickness atypia heralds the development of squamous cell carcinoma in situ.

Malignant Epidermal Tumors

SQUAMOUS CELL CARCINOMA

Squamous cell carcinoma is *the most common tumor arising on sun-exposed sites in older people.* Except for lesions on the lower legs, these tumors have a higher incidence in men than in women. Implicated as predisposing factors, in addition to sunlight, are industrial carcinogens (tars and oils), chronic ulcers and draining osteomyelitis, old burn scars, ingestion of arsenicals, ionizing radiation, and (in the oral cavity) tobacco and betel nut chewing. Indeed, the incidence of oral squamous cell carcinomas is quite high in certain regions of India, where betel nut chewing is fairly common.

Squamous cell carcinomas that have not invaded through the basement membrane of the dermoepidermal junction *(in situ carcinoma)* appear as sharply defined, red, scaling plaques. More advanced, invasive lesions are nodular, show variable keratin production appreciated clinically as hyperkeratosis, and may ulcerate (Fig. 22–14*B*).

MORPHOLOGY. Unlike actinic keratoses, squamous cell carcinoma in situ is characterized by highly atypical cells at **all levels** of the epidermis (see Fig. 22–13*B*). When these cells break through the basement membrane, the process has become invasive. Invasive squamous cell carcinomas (Fig. 22–14*A*) exhibit variable differentiation, ranging from tumors formed by polygonal squamous cells arranged in orderly lobules that exhibit numerous large zones of keratinization, to neoplasms formed by highly anaplastic, rounded cells with foci of necrosis and only abortive, single-cell keratinization (dyskeratosis).

Invasive squamous cell carcinomas of the skin are usually discovered while small and resectable; less than 5% have metastases to regional nodes at diagnosis.

The most commonly accepted exogenous cause of squamous cell carcinoma is exposure to ultraviolet light, with subsequent unrepaired DNA damage (see Chapter 6). Individuals who are immunosuppressed as a result of chemotherapy or organ transplantation, or who have *xeroderma pigmentosum,* are at increased risk for developing these tumors. In addition to their effect on DNA, ultraviolet rays in sunlight also seem

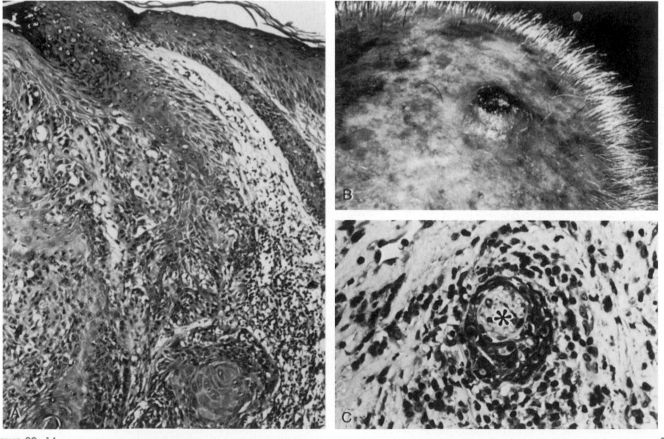

Figure 22–14 ■

Invasive squamous cell carcinoma. *A,* Tongues of atypical squamous epithelium have transgressed the basement membrane, invading deeply into the dermis. *B,* Such lesions are often nodular and ulcerated clinically. *C,* Tumor cells highlighted by staining with labeled antibodies to keratin surround a dermal nerve twig (*), indicative of the locally aggressive nature of this neoplasm.

to exert at least a transient immunosuppressive effect on skin by impairing antigen presentation by Langerhans cells. This may contribute to tumorigenesis by impairing immunosurveillance.

BASAL CELL CARCINOMA

Basal cell carcinomas are common, *slow-growing tumors that rarely metastasize*. They have a tendency to occur at sites subject to chronic sun exposure and in lightly pigmented people. As with squamous cell carcinoma, the incidence of basal cell carcinoma rises sharply with immunosuppression and in patients with inherited defects in DNA replication or repair (xeroderma pigmentosum, Chapter 6).

Clinically, these tumors present as *pearly papules, often containing prominent, dilated subepidermal blood vessels (telangiectasias)* (Fig. 22–15A). Some tumors contain melanin pigment and thus appear similar to nevocellular nevi or melanomas. Advanced lesions may ulcerate, and extensive lo-

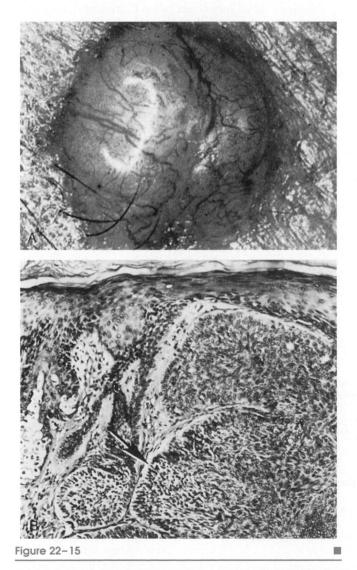

Figure 22–15   ■

Basal cell carcinoma. Pearly, telangiectatic nodules *(A)* are composed of nests of basaloid cells within the dermis *(B)* that are often separated from the adjacent stroma by thin clefts *(arrow)*.

cal invasion of bone or facial sinuses may occur after many years of neglect, justifying the past designation "rodent ulcers."

> **MORPHOLOGY.** Histologically, tumor cells resemble those in the normal basal cell layer of the epidermis. Because they arise from the epidermis or follicular epithelium, they are not encountered on mucosal surfaces. Two patterns are seen, either **multifocal growths** originating from the epidermis and extending over several square centimeters or more of skin surface (multifocal superficial type), or **nodular lesions** growing downward deeply into the dermis as cords and islands of variably basophilic cells with hyperchromatic nuclei, embedded in a mucinous matrix, and often surrounded by many fibroblasts and lymphocytes (Fig. 22–15B). The cells forming the periphery of the tumor cell islands tend to be arranged radially with their long axes in approximately parallel alignment (palisading). The stroma shrinks away from the epithelial tumor nests, creating clefts or separation artifacts that assist in differentiating basal cell carcinomas from certain appendage tumors.

Tumors and Tumor-Like Lesions of Melanocytes

NEVOCELLULAR NEVUS (PIGMENTED NEVUS, MOLE)

Strictly speaking, the term "nevus" denotes any congenital lesion of the skin. "Nevocellular" nevus, however, refers to any congenital or acquired neoplasm of melanocytes.

Clinically, common acquired nevocellular nevi are tan-to-brown, uniformly pigmented, small (usually 5 mm or less across), solid regions of elevated skin (papules) with well-defined, rounded borders (Fig. 22–16A, inset). There are numerous clinical and histologic types of nevocellular nevi, and the clinical appearance may be variable. Table 22–2 provides a comparative summary of salient clinical and histologic features of the more commonly encountered forms of melanocytic nevi.

> **MORPHOLOGY.** Nevocellular nevi are formed by melanocytes that have been transformed from highly dendritic single cells normally interspersed among basal keratinocytes to round-to-oval cells that grow in aggregates, or "nests," along the dermoepidermal junction (Fig. 22–16B). Nuclei of nevus cells are uniform and rounded in contour, contain inconspicuous nucleoli, and show little or no mitotic activity. Such lesions, believed to represent an early developmental stage in nevocellular nevi, are called **junctional nevi**. Eventually, most junctional nevi grow into the underlying dermis as nests or cords of cells **(compound nevi)**, and in older lesions the epidermal nests may be lost en-

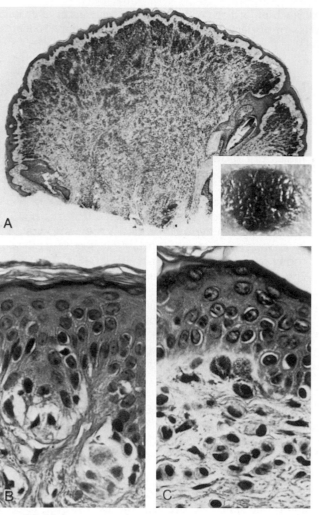

Figure 22–16

Nevocellular nevus. Lesions are symmetric and uniform in clinical *(A, inset)* and histologic *(A)* appearance. Junctional nevi *(B)*, characterized by rounded nests of nevus cells at the dermoepidermal junction, may progress in time to become compound and pure dermal nevi *(C)*, exhibiting migration of nevus cells into the underlying dermis.

tirely to form pure **dermal nevi** (Fig. 22–16A and C). Clinically, compound and dermal nevi are often more elevated than are junctional nevi.

Progressive growth of nevus cells from the dermoepidermal junction into the underlying dermis is accompanied by a process termed "maturation." Whereas less mature, more superficial nevus cells are larger, tend to produce melanin pigment, and grow in nests, more mature, deeper nevus cells are smaller, produce little or no pigment, and grow in cords. This *sequence of maturation of individual nevus cells is of diagnostic importance in distinguishing some benign nevi from melanomas, which usually show little or no maturation.*

Although nevocellular nevi are common and benign, it is important to recognize their distinctive features, lest they become confused with other skin conditions, notably malignant melanoma.

DYSPLASTIC NEVI

Dysplastic nevi, sometimes called Clark's nevi, may occur *sporadically or in a familial form.* The hereditary forms are inherited in an autosomal dominant fashion and are considered precursors of malignant melanoma. In the sporadic form, the risk of malignant transformation appears low.

Clinically, *dysplastic nevi are larger than most acquired nevi* (often more than 5 mm across) and may occur as hundreds of lesions on the body surface (Fig. 22–17A). They are flat macules to slightly raised plaques, with a "pebbly" surface. They usually show *variability in pigmentation* (variegation) and borders that are irregular in contour. Unlike ordinary moles, *dysplastic nevi have a tendency to occur on non–sun-exposed as well as sun-exposed body surfaces.* Dysplastic nevi have been documented in multiple members of families prone to the development of malignant melanoma (the heritable melanoma syndrome).

MORPHOLOGY. Histologically (Fig. 22–17B), dysplastic nevi consist of compound nevi with both architectural and cytologic evidence of abnormal

Table 22–2. VARIANT FORMS OF NEVOCELLULAR NEVI

Nevus Variant	Diagnostic Architectural Features	Diagnostic Cytologic Features	Clinical Significance
Congenital nevus	Deep dermal and sometimes subcutaneous growth around adnexae, neurovascular bundles, and blood vessel walls	Identical to ordinary acquired nevi	Present at birth; large variants carry increased melanoma risk
Blue nevus	Non-nested dermal infiltration, often with associated fibrosis	Highly dendritic, heavily pigmented nevus cells	Black-blue nodule; often confused with melanoma clinically
Spindle and epithelioid cell nevus (Spitz's nevus)	Fascicular growth	Large, plump cells with pink-blue cytoplasm; fusiform cells	Common in children; red-pink nodule; often confused with hemangioma clinically
Halo nevus	Lymphocytic infiltration surrounding nevus cells	Identical to ordinary acquired nevi	Host immune response against nevus cells and surrounding normal melanocytes
Dysplastic nevus	Large, coalescent intraepidermal nests	Cytologic atypia	Potential precursor of malignant melanoma

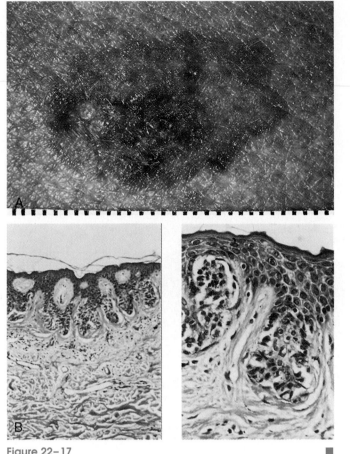

Figure 22–17

Dysplastic nevus. *A,* The nevus has an irregular contour, variegated color, and a typical center of darker pigment with a "pebbly" surface. *B,* Low *(left)* and high *(right)* magnification of the histologic appearance of a dysplastic nevus, showing poorly formed and coalescent nests of nevus cells associated with eosinophilic linear fibrosis forming concentric lamellae within the underlying papillary dermis.

growth. **Nevus cell nests within the epidermis may be enlarged and exhibit abnormal fusion or coalescence with adjacent nests. As part of this process, single nevus cells begin to replace the normal basal cell layer along the dermoepidermal junction, producing so-called lentiginous hyperplasia.** Cytologic atypia consisting of irregular, often angulated, nuclear contours and hyperchromasia is frequently observed. Associated alterations also occur in the superficial dermis. These consist of a usually sparse lymphocytic infiltrate, loss of melanin pigment from presumably destroyed nevus cells, phagocytosis of this pigment by dermal macrophages (melanin pigment incontinence), and a peculiar linear fibrosis surrounding the epidermal rete ridges that are involved by the nevus.

The evidence that some dysplastic nevi are precursors of malignant melanoma is impressive. In individuals with a fam-

ily history of malignant melanoma, the melanomas occur only in individuals who first develop dysplastic nevi. In these cases, the lifetime risk of malignant degeneration in dysplastic nevi is close to 100%.

MALIGNANT MELANOMA

Malignant melanoma is a relatively common neoplasm that not long ago was considered almost uniformly deadly. Today, as a result of increased public awareness of the earliest signs of skin melanomas, most are cured surgically. Nonetheless, the incidence of these lesions is on the rise, necessitating vigorous surveillance for their development.

Although most of these lesions arise in the *skin,* other sites of origin include the *oral* and *anogenital mucosal surfaces,* the *esophagus,* the *meninges,* and notably the *eye.* The following comments apply to cutaneous melanomas; intraocular melanomas are briefly discussed later.

As with other cutaneous malignancies, sunlight plays an important role in the development of malignant melanoma. The incidence is highest in sun-exposed skin and in geographic locales such as New Zealand and Australia, where sun exposure is high. Sunlight, however, does not seem to be the only predisposing factor, and the presence of a preexisting nevus (e.g., a dysplastic nevus), hereditary factors, or even exposure to certain carcinogens may play a role in lesion development and evolution. As with several other common neoplasms (e.g., of the breast or colon), melanomas occur sporadically, but a small fraction are hereditary and familial. Recently, a tumor suppressor gene called MTS (melanoma tumor suppressor) mapped on chromosome 9 has been implicated in familial melanomas.

Clinically, malignant melanoma of the skin is usually asymptomatic, although itching may be an early manifestation. *The most important clinical sign of the disease is a change in the color in a pigmented lesion.* Unlike benign (nondysplastic) nevi, melanomas exhibit striking variations in pigmentation, appearing in shades of black, brown, red, dark blue, and gray (Fig. 22–18*A*). The borders of melanomas are irregular and often "notched." In summary, the clinical warning signs of melanoma are (1) enlargement of a preexisting mole, (2) itching or pain in a preexisting mole, (3) development of a new pigmented lesion during adult life, (4) irregularity of the borders of a pigmented lesion, and (5) variegation of color within a pigmented lesion.

Central to an understanding of the complicated histology of malignant melanoma is the concept of radial and vertical growth. Simply stated, *radial growth* indicates the tendency of a melanoma to grow horizontally within the epidermal and superficial dermal layers, often for a prolonged period. During this stage of growth, melanoma cells do not have the capacity to metastasize. With time, the pattern of growth assumes a *vertical component,* and the melanoma now grows downward into the deeper dermal layers as an expansile mass lacking cellular maturation, without any tendency for the cells to become smaller as they descend into the reticular dermis (Fig. 22–18*B*). This event is heralded clinically by the development of a nodule in the relatively flat radial growth phase, and correlates with the emergence of a clone of cells with metastatic potential. Interestingly, the probability of metastasis in such a lesion may be predicted by simply measuring in millimeters

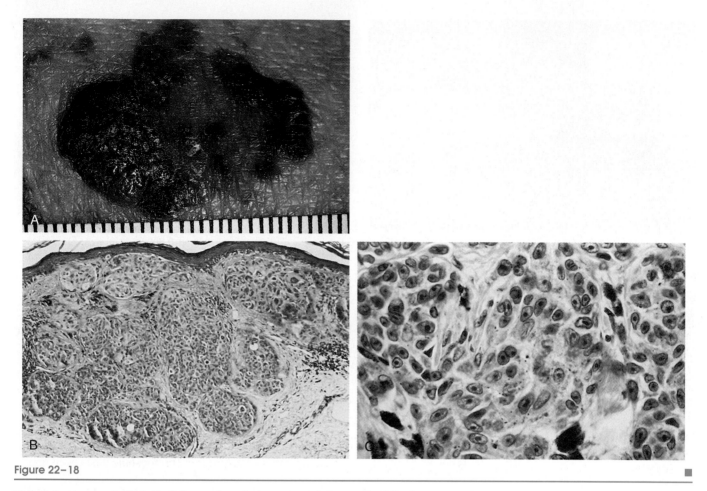

Figure 22-18

Malignant melanoma. *A,* Clinically, lesions are irregular in contour and pigmentation. Macular areas correlate with the radial growth phase, while raised areas usually correspond to nodular aggregates of malignant cells in the vertical phase of growth. *B,* Photomicrograph of a lesion in the vertical phase of growth, demonstrating nodular aggregates of infiltrating cells. *C,* High-power view of malignant melanoma cells.

the depth of invasion of this vertical growth phase nodule below the granular cell layer of the overlying epidermis. *Metastases involve not only regional lymph nodes but also liver, lungs, brain, and virtually any other site that can be seeded by the hematogeneous route.* Remarkably, in some cases, metastases may appear for the first time many years after surgical excision of the primary tumor, suggesting a long phase of dormancy.

MORPHOLOGY. Individual melanoma cells are usually considerably larger than nevus cells. They contain large nuclei with irregular contours having chromatin characteristically clumped at the periphery of the nuclear membrane and prominent red (eosinophilic) nucleoli (Fig. 22-18*C*). These cells grow as poorly formed nests or as individual cells at all levels of the epidermis and, in the dermis, as expansile, balloon-like nodules (Fig. 22-18*B*). **The nature and extent of the vertical growth phase determine the biologic behavior of malignant melanomas,** and thus it is important to observe and record vertical growth phase parameters.

Melanoma of the eye is about one twentieth as common as melanoma of the skin. Most intraocular melanomas arise in the melanocytes of the uvea (iris, ciliary body, and choroid), but they can also originate in the pigmented epithelium of the retina.

Unlike the cutaneous type, ocular melanomas are composed of two distinctive cell types, spindle and epithelioid, having differing clinical implications. Lesions composed completely or predominantly of spindle cells are of low aggressiveness, do not tend to metastasize, and permit about a 75% 15-year survival. In contrast, epithelioid melanomas provide only about 35% survival at 15 years despite early enucleation, owing to late metastasis.

The Nervous System

DENNIS K. BURNS, MD

The nervous system represents the major communications network in the human body. As in other vertebrates, its normal function in humans is exquisitely dependent on the maintenance of structural integrity and a host of metabolic processes. Accordingly, influences that disrupt normal structure, metabolism, or both, are capable of producing neurologic disease.

Disorders of the nervous system are often regarded as more complex or arcane than those in other organ systems. When allowances are made for the unique structural and cellular characteristics of the nervous system, however, neuropathologic processes can be understood in the context of the principles introduced in the general pathology sections of the text.

To gain an understanding of disorders affecting the nervous system, it is appropriate to review some of the important structural features of the central and peripheral nervous systems and their cellular composition. At the outset, it is important to recall that bodily functions are regulated by specific areas within the nervous system. This renders the nervous system vulnerable to focal lesions that in other organ systems might produce no significant dysfunction. As an example, an isolated renal infarct would not be expected to have a significant effect on renal function. An infarct of comparable size in the internal capsule of the brain, in contrast, might leave a patient with contralateral hemiplegia. Moreover, a particular focal lesion might produce highly variable neurologic deficits, depending on its location.

The nervous system has anatomic features that confer protection against some insults while rendering it more vulnerable to others. As an example, while the rigid confines of the skull serve to protect the brain from trauma, they also render the organ vulnerable to processes that produce elevated intracranial pressure.

The brain parenchyma is composed of neurons supported by a framework of glial cells (astrocytes, oligodendrocytes, and ependyma), bloods vessels, and microglia. The processes of these cells combine to form a delicate fibrillar background termed the *neuropil*.

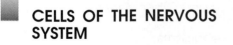

CELLS OF THE NERVOUS SYSTEM

Neurons

The neurons are a heterogeneous family, both morphologically and functionally, ranging from the small round cells that populate the internal granular layer of the cerebellum to the large, pyramidal Betz cells of the primary motor cortex. A variety of morphologic alterations may be encountered in neurons, one of the most common of which is necrosis. As in the case of coagulation necrosis in other sites, neuronal necrosis is characterized by cytoplasmic eosinophilia and nuclear changes, including contraction (pyknosis), fragmentation (karyorrhexis), and loss of staining (karyolysis). In addition, a number of neuronal alterations occur in degenerative diseases that are unique to the nervous system, such as neurofibrillary tangle and Lewy body formation. Chromatolysis, a common reaction of the neuron to axonal injury, is characterized by dispersion of the Nissl substance and swelling of the neuronal cell body. Finally, a number of infectious agents may produce characteristic nuclear or cytoplasmic inclusions. These changes specific to the neurons are discussed more fully in the discussions of the diseases in which they occur.

Astrocytes

Astrocytes represent the major supporting cell in the brain and show some of the most common reactive changes. In cases of brain parenchymal injury, astrocytes respond by producing a dense network of processes, somewhat analogous to a fibrous scar occurring elsewhere in the body. In contrast to the fibroblasts, however, astrocytes do not produce collagen. The glial "scar," accordingly, is made up predominantly of cytoplasmic processes, with little or no extracellular protein. The cytoplasm of astrocytes may swell in response to injury, often in association with increased synthesis of glial fibrillary acidic protein (GFAP), the astrocyte's major cytoskeletal protein. The cytoplasm around the nucleus of such cells, termed *gemistocytic astrocytes* (Greek, *gemistos* = "full"), is eosinophilic and readily visualized in routine sections. *Rosenthal fibers* represent yet another distinctive structure and are encountered in slowly growing neoplasms and some non-neoplastic disorders, such as chronic cavitary lesions and vascular malformations. Rosenthal fibers are dense aggregates within astrocytic cell processes that appear as brightly eosinophilic structures with an almost refractile quality. Certain metabolic disturbances, notably liver failure, produce astrocytes with enlarged, pale nuclei, termed *Alzheimer type II glia.* Finally, glycoprotein-rich materials, termed *corpora amylacea,* commonly accumulate in astrocytic processes with age. In hematoxylin-and-eosin (H & E) sections corpora amylacea appear as spherical basophilic bodies in regions rich in astrocytic foot processes (e.g., the subependymal, subpial, and perivascular regions), as well as within the dorsal columns of the spinal cord.

Oligodendrocytes

Oligodendroglial cytoplasmic processes wrap around the axons of neurons to form myelin in a manner analogous to the Schwann cells of the peripheral nervous system. In routine sections, oligodendroglia are recognizable by their small, rounded, lymphocyte-like nuclei, often arranged in linear arrays. Injury to oligodendroglial cells is a feature of acquired demyelinating disorders (e.g., multiple sclerosis) and is also seen in the leukodystrophies. Oligodendroglial nuclei may harbor inclusions in certain conditions such as progressive multifocal leukoencephalopathy.

Ependymal Cells

Ependymal cells line the cerebral ventricles and are closely related to the cuboidal cells lining the choroid plexus. Disruption of ependymal cells is often associated with a local proliferation of subependymal astrocytes to produce small irregularities termed *ependymal granulations* on the ventricular surfaces. Certain infectious agents, particularly cytomegalovirus (CMV), may produce extensive ependymal injury, with prominent associated viral inclusions, in ependymal cells.

Microglia

Despite their name, microglia are in all likelihood derived from circulating monocytes rather than from the neural tube. The major phagocytic cells in the central nervous system (CNS), microglia may accumulate abundant intracellular lipids to form foamy macrophages, termed *gitter cells*. In other conditions, the nuclei of microglia may elongate to form so-called rod cells. Microglia may also aggregate in response to various insults (e.g., viral infections) to form microglial nodules.

EDEMA, HERNIATION, AND HYDROCEPHALUS

The brain and spinal cord exist within a rigid compartment defined by the skull, vertebral bodies, and dura mater. The advantage of housing as vital and delicate a structure as the CNS in a protective environment is obvious. On the other hand, such rigid confines provide very little room for brain parenchymal expansion. A number of disorders may upset the delicate balance between brain parenchymal mass and the fixed boundaries of the intracranial vault. These include generalized brain edema, hydrocephalus, and more localized expanding mass lesions.

Cerebral Edema

Cerebral edema or, more appropriately, brain parenchymal edema, may arise in the setting of a number of diseases. Broadly speaking, it may be categorized as vasogenic edema and cytotoxic edema.

Vasogenic edema occurs when the integrity of the normal blood-brain barrier is disrupted, allowing fluid to escape from the vasculature into the interstitial space of the brain (interstitial edema). The paucity of lymphatics in the brain greatly impairs the resorption of excess intercellular fluid. The edema may be localized, as in the case of the abnormally permeable vessels encountered adjacent to abscesses and neoplasms, or more generalized.

Cytotoxic edema, in contrast, implies an increase in intracellular fluid (intracellular edema) secondary to cellular injury, as might be encountered in a patient with a generalized hypoxic-ischemic insult. In practice, conditions associated with generalized edema are usually associated with elements of vasogenic and cytotoxic edema.

> The edematous brain is softer than normal and often appears to "overfill" the cranial vault. In generalized edema, the gyri are flattened, the intervening sulci narrowed, and the ventricular cavities compressed (Fig. 23–1). As the brain expands herniation may occur.

Herniation

The cranial sutures in infants and young children permit some accommodation to increases in intracranial pressure. In older children and adults, however, increases in intracranial pressure are poorly tolerated owing to the rigid nature of the

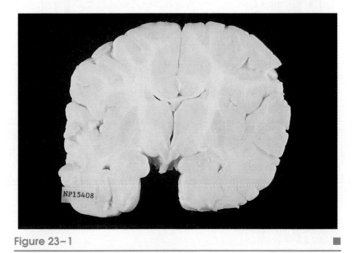

Figure 23–1   ■

Generalized brain edema. The surfaces of the gyri are flattened as a result of compression of the expanding brain by the dura mater and inner surface of the skull. Such changes are associated with a dangerous increase in intracranial pressure.

cranial vault. As noted previously, for example, the surface of the edematous brain is typically flattened, because of pressure of the brain on the inner table of the skull. In addition, as expanding brain parenchyma encounters other unyielding structures, such as dural reflections or the foramen magnum, one or more different patterns of herniation may occur. The three most common forms are illustrated in Figure 23–2 and are described as follows:

1. *Transtentorial (uncinate, mesial temporal) herniation* occurs when the medial aspect of the temporal lobe is compressed against the free margin of the tentorium cerebelli. As displacement of the temporal lobe extends, the third cranial nerve is compressed, resulting in pupillary dilation and impairment of ocular movements on the side of the lesion. The posterior cerebral artery is also often compressed, resulting in ischemic injury to the territory supplied by that vessel, including the primary visual cortex.
2. *Subfalcine (cingulate gyrus) herniation* occurs when unilateral or asymmetric expansion of the cerebral hemisphere displaces the cingulate gyrus under the falx cerebri. This is often associated with compression of branches of the anterior cerebral artery.
3. *Tonsillar herniation* refers to displacement of the cerebellar tonsils through the foramen magnum. This pattern of herniation is life threatening because it causes brain stem compression and compromises vital respiratory centers in

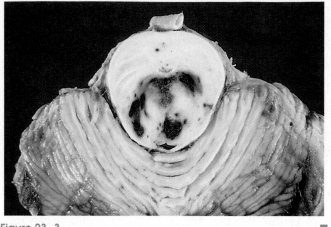

Figure 23–3 ■

Duret's hemorrhage. Herniation of the brain stem through the foramen magnum compromises the flow of blood in small branch vessels supplying the brain stem, resulting in areas of hemorrhage and necrosis.

the medulla oblongata. Brain stem herniation is often accompanied by hemorrhagic lesions in the midbrain and pons, termed *secondary brain stem,* or *Duret's, hemorrhages* (Fig. 23–3). These linear or fountain-shaped lesions usually occur in the midline and paramedian regions, and actually represent hemorrhagic infarcts caused by kinking of branches of the basilar artery during herniation.

Hydrocephalus

In the normal brain, cerebrospinal fluid (CSF) is produced by the choroid plexus within the lateral and fourth ventricles. The CSF normally circulates through the ventricular system, enters the cisterna magna at the base of the brain stem via the foramina of Luschka and Magendie and then bathes the superior cerebral convexities, where it is absorbed by the arachnoid granulations. *Hydrocephalus* refers to the accumulation of excessive CSF within the ventricular system of the brain. Most such cases occur as a consequence of decreased resorption of CSF, although in rare instances (e.g., tumors of the choroid plexus), overproduction of CSF may be responsible. Whatever its origin, increases in CSF within the ventricles expands them and causes an elevation in intracranial pressure. The term *noncommunicating hydrocephalus* is used when obstruction to the flow of CSF occurs within the ventricular system. If the obstruction occurs outside of the ventricular system (e.g., in the subarachnoid space or at the arachnoid granulations), the process is referred to as *communicating hydrocephalus.*

If hydrocephalus develops before closure of the cranial sutures, there is enlargement of the head, manifested by an increase in head circumference. Hydrocephalus developing after fusion of the sutures, in contrast, is associated with expansion of the ventricles and increased intracranial pressure, without a change in head circumference (Fig. 23–4).

The term *hydrocephalus ex vacuo* refers to dilation of the ventricular system with a compensatory increase in CSF volume secondary to a loss of brain parenchyma. There is no

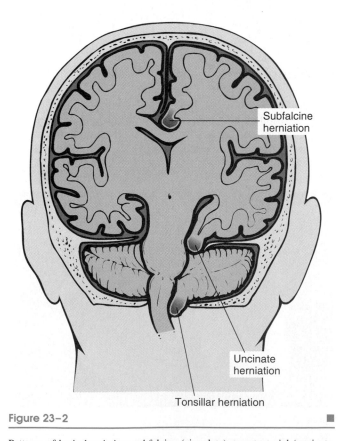

Subfalcine
herniation

Uncinate
herniation

Tonsillar herniation

Figure 23–2 ■

Patterns of brain herniation: subfalcine (cingulate), transtentorial (uncinate, mesial temporal), and tonsillar. (Adapted from Fishman RA: Brain edema. N Engl J Med 293:706, 1975. Adapted, with permission, from The New England Journal of Medicine.)

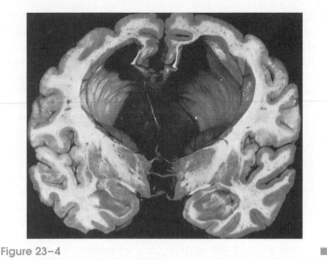

Figure 23–4

Hydrocephalus. Obstruction of the flow of cerebrospinal fluid has caused the ventricles to expand, with a resultant increase in intracranial pressure. Obstructive hydrocephalus must be distinguished from hydrocephalus ex vacuo, in which the ventricles expand to compensate for a loss of brain parenchyma.

sures, constricting in response to abnormally high pressures and dilating in response to hypotension. Below a systolic pressure of approximately 50 mm Hg, however, autoregulatory mechanisms are inadequate to compensate for the reduction in blood flow, and parenchymal injury may occur. The term *hypoxia* refers to a decrease in the oxygen available to tissues, while *ischemia* refers to a decrease in tissue perfusion. In practice, the effects of pure hypoxia are difficult to separate from those of ischemia—cardiopulmonary arrest, for example, is associated with both hypoxemia and decreased perfusion pressure—and the two are usually considered together. Within the CNS, certain regions and cell populations are more susceptible than others to hypoxic-ischemic injury. For example, neurons, as a group, are far more vulnerable to ischemic injury than are glial cells. Among the neuronal elements, certain subpopulations, such as the pyramidal cells of the hippocampus and the Purkinje cells of the cerebellum, are particularly sensitive to anoxia and are often sites of selective injury. Areas of the brain located at the junctions of arterial territories (i.e., arterial border zones, sometimes termed *watershed areas*) are also particularly susceptible.

increase in the rate of CSF fluid production, and the flow of CSF remains normal. Hydrocephalus ex vacuo is often associated with other evidence of parenchymal atrophy, such as thinning of cortical gyri and widening of sulci.

VASCULAR DISEASES

Under normal circumstances, the brain receives 15% of the cardiac output and utilizes roughly 20% of the oxygen consumed by the body. Interruption of normal blood flow to the brain and spinal cord may produce irreversible parenchymal injury within a very brief time. Hence, the brain is exquisitely sensitive to changes in cerebral blood flow and is capable of regulating the flow of blood over a wide range of perfusion pressures, a process termed *autoregulation*.

Although the incidence of cerebrovascular disease has decreased in recent decades, vascular insults remain the third most common cause of death in the United States, exceeded only by heart disease and cancer. Cerebrovascular diseases fall into the following three major categories:

■ Parenchymal injuries associated with a *generalized reduction in blood flow*, including global hypoxic-ischemic encephalopathy
■ *Infarcts* caused by local vascular obstruction
■ *Hemorrhages* within the brain parenchyma or the subarachnoid space

Of the three, infarcts are the most common, accounting for roughly 80% of the total.

Global Hypoxic-Ischemic Encephalopathy

The cerebral vasculature has a remarkable capacity to maintain normal blood flow over a wide range of perfusion pres-

MORPHOLOGY. In the period immediately after a global hypoxic-ischemic insult (e.g., cardiac arrest), the brain may appear normal, both grossly and microscopically. In patients who survive the acute insult, within 24 to 48 hours, the brain is softened and edematous. Irregular, mottled discoloration is often visible in gray matter; in some areas, such as arterial border zones, areas of hemorrhage may be present. The cortical mantle may be interrupted by an irregular, linear zone of softening and discoloration; this pattern, termed **laminar cortical necrosis,** reflects the vulnerability of specific cortical layers to hypoxic-ischemic injury. The demarcation between gray and white matter is usually blurred. Fragments of soft, necrotic cerebellar parenchyma may be present in the spinal subarachnoid space. The brains of patients maintained on respiratory support after cessation of brain activity ("brain death") appear swollen, dusky, and soft, even after formalin fixation. The term **respirator brain** is sometimes used to designate such cases, but it should be understood that the use of artificial ventilatory support is not the cause of the changes noted. Microscopic changes are apparent within 12 to 24 hours and include neuronal shrinkage or swelling, followed by the development of cytoplasmic eosinophilia, nuclear pyknosis, and cytologic features of necrosis. The parenchyma is often vacuolated, with widened perivascular and pericellular spaces (vasogenic edema), and the endothelial cells may show some swelling. In contrast to localized infarcts, there is little host inflammatory reaction. In cases associated with prolonged survival, neurons disappear, and the intervening neuropil becomes cystic and gliotic.

Clinical Features. Hypoxic-ischemic encephalopathy may occur under any circumstance that results in a global decrease in the amount of oxygen available to the brain, including cardiac dysrhythmias, shock, and large increases in intracranial pressure. A number of factors may modify the degree of parenchymal injury, including the age of the patient (young patients tolerate global insults better than do the elderly), duration of the circulatory disturbance, and temperature (hypothermia increases the resistance of the brain to hypoxic-ischemic injury). The resulting deficits range from transient neurologic disturbances to "brain death," with a global cessation of electrical activity.

Infarcts

Infarcts are caused by local circulatory disturbances. Such lesions represent the most common form of cerebrovascular disease, accounting for roughly 80% of all cerebrovascular accidents, or "strokes." They occur most commonly in the seventh decade of life and are more common in males than in females. Cerebral atherosclerosis is the most common cause of brain infarcts, and factors that predispose individuals to atherosclerosis (e.g., hypertension, diabetes mellitus, and smoking) increase the risk of infarcts. The most severe atherosclerosis typically affects larger vessels, such as the internal carotid arteries, the proximal middle cerebral arteries, and the basilar artery. An important cause of vascular occlusion in patients with cerebral atherosclerosis is thrombosis of an atherosclerotic arterial segment, occurring most commonly near the carotid bifurcation or in the basilar artery. Other causes of vascular occlusion include emboli, often originating from the heart and proximal segments of the carotid arteries. With the exception of the basilar arterial system, embolic occlusion most frequently affects intracranial blood vessels, especially the middle cerebral artery. Vasculitis and trauma are less common causes of cerebrovascular occlusion.

The location and distribution of cerebral infarcts is influenced by a number of factors, including the site of arterial occlusion, the time over which an occlusive event develops, the presence or absence of arterial anastomoses (e.g., the circle of Willis), and systemic perfusion pressure. For example, individuals with well-developed arterial anastomoses might tolerate gradual thrombotic occlusion of the internal carotid artery with minimal symptoms, whereas embolic occlusion of the middle cerebral artery might result in a massive hemispheric infarct. Collateral circulation is, in general, less well developed in more distal arterial branches; therefore, occlusion of a distal arterial branch almost always results in the development of an infarct. Patients with significant atherosclerosis may develop infarcts even in the absence of vascular occlusion if blood pressure drops significantly.

MORPHOLOGY. Although cell death occurs within minutes of arterial occlusion, the gross and histologic appearance of the brain is normal for the first 8 to 12 hours. The first alterations are apparent microscopically and consist of ischemic neuronal changes (described earlier), and a neutrophilic in-

flammatory reaction. By 36 to 48 hours, the necrotic area becomes swollen and softer than the adjacent, unaffected brain parenchyma. Demarcation between gray and white matter becomes blurred owing to interstitial and intracellular edema. Areas of hemorrhage may be seen, particularly in infarcts involving arterial border zones or those resulting from transient occlusion by emboli or by external compression of the vessel. Over the next several days, macrophages infiltrate the lesion and phagocytose necrotic parenchyma, resulting in progressively sharper demarcation of the infarct. By 1 month, extensive phagocytosis of necrotic parenchyma results in further softening and liquefaction of the infarct, with cavitation. By about 6 months, most infarcts are completely cavitated (Fig. 23–5). In the case of infarcts involving cerebral cortex, a thin rim of subpial parenchyma, supplied by small superficial leptomeningeal blood vessels, is preserved over the infarct, a feature that may be helpful in differentiating remote infarcts from old contusions (discussed later).

Clinical Features. Typically, the onset of brain infarction is fairly sudden but is often preceded by transient episodes of neurologic dysfunction lasting from several minutes to several hours. Such episodes, termed *transient ischemic attacks (TIAs)*, are caused by self-limited episodes of vascular obstruction by atheromatous emboli and/or platelet-fibrin aggregates. TIAs are an important predictor of subsequent infarcts, because approximately one third of patients with TIAs develop clinically significant infarcts within 5 years. Predictably, the neurologic deficits associated with brain infarction are related to the location and amount of brain damage. In addition to the deficits directly related to loss of brain parenchyma, edema of adjacent brain during the early stages also contributes to local neurologic deficits and, in the case of large infarcts, to life-threatening mass effect and brain herniation.

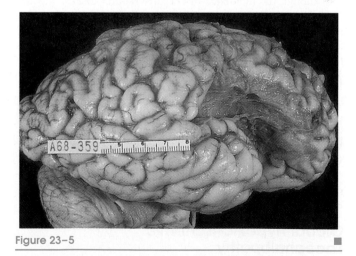

Figure 23–5 ■

Remote infarct. Necrotic tissue has liquefied over a period of approximately 6 months, leaving behind a permanent, fluid-filled, cystic defect in the right lateral frontal area.

Infarcts occur most commonly in areas supplied by branches of the middle cerebral artery. They result, in most cases, from embolic occlusion and are manifested by contralateral hemiparesis and spasticity; loss of sensation on the side of the body opposite the infarct; visual field abnormalities; and in the case of infarcts involving the dominant cerebral hemisphere, speech abnormalities (aphasias). *Occlusion of the internal carotid artery* (resulting from thrombosis) is less common than occlusion of the middle cerebral artery. In extreme cases, internal carotid occlusion may result in massive infarction of the ipsilateral cerebral hemisphere, accompanied by monocular blindness secondary to the loss of flow to the ophthalmic artery. In most cases, however, arterial anastomoses, particularly at the base of the brain (circle of Willis) continue to supply blood to the internal carotid territory, and hence the resultant deficits are smaller than might be expected. Branches of the *vertebrobasilar system* are also affected by atherosclerosis and are therefore sites of thrombosis. Occlusion of these vessels may produce lesions ranging from large, rapidly fatal infarcts involving vital brain stem areas, to small, clinically silent infarcts.

Intracranial Hemorrhages

Hemorrhages may occur at any site within the CNS. In some instances they may be a secondary phenomenon occurring, for example, within infarcts in arterial border zones or in infarcts caused by only partial or transient vascular obstruction. Primary hemorrhages within the epidural or subdural space are typically related to trauma and will be discussed later with traumatic lesions. Hemorrhages within the brain parenchyma and subarachnoid space, in contrast, are often a manifestation of underlying cerebrovascular disease, although trauma may also cause hemorrhage in these sites.

PRIMARY BRAIN PARENCHYMAL HEMORRHAGE

Spontaneous (nontraumatic) intraparenchymal hemorrhages occur most commonly in mid- to late adult life, with a peak incidence at about age 60. Most are caused by rupture of a small intraparenchymal vessel. *Hypertension is the most common underlying cause of primary brain parenchymal hemorrhage,* accounting for more than 50% of cases of clinically significant hemorrhage. Conversely, brain hemorrhage accounts for roughly 15% of deaths among patients with chronic hypertension. Hypertension causes a number of abnormalities in vessel walls, including accelerated atherosclerosis in larger arteries; hyaline arteriolosclerosis in smaller vessels; and in severe cases, proliferative changes and frank necrosis of arterioles. Arteriolar walls affected by hyaline change are presumably weaker than are normal vessels and are therefore more vulnerable to rupture. In some instances chronic hypertension is associated with the development of minute aneurysms, termed *Charcot-Bouchard microaneurysms,* which may be the site of rupture in some cases of hypertensive intracranial hemorrhage. Charcot-Bouchard aneurysms, not to be confused with saccular aneurysms of larger intracranial vessels, occur in vessels that are less than 300 μm

in diameter, most commonly within the basal ganglia. In addition to hypertension, other local and systemic factors may cause or contribute to nontraumatic hemorrhage, including systemic coagulation disorders, open heart surgery, neoplasms, amyloid angiopathy, vasculitis, saccular aneurysms, and vascular malformations. Vascular malformations and saccular aneurysms are discussed later in this section.

> **MORPHOLOGY. Parenchymal hemorrhages occur most commonly in the basal ganglia, particularly in the region of the putamen and external capsule, followed by the thalamus, cerebral white matter, pons, and cerebellum.** Multiple hemorrhages are seen in a minority of cases. With a massive hemorrhage, the site of origin of the hematoma may be impossible to determine with certainty. Externally, the brain is asymmetrically distorted by the mass effect caused by the hematoma and associated edema. Various herniation patterns, described previously, are almost invariably present. On cut surface, primary intraparenchymal hemorrhages take the form of fairly well demarcated hematomas, which may dissect through adjacent parenchyma into the ventricles and/or subarachnoid space (Fig. 23–6). Some degree of softening of the adjacent neuropil is often present, although, in contrast to infarcts with secondary hemorrhage, large areas of necrosis are not seen. Large hemorrhages occurring above the tentorium cerebelli usually cause herniation of cerebellar tonsils and brain stem, with associated secondary brain stem (Duret's) hemorrhages. In patients surviving the acute hemorrhage, the hematoma is resorbed over time, ultimately leaving a fluid-filled cavity lined by gliotic neuropil and hemosiderin-laden macrophages.

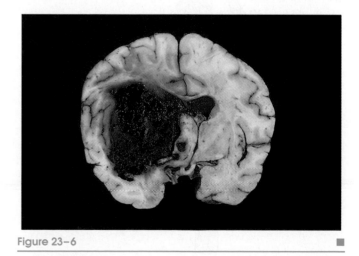

Figure 23–6 ■

Acute intracerebral hemorrhage. A fresh hematoma has disrupted and expanded the left cerebral hemisphere, causing the midline structures to shift to the right. Uncontrolled hypertension is an important cause of this catastrophic lesion.

Clinical Features. The onset of a primary brain parenchymal hemorrhage is almost always abrupt and is accompanied by evidence of increased intracranial pressure, including severe headache, vomiting, and rapid loss of consciousness. Localizing signs may be present but are often difficult to detect in the setting of a massive elevation in intracranial pressure and coma. Progression of mass effect is associated with evidence of brain stem compression, including deep coma; irregular, intermittent respirations (Cheyne-Stokes respiration); dilated, nonresponsive pupils; and spasticity.

SACCULAR ANEURYSMS AND SUBARACHNOID HEMORRHAGE

The subarachnoid space may also be the site of nontraumatic intracranial hemorrhage. *The most common cause of spontaneous subarachnoid hemorrhage is rupture of a saccular aneurysm.* Saccular, or berry, aneurysms are present in approximately 1% of the general population. Their incidence is higher in patients with certain disorders, including polycystic kidney disease, fibromuscular dysplasia, coarctation of the aorta, and arteriovenous malformations of the brain. They must be distinguished from the fusiform dilations of intracranial vessels that may be seen in atherosclerosis, from infectious ("mycotic") aneurysms, and from the occasional dissecting aneurysms that may also be encountered in the intracranial compartment. Most saccular aneurysms (80%) arise at arterial bifurcations in the territory of the internal carotid artery. Common sites include branches of the middle cerebral artery, intracranial branches of the internal carotid artery, and the junction between the anterior cerebral and anterior communicating arteries (Fig. 23–7). Approximately 15% to 20% occur within the posterior (vertebrobasilar) cir-

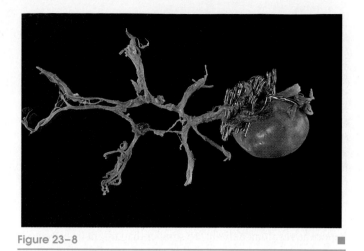

Figure 23–8 ■

Gross view of a massive saccular aneurysm arising at the junction of the vertebral and basilar arteries. The vessels have been dissected from the brain. Multiple surgical clips, visible in the photograph, were placed on the aneurysm before death in an attempt to prevent further bleeding.

culation. Saccular aneurysms are thought to arise as a result of congenital defects in the media of arteries at branch points. However, they are distinctly rare in infancy and childhood. They enlarge with time and are at greatest risk for rupture once they reach diameters of 4 to 7 mm. Beyond this size, interestingly, the likelihood of rupture decreases, and symptoms referable to their mass effects predominate.

MORPHOLOGY. Asymptomatic saccular aneurysms are usually small, with diameters of less than 3 mm. They appear as rounded bulges in the arterial wall, usually at arterial bifurcations (Fig. 23–8). Multiple aneurysms are present in about 25% of patients. The wall of the saccular aneurysm is composed of dense, collagen-rich tissue derived from the intima and adventitia of the parent vessel. The media typically ends abruptly at the neck of the aneurysm. The lumen of the aneurysm may contain a laminated thrombus. Aneurysms may compress adjacent structures and produce symptoms referable to local mass effects. Rupture of a saccular aneurysm usually occurs at the thin-walled fundus. Depending on its location, rupture may result in bleeding into the subarachnoid space and, in many cases, into adjacent brain parenchyma. **Infarcts of brain parenchyma** may also develop in patients with subarachnoid hemorrhage, probably because of **arterial spasm,** a phenomenon demonstrable radiographically in 40% of cases.

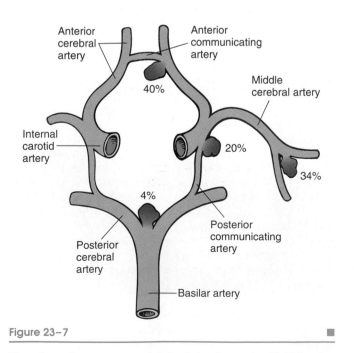

Figure 23–7 ■

Sites of saccular aneurysms and their relative frequencies. Multiple aneurysms may be present in an individual patient.

Clinical Features. Subarachnoid hemorrhage resulting from a ruptured saccular aneurysm is less common than is primary cerebral hemorrhage. Females are affected somewhat more commonly than males, with most cases occurring before the age of 50. As in the case of primary intraparenchymal hemorrhages, the onset of subarachnoid hemorrhage is abrupt and is associated with severe headache, vomiting, and loss of consciousness. No obvious precipitating factor is usually apparent. Meningeal signs, including neck rigidity, are usually present, and the CSF is grossly bloody. Roughly 50% of patients with subarachnoid hemorrhage due to ruptured saccular aneurysm die within several days of the onset of symptoms. Other acute complications include cerebral infarcts, usually developing within 4 to 9 days after the onset of symptoms, acute hydrocephalus, and herniation. Chronic hydrocephalus may occur in patients surviving the acute insult, owing to organization of blood in the leptomeninges and/or arachnoid granulations, with resultant obstruction of CSF flow.

VASCULAR MALFORMATIONS

Vascular malformations are another important cause of intracranial hemorrhage. Most result from abnormalities in angiogenesis in the developing brain; they range from small, incidental abnormalities identified only at autopsy, to large lesions associated with variable neurologic deficits and catastrophic intracranial hemorrhage. Four major types are usually recognized: arteriovenous malformations, capillary telangiectasias, venous angiomas, and cavernous angiomas.

Arteriovenous malformations (AVMs) are the most common congenital vascular abnormalities in the brain and are the type most likely to be associated with clinically significant hemorrhage. They occur most commonly in the cerebral hemispheres and are often supplied by branches of the middle cerebral artery. Grossly, the AVM appears as a conglomerate of tortuous vessels, most dramatically visualized while still engorged with blood (Fig. 23–9). The microscopic appearance is that of haphazardly arranged vessels of variable caliber that include arteries, veins, and transitional forms that are neither clearly venous nor clearly arterial. The vascular channels are separated by brain parenchyma. Secondary changes, including recent and remote hemorrhages, calcification, and reactive gliosis, are common. The most common clinical manifestation of AVMs is spontaneous hemorrhage, which usually occurs after the first decade of life. Saccular aneurysms have been identified in up to 10% of people with AVMs.

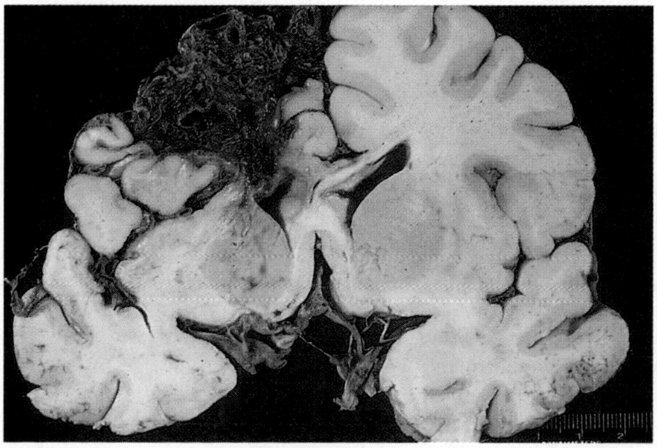

Among the other types of vascular malformations, *cavernous angiomas* are another significant cause of spontaneous intracranial hemorrhage and seizures. They are composed of ectatic, thick-walled venous channels separated by dense fibrous stroma. *Capillary telangiectasias* are small, punctate lesions found most commonly in the pons and cerebral white matter. These delicate capillary channels, usually encountered as incidental lesions at the time of autopsy, may leak occasionally. *Venous angiomas* occur most commonly in the meninges and spinal cord, where they appear as dilated, thin-walled veins. They are usually asymptomatic.

CENTRAL NERVOUS SYSTEM TRAUMA

Traumatic injury to the nervous system is an important cause of death and long-term disability in Western society, accounting for some 500,000 hospital admissions and 100,000 deaths annually in the United States. Among survivors of head injury, more than 70% are permanently disabled, and a significant number remain in a permanent vegetative state. Most fatal or debilitating head injuries are caused by blunt trauma associated with motor vehicle accidents, falls, and criminal assaults, including child abuse. Factors that increase the risk of head trauma include alcohol abuse, previous head injury, mental retardation, and seizure disorders. Traumatic injuries to the nervous system include three important groups: (1) epidural hematoma, (2) subdural hematoma, and (3) parenchymal injuries. Combinations of various patterns are quite common.

Epidural Hematoma

Epidural hematomas are caused by *rupture of a meningeal* artery, usually in association with a skull fracture (Fig. 23–10). The most common site of arterial disruption is a branch of the middle meningeal artery as it courses between the dura mater and squamous portion of the temporal bone. This artery is firmly attached to the periosteum of the temporal bone and hence is easily torn whenever a fracture occurs at that site. Epidural hematomas compress the subjacent dura and flatten the underlying brain parenchyma. If not immediately drained, they produce uncal, gyral, and cerebellar tonsillar herniation; brain stem compression; and death. *A significant number of patients with epidural hematomas have a "lucid interval" immediately after injury, followed by progressive loss of consciousness.* Because the bleeding is arterial in origin, cranial epidural hematomas expand rapidly, necessitating prompt surgical intervention.

Figure 23–9 ■

Arteriovenous malformation. These are the most dangerous type of vascular malformation in the brain because of the associated risk of massive bleeding.

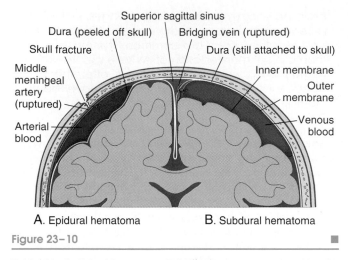

Figure 23–10

Epidural and subdural hematomas. Epidural hematomas are caused by disruption of the middle meningeal artery as it courses through the epidural space; subdural hematomas result from tearing of "bridging" veins between the brain and dural sinuses.

Subdural Hematoma

Subdural hematomas are caused by *disruption of bridging veins* that extend from the surface of the brain to the dural sinuses (Fig. 23–10). Any condition associated with rapid changes in head velocity (e.g., whiplash injury; blows to the head; and, in the case of infants, violent shaking of the head) may produce tears in the delicate bridging veins as they penetrate the overlying dura mater, with resultant subdural hemorrhage. Subdural hematomas occur most often over the cerebral convexities and vary from small hemorrhages to massive lesions with substantial mass effect. They are traditionally classified as acute or chronic, depending on whether the contents of the hematoma consist predominantly of clotted blood or liquefied blood clots respectively.

Acute subdural hematomas are usually associated with a clear history of trauma. They may be unilateral or, particularly in infants, bilateral and are frequently associated with other traumatic lesions. Acute subdural hematomas contain clotted blood, most frequently in the frontoparietal region. The underlying gyral convexities are usually preserved, in contrast to the flattening of the convexities seen in epidural hematomas. There may be considerable swelling of the cerebrum on the side of the hematoma, as well as compression of the contralateral hemisphere against the inner table of the skull and various forms of herniation. Because the blood is of venous origin, the onset of symptoms is somewhat slower than with epidural hematomas. With time, nonfatal untreated hematomas are gradually liquefied and demarcated from the underlying brain by a reactive "neomembrane" to form chronic subdural hematomas.

Chronic subdural hematomas are less commonly associated with a well-defined history of trauma than are acute lesions. They are often associated with brain atrophy, which in turn increases the mobility of the brain within the cranial vault and renders bridging veins even more susceptible to tearing. Accordingly, traumatic episodes causing chronic subdural hematomas may be so trivial as to escape notice. Chronic sub-

dural hematomas are composed of liquefied blood or yellow-tinged fluid separated from the inner surface of the dura mater and the underlying brain by "neomembranes" composed of granulation tissue and mature collagen, derived from the dura mater. Blood vessels within the neomembranes are abnormally permeable owing to an incompletely developed endothelial layer, contributing to progressive accumulation of fluid and recurrent hemorrhage within the hematoma. Clinical symptoms include altered mental status, sometimes accompanied by focal neurologic deficits. Because of the slowly evolving nature of the deficits, chronic subdural hematomas may be confused clinically with dementias such as Alzheimer's disease. Appropriate imaging studies of the head (e.g., computed tomography [CT] or magnetic resonance imaging [MRI] scans) are invaluable in excluding the possibility of subdural hematomas in patients with slowly evolving neurologic abnormalities.

Traumatic Parenchymal Injuries

Traumatic injuries to the brain parenchyma include concussions, contusions and lacerations, diffuse axonal injury, traumatic intracerebral hemorrhage, and generalized brain swelling.

The term *concussion* refers to a transient loss of consciousness and widespread paralysis, sometimes accompanied by seizures, followed by recovery over a period of hours to days. Patients recover without sequelae, save for loss of memory about the injury. Isolated concussions are not associated with any anatomic lesions in the brain; transient injury to the reticular activating system in the brain has been proposed as the mechanism for loss of consciousness in such cases. In more severe cases, the pattern of injury is similar to that of diffuse axonal injury, discussed below.

Diffuse axonal injury is the cause of most cases of post-traumatic dementia and, along with hypoxic injury, is responsible for most cases of persistent vegetative state. The lesions of diffuse axonal injury result from sudden angular deceleration or acceleration forces sufficient to stretch or shear nerve cell process within the cerebral white matter. Grossly, diffuse axonal injury may produce only minimal changes, but sometimes multiple areas of hemorrhage may be seen.

Contusions are hemorrhages in the superficial brain parenchyma caused by blunt trauma. They may occur at any place where the brain comes in contact with the skull or an unyielding dural reflection but are most common in the frontal poles, orbital surfaces of the frontal lobes, temporal poles, occipital poles, and posterior cerebellum. The overlying skull may contain a fracture but is often intact. When blunt force is applied to an immobile head, contusions are most pronounced in the area of brain immediately underneath the point of impact, a configuration referred to as a *coup contusion*. In contrast, when contusions are produced by a rapidly moving head that impacts against an immobile surface, such as a floor, the severest injuries occur in the areas of brain farthest removed from the site of impact, a so-called *contrecoup contusion*. It is impossible to distinguish coup from contrecoup lesions morphologically, without information about the circumstances of the injury. Cerebral contusions, particularly if accompanied by tearing of the superficial layers of the brain

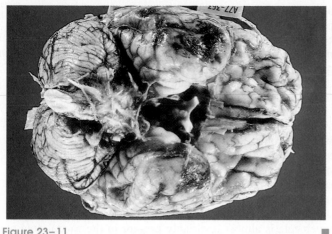

Figure 23–11

Cerebral contusions. The temporal poles are discolored by areas of hemorrhage. Such lesions represent "bruises" of the surface of the brain caused by violent contact between the delicate brain parenchyma and the hard inner surface of the skull.

(lacerations), are an important cause of traumatic subarachnoid hemorrhage. In the acute phase, contusions appear as hemorrhagic lesions involving the superficial gray matter and, on occasion, the subjacent white matter (Fig. 23–11). Microscopically, the brain parenchyma within the contusion is hemorrhagic, fragmented, and necrotic. In contrast to infarcts, which may also produce superficial hemorrhagic gray matter lesions, the subpial molecular layer is also disrupted in contusions. Healed lesions appear as depressed, firm areas on the surface of the brain. A golden brown discoloration is usually evident as a result of associated hemosiderin deposits. Remote contusions are a common cause of focal seizure activity.

Traumatic intracerebral hemorrhages are usually multiple and are most common in the frontal lobes, temporal lobes, and deep gray matter. They are caused by mechanical shearing of intraparenchymal vessels. Traumatic hemorrhages are usually accompanied by other traumatic lesions but may be difficult, in some cases, to distinguish from spontaneous intracranial hemorrhages.

Brain swelling may occur as an isolated manifestation of traumatic injury or may coexist with other traumatic lesions. It may be localized, as in the case of edema associated with an adjacent contusion or subdural hematoma, or generalized. Diffuse brain swelling occurs most commonly in children and adolescents and may follow a lucid interval immediately after trauma. Cerebral congestion probably plays an important role in its development.

CONGENITAL MALFORMATIONS AND PERINATAL BRAIN INJURY

Major congenital malformations occur in about 3% of newborns. Of these, malformations of the CNS account for approximately one third, and they are an important cause of infant mortality. The development of the mammalian CNS is a complex process that may be disrupted by a number of factors, including intrinsic genetic abnormalities, exogenous factors such as toxins and infections, and various combinations of the two. As discussed in Chapter 7, the timing of the insult is critical in terms of the effects on the developing nervous system. Like other systems, the developing CNS is most susceptible to teratogenesis early during embryogenesis.

The most common congenital malformations of the nervous system include neural tube defects, malformations associated with hydrocephalus, and primary forebrain abnormalities. Another group of conditions, the so-called neurocutaneous syndromes, are also associated with a wide range of abnormalities in the nervous system. In addition, perinatal injury is responsible for a significant proportion of CNS abnormalities in the neonatal period. Many changes, such as hemorrhages and infarcts, are clearly acquired disorders and traditionally have been distinguished from congenital malformations. As will be discussed below, the distinction between "acquired" abnormalities and those regarded as "intrinsic" developmental abnormalities is often somewhat arbitrary.

Neural Tube Defects

The brain and spinal cord are derived from ectodermal elements that differentiate and proliferate to form the neural tube. Closure of the neural tube begins on approximately the 22nd day of gestation and is complete between the 26th and 28th day. *Disorders related to abnormal closure of the neural tube are the most common CNS malformations.* Such developmental aberrations, broadly designated as *neural tube defects* or *dysraphic states*, may involve the brain, spinal cord, or both. Examples include anencephaly, cranial meningoceles and encephaloceles, and the various forms of spinal bifida.

Anencephaly is the most common congenital brain malformation, occurring with a frequency of about one in 500 births; a higher incidence has been noted in certain parts of the world, notably Ireland and Wales. As with all neural tube defects, it is more common among lower socioeconomic groups and in infants of women older than 40. The cranial vault in the anencephalic fetus is hypoplastic or absent, and the bones at the base of the skull are thickened. The orbits are shallow, resulting in characteristic protrusion of the eyes and a "froglike" facies (Fig. 23–12). The neurohypophysis is absent, and the anterior pituitary is smaller than normal, reflecting an absence of trophic hormones from the hypothalamus. Abnormalities in the vertebral bodies or spinal cord may also be present. Other organs, including the lungs and adrenal glands, are hypoplastic. Anencephaly is incompatible with prolonged extrauterine survival, and most fetuses die within minutes to hours after birth. The diagnosis of anencephaly can be made prenatally. Hydramnios is common in anencephalic gestations, and concentrations of α-fetoprotein and acetylcholinesterase are increased in amniotic fluid. Sonography can detect the presence of anencephaly in the later stages of the first trimester.

Encephaloceles and cranial meningoceles represent less severe examples of cranial neural tube defects. Encephaloceles are the more common of the two conditions and are characterized by protrusion of a variable amount of brain paren-

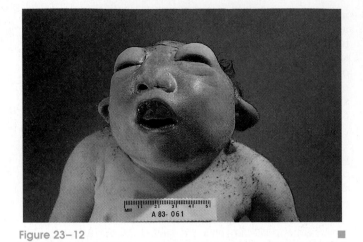

Figure 23–12 ■

Anencephaly, the most common and most severe of cranial neural tube defects. The orbital bones are of nearly normal size, despite absence of the brain and cranial bones, resulting in a froglike facial appearance.

chyma through a defect in the cranial bones. This occurs most commonly in the occipital region, although any portion of the skull may be affected. Anterior encephaloceles are particularly prevalent in southeast Asia. Cranial meningoceles are uncommon and are distinguished from encephaloceles by the presence of only meninges and CSF in the herniated tissue.

Spinal neural tube defects (spina bifida) may occur at any level but are most common in the lumbosacral region. In all cases there is absence or hypoplasia of one or more vertebral arches, with variable abnormalities in the underlying meninges and/or spinal cord. Four patterns are seen:

1. *Myelocele*, the most severe form of spinal neural tube defect, is characterized by an exposed plaque of flattened neuroectodermal tissue.
2. *Spinal meningoceles* present as cystic masses filled with CSF. The wall of the cyst contains meninges without accompanying spinal cord elements.
3. *Meningomyeloceles* are more common than myeloceles or meningoceles. They are characterized by herniation of spinal meninges and spinal cord through a posterior vertebral defect (Fig. 23–13). The meninges may be exposed to the external environment or covered by skin. Meningomyeloceles are frequently associated with hydrocephalus and the Arnold-Chiari malformation (see below).
4. *Spina bifida occulta* is the mildest form of spinal neural tube defect. It is characterized by defective closure of the posterior vertebral arches, with intact meninges and spinal cord. This site of the defect may be marked by a small skin dimple or tuft of hair. The abnormality, which occurs in about 20% of the general population, is asymptomatic.

Malformations Associated With Hydrocephalus

A number of disorders may be associated with the development of hydrocephalus. In many instances it is caused by

acquired lesions (e.g., tumors, hemorrhage, and inflammatory processes) that interfere with the normal flow and resorption of CSF. In other cases, primary developmental abnormalities may give rise to hydrocephalus. The more common primary malformations involve the cerebellum and are exemplified by the Arnold-Chiari malformation and the Dandy-Walker malformation.

The Arnold-Chiari malformation is characterized by extension of the medulla oblongata and caudal portions of the cerebellum through the foramen magnum. The lower brain stem appears elongated and compressed, with a thin layer of herniated, gliotic cerebellar parenchyma overlying the dorsal surface of the medulla. Abnormalities of the cranial vault are usually present, reflecting the close relationship between the developing brain and its coverings. An associated meningomyelocele is almost invariably present in the caudal area of the cord. The malformation is frequently, although not invariably, associated with hydrocephalus. While the pathogenesis of the hydrocephalus in the Arnold-Chiari malformation is not completely understood, it is now reasonably clear that the hydrocephalus is secondary and not the cause of the Arnold-Chiari defect, as was once postulated.

The Dandy-Walker malformation consists of aplasia or hypoplasia of the cerebellar vermis, associated with balloon-like dilation of the fourth ventricle. The lesion is usually associated with hydrocephalus. Other abnormalities, including agenesis of the corpus callosum, occipital encephalocele, and lesions reflecting abnormal cellular migration during CNS development, may also be present.

Disorders of Forebrain Development

Given the complexity of normal forebrain development, it is not surprising that a large number of malformations may be

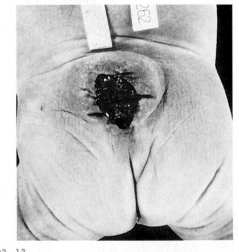

Figure 23–13 ■

Meningomyelocele. These defects occur because the caudal neural tube fails to close properly. In meningomyelocele, both the meninges and spinal cord parenchyma are included in the cystlike structure visible just above the buttocks. Because such lesions expose the central nervous system to the outside environment, infection is a common complication.

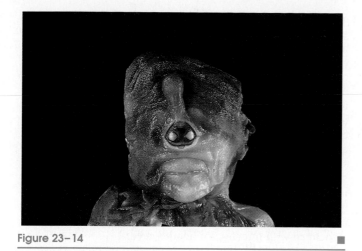

Figure 23–14 ■

Cyclopia, the most severe of the facial abnormalities associated with holo-prosencephaly. The term *cyclopia* is based on the presence of a single eye structure in the center of the face, reminiscent of the Cyclops in Greek mythology. A blind-ending structure termed a proboscis is visible just above the nonfunctional eye.

Neurocutaneous Syndromes

The neurocutaneous syndromes, or phakomatoses, are a group of disorders characterized by malformations and a variety of non-neoplastic and neoplastic proliferations involving the nervous system, skin, eyes, and other organ systems. With the exception of the Sturge-Weber syndrome, most are inherited as autosomal dominant traits with variable expression. The major neurocutaneous syndromes are summarized in Table 23–1. Some, such as neurofibromatosis type I and von Hippel-Lindau disease are also described elsewhere in the text (Chapters 6 and 7).

Perinatal Injury

A variety of exogenous factors may injure the developing brain. Injuries that occur early in gestation may destroy brain without evoking the usual "reactive" changes in the parenchyma and may be difficult to distinguish from malformations. Brain injury occurring in the perinatal period is an important cause of childhood neurologic disability. Some of the more important patterns of perinatal brain injury are described below.

Germinal matrix hemorrhage is the most common cause of intraventricular hemorrhage in premature infants. The germinal matrix persists in the developing human brain until approximately 35 weeks of gestation, particularly in the subependymal region of the caudate nucleus and thalamus. It is composed of primitive cells nourished by delicate, thin-walled vessels consisting of little more than an endothelial layer and basal lamina. Insults such as hypoxemia, hypercarbia, and acidosis, which are fairly common in premature infants, may injure the endothelial cells within the germinal matrix, causing hemorrhage into the matrix. Large hemorrhages easily disrupt the ependymal layer and enter the ventricular system (Fig. 23–15). Many infants with matrix hemorrhage succumb in the neonatal period. In those surviving the acute episode, organization of the hemorrhage may cause scarring and reactive

encountered in the cerebral hemispheres. Examples of such malformations include holoprosencephaly and cerebral cortical malformations. *Holoprosencephaly* refers to a range of malformations associated with abnormal division of the cerebral hemispheres. Such abnormalities may be seen in patients with trisomies 13 and 15 but may also occur in the absence of a specific chromosomal abnormality. In the severest form of holoprosencephaly, hemispheric development does not occur, and a rudimentary forebrain overlies a common ventricular cavity. The forebrain abnormalities are accompanied by facial abnormalities ranging in severity from cyclopia to mild facial clefts (Fig. 23–14). Cerebral cortical malformations may result in absence of gyral development, or the formation of numerous abnormally complex small gyri (polymicrogyria).

■

Table 23–1. NEUROCUTANEOUS SYNDROMES

Syndrome	Frequency	Genetic Abnormality	Features
Neurofibromatosis, type I	1:3000	Chromosome 17 (17q11.2)	Neurofibromas, schwannomas, malignant peripheral nerve neoplasms, meningiomas, gliomas, hyperpigmented skin lesions (café-au-lait spots), pigmented nodules of iris (Lisch nodules)
Neurofibromatosis, type II	1:40,000	Chromosome 22 (22q12)	Schwannomas of eighth cranial nerve (often bilateral), meningiomas, spinal neurofibromas
Tuberous sclerosis	1:100,000 to 1:200,000	Chromosomes 9 (9q34) or 16 (16p13.3)	Cerebral cortical malformations, subependymal tumors, seizures, mental retardation, cardiac rhabdomyomas, renal angiomyolipomas
von Hippel–Lindau disease	1:36,000	Chromosome 3 (3p25–26)	Cerebellar hemangioblastomas, retinal angiomas, renal cell carcinomas, pheochromocytomas, visceral cysts, epididymal tumors
Sturge-Weber disease	1:10,000	Sporadic; defect unknown	Cutaneous angiomas in distribution of seventh cranial nerve, meningeal angiomatosis, cerebral calcification, seizures, mental retardation

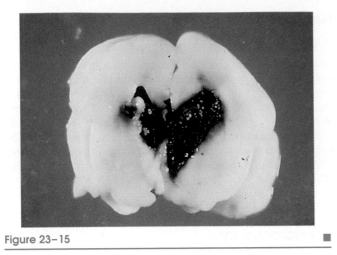

Figure 23-15 ■

Germinal matrix hemorrhage. Premature infants suffering from hypoxia and related metabolic problems are susceptible to hemorrhage within the delicate germinal matrix, located just beneath the ependymal lining of the lateral ventricles. These hemorrhages commonly extend into the ventricles, as was the case in this patient, and are sometimes designated *intraventricular* hemorrhages. (Courtesy of Linda Margraf, MD, Department of Pathology, University of Texas Southwestern Medical School, Dallas, TX.)

gliosis, interference with CSF drainage, and obstructive hydrocephalus.

White matter necrosis, also termed *periventricular leukomalacia*, is another important perinatal brain injury; it may be fatal or cause developmental delay and quadriplegia. In contrast to germinal matrix hemorrhages, white matter necrosis may occur in term infants as well as in premature infants. Conditions associated with cardiorespiratory dysfunction, including hyaline membrane disease, shock, sepsis, and congenital heart disease, increase the risk of white matter necrosis, presumably by potentiating hypoperfusion of the brain. The lesions of white matter necrosis appear as areas of chalky discoloration, sometimes associated with cavitation and hemorrhage in white matter. They are particularly common adjacent to the lateral cerebral ventricles.

Gray matter injury, resulting from hypoxia or sometimes infections, may assume the form of a typical infarct involving a well-defined vascular territory, or it may occur in areas of special vulnerability, such as the thalamus, basal ganglia, and certain brain stem nuclei. *Gray matter injury may give rise to long-term neurologic impairment and is responsible for a significant number of cases of cerebral palsy, an etiologically heterogeneous group of disorders characterized by nonprogressive neurologic deficits.*

INFECTIONS OF THE NERVOUS SYSTEM

The development of infections within the CNS is influenced by at least two factors, acting alone or in concert: the nature of the infectious agent and the integrity of normal host defenses. For example, disruption of normal barriers, such as might be encountered in a patient with a skull fracture and

meningeal tear, allows organisms of even low virulence to gain access to brain parenchyma. At the other end of the spectrum, certain organisms, because of either their highly virulent nature or their selective neurotropism (e.g., rabies virus or herpes simplex type I) are capable of producing CNS infection even in the presence of normal host defenses. Any part of the nervous system may be the site of active infection. In some instances infections rapidly become generalized, as in the case of acute bacterial infections in the leptomeninges. In other cases infections may be more localized, as in the case of abscesses caused by pyogenic bacteria, or infections caused by viruses such as poliovirus that affect neuronal subpopulations in a selective manner. Infections of the nervous system will be discussed on a regional basis, recognizing that infections affecting one compartment of the nervous system are often associated with infection of another area.

Epidural and Subdural Infections

Epidural abscesses and subdural empyemas are relatively rare but have a high rate of mortality. Within the skull, such lesions usually occur as a complication of primary infections in the paranasal sinuses or mastoid or as a consequence of trauma. Because the dura mater is firmly attached to the inner table of the skull, epidural infections in this region tend to remain localized, while those involving the subdural space may spread widely. They are caused most commonly by virulent agents such as staphylococci and streptococci. Spinal epidural infections are more common than cranial infections owing to the presence of intervertebral foramina connecting the epidural space with the pleura and retroperitoneum.

Leptomeningitis

Leptomeningitis or *meningitis,* as it is often called, refers to inflammation of the leptomeninges and subarachnoid space. Most cases result from infection, although certain chemical agents introduced into the subarachnoid space may also cause meningitis. Infectious meningitis can be divided into acute purulent meningitis, usually caused by bacteria; acute lymphocytic meningitis, usually caused by viruses; and chronic meningitis, which may be caused by a number of different infectious agents.

ACUTE (PURULENT) LEPTOMENINGITIS

Acute meningitis is an important cause of morbidity and mortality at all ages. Acute leptomeningitis in the neonatal period is caused most often by group B streptococci, *Escherichia coli*, and *Listeria monocytogenes*. Although any infant may be affected, those with open neural tube defects are particularly at risk.

■ Among children older than 6 months of age, *Haemophilus influenzae* formerly accounted for most cases of acute meningitis; its frequency has declined in recent years owing to the introduction of an effective vaccine. *Streptococ-*

cus pneumoniae currently accounts for most cases of acute meningitis in young children.

■ *Neisseria meningitidis* is the most common cause of epidemics of acute leptomeningitis and the most common cause of acute meningitis in older children, adolescents, and young adults.

■ Among older adults, most cases of acute meningitis are caused by *S. pneumoniae* and various gram-negative bacilli.

■ *L. monocytogenes* is an important cause of acute leptomeningitis in the elderly, certain immunocompromised patients, and neonates.

MORPHOLOGY. In the usual case of acute leptomeningitis, the meninges are intensely congested and opaque owing to the presence of a variable amount of creamy exudate in the subarachnoid space. The distribution of the exudate varies somewhat with the cause of the meningitis (Fig. 23–16). In cases of pneumococcal meningitis, for example, exudate is usually most pronounced over the cerebral convexities, while *H. influenzae* often causes a more pronounced basilar exudate. The underlying brain and spinal cord are congested and edematous. Microscopically, the leptomeninges are intensely congested and contain neutrophils and fibrin in the acute phase. Bacteria may be apparent even in tissue sections but are most reliably demonstrated in smears of the exudate. Variable numbers of lymphocytes and other mononuclear cells may be seen in partially resolved cases.

The clinical features of acute leptomeningitis include fever, headache, stiff neck, and altered mental status. The CSF, which is often turbid, contains predominantly neutrophils. CSF protein is elevated owing to increased vascular permeability, and glucose levels are markedly decreased (relative to serum levels) because of impaired transport of glucose into the CSF and the metabolic activity of the neutrophils. Organisms may be visible in gram-stained preparations of CSF in severe cases and are usually readily isolated if cultures are obtained before the initiation of antibiotic therapy. The prognosis of acute leptomeningitis is largely dependent on the rapidity with which appropriate antimicrobial therapy is initiated. Hence, rapid diagnosis is of paramount importance. Although isolation of the offending organism is always desirable, treatment of meningitis must be initiated promptly, before the results of cultures are available. Some knowledge of the clinical setting in which the meningitis occurs provides important clues to the identity of the causative agent.

ACUTE LYMPHOCYTIC (VIRAL) MENINGITIS

Most cases of acute lymphocytic meningitis are caused by viruses. Because routine cultures are negative, viral meningitis is also referred to as *aseptic meningitis*. In contrast to acute bacterial meningitis, most cases of viral meningitis are self-limited, and patients have, in general, a much better prognosis. Meningitis can occur in the course of any viral infection. In some instances viral meningitis is associated with concurrent parenchymal infection (encephalitis), but often it is the only manifestation of CNS infection. Common causative agents include mumps virus, echovirus, coxsackievirus, and Epstein-Barr virus.

The clinical features of viral meningitis are similar to those of acute bacterial meningitis but are usually less severe. The *CSF contains predominantly lymphocytes. CSF protein concentrations are usually elevated to a modest degree, but in contrast to acute bacterial meningitis, CSF glucose levels are usually normal.*

CHRONIC MENINGITIS

Chronic leptomeningitis is most often caused by bacteria and fungi. Important etiologic agents include *Mycobacterium tuberculosis, Cryptococcus neoformans,* and, less commonly, *Brucella* species and *Treponema pallidum.* Cryptococcal meningitis is an especially important cause of leptomeningitis in patients with the acquired immunodeficiency syndrome (AIDS).

MORPHOLOGY. The gross and microscopic features of chronic leptomeningitis vary depending on the cause of the meningitis. In general, however, the leptomeninges and occasionally the dura mater are thickened and contain a dense exudate in the subarachnoid space. In some cases, notably tuberculous meningitis, the exudate is particularly abundant around the base of the brain. Dense arachnoid adhesions are often present and may cause obstructive hydrocephalus. The host inflammatory reaction depends on the cause of the meningitis. In contrast to acute lep-

---

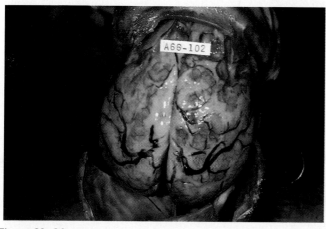

A66-102

Figure 23–16 ■

Acute leptomeningitis. The leptomeninges contain abundant creamy, purulent exudate, most prominently over the superior surface of the cerebrum. The underlying brain is swollen and the vessels are congested.

tomeningitis, however, the infiltrate is usually dominated by lymphocytes, plasma cells, and epithelioid histiocytes. In cases of tuberculous meningitis (discussed later), well-developed areas of caseous necrosis and a granulomatous inflammatory reaction may be present. In other forms of chronic meningitis, notably cryptococcal meningitis, inflammatory cells may be inconspicuous. Leptomeningeal blood vessels are often infiltrated by inflammatory cells that may cause proliferative changes in the vessel wall, thus compromising the vascular channels sufficiently to produce infarcts in the underlying brain.

The clinical features of chronic meningitis include headache, sometimes associated with stiff neck and other signs of meningeal irritation. In many cases, however, classic "meningeal" signs may be absent. *The CSF contains increased numbers of mononuclear cells, significantly increased levels of protein, and decreased levels of glucose.*

Infections of the CNS in syphilis deserve special mention. *Treponema pallidum* can cause nervous system disease in both congenital and acquired syphilis. The organism frequently gains access to the nervous system during the early stages of syphilis and may cause an acute lymphocytic leptomeningitis during the secondary phase of infection. Tertiary neurosyphilis may involve the meninges, vessels, or CNS parenchyma. The morphologic features of meningeal syphilis are nonspecific and include meningeal thickening and a mononuclear inflammatory infiltrate. The presence of significant numbers of plasma cells in the infiltrates should raise the possibility of syphilis. Proliferative changes are often present in the meningeal vessels and may cause ischemic damage in the underlying brain parenchyma. Meningovascular lesions involving the subarachnoid portions of the dorsal nerve roots may cause degeneration of ascending sensory fibers in the posterior columns of the spinal cord, with resultant sensory and gait abnormalities, a condition known as *tabes dorsalis*. Treponemal infection of the brain parenchyma may accompany meningeal infection, producing a condition known as *general paresis* or *general paresis of the insane*. This is characterized by cortical atrophy, neuronal loss, and proliferation of elongated microglial cells termed *rod cells*. Special stains may demonstrate the presence of spirochetes within the brain parenchyma in such cases.

Parenchymal Infections (Including Encephalitis)

Infection of the brain parenchyma is termed *encephalitis*. Parenchymal infections may be localized, as in the case of bacterial abscesses, tuberculomas, and most cases of toxoplasmosis, or be more generalized, as in the case of many viral infections. The discussion of parenchymal infections will be divided into brain abscesses and other localized infections, viral encephalitis, and spongiform encephalopathies caused by unconventional agents.

BRAIN ABSCESSES AND OTHER LOCALIZED INFECTIONS

Brain abscesses may be caused by a wide variety of bacteria, including staphylococci, streptococci, and a number of anaerobic organisms. The infecting organisms may reach the brain parenchyma by *hematogenous spread* from an infection elsewhere in the body, by *contiguous spread* from adjacent foci of infection (e.g., sinusitis or chronic suppurative otitis media), or by *direct implantation* during trauma. Common sources of hematogenous spread include bacterial endocarditis, lung abscesses, and bronchiectasis. Patients with cyanotic congenital heart diseases associated with right-to-left shunts are at higher risk for the development of brain abscesses owing to the fact that infectious material in the venous circulation may bypass the lungs and directly enter the systemic arterial circulation ("paradoxic" embolism).

Brain abscesses may occur anywhere, but they are most common in the cerebral hemispheres. They are frequently solitary but may be multiple, particularly when the organisms arrive by the hematogenous route. The temporal and frontal lobes are particularly common sites of involvement when abscesses arise as complications of infections of the middle ear and paranasal sinuses, respectively. The lesion begins as an area of softening (cerebritis), which gradually liquefies. The resultant cavity usually contains yellow-green pus, which may become quite thick. Over the next few weeks, the abscess is delimited from the adjacent brain by proliferating fibroblasts and collagen derived from blood vessels in the adjacent brain (Fig. 23–17). The surrounding brain is edematous and congested, containing reactive astrocytes and, frequently, perivascular inflammatory cells.

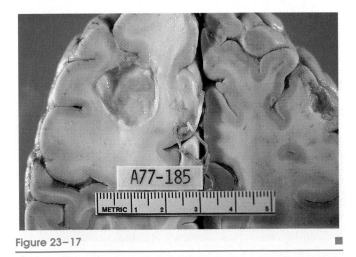

Figure 23–17 ■

Brain abscess that is sharply demarcated, indicating that it has been present for some time. Purulent exudate is visible in the center of the abscess. Because antibiotics penetrate very poorly into abscesses, surgical drainage is often necessary to treat such lesions.

The clinical features of brain abscesses are fever, evidence of increased intracranial pressure, and variable focal neurologic deficits. The CSF contains only scanty cells, increased protein, and normal levels of glucose. Complications of cerebral abscess include brain herniation and rupture of the abscess into the ventricles or subarachnoid space.

Tuberculosis may involve the brain parenchyma as well as the meninges. CNS tuberculosis is virtually always secondary to a pulmonary infection. Organisms reach the brain and/or meninges from active pulmonary lesions via the bloodstream to establish focal lesions known as **tuberculomas.** Tuberculomas may appear as small, single or multiple firm nodules or as larger, irregular lesions with a central area of caseous ("cheeselike") necrosis. Histologically, they are composed of aggregates of epithelioid histiocytes and giant cells, often associated with areas of necrosis. Stains for acid-fast bacilli are necessary to demonstrate the organisms, which may be quite scanty. Rupture of tuberculomas into the subarachnoid space results in the development of tuberculous meningitis, which may present as an acute or chronic meningitis.

Toxoplasmosis deserves special mention because of its occurrence in patients with AIDS. In the CNS, toxoplasmosis presents with multiple focal lesions, usually within gray matter. Histologically, untreated lesions often contain areas of necrosis associated with a variable mononuclear cell inflammatory infiltrate. *Toxoplasma gondii* organisms, in the form of pseudocysts or individual tachyzoites, are best visualized in tissue sections at the margins of necrotic areas. They may be extremely difficult to demonstrate in previously treated cases. Other important parasitic diseases responsible for focal brain lesions include cysticercosis, echinococcosis, and encephalitis caused by free-living amebae (e.g., *Naegleria* species).

VIRAL ENCEPHALITIS

Although a number of organisms are capable of producing generalized infection of the brain parenchyma (see the discussion of syphilis, above), viral infections are the most common cause. A large number of viruses can infect the CNS. In some instances CNS infection occurs as a minor component of systemic infection, while in other cases CNS disease represents the sole, or predominant, manifestation of infection. CNS involvement may be somewhat localized, e. g., temporal lobe encephalitis caused by herpes simplex virus (HSV), or generalized. Selective infection of certain cell populations is a feature of some forms of viral encephalitis. For example, rabies virus selectively infects neurons, while oligodendroglial cells are targets in progressive multifocal leukoencephalopathy (PML). Many forms of viral encephalitis occur in previously healthy individuals. In other infections, such as PML and CMV encephalitis, viral infection occurs as a consequence of host immunosuppression.

The morphologic features of viral encephalitis depend to some degree on the cause of the encephalitis. However, certain general features are shared by most forms, including perivascular inflammatory infiltrates; microglial nodules; and in some cases, inclusion bodies. The **perivascular inflammatory infiltrates** consist of mononuclear cells, including lymphocytes, plasma cells, and macrophages. Similar inflammatory infiltrates are often present in the meninges (see "Acute Lymphocytic (Viral) Meningitis," above). **Microglial nodules** are usually present and are sometimes associated with phagocytosis of a neuron **(neuronophagia).** Although not seen in all cases of viral encephalitis, a number of viruses produce characteristic **inclusion bodies** within the nuclei or cytoplasm of infected cells. Examples include the intracytoplasmic Negri bodies of rabies and the prominent intranuclear inclusions of CMV. The clinical and morphologic feature of some of the more common viral encephalitides are discussed below.

Arbovirus Encephalitides. Encephalitis caused by arthropod-borne viruses is the most common cause of epidemic encephalitis in the United States. Examples include eastern and western equine, Venezuelan, St. Louis, and California encephalitis. Most cases of arbovirus encephalitides occur in late summer, when the vectors (mosquitoes) are most abundant. Histologically, nonspecific perivascular inflammation and microglial nodules, which are sometimes most pronounced in the brain stem are seen. The prognosis varies, depending on the specific virus responsible for the encephalitis and the general health of the infected individual.

Herpes Simplex Encephalitis. HSV type I is the most common cause of sporadic viral encephalitis in the United States. The disease usually presents abruptly in previously healthy individuals. *An important feature of HSV I encephalitis is its proclivity to involve the temporal lobes and orbital frontal areas,* where it produces a hemorrhagic, necrotizing encephalitis (Fig. 23–18). Microscopic features include the usual perivascular mononuclear inflammatory infiltrates, microglial nodules, and smudgy inclusion bodies within the nuclei of infected glial cells and neurons. Herpesviruses can be detected in most cases by immunohistochemical stains, viral culture, or electron microscopy. Prompt treatment with effective antiviral agents such as acyclovir has greatly reduced morbidity and mortality. HSV type II is a less common cause of encephalitis in adults than HSV I, but it may produce a devastating, generalized encephalitis in neonates born to women with genital HSV II infection.

Cytomegalovirus Encephalitis. CMV, another member of the herpesvirus group, is an important cause of encephalitis in neonates and immunocompromised patients. Its frequency has increased substantially in recent years, particularly in patients with AIDS. Although CMV may infect any portion of the brain or spinal cord, in a significant number of cases, *it affects the ependyma, causing the ependymal surfaces of the cerebral ventricles to appear frankly hemorrhagic.* Microscopically, the virus evokes a typical perivascular and mi-

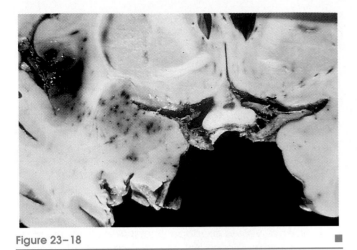

Figure 23–18 ■

Herpes simplex encephalitis. The typical necrotizing, hemorrhagic lesions of herpes encephalitis are visible in the medial aspect of the left temporal lobe, and more laterally in the insular cortex. (Courtesy of Beverly Rogers, MD, and Charles L. White III, MD, Department of Pathology, University of Texas Southwestern Medical School, Dallas, TX.)

croglial nodule inflammatory reaction, associated with enlarged cells bearing prominent, well-defined, intranuclear and occasionally cytoplasmic inclusions. The full spectrum of CMV-induced diseases is described in Chapter 13.

Human Immunodeficiency Virus Encephalitis. HIV type I is an important cause of progressive neurologic disease in AIDS, sometimes termed AIDS-dementia complex or HIV-1 encephalitis. Early in the course of HIV disease, there is a self-limited lymphocytic meningitis. Symptoms of progressive encephalopathy, however, characteristically develop in the later stages of HIV infection. The brain in HIV I encephalitis is often atrophic. Morphologic changes are usually most pronounced within white matter and basal ganglia and include variable degrees of myelin pallor associated with macrophages, scanty perivascular mononuclear inflammatory infiltrates, microglial nodules, and multinucleate giant cells (Fig. 23–19). The multinucleate giant cells, derived from fusion of HIV-infected mononuclear cells, contain viral proteins or maturing virions. HIV I encephalopathy is often associated with vacuolar myelopathy, a condition characterized by vacuolation and myelin breakdown in the dorsal and lateral columns of the spinal cord that bears a striking resemblance to the subacute combined degeneration of vitamin B_{12} deficiency (see discussion of vitamin B_{12} deficiency in "Nutritional Diseases," below). Despite its frequent association with HIV I encephalitis, the pathogenesis of vacuolar myelopathy remains obscure.

Progressive Multifocal Leukoencephalopathy. PML is a slowly evolving encephalopathy caused by a member of the papovavirus group, the JC virus (JC designates the initials of the patient from whom the virus was first isolated, and bears no relationship to Creutzfeldt-Jakob disease [CJD], discussed later). PML strikes the immunocompromised and, like CMV and *Toxoplasma* encephalitis, has become increasingly common with the emergence of AIDS. In PML, *the virus infects oligodendroglia, resulting in areas of demyelination,* which appear grossly as irregular, gelatinous foci, most pronounced

at the junction between gray and white matter. Histologic features include demyelination; enlarged, atypical astrocytes; and enlarged oligodendroglial nuclei containing smudgy, light purple inclusions.

SPONGIFORM ENCEPHALOPATHIES

The spongiform encephalopathies represent a group of diseases that includes Creutzfeldt-Jacob disease (CJD) and a number of other exceedingly rare conditions (kuru; Gerstmann-Sträussler syndrome and fatal familial insomnia; and, in some animals, scrapie and the much publicized "mad cow" disease in Great Britain). These diseases are transmitted by a unique category of proteinaceous infectious particles termed *prions* that lack DNA or RNA. *Infectious prions are a modified form of a normal structural protein found in the mammalian nervous system.* The major difference between normal prion proteins and pathogenic prions is in their conformation. Apparently, the pathogenic prions propagate themselves by contacting their normal counterparts and inducing them to refold in the pathogenic conformations. As this cycle continues, an ever-increasing population of normal prion proteins is converted into the disease-causing form. The mechanism of this fascinating process is still unclear. The notion of a protein-based infectious agent capable of initiating its own replication and causing disease represents a radical departure from the traditional concept of an "organism." Because they lack nucleic acids, prions are remarkably resistant to many agents that normally inactivate viruses, such as ultraviolet light and standard disinfectants. CJD is probably the best characterized of the human spongiform encephalopathies. Both sporadic and familial cases of CJD occur, and rare instances of iatrogenic transmission have occurred in patients who have received corneal transplants and human pituitary extract.

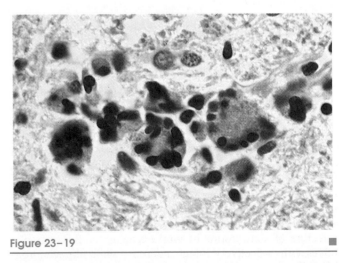

Figure 23–19 ■

Human immunodeficiency virus (HIV) encephalopathy. HIV infection in the brain is associated with the formation of characteristic multinucleate giant cells, created by fusion of HIV-infected macrophages. (Adapted from Burns DK, et al: The neuropathology of human immunodeficiency virus infection. Arch Pathol Lab Med 115:1112, 1991. Copyright 1991, American Medical Association.)

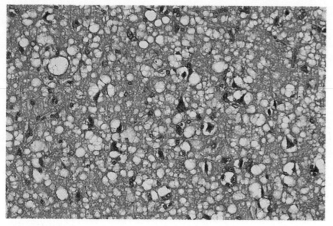

Figure 23-20   ■

Creutzfeldt-Jakob disease. This and related disorders are designated *spongiform encephalopathies* because of their tendency to produce extensive vacuolation, or "spongy" change, within the neuropil.

In the early stages of CJD, the brain is grossly normal. Atrophy is present in cases of long duration and may be severe. The hallmark of CJD and other spongiform encephalopathies is the presence of vacuoles within neuropil and cell bodies in gray matter **(spongiform change)** (Fig. 23-20). The vacuolation is accompanied by a variable degree of neuronal loss and reactive gliosis, the degree of which increases with the duration of the disease. Inflammatory infiltrates are usually absent.

CJD is characterized by rapidly progressive dementia, often accompanied by gait abnormalities and startle myoclonus. The disease is invariably fatal, with most patients succumbing within about a year after the onset of symptoms.

NEOPLASMS OF THE CENTRAL NERVOUS SYSTEM

Neoplasms of the CNS include not only those originating within the brain, spinal cord, or meninges, but also metastatic tumors originating in other sites. Primary CNS neoplasms are somewhat different from neoplasms arising in other sites, in the sense that even histologically benign lesions may result in death owing to compression of vital structures. Furthermore, in contrast to neoplasms arising outside the CNS, even histologically malignant primary tumors of the brain rarely disseminate to other parts of the body. The discussion of primary CNS tumors will focus on the more common neuroglial tumors (astrocytomas, oligodendrogliomas, and ependymomas), primitive neuroectodermal tumors (PNETs), and meningiomas.

Primary Neuroglial Tumors (Gliomas)

ASTROCYTOMAS

Astrocytomas represent the most common group of primary CNS tumors. They comprise a heterogeneous group of neoplasms, ranging from circumscribed, slow-growing lesions typified by pilocytic astrocytoma to highly malignant, infiltrating neoplasms such as the glioblastoma multiforme. For purposes of classification, astrocytic tumors can be subdivided into fibrillary (infiltrating) astrocytic neoplasms, pilocytic astrocytomas, and a few uncommon variants that will not be discussed in this brief overview.

Fibrillary astrocytic neoplasms, sometimes termed *diffuse astrocytomas,* are characterized by an infiltrative growth pattern. Although most commonly encountered in adults, they may occur at any age. Tumors of this type occur most often in the cerebral hemispheres but may be found anywhere in the neuraxis. These neoplasms are subdivided into histologic grades based on their degree of differentiation. As with other neoplasms, histologic grade is an important predictor of biologic behavior. A number of grading schemes have been proposed over the years, based on features such as nuclear pleomorphism, mitotic activity, vascular proliferation, and necrosis. One scheme in common use is a three-tiered system, which divides these tumors into three grades: well-differentiated lesions, designated *astrocytoma*; intermediate-grade tumors, termed *anaplastic astrocytoma*; and the most aggressive lesions, designated *glioblastoma multiforme*. It should be noted that fibrillary astrocytic neoplasms have a tendency to become progressively less well differentiated over time.

MORPHOLOGY.   Well-differentiated astrocytomas are usually poorly defined, infiltrative lesions that expand the parenchyma and obliterate normal gray matter–white matter boundaries (Fig. 23–21).

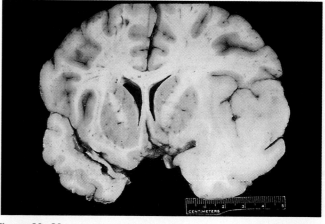

Figure 23-21   ■

Well-differentiated infiltrating astrocytoma. The right temporal lobe contains an infiltrative, homogeneous lesion that has expanded the lobe and obscured the normal boundaries between gray and white matter. Because of the ill-defined borders, surgical resection seldom removes all the tumor in such cases.

Microscopically, well-differentiated astrocytomas are characterized by the presence of increased numbers of irregularly distributed astrocytes, which tend to infiltrate around native cells such as neurons. The nuclei of the neoplastic astrocytes are mildly atypical. The cells often have discernible fibrillar processes, in keeping with their astrocytic differentiation, and may be accompanied by small accumulations of intercellular fluid, termed **microcysts**. The distinction between low-grade astrocytoma and reactive gliosis may be quite difficult in some cases.

Anaplastic astrocytomas are grossly indistinguishable from their better differentiated counterparts. Radiographic imaging studies, however, may provide a clue to their identity by the presence of proliferating blood vessels within the tumor. Such vessels are abnormally permeable, permitting injected contrast material to leak out of the vasculature, manifested radiographically as **contrast enhancement**. Histologically, anaplastic astrocytomas are distinguished from well-differentiated lesions by greater cellularity, nuclear pleomorphism, mitotic activity, and vascular endothelial proliferation.

Glioblastoma multiforme presents radiographically as irregular, contrast-enhancing lesions, usually associated with considerable edema in the adjacent brain parenchyma. Grossly, they are infiltrative lesions with irregular areas of hemorrhage, necrosis, and cystic change (Fig. 23–22). **They are distinguished histologically from anaplastic astrocytomas by areas of necrosis that are often surrounded by a dense cluster of tumor cells with prominent nuclei.** Such an array of nuclei around necrotic areas is described as nuclear pseudopalisading (Fig 23–23).

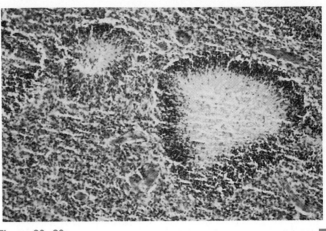

Figure 23–23 ■

Photomicrograph of glioblastoma multiforme. Glioblastomas are characterized by hypercellularity and necrosis. The necrotic areas in this example are surrounded by a dense border of tumor cells giving rise to an appearance termed nuclear *pseudopalisading*. (Courtesy of Elisabeth Rushing, MD, Department of Pathology, University of Texas Southwestern Medical School, Dallas, TX.)

Clinically, fibrillary astrocytic neoplasms may present with evidence of increased intracranial pressure or with focal abnormalities related to their location. Their prognosis is influenced by several factors, including location, the histologic grade of the tumor, and age. Elderly patients generally fare worse than do younger patients with tumors in similar locations. Treatment is influenced by the grade of the neoplasm and currently involves surgical resection, sometimes followed by radiation therapy and/or chemotherapy.

Pilocytic astrocytomas are more common in children, although they may occur at any age. Common sites include the cerebellum, third ventricle, and optic nerves, but as in the case of fibrillary astrocytomas, any part of the CNS may be involved. In general, they are distinguished from fibrillary astrocytic neoplasms by their more discrete nature and more indolent behavior.

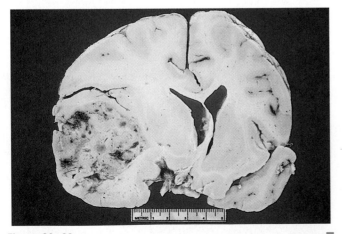

Figure 23–22 ■

Glioblastoma multiforme. In contrast to the well-differentiated infiltrating astrocytoma in Figure 23–21, this glioblastoma contains irregular areas of discoloration and cystic change, reflecting the presence of necrosis and hemorrhage. These lesions are widely infiltrative and associated with considerable mass effect. Note the shift of midline structures to the right.

MORPHOLOGY. Pilocytic astrocytomas are usually fairly well defined lesions. Often, they are cystic and contain a mural nodule. Pilocytic astrocytomas derive their name from the presence of astrocytes with elongated, "hairlike" cell processes (Fig. 23–24). Cystic areas and brightly eosinophilic structures termed **Rosenthal fibers** are often present. Although the cells may be somewhat atypical, frank malignancy is rarely seen.

The prognosis of patients with pilocytic astrocytomas is influenced primarily by location. Patients with surgically resectable tumors, such as those in the cerebellar hemispheres, usually have an excellent prognosis, while tumors in less accessible sites, such as the hypothalamus, may cause death even in the absence of histologic evidence of malignancy.

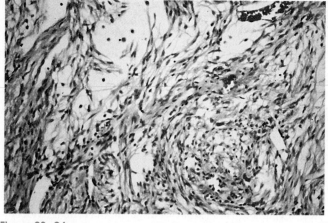

Figure 23–24   ■

Pilocytic astrocytoma. These lesions are characterized by presence of cells with elongated processes reminiscent, to some observers, of hair—hence the term *pilocytic*. Pilocytic astrocytomas are distinguished from infiltrating astrocytomas by their more circumscribed nature and, in most cases, a more favorable prognosis.

OLIGODENDROGLIOMAS

Oligodendrogliomas are most common during adulthood, where they usually occur within the cerebral hemispheres.

MORPHOLOGY. Grossly, oligodendrogliomas are usually soft and gelatinous, and they are often better circumscribed than are infiltrating astrocytomas. **Calcification is common** and, when detected radiographically, may provide an important clue to the diagnosis. Microscopically, the classic oligodendroglioma is distinguished by the presence of infiltrating cells with rounded, uniform nuclei, often surrounded by a clear perinuclear halo. The neoplastic cells tend to cluster around native neurons, a phenomenon referred to as **satellitosis.** In some cases, the tumor may extend into the subarachnoid space. Anaplastic change, characterized by increasing nuclear pleomorphism, mitotic activity, and necrosis, may be seen.

The prognosis for patients with oligodendrogliomas is less predictable than that for patients with infiltrating astrocytomas but depends, to some degree, on the histologic grade of the lesion.

EPENDYMOMAS

Ependymomas may occur at any age. Most arise within one of the ventricular cavities or in the area of the central canal in the spinal cord. Intracranial ependymomas, in general, are most common in the first two decades of life, while intraspinal lesions predominate in adults. Intracranial ependymomas occur most commonly in the fourth ventricle, where they may obstruct CSF outflow and lead to hydrocephalus and increased intracranial pressure.

MORPHOLOGY. Ependymomas are generally well-demarcated lesions arising from either ventricular walls or, in the case of intraspinal lesions, from remnants of the central canal. Intracranial lesions typically project into the ventricular cavities as solid masses, sometimes with a discernible papillary architecture (Fig. 23–25). The microscopic picture, although variable, is often dominated by elongated cells with processes radiating around blood vessels **(perivascular "pseudorosettes")** or lumina **(ependymal rosettes),** the latter recapitulating the structure of normal ependyma. Some tumors may contain clear cells reminiscent of oligodendroglioma. Most tumors are well differentiated, although a spectrum of anaplastic changes may be encountered.

The clinical manifestations of ependymoma depend on the location of the neoplasm. Intracranial tumors are often associated with hydrocephalus and evidence of increased intracranial pressure. Because of their location within the ventricular system, some tumors, particularly anaplastic variants, may disseminate within the subarachnoid space.

Primitive Neuroectodermal Tumors

The term primitive neuroectodermal tumor (PNET) refers to a group of neoplasms composed of embryonal (primitive) small cells. Such neoplasms may be undifferentiated, or may show varying degrees of neuronal, glial, or even mesenchymal differentiation. Considerable controversy exists about the proper classification of this group of neoplasms, with some authorities arguing that the "PNET" designation represents an

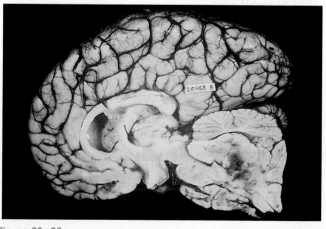

Figure 23–25   ■

Ependymoma. These may arise in both the intracranial compartment and the spine. Intracranial tumors typically originate from a ventricular surface, as in the case of this large lesion arising in the fourth ventricle.

artificial amalgamation of biologically distinct lesions. The histologic similarities between the various neoplasms in this group, however, have led many to regard these as members of a common family of neoplasms. PNETs occurring within the CNS include medulloblastomas, neuroblastomas, pineoblastomas, and ependymoblastomas. Only medulloblastomas, the most common of these tumors, will be considered here. Neuroblastomas are described in Chapter 7. Ewing's tumor a non-neuronal PNET tumor is described in Chapter 21.

Medulloblastomas are lesions of the cerebellum that occur predominantly within the first two decades of life. The cerebellar vermis is the usual site of origin in young children, while those occurring in older patients often originate in the cerebellar hemispheres. The lesions obliterate normal cerebellar architecture and may project into the ventricular system, where they may mimic ependymomas. Like ependymomas, medulloblastomas may disseminate through CSF, sometimes encasing the neuraxis in sheathlike metastatic deposits. Microscopically, medulloblastomas are composed of small, primitive cells with scant cytoplasm, reminiscent of other small blue cell tumors encountered in the pediatric population (Chapter 7). The neoplastic cells often form small rosettes, termed **Homer Wright rosettes,** around a central fibrillar core (Fig. 23–26). Some evidence of neuronal differentiation may be present.

Most patients with medulloblastoma present with evidence of increased intracranial pressure and gait abnormalities, reflecting CSF obstruction and cerebellar injury, respectively. With multimodality therapy, including radiation and chemotherapy, a majority of patients survive 5 years or more.

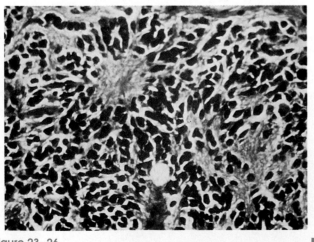

Figure 23–26 ■

Photomicrograph of a medulloblastoma. These cerebellar neoplasms are composed of primitive neuroectodermal cells, which sometimes surround small, acellular fibrillar areas to form the so-called Homer Wright rosettes. (Courtesy of Elisabeth Rushing, MD, Department of Pathology, University of Texas Southwestern Medical School, Dallas, TX.)

Other Primary Intraparenchymal Neoplasms

Primary CNS lymphomas have increased in frequency in recent years, particularly in association with the emergence of AIDS; indeed lymphoma of the brain is considered an AIDS defining condition in HIV positive individuals (Chapter 5). The lesions of primary CNS lymphoma may be solitary or multiple. They are often hemorrhagic and may be necrotic, even in the absence of treatment. Microscopically, their appearance is similar to that of non-Hodgkin's malignant lymphomas arising in other sites, with a predominance of large cell, aggressive lesions. Like most peripheral large cell lymphomas, CNS lymphomas are usually tumors of B lymphocytes. A characteristic feature of these tumors is their tendency to grow around and within the walls of blood vessels (angiocentric growth).

A number of *germ cell neoplasms* may arise primarily within the intracranial compartment. Most such lesions occur in the suprasellar and pineal areas, particularly in children and young adults. The microscopic appearance of these neoplasms is identical to that of germ cell neoplasms occurring in the gonads. Intracranial germinomas, which are morphologically identical to testicular seminomas and ovarian dysgerminomas, and teratomas are the most commonly encountered variants.

Neuronal neoplasms may also occur in the CNS. Of these, the most common type is the *ganglion cell tumor* (ganglioglioma), composed of mature but dysplastic ganglion cells admixed with variable numbers of glial cells. Most occur in children and young adults and arise within the temporal lobes, where they are an important cause of seizures.

Hemangioblastomas occur in the cerebellum and, less commonly, in the meninges. In the former site, they usually present as circumscribed, cystic lesions with a mural nodule. Microscopically, they are composed of a mixture of delicate vascular channels and intervening lipid-laden, foamy stromal cells of uncertain derivation. They may occur as solitary lesions, or they may be a component of the von Hippel-Lindau syndrome (see Table 23–1).

Meningiomas and Other Meningeal Neoplasms

Meningiomas are tumors derived from the meningothelial cells that invest the arachnoid mater. Accordingly, most lesions occur outside the brain parenchyma. Meningiomas usually occur in adults and may arise in both the cranial vault and the spinal cord. A female predominance has been noted consistently, particularly among lesions occurring in the spinal cord. This may be related to the presence of progesterone receptors on meningothelial cells and a trophic response to that hormone. Their frequency is also increased in patients with neurofibromatosis type 2, in whom they are often multiple.

MORPHOLOGY. Meningiomas usually present as firm, lobulated lesions attached to the dura mater.

A sharp interface is usually present between the tumor and the adjacent brain or spinal cord (Fig. 23–27). The overlying skull may be thickened and is sometimes invaded by tumor. A variety of microscopic patterns may be seen in meningiomas, but there is often some recapitulation of the compact cellular whorls seen in the normal arachnoid mater. Common histologic types include **syncytial** and **fibroblastic** variants; neoplasms containing a mixture of these two patterns are designated **transitional meningiomas**. Calcification, if present, usually takes the form of concentrically laminated, calcified granules termed **psammoma bodies**. Other histologic patterns may occur, but most are of no prognostic significance. Some meningiomas may become histologically malignant, as manifested by increasing cellularity and nuclear pleomorphism; mitotic activity; necrosis; papillary architecture; and, most importantly, invasion of underlying brain parenchyma.

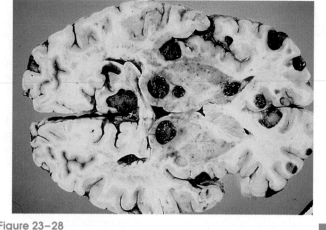

Figure 23–28 ■

Metastatic melanoma. Metastatic lesions are distinguished grossly from most primary central nervous system tumors by their multicentricity and well-demarcated margins. The dark pigment in the tumor nodules in this case is characteristic of most malignant melanomas.

Like many other expanding intracranial masses, intracranial meningiomas present with evidence of increased intracranial pressure, sometimes accompanied by seizures and focal neurologic deficits. The prognosis for patients with meningiomas is influenced by the size and location of the lesion, surgical accessibility, and histologic grade.

Other primary meningeal neoplasms include hemangioblastomas (discussed above), the aggressive meningeal hemangiopericytoma, and rare meningeal sarcomas.

Metastatic Neoplasms

The brain is a common site for metastatic lesions. These occur predominantly in the elderly, paralleling the increase in solid visceral tumors with increasing age. However, hemato-

poietic neoplasms such as lymphomas and leukemias, which occur in children as well as in adults may also metastasize to the CNS. Metastatic neoplasms may involve the meninges as well as brain parenchyma. Excluding leukemias and lymphomas, the most common primary sites, in descending order of frequency, are carcinomas of the lung and breast and malignant melanomas. Neurologic abnormalities may be the first clue to the presence of a visceral carcinoma, particularly in the case of carcinomas arising in the lung.

MORPHOLOGY. Carcinomas and melanomas metastatic to the brain parenchyma are well-demarcated, roughly spherical lesions that may be solitary or multiple (Fig. 23–28). A sharp interface is present between the focus of metastatic carcinoma and the adjacent parenchyma. Considerable edema may be present around some lesions, which contributes to their mass effect. Microscopically, the morphology of metastatic carcinomas usually recapitulates the morphology of the primary lesion. Less commonly, carcinomas may metastasize to the leptomeninges. **Leptomeningeal carcinomatosis** produces a vague opacification of the leptomeninges. Malignant cells are usually demonstrable in the CSF of such patients, and concomitant metastatic lesions are sometimes present in the brain parenchyma. Carcinomas metastatic to the **dura mater** may be encountered, particularly in patients with primary lesions in the prostate, breast, or lung.

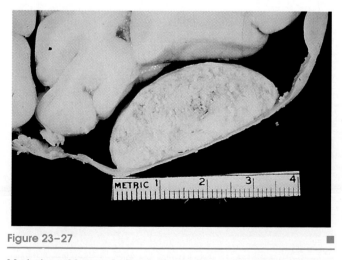

Figure 23–27 ■

Meningioma. Most meningiomas originate from meningothelial cells in intimate association with dura mater. Like this tumor they push, rather than infiltrate, the adjacent brain parenchyma. (Adapted from Burns DK: The central nervous system. In Henson DE, Albores-Saavedra J (eds): Pathology of Incipient Neoplasia, 2nd ed. Philadelphia, WB Saunders, 1993, p 528.)

Clinical features of metastatic carcinomas include evidence of increased intracranial pressure and variable focal neurologic deficits. Cranial nerve palsies are particularly common in patients with leptomeningeal carcinomatosis.

PRIMARY DISEASES OF MYELIN

In the CNS the myelin sheath is derived from the cytoplasmic processes of oligodendroglial cells, which wrap concentrically around neuronal processes in the same fashion as do Schwann cells in the peripheral nervous system. The purpose of myelin in the CNS, as in the peripheral nervous system, is to provide "insulation" for neuronal cell processes, permitting rapid conduction of electrical impulses along cell membranes. A number of disorders may interfere with the integrity of the myelin sheath, thereby disrupting the normal transmission of electrical activity within the brain and causing neurologic disease. Such processes may affect the myelin primarily, the oligodendroglial cell body, or both. For purposes of discussion, diseases of myelin will be divided into *acquired demyelinating diseases,* typified by multiple sclerosis, in which normally formed myelin is injured, and the so-called *leukodystrophies,* in which an inborn metabolic error interferes with normal myelin development.

Multiple Sclerosis

Multiple sclerosis (MS) is the most common demyelinating disease of the CNS. It is more frequent in temperate climates and in people of European extraction. MS affects young adults, with a peak incidence between the ages of 18 and 40 years. Most cases are characterized by waxing and waning neurologic abnormalities involving different regions of the CNS, occurring over a number of years. The cause and pathogenesis of MS are not fully understood. However, it is highly likely that it is an autoimmune disease in which T cells reactive against myelin components develop. Both CD4+ and CD8+ cells are present within the lesions, and many are reactive against myelin basic protein. A similar disease, called *experimental allergic encephalomyelitis,* can be induced in mice by immunization with myelin basic protein and can be transferred into naive animals by sensitized T cells. Current evidence suggests that both environmental (infectious?) and hereditary factors contribute to the development of autoimmunity in this disease. People migrating from high-risk to low-risk geographic areas, and vice versa, retain the risk of MS associated with their birthplace if migration occurs after the age of 15; if migration occurs before the age of 15, however, individuals assume the risk of MS associated with their new homes, suggesting that exposure to an environmental agent early in life contributes to the development of MS. A genetic component, in addition, is suggested by the increased risk of MS in association with certain class II human leukocyte antigen (HLA) genes and a higher rate of concordance in identical twins than dizygotic twins. Presumably, class II HLA genes regulate the autoimmune response (Chapter 5).

MORPHOLOGY. The external appearance of the brain and spinal cord is usually normal. On cut surface MS is characterized by the presence of multiple areas of demyelination, termed **plaques.** MS plaques may occur anywhere in the brain or spinal cord, accounting for the wide range of clinical manifestations associated with the disease. Common sites include the periventricular white matter, the optic nerves, and the white matter of the spinal cord. Plaques are usually well-demarcated lesions ranging from a few millimeters to several centimeters in diameter. Acute lesions are often soft and slightly pink, while older lesions tend to be firm and pearly gray to pink (Fig. 23–29). Microscopically, plaques are characterized by areas of demyelination, initially in a perivenous distribution, accompanied by a variable perivascular lymphocytic inflammatory infiltrate. In active lesions, there is evidence of myelin breakdown, manifested by the presence of lipid-laden macrophages. Residual axonal processes are usually present in the areas of demyelination but are reduced in number, particularly in chronic lesions. The peripheral nervous system is spared.

Clinical Features. The onset of MS may be acute or insidious. In keeping with the highly variable distribution of MS plaques, the clinical manifestations of the disease are protean. *Common manifestations include visual disturbances (blurred vision, diplopia, scotomata), paresthesias, spasticity of one or more extremities, speech disturbances, and gait abnormalities.* Various emotional disturbances may be seen, but intellectual function is typically preserved. Examination of the CSF usually reveals slightly increased protein levels and a small number of lymphocytes. The proportion of gamma globulin is increased and CSF electrophoresis reveals oligoclonal bands of immunoglobulins in most patients with MS. However, these antibodies are believed to arise after damage to myelin by sensitized T cells and are not thought to play a primary role in the myelin injury. Myelin basic protein may

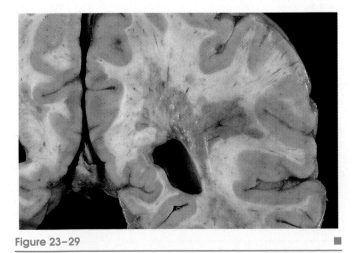

Figure 23–29 ■

Multiple sclerosis (MS). The typical MS plaque is a well-demarcated, firm, gray pink lesion. The periventricular white matter is a common site for these lesions, although they may occur in any part of the brain or spinal cord.

Table 23-2. LEUKODYSTROPHIES

Disorder	Inheritance	Metabolic Abnormality
Metachromatic leukodystrophy	Autosomal recessive	Arylsulfatase A deficiency
Krabbe's disease	Autosomal recessive	Galactocerebroside β-galactosidase deficiency
Adrenoleukodystrophy	X-linked and autosomal recessive	Peroxisomal defect; elevated levels of very-long-chain fatty acids

be present in the CSF during periods of active demyelination. The course of MS is somewhat unpredictable, with some patients dying within weeks to months of onset and others experiencing a normal life span, with few or no chronic sequelae. In most cases, however, the disease is characterized by multiple exacerbations and remissions, with cumulative neurologic deficits developing over the course of several years.

Other Acquired Demyelinating Diseases

Acute disseminated encephalomyelitis is an immune-mediated demyelinating disease that may follow certain infections (measles, chickenpox, rubella, and others) and vaccination. This disorder is believed to represent an allergic reaction, possibly triggered by exposure to selected foreign antigens; attempts to isolate virus from CNS tissues of affected patients have been unsuccessful. In contrast to the usual case of MS, acute disseminated encephalomyelitis is typically a monophasic illness of abrupt onset. Signs and symptoms include fever, seizures, coma, spinal cord dysfunction, and other focal neurologic deficits. Histologically, this reaction is characterized by areas of perivascular demyelination and mononuclear cell infiltration. The disease is fatal in 15% to 20% of cases.

Central pontine myelinolysis is a condition characterized by demyelination within the basis pontis. This condition has been associated with a number of factors, including alcoholism. Hyponatremia has been noted in a significant number of patients who subsequently develop central pontine myelinolysis, and excessively rapid correction of hyponatremia has been implicated as one possible cause of the disorder. The basis of this association with rapid correction of hyponatremia is unclear.

A number of infections may be associated with demyelination, the most well known of which is PML, discussed previously in the section "Viral Encephalitis." Herpes zoster encephalitis and CMV encephalitis may also produce areas of demyelination.

Leukodystrophies

The leukodystrophies represent a group of disorders in which an intrinsic defect interferes with the generation and/ or maintenance of myelin. Most are hereditary, with both au-

tosomal recessive and X-linked patterns of inheritance. In some, but not all, cases a specific lysosomal enzymatic defect has been associated with the myelin abnormality. In contrast to MS, the leukodystrophies are usually diseases of infancy and childhood, and are characterized by a relentlessly progressive course. They may involve peripheral nerves as well as the CNS. The most common leukodystrophies are listed in Table 23–2, along with their inheritance patterns and underlying biochemical defects, if known.

MORPHOLOGY. Leukodystrophies are characterized by a widespread, symmetric loss of myelin throughout the brain, and often the spinal cord as well. The brain is usually atrophic, and the centrum ovale and other central white matter areas appear shrunken, gray, and translucent. Some sparing of subcortical myelin ("U fibers") may be evident (Fig. 23–30). Microscopic features vary with the type of leukodystrophy but include widespread loss of myelin, accompanied in some cases by accumulations of abnormal myelin breakdown products.

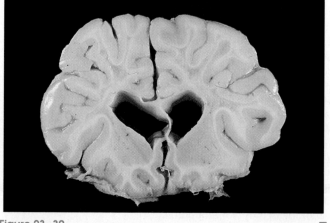

Figure 23-30 ■

Leukodystrophy. These are characterized by extensive, fairly symmetric loss of white matter, in contrast to the multifocal, demarcated areas of demyelination seen in MS. Sparing of the white matter immediately beneath the cerebral cortex (subcortical U fibers), as is present in this case, is seen in many leukodystrophies.

ACQUIRED METABOLIC AND TOXIC DISTURBANCES

The delicate circuitry of the nervous system may be disrupted by a number of toxic and metabolic disturbances. In some cases the changes in the nervous system are largely functional, with only subtle attendant structural abnormalities. In other instances, however, striking and sometimes highly characteristic morphologic changes are produced by the toxin or underlying metabolic abnormality. The list of acquired toxic and metabolic diseases in the nervous system is formidable; hence, only some of the more common examples will be reviewed here.

Nutritional Diseases

Thiamine and vitamin B_{12} (cobalamin) deficiencies are two of the most common nutritional disorders associated with nervous system abnormalities.

Thiamine deficiency causes the *Wernicke-Korsakoff syndrome* and is an important cause of peripheral neuropathy as well. Thiamine deficiency may occur in a number of settings, but in the United States it is most commonly encountered in chronic alcoholics. Indeed, abnormalities referable to thiamine deficiency are second only to traumatic lesions as a cause of pathologic alterations in the brains of alcoholics. *Wernicke's encephalopathy* is characterized by fairly rapid onset of confusion, paralysis of extraocular muscles (particularly the lateral rectus), and ataxia. The syndrome may progress to coma and death if untreated, but responds well to the administration of thiamine in the early stages.

> The morphologic changes of Wernicke's encephalopathy are most evident in the mammillary bodies of the hypothalamus, the dorsal medial areas of the thalamus, and the gray matter around the cerebral aqueduct, the last correlating with the eye movement abnormalities noted clinically. The earliest change is capillary endothelial proliferation associated with abnormal vascular permeability. The hemorrhages result from leakage of red cells from these abnormal capillaries. (Fig. 23–31).

If Wernicke's encephalopathy is not treated promptly, a permanent memory deficit known as *Korsakoff's psychosis* may result. Korsakoff's psychosis is characterized by an inability to either form new memories or retrieve old ones, often accompanied by confabulation.

> Morphologic changes associated with this chronic state are present in the same areas as those involved in Wernicke's encephalopathy and include gliosis and hemosiderin deposits resulting from pre-

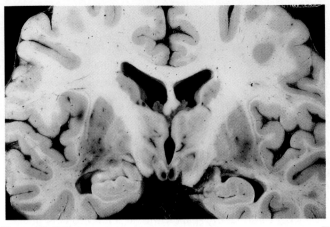

Figure 23–31 ■

Wernicke's encephalopathy. Thiamine deficiency in the central nervous system is associated with the development of hemorrhagic gray matter lesions, depicted here in the mamillary bodies of the hypothalamus.

> vious hemorrhage. In contrast to changes after ischemic injury, neurons are relatively spared but are often somewhat shrunken.

Thiamine deficiencies has also been implicated in the development of atrophy of the superior vermis often seen in alcoholics, termed *alcoholic cerebellar degeneration*. In the peripheral nervous system, thiamine deficiency causes a peripheral axonal neuropathy (discussed later).

Deficiency of vitamin B_{12} (cobalamin) causes pernicious anemia (Chapter 12). In the nervous system, vitamin B_{12} deficiency is associated with the development of *subacute combined degeneration of the spinal cord,* a condition characterized by myelin vacuolation in the dorsal and lateral white matter columns of the spinal cord. In keeping with the distribution of the lesions, subacute combined degeneration is characterized by both motor and sensory abnormalities, including spasticity, weakness, and loss of proprioception. Deficiency of vitamin B_{12} may also produce a confusional state, sometimes termed "megaloblastic madness."

Acquired Metabolic Disorders

Patients with a number of systemic conditions may develop varying degrees of CNS dysfunction. Probably the best characterized is that associated with hepatic failure. Hepatic encephalopathy is characterized by altered levels of consciousness and a characteristic "flapping" tremor termed *asterixis* (Chapter 16). Grossly, the brain may be normal or edematous. Microscopically this condition is characterized by increased numbers of large, "naked," pale-staining astrocytic nuclei, termed *Alzheimer type II glia,* within gray matter. The astrocytic changes are likely related in some way to high levels of ammonia, the detoxification of which occurs predominantly within astrocytes. Identical changes are encountered in patients with Wilson's disease, an entity considered more fully in the discussion of diseases of the liver.

Toxic Disorders

The list of environmental neurotoxins is so large that not even a basic outline can be given here. Among the major categories of neurotoxic substances are *metals,* examples of which are arsenic, mercury, and lead; a wide variety of *industrial chemicals,* including organophosphates and methyl alcohol; and a range of *environmental pollutants* such as carbon monoxide. The most important of these were discussed in Chapter 8.

Therapeutic agents are an additional important and expanding category of neurotoxins; some of the many types of adverse effects are *peripheral neuropathies* (vinca alkaloids, isoniazid) and *convulsions* (metronidazole). Many neurotoxic effects have occurred after antitumor treatment. *Methotrexate,* an important antineoplastic agent, may cause CNS injury, particularly in patients receiving intrathecal or high-dose systemic therapy in conjunction with radiation therapy. The morphologic changes associated with methotrexate toxicity are most prominent in white matter and consist of necrosis, demyelination, gliosis, and calcification. *Ionizing radiation,* as it does in other organs, can cause a vasculopathy leading to tissue ischemia and infarction.

DEGENERATIVE DISEASES

The term *degenerative disease of the CNS* embraces a heterogeneous group of disorders characterized by spontaneous, progressive degeneration of neurons in a specific region or system in the brain, spinal cord, or both. Degenerative diseases may be sporadic or familial. They show considerable clinical variability, and often there is overlapping of clinical features that clouds distinction between the various types. Our comments will focus on some of the more common degenerative diseases, including Alzheimer's disease, parkinsonism, Huntington disease, and amyotrophic lateral sclerosis (motor neuron disease).

Alzheimer's Disease

Alzheimer's disease (AD) is the most common cause of dementia in the elderly, with cerebrovascular disease accounting for most of the remaining cases. Most cases of AD occur after the age of 50, with a progressive increase in incidence with increasing age. Most cases are sporadic, but in roughly 10% of patients, there is a family history of dementia. The term Alzheimer's disease embraces the two conditions previously designated *senile dementia* and *presenile dementia.* Morphologic changes identical to those seen in AD are almost invariably present in patients with Down syndrome who survive beyond the age of 40. Despite extensive research in recent years, the cause of AD remains unknown, although many factors associated with the development of the disease have been identified:

■ *Genetic factors* play a role in the development of some cases of AD, as evidenced by the occurrence of familial cases. A number of investigations have implicated genetic abnormalities on chromosomes 21, 19, 14, and 1 in the pathogenesis of both sporadic and familial AD. Most familial cases are linked to a mutation on chromosome 14. The functions of this gene product are not known. The genetic heterogeneity noted thus far suggests that no single genetic defect is likely to be responsible for all cases of AD.

■ *Deposition of amyloid,* derived from breakdown of a protein known as amyloid precursor protein (APP), is a consistent feature of AD. The breakdown product, known as β-amyloid, is a prominent component of both the neurofibrillary tangles and senile plaques found in the brains of AD patients (discussed below), and it is usually present within the walls of cerebral blood vessels as well. In some familial cases of AD, various mutations in the gene coding for APP have been identified. β-amyloid has also been shown to be toxic to neurons in cell cultures, although the relationship between such in vitro activity and the pathogenesis of AD is unclear. Whether amyloid deposition plays a primary role in the development of AD or represents a secondary phenomenon is a hotly debated topic.

■ *Expression of specific alleles of apoprotein E* (apoE) has been demonstrated in both sporadic and familial AD. Retrospective and prospective studies have demonstrated that the ϵ_4 allele of apoE, in particular, is expressed with increased frequency in patients with late-onset AD. It has been suggested that apoE may be involved in the transport or processing of the β-amyloid precursor protein. ApoE-ϵ_4 is reported to bind better to β-amyloid than other forms of apoE and may thus contribute to enhanced amyloid fibril formation. However, the fact that a significant percentage of patients with documented AD do not express the apoE ϵ_4 allele, as well as the observation that ϵ_4 is expressed in some elderly individuals without AD, suggest that while apoE-ϵ_4 may contribute to AD, it is neither sufficient nor essential in the pathogenesis of AD.

MORPHOLOGY. Although the brain in AD is often atrophic, it may be grossly normal in the earlier stages of the disease. The atrophy is most evident in the frontal, temporal, or parietal lobes but usually involves all cortical areas to some degree (Fig. 23–32). Examination of the cut surface reveals that the cerebral ventricles are symmetrically dilated in most cases, reflecting a generalized loss of parenchyma (hydrocephalus ex vacuo). Microscopic changes include the presence of **neurofibrillary tangles**, which appear as coarse, filamentous aggregates within the cytoplasm of neurons. They are found in the neocortex, hippocampus, basal forebrain and some parts of the brain stem. The neurofibrillary tangles are composed of insoluble, protein-rich paired helical filaments (PHFs). Additional accumulations of PHFs occur within distal neuronal cell processes (neurites) to form characteristic **senile plaques**, which appear as aggregates of coarse, tortuous neurites in the neuropil of the cerebral cortex (Fig. 23–33). The senile

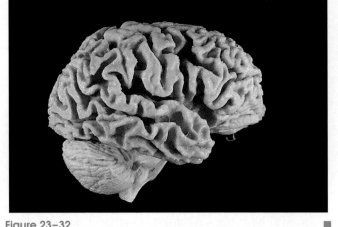

Figure 23–32 ■

Alzheimer's disease. Generalized loss of brain parenchyma has resulted in narrowing of the cerebral cortical gyri and widening of sulci. Compensatory enlargement of the ventricles (hydrocephalus ex vacuo) is usually apparent in such cases.

plaques contain a central **amyloid core** composed of β-amyloid. β-amyloid deposits are usually present in leptomeningeal and parenchymal vessels, as well, a pattern referred to as **amyloid angiopathy.** These amyloid deposits are unrelated to those encountered in other forms of systemic or localized amyloidosis (Chapter 5). The simple presence of plaques and/or tangles is not, by itself, specific for AD, because such structures are also frequently present in the brains of otherwise normal elderly individuals. It is rather the **number of plaques and tangles** in neocortical areas in the

setting of dementia that allows one to make a diagnosis of AD.

Clinical features of AD include a progressive impairment of memory and other cognitive functions. Symptoms may be subtle at first and can be easily confused with depression, another clinically important disease in the elderly. Cognitive impairment continues inexorably, usually over the course of 5 to 15 years, resulting in complete disorientation and loss of language and other higher cortical functions. Death usually results from intercurrent bronchopneumonia or other infections.

Parkinsonism

Parkinsonism is a disturbance in motor functions characterized by rigidity, expressionless facies, stooped posture, gait disturbances, slowing of voluntary movements, and a characteristic "pill-rolling" tremor. Parkinsonism is not a single disease, but rather a clinical manifestation of a disturbance in the dopaminergic pathways connecting the substantia nigra to the basal ganglia. Such disturbances occur in a number of other degenerative diseases and may also be caused by trauma, certain toxic agents, vascular diseases, encephalitis, and a number of other conditions.

Perhaps the best known form of parkinsonism is that associated with Parkinson's disease, also known as *idiopathic parkinsonism* or *paralysis agitans.* Parkinson's disease is a degenerative disorder involving the dopamine-secreting neurons of the substantia nigra, as well as the locus ceruleus. It is a disease of adulthood, with most cases becoming manifest by the sixth decade. The disease is usually sporadic.

MORPHOLOGY. The brain may be externally normal or mildly atrophic, particularly in older individuals. The **substantia nigra** and **locus ceruleus** are depigmented in most cases (Fig. 23–34) as a result of loss of neuromelanin-containing neurons in the substantia nigra, locus ceruleus, and dorsal motor

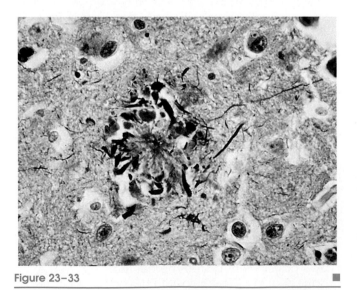

Figure 23–33 ■

Photomicrograph of a senile plaque (Bielschowsky silver stain). Enlarged, tortuous, darkly stained neuronal cell processes, sometimes referred to as *dystrophic neurites,* surround a central amyloid-rich core. (Courtesy of Eileen Bigio, MD, Department of Pathology, University of Texas Southwestern Medical School, Dallas, TX.)

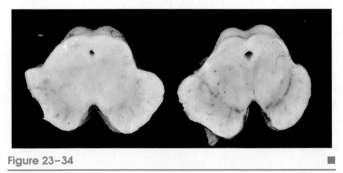

Figure 23–34 ■

Parkinson's disease, or idiopathic parkinsonism, is characterized by a loss of neurons from the substantia nigra and other pigmented nuclei. Such neuronal loss is responsible for the pallor of the substantia nigra on the left, compared with the normal midbrain on the right. (Courtesy of Eileen Bigio, MD, Department of Pathology, University of Texas Southwestern Medical School, Dallas, TX.)

nucleus of the vagus nerve. Microscopically, the neuropil in these areas is gliotic and contains scattered accumulations of neuromelanin pigment. Some of the remaining neurons in these areas contain concentrically laminated, eosinophilic, intracytoplasmic inclusions known as **Lewy bodies.**

The clinical onset of Parkinson's disease is usually insidious. The course of the disease is one of steady progression, usually over a period of about 10 years. In addition to the motor disturbances noted previously, dementia may occur in a minority of cases. Whether such dementia represents an intrinsic element of Parkinson's disease, concomitant AD, or a combination of factors remains unclear. Death is usually the result of intercurrent infection or trauma from frequent falls caused by postural instability.

Huntington Disease

Huntington disease is a hereditary, progressive, fatal *disorder involving the "extrapyramidal" motor system, characterized by involuntary movements (chorea) and dementia.* The disease is inherited as an autosomal dominant trait with complete penetrance. It usually does not become apparent until adulthood, often after affected individuals have had children. The responsible gene has been localized to chromosome 4, and the encoded gene product is called *huntingtin.* The disease is caused by trinucleotide repeat mutations in the Huntington gene (Chapter 7). At the Huntington locus, the normal chromosomes contain between 11 and 34 copies of the cytosine-adenine-guanine (CAG) sequence. In Huntington disease, the number of triplet repeats is increased, and the larger the number, the earlier the onset of disease. Unlike fragile X syndrome, another trinucleotide repeat disorder, expansion of the trinucleotide repeats occurs during spermatogenesis rather than oogenesis, and hence asymptomatic carrier fathers can transmit the disease to their offspring. Affected individuals can be identified before the development of symptoms by analysis for the presence of excessive CAG triplet repeats in the responsible gene.

The molecular pathogenesis of Huntington disease is not fully understood. It seems, however, that the disease is not caused by a loss of function of the huntingtin protein. To the contrary, several lines of evidence suggest that *mutant huntingtin acquires the ability to bind to and inactivate some other normal protein* that is critical for the normal functioning of neurons in the extrapyramidal motor system. In genetic parlance this phenomenon is referred to as a *gain of function mutation,* because the mutant protein acquires new properties that are deleterious. The precise identity of the normal proteins that are disabled by the mutant huntingtin continues to be an active area of investigation.

MORPHOLOGY. The brain in Huntington disease is usually small, often weighing less than 1100 gm. The most distinguishing feature of the disorder is striking **atrophy of the caudate nucleus, putamen,** **and globus pallidus,** with the caudate often reduced to a thin band adjacent to the lateral ventricles. The ventricles are symmetrically dilated, with a concave lateral wall, reflecting atrophy of the caudate nucleus. Some atrophy of other subcortical nuclei and cerebral cortex may be present, although it is seldom as striking as that seen in the caudate and putamen. Microscopically, this disease is characterized by a severe loss of neurons within the caudate and putamen, accompanied by fibrillary gliosis in these areas. The smaller neurons in the corpus striatum are preferentially affected, but there is often some loss of larger neurons as well. Cortical neuronal loss is often present and correlates with the degree of dementia.

The clinical onset of Huntington disease is usually in the fourth or fifth decades, although rare cases present in childhood. The initial manifestations include involuntary, writhing movements known as *choreiform movements.* In cases with earlier onset, seizures and rigidity may be prominent. Neuropsychiatric disturbances, including depression and cognitive impairment, typically develop after the onset of motor abnormalities but may be the presenting manifestations. Symptoms progress inexorably, typically over a period of 15 to 20 years. Common causes of death include suicide and intercurrent infections. The risk of suicide, in particular, mandates the availability of proper counseling in the evaluation of presymptomatic carriers of the disease.

Diseases of Motor Neurons

Amyotrophic lateral sclerosis (ALS), more popularly known as *Lou Gehrig's disease,* is a progressive degenerative disorder involving the upper and lower motor neurons of the pyramidal system, with resultant progressive muscle weakness, atrophy, and spasticity. Most cases of ALS are sporadic, although familial forms with an autosomal dominant inheritance pattern are also encountered. The cause and pathogenesis of most cases of ALS remain unknown, although some familial cases have been associated with mutations in the gene coding for the enzyme superoxide dismutase.

ALS is characterized by a **loss of motor neurons** in the anterior horns of the spinal cord, brain stem motor nuclei, and the primary motor cortex of the cerebrum. Grossly, the brain and cord are usually normal, although some atrophy of the anterior spinal roots may be apparent. Microscopically, in addition to neuronal loss and gliosis in the motor areas noted above, degeneration and loss of neurons in the primary motor cortex often cause a **loss of corticospinal fibers** in the cerebral peduncles, basal pons, medullary pyramids, and especially within the lateral and anterior columns of the spinal cord. Peripheral nerves carrying motor fibers are depopulated; affected skeletal muscles show evidence of denervation atrophy (Chapter 21).

The onset of ALS is insidious, marked by weakness, clumsiness, and speech difficulties. Muscle weakness, which progresses with time, is accompanied by atrophy and small involuntary contractions termed *fasciculations*. Extraocular muscles are not affected. Spasticity, reflecting involvement of upper motor neurons, is present in most cases. It is manifested by hyperactive deep tendon reflexes and a Babinski reflex. The degree of involvement of upper and lower motor neurons varies from case to case, although most patients have evidence of both lower and upper motor neuron disease. ALS is a progressive disease, with a median survival of about 5 years after the onset of symptoms. Death usually results from a combination of respiratory insufficiency and infections.

Other forms of progressive motor neuron diseases include the progressive spinal muscular atrophies of infancy and childhood. The best known of these is infantile spinal muscular atrophy, or Werdnig-Hoffmann disease. This is an autosomal recessive disorder manifested by congenital hypotonia ("floppy infant" syndrome). It is characterized by a loss of motor neurons in the anterior horns of the spinal cord, resulting in atrophy of anterior spinal roots and peripheral motor nerves and denervation in multiple skeletal muscle groups, including those controlling respiration. Generalized hypotonia, often present at birth, may even be evident in utero. The course of Werdnig-Hoffmann disease is relentlessly progressive, with most patients dying within the first year of life.

DISEASES OF THE PERIPHERAL NERVOUS SYSTEM

The peripheral nervous system begins a few millimeters from the pial surface of the brain and spinal cord, where Schwann cell processes replace oligodendroglial processes as the source of myelin. Myelinated axons are invested by concentric laminations of Schwann cell cytoplasm. The myelin sheath contributed by each Schwann cell is termed a *myelin internode*. In the case of the smaller unmyelinated axons, in contrast, multiple axons are embedded within the cytoplasm of a single Schwann cell, with no concentric laminations of the Schwann cell cytoplasm. The peripheral nervous system, then, is composed of axons, associated Schwann cells, blood vessels, and nerve sheath elements that provide structural support for the axons. Axons are insulated from the interstitial fluids of the body by a "blood-nerve" barrier, somewhat analogous to the blood-brain barrier, formed by the tight junctions in vessels supplying the nerve twigs, and by the perineurial cells surrounding individual bundles (fascicles) of axons. Disorders of the peripheral nervous system include peripheral neuropathies and neoplasms arising from Schwann cells and other nerve sheath elements.

Peripheral Neuropathies

A number of disorders may disrupt the normal conduction of electrical impulses in the peripheral nerves. Some of the more common causes of peripheral neuropathy are listed in Table 23–3. Broadly speaking, peripheral neuropathies may be subdivided into three basic categories: wallerian degeneration, axonal degeneration, and segmental demyelination. Mixtures of axonal degeneration and segmental demyelination are often encountered.

Wallerian degeneration refers to degeneration of axons distal to a point of transection, as might occur if a nerve is cut by a knife. Distal to the point of injury, both axons and their myelin sheaths disintegrate to form coarse globules, termed *myelin ovoids.* Subsequently, axons may regenerate to some degree, a process manifested by the presence of axonal sprouts, which are invested by new myelin sheaths. Axonal regeneration may be accompanied by recovery of function in the denervated area, often incomplete. In addition to traumatic injuries, vascular diseases such as vasculitis, with resultant ischemic injury to a segment of peripheral nerve, are an important cause of peripheral Wallerian degeneration.

Primary axonal degeneration is the most common type of peripheral neuropathy. It is caused by a derangement of the neuron giving rise to axon degeneration and is characterized by a "dying back" of the axon from its distal end. Myelin ovoids, a feature of primary axonal degeneration, are generally less conspicuous than those seen in wallerian degeneration. If the neuronal derangement is corrected, some regeneration of the distal axons may occur, with concomitant

■

Table 23–3. CAUSES AND TYPES OF PERIPHERAL NEUROPATHIES

Nutritional and Metabolic Neuropathies
Diabetes, thiamine deficiency, pyridoxine deficiency, alcoholism, renal failure
Toxic Neuropathies
Lead, arsenic, cisplatin, vincristine, organic solvents
Inflammatory Neuropathies
Guillain-Barré syndrome, chronic inflammatory demyelinating neuropathy, vasculitic neuropathy, leprosy, sarcoidosis
Hereditary Neuropathies
Hereditary motor and sensory neuropathies (Charcot-Marie-Tooth disease, Refsum's disease, Dejerine-Sottas disease), hereditary sensory neuropathies, leukodystrophies
Miscellaneous
Amyloid neuropathy, paraneoplastic neuropathies, neuropathies associated with immunoglobulin abnormalities

recovery of function. A wide range of disorders, including many nutritional deficiencies and intoxications, may produce primary distal axonal degeneration.

Segmental demyelination is characterized by primary injury to the myelin sheath, with relative preservation of axons. In practice, segmental myelin injury is often accompanied by some degree of distal axonal injury. The leukodystrophies and acute inflammatory demyelinating neuropathy (Guillain-Barré syndrome) are important causes of demyelinating neuropathies. In some neuropathies, including some forms of diabetic neuropathy, combinations of axonal degeneration and demyelination are common.

The clinical manifestations of peripheral neuropathies include some combination of motor, sensory, and occasionally autonomic deficits. The presentations vary, however, depending on the cause and type of the neuropathy. *Most neuropathies, particularly axonal disorders, present with slowly evolving symmetric sensory loss, often in a "glove-and-stocking" distribution, reflecting injury of distal axonal processes.* Motor deficits, if present, are manifested by weakness. Deep tendon reflexes are diminished or absent. Involvement of the autonomic nervous system may produce changes such as postural hypotension and constipation. In other cases the presentation may be that of asymmetric neurologic deficits. This is particularly the case in neuropathies caused by vasculitis, which may affect multiple nerves in a random distribution, a presentation termed *mononeuropathy multiplex*.

Guillain-Barré syndrome is one of the most common life-threatening diseases of the peripheral nervous system. Its etiology is unknown, and it may develop spontaneously or after a "viral" prodrome, *Mycoplasma* infection, allergic reaction, or surgical procedure; an immunologic basis is considered most likely. Patients with the Guillain-Barré syndrome present with rapidly progressive, ascending motor weakness that may lead to death owing to failure of respiratory muscles. The dominant histopathologic finding is inflammation of peripheral nerves, with segmental demyelination. The CSF usually contains increased levels of protein but only a minimal cellular reaction.

Neoplasms of the Peripheral Nervous System

Neoplasms of peripheral nerve arise from Schwann cells and other elements of the peripheral nerve sheath, such as fibroblasts. The two most common primary peripheral nerve sheath neoplasms are neurofibromas and schwannomas. The frequency of both neoplasms is dramatically increased in patients with type I neurofibromatosis (von Recklinghausen's disease), in whom such tumors may develop in childhood.

Schwannomas present as well-circumscribed masses attached to peripheral nerves, cranial nerves, or spinal nerve roots. The eighth cranial nerve is a particularly common site for schwannomas (also termed **acoustic neuromas**), where they present as well-demarcated masses in the angle between the cerebellum and pons. Microscopically, schwannomas classically contain areas of densely packed spindle cells, termed **Antoni A tissue,** intermixed with looser, myxoid regions termed **Antoni B tissue.** In the denser areas, cell nuclei may form orderly palisades, termed **Verocay bodies.** Degenerative changes, including vascular hyalinization and lipid-laden macrophages, are quite common. Scattered enlarged, hyperchromatic nuclei are often present and, in the absence of mitotic activity, usually represent another degenerative change. Native (non-neoplastic) peripheral nerve elements are sometimes identifiable at the periphery of the neoplasm.

In contrast to schwannomas, **neurofibromas** typically produce a fusiform enlargement of the involved nerve, which tends to be less well defined than a schwannoma. They may be solitary or multiple. Microscopically, neurofibromas are composed of interlacing bundles of delicate, elongated cells with slender, frequently wavy nuclei. Native axons are usually intermingled with the neoplastic cells rather than displaced to the periphery, as in the case of schwannomas. A variety of degenerative changes similar to those seen in schwannomas may also be present in neurofibromas. Areas of increased cellularity and mitotic activity should raise concern about the possibility of malignant transformation, particularly in neurofibromas occurring in patients with **type I neurofibromatosis** (von Recklinghausen's disease), a disorder tragically exemplified by the "Elephant Man."

Schwannomas and neurofibromas are most common in adults, except in patients with type I neurofibromatosis. Most sporadic lesions are solitary. The tumors may present as asymptomatic masses, or they may produce neurologic deficits, depending on their location. Schwannomas of the eighth cranial nerve are common intracranial neoplasms; they may be difficult to distinguish from meningiomas on clinical grounds. The possibility of von Recklinghausen's disease should be entertained if multiple peripheral nerve sheath tumors are present. Malignant transformation occurs much more often in neurofibromas than in schwannomas. Most cases of malignant transformation occur in patients with type I neurofibromatosis. Malignant lesions are manifested by aggressive local growth and distant metastases, particularly to lung.

BIBLIOGRAPHY

Bell JE, Ironside JW: Neuropathology of spongiform encephalopathies in humans. Br Med Bull 49:738, 1993. (A comprehensive review of the history, classification, and pathology of Creutzfeldt-Jakob disease and related disorders.)
Dyck PJ: Diseases of peripheral nerves. In Engel AG, Franzini-Armstrong C (eds): Myology, 2nd ed. New York, McGraw-Hill, 1994, pp 1870–1905. (A thorough review of the clinical and pathologic aspects of human peripheral nerve disease.)
Forno LS: Neuropathology of Parkinson's disease. J Neuropathol Exp Neurol

55:259, 1996. (An informative review of some of the important historical and clinicopathologic aspects of Parkinson's disease and related disorders.)

Garcia JH: Pathophysiology of ischemic injury to the brain. In Nelson JS, et al (eds): Principles and Practice of Neuropathology. St. Louis, Mosby, 1993, pp 456–469. (A concise review of the causes, pathogenesis, and morphology of brain infarcts and related conditions.)

Graham DI, et al: The nature, distribution and causes of traumatic brain injury. Brain Pathol 5:397, 1995. (A concise overview of the current classification and mechanisms of traumatic brain injury.)

Gusella JF, MacDonald ME: Huntington's disease. Semin Cell Biol 6:21, 1995. (A review of the molecular aspects of this disease.)

Hafler DA, Weiner HL: Immunologic mechanisms and therapy in multiple sclerosis. Immunol Rev 144:75, 1995. (A detailed analysis of the immunologic basis of multiple sclerosis and potential therapeutic applications.)

Janus TJ, et al: Biology and treatment of gliomas. Ann Oncol 3:423, 1992. (A review of recent developments in prognostic indicators and treatment of gliomas.)

Norman MG: Malformations of the brain. J Neuropathol Exp Neurol 55:133, 1996. (An excellent overview of the classification, morphology, and pathogenesis of major CNS malformations.)

Parisi JE, Scheithauer BW: Glial Tumors. In Nelson JS, et al (eds): Principles and Practice of Neuropathology. St. Louis, Mosby, 1993, pp 123–183. (A comprehensive review of the pathology and behavior of the diverse spectrum of glial neoplasms.)

Prusiner SB: Human prion disease and neurodegeneration. Curr Topics Microbiol Immunol 207:1, 1996. (An account of how prion proteins are propagated and cause human disease, by the discoverer of prions.)

Roses AD: From genes, to mechanisms to therapies: Lessons to be learned from neurologic disorders. Nat Med 2:269, 1996. (An excellent commentary on the molecular basis of Huntington disease and Alzheimer's disease.)

Ransohoff RM: Multiple sclerosis: new concepts of pathogenesis, diagnosis, and treatment. Compr Ther 15:39, 1989. (An informative discussion of the development of morphologic changes in MS, with excellent clinical correlation.)

Rewcastle NB: Degenerative diseases of the central nervous system. In Davis RL, Robertson DM (eds): Textbook of Neuropathology, 2nd ed. Baltimore, Williams & Wilkins, 1991, pp 904–961. (A comprehensive summary of the morphology of Alzheimer's disease and other degenerative conditions of the CNS.)

Scaravilli F, et al: Pathology of the nervous system. In Scaravelli F (ed): The Neuropathology of HIV Infection. London, Springer-Verlag, 1993, pp 99–156. (A comprehensive discussion of the pathology of primary HIV encephalopathy and opportunistic CNS diseases associated with HIV infection.)

Steinman L: Multiple sclerosis: a coordinated immunologic attack against myelin in the central nervous system. Cell 85:299, 1996. (A brief but excellent summary of the immunopathogenesis of multiple sclerosis.)

Tienari PJ: Multiple sclerosis: multiple etiologies, multiple genes? Ann Med 26:259, 1994. (A review of work on the identification of genetic factors that might contribute to susceptibility to MS.)

Van Broeckhoven CL: Molecular genetics of Alzheimer disease: identification of genes and gene mutations. Eur Neurol 35:8, 1995. (A review of work on the role of abnormalities involving chromosomes 21, 19, and 14 in the pathogenesis of Alzheimer's disease.)

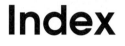

Index

Note: Page numbers in *italics* refer to illustrations; page numbers followed by t refer to tables.

A

Erythrocyte(s), disorders of, 341–358. See also specific diseases.
Erythrocytosis, 358
Erythroplasia, 473
Erythroplasia of Queyrat, 578
Escherichia coli, and acute pyelonephritis, 455
  in enterocolitis, 494, 495t
  in leptomeningitis, 726
Esophagus, 476–481
  achalasia of, 477
  Barrett's, 479, *479, 480*
  cancer of, 480–481, *481*
  candidiasis of, 427t
  diverticulae of, 476t
  hiatal hernia of, 476–477,*477*
  inflammation of, 478–479, *479*
  motor disorders of, 476–478
  reflux and, 479, *479*
  systemic sclerosis involving, 114
  varices of, 478, *478, 524*
Essential hypertension, 290
Estrogen(s), adverse effects of, 230–231
  and breast cancer, 630
  and endometrial carcinoma, 612
  and endometrial hyperplasia, 602
  and gallstones, 551
  and vaginal carcinoma, 601–602
  deficiency of, and osteoporosis, 670
Ethanol, toxic effects of, 234–236
Euploidy, definition of, 191
Ewing's sarcoma, 211t, 675t, 679–680
Excision repair, of DNA, 157
Excoriation, definition of, 698
Exocrine pancreas, 558–562. See also *Pancreas.*
Exophthalmos, Graves' disease and, 646
Exostoses, 677
Exotoxins, bacterial, 273–274
Extracellular matrix (ECM), 52–53, *53, 54*
  in spread of cancer, 161–162
Extractable nuclear antigen (ENA), 103
Extrahepatic biliary atresia, 553–554
Extramedullary hematopoiesis, and erythroblastosis fetalis, 206
Extravascular hemolysis, 343
Extrinsic asthma, 395
Exudate, 27, 61
Eye(s), in diabetes mellitus, 571
  in galactosemia, 185
  in Marfan syndrome, 181
  in mucopolysaccharidoses, 188
  in neurofibromatosis, 190
  in Sjögren's syndrome, 112
  in vitamin A deficiency, 248
  retinoblastoma in, 212
  sarcoidosis involving, 410

F

FAB classification, of acute myeloblastic leukemia, 376t
Factor V, mutations in, and thrombosis, 69, 231
Factor VIII, deficiency of (hemophilia A), 389
Factor VIII-von Willebrand factor complex, 388–389, *388*
Factor IX, deficiency of (Christmas disease), 389
Factor XII (Hageman factor), activation of, 34, *35*
Fallopian tubes, 613
  and ectopic pregnancy, 620
  inflammation of, 613
Familial adenomatous polyposis, 507, *508*
Familial hypercholesterolemia (FH), 182–184, *183*
Familial Mediterranean fever, 129
Fanconi's anemia, 145t, 157
Farmer's lung, 94, 410t

Fasciitis, nodular, 692, *692*
Fat embolism, 74
Fat necrosis, 13, *13*
  enzymatic, of pancreas, 558, *558*
  traumatic, of breast, 628
Fatty change, 11, 17, *18*
  in liver, alcohol induced, 535, *536, 537*
  in Reye's syndrome, 542
Fatty streak, in atherosclerosis, 286–287, *286, 287*
Female genital system, 598–619. See also specific parts.
Ferritin, 353
  in anemia of chronic disease, 354
  in iron deficiency anemia, 353
Fetal alcohol syndrome, 202
Fetor hepaticus, liver failure and, 522
Fever, blackwater, 352
  familial Mediterranean, 129
  in inflammation, 45
Fibrillin, in Marfan syndrome, 181, 181t
Fibrinoid necrosis, in malignant hypertension, 462, *462*
  in immune complex vasculitis, 93, *92, 93*
Fibrinolytic system, 68
  in inflammation, 35
Fibrinous inflammation, 44–45, *44*
Fibroadenoma, of breast, 134, *138*, 628–629, *628*
Fibroblast growth factors 51, 51t
Fibrocystic changes, in breast, 624–627, *625*
Fibrocystic disease of pancreas. See *Cystic fibrosis (CF).*
Fibroids, uterine, 611
Fibrolipoma, 692
Fibroma, 133
Fibromatosis, 692–693
Fibronectin, 52, *52*
Fibroplasia, 48, 54–55
Fibrosarcoma, 133, 693
Fibrosis (scarring), bone marrow, 379
  hepatic, in cirrhosis, 523
  in inflammation, 40–41
  progressive massive pulmonary, 225, *226*
  pulmonary, idiopathic, 407–409, *408*
  repair by, 53–55, 58
Fibrous dysplasia, of bone, 680, *680*
Fibrous histiocytoma, 693, *694*
Filariasis, 62
Fingers, clubbing of, 171, 434
Flapping tremor (asterixis), 522
Flat condyloma, 605
Flexner-Wintersteiner rosettes, 212, *213*
Floppy infant syndrome, 688, *742*
Floppy mitral valve syndrome, 325
Floppy valve syndrome, in Marfan syndrome, 182
FMR-1 gene, 177, 198–199
Foam cells, 18
  in atherosclerosis, *286, 287*
Focal nodular hyperplasia, of liver, 548
Focal segmental glomerulosclerosis, 449, *449*
Folate (folic acid), 247t
  deficiency of, 355–356
Follicle cysts, of ovary, 614
Follicular adenoma, of thyroid gland, 649–650, *650*
Follicular carcinoma, of thyroid gland, 651–652
Follicular dendritic cells (FDCs), in AIDS, 122
Follicular hyperplasia, of lymph nodes, 361
Follicular (nodular) lymphoma, 363, *364*, 366, 369t
Follicular small cleaved lymphoma, *365,* 366
Forebrain, malformations of, 724–725
Foreign body granulomas, 43
Fragile X syndrome, 181t, 197–199, *198, 218*
Free radicals, in cell injury, *7,* 8–9, 9–11, *10,* 23
  in inflammation, 38–39
French-American-British classification, of acute myeloblastic leukemia, 376t
Friedreich ataxia, 180t
Frontal bossing, 251

M